Core Curriculum for
Maternal-Newborn Nursing

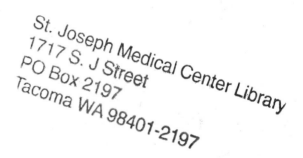

Core Curriculum for Maternal-Newborn Nursing

Fourth Edition

Edited by:

Susan Mattson, RNC-OB, CTN, PhD, FAAN

Professor Emerita
College of Nursing and Healthcare Innovation
Arizona State University
Tempe, Arizona

Judy E. Smith, PhD, RNC-WHNP

Professor
School of Nursing
California State University—Long Beach
Long Beach, California

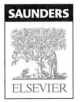

SAUNDERS

ELSEVIER

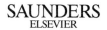

SAUNDERS
ELSEVIER

3251 Riverport Lane
Saint Louis, MO 63043

Notice

Knowledge and best practice in this field are constantly changing. As new research and experience broaden
our knowledge, changes in practice, treatment and drug therapy may become necessary or appropriate.
Readers are advised to check the most current information provided (i) on procedures featured or (ii) by the
manufacturer of each product to be administered, to verify the recommended dose or formula, the method and
duration of administration, and contraindications. It is the responsibility of the practitioner, relying on their
own experience and knowledge of the patient, to make diagnoses, to determine dosages and the best treatment
for each individual patient, and to take all appropriate safety precautions. To the fullest extent of the law,
neither the Publisher nor the Editors assumes any liability for any injury and/or damage to persons or
property arising out of or related to any use of the material contained in this book.

Library of Congress Cataloging-in-Publication Data

Core curriculum for maternal-newborn nursing/edited by Susan Mattson, Judy E.
Smith. – 4th ed.
      p. ; cm.
 Includes bibliographical references and index.
 ISBN 978-1-4377-1576-7 (hardcover : alk. paper)
 1. Maternity nursing—Outlines, syllabi, etc. 2. Nursing—Study and teaching—Outlines, syllabi, etc.
 I. Mattson, Susan. II. Smith, Judy E.
 [DNLM: 1. Maternal-Child Nursing—Outlines. 2. Curriculum—Outlines. WY 18.2 C7965
2011]
 RG951.N33 2011
 618.2'0231—dc22   2010005124

Executive Editor: Robin Carter
Managing Editor: Laurie K. Gower
Publishing Services Manager: Jeff Patterson
Project Manager: Jeanne Genz
Design Direction: Charlie Seibel

Printed in the United States of America

Last digit is the print number: 9 8 7 6 5 4 3 2 1

Contributors

Linda Bond, PhD, RNC
Professor Emerita, Kirkhof College of
  Nursing
Grand Valley State University
Allendale, Michigan

Beverly Bowers, PhD, RN, CNS
Associate Professor, College of Nursing
University of Oklahoma Health Sciences
  Center
Oklahoma City, Oklahoma

Linda Callahan, CRNA, PhD
Professor, School of Nursing
California State University—Long Beach
Long Beach, California

**Natalie Diane Cheffer, PhD, RN,
  CPNP**
Associate Professor, Department of
  Nursing
California State University—Long Beach
Long Beach, California

Catherine R. Coverston, PhD, RNC
Associate Professor, College of Nursing
Brigham Young University
Provo, Utah

Dustine Dix, RN, MSN
Clinical Assistant Professor, School of
  Nursing
University of North Carolina—Chapel Hill
Chapel Hill, North Carolina

**Makeba B. Felton, RN, MSN, FNPC,
  WHNP**
Clinical Assistant Professor
College of Nursing and Healthcare
  Innovation
Arizona State University
Phoenix, Arizona

**S. Kim Genovese, PhD, MSN, MSA,
  RN-BC**
Executive Director, Nursing 2000 North,
  Inc.
La Porte, Indiana

**Elizabeth Gilbert, RNC, MS, FNP-BC,
  CNS**
Director of Professional Practice
Banner Thunderbird Medical Center
Glendale, Arizona

Whitney Hardy, RN, BS
Staff Nurse, Neonatal Intensive Care Unit
CJW Medical Center, Chippenham
  Campus
Richmond, Virginia

**Denise G. Link, PhD, WHNP, CNE,
  FNAP**
Associate Dean, Clinical Practice and
  Community Partnerships
College of Nursing and Healthcare
  Innovation
Arizona State University
Phoenix, Arizona

**Susan Mattson, RNC-OB, CTN, PhD,
  FAAN**
Professor Emerita
College of Nursing and Healthcare
  Innovation
Arizona State University
Phoenix, Arizona

**Jacqueline M. McGrath, PhD, RN,
  FNAP, FAAN**
Associate Professor, School of Nursing
Department of Family and Community
  Health
Virginia Commonwealth University
Richmond, Virginia

Barbara A. Moran, PhD, CNM, FACCE
Assistant Professor, School of Nursing
The Catholic University of America
Washington, DC

Susan Saffer Orr, PT, PCS, IBCLC
Lactation Consultant
Torrance Memorial Medical Center
Torrance, California;
Columbia Pediatrics
Long Beach, California

Debra Ann Rannalli, RN, MSN, CPNP
Lecturer
California State University—Long Beach
Long Beach, California
Children's Hospital—Los Angeles
Los Angeles, California

Kathryn Records, PhD, RN
Associate Professor
Core Director, Research Mentoring and
Collaboration
College of Nursing and Healthcare
Innovation
Arizona State University
Phoenix, Arizona

Mary Ann Rhode, RN, MS, CNM
Clinical Practice Coordinator
Exempla Certified Nurse-Midwives
Exempla Saint Joseph Hospital
Denver, Colorado

Charlotte Stephenson, RN, DSN, CLNC
Clinical Professor, Nelda C. Stark College
of Nursing
Texas Woman's University
Houston, Texas

Judy E. Smith, PhD, RNC-WHNP
Professor, Department of Nursing
California State University—Long Beach
Long Beach, California

Keiko L. Torgersen, BSN, MS, RNC
Perinatal Educator
MatSu Regional Medical Center
Palmer, Alaska

Gail M. Turley, MSN, RNC-OB, NEA-BC
Administrative Director, Nursing Services
Crozer-Chester Medical Center
Upland, Pennsylvania

Lucy R. Van Otterloo, RNC, MSN
Assistant Professor, Department of
Nursing
California State University—Long Beach
Long Beach, California

Connie Sampson von Köhler, RNC-OB, MSN, C-EFM, CPHQ
Clinical Nursing Instructor
Long Beach Memorial Medical Center/
Miller Children's Hospital
Adjunct Faculty, School of Nursing
California State University—Long Beach
Long Beach, California

Tamara Whitmer, MS, NPD, RN-BC
Clinical Educator, Women's Center
Banner Desert Medical Center
Mesa, Arizona

Margaret Yancy, RN, MS, WHNP, ANP-C
Clinical Associate Professor
Advanced Practice Nursing of Adults in
Primary Care
College of Nursing and Healthcare
Innovation
Arizona State University
Phoenix, Arizona

Reviewers

Beverly Bowers, PhD, RN, CNS
Associate Professor, College of Nursing
University of Oklahoma Health Sciences
  Center
Oklahoma City, Oklahoma

Kathleen Haubrich, PhD, RN
Associate Professor, Department of
  Nursing
Miami University—Hamilton Campus
Hamilton, Ohio

Janet Massoglia, BSN, MSN, FNP
Instructor, Department of Nursing
Delta College
University Center, Michigan
Administrator, VA Health Care
Saginaw, Michigan

Barbara Pascoe, RN, BA, MA
Director, The Family Place
Concord Hospital
Concord, New Hampshire

Danielle Patrick, MSN, RN, WHCNP
OB/GYN Nurse Practitioner
Today's Women's Health Specialists
Chandler, Arizona

JoAnne M. Pearce, RNC, MS, FNP-C
ADRN Instructor, College of Technology
Idaho State University
Pocatello, Idaho

Elizabeth J.W. Scott, RN, MSN
Lead Clinical Development Specialist
Erlanger Health System
Chattanooga, Tennessee

Charlotte Stephenson, RN, DSN, CLNC
Clinical Professor, Nelda C. Stark College
  of Nursing
Texas Woman's University
Houston, Texas

Sandra L. Walker, PhD, RN
Instructor, ADN Program
Southwest Georgia Technical College
Thomasville, Georgia

Sarah E. Whitaker, DNS, RN
Program Director, Nursing
Dona Ana Community College at New
  Mexico State University
Las Cruces, New Mexico

Preface

This book is intended to be used by practicing nurses for several purposes. First, it can be a study guide for those wishing to sit for certification examinations in maternal-newborn nursing. Basic and complex information is presented and accompanied by an extensive reference list to augment the knowledge base.

Second, the text may be used by development personnel and educators as an orientation for new staff, a source of information for nurses entering or returning to maternal-newborn nursing, and a reference for nurses on those units.

Third, this book can be a classroom text, particularly for students requiring a resource or reference. It is not designed to be a primary text for undergraduate students, but it could be a resource for those graduate students in women's health nurse practitioner programs who want to review some of the material relating to pregnancy that will be needed for their practice.

This edition has several significant changes that should make the book more usable for a wider audience yet keep the content directed toward the original audience. We carried forward the changes regarding complications of the newborn from the 3rd edition, in that most of the content is integrated into those chapters dealing with maternal complications, with reference to how the condition affects the fetus or neonate.

This will make it easier for the maternal-newborn or LDR nurse to identify the high-risk infant and the care required until the baby stabilizes or can be transferred (if necessary). Theoretical information about the continued care of high-risk neonates with selected conditions has also been reconfigured into one chapter titled "The Newborn at Risk." The information is included to provide a basis from which the maternal-newborn nurse may give answers to parents' questions and provide anticipatory guidance to new parents of sick neonates.

A change for the 4th edition has been the deletion of nursing diagnoses as a basis for interventions. It became apparent that using that approach led to repetitiveness in each chapter. Additionally, certain terminology fits more appropriately in some settings than in others and can be used to express the needs of a particular client at that time. Core curriculum for acute care maternity nursing did not seem to be one of those settings in most cases. The new format of the book is one of assessment/clinical practice and interventions, with continued use of a section for health education, and the case studies and questions.

We hope this text will be helpful to those of you using it for all purposes. Its editing continues to be an educational and a character-building experience for us both.

Susan Mattson
Judy E. Smith

Acknowledgments

We would like to acknowledge the contributors to the previous edition:

Linda Bond, PhD, RNC
Physiology of Pregnancy

Linda Callahan, CRNA, PhD
Genetics
Fetal and Placental Development and Functioning
Surgery in Pregnancy

Natalie Diane Cheffer, RN, CPNP, PhD
Adaptation to Extrauterine Life and Immediate Nursing Care
Newborn Biologic/Behavioral Characteristics and Psychosocial Adaptations

Diana E. Clokey, MS, RD, RPh, CDE
Endocrine and Metabolic Disorders

Catherine R. Coverston, PhD, RNC
Psychology of Pregnancy

Sandra L. Gardner, RN, MS, CNS, PNP
Ethics

Elizabeth Gilbert, RNC, MS, CFNP
Labor and Delivery at Risk

Starre Haney, RN, MS, TNCC-I, ENPC
Trauma in Pregnancy

Patricia Grant Higgins, PhD, RN, BSHEd, BSN, MN
Postpartum Complications

Marcia Liden Jasper, BSN, MS, RNC
Antepartum Fetal Assessment

Denise G. Link, RNC, DNSc
Reproductive Anatomy, Physiology, and the Menstrual Cycle
Family Planning

Susan Mattson, PhD, RNC-OB, CTN, FAAN
Ethnocultural Considerations in the Childbearing Period
Intimate Partner Violence

Jacqueline M. McGrath, PhD, RN, NNP, CCNS
Identification of the Sick Newborn

Barbara A. Moran, MS, MPH, CNM
Maternal Infections
Substance Abuse in Pregnancy

Susan Saffer Orr, PT, CLC, IBCLC
Breastfeeding

Judith H. Poole, PhD, BSN, BA, MN
Hypertensive Disorders in Pregnancy
Hemorrhagic Disorders

Margaret A. Putman, RN, MS, NNP
Risks Associated with Gestational Age and Birth Weight

Debra Ann Rannalli, RN, PNP, MSN
Newborn Biologic/Behavioral Characteristics and Psychosocial Adaptations

Janet Scoggin, PhD, CNM
Physical and Psychologic Changes

Judy E. Smith, PhD, RNC-WHNP
Age-Related Changes

Kathleen V. Smith, RNC, BSN, MSN
Normal Childbirth

Keiko L. Torgersen, BSN, MS, RNC
Intrapartum Fetal Assessment

Gail M. Turley, RNC, MSN, CNAA
Essential Forces and Factors in Labor

Cheryl Wallerstedt, MS, RNC, IBLCE, FACCE
Endocrine and Metabolic Disorders

Roxena Wotring, RN, MS
Environmental Hazards

Margaret Yancy, RN, MS, WHNP, ANP-C
Other Medical Complications

Contents

SECTION ONE

REPRODUCTION: FETAL AND PLACENTAL DEVELOPMENT, *1*

1 Reproductive Anatomy, Physiology, and the Menstrual Cycle, *3*
DENISE G. LINK

2 Genetics, *20*
LINDA CALLAHAN

3 Fetal and Placental Development and Functioning, *35*
LINDA CALLAHAN

SECTION TWO

NORMAL PREGNANCY, *59*

4 Ethnocultural Considerations in the Childbearing Period, *61*
SUSAN MATTSON
Appendix 4-1
Quick Reference Guide to Ethnocultural Differences, *75*

5 Physiology of Pregnancy, *80*
LINDA BOND

6 Psychology of Pregnancy, *101*
CATHERINE R. COVERSTON

SECTION THREE

MATERNAL-FETAL WELL-BEING, *115*

7 Age-Related Concerns, *117*
CONNIE SAMPSON VON KÖHLER

8 Antepartum Fetal Assessment, *128*
KEIKO L. TORGERSEN

9 Environmental Hazards, *163*
BEVERLY BOWERS

SECTION FOUR

INTRAPARTUM PERIOD, *189*

10 Essential Forces and Factors in Labor, *191*
GAIL M. TURLEY

11 Normal Childbirth, *225*
MAKEBA B. FELTON

12 Intrapartum Fetal Assessment, *248*
KEIKO L. TORGERSEN

SECTION FIVE

POSTPARTUM PERIOD, *299*

13 Physical and Psychologic Changes, *301*
TAMARA WHITMER

14 Breastfeeding, *315*
SUSAN SAFFER ORR

15 Contraception, *335*
DENISE G. LINK

SECTION SIX

THE NEWBORN, *343*

16 Transitional Care of the Newborn, *345*
NATALIE DIANE CHEFFER AND DEBRA ANN RANNALLI

17 The Infant at Risk, *362*
JACQUELINE M. McGRATH AND WHITNEY HARDY

SECTION SEVEN

COMPLICATIONS OF CHILDBEARING, *415*

18   Intimate Partner Violence, *417*
KATHRYN RECORDS

19   Hypertensive Disorders in
Pregnancy, *432*
DUSTINE DIX

20   Maternal Infections, *449*
BARBARA A. MORAN

21   Hemorrhagic Disorders, *478*
S. KIM GENOVESE

22   Endocrine and Metabolic
Disorders, *500*
LUCY R. VAN OTTERLOO

23   Trauma in Pregnancy, *535*
LUCY R. VAN OTTERLOO

24   Surgery in Pregnancy, *556*
LINDA CALLAHAN

25   Substance Abuse
in Pregnancy, *573*
BARBARA A. MORAN

26   Other Medical
Complications, *587*
MARGARET YANCY

27   Labor and Delivery at Risk, *624*
ELIZABETH GILBERT

28   Postpartum Complications, *650*
MARY ANN RHODE

SECTION EIGHT

ETHICS AND ISSUES, *667*

29   Ethics, *669*
CHARLOTTE STEPHENSON

Core Curriculum for
Maternal-
Newborn
Nursing

REPRODUCTION: FETAL AND PLACENTAL DEVELOPMENT

1 Reproductive Anatomy, Physiology, and the Menstrual Cycle

Denise G. Link

OBJECTIVES

1. Identify and locate the female organs of reproduction.
2. Describe the physiologic functioning of the female reproductive system.
3. Identify the parameters of sexual maturation and menstruation, including cycle interval, duration of menstrual flow, and perimenopause.
4. Describe the physiologic changes in the ovaries, uterus, and cervix that occur during the menstrual cycle.
5. Explain the physiologic pathways of the hypothalamic-pituitary-ovarian axis and their relationship to the normal menstrual cycle.
6. Describe variations in anatomy that affect reproduction.
7. Describe variations in physiology that affect reproduction.
8. Identify the common variations in the menstrual cycle.
9. Analyze the data from a reproductive history and physical examination to determine overt and covert anatomic and physiologic factors that could affect pregnancy.
10. Prepare a set of nursing interventions for teaching pertinent concepts of anatomy and physiology to clients.

INTRODUCTION

Female Organs of Reproduction

A. **External genitalia: Vulva** (Figure 1-1)
   1. Mons pubis (or mons veneris)
      a. A rounded pad of subcutaneous fatty tissue over the symphysis pubis; covered with pubic hair
      b. Function is the protection of the symphysis pubis during intercourse.
   2. Labia majora
      a. Two rounded folds of fatty and connective tissues, covered with pubic hair, that extend from the mons pubis to the perineum
      b. Function is the protection of the vaginal introitus.
   3. Labia minora
      a. Narrow folds of hairless skin located within the labia majora; begin beneath the clitoris and extend to the fourchette.
      b. Highly vascular and rich in nerve supply; glands lubricate the vulva
      c. Function is erotic; swell in response to stimulation and are highly sensitive.
   4. Prepuce of clitoris is a hoodlike covering over the clitoris.
   5. Clitoris
      a. An erectile organ located beneath the pubic arch that consists of shaft and glans
      b. Secretes smegma, a pheromone (olfactory erotic stimulant)
      c. Extremely sensitive to touch, pressure, and temperature
      d. Function is sexual stimulation.

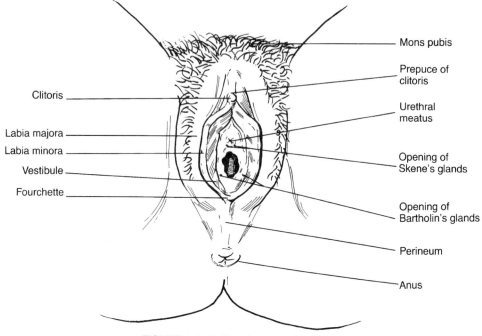

Clitoris

Labia majora

Labia minora

Vestibule

Fourchette

Mons pubis

Prepuce of clitoris

Urethral meatus

Opening of Skene's glands

Opening of Bartholin's glands

Perineum

Anus

FIGURE 1-1 ■ Female external genitals.

6. Vestibule
   a. An oval-shaped area whose boundaries are the clitoris, fourchette, and labia minora; contains the following:
      (1) Urethral meatus
         (a) The terminal portion of the urethra, with puckered or slit appearance
         (b) Located 2.5 cm (1 inch) below the clitoris
      (2) Skene's glands
         (a) Located inside the urethral meatus
         (b) Produce mucus for lubrication
      (3) Hymen
         (a) Tough, elastic, perforated, mucosa-covered tissue that forms a rim around the internal perimeter of the vaginal introitus
         (b) Hymenal opening might be absent or small, impeding menstrual flow and intercourse.
         (c) Characteristics of the hymen vary widely among women; the presence or absence of the hymen can neither confirm nor rule out sexual experience.
      (4) Bartholin's glands
         (a) Located at the base of each of the labia minora, just inside the vaginal orifice
         (b) During coitus, secrete mucus that creates a favorable environment for sperm
7. Fourchette is a point located midline below the vaginal opening where the labia majora and labia minora merge.
8. Perineum
   a. Skin-covered muscular tissue located between the vaginal opening and the anus
   b. The area of a midline episiotomy
   c. Might be lacerated during childbirth.
B. **Internal organs** (Figure 1-2)
   1. Vagina
      a. A hollow tubular structure located behind the bladder and in front of the rectum; extends from the introitus to the cervix
      b. Thin-walled; composed of smooth muscle; capable of great distention as well as collapse
      c. Lined with a glandular mucous membrane that is arranged in folds called rugae

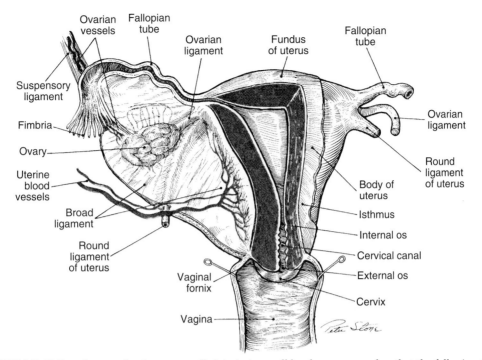

FIGURE 1-2 ■ Female reproductive organs. Front uterine wall has been removed so that the fallopian tube, uterus, cervical canal, and vagina are seen as a continuous channel. (From Langley, L.L., Telford, I.R., & Christensen, J.B. [1980]. *Dynamic anatomy and physiology.* New York: McGraw-Hill.)

   d. Highly vascular and relatively insensitive; adds little sensation for the female during coitus
   e. Functions as the outflow track for menstrual fluid and for vaginal and cervical secretions, the birth canal, and the organ for coitus
 2. Uterus
   a. Located behind the symphysis pubis between the bladder and the rectum
   b. Muscular, hollow, smooth, mobile, nontender, firm, and symmetric
   c. In a woman who has not been pregnant, uterine size ranges from 5.5 to 8 cm (2.2 to 3.2 inches) long, 3.5 to 4 cm (1.4 to 1.6 inches) wide, and 2 to 2.5 cm (0.8 to 1 inch) deep; size increases after childbirth.
   d. Is similar in shape to a light bulb or pear
   e. Is a single organ composed of four distinct areas:
      (1) Fundus
         (a) The upper, rounded portion above the insertion of the fallopian tubes
         (b) Beginning at the 20th week of pregnancy, uterine size is measured in centimeters from the height of the fundus to the top of the symphysis pubis.
      (2) Corpus (or body) is the main portion of the uterus, located between the cervix and the fundus.
      (3) Isthmus
         (a) Also called the lower uterine segment during pregnancy
         (b) Joins the corpus to the cervix
      (4) Cervix (or opening of the uterus)
         (a) Divided into two portions: the portion above the site of attachment of the cervix to the vaginal vault is called the supravaginal portion; the portion below the attachment site that protrudes into the vagina is called the vaginal portion.
         (b) Composed of fibrous connective tissue
         (c) Diameter varies from 2 to 5 cm (0.8 to 2 inches), depending on childbearing history.
         (d) Length is usually 2.5 to 3 cm (1 to 1.2 inches) in a nonpregnant woman.
         (e) Vaginal portion is smooth, firm, and doughnut shaped, with visible central opening called the external os.

       (f) Internal os is the opening of the cervix inside the uterine cavity.
       (g) Cervical canal forms the passageway between the external os of the cervix and the uterine cavity; major feature is the ability to stretch to a diameter large enough to allow passage of an infant's head and then to return to a closed position.
       (h) Produces mucus in response to cyclic hormones; thickened cervical mucus can impede the passage of sperm and bacteria; thin cervical mucus facilitates the movement of sperm and prolongs sperm life; observation of changes in cervical mucus is important in fertility awareness methods of family planning.
       (i) At maturity the cervical vaginal surface is covered with squamous epithelium; cervical canal is lined with columnar epithelium.
         [i] Area where two types of epithelium meet is called the squamocolumnar (SC) junction; also called the transformation zone or T-zone.
         [ii] Prior to puberty, the cervix is covered with columnar epithelium, and the SC junction is located on the outer surface of the cervix.
         [iii] Beginning at puberty, under the influence of estrogen, the SC junction gradually recedes back toward the external os, with squamous epithelium replacing the columnar epithelium.
         [iv] The SC junction is the most frequent site of changes associated with the development of cervical cancer; cells from the SC junction and other areas of the cervix are assessed via the Papanicolaou (Pap) test.
  f. Uterine position (Figure 1-3)
    (1) Five positions are possible
      (a) Anteflexed
      (b) Anterior (anteverted)
      (c) Midposition
      (d) Posterior (retroverted)
      (e) Retroflexed
  g. Uterine support (see Figure 1-2)
    (1) Anterior ligament extends from the anterior cervix to the bladder.
    (2) Cardinal (transverse) ligaments
      (a) Portion of the broad ligaments
      (b) Contain uterine blood vessels and ureters
      (c) Connected to the lateral margins of the uterus
    (3) Posterior ligament extends from the posterior cervix to the rectum.
    (4) Uterosacral ligaments
      (a) Extend from the cervix over the rectum to the sacral vertebrae
      (b) Maintain traction on the cervix to hold the uterus in position
  h. Uterine wall
    (1) Composed of three layers
      (a) Endometrium is a highly vascular mucous membrane that responds to hormone stimulation first by hypertrophy and then by secretion to prepare to receive the developing ovum; sloughs if pregnancy does not occur, resulting in menstruation; if pregnancy occurs, sloughs after delivery.
      (b) Myometrium is composed of smooth muscle in layers.

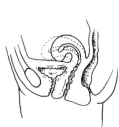
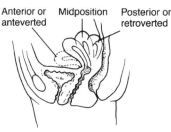
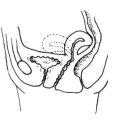

FIGURE 1-3 ■ Uterine positions.

[i] Outer layer is composed of longitudinal fibers, which predominate in the fundus and provide power to expel the fetus.

[ii] Middle layer is composed of fibers interlaced with blood vessels in a figure-eight pattern; contraction following childbirth helps control blood loss.

[iii] Inner layer is composed of circular fibers concentrated around the internal cervical os; provides sphincter action to help keep the cervix closed during pregnancy.

(c) Parietal peritoneum covers most of the uterus, except for the cervix and a portion of the anterior corpus.

3. Fallopian tubes or oviducts (see Figure 1-2)
    a. Attached to the uterine fundus and curve around each ovary
    b. Provide a passageway for the ovum into the uterus
    c. 10 cm (4 inches) in length and 0.6 cm (0.25 inch) in diameter
    d. Composed of four parts
        (1) Infundibulum: the most distal portion; funnel-shaped; covered with fimbriae that guide the ovum into the tube by creating a wavelike motion
        (2) Ampulla: next most distal portion of the fallopian tube and site of fertilization
        (3) Isthmus: narrowed part of the fallopian tube; closest to the uterus
        (4) Interstitial: narrowest portion, which passes through the uterine myometrium and opens into the uterine cavity
    e. Functions
        (1) Capture of the ovum
        (2) Transport of the ovum into the uterus via peristaltic activity and wavelike motion of the cilia that line the fallopian tube
        (3) Secretion of nutrients to support the ovum during transport
4. Ovaries (female gonads) (see Figure 1-2)
    a. Comparable with the testes in the male
    b. Located on either side of the uterus, below and behind the fimbriated ends of the oviducts
    c. Supported by the ovarian ligaments and the mesovarian portion of the broad ligament
    d. Similar to shelled almonds in size and shape; smooth, mobile, slightly tender, and firm
    e. Functions include ovulation and production of hormones (estrogen, progesterone, and androgens).

C. **Support for organs of reproduction**
    1. Circulation
        a. Blood is supplied to the pelvis by arteries branching from the hypogastric artery (which branches from the iliac artery, a division of the aorta).
        b. Major pelvic arteries include the uterine, vaginal, pudendal, and perineal arteries.
        c. Ovarian arteries branch directly from the aorta.
        d. Lymphatic drainage is accomplished from the uterus, ovaries, and fallopian tubes to nodes around the aorta, with some use of the femoral, iliac, and hypogastric nodes.
    2. Pelvic floor and perineum
        a. Functions
            (1) Support of the suspended internal organs of reproduction
            (2) Support for sphincter control, allowing for expansion of the vagina with expulsion of the fetus, and closure of the vagina after delivery
        b. Pelvic diaphragm (Figure 1-4)
            (1) Levator ani muscles
                (a) Puborectalis
                (b) Iliococcygeus
                (c) Pubococcygeus
            (2) Coccygeal muscles
        c. Urogenital diaphragm (see Figure 1-4): transverse perineal muscles
        d. Perineum (see Figure 1-4)
            (1) Bulbocavernosus muscle
            (2) Ischiocavernosus muscle
            (3) Anal sphincter muscle
            (4) Perineal strength can be increased through pelvic floor (Kegel) exercises.

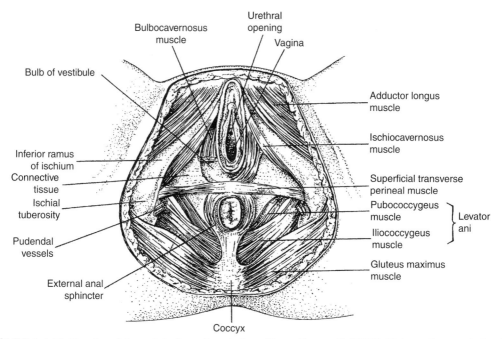

FIGURE 1-4 ■ Muscles of the pelvic floor, from below. (From Sloane, E. [2002]. *Biology of women* [4th ed.]. Albany, NY: Delmar.)

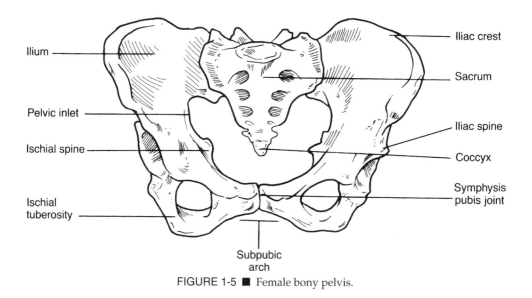

FIGURE 1-5 ■ Female bony pelvis.

  e. Perineal body
   (1) Wedge-shaped area between the vagina and the rectum
   (2) Anchor point for muscles, ligaments, and fascia of the pelvis
 3. Bony pelvis (Figure 1-5)
  a. Functions include support and protection of pelvic structures, and support for a growing fetus during gestation.
  b. Components include:
   (1) Ilium
    (a) Iliac crests
    (b) Anterior, superior iliac spines

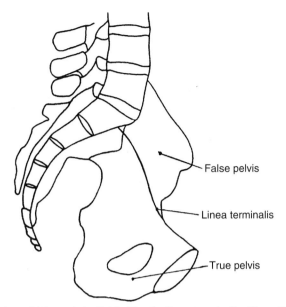

FIGURE 1-6 ■ True pelvis and false pelvis divided by the linea terminalis. (From Ross Laboratories. *Clinical Education Aid No. 18*, Columbus, OH.)

          (2) Ischium
             (a) Ischial spines
             (b) Ischial tuberosities
          (3) Pubic bone
             (a) Symphysis pubis joint
             (b) Subpubic arch
          (4) Sacrum; sacral promontory
          (5) Coccyx
      c. Ilium, ischium, and pubic bones fuse after puberty; the pelvic bone then is called the right or left innominate bone.
      d. False pelvis (Figure 1-6)
          (1) Area of the pelvis above the anterior, superior iliac spines
          (2) Provides no useful data for estimating the size of the birth canal
      e. True pelvis (see Figure 1-6)
          (1) Composed of three pelvic planes
             (a) Pelvic inlet is bordered by anterior and superior iliac spines and the sacral promontory.
             (b) Midpelvis is the area between the inlet and the outlet.
             (c) Pelvic outlet is bordered by ischial tuberosities and the coccyx.
  4. Nervous innervation
      a. Motor nerves
          (1) Parasympathetic fibers from the sacral nerves stimulate pelvic vasodilation and inhibit uterine contractions.
          (2) Sympathetic motor nerves from ganglia between T-5 and T-10 stimulate pelvic vasoconstriction and uterine contractions.
      b. Sensory nerves
          (1) Fibers from ovaries and uterus transmit pain sensations to the spinal cord at T-11 to L-1.
          (2) Pain in ovaries, oviducts, and uterus is difficult to differentiate; might be felt in flank, inguinal, vulvar, or suprapubic area.
D. Menstruation
  1. Menarche (onset of the first menstrual period) normally occurs between the ages of 9 and 16 years, with a mean age of 12.8 years in the United States.
  2. Menstrual cycles in the first 2 years postmenarche tend to be irregular; irregular menstrual cycles are associated with irregular ovulation.

3. Menstrual cycles are timed from the first day of menstrual bleeding; the first day of bleeding is marked as day 1 of the cycle.
4. Menstrual cycle length ranges normally from 21 to 36 days; 95% of women have a cycle length between 25 and 32 days.
5. Duration of bleeding ranges from 1 to 8 days; most women report a menstrual flow that lasts from 3 to 5 days.
6. Amount of blood lost averages 30 mL (1 ounce) per menstrual period; a normal range is between 20 and 80 mL (⅔ and 2⅔ ounces).
7. The perimenopausal transition occurs between the ages of 35 and 60 years. Cessation of menses (menopause) is one event that occurs during the perimenopausal transition. The average age for menopause in the United States is 51 years.
8. The menstrual cycle is divided into two phases
   a. Follicular phase
      (1) Starts with day 1 of menses
      (2) Multiple follicles are maturing in the ovary; the terms *primary* or *dominant* describe the follicle selected for maturation during this cycle.
      (3) Maturing follicle is called a graafian follicle.
      (4) Estrogen is produced in the follicles.
      (5) Follicular phase ends with the release of the egg from the mature follicle (ovulation).
      (6) Normal variation in length of this phase is 7 to 22 days (e.g., it would be 14 days in a 28-day cycle).
      (7) The endometrium is in the proliferative phase and thickens during this period of rapid growth.
      (8) At the end of this phase the external cervical os dilates slightly to admit sperm; the cervix becomes softer.
      (9) Cervix produces mucus that is thin, clear, slippery, stretchy, copious in quantity, and designed to aid sperm in passage through the cervix; the stretching property is called spinnbarkeit.
      (10) Ovulation usually occurs within 24 hours before, during, or after the last day of this slippery discharge.
   b. Luteal phase
      (1) Starts with ovulation
      (2) Follicle that releases the ovum becomes the corpus luteum.
      (3) Corpus luteum produces estrogen and progesterone.
      (4) Function ends in 14 days if conception does not occur.
      (5) Endometrium is in the secretory phase; increasingly vascular and filled with glandular secretions, ready to support a fertilized ovum.
      (6) If no conception occurs, the corpus luteum deteriorates, and levels of estrogen and progesterone decrease.
      (7) Menstruation begins, signaling the start of a new cycle.
9. Common deviations from normal in the menstrual cycle
   a. Amenorrhea: absence of menstrual periods; pregnancy is a common cause.
      (1) Primary amenorrhea
         (a) Failure of the onset of menstruation
            [i] By age 14 in the absence of secondary sex characteristics
            [ii] By age 16 in the presence of secondary sex characteristics
         (b) Might be due to chromosomal defects
            [i] Congenital agenesis of the ovaries or uterus
            [ii] "Streak" ovaries: nonfunctional; will not produce ova or the hormones necessary to initiate puberty
      (2) Secondary amenorrhea
         (a) Interruption of menses prior to age 40 in a previously menstruating woman
         (b) Absence of menses for 6 months or the equivalent of three cycles in a woman who does not menstruate every month.
      (3) Menarche usually requires a minimum height of 152.4 cm (5 feet) and a minimum weight of 47.5 kg (105 pounds), with a fat-to-lean ratio of 1:3; females with body fat levels less than 16% seldom menstruate.

(4) Menarche delay is common in girls who are competitive athletes, who have eating disorders such as anorexia nervosa, or who participate in activities in which extreme thinness is valued, such as ballet and gymnastics; might lead to the development of osteoporosis if estrogen levels are consistently low for a prolonged period of time.

  b. Anovulatory cycles

    (1) Common in the early years following menarche and the years immediately preceding menopause

    (2) A graafian follicle matures and estrogen is produced, but ovulation does not occur.

      (a) Corpus luteum does not form and progesterone is not available.

      (b) Uterine lining thickens in response to estrogen.

      (c) Progesterone-induced signal to start and stop the menstrual flow is absent.

    (3) Might result in light, irregular menses, and difficulty in conceiving, or might result in frequent, prolonged, heavy menstrual flow.

  c. Inadequate (short) luteal phase

    (1) Corpus luteum stops producing hormones prematurely or produces inadequate levels of estrogen and progesterone.

    (2) Can lead to infertility

    (3) Can cause early pregnancy losses when progesterone levels are too low to support the pregnancy until the placental formation is complete

E. The hypothalamic-pituitary-ovarian axis

  1. Responsible for the control of the hormones that regulate function of the reproductive system

  2. Sphenoidal sinus in the brain houses the pituitary gland; the hypothalamus is located directly above the pituitary gland.

  3. Pituitary gland is divided into two parts: the anterior and the posterior; function and control of the two sections are separate and distinct.

  4. Hypothalamus releases hormones (called releasing factors) into the hypophysial portal system that supplies the anterior pituitary; these hormones provide instructions to the anterior pituitary.

  5. Releasing factors signal the anterior pituitary to produce hormones, which in turn stimulate certain target organs to produce hormones.

  6. Releasing factors are produced by the hypothalamus in response to the decreasing levels of hormones being produced by the target organs; when the levels of hormones from the target organs increase, the hypothalamus responds by decreasing the releasing factor hormones sent to the anterior pituitary.

  7. This type of system is called a feedback loop; when rising levels of target organ hormones result in a decrease in the releasing factor and stimulating hormones, the system is called a negative feedback loop.

  8. Target organs include the ovaries, the thyroid, and the adrenal cortex.

  9. Feedback loop functioning for the ovary

    a. During menstruation a message is sent through the central nervous system to the hypothalamus that circulating levels of estrogen are low.

    b. Hypothalamus responds by sending gonadotropin-releasing hormone to the anterior pituitary.

    c. Anterior pituitary responds by sending first follicle-stimulating hormone (FSH) and then luteinizing hormone (LH) to the ovary.

    d. Ovary responds to FSH by selecting a follicle for maturation and choosing from among several follicles that are undergoing early development and producing estrogen; the chosen follicle that begins to mature is called the graafian follicle.

    e. LH stimulates the graafian follicle to release the egg, and ovulation occurs; the graafian follicle becomes a corpus luteum, which produces estrogen and progesterone.

    f. There are now high circulating levels of estrogen and progesterone.

      (1) If conception does not occur, circulating levels of estrogen and progesterone gradually decrease as the corpus luteum disintegrates.

      (2) When estrogen levels are again low, menstruation begins, another message is sent to the hypothalamus, and the cycle begins again.

CLINICAL PRACTICE

A. Assessment

1. Subjective assessment (health interview or history)
    a. Health history, including previous or current factors that might affect reproductive function or affect pregnancy
        (1) Endocrine disorders
            (a) Hypothyroidism or hyperthyroidism
            (b) Hypertension
            (c) Diabetes mellitus (types 1 and 2; gestational diabetes)
            (d) Hyperparathyroidism
            (e) Adrenal disorders
        (2) Pelvic infection
            (a) Interferes with conception secondary to the formation of scar tissue in the fallopian tubes in response to inflammation
            (b) Can be asymptomatic
            (c) Infection and resultant scarring of the fallopian tubes, which leaves the oviducts blocked, is a major cause of infertility.
        (3) Endometriosis
            (a) May cause significant pain with menstruation and interfere with conception
            (b) Scar tissue is formed in response to inflammation and/or bleeding from ectopic endometrial implants (functioning endometrial tissue that has migrated outside of the uterus).
        (4) Uterine fibroids
            (a) Benign tumors that alter the shape of the uterus and its ability to expand
            (b) Might cause excessive menstrual bleeding
            (c) More common in women older than 35
    b. Surgical history
        (1) Pelvic surgery (i.e., ovarian cystectomy or uterine myomectomy) increases risk of formation of adhesions that interfere with conception or maintenance of a pregnancy.
        (2) Repetitive dilation and curettage procedures in the uterus for diagnosis or pregnancy termination might result in the following:
            (a) Asherman syndrome
                [i] Uterine scar tissue forms, usually as a result of aggressive curettage.
                [ii] Scar tissue interferes with the normal cyclic changes in the endometrium (uterine lining)
            (b) Incompetent cervix
                [i] Due to repetitive, forced dilation of the cervix
                [ii] Cervix is unable to remain closed during pregnancy, which leads to spontaneous abortion or preterm labor (see Chapter 24 for discussion of surgery as treatment for incompetent cervix).
        (3) A cone biopsy/cryosurgery, laser surgery to cervix, and loop electrosurgical excision procedure (LEEP)
            (a) Risk of scarring, which prevents conception
            (b) Risk of incompetent cervix
    c. Reproductive history
        (1) Puberty is characterized by developmental milestones that provide evidence that ovaries and uterus are present and functioning, such as the following:
            (a) Secondary sex characteristics, including breast development and the appearance of axillary and pubic hair (Tanner scale)
            (b) Menarche occurring before the age of 16 years
        (2) Menstrual history
            (a) Age at menarche
            (b) Date of the last menstrual period and determination of whether the last menstrual period was a normal one for the woman
            (c) The usual cycle length and the cycle length for this period
            (d) The usual duration of bleeding and the duration of bleeding for this cycle
            (e) Cramps

[i] Present or absent
[ii] Degree of interference with normal activities
(f) Clots
(g) Molimina symptoms
[i] Defined as cyclic symptoms associated with menses
[ii] Examples: premenstrual bloating, breast tenderness, and irritability
[iii] Presence is due to estrogen and progesterone
[iv] Molimina symptoms plus regular and normal menses imply a pattern of normal ovulation.
(3) Reproductive functioning
(a) Pregnancy history
[i] Number of confirmed pregnancies: gravida
[ii] Number of term pregnancies (pregnancies that lasted at least 37 weeks)
[iii] Number of preterm pregnancies (confirmed pregnancies that ended between 20 and 37 weeks' gestation)
[iv] Number of confirmed pregnancies that ended before 20 weeks' gestation: spontaneous and induced abortions
[v] Number of children who are currently living
[vi] Difficulty in conceiving
[vii] Causes of pregnancy losses
[viii] Problems in perinatal period
[ix] Labor: preterm or prolonged
[x] Delivery: type of anesthesia, episiotomy, vacuum extraction, or forceps used; cesarean birth
[xi] Postpartum period: hemorrhage, infection, difficulty with healing of lacerations or episiotomy (e.g., fistula formation)
d. Sociocultural history
(1) Attitudes and values toward menstruation
(a) Common cultural attitudes include menstruation as illness, as a state of uncleanliness, as a time of decreased competence, and as a time associated with fear of contamination.
(b) Some American Indian cultures isolate a menstruating woman.
(c) Orthodox Judaism requires a ritual bath after menstruation.
(d) In post–World War II Japan, a policy of menstrual leave for "incapacitated" women was enacted.
(e) In the United States and the United Kingdom, criminal court cases have been tried with defenses of diminished capacity from premenstrual syndrome as a plea for women accused of acts of violence.
(2) Sexual practices that can lead to increased risk of pelvic infection and affect fertility
(a) Multiple partners
(b) Recent change in sexual partners
(c) Failure to use a condom when indicated
2. Objective assessment (physical examination)
a. General survey
(1) Secondary sex characteristics: Tanner stages of development (Figure 1-7)
(2) Pelvic examination
(a) External genitalia
[i] Structural abnormalities (i.e., evidence of female circumcision procedure common in some cultures)
[ii] Evidence of infection, as signaled by discharge from glands
[iii] Hymenal opening
(b) Internal organs
[i] Vagina
• Color, integrity, and presence of discharge
• Rectocele or cystocele is the herniation of the vaginal wall with the rectum or the bladder protruding into the vagina.
• Uterine prolapse is the relaxation of vaginal support, with the uterus in the vagina.

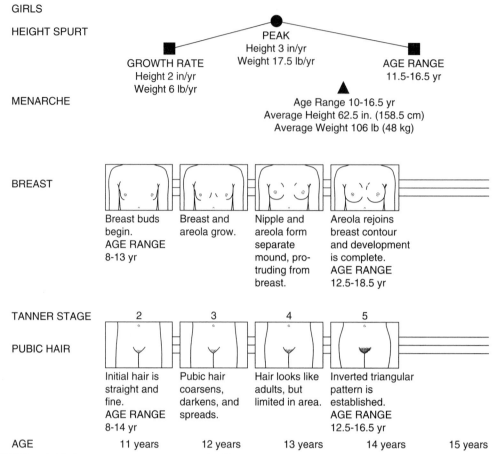

GIRLS

HEIGHT SPURT

PEAK
Height 3 in/yr
Weight 17.5 lb/yr

GROWTH RATE
Height 2 in/yr
Weight 6 lb/yr

AGE RANGE
11.5-16.5 yr

MENARCHE

Age Range 10-16.5 yr
Average Height 62.5 in. (158.5 cm)
Average Weight 106 lb (48 kg)

BREAST

| Breast buds begin. AGE RANGE 8-13 yr | Breast and areola grow. | Nipple and areola form separate mound, protruding from breast. | Areola rejoins breast contour and development is complete. AGE RANGE 12.5-18.5 yr |

TANNER STAGE

| 2 | 3 | 4 | 5 |

PUBIC HAIR

| Initial hair is straight and fine. AGE RANGE 8-14 yr | Pubic hair coarsens, darkens, and spreads. | Hair looks like adults, but limited in area. | Inverted triangular pattern is established. AGE RANGE 12.5-16.5 yr |

| AGE | 11 years | 12 years | 13 years | 14 years | 15 years |

FIGURE 1-7 ■ Tanner maturity rating scale (female). (From Tanner, J.M. [1962]. *Growth at adolescence* [2nd ed.]. Oxford, UK: Blackwell Scientific Publications.)

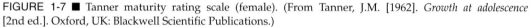

[ii] Cervix: parity and appearance
 • Structural abnormalities
 • Patency
 • Evidence of infection
 [iii] Uterus
 • Size, shape, consistency, and mobility
 • Position
 [iv] Adnexa
 • Size, shape, consistency, and mobility of ovaries
 • Oviducts usually not palpable.
 (c) Bony pelvis
 [i] Estimate of anteroposterior diameter of the pelvic inlet (i.e., the distance between sacral promontory and subpubic arch [12.5 to 13 cm])
 [ii] Prominence of ischial spines and bispinous diameter (11 cm)
 [iii] Prominence of coccyx (see Chapter 10 for a complete discussion of pelvic measurements)
3. Diagnostic procedures
 a. Menstrual calendar
 b. Blood chemistry, including lipid levels
 c. Hemoglobin and hematocrit
 (1) Anemia might result from excessive menstrual blood loss.
 (2) Anemia is usually when hemoglobin levels are less than 12 g/dL and hematocrit levels are less than 37%.

    d. FSH and LH levels
- (1) Elevated when ovaries are not functioning normally with cyclic ovulation
- (2) FSH levels higher than 40 mIU/mL and LH levels higher than 25 mIU/mL are diagnostic for anovulation.
- (3) Normal levels of FSH are 5 to 30 mIU/mL and normal LH levels are 5 to 20 mIU/mL.
- (4) FSH level is a better indicator of ovarian function than gonadal hormone levels.

    e. Prolactin
- (1) Elevated levels block the action of estrogen.
- (2) Normal levels are 0 to 23 mg/dL.

    f. Thyroid function tests
- (1) Identify hyperthyroidism and hypothyroidism.
- (2) Normal nonpregnant values
  - (a) Serum thyroxine (T_4), 5 to 12 mcg/dL
  - (b) Serum triiodothyronine (T_3), 80 to 200 mg/dL
  - (c) Thyroid-stimulating hormone, 2 to 5.4 mIU/mL

    g. Progesterone
- (1) Level is tested on menstrual cycle days 21 to 23 (28-day cycle).
- (2) Provides evidence of ovulation
- (3) Low levels after conception might lead to a spontaneous abortion.

    h. Testosterone and dehydroepiandrosterone sulfate (DHEAS)
- (1) Androgens are produced by the normal ovary and the adrenal gland.
- (2) High levels usually are associated with anovulation and amenorrhea.

    i. Endometrial biopsy
- (1) Evaluates the influences of hormones on the uterine lining
- (2) Is performed on days 21 to 23 of a 28-day cycle
- (3) Estrogen and progesterone, which are present after ovulation, produce the characteristic changes in the microscopic lining of the uterus.

4. Potential psychosocial responses to the reproductive assessment

    a. Concerns
- (1) Modesty
- (2) Feelings of invasion of privacy
- (3) Strangers invading privacy
- (4) Gender of examiner; same or different

    b. Meaning of examination for the woman

    c. Desire for assurances that all structures appear normal

B. Interventions/Outcomes

1. Not knowledgeable about normal anatomy and physiology of the female reproductive system

    a. Interventions
- (1) Assess current level of understanding.
- (2) Identify inaccuracies or gaps in knowledge.
- (3) Identify the woman's interest in increasing her knowledge.
- (4) Formulate a teaching plan.
- (5) Evaluate the effectiveness of the implemented plan.

    b. Outcomes
- (1) The woman will be able to explain anatomic or physiologic functioning in the areas in which previous inaccuracies or gaps were identified.
- (2) The woman will state that her learning needs were met.

2. Abnormal anatomic or physiologic status of the female reproductive system

    a. Interventions
- (1) Identify the specific alteration in function.
- (2) Identify the physiologic basis for the alteration in function.
- (3) Formulate a management plan with the woman.
- (4) Assess the woman's level of understanding of the problem and plan of management.
- (5) Formulate a teaching plan to increase understanding.
- (6) Implement the management plan and the teaching plan.
- (7) Evaluate the effectiveness of the implemented plans.
- (8) Communicate the effectiveness to other members of the health care team.

   b. Outcomes
       (1) The woman will repeat an accurate description of the specific problem of alteration in functioning.
       (2) The woman will describe the proposed management plan accurately.
       (3) The woman will state that her health care needs were met.
3. Not knowledgeable about physical changes that occur during the normal menstrual cycle
   a. Interventions
       (1) Assess the current level of knowledge of the cyclic physical changes that occur in a normal menstrual cycle.
       (2) Provide necessary instruction for learning gaps that have been identified.
       (3) Reassess the level of knowledge of physical changes attributed to the menstrual cycle after instruction.
   b. Outcomes
       (1) The woman will be able to describe the timing of the physical changes that commonly occur during her menstrual cycle.
       (2) The woman will be able to identify whether those changes are within the normal range.
       (3) The woman will be able to identify changes in her menstrual cycle that require the attention of a health care professional.

HEALTH EDUCATION

Appropriate, age-specific, individualized instruction regarding reproductive anatomy and physiology should be presented by the health care provider. Health education about the menstrual cycle should also be provided according to an assessment of the current level of knowledge of the woman as well as her current level of understanding of the subject. The teaching plan should use the particular concerns of the woman or the particular details of her diagnosis to help her understand her own situation as well as the parameters of normal functioning.

A. **Identify the purpose of the instruction.**
B. **Identify the characteristics of the learner.**
   1. Assess the current level of understanding.
   2. Identify learning needs and preferred learning style of the woman.
   3. Identify the woman's level of comfort with the subject matter.
   4. If in a group educational setting, identify the level of comfort of members of the group with each other.
C. **Choose an instructional method appropriate to the learning needs and comfort level of the participants.**
D. **Develop a teaching plan.**
E. **Implement the teaching plan.**
F. **Evaluate the effectiveness of the teaching plan in terms of meeting the learning needs of the participants.**
G. **Alter the teaching plan.**
H. **Implement the alterations.**
I. **Reevaluate the teaching plan.**

CASE STUDIES AND STUDY QUESTIONS

An 18-year-old girl has decided to see a health care provider to find out "why I'm so slow in developing." Her last physical examination was 5 years ago; she reports no serious illnesses and no operations. Her chief complaints are lack of breast development and delayed onset of menstruation. She is 156 cm (5 feet, 1 inch) tall and weighs 48 kg (105 pounds). She states that she has never had a menstrual period, does not have to shave her underarms and legs, and has never had acne. Pertinent physical findings include an absence of secondary sex characteristics, including a lack of breast development and of axillary hair and pubic hair. A vaginal examination was attempted but not completed because of an imperforate hymen. The primary diagnosis is delayed puberty.

1. Further assessment and intervention for this client:
   a. Should be delayed because there is a wide variation in the onset of menses and breast development among young girls.
   b. Are necessary because the development of secondary sex characteristics and the onset of menstruation normally occur by the age of 16 years.
   c. Are not essential because breast development normally precedes menstruation by several years.
   d. Should focus on treatment of her imperforate hymen.
2. Further studies reveal a chromosomal karyotype of XX, the presence of a very small uterus, and "streak" ovaries. Exogenous sources of estrogen and progesterone are recommended to trigger the onset of puberty for this young woman. She will need to take these hormones:
   a. Only until her own ovaries are stimulated to begin producing hormones
   b. Only until she decides to become pregnant
   c. Until well past the normal time for menopause because "streak" ovaries are nonfunctioning and will never produce the necessary hormones
   d. She will not need to take these hormones because her ovaries will begin functioning soon.
3. The imperforate hymen:
   a. Must be treated because menstrual flow started by the use of hormone therapy can be trapped and prevented from exiting the vagina

   b. Should be treated when she decides to become sexually active
   c. Should be treated when she decides to become pregnant
   d. Does not require treatment because it will be broken when she has sexual intercourse
4. This girl wants to know about her childbearing capabilities. She will:
   a. Be able to have as many children as she wishes as long as she takes the necessary hormones
   b. Need to use birth control to prevent unwanted pregnancies
   c. Not be able to become pregnant without donor eggs because "streak" ovaries are nonfunctioning and do not contain ova
   d. Not be able to become pregnant because of her imperforate hymen

Mrs. A., 25 years old and married, wants to use the techniques of natural family planning to help her conceive. She had her first menstrual period at the age of 12 years. Her periods are regular, occur every 28 days, and last 4 to 5 days. She has no trouble with cramping or excessive flow. She has noticed breast tenderness, feelings of heaviness and bloating, and irritability in the few days before each period. She also notices an increase in her vaginal discharge in the middle of her cycle; the discharge is thin, slippery, stretchy, and clear.

5. She is probably experiencing:
   a. Regular ovulation because her periods are regular and she is experiencing normal moliminal symptoms
   b. A vaginal infection because of the repetitive discharge
   c. Anovulatory cycles because she is not having trouble with cramps or clots
   d. Some anovulatory cycles because her cycle length varies by a few days and is not always consistent
6. The breast tenderness, bloating, and irritability are due to:
   a. The effects of falling levels of estrogen during this phase of the cycle
   b. The effects of progesterone produced by the corpus luteum after ovulation occurs
   c. The effects of rising levels of testosterone during this phase of the cycle
   d. These symptoms have no relationship to the levels of hormones in the body.

7. Clear, slippery cervical mucus that occurs at midcycle has a quality of stretchiness called spinnbarkeit. This quality is associated with cervical changes, including:
   a. The opening of the cervical os to aid the sperm in moving into the uterus
   b. The closing of the cervical os to become more hostile to sperm
   c. The shortening of the cervix to prepare for cervical dilation in labor
   d. A maturation of the cervix that occurs after puberty

ADDITIONAL STUDY QUESTIONS

8. All of the following are components of the external female genitalia except the:
   a. Vulva
   b. Vestibule
   c. Fourchette
   d. Vagina
9. The middle layer of the uterine myometrium is composed of smooth muscle fibers in figure-eight patterns around major blood vessels. This is called a living ligature because:
   a. Contraction of these fibers after childbirth or an abortion helps prevent massive blood loss.
   b. These fibers provide support for the major blood vessels that innervate the uterus.
   c. These fibers contract before the placenta detaches from the uterine wall, thus preventing blood loss from the umbilical cord.
10. Which statement is *not* true for ovaries?
   a. Normally are the size of almonds in women during the reproductive years
   b. Are comparable to the testes in the male
   c. On examination, should be fixed and nonmobile
   d. Are responsible for the production of estrogen, progesterone, and the androgens
11. Which of the following uterine positions is considered abnormal?
   a. Anteflexed
   b. Anterior
   c. Posterior
   d. Retroflexed
   e. None of the above
12. Blocked oviducts are a major cause of infertility. They are most often the result of:
   a. Pelvic inflammatory disease
   b. Congenital abnormality
   c. Exposure to diethylstilbestrol (DES)
   d. Cone biopsy
13. Which of the following describes a menstrual cycle that is within the normal parameters?
   a. Age at menarche: 11 years; cycle length, 42 days; duration of menses, 3 days; blood loss, light
   b. Age at menarche: 8 years; cycle length, 28 days; duration of menses, 4 days; blood loss, heavy
   c. Age at menarche: 12 years; cycle length, 26 to 28 days; duration of menses, 5 days; blood loss, moderate
   d. Age at menarche: 12 years; cycle length, 14 days; duration of menses, 8 days; blood loss, heavy
14. During the menstrual cycle, the hormone progesterone is produced:
   a. Throughout the cycle
   b. From days 1 to 14 by the graafian follicle
   c. From days 14 to 28 by the graafian follicle
   d. Beginning just after ovulation by the corpus luteum

ANSWERS TO STUDY QUESTIONS

1. b	6. b	11. e
2. c	7. a	12. a
3. a	8. d	13. c
4. c	9. a	14. d
5. a	10. c	

BIBLIOGRAPHY

Berak, J. (Ed.). (2006). *Berek & Novak's gynecology* (14th ed.). Philadelphia: Lippincott Williams & Wilkins.

Bickley, L. S., & Szilagyi, P. G. (2008). *Bates's guide to physical examination and history taking* (10th ed.). Philadelphia: Lippincott Williams & Wilkins.

Guyton, A. C., & Hall, J. E. (2006). *Textbook of medical physiology* (11th ed.). Philadelphia: Saunders.

Lowdermilk, D. L., & Perry, S. E. (2007). *Maternity & women's health care* (9th ed.). St. Louis: Mosby.

Speroff, L., & Fritz, M. (2004). *Clinical gynecologic endocrinology and infertility* (7th ed.). Philadelphia: Lippincott Williams & Wilkins.

Thibodeau, G. A., & Patton, K. (2006). *Anatomy and physiology* (6th ed.). St. Louis: Mosby.

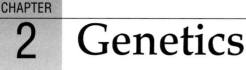

2 Genetics

Linda Callahan

OBJECTIVES

1. Discuss the potential importance of the National Human Genome Project on patient care.
2. Define the terms commonly used in genetic conditions.
3. Describe the implications of an increased amount of chromosomal material, the deletion of genetic material, and the translocation process in chromosomal disorders.
4. Explain the basic mendelian modes of inheritance.
5. Identify client situations that indicate the need for a chromosomal analysis.
6. Assess the emotional effect on couples of the birth of an infant with a genetic disorder.
7. Discuss the responsibility and needed competencies of the nurse in initial counseling and referral of patients for further genetic testing and counseling.

INTRODUCTION

A. **The National Human Genome Project**
   1. First discussed in the 1980s; officially completed in 2003
   2. Goals included sequencing the entire human genome (achieved in April 2003), identifying human deoxyribonucleic acid (DNA) sequence variations, identifying and determining the function of individual genes, and studying the ethical, legal, and social implications of information and technologic outcomes of the Human Genome Project on human beings and society.
   3. Increased understanding of the genotype has allowed:
      a. Development of targeted health promotion strategies
      b. Potential disease prevention
      c. Genotype-tailored drugs to optimize therapeutic effects while minimizing negative drug interactions and side effects
      d. Eventual correction of disease states by development of gene transfer technology (gene therapy)
B. **Definition: Genetics is a medical science concerned with the transmission of characteristics from parent to child** (Nussbaum, McInnes, & Willard, 2007)
   1. Gene: the basic hereditary unit; a DNA sequence required for production of a functional product, usually a protein
   2. Genotype: an individual's genetic makeup
   3. Phenotype: the outward appearance or expression of the genes
   4. Allele: an alternative form of a gene; the wild type, or major sequencing allele is the most common form of a gene found within a population
   5. Mutation: a rare alternative form of an allele; occurs in less than 1% of the population
   6. Polymorphism: a common alternative form of an allele; occurs in more than 1% of the population
   7. Genome: complete DNA sequence containing all of the genetic information for an individual
C. **Foundation of inheritance**
   1. Cell division: all beings begin life as a single cell (zygote). The single cell continues to reproduce itself by the process of either mitosis or meiosis.
      a. Mitosis is the process of cell division in which new cells are made. The new cells have the same number and pattern of chromosomes as the parent cell (46 chromosomes comprising 44 autosomes and 2 sex chromosomes); mitosis occurs in five stages (Figure 2-1).

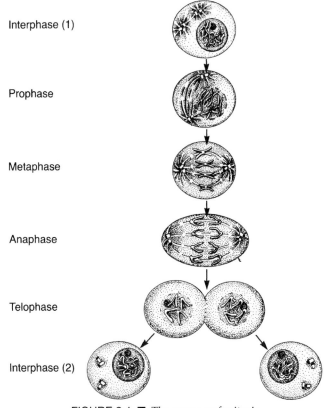

Interphase (1)

Prophase

Metaphase

Anaphase

Telophase

Interphase (2)

FIGURE 2-1 ■ The process of mitosis.

(1) Interphase: before cell division, the DNA replicates itself
(2) Prophase: the strands of chromatin shorten and thicken; the chromosomes reproduce; spindles appear, and the centrioles migrate to the opposite poles of the cell; the membrane separating the nucleus from the cytoplasm disappears
(3) Metaphase: the chromosomes line up along the poles of the spindle
(4) Anaphase: the two chromatids separate and move to the opposite ends of the spindle
(5) Telophase: a nuclear membrane forms, the spindles disappear, and the centrioles relocate to the outside of the new nucleus; toward the end of this phase, the cells divide into two new cells, each with its own nucleus and each having the same number of chromosomes as the parent cell
b. Meiosis is a process of cell division that occurs involving the sperm and ova and is known as gametogenesis; this process decreases the number of chromosomes by 50% (from 46 to 23 per cell) and occurs in two successive cell divisions (Figure 2-2)
  (1) The first division consists of four phases.
    (a) Prophase: the chromosomes move close together
      [i] Crossover of genetic material from each parent takes place at this time.
      [ii] Crossover accounts for the wide individual variation of features seen within same-parent siblings.
    (b) Metaphase: spindle fibers attach to separate chromosomes
    (c) Anaphase: intact chromosome pairs migrate to opposite ends of the cell (the distribution of maternal and paternal chromosomes is random)
    (d) Telophase: the cell divides into two cells, each with 50% (23) of the usual number of chromosomes (22 autosomes and 1 sex chromosome)
  (2) Second division
    (a) The chromatids of each chromosome separate and move to the opposite poles of each of the daughter cells.

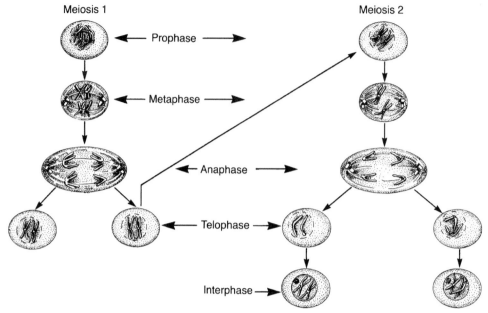

FIGURE 2-2 ■ The process of meiosis.

(b) This is followed by each of the cells dividing into two cells, which results in four cells (spermatogenesis and oogenesis).
  [i] Spermatogenesis is continuous from puberty to senescence.
  [ii] Oogenesis is noncontinuous.
    • Begins in utero, and by the fifth intrauterine month, a full complement of primary oocytes has been produced.
    • Primary oocytes are dormant until puberty, at which time one or two will complete the meiotic cycle each month during a woman's reproductive years.
(c) During the meiotic division, two of the chromatids might not move apart when the cell divides; this lack of separation is called autosomal nondisjunction; this is also the stage at which breakage can occur, resulting in abnormalities of chromosomal structure such as that producing cri du chat syndrome and Down syndrome
(d) Thus meiosis mixes up the chromosomes and crossing over mixes up the genes within a chromosome.
2. Genetic information is present on the chromosomes (Jarvi & Chitzyat, 2008; Lashley, 2007; Nussbaum et al., 2007).
  a. Chromosomes are composed of DNA, a complex protein that carries the genetic information.
  b. DNA occurs as a double-stranded helix found in the cell nucleus.
    (1) Two long strands of DNA molecules are wound around each other.
    (2) The strands are linked by chemical bonds.
    (3) The strands are complementary.
    (4) The chains comprise sequences of four nitrogen base subunits (adenine, guanine, thymine, and cytosine).
  c. Genes are the smallest known unit of heredity.
    (1) Genes are present on the chromosomes and are made up of coding exons and noncoding introns.
    (2) Each gene codes for a particular cellular function, such as specific protein structure.
    (3) Genes occur in pairs (alleles) derived from the mother and father during reproduction.
    (4) Each gene has a specific location on the chromosomes.
    (5) Genetic errors often occur when there are changes, such as deletions, substitutions, or duplications in the location of the gene.

3. Chromosomes form a genetic blueprint that is composed of tightly coiled structures of DNA.
    a. Chromosomes are threadlike structures within the nucleus of the cell that carry the genes.
    b. Humans have 46 chromosomes in each body cell (22 pairs of autosomes and 1 pair of sex chromosomes [diploid]).
    c. Chromosomes have a primary central constriction called the centromere (Figure 2-3).
        (a) The short arm of the chromosome is designated by the letter p.
        (b) The long arm of the chromosome is designated by the letter q.
    d. The sex cells contain 23 chromosomes (haploid).
    e. Abnormalities of chromosome number are as follows (Lashley, 2005, 2007; Nussbaum et al., 2007):
        (1) Paired chromosomes fail to separate during cell division (nondisjunction).
        (2) If nondisjunction occurs during meiosis (before fertilization), the fetus usually will have abnormal numbers of chromosomes in every cell (trisomy or monosomy).
            (a) Trisomy is a product of the union between a normal gamete (egg or sperm) and a gamete that contains an extra chromosome.
                [i] The individual will have 47 chromosomes; one "pair" will have three chromosomes instead of two.
                [ii] Examples of trisomies are Down syndrome (47, XY, +21 [the extra chromosome is in the 21st pair]); trisomy 18 (47, XX, +18); and trisomy 13 (47, XY, +13).
            (b) Monosomy is the product of a union between a normal gamete and a gamete with a missing chromosome.
                [i] The individual will have 45 chromosomes instead of 46.
                [ii] Monosomy of an entire autosome is incompatible with life.
                [iii] Complete monosomy of a sex chromosome is compatible with life; an example is a female with only one X chromosome (45, XO); known as Turner syndrome.
        (3) If nondisjunction occurs after fertilization, the fetus might have two or more chromosomes that evolve into more than one cell line (mosaicism), each with a different number of chromosomes (Lashley, 2007).
            (a) Different body tissues may have different chromosome numbers or a mixture of cells, depending on when the nondisjunction occurred.
            (b) Clinical signs and symptoms vary in mosaicism; they can be severe or inapparent, depending on the number and location of the abnormal cell line.
    f. Abnormalities in chromosome structure are as follows:
        (1) Abnormalities of the chromosomes involving only a part of the chromosome

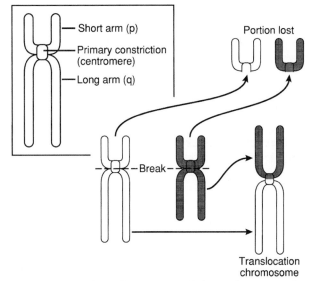

FIGURE 2-3 ■ The process of translocation. Detail shows chromosomal representation.

(2) Abnormalities that can occur by translocation, by deletions, or by additions (Lashley, 2007)

    (a) Translocation occurs when the individual has 45 chromosomes, with one of the chromosomes fused to another chromosome (usually number 21 fused to number 14) (see Figure 2-3).

      [i] The person has the correct amount of chromosomal material (45, t[14q21q]), but it has been rearranged; this individual is known as a balanced translocation carrier.

      [ii] When such an individual and a structurally normal mate have a child, there is a possibility that the offspring:

        • Will receive the carrier parent's abnormal 21/14 chromosome and a normal 14 and 21 from the other parent; thus the child will be a carrier.

        • Will receive the abnormal chromosome, plus a normal 21 from the carrier parent; this will result in an extra amount of chromosomal material for the 21 pair (unbalanced translocation), and the child will have Down syndrome (46,14,t[14q21q]).

    (b) Additions and/or deletions: a portion of a chromosome can be added or lost, which will result in adverse effects on the infant

      [i] Deletions and additions result from a small breakage in the chromosomal structure during early cell division.

      [ii] An example of the consequences of a deletion is the cri du chat syndrome, in which a small amount of chromosomal material is missing from the short arm of chromosome 5 (5p–).

D. Modes of inheritance (mendelian)

  1. Many diseases are caused by an abnormality of a single gene or a pair of genes.

  2. Autosomal dominant inheritance: autosomal dominant disorders occur when an individual has a gene that produces an effect whenever it is present (homozygous or heterozygous); this gene overshadows the other gene of the pair

    a. Mode of transmission (Figure 2-4)

    b. Characteristics

      (1) Affected individuals generally have an affected parent; the family tree (genogram) might show several generations of individuals with the condition

      (2) The affected individual has a one in two (50%) chance with each pregnancy of passing the abnormal gene on to his or her child.

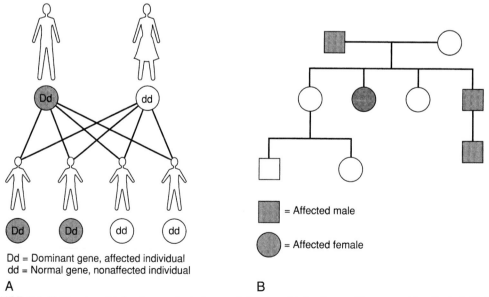

Dd = Dominant gene, affected individual
dd = Normal gene, nonaffected individual

A   B

■ = Affected male

● = Affected female

FIGURE 2-4 ■ Dominant inheritance. **A,** Autosomal dominant inheritance. One parent is affected. Statistically, the offspring have a one in two chance of being affected, regardless of gender. **B,** Autosomal dominant genogram.

(3) Males and females are equally affected.

(4) An unaffected individual cannot transmit the disorder to his or her children.

(5) A mutation (a gene that has been spontaneously altered) can result in a new case.

(6) Autosomal dominant disorders vary greatly in the degree of characteristics that are seen within a family (e.g., in Marfan syndrome, the parent might have only elongated extremities but the child might have a more involved condition, including dislocation of the lens of the eye and severe cardiovascular abnormalities).

3. Autosomal recessive inheritance: an individual has an autosomal recessive disorder if he or she has a gene that produces its effects only when there are two genes on the same chromosome pair (homozygous trait).

   a. A carrier state can occur (heterozygote).

      (1) An individual with the abnormal gene does not manifest obvious symptoms.

      (2) When two carriers pass on the same abnormal gene, the condition might appear.

   b. Mode of transmission (Figure 2-5)

   c. Characteristics

      (1) An affected individual has clinically normal parents, but the parents are both carriers for the abnormal gene.

      (2) The carrier parents have a one in four (25%) chance with each pregnancy of passing the abnormal gene on to their offspring; in this case, when a recessive gene is received from each parent, the child will have the disorder.

      (3) If the offspring of two carrier parents is clinically normal, there is a one in two (50%) chance that he or she will be a carrier, like the parents.

      (4) Males and females are affected equally.

      (5) The family genogram usually shows siblings affected in a horizontal pattern.

      (6) There is an increased risk if intermarriage occurs (consanguineous matings); individuals who are closely related are more likely to have the same genes in common.

      (7) Recessive disorders tend to be more severe in their clinical manifestations.

      (8) The presence of certain autosomal recessive genes can be detected in the normal carrier parent; examples of diseases for which carrier screening is available are sickle cell anemia, Tay-Sachs disease, and cystic fibrosis.

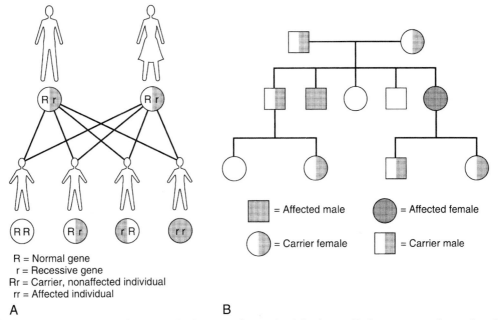

R = Normal gene
r = Recessive gene
Rr = Carrier, nonaffected individual
rr = Affected individual

= Affected male   = Affected female

= Carrier female   = Carrier male

A   B

FIGURE 2-5 ■ Recessive inheritance. **A,** Autosomal recessive inheritance. Both parents are the carriers. Statistically, the offspring have a one in four chance of being affected, regardless of gender. **B,** Autosomal recessive genogram.

4. Sex-linked dominant inheritance
   a. The gene is located on the X chromosome of either the mother or the father.
   b. The gene only needs to be present on one X chromosome for symptoms to be manifested.
   c. Mode of transmission—similar to dominant inheritance (see Figure 2-4), but the gene in question is carried only on the X chromosome.
   d. Characteristics
      (1) All individuals with the gene exhibit the disorder.
      (2) It appears in every generation.
      (3) There is a one in two chance of the female child being affected if the mother is affected.
      (4) All the female children are affected if the father has the affected gene.
      (5) None of the male children is affected if the father has the affected gene.
   e. Examples of sex-linked dominant conditions are vitamin D–resistant rickets, polydactyly, and polycystic renal disease (adult).
5. Sex-linked recessive inheritance
   a. Sex-linked or X-linked disorders are those for which the gene is carried on the X chromosome.
   b. A female might be heterozygous or homozygous for a trait carried on the X chromosome because she has two X chromosomes.
   c. A male has only one X chromosome, and there are some traits for which no comparable genes are located on the Y chromosome; in this case, the gene will be expressed.
   d. The X-linked recessive disorders are manifested only in the male who carries the gene.
   e. Mode of transmission (Figure 2-6).
   f. Characteristics
      (1) There is no male-to-male transmission; fathers pass on their Y chromosome to their sons and their X chromosome to their daughters.
      (2) Affected males are related through the female line.
      (3) There is a one in two (50%) chance with each pregnancy that a carrier mother will pass the abnormal gene on to her son, who will then be affected.
      (4) There is a one in two (50%) chance with each pregnancy that a mother will pass the abnormal gene to her daughter, who will then be a carrier like herself.
      (5) A father affected with an X-linked condition cannot pass the disorder on to his sons, but all of his daughters will be carriers.

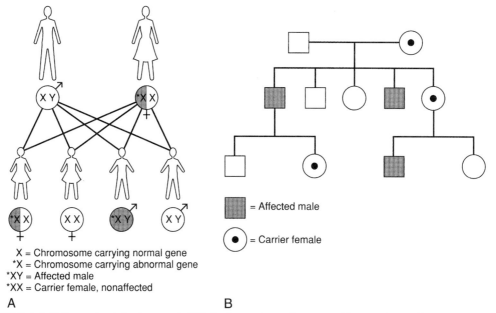

X = Chromosome carrying normal gene
*X = Chromosome carrying abnormal gene
*XY = Affected male
*XX = Carrier female, nonaffected

A

B

■ = Affected male

● = Carrier female

FIGURE 2-6 ■ Recessive inheritance. **A,** X-linked recessive inheritance. The mother is the carrier. Statistically, the male offspring have a one in two chance of being affected, and none of the females will be affected. The female offspring have a one in two chance of being carriers. **B,** X-linked genogram.

(6) Occasionally a female carrier demonstrates the symptoms of an X-linked disorder; this situation is probably due to the random inactivation of the second X chromosome.

    g. Examples of X-linked recessive disorders are color blindness (red-green), Duchenne's muscular dystrophy, and hemophilia A and B.

E. Polygenic or multifactorial disorders

    1. Many common congenital malformations are caused by the interaction of multiple genes and environmental factors, such as health status, age of the parents, and/or exposure to pollutants and viruses.

    2. Characteristics

        a. Malformations vary from mild to severe.

        b. The more severe the defect, the greater the number of genes involved.

        c. There is often a gender bias in occurrence rates for specific malformations.

            (1) Congenital hip dysplasia occurs more frequently in females.

            (2) Pyloric stenosis occurs more frequently in males.

            (3) When a member of the less commonly affected gender manifests the condition, more genes must be present to cause the defect.

        d. In the presence of environmental influences, the appropriate sequence of genes may be affected to manifest the disease.

        e. In contrast with gene disorders, in multifactorial inheritance an additive effect occurs:

            (1) When more than one family member is affected

            (2) In proportion to the severity of the condition in the child

        f. Risk factors are determined by the distribution of cases found in the general population.

        g. The risk of occurrence is usually 2% to 5% for all first-degree relatives but is higher (10% to 15%) if more than one member is affected.

F. Complex disorders occur when:

    1. Multiple genes specify proteins whose effects, when expressed, combine to produce a particular phenotype.

    2. Expression of these specific proteins is environmentally influenced to variable degrees throughout individual development, maturation, and aging.

    3. Some examples of complex disorders include hypercholesterolemia, depression, schizophrenia, essential hypertension, and type 2 diabetes mellitus.

    4. The prevalence of such disorders is generally high in the population.

    5. Individual disease occurrence is not easily traced through the pedigree; there generally is not a clear path of inheritance or segregation.

    6. The age at disease onset is often during adult years when reproduction has already occurred.

    7. The threshold for disease expression can be affected by a number of different variables; such variables are often controlled to decrease risk of disease expression (e.g., weight control to decrease the incidence of type 2 diabetes mellitus onset).

CLINICAL PRACTICE

A. The health care professional, at a minimum, should:

    1. Appreciate his/her personal limitations of genetic expertise

    2. Understand the social and psychologic implications of genetic services

    3. Know how and when to make a referral to a genetics professional

    4. Strive to meet the knowledge, skill, and attitude competencies as outlined by the National Coalition for Health Professional Education in Genetics (NCHPEG) most recently in 2007 (Competencies are available at www.nchpeg.org.)

B. Assessment

    1. Family history: take a thorough family history going back at least three generations (genogram) (Figure 2-7) (Lashley, 2007). Competencies in Family History (2008) is a program that lays out health care professional competencies for taking and interpreting a family history (available at www.nchpeg.org).

    2. Information to be gathered about all three generations should include:

        a. Legal names, including maiden names of all family members

        b. Racial, ethnic background, and country of origin

        c. Place and date of birth

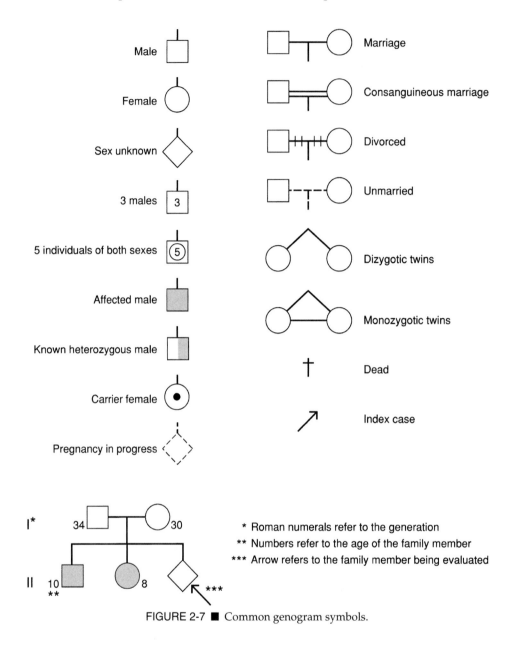

FIGURE 2-7 ■ Common genogram symbols.

d. Occupation
e. Current and past health status
f. Age and cause of death
g. Presence of birth defects, retardation, or repetitive family traits
h. Any miscarriages, stillbirths, or severe childhood illnesses/deaths
i. Environmental, occupational exposures, and social history
j. Medication and drug use history

3. Physical findings: evaluate all systems; chromosomal disorders affect multiple body systems, and many gene disorders have subtle signs that will be detected only through careful assessment of, for example, skin pigmentation, color of sclera, fingernail patterns, texture of hair, and neurologic responses

4. Diagnostic tests that might be performed are:
   a. Maternal serum alpha-fetoprotein (AFP) to screen for neural tube defects (elevated) or Down syndrome (low) in the fetus
      (1) AFP alone detects only 20% of Down syndrome fetuses.

(2) AFP in combination with human chorionic gonadotropin (hCG) levels and assessing for levels of unconjugated estriol can improve the rate of detection.

(3) If AFP, hCG, and unconjugated estriol levels are indicative, the mother can be counseled to undergo chromosome analysis to verify the diagnosis.

b. Chromosomal and biochemical analyses via chorionic villi sampling or amniocentesis

c. DNA analysis can be performed on the fetus.

d. Developmental assessment of parents or siblings as indicated by possible risk status established by a family history (such as fragile X syndrome)

e. Fetal ultrasonography for suspected structural disorders (e.g., omphaloceles, renal agenesis)

f. Newborn screening tests (phenylketonuria [PKU], galactosemia, hypothyroidism)

g. Other laboratory tests as indicated by physical signs and symptoms.

5. 10% to 25% of birth defects are due to classical gentics abnormalitites; 65% to 80% are classified as multifactorial (Rappaport, 2008). Some indications for prenatal diagnostic testing include the following (Lashley, 2007; Nussbaum et al., 2007):

a. Pregnancy at risk for chromosomal aberration
(1) Maternal age older than 35 years
(2) Known chromosomal abnormality in the parent
(3) Previous pregnancy with recognized chromosomal abnormality or observable malformation
(4) Previous stillbirth or perinatal death in which the cause is unknown
(5) History of infertility in either parent
(6) Family history of a genetic disorder that may be diagnosed or ruled out by biochemical or DNA testing
(7) Family history of an X-linked disorder for which there is no specific prenatal diagnostic test
(8) Diagnostic tools—amniocentesis, chorionic villus sampling. Obvious malformations often can be observed using ultrasound.

b. Pregnancy at risk for neural tube defects
(1) High maternal blood levels of AFP
(2) Previous child with neural tube defect
(3) Presence of neural tube defect in either parent or a close relative
(4) Diagnostic tools—amniocentesis, ultrasound (see Chapter 24 for information on intrauterine fetal surgery for neural tube defect repair)

c. Pregnancy at risk for X-linked inherited disorder
(1) Mother known to be a carrier
(2) Presence of a close maternal male relative who is affected
(3) Diagnostic tools—amniocentesis, chorionic villus sampling

d. Pregnancy at risk for detectable, inherited, biochemical disorders
(1) Parents are known carriers or are affected.
(2) Previous children born with a biochemical disorder
(3) Close family members with a known inherited biochemical disorder
(4) Diagnostic tools—amniocentesis, chorionic villus sampling

e. Miscellaneous
(1) Extreme parental anxiety
(2) Significant exposure to radiation, infection, drugs, or chemicals
(3) Presence of diabetes mellitus in the mother
(4) Birth of a previous child with a structural abnormality
(5) Family history of structural abnormality
(6) Diagnostic tools—amniocentesis, chorionic villus sampling, ultrasound (exception: chorionic villus sampling is not indicated in mothers with diabetes mellitus)

f. Preconception carrier screening allows carrier couples the ability to consider a full range of reproductive options, including decisions against reproduction, the possibility of adoption, accepting gamete donations, or accepting genetic risk without further testing. Preimplantation testing with in vitro fertilization can ensure that only unaffected embryos are implanted (Bick & Lau, 2006; Rappaport, 2008; Solomon, Jack, & Feero, 2008).

g. First-trimester screening using nuchal tanslucency detects 75% of Down syndrome fetuses; if combined with serum markers PAPP-A and free B-hCG, the detection rate is 82% to 87% (Rappaport, 2008).

6. Social, legal, and ethical implications associated with prenatal diagnosis
   a. Option of pregnancy termination/selective reduction for certain conditions
   b. Right of individual to refuse prenatal diagnostic procedures or termination should a defect be found (Nussbaum et al., 2007)
   c. Right to privacy and ownership of sample taken (Minkoff & Ecker, 2008; Slaughter, 2008)
   d. Possibility of an ambiguous finding with a resultant dilemma regarding the proper course of action to be taken

C. **Interventions/Outcomes**
   1. Lack of knowledge about heredity, potential effects on offspring, and community resources
      a. Interventions
         (1) Explain appropriate genetic information to the family.
         (2) Discuss implications of the condition for the parent, the infant, and the siblings.
         (3) Provide written educational material or refer the family to the appropriate agency (such as the March of Dimes National Foundation) for educational materials. A list of websites dealing with genetics may be viewed in Table 2-1.
         (4) Refer the family to a genetics center for a complete evaluation with appropriate genetic counseling.
         (5) Maintain a supportive attitude toward the family's questions, need for clarification, and final decision about actions to be taken.
         (6) Explain diagnostic procedures and emphasize the purpose, anticipated findings, and possible side effects.
      b. Outcomes
         (1) The family demonstrates an understanding of the information provided through feedback and appropriate questions.
         (2) The family has obtained the appropriate diagnostic tests.
   2. Effective family coping mechanisms
      a. Interventions
         (1) Assure family members that they do not need to rush into a decision.
         (2) Provide the necessary information and resources for the family to make an informed decision.

■ TABLE 2-1
■ ■ **Useful Internet Genetic Reference Sites**

Web Address	Database
www.ncbi.nlm.nih.gov	General reference maintained by National Library of Medicine
www.ncbi.nlm.nih.gov/Omim	Online Mendelian Inheritance in Man (extremely useful for clinicians—more than 10,000 entries of genetic traits indexed by gene name, symptoms, and so forth)
www.ncbi.nlm.nih.gov/genemap	General reference to current efforts to map the human genome
www.ncbi.nlm.nih.gov/Web/GenBank	Searchable repository of all DNA sequence data
www.ncbi.nlm.nih.gov/ncicgap	Cancer Genome Anatomy Project (National Cancer Institute)
www.nhgri.nih.gov	National Human Genome Research Institute website (useful information about human genetics and ethical issues)
www.hgmd.cf.ac.uk/	Human Gene Mutation Database (searchable index of all described mutations in human genes with phenotypes and references)
www.genetests.org	Directory of clinics and labs for testing of genetic disorders
www.geneletter.com	Health, clinical, legal, social, and ethical issues
www.ashg.org	American Society of Human Genetics site
www.aap.org/VISIT/cmte18.htm	Committee on Genetics of the American Academy of Pediatrics site. Educational Genetics Compendium. Health supervision guidelines for common genetic disorders.

From Korf, B.R. (2007). The genetic approach in pediatric medicine. In Kliegman R.M., Behrman, R.E., Jenson, H.B., & Stanton, B.M. (Eds.). *Nelson textbook of pediatrics* (18th ed.). Philadelphia: Saunders.

           (3) Encourage family members to verbalize their feelings.
           (4) Interact with family members to encourage individual feelings of self-worth.
           (5) Recognize that grief is appropriate during a difficult decision-making process.
       b. Outcomes
           (1) The family is able to make appropriate decisions.
   3. Effects on the family due to diagnosis of a genetic disorder in the fetus or newborn
       a. Interventions
           (1) Explain that grief is appropriate during a difficult decision-making process.
           (2) Encourage family members to verbalize their feelings.
           (3) Interact with family members to encourage individual feelings of self-worth.
           (4) Refer family members to appropriate resources to deal with current crises.
       b. Outcomes
           (1) The family is able to make appropriate decisions.
           (2) Family members are able to provide each other with the necessary emotional and physical support and care.
   4. Mechanisms for improved parenting of a newborn with a genetic disorder
       a. Interventions
           (1) Explain appropriate genetic information to the family.
           (2) Discuss implications of the condition.
           (3) Interact with the family to encourage feelings of self-worth.
           (4) Explain that grief is appropriate during a difficult decision-making process.
           (5) Refer the family to the appropriate agency to assist in the parenting of an affected child.
       b. Outcomes
           (1) Family members have obtained needed services.
           (2) Family members are able to make appropriate decisions.
   5. Dealing with the loss of a normal child
       a. Interventions
           (1) Assure family members that they do not need to rush into a decision.
           (2) Provide privacy and encourage family members to verbalize their feelings.
           (3) Explain that grief is a normal response.
           (4) Provide the necessary information and resources.
       b. Outcomes
           (1) Family members verbalize grief and feelings of loss.
           (2) Family members make the appropriate decisions.
   6. Avoidance of social isolation of the family due to a child's genetic disorder
       a. Interventions
           (1) Explain appropriate genetic information to the family.
           (2) Discuss the implications of the condition and the resources available to the family.
           (3) Maintain a supportive attitude toward the family.
           (4) Encourage family members to verbalize their feelings.
           (5) Refer family members to appropriate agencies to deal with their concerns.
       b. Outcomes
           (1) The family is able to provide necessary care for the affected infant.
           (2) The family has obtained services from referral agencies.
           (3) The family is able to make the appropriate decisions.

HEALTH EDUCATION

A. Explain the known causes for the condition (the genetics of the disorder) in terminology understood by the parents.
B. Describe the referral agencies that are available for follow-up and support.
C. Explain the reproductive options and recurrence risks.
D. Discuss available treatment options.
E. Discuss the prognosis of the condition.
F. Discuss the measures to be taken to prevent the condition in future offspring.

CASE STUDIES AND STUDY QUESTIONS

Mrs. C., 43 years old, gravida 3, para 2 (G3, P2) is at 16 weeks' gestation. She underwent a prenatal diagnostic test for chromosomal abnormalities. She received the result of the test, which was 47,XY,+21 (male with Down syndrome). Otherwise the pregnancy has been normal with no complications to date.

1. What information would you need to know to assist Mr. and Mrs. C. in understanding the cause of chromosomal abnormalities?
   a. A history of maternal substance use during pregnancy
   b. The level and quality of prenatal care received to date
   c. The family history of chromosomal abnormalities
   d. The delivery history of previous children
2. Mr. and Mrs. C. do not understand what 47,XY, +21 means. What is the correct interpretation?
   a. The 47th chromosome has 21 extra genes and XY refers to gender.
   b. There is an extra chromosome in the 21st pair and XY refers to gender.
   c. The 21st chromosome has additional genetic material and XY refers to location on the gene.
   d. The number 47 refers to the type of test and 21 refers to the number of abnormal cells identified.
3. Mr. and Mrs. C. believe that they must have done something that caused this abnormality in their fetus. You can tell them:
   a. They are not responsible because this was an accident that occurred in early cell division before fertilization.
   b. Mrs. C. might have had a viral infection in the first few days after conception.
   c. Mr. C. might have been exposed to an environmental toxin during adolescence, thus altering his ability to produce normal sperm.

   d. Mrs. C. might have exposed the embryo to an environmental toxin that altered the basic cell structure.
4. Mr. and Mrs. C. are concerned about the potential risks to their future grandchildren. What is an appropriate response?
   a. With each occurrence of a chromosomal abnormality, there is an increased risk of recurrence of 2% to 5%.
   b. Recommend that their children undergo regular chromosomal monitoring to rule out a future translocation.
   c. Recommend that only male children should consider future pregnancies because they would not be at risk.
   d. The recurrence risk should not be higher than that for the general population. Mrs. K is a 29-year-old white woman. She is a G1, P1 and has delivered an infant boy. The child was diagnosed as having achondroplasia (a type of dwarfism that is inherited via the autosomal dominant mode [Figure 2-8]). The child weighs 2722 g (6 pounds) and is in no apparent distress. On further questioning, you learn that Mr. K. is 45 years old and has achondroplasia. Mrs. K. has three sisters with no health problems, and her parents are living and well. Mr. K. has one brother and one sister; both are normal. Mr. K.'s mother is living and well; Mr. K.'s father is dead and he, too, had achondroplasia. Both Mr. and Mrs. K are interested in future pregnancies.
5. The couple does not understand what autosomal dominant means. You tell the couple that an autosomal dominant condition is:
   a. A disorder that is caused by a single gene that overshadows a gene that is at the same location on the other chromosome pair
   b. A condition that occurs when each parent contributes a gene for the particular disorder
   c. A condition that produces a result that is severe and usually is not correctable

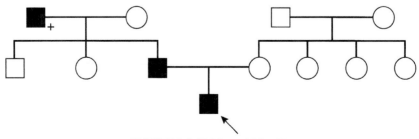

FIGURE 2-8 ■ Mr. and Mrs. K.

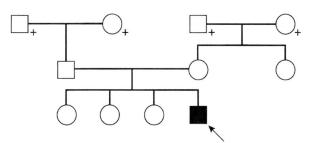

FIGURE 2-9 ■ Mr. and Mrs. Y.

d. A condition that is caused by a combination of many genes and an environmental factor

6. Because they would like to have other children, they are interested in knowing the recurrence risk for this condition. The estimated risk is:
   a. Quite small
   b. 10% to 15%
   c. 25%
   d. 50%

7. Mr. and Mrs. K. note that two individuals with achondroplasia in their family were males, and they would like to know if boys are at a greater risk. You advise them that this dominant condition:
   a. Has a 25% increased risk for males
   b. Occurs in males and females
   c. Occurs more frequently when the woman is older than 35 years
   d. Has a 50% increased risk for males

Mr. and Mrs. Y. were contacted by their pediatrician because their newborn son's screening PKU test results were abnormal (the PKU level was elevated). The infant is now 5 days old and appears normal, although a little colicky. Further testing verified the diagnosis of PKU. Mr. and Mrs. Y. are in their late 20s; they have three normal daughters, and Mr. Y. is convinced that if their next child is a girl, she will be normal. Mrs. Y. has one sister who has three normal children. Her parents died in an automobile accident when she was small. Mr. Y. is an only child, and his parents died when he was a young child (Figure 2-9).

8. The couple does not understand what autosomal recessive means. You could tell them that an autosomal recessive condition is:

a. A disorder that is caused by a single gene that overshadows a gene that is at the same location on the other chromosome pair
b. A condition that occurs when each parent contributes a gene for the particular disorder
c. A condition that produces a result that is not severe and usually is correctable

9. Because they would like to have other children, they are interested in knowing that the recurrence risk for this condition is:
   a. Extremely small
   b. 10% to 15%
   c. 25%
   d. 50%

10. Mr. and Mrs. Y. do not understand why the girls were normal and the boy was not; they would like to know if only a boy would be at risk. You advise them that this recessive condition:
   a. Has a 25% increased risk for males
   b. Occurs in males and females
   c. Occurs more frequently in women older than 35 years
   d. Has a 50% increased risk for males

11. The couple has difficulty believing that the condition is inheritable in their family, because no one else has a similar problem. You can explain to them that recessive disorders:
   a. Occur among siblings versus occurring from generation to generation
   b. Occur in a random pattern in the first two or three generations
   c. Have a high frequency of mutations in the original case
   d. Usually skip a generation before they manifest themselves

ANSWERS TO STUDY QUESTIONS

1. c	4. d	7. b	10. b
2. b	5. a	8. b	11. a
3. a	6. d	9. c	

REFERENCES

Bick, D. P., & Lau, E. C. (2006). Preimplantation genetic diagnosis. *Pediatric Clinics of North America, 53,* 559–577.

Jarvi, K., & Chitzyat, D. (2008). The genetics you never knew: A genetics primer. *Urological Clinics of North America, 35,* 243–256.

Lashley, F. R. (2005). *Clinical genetics in nursing practice* (3rd ed.). New York: Springer.

Lashley, F. R. (2007). *Essentials of clinical genetics in nursing practice.* New York: Springer.

Minkoff, H., & Ecker, J. (2008). Genetic testing and breach of patient confidentiality: law, ethics, and pragmatics. *American Journal of Obstetrics and Gynecology,* 198(5), *498,* e1–498, e1–4.

Nussbaum, R. L., McInnes, R. R., & Willard, H. F. (2007). *Thompson & Thompson genetics in medicine* (7th ed.). Philadelphia: Saunders.

Rappaport, V. J. (2008). Prenatal diagnosis and genetic screening—Integration into prenatal care. *Obstetrics and Gynecology Clinics of North America, 35,* 435–458.

Slaughter, L. M. (2008). The genetic information nondiscrimination act: Why your personal genetics are still vulnerable to discrimination. *Surgical Clinics of North America, 88,* 723–738.

Solomon, B. D., Jack, B. W., & Feero, W. G. (2008). The clinical content of preconception care: Genetics and genomics. *American Journal of Obstetrics and Gynecology, December,* S340–344.

Wright, A., & Hastie, N. (2007). *Genes and common diseases.* Cambridge, UK: Cambridge University Press.

3

Fetal and Placental Development and Functioning

Linda Callahan

OBJECTIVES

1. Describe the process of fertilization.
2. Discuss the stages of placental development.
3. Describe the functions of the placenta.
4. Explain the implications of ineffective placental development on fetal development.
5. Describe the functions of the amniotic fluid.
6. Identify the important milestones for the development of fetal organs, such as the heart, lungs, kidney, and brain.
7. Identify the periods when the developing body systems of the fetus are most susceptible to teratogenic influences.

INTRODUCTION

A. Pregenesis
   1. Encompasses the time after formation of the germ cells and before union of sperm and egg
   2. Begins with differentiation and migration of primitive germ cells to the genital ridge and ends with the formation of the gametes (karyogamy)
   3. Aneuploidies (abnormal numbers of chromosomes) might occur as a consequence of abnormal meiotic division of chromosomes during gamete formation.
B. Conception
   1. Fertilization usually occurs in the ampulla of the fallopian tube.
   2. Estrogen levels increase during ovulation, aiding fertilization and easing transit of the ovum down the fallopian tube.
   3. The ovum membrane is surrounded by two layers of tissue.
      a. An inner layer called the zona pellucida
      b. An outer layer called the corona radiata (Figure 3-1)
   4. In a single ejaculation, 400 million spermatozoa are deposited in the vagina, reaching the fallopian tubes within 5 minutes by frantic movement of their flagellar tails.
      a. A sperm undergoes two processes before it is able to penetrate the ovum.
         (1) Capacitation: structural changes occur once in the female genital tract.
         (2) Acrosomal reaction: the sperm releases enzymes (see Figure 3-1).
            (a) Hyaluronidase causes separation of the corona radiata.
            (b) Acrosin and neuraminidase allow the sperm to enter the zona pellucida.
      b. Ova are considered fertile for approximately 24 hours after ovulation, whereas sperm, although viable for 72 hours, are believed to be fertile for only 24 hours.
      c. At the moment of penetration, the oocyte completes the second meiotic division (see Figure 3-1), whereas cellular changes prevent other sperm from entering the ovum (zona reaction).
   5. With fertilization, the diploid number (46) of chromosomes is restored, and cell division begins.
      a. Within the cell the nuclei of the spermatozoon and oocyte unite, and their nuclear membranes disappear.
      b. The chromosomes pair up, and a new cell, the zygote, which contains a new combination of genetic material, is formed.

C. Pre-embryonic stage: The first 2 weeks after fertilization; the blastogenetic period is the first 4 weeks of human development
  1. This stage is characterized by rapid cell division, cell differentiation, and the development of embryonic membranes and germ layers.
     a. First week (Figure 3-2)
        (1) Division of the zygote occurs within the first 30 hours.
        (2) The zygote continues to divide into a solid ball of cells (the morula).
        (3) The morula floats inside of the uterus for 2 or 3 days obtaining nourishment from the mucous lining of the uterus and the fluid in the uterine cavity.
        (4) Two distinct layers of cells develop as the morula hollows out.
           (a) The inner cell mass (blastocyst), which will form the embryo, the amnion, and the yolk sac membrane
           (b) The outer cell layer (trophoblast), which becomes the fetal side of the placenta and chorion

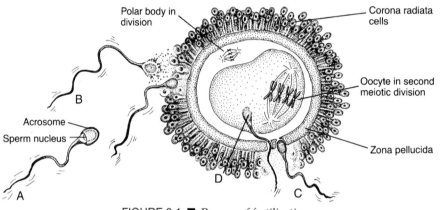

FIGURE 3-1 ■ Process of fertilization.

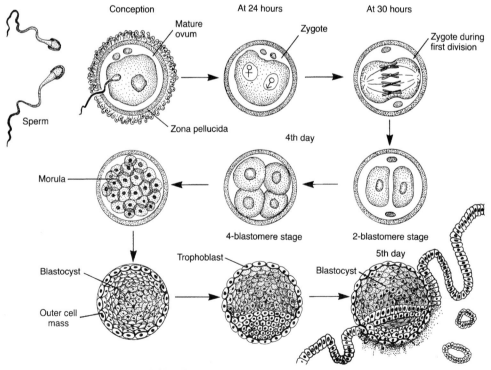

FIGURE 3-2 ■ Process of implantation.

(5) Zona pellucida disappears at about 5 days.
   (a) The blastocyst enlarges.
   (b) The trophoblast attaches to the endometrial epithelium and begins the process of implantation.
(6) The attached portion of the trophoblast develops into two layers.
   (a) The internal cellular layer is called the cytotrophoblast.
   (b) The outer layer is called the syncytiotrophoblast, which invades the endometrial epithelium by the end of the 7th day.
   (c) Embedding is completed by the 11th day, with the site of attachment usually being the upper part of the posterior uterine wall. Attachment can occur anywhere, even extrauterine.

b. Second week
   (1) The inner cell mass differentiates into two cell layers: the endoderm (the inside of the embryo) and the ectoderm (the outside of the embryo).
      (a) The amniotic cavity appears as a space between the inner cell mass and the trophoblast.
      (b) When the embryo becomes a cylinder, the amnion surrounds it and forms the amniotic sac.
   (2) By the end of the second week, the embryonic cells and the amniotic and yolk sacs are attached to the chorionic sac by a slender band, which becomes the umbilical cord.
   (3) Malformations that occur during the pre-embryonic stage seldom result in a viable fetus.

c. Placental development
   (1) Description: the placenta is a temporary disk-shaped organ that connects the fetus to the uterine wall and provides for fetal respiration as well as metabolic and nutrient exchanges between the maternal and fetal circulations.
   (2) Approximately 5 to 6 days after fertilization, the blastocyst adheres to the endometrium.
   (3) Blastocyst penetrates toward the maternal capillaries by eroding the uterine epithelium; this erosion process continues until the blastocyst is completely embedded in the uterine wall.

d. Decidua: the portion of the endometrium enveloping the developing fertilized ovum (Figure 3-3)
   (1) On approximately the 14th day, the endometrium changes at the site of implantation and becomes the decidua.
   (2) Implantation causes the adjacent decidual cells to engorge with glycogen and lipids (decidual reaction).
   (3) The swollen decidual cells release their contents during the erosion process to provide nourishment to the embryo.

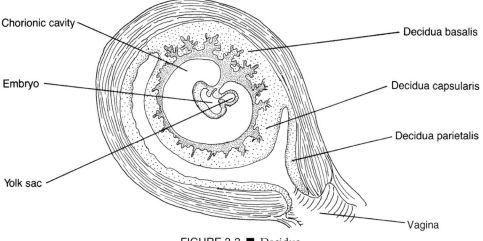

FIGURE 3-3 ■ Decidua.

(4) The decidua divides into three layers:
   (a) Decidua capsularis—covers the embryoblast
   (b) Decidua basalis—maternal portion of the placenta that supplies vessels to nourish the intervillous spaces
   (c) Decidua parietalis—lines the remainder of the uterine cavity
   e. Placenta
(1) When the embryoblast is partially embedded in the decidua, two distinct layers of cells can be seen in the trophoblast.
   (a) Inner layer (cytotrophoblast) is made of mononuclear cells.
   (b) Outer layer (syncytiotrophoblast) consists of multinucleated cells and is responsible for the erosive ability of the trophoblast.
(2) The cytotrophoblast and the syncytiotrophoblast separate the maternal and fetal circulations and are called the placental barrier.
(3) On approximately the 9th day, spaces (vacuoles) appear in the syncytium; these fuse together to form lacunae (intervillous spaces), which develop into an interconnecting system.
(4) On approximately the 11th day:
   (a) Invading syncytium encounters the congested capillaries of the decidua.
   (b) Syncytium enzymes break down the vessel walls, releasing blood into the lacunae.
   (c) Eventually the syncytium encounters the larger arteries and veins and establishes a directional flow of blood.
   (d) Blood enters the lacunae.
      [i] The embryo experiences rapid growth because of a high concentration of nutrients.
      [ii] This growth results in an increase in the distance that nutrients must travel by diffusion to reach the embryo.
(5) Chorionic villi develop between the 9th and 25th days (Figure 3-4).
   (a) The chorion (trophoblastic cells) is the first placental membrane to form, enclosing the embryo, amnion, and yolk sac and growing outward, forming finger-like projections called villi within which blood vessels develop.
   (b) Initially the chorion covers the whole chorionic surface, but with fetal growth the intraluminal villi become compressed and degenerate.
   (c) Villi located below the embryo continue to grow, forming a large surface for exchange with villi that contact the decidua basalis to become anchoring villi.
      [i] Decidual septa form between anchoring villi, which results in 15 to 20 lobes (cotyledons).
      [ii] Exchange of gases and nutrients occurs in this vascular system.
   (d) Other villi float free and conduct most of the exchange between mother and developing fetus.
   (e) No further villi are formed after the 12th week.

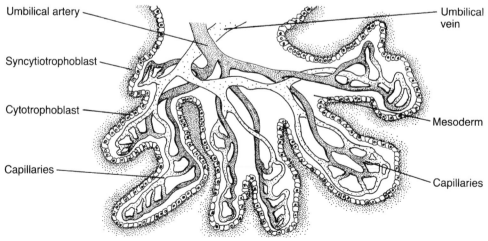

FIGURE 3-4 ■ Chorionic villi.

D. Embryonic stage: Begins with the folding of the disk in week 2 of development
  1. Third week
   a. Gastrulation
     (1) The embryonic disk converts into a trilaminar embryonic disk comprising three germ layers: ectoderm (to become the epidermis and the nervous system); mesoderm (to become the smooth muscle); and endoderm (to become the epithelial lining of the respiratory and digestive tracts).
     (2) The process is completed in the third week with the formation of intraembryonic mesoderm by the primitive streak.
   b. Proliferation and migration of cells from the primitive streak give rise to mesenchyme
     (1) Cells spread cranially and caudally.
     (2) Cells begin to form the embryonic endoderm, which gives rise to the lining of the digestive and respiratory tracts.
     (3) The cells that remain on the surface of the embryonic disk form the layer of cells called the embryonic ectoderm, which develop into the nervous system (i.e., the sensory epithelium of the eye, ear, and nose).
   c. The mesenchymal cells migrate cephalad under the embryonic ectoderm and form the notochordal process.
     (1) These cells grow until they reach the prochordal plate, the future site of the mouth.
     (2) Caudal to the primitive streak is a circular area called the cloacal membrane, which becomes the anus.
     (3) The primitive streak continues to form mesoderm until the end of the fourth week.
     (4) The notochord develops by transformation of the notochordal process by the end of the third week of gestation.
   d. Neurulation is the process of developing the neural plate, neural folds, and neural tube.
     (1) Neural plate
       (a) Embryonic ectoderm lying over the notochord thickens to form the neural plate.
       (b) It first appears near the primitive knot and enlarges to form a neural groove, which becomes bounded by the neural folds on each side.
     (2) Neural tube
       (a) By the third week the neural folds begin to fuse, forming the neural tube.
       (b) This occurs near the middle of the embryo and progresses toward the cranial and caudal ends.
     (3) Neural crest
       (a) Cells lying along the neural fold migrate ventrolaterally on each side of the neural tube forming an irregular mass called the neural crest.
       (b) These cells migrate throughout the embryo and give rise to the spinal ganglia.
       (c) The neural crest cells also form the meninges of the brain and spinal cord, the adrenal medulla, and several components of the skeletal and muscular parts of the head.
   e. Somite development
     (1) Some of the mesoderm forms columns that divide into paired cuboidal bodies (somites).
     (2) Mesenchymal cells from the somites will become the vertebral column, the ribs, the sternum, the skull, and associated muscles.
   f. Intraembryonic coelom
     (1) Cavities in the lateral mesoderm form a horseshoe-shaped cavity called the intraembryonic coelom.
     (2) The intraembryonic coelom divides the lateral mesoderm into two layers.
       (a) Somatic layer is continuous with the extraembryonic mesoderm covering the amnion.
       (b) Visceral layer is continuous with the extraembryonic mesoderm covering the yolk sac.
     (3) During the second month the intraembryonic coelom will become the pericardial, the pleural, and the peritoneal cavities.
   g. Primitive cardiovascular system (Figure 3-5)
     (1) Blood vessels start forming in the extraembryonic mesoderm of the yolk sac, connecting stalk and chorion at the end of the third week.
     (2) Mesenchymal cells (angioblasts) aggregate to form blood islands.

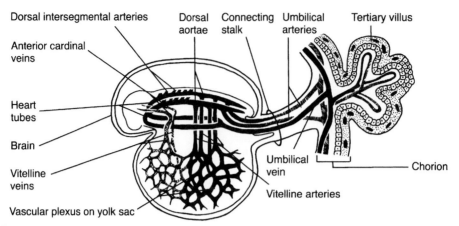

FIGURE 3-5 ■ Primitive cardiovascular system (at about 20 days). (Adapted from Moore, K.L. [1988]. *Essentials of human embryology* [p. 61]. Philadelphia: B.C. Decker.)

    (3) Mesenchymal cells arrange around cavities in the blood islands to form the endothelium of primitive blood vessels, which go on to develop into a series of vascular networks.

    (4) Primitive blood cells develop from the endothelial cells of the vessels in the walls of the yolk sac; blood formation does not begin in the embryo until the fifth week.

    (5) The primitive heart is a tubular structure formed from the mesenchymal cells in the cardiogenic area.

        (a) Paired endocardial heart tubes develop and fuse to form a primitive heart.

        (b) The heart tubes join blood vessels in the embryo, connective stalk, chorion, and yolk sac, forming a primitive cardiovascular system.

        (c) The primitive blood cells begin to circulate at the end of the third week as the tubular heart begins to beat.

  h. Malformations that might occur during this stage:

    (1) Anencephaly, as a result of a defect in the closure of the anterior neural tube, which results in the degeneration of the forebrain

    (2) Cyclopia, as a result of an alteration in the prechordal mesodermal development, and producing secondary defects of the midface and forebrain

    (3) Ectromelia (congenital absence of a limb)

    (4) Ectopia cordis (heart remains outside of the thoracic cavity)

2. Fourth week

  a. The neural tube is open at the rostral and caudal neuropores, and the embryo is almost straight (Figure 3-6, *A* and *B*).

  b. The first and second pairs of the branchial arches (future head and neck) are visible.

  c. The otic placodes (primordia of the internal ears) are developed.

  d. By the middle of the fourth week, the embryo is cylindric and curved because of the folding of the median and horizontal planes.

    (1) The rostral neuropore closes.

    (2) The upper limb buds appear as small swellings on the lateral wall (see Figure 3-6, *C*).

    (3) The heart is a distinct prominence on the surface of the embryo.

    (4) The otic pits are formed.

  e. By the end of the fourth week, the embryo is C-shaped.

    (1) The oral cavity begins while the esophagotracheal septum begins to divide into the esophagus and the trachea.

    (2) The stomach, the pancreas, and the liver begin to form.

    (3) Upper limb buds have a flipper shape (see Figure 3-6, *D*).

    (4) Lower limb buds appear as small swellings (Figure 3-7, *A*).

    (5) Four pairs of branchial arches and lens placodes (the lens of the eye) have developed.

    (6) A tail is prominent.

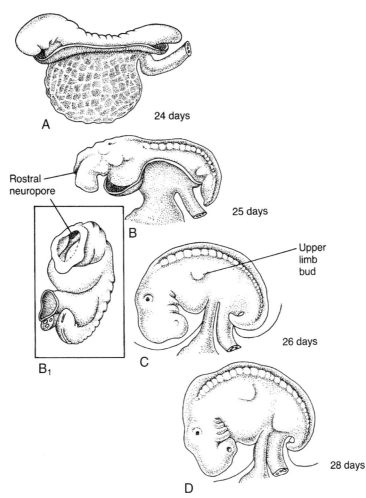

FIGURE 3-6 ■ Development of head to tail regions. (Adapted from Moore, K.L. [1988]. *Essentials of human embryology* [p. 29]. Philadelphia: B.C. Decker.)

    f. Malformations that might occur during this stage of development:
       (1) Myelomeningocele results from a defect in the closure of the posterior neural tube.
       (2) Esophageal atresia and tracheoesophageal fistulas can occur as a result of the lateral septation of the foregut.
       (3) Extravasation of the bladder occurs if the infraumbilical mesenchyme does not migrate effectively.
  3. Fifth week (see Figure 3-7, *B*)
    a. The embryo is approximately 8 mm (⅜ inch) long.
    b. The head grows because of the rapid development and differentiation of the brain.
    c. The cranial nerves have developed.
    d. Atrial division in the heart begins.
    e. Upper limbs become paddle-shaped.
    f. Malformations can occur during this stage.
       (1) Cleft lip and other facial clefts result from a defect in the closure of the lip.
       (2) Transposition of the great vessels can occur if the aorticopulmonary septum fails to spiral.
       (3) Nuclear cataracts
       (4) Microphthalmia (small eyeballs)
       (5) Carpal and pedal ablation
  4. Sixth week (see Figure 3-7, *C* and *D*)
    a. The embryo is 12 mm (½ inch) long.
    b. The fissures of the brain are obvious.

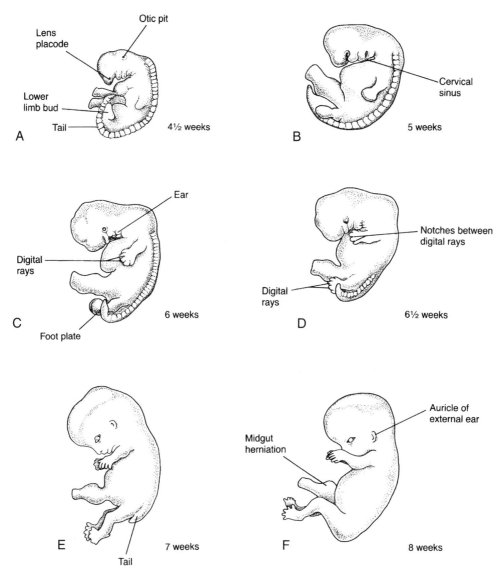

FIGURE 3-7 ■ Embryo from 4 weeks to 8 weeks. (Adapted from Moore, K.L. [1988]. *Essentials of human embryology* [p. 37]. Philadelphia: B.C. Decker.)

   c. The heart begins to divide into chambers, and the liver begins to form red blood cells.
   d. The trachea and lung buds appear, and the oral and nasal cavities are formed.
   e. The upper and lower jaw begin to form; upper lip and palate development also occur.
   f. Embryonic sex glands appear.
   g. Skeletal and muscular systems
      (1) Ossification of the jaw and skull begins.
      (2) The wrist and elbow are identifiable.
      (3) Ridges called digital rays (future fingers and thumb) form on the paddle-shaped hands.
      (4) Muscle begins to develop.
   h. The primordia of the external acoustic meatus and external ear are present; the external, middle, and inner ears continue to form.
   i. Malformations can occur during this period.
      (1) Rectal atresia with fistula occurs if there is a defect in the lateral septation of the cloaca into the rectum and urogenital sinuses.
      (2) Diaphragmatic hernia occurs when there is a defect in the closure of the pleuroperitoneal canal.

(3) Ventricular septal defect results during the closure of the ventricular septum.

5. Seventh week (see Figure 3- 7, *E*)
   a. The embryo is approximately 18 mm (¾ inch) long.
   b. Fetal heartbeat can be heard and fetal circulation begins.
   c. Gastrointestinal system
      (1) The tongue separates, and the palate begins to fold inward.
      (2) The stomach assumes its final shape.
      (3) The diaphragm separates the abdominal and thoracic cavities.
   d. Genitourinary system
      (1) The bladder and the urethra separate from the rectum.
      (2) The sex glands begin to differentiate into testes or ovaries.
   e. Skeletal and muscular systems
      (1) Notches develop between the digital rays of the hand.
      (2) Digital rays appear in the developing feet.
   f. The optic nerve forms, the eyelids appear, and the eye lenses begin to thicken.
   g. Malformations that can occur during this period:
      (1) Duodenal atresia resulting from an error in the recanalization of the duodenum
      (2) Pulmonary stenosis
      (3) Brachycephalism (shortening of the head)
      (4) Alteration in sexual characteristics
      (5) Cleft palate
6. Eighth week (see Figure 3-7, *F*)
   a. The embryo is 2.5 to 3 cm (1 inch) long and weighs 8 g (0.25 ounce).
   b. Sensory and motor neurons have functional connections, and the embryo is able to contract large muscles.
   c. Development of the heart is complete, and the circulatory system through the umbilical cord is formed.
   d. Gastrointestinal system
      (1) Abdomen protrudes because the intestines are in the proximal part of the umbilical cord.
      (2) Anal membrane perforates, and rectal passage opens.
      (3) Lips are fused.
   e. External genitalia begin to differentiate.
   f. Skeletal and muscular systems
      (1) Distinct notches are present between the toes.
      (2) The fingers and toes are distinct and separated.
      (3) Differentiation of the cells occurs in the primitive skeleton.
      (4) Cartilaginous bones begin to ossify.
      (5) Muscle development begins in the trunk, limbs, and head.
   g. The eyes are open but fuse at the end of the eighth week, and the auricles of the external ear assume their final appearance.
   h. Malformations that can occur during this period:
      (1) Persistent opening of the atrial septum
      (2) Digital stunting
E. **Fetal stage: Every organ system and external structure is present, and the remainder of gestation is devoted to refining the function of the organs**
   1. Placental growth continues until the 20th week; beyond 20 weeks the placenta increases only in thickness.
      a. At term
         (1) Placenta is round and flat; approximately 15 to 20 cm (6 to 8 inches) in diameter and 2.5 cm (1 inch) thick.
         (2) Placenta weighs approximately one sixth of the weight of the infant.
         (3) Maternal surface (red and blue)
            (a) Arises from the decidua basalis
            (b) Has multiple lobules (cotyledons)
         (4) Fetal surface (smooth, white, and shiny in appearance):
            (a) Develops from the chorionic villi
            (b) Contains branches of umbilical veins and arteries
            (c) Is covered with the chorionic and the amniochorionic membranes

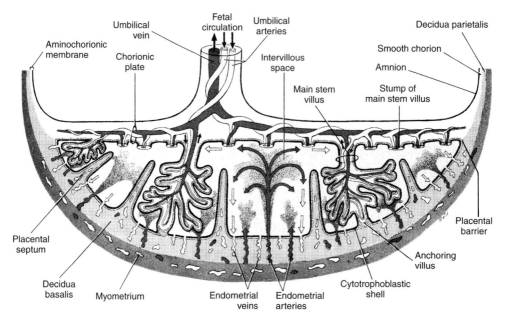

Maternal circulation

FIGURE 3-8 ■ Placental circulation. Arrangement of the placental blood vessels. Blood of the fetus flows through the umbilical arteries into the fetal capillaries in the villi and then back to the fetal circulation through the umbilical vein. Maternal blood is transported by the uterine arteries to the intervillous space and leaves by the uterine veins to go back to the maternal circulation. (From Moore, K.L. & Persaud, T.V. [2007]. *The developing human: Clinically oriented embryology* [8th ed.]. Philadelphia: Saunders.)

    b. Circulation (Figure 3- 8)
        (1) Maternal placental circulation
            (a) Oxygenated blood enters the intervillous spaces from the decidua basalis.
            (b) Maternal blood pressure directs the blood toward the chorionic villi.
            (c) Deoxygenated blood leaves the intervillous spaces through openings in the cytotrophoblast and enters the endometrial veins.
            (d) Uterine contractions compress intervillous spaces, forcing the blood into the uterine veins.
        (2) Fetal placental circulation
            (a) Deoxygenated blood leaves the fetus through the two umbilical arteries.
            (b) Umbilical arteries divide into multiple branches as they enter the chorionic villi.
            (c) Oxygenated blood returns via venules and veins in the chorionic villi.
            (d) The veins in the chorionic villi join to form the umbilical vein.
  2. Mechanism of placental transfer (Table 3-1)
    a. The passage of substances from mother to fetus against a concentration gradient (active transport) requires expenditure of energy by the cells and can be inhibited by substances that interfere with energy production. Amino acids, iron, calcium, iodine, and water-soluble vitamins are transported by this process.
    b. Defects or breaks in the placental membrane allow for the transfer of large cells, such as red blood cells.
        (1) This process is responsible for Rh sensitization.
        (2) This can only occur when the mother is Rh negative and the fetus is Rh positive.
        (3) Rh-positive fetal cells enter the maternal system through a break or defect in the placenta.
        (4) Maternal system develops antibodies to the Rh-positive fetal cells.
        (5) Process occurs most frequently during delivery.
    c. Bulk flow
        (1) Transfers substances by osmosis through micropores in the membrane.
        (2) This process maintains the maternal-fetal exchange of water.

■ TABLE 3-1
■ ■ **Placental Transfer**

Type of Transfer	Products Transferred
Active transport	Amino acids
	Iron
	Calcium
	Iodine
	Water-soluble vitamins
Breaks in membrane	Rh factors that result in isoimmunization
Bulk flow	Water
Diffusion	Oxygen
	Carbon dioxide
	Electrolytes
	Lipid-soluble vitamins
Facilitated diffusion	D-Glucose
Pinocytosis	Some immunoglobulins

      d. Diffusion
         (1) The process by which molecules that present at higher levels of concentration move more rapidly toward areas of lower concentrations across a membrane.
         (2) Molecular size determines rate of movement; also the higher the temperature, the greater the activity.
         (3) Provides the mechanism for the transfer of respiratory gases (oxygen and carbon dioxide), electrolytes, and some lipid-soluble vitamins.
         (4) Limitations in diffusion are a major factor in placental failure.
      e. Facilitated diffusion
         (1) Occurs on a maternal-to-fetal concentration gradient without an expenditure of energy
         (2) Occurs at a rate greater than that of simple diffusion
         (3) D-Glucose, galactose, and some oxygen are transported.
         (4) Substances that are highly fat soluble cross the placenta at a faster rate.
      f. Pinocytosis
         (1) The transfer by invagination into the cell membrane of a molecule, which then crosses to the opposite side. Examples:
            (a) Microdrops of plasma are taken up by the trophoblasts.
            (b) Trophoblasts transport immunoglobulins from the plasma to the fetus.
   3. Transfer disorders
      a. Separation of the placenta from the uterine wall
         (1) Placenta previa
         (2) Placental infarcts
         (3) Abruptio placentae
      b. Intervillous coagulation and ischemic necrosis
      c. Alterations in the membrane as a result of calcifications, thickening, and degeneration can alter permeability.
      d. Usually result from a problem in maternal circulation
         (1) Hypertensive disorders in pregnancy
         (2) Diabetes mellitus
         (3) Severe maternal malnutrition
      e. For placental insufficiency to occur, a major portion of the placenta must be involved.
   4. Placental function
      a. Respiration
         (1) Oxygen in the maternal blood crosses the placental membrane and enters the fetal blood supply by diffusion.
         (2) Carbon dioxide returns to the maternal system across the placental membrane.
         (3) Actual fetal pulmonary respiration does not take place in utero.

    b. Nutrition

        (1) Water, inorganic salts, carbohydrates, fats, proteins, and vitamins pass from the maternal blood through the placental membrane into the fetal system via enzymatic carriers.

        (2) The placenta metabolizes glucose and stores it in the form of glycogen until the fetal liver is able to function.

    c. Excretion

        (1) Waste products cross the placental membrane and enter the maternal blood.

        (2) Waste products produced by the fetus are minimal due to the dominance of anabolic (building rather than breaking down activities) metabolism.

    d. Protection

        (1) Placental barrier prevents the transfer of many harmful substances from the maternal blood system.

        (2) Maternal immunity is transferred to the fetus across the placenta.

    e. Storage: placenta stores carbohydrates, proteins, calcium, and iron.

    f. Hormonal production

        (1) The placenta secretes and synthesizes hormones necessary for the maintenance of the pregnancy and for fetal development.

        (2) These hormones are the steroid hormones, estrogen and progesterone; the protein hormones, human chorionic gonadotropin, and human chorionic somatomammotropin (also known as human placental lactogen); and thyrotropin.

5. At 9 to 12 weeks

    a. By 12 weeks the fetus is 8 cm (3 inches) in length and weighs about 45 g (1.6 ounces).

    b. Brain and neurologic system

        (1) Divisions of the brain begin to develop.

        (2) The head is large and constitutes almost half of the fetus's size.

        (3) The neck is distinct from the head and body.

        (4) Neurons appear at the caudal end of the spinal cord.

        (5) By the 12th week spontaneous movements of the fetus occur; lip movements indicate the development of the sucking reflex.

    c. Heart and circulatory system

        (1) Red blood cells are produced in the liver by the 9th week.

        (2) By the 12th week the spleen begins to produce red blood cells.

    d. Gastrointestinal system

        (1) The buccopharyngeal and anal membranes open (the intestinal system from mouth to anus is patent).

        (2) Intestinal loops are visible in the proximal end of the umbilical cord and reenter the abdomen during the 11th week.

        (3) By the 12th week the face is well formed and broad.

            (a) The nose begins to protrude.

            (b) The chin is small and receding.

            (c) Tooth buds appear.

            (d) The palate is complete.

        (4) Bile secretions begin.

    e. Genitourinary system

        (1) The kidneys begin to produce urine (amniotic fluid volume increases).

        (2) Well-differentiated genitals appear.

        (3) Urogenital tract is developed.

    f. Skeletal and muscular systems

        (1) The limbs are long and slender.

        (2) The digits are well formed, and the fetus can curl the fingers and make a tiny fist.

        (3) The legs are still shorter and less developed than the arms.

        (4) Primary ossification centers appear, and ossification begins in the skull and long bones.

        (5) Involuntary muscles in the viscera begin to appear.

    g. Eyes and ears

        (1) Eyes are widely spaced and fused.

        (2) Ears are set low and beginning to acquire an adult shape.

    h. Endocrine and immunologic systems

        (1) The thyroid begins to secrete hormones.

        (2) Lymphoid tissue develops in the fetal thymus.

    i. Malformations that can occur during this period:

        (1) Cleft palate

        (2) Malrotation of the gut

        (3) Omphalocele

        (4) Meckel's diverticulum

6. Between 13 and 16 weeks there is a period of rapid growth.

    a. At 13 weeks the fetus is about 9 cm (3.6 inches) long and weighs between 55 and 60 g (about 2 ounces).

    b. Brain and neurologic system

        (1) Fetal movements are present.

        (2) Thumb sucking can be detected by ultrasonography.

    c. Respiratory system

        (1) Bronchial tubes are branching out in the primitive lungs.

        (2) Lungs are fully shaped.

    d. Gastrointestinal system

        (1) Hard and soft palates are developed.

        (2) Fetus begins to swallow amniotic fluid.

        (3) Fetus is able to produce meconium in the intestinal tract.

        (4) Liver and pancreas begin to produce secretions.

        (5) Gastric and intestinal glands begin to form.

    e. Genitourinary system

        (1) The ovaries have differentiated.

        (2) Primordial follicles containing primitive oocytes and ova (oogonia) are visible.

        (3) External genitalia are formed.

        (4) Kidneys assume the normal shape.

    f. Skeletal and muscular systems

        (1) More muscle tissue develops.

        (2) Ossification of the skeleton occurs.

        (3) By the 16th week skeletal structure is identifiable.

        (4) Lower limbs are longer than the upper limbs.

        (5) Hard tissue in the jaw begins to form.

    g. Eyes, ears, skin, and hair

        (1) Downy lanugo hair begins to develop.

        (2) Fetal skin is transparent and the blood vessels are visible.

        (3) Eyes move to the front of the face.

        (4) Ears migrate upward and are fully formed.

7. At 17 to 20 weeks

    a. At 20 weeks the fetus measures 19 cm (8 inches) and weighs between 435 and 465 g (1 pound, 3 ounces).

    b. Myelination of the spinal cord begins.

    c. Heart tones are audible with a fetoscope.

    d. Respiratory system

        (1) Lung development continues.

        (2) Gas exchange does not occur at this stage, although primitive respiratory-type movements begin.

        (3) Bronchial branching is complete, and pulmonary capillary beds are forming.

        (4) Terminal sacs (alveoli) are developing.

    e. Gastrointestinal system

        (1) Fetus is able to suck and swallow amniotic fluid.

        (2) Peristaltic movements begin.

    f. Skin and hair

        (1) Subcutaneous deposits of brown fat make the skin less transparent.

        (2) Nipples begin to develop over the mammary glands.

        (3) The head has wool-like hair; the eyebrows and eyelashes form.

        (4) Nails are present on fingers and toes.

- (5) Muscles develop and fetal movements are felt by the mother.
- (6) The sebaceous glands become active and produce a greasy substance called vernix caseosa that covers and protects the fetus from the effects of the amniotic fluid by preventing the skin from becoming chapped and hardened.
- **g.** Endocrine and immunologic systems
  - (1) Detectable levels of fetal antibodies are present.
  - (2) The fetus stores iron, and the bone marrow begins to function.
8. At 21 to 24 weeks
   - **a.** At 24 weeks the fetus is 28 cm (11.2 inches) long and weighs approximately 780 g (1 pound, 10 ounces).
   - **b.** Brain and neurologic system
     - (1) The fetus has a reflex hand grip.
     - (2) By the sixth month the fetus will exhibit a startle reflex.
     - (3) The brain structure is mature.
   - **c.** Heart and circulatory system
     - (1) The fetal heartbeat is audible through a stethoscope.
     - (2) The blood in the capillaries is visible.
   - **d.** Respiratory system
     - (1) The alveoli of the lungs are beginning to form.
     - (2) Secretory epithelial cells in the interalveolar walls begin to secrete surfactant.
       - (a) Surfactant facilitates expansion of the alveoli, but not in a quantity sufficient to prevent respiratory distress syndrome (RDS).
       - (b) A fetus born at this stage might survive.
     - (3) Lecithin can be detected in the amniotic fluid.
     - (4) Respiratory movements might occur, and gas exchange is possible.
     - (5) The nostrils reopen.
   - **e.** Genitourinary system: the testes descend to the inguinal ring.
   - **f.** Skeletal and muscular systems: the muscles are developed and the fetus is more active.
   - **g.** Eyes, ears, skin, and hair
     - (1) The eyes are fully developed and will open.
     - (2) The hair is growing longer.
     - (3) Eyebrows and eyelashes have formed.
     - (4) The ears are flat and shapeless, but the fetus can hear.
     - (5) The skin is red and wrinkled, with little subcutaneous fat.
     - (6) Skin ridges on the palms and soles of the feet are forming.
     - (7) The skin is less transparent because of deposits of brown fat.
     - (8) Vernix caseosa covers the entire body.
     - (9) Fingernails are well developed.
   - **h.** Endocrine and immunologic systems: immunoglobulin G (IgG) levels in the fetus reach maternal levels.
9. At 25 to 29 weeks
   - **a.** The fetus is now between 35 and 38 cm (14 and 15 inches) long and weighs about 1200 g (2 pounds, 10.5 ounces).
   - **b.** Brain and neurologic system
     - (1) The brain continues to mature and grow in size.
     - (2) The nervous system is complete enough to provide some regulation of the body functions and body temperature.
   - **c.** Heart and circulatory system: erythropoiesis ends in the spleen and begins in the bone marrow.
   - **d.** Respiratory system
     - (1) Respiratory system is developed enough to provide gaseous exchange.
     - (2) Lungs are capable of breathing air, but the fetus will need intensive care to survive.
     - (3) Surfactant forms on the alveolar surfaces.
   - **e.** Genitourinary system
     - (1) In the male, the testes descend into the scrotal sac.
     - (2) In the female, the clitoris is prominent, and the labia majora are small and do not cover the labia minora.

   f. Skin and hair
      (1) Adipose tissue begins to accumulate.
      (2) Eyebrows and eyelashes develop.
10. At 30 to 34 weeks
   a. The fetus is gaining weight from an increase in muscle and fat.
   b. The fetus will grow from about 1200 g (2 pounds, 10.5 ounces) and a length of about 38 cm (15 inches) to 2000 g (4 pounds, 6.5 ounces) and a length of 40 cm (16 inches).
   c. Brain and neurologic system
      (1) The central nervous system has matured enough to direct breathing movements and partially control body temperature.
      (2) Reflexes are present.
   d. Respiratory system
      (1) The lungs are not fully developed, but the fetus can survive if born at this stage.
      (2) The lecithin/sphingomyelin (L/S) ratio is approximately 1.2:1 at 30 weeks, increasing to greater than 2:1 by 38 weeks.
   e. Genitourinary system
      (1) The testes descend into the scrotum; scrotum is small and rugae are present anteriorly.
      (2) Clitoris is covered and labia majora increase in size.
   f. Skeletal and muscular systems: distal femoral ossification centers develop.
   g. Eyes, ears, skin, and hair
      (1) Pinna is still folded and soft.
      (2) Skin is less wrinkled, and the fetus is more filled out.
      (3) Fingernails extend to the ends of the fingertips.
11. At 35 to 38 weeks
   a. The fetus is 46 cm (17.5 inches) in length and weighs 2600 g (6 pounds).
   b. A fetus born at this time has a fairly good chance of surviving.
   c. Respiratory system: the L/S ratio is greater than 2:1 by 38 weeks.
   d. Genitourinary system
      (1) Scrotum is small, and rugae are present anteriorly.
      (2) Clitoris is covered, and labia majora increase in size.
   e. Skeletal and muscular systems: distal femoral ossification centers develop.
   f. Eyes, ears, skin, and hair
      (1) The body and extremities are filling out.
      (2) The fetus is less wrinkled.
      (3) Lanugo is disappearing.
      (4) The fetus has a firm grasp and begins to orient to light.
12. At 39 to 40 weeks the fetus is considered full-term.
   a. The fetus is approximately 50 cm (20 inches) in length and weighs between 3000 and 3600 g (6 pounds, 10 ounces and 7 pounds, 15 ounces).
   b. Genitourinary system
      (1) The testes should be palpable in the inguinal canals.
      (2) The labia majora are well developed.
   c. Ears, skin, and hair
      (1) The skin is smooth and has a polished look.
      (2) Vernix caseosa is present, with the heaviest deposits in the creases and folds of the skin.
      (3) The chest is prominent and slightly smaller than the head.
      (4) The mammary glands protrude in both sexes.
      (5) The fetal body fills most of the uterine cavity, and the amniotic fluid volume diminishes to about 500 mL.
      (6) Lanugo remains on shoulders and upper back only.
      (7) Earlobes become firm as the cartilage thickens.
   d. Malformations that might occur during this period
      (1) Patent ductus arteriosus
      (2) Cryptorchidism (failure of the testes to descend into the scrotum)
13. Postterm (42 weeks and beyond)
   a. Fetuses might gain weight, thus increasing the difficulty of labor or might lose weight because parts of the placenta fail to function.

  b. Fetus might pass meconium due to hypoxia from placental insufficiency.

  c. Nails and hair continue to grow.

14. Congenital malformations

 a. Approximately 3% to 4% of all live-born infants have obvious malformations.

 b. Genetic factors are involved in more than 33% of all congenital malformations.

 c. Environmental factors cause approximately 7% of malformations.

  (1) Organs and parts of the embryo affected will be determined by the time of ingestion or exposure to teratogens (an environmental agent that causes malformations) (Figure 3-9). (See Chapter 9 for a complete discussion of environmental hazards.)

  (2) The organs and fetal system are most sensitive to teratogens during periods of rapid growth in the first trimester.

F. Placental abnormalities

1. Extrachorial placentas: situation in which the membrane is 1 cm or more central to the chorionic plate

 a. Causes

  (1) Might be the result of lateral placental growth or implantation that was too deep, causing an undermining of the membranes.

  (2) Hemorrhage and separation with resealing

 b. Common in the placentas of extramembranous pregnancies

  (1) Associated rare occurrence: amniotic fluid might leak throughout the pregnancy because of rupture of the membranes.

  (2) The ruptured membrane might retract to such an extent that the pregnancy is extramembranous and the fetus is no longer contained within the amniotic sac.

  (3) The newborn can have pulmonary hypoplasia because of a lack of amniotic fluid and a resultant inability to inspire in utero.

 c. Possibly exists in 20% of placentas

  (1) More common in multigravid pregnancies

  (2) Familial occurrence has been noted.

  (3) Not related to maternal age

 d. Are usually of no major fetal consequence but, if severe, can cause:

  (1) Prematurity

  (2) Hemorrhage

  (3) Fetal growth restriction

2. Amniotic bands (Table 3-2)

 a. Believed to arise from ruptures in the amnion, resulting in floating strands and cords of the amnion

 b. Etiology is unknown, but ruptures usually occur near the cord insertion site.

  (1) Inflammation and trauma are possible causes.

  (2) Amniotic bands have occurred in some pregnancies after amniocentesis has been performed.

  (3) Oligohydramnios might be present.

 c. The floating amniotic strands are sticky and can adhere to the fetus.

  (1) The bands might restrict embryonic development; facial defects, such as clefts and encephaloceles, and thoracic and abdominal defects, such as gastroschisis, can result.

  (2) If the bands constrict the extremities, amputation and constriction bands on limbs and digits can result.

G. Cord

1. Description: the cord is the connecting link between the fetus and the placenta; it usually contains one large vein and two smaller arteries.

2. Development

 a. Formed from the union of the amnion, yolk, and connecting stalk

 b. First trimester

  (1) The body stalk, which attaches the embryo to the yolk sac, contains blood vessels that extend into the chorionic villi.

  (2) The body sac fuses with the embryonic portion of the placenta to provide a circulatory pathway from the chorionic villi to the embryo.

  (3) The body stalk elongates and becomes the umbilical cord.

   (a) The vessels of the cord decrease to one large vein and two smaller arteries.

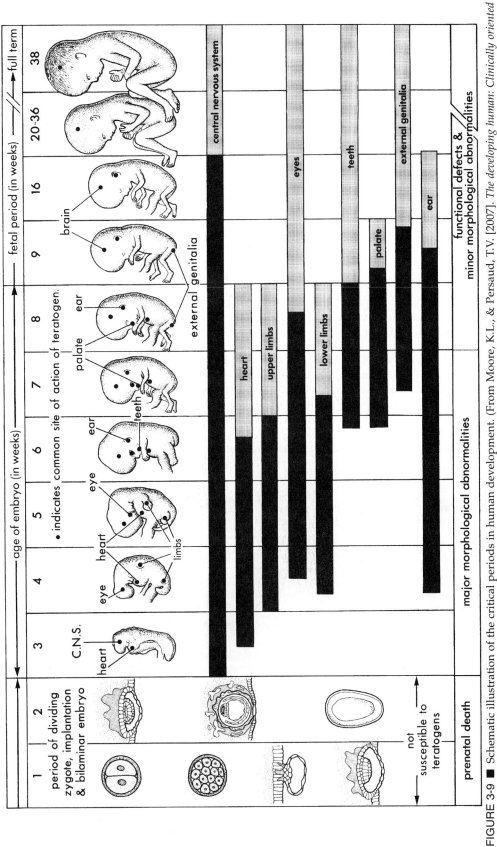

FIGURE 3-9 ■ Schematic illustration of the critical periods in human development. (From Moore, K.L., & Persaud, T.V. [2007]. *The developing human: Clinically oriented embryology* [8th ed., p.143]. Philadelphia: Saunders.)

■ TABLE 3-2
■ ■ **Abnormalities Resulting from Amniotic Bands**

Fetal Age	Abnormality Most Likely Seen
3 weeks	Anencephaly Facial distortions Facial clefting Encephaloceles
5 weeks	Cleft lip Choanal atresia Limb reduction Syndactyly Abdominal wall defects Thoracic wall defects Scoliosis
7 weeks and after	Ear deformities Amputations Distal lymphedema Foot deformities Omphaloceles

Adapted from Smith, D.W. (1982). *Recognizable patterns of human malformation: Genetic, embryologic, and clinical aspects* (3rd ed.). Philadelphia: Saunders.

[i] The umbilical vein contains placental oxygenated blood that returns to the fetus.
[ii] The arteries carry unoxygenated blood to the placenta.
(b) Approximately 1% of umbilical cords have only two vessels—an artery and a vein; this condition is frequently associated with congenital malformations.
[i] Sirenomelia, in which the lower limbs are fused, giving the infant a "mermaid" appearance
[ii] VATERS syndrome, which can comprise any or all of the following:
• **V**ertebral and ventricular septal defects
• **A**nal atresia
• **T**racheoesophageal fistula
• **E**sophageal atresia
• **R**adial and renal dysplasia
• **S**ingle umbilical artery
[iii] Trisomies 13 and 18
(c) The cord has no nerves.
(4) Specialized gelatinous connective tissue, called Wharton jelly, surrounds the blood vessels and prevents compression of the cord.
(5) At term, the average cord is about 55 cm (22 inches) long.
(a) A cord shorter than 32 cm (13 inches) might indicate problems with the fetus.
[i] There can be renal agenesis.
[ii] A short cord is often associated with pulmonary hypoplasia.
[iii] May predispose to abruptio placentae or cord rupture
(b) An unusually long cord is associated with cord prolapse and fetal entrapment.
(6) The cord can attach itself to the placenta at various sites, but central insertion into the placenta is considered normal; abnormalities include:
(a) Velamentous insertion, in which the cord is implanted at the edge of the placenta, and fetal vessels separate in the membranes before reaching the placenta.
[i] Increased incidence of structural defects in the fetus occurs.
• Congenital hip dislocation
• Asymmetric head shape
[ii] Can increase risk for intrauterine growth restriction and preterm birth
(b) Vasa previa is associated with velamentous insertion of the cord, in which the vessels lie over the internal cervical os in front of the fetus.
[i] The vessels might be compressed, compromising oxygen exchange in the fetus.

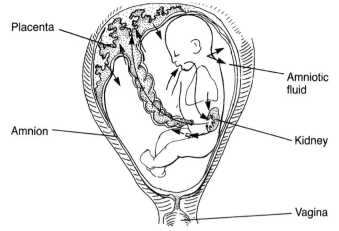

Placenta

Amniotic fluid

Amnion

Kidney

Vagina

FIGURE 3-10 ■ Circulation of amniotic fluid.

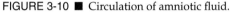

[ii] If the vessels rupture, the fetus might experience severe blood loss, which can occur when membranes rupture.
   (c) Marginal insertion (battledore)
     [i] Occurs in 2% to 15% of gestations.
     [ii] Is associated with a higher-than-normal frequency of preterm labor and birth
  (7) The cord can appear twisted or spiraled.
   (a) This is most likely caused by fetal movement.
   (b) A true knot in the cord rarely occurs; when there is a true knot in the cord, the cord is usually longer than normal, allowing the fetus to pass through a loop in the cord.
   (c) So-called false knots are more common.
     [i] False knots are caused by the folding of the cord vessel.
     [ii] False knots are not usually a problem for the developing fetus.
  (8) When the umbilical cord is around the neck of the fetus, it is called a nuchal cord.

H. Amniotic fluid: the pale straw-colored fluid in which the fetus floats
  1. Development
   a. Early pregnancy
    (1) Shortly after fertilization, a cleft forms in the morula.
    (2) As the cleft enlarges, it becomes fused with the surrounding amnion, creating the amniotic sac.
    (3) The sac then fills with colorless fluid, which increases in volume to 50 mL at 12 weeks' gestation.
    (4) The fluid is produced by the amniotic membrane.
   b. Second trimester to delivery (Figure 3-10)
    (1) Fetus modifies amniotic fluid through the processes of swallowing and urinating.
    (2) The volume can also be modified through movement of fluid through the fetal respiratory tract.
  2. Volume
   a. There is a wide range of amniotic fluid volume during pregnancy.
   b. Normal approximations of volume
    (1) At 12 weeks there is approximately 50 mL.
    (2) At 20 weeks there is approximately 400 mL.
    (3) At 36 to 38 weeks there is approximately 1 L.
    (4) Volume decreases after 38 weeks.
  3. Function
   a. Provides a medium for fetal movement
   b. Protects the fetus against injury from external causes
   c. Assists in maintaining temperature
   d. Provides nourishment to fetus
   e. Might be an important factor in dilating the cervical canal
   f. Prevents the amnion from adhering to the developing fetus

4. Composition
    a. Consists of approximately 98% water
    b. Is alkaline in reaction (pH is 7.0 to 7.25)
    c. Early pregnancy
        (1) Is similar in composition to maternal plasma
        (2) Contains a lower protein concentration than maternal plasma
        (3) Is nearly devoid of particulate matter
    d. Second trimester to delivery (see Figure 3-10)
        (1) As pregnancy progresses, phospholipids (from the lung) accumulate.
        (2) Variable amounts of particulate matter occur from the shedding of fetal cells, lanugo, scalp hair, and vernix caseosa into the fluid.
        (3) Osmolality decreases.
        (4) Fluid becomes hypotonic as a result of fetal urination.
        (5) Fluid contains higher levels of urea, creatinine, and uric acid than the plasma.
5. Abnormalities in volume
    a. Oligohydramnios (decreased amounts of amniotic fluid)
        (1) Less than 500 mL, between 32 and 36 weeks
        (2) Common causes
            (a) Amniotic leakage
            (b) Abnormalities of the fetal kidneys (e.g., renal agenesis)
        (3) Primary oligohydramnios associated with fetal abnormalities
            (a) Renal agenesis
            (b) Polycystic kidneys
            (c) Urinary tract obstructions
        (4) Oligohydramnios that occurs during or before the second trimester; usually associated with a poor pregnancy outcome
            (a) Compression of the fetus
            (b) Fetal death due to respiratory insufficiency and a lack of lung development
    b. Hydramnios (increased amounts of amniotic fluid)
        (1) Exceeds 2 L of fluid between 32 and 36 weeks.
        (2) Is often associated with poor fetal outcomes because of tendency toward:
            (a) Preterm delivery
            (b) Fetal malpresentation
            (c) Cord prolapse
        (3) Hydramnios that occurs during or before second trimester spontaneously resolves in 45% of the cases, resulting in normal outcomes.
        (4) Pathogenesis is usually unclear.
            (a) Is possibly caused by defective regulation of fluid transfer across the amniochorion
            (b) Occurs more frequently with Rh-sensitized pregnancies, monozygotic multiple pregnancy, and gestational or type 1 diabetes mellitus
            (c) Occurs frequently with fetal gastrointestinal obstructions or atresias

CLINICAL PRACTICE

A. Assessment
    1. History
        a. Ascertain the date of day 1 of the last menstrual period to monitor fetal development.
        b. It is important to ascertain the dates of maternal immunizations for rubella, rubeola, and mumps.
        c. Knowledge of any infections during pregnancy is important because viruses are known to cross the placental barrier and the timing of viral infections might determine the type and extent of fetal injury.
        d. A thorough family history is needed to detect potential inheritable diseases.
        e. A complete medical history can identify maternal high-risk conditions, such as diabetes mellitus, that might adversely affect fetal development.

    f. A comprehensive assessment of drug intake should include prescription, over-the-counter, and illicit drugs; alcohol; and nicotine. Teratogenic effects of chemical substances will be determined by the stage of fetal development at the time of drug consumption.

    g. Previous pregnancies and outcomes

    h. Known uterine infections

    i. Episodes of bleeding, hypertension, and trauma

2. Physical findings

    a. Excessive weight gain or lack of weight gain during pregnancy

    b. Delayed or accelerated uterine growth related to gestational age might indicate problems with fetal development.

    c. Physical signs of placental risk

        (1) Bleeding

        (2) Sudden and severe abdominal pain

        (3) Uterine rigidity

        (4) Fundal height not appropriate for gestational age

3. Diagnostic procedures

    a. Monitoring of uterine growth by measuring fundal heights

    b. Ultrasonography

        (1) Monitors fetal growth and development. Fetus can be first identified by transvaginal sonography 4 weeks from the last period. The mean sac diameter increases 1 mm/day. Gestational age can be figured by adding 30 to the mean sac diameter (in mm) during the first 6 weeks.

        (2) Can identify major congenital malformations such as hydrocephalus, renal agenesis, neural tube defects (3-dimensional approached is preferrred), cleft lip and palate, abdominal and skeletal abnormalities, and anencephaly

        (3) Location of the placenta

        (4) Placental grading

        (5) Amniotic volume

    c. Maternal serum alpha-fetoprotein (MS-AFP)

        (1) Lower-than-normal results might indicate a chromosomal abnormality such as trisomy 21 (Down syndrome).

        (2) Elevated AFP level might indicate a neural tube defect but is also normally associated with multiple pregnancy.

    d. Amniocentesis is the withdrawal of fluid from the amniotic cavity.

        (1) Identifies chromosomal abnormalities.

        (2) Assesses the fluid for AFP levels to rule out open-neural tube defects.

    e. Chorionic villus sampling is performed for chromosome analysis and selected metabolic tests on the fetus (see Chapter 8 for a complete discussion of antenatal testing).

    f. Kleihauer-Betke test is used to determine if vaginal bleeding is of maternal or fetal origin.

B. Interventions/Outcomes

1. Congenital malformation due to exposure to teratogens

    a. Interventions

        (1) Assess for exposure to infection, chemicals, or environmental factors.

        (2) Identify the stage of fetal development at which exposure occurred.

        (3) Provide parents with the information they need to understand risks and make appropriate medical and health decisions about the pregnancy.

        (4) Refer parents to appropriate resources to assess the effects of exposure (e.g., to a genetic center or tertiary high-risk obstetric services).

        (5) Maintain an accepting and supportive approach toward the parents.

        (6) Listen to their fears and concerns, and provide health information that is appropriate to their level of understanding.

    b. Outcomes

        (1) Parents are able to express an understanding of the risks from exposure.

        (2) Parents have obtained appropriate services from referral agencies.

        (3) Parents have made an appropriate decision regarding the outcome of the pregnancy that is based on their values and needs.

2. Delayed growth and development due to inadequate maternal nutrition
   a. Interventions
      (1) Assess maternal nutritional intake to identify deficiencies.
      (2) Assess maternal understanding of nutritional needs for fetal development.
      (3) Educate the mother about healthy nutritional intake.
      (4) Provide supplements for nutritional deficiencies, as indicated.
         (a) Supplement the mother's diet with vitamins and iron.
         (b) Refer the parents to a nutritionist for further counseling or to Women, Infants, and Children (WIC) nutritional supplement program, if eligible.
   b. Outcomes
      (1) Maternal nutritional intake improves.
      (2) Fetus continues to grow.
      (3) Mother obtains services from referral sources.
3. Developmental defects due to genetic disorders
   a. Interventions
      (1) Assess parents for a genetic history.
      (2) Interpret risks, as indicated.
      (3) Refer the parents for genetic counseling, as indicated.
      (4) Provide appropriate information to assist the couple in making decisions about the outcome of pregnancy.
      (5) Maintain a nonjudgmental attitude toward the couple, and allow the couple to discuss fears and concerns.
   b. Outcomes
      (1) Parents have made an appropriate decision about the outcome of the pregnancy, based on their values and needs.
      (2) Parents have obtained the necessary services from referral sources.
4. Altered amniotic fluid volume due to impaired placental transport
   a. Interventions
      (1) Explain diagnostic tests (ultrasonography and amniocentesis) to the woman and her family.
      (2) Remain with the woman during procedure, if possible.
      (3) Clarify misconceptions and allow the woman and her family to discuss fears and concerns.
      (4) Ensure that the woman and her family understand the test results and the test's implications.
   b. Outcomes
      (1) The woman and her family can explain the reason for the diagnostic procedure.
      (2) The woman reports an understanding of test results.
      (3) The woman and her family report decreased fear and anxiety.
5. Inadequate fetal growth due to poor nutritional placental transport
   a. Interventions
      (1) Explain the importance of adequate nutritional intake.
      (2) Discuss the possible consequences of poor nutritional intake.
      (3) Evaluate maternal nutritional intake.
   b. Outcomes
      (1) The woman complies with proposed nutritional program.
      (2) The woman can explain the possible negative consequences to the fetus resulting from poor maternal nutritional intake.
6. Impaired fetal gas exchange due to poor placental transport
   a. Interventions
      (1) Explain the possible outcome of poor fetal gas exchange.
      (2) Explain the importance of compliance with the testing regimen.
      (3) Reinforce the need for lateral position (left is preferable) to improve uteroplacental circulation when the client is recumbent.
   b. Outcomes
      (1) The woman can explain the possible outcome to fetus of poor gas exchange.
      (2) The woman agrees to comply with recommended antepartal testing.
      (3) The woman agrees to lie in the lateral position when recumbent during the remainder of the pregnancy.

HEALTH EDUCATION

A. Nutritional needs for adequate fetal development
   1. Calories: 2300 to 2400 per day
   2. Protein: 74 to 76 g/day
   3. Carbohydrates: increased requirement to allow for protein uptake for fetal development
   4. Fat: provides energy, and fat deposits increase in the fetus from 2% at midpregnancy to 12% at term
   5. Vitamins and minerals: a slight increase in intake is needed to provide for the growth of new tissue in the fetus
B. Effects of chemical use (smoking, alcohol, and drugs) on the fetus
   1. Timing of ingestion and amount of chemical consumed
   2. Effect on fetus (teratogenic)
      a. Intrauterine growth restriction
      b. Premature birth
      c. Congenital malformations, determined by the effects on developing systems
      d. Newborn withdrawal
   3. Importance of eliminating chemical use during pregnancy
C. Reasons for and the procedures used in ultrasonography and amniocentesis
D. Importance of prenatal visits for assessing fetal well-being
E. Importance of relating any unusual symptoms to health care provider
F. Implications of any symptoms
G. Review of the stages of fetal development and the role of the placenta and amniotic fluid

STUDY QUESTIONS

1. The most critical stage of physical development for the unborn child occurs:
   a. During the pre-embryonic stage
   b. From the 3rd to the 8th week of development
   c. From the 9th to the 20th week of development
   d. From the 20th week to delivery
2. The major function of vernix caseosa is to:
   a. Protect fetal skin from the amniotic fluid
   b. Prevent adhesions to the amniotic sac
   c. Enhance the nutrient balance of the amniotic fluid
   d. Prevent the excessive shedding of fetal tissue
3. During which weeks of development is the fetus first able to provide some regulation of its own body functions and body temperature?
   a. At 17 to 20 weeks
   b. At 21 to 24 weeks
   c. At 25 to 29 weeks
   d. At 30 to 34 weeks
4. The main function of the placenta is to:
   a. Provide a nutrient exchange between maternal and fetal circulations
   b. Ensure that the fetus is protected from trauma
   c. Provide a mechanism for the direct exchange of oxygen and carbon dioxide
   d. Allow for the elimination of excess fetal hormones

5. Which statement best describes placental development?
   a. It develops rapidly, with limited changes after the first month.
   b. It continues to develop and grow throughout pregnancy.
   c. Major growth and development occur in the first trimester.
   d. There are two major stages of development; these are in the first and third trimesters.
6. What is the major reason for monitoring placental growth and function?
   a. To predict fetal positioning at time of birth
   b. To evaluate fetal well-being
   c. To predict gestational age at delivery
   d. To indicate risk factors for chromosomal abnormalities
7. What are the major functions of amniotic fluid?
   a. Provides respiratory and nutritional exchange between fetal and maternal circulation
   b. Is a major component of fetal blood circulation and hormone production
   c. Protects the fetus from injury by cushioning it from trauma, and maintains a constant temperature
   d. Is an important component in monitoring and altering fetal biochemical status

ANSWERS TO STUDY QUESTIONS

1. b
2. a
3. c
4. a

5. c
6. b
7. c

BIBLIOGRAPHY

Achildi, O., & Grewal, H. (2007). Congenital anomalies of the esophagus. *Otolaryngology Clinics of North America, 40,* 219–244.

Bernstein, D. (2007). The cardiovascular system: developmental biology of the cardiovascular system. In R. M. Kliegman, R. R. Behrman, H. B. Jenson, & B. M. Stanton (Eds.), *Nelson textbook of pediatrics* (18th ed.). Philadelphia: Saunders.

Burton, G. J., Sibley, C. P., & Jauniaux, E. R. M. (2007). Placental anatomy and physiology. In S. G. Gabbe, J. R. Niebyl, & J. L. Simpson (Eds.), *Obstetrics: Normal and problem pregnancies* (5th ed., pp. 3–19). London: Churchill Livingstone.

Cheng, E., & Katz, V. L. (2007). Fertilization and embryogenesis: meiosis, fertilization, implantation, embryonic development, sexual differentiation. In V. L. Katz (Ed.), *Comprehensive gynecology* (5th ed., pp. 1–8). Philadelphia: Mosby.

Guercio, J. R., & Martyn, L. J. (2007). Congenital malformation of the eye and orbit. *Otolaryngology Clinics of North America, 40,* 113–140.

Kanev, P. M. (2007). Congenital malformations of the skull and meninges. *Otolaryngology Clinics of North America, 40,* 9–26.

Lazebnik, N., Bornstein, E., & Timor-Tritsch, I. E. (2008). The utility of volume sonography for the detection of fetal spine abnormalities. *Ultrasound Clinics, 3,* 529–539.

Lee, M. C., & Eberson, C. P. (2006). Growth and development of the child's hip. *Orthopedic Clinics of North America, 37,* 119–132.

Lee, W., & Comstock, C. H. (2006). Prenatal diagnosis of congenital disease: Where are we now? *Ultrasound Clinics, 1,* 273–291.

Moore, K. L., & Persaud, T. V. (1998). *Before we are born: Essentials of human embryology and birth defects* (5th ed.). Philadelphia: Saunders.

Niebyl, J. R., & Simpson, J. L. (2007). Drugs and environmental agents in pregnancy and lactation: Embryology, teratology, epidemiology. In S. G. Gabbe, J. R. Niebyl, & J. L. Simpson (Eds.), *Obstetrics: Normal and problem pregnancies* (5th ed., pp. 184–206). London: Churchill Livingstone.

Richard, D. S. (2007). Ultrasound for pregnancy dating, growth, and diagnosis of fetal malformations. In S. G. Gabbe, J. R. Niebyl, & J. L. Simpson (Eds.), *Obstetrics: Normal and problem pregnancies* (5th ed., pp. 216–240). London: Churchill Livingstone.

Ross, M. G., Ervin, M. G., & Novak, D. (2007). Fetal physiology. In S. G. Gabbe, J. R. Niebyl, & J. L. Simpson (Eds.), *Obstetrics: Normal and problem pregnancies* (5th ed., pp. 26–43). London: Churchill Livingstone.

NORMAL PREGNANCY

4 Ethnocultural Considerations in the Childbearing Period

Susan Mattson

OBJECTIVES

1. State the need for a cultural assessment of the childbearing family.
2. Describe data to be collected through a cultural assessment.
3. Perform a cultural assessment of a childbearing family.
4. Analyze data obtained from a cultural assessment for potential problem areas.
5. Formulate nursing interventions to address problem areas identified from the assessment.
6. Identify barriers to care that are frequently encountered by the culturally diverse client.
7. Identify ways to decrease barriers to care encountered by the culturally diverse client.

INTRODUCTION

A. **Transcultural nursing is concerned with the provision of nursing care in a manner that is sensitive to the needs of individuals, families, and groups.**
   1. A major aim of transcultural nursing is to understand and assist members of diverse cultural groups with their nursing and health care needs.
   2. Nursing interventions that are culturally relevant to the needs of the client decrease the possibility of conflict or misunderstanding arising from people from different backgrounds (Andrews, 1995).
   3. The goal of transcultural nursing is "to develop a scientific and humanistic body of knowledge to provide culture-specific and culture-universal nursing care practices" (Andrews, 2003).
      a. Culture-specific refers to particular values, beliefs, and patterns of behavior that tend to be special or unique to a group and that do not tend to be shared with members of other cultures.
      b. Culture-universal refers to the commonly shared values, norms of behavior, and life patterns that are similarly held among cultures about human behavior and lifestyles (Leininger & McFarland, 2002).
   4. Applying transcultural concepts to nursing practice includes:
      a. Identifying cultural needs
      b. Understanding the cultural context of the client and family
      c. Using culturally sensitive strategies to meet mutually satisfying goals
   5. A common problem faced by nurses who want to use cultural data is knowing what data to collect and how to use the data effectively.
      a. A major purpose of collecting cultural data is to give the nurse greater insight into and understanding of:
         (1) The nature and behavior of clients
         (2) The problems that clients encounter in health promotion and maintenance
         (3) Clients' ways of coping with illness
      b. These data should be relevant to potential or actual nursing problems.
      c. Transcultural knowledge is used to augment, clarify, explain, or assist in attaining client-centered goals.

B. **The overall goal is to develop and sustain cultural (and linguistic) competence among health care professionals.**
   1. The concept refers to a complex integration of knowledge, attitudes, and skills that enhance cross-cultural communication and appropriate/effective interactions with others (American Academy of Nursing, 1992, 1993; Campinha-Bacote, 2000, 2003; Geron, 2002).
   2. Cultural competence has been defined as a process, as opposed to an end point, in which the nurse continually strives to work effectively within the cultural context of individuals, families, or communities from diverse cultural backgrounds (Andrews & Boyle, 1997; Campinha-Bacote, 2000, 2003; Purnell & Paulanka, 2008; Wells, 2000).
   3. Cultural and linguistic competence have been defined and issued as standards from the Office of Minority Health at the U.S. Department of Health & Human Services (1999) as the ability of health care providers and organizations to understand and effectively respond to the cultural and linguistic needs brought by the clients to the health care encounter.
C. **Childbearing is a time of transition and social celebration of great importance in any society** (Lauderdale, 2008).
   1. Many cultures have particular customs and beliefs that dictate activities and behavior during this time.
      a. Some might be considered prescriptive in nature: phrased positively, and describing expectations of behavior.
         (1) Might involve wearing special articles of clothing
         (2) Might involve ceremonies
         (3) Might be recommendations for physical activity and/or diet
      b. Others are restrictive: phrased negatively, and limiting choices or behaviors; usually directed toward:
         (1) Activity—physical and sexual
         (2) Work and environment
         (3) Emotions
      c. A third area of beliefs is the taboo—restrictions with serious supernatural consequences.
         (1) Often involve exposure to moon and sun at certain times of the day
         (2) Might refer to witchcraft as a mechanism, or avoidance of some types of people (widows, people in mourning)
         (3) Often refer to food choices (Lauderdale, 2008)
   2. The labor and delivery and postpartum periods might also be governed by unique customs.
      a. Cultural factors influencing labor and delivery center on a general attitude toward:
         (1) Birth
         (2) Methods of dealing with the pain of labor
         (3) Preferred positions during delivery
         (4) The role of support persons and health practitioners
      b. Many cultures consider the postpartum period to be one of increased vulnerability for both mother and infant.
         (1) Dietary and activity prescriptions are common at this time and might be in conflict with the usual Western methods of obstetric care.
         (2) Infant care also varies from culture to culture in regard to:
            (a) Bathing
            (b) Swaddling
            (c) Feeding
            (d) Care of the umbilical cord
            (e) Circumcision
D. **The different ways in which a particular society views this transitional period and manages childbirth depend on the culture's beliefs about health, medical care, reproduction, and the role and status of women** (Figure 4-1).
   1. Pregnancy and childbirth practices in Western society have changed dramatically during the past two decades. A few of the trends that require nurses to examine and rethink how we can better care for our clients include:
      a. An increase in the number of women in the workforce
      b. Advances in reproductive technology
      c. Self-care
      d. Alternative therapies

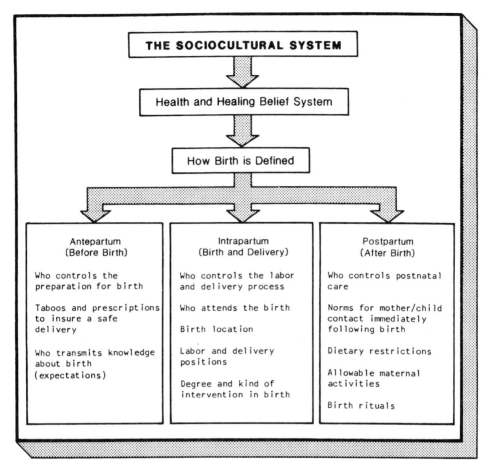

THE SOCIOCULTURAL SYSTEM

Health and Healing Belief System

How Birth is Defined

Antepartum (Before Birth)	Intrapartum (Birth and Delivery)	Postpartum (After Birth)
Who controls the preparation for birth	Who controls the labor and delivery process	Who controls postnatal care
Taboos and prescriptions to insure a safe delivery	Who attends the birth	Norms for mother/child contact immediately following birth
Who transmits knowledge about birth (expectations)	Birth location	Dietary restrictions
	Labor and delivery positions	Allowable maternal activities
	Degree and kind of intervention in birth	Birth rituals

FIGURE 4-1 ■ Components of the childbearing system. A culturally diverse woman, familiar with her own ethnic group's childbearing system, might feel estranged by the dominant culture's birth practices. (From Mattson, S., Galanti, G., Lettieri, C., & Kellogg, J. [1986]. *Culture and health module 2: The family and life cycle in transcultural perspective* [p. 60]. Long Beach, CA: Statewide Nursing Program, Consortium of the California State University.)

    e. Increase in health information available to consumers on the Internet
    f. The large influx of refugees and immigrants (Tiedje, 2000)
2. Subcultures within the United States and Canada have very different practices, values, and beliefs about childbirth and the roles of men, women, social support networks, and health care practitioners.
3. Additionally, religious background, regional variations, age, urban or rural background, sexual preferences, and other individual characteristics all contribute to cultural differences surrounding the childbearing period.
4. Great variations exist in the social class, ethnic origin, family structure, and social support networks of women and their families. One must keep in mind the individual differences that are present within cultures as well as those found between cultures.
5. Culturally competent care for ethnic minority women requires a delicate balance in assumptions that drive the assessment process and the resultant care.
    a. One must balance the assumption that those women who immigrated from a similar region share similar values and beliefs that influence how they will respond to the childbirth experience with the assumption of diversity among women from the same area (Meleis, 2003).
    b. Women's experiences that profoundly influence their childbirth experience include all of the individual characteristics described previously; therefore, the descriptions of the various "populations" in this chapter must be viewed within the context of diversity within each group.

CLINICAL PRACTICE

A. Introduction
   1. Cultural assessment is defined as assessment of:
      a. Shared beliefs
      b. Values
      c. Customs that have relevance to health behaviors (Tripp-Reimer, Brink, & Saunders, 1984)
   2. It is performed to identify patterns that might assist or interfere with a nursing intervention or planned treatment regimen.
   3. To understand why birth is managed in a particular way, it is necessary to view the process in terms of the society's:
      a. Social organization
      b. Political and economic system
      c. Medical theory
      d. In addition, Kay (1982) delineated specific cultural data for the four periods during childbearing: antepartum, intrapartum, postpartum, and newborn. In this chapter assessment needs during each of these four periods are discussed. (For specific details about particular cultural groups, see the material referenced in appropriate chapters and sections; see also the appendix at the end of this chapter.)

B. Assessment
   1. Antepartum period
      a. Determinants of the society's acceptance of the pregnancy
         (1) Acceptable age
         (2) Marriage requirements
         (3) Acceptable father
         (4) Pregnancy frequency
      b. Consideration of pregnancy as a state of illness or of health. Many cultural groups perceive pregnancy as a normal physiologic process or state, and don't believe that pregnant women are ill or in need of "curative services." These women often delay or do not receive any prenatal care from a health care provider (Lauderdale, 2008).
         (1) Latinos in particular consider pregnancy a natural condition that usually doesn't require medical care, unless there is a problem, until late in the pregnancy. However, the mother and fetus are vulnerable to outside influences and will take protective measures (Mattson, 2003).
         (2) In one study, Amish women used perinatal care based on their beliefs about pregnancy and childbirth, and in relation to cost, transportation, and child care. The women initiated prenatal care earlier for first pregnancies, and later with subsequent ones, knowing that pregnancy was a "nonproblematic" condition. They did seek immediate attention if a serious problem arose (bleeding, for example) (Campanella, Korbin, & Acheson, 1993).
      c. Behavioral expectations
         (1) Dietary prescriptions or restrictions
            (a) Adherence to the hot or cold theory of health and diet (especially with Hispanic and Asian clients). This theory describes the intrinsic properties of foods, beverages, medicines, and their effects on the body.
               [i]   Health is maintained through a balance of these forces.
               [ii] If an imbalance occurs, illness results.
               [iii] To produce balance (and restore or maintain health), illness and conditions such as pregnancy are treated with substances having the opposite property of the illness (i.e., pregnancy is considered to be a hot state; thus any treatments must be of a cold nature).
                  • Temperature and spiciness do not determine classification; however, this varies among cultural groups.
                  • Generally, warm or hot foods are believed to be easier to digest than cold or cool foods.
               [iv] These properties of hot and cold are also part of the yin-yang belief system prevalent among Asian approaches to health and diet (Andrews, 2008b).

        (b) Another somewhat unfamiliar practice is that of pica, or the ingestion of nonfood substances, especially clay or starch
            [i] Pica is often practiced by African-American women, usually in the rural southern United States.
            [ii] There are many explanations for why this occurs.
- A result of an iron deficiency that leads to the craving
- A carryover from behaviors practiced in Africa

            [iii] Some Hispanic women prefer the solid milk of magnesia, whereas others eat the ice or frost that forms inside refrigerator/freezer units (Boyle & Mackey, 1999).

   (2) Activity restrictions or prescriptions, including the use of massage as a treatment for the various ills experienced during pregnancy; many people believe that the activities of the mother influence the outcome of pregnancy and the well-being of the newborn.

   (3) Expression of emotions, including anger, fear, and anxiety
        (a) Pueblo and Navajo Indians, Mexicans, and Japanese believe the mother should remain happy to bring the baby joy and good fortune (Waxler-Morrison, Andrews, & Richardson, 1990).
        (b) Hispanics believe experiencing *susto* in pregnancy is bad for the mother and baby (Mattson, 2003).
        (c) One major consideration at this time is intimate partner violence (IPV) that may escalate or begin during pregnancy. IPV of pregnant women has been associated with adverse pregnancy outcomes for mother and infant (Taggart & Mattson, 1996). (See Chapter 18 for further discussion.)

   (4) People from whom to seek advice, and the appropriate time to do so
        (a) Women from many cultures might refuse to seek early prenatal care because they consider pregnancy a normal and healthy state.
        (b) Fear, modesty, and a wish to avoid a physical examination by a male care provider might also prevent some women from seeking care from Western providers (Andrews, 2008b).

2. Intrapartum period
  a. Appropriate setting for labor and delivery to occur
   (1) There are often cultural differences between laboring women and nurses in a highly biotechnologic Western birthing unit related to the application of technology and pain management (Carlton, Callister, & Stoneman, 2005)
  b. Appropriate attendants for support and as a "practitioner"
   (1) Most non-Western cultures see childbearing as being within the woman's domain.
   (2) Support during labor and assistance after delivery are usually provided by women relatives or friends.
        (a) It is unusual, and should not be expected, for a father from a non-Western culture to provide this support and caretaking.
        (b) Male caregivers may be refused, or may cause distress (Asian, Arab, many Hispanic groups). Practices followed by women of Islamic, Chinese, and Asian Indian backgrounds might include strict religious and cultural prohibitions against viewing the woman's body by *either* the husband or any other man (Lauderdale, 2008).
        (c) For an Orthodox Jewish woman in labor, and for reasons of modesty, the support person of choice may be a woman of her community (Lewis, 2003)
  c. Pain control, including what expressions of discomfort are permitted and expected
  d. Restrictions and prescriptions for activity, including ambulation and massage
  e. Dietary recommendations, including the continuation of intake of food and drink; possible preference for herbal teas (Hispanic and Asian women especially).
  f. Expected length of labor
   (1) Behaviors that are necessary to ensure the appropriate length, including diet and activity; Hispanics in particular like to walk around rather than remain lying in bed, and also believe that drinking *manzanilla* tea makes the contractions stronger.
   (2) Expected interventions if the time is prolonged. Despite the growing number of Cesarean births occurring across the world, there is little in the literature documenting the beliefs of women about this growing surgery.

(a) However, it is known that there are many cultures in which women are reluctant or fearful of having a cesarean birth (Callister, 2008; Zlot, Jackson & Korenbrot, 2005).

(b) Who makes the decision as to whether the recommendation for a cesarean birth will be accepted is also culturally based; it might be the husband, a religious leader, or community or family elders.

  g. Expected and ideal positions for facilitating pushing and delivery

    (1) Squatting

    (2) Sitting

    (3) Side-lying

  h. Appropriate disposition of placenta and umbilical cord after delivery

    (1) Some cultural groups believe that burying the placenta, the umbilical cord, or both in a particular place will bring good fortune to the child and family.

    (2) Others wish to preserve the cord through drying to use it medicinally at a later time.

3. Postpartum period

  a. Postpartum practices provide social support, adaptation to the maternal role, care of the newborn and physical recovery, with many culturally derived variations.

  b. Activity restrictions and prescriptions

    (1) The postpartum period is viewed by many as one that is fraught with dangers for mother and infant.

      (a) One way to protect against danger is for the mother to remain quietly in bed, with little activity to disturb her.

      (b) This includes a restriction on:

        [i] Ambulating

        [ii] Bathing (especially showering)

        [iii] Infant caretaking

        [iv] Other activities seen as normal from a Western medical perspective

      (c) Alter Western expectations for activity and hygiene during the postpartum period to allow comfort for the new mother.

    (2) In some cultures, women are considered to be in a state of impurity during the puerperium, which often coincides with the period of lochial flow. Common behaviors include:

      (a) Seclusion and avoidance of contact with others

      (b) Avoidance of sexual relations

  c. Dietary restrictions and prescriptions

    (1) Many of the same requirements that are based on a theory of hot and cold also affect postpartum guides.

    (2) The puerperium is a cold time (heat is lost at time of delivery) so foods should be hot in nature; women will avoid fruits and vegetables that are considered cold.

  d. Appropriateness of therapeutic heat and cold

    (1) Western practitioners often use cold packs or sitz baths for perineal comfort and healing.

    (2) These practices are not acceptable to women from many cultures.

      (a) Cold air and water are frequently believed to be harmful.

      (b) They are believed to cause uterine problems and even infertility when they enter the uterus through the vagina, along with headaches and other chronic illnesses such as arthritis (Greener, 1989; Moore, Moos, & Callister, 2009).

  e. Expression of emotions

    (1) Postpartum depression (PPD) seems to occur in most cultures throughout the world, with similar levels of prevalance (13%) (Beck, 2008).

    (2) Risk factors are similar, but some specific to particular cultures may include:

      (a) Higher value placed on birth of a male child

      (b) The family's immigrant or refugee status

      (c) Distress from not being able to practice expected postpartum rituals

      (d) Lack of an effective social support system (Callister & Birkhead, 2007; Chaudron et al, 2005; Goldbort, 2005)

    (3) Reporting of the phenomenon in non-Western culture may be hindered by culturally unacceptable labeling of the disorder, variance of symptoms from group to group, or differences in diagnostic standards (Lauderdale, 2008).

(4) Women may report somatic symptoms rather than psychologic ones, especially in cultures that have no name or definition for PPD, such as the Korean and other Asian cultures (Mattson, 1993; Posmontier & Horowitz, 2004).

4. Newborn period
   a. Feeding of the infant, including the method and timing of the first feeding
       (1) A society's advocacy of breastfeeding varies, and many influences must be considered.
       (2) Although American women are choosing to breastfeed in increasing numbers, immigrants from developing and poorer countries see bottle-feeding as the modern way to provide nourishment to their infants.
           (a) This may be an issue with immigrants from areas of the world where human immunodeficiency virus (HIV) and acquired immunodeficiency syndrome (AIDS) is prevalent. Current recommendations in developed countries are to *not* breastfeed if the mother has AIDS (see Chapter 20), but due to the problem with safe water in developing countries, those mothers *are* told to breastfeed, even with the small chance of HIV transmission through breast milk
       (3) Several cultural groups, Hispanic and Arab in particular, believe that colostrum is bad for the infant and prefer to bottle-feed until their milk comes in.
   b. Bathing of the infant, including:
       (1) Time of the first bath
       (2) Appropriate person to perform the bath
       (3) Measures used to protect the infant during the procedure
           (a) Traditional Hispanics believe that both the head and feet should be wet.
           (b) Water will be placed on the head at the same time that the body is immersed in the bath (Clark, 1978).
   c. Sleeping arrangements provided for the infant and what is done to promote sleeping
       (1) Women often keep the infant physically as close as possible, often sharing the same bed. This is true in Vietnam even in the immediate post-birth time in the hospital (Mattson, personal communication/observations, 2008).
       (2) This is particularly true if ritual seclusion and limited activity are enforced.
   d. Swaddling practices. Swaddling the infant is good protection against "bad air" and wind for Hispanics and Southeast Asians in particular (Mattson, 1995, 2003).
   e. Circumcision
       (1) Cultures vary greatly in their beliefs about this practice.
       (2) Ritual circumcision is frequently practiced in traditional Judaism and among followers of Islam.
   f. Caretaking of the infant at home
       (1) Appropriate person to do so. In Asian and Asian Indian cultures, it is still considered inappropriate for the mother to care for the child immediately and/or show attention to the child; the grandmother or other female relative performs this task (Choudhry, 1997; Mattson, personal communication/observation 2008).
       (2) Length of time that the infant is allowed to cry before being attended to
           (a) Some cultures expect that infants will be picked up and attended to (usually breastfed) immediately.
           (b) Others believe that the infant should be allowed to cry for a certain period.
       (3) Care of the umbilical cord
           (a) Hispanic, Filipino, and African-American women might use an abdominal binder or "belly band" to protect the umbilical area against dirt, injury, or hernia.
           (b) These binders are usually not seen by the Western care provider because they are removed before office or clinic visits.
           (c) Oils might also be applied to the umbilical cord stump (Greener, 1989).
   g. Ritual beautification varies according to cultural interpretation and might be done to avoid the evil eye. Navajo infants undergo piercing of their ears and insertion of turquoise earrings to provide protection from evil forces (Kay, 1982).
   h. Attachment behaviors toward the infant
       (1) Asian and Middle Eastern women, in particular, might be erroneously assessed as demonstrating maladaptive attachment behaviors.
       (2) Asian women maintain a distance and do not praise their infants because of a fear of evil influences harming the infant if he or she were seen to be joyfully received.

(3) Middle Eastern women believe that the mother is the one deserving of praise for her great work in producing the infant (Meleis & Sorrell, 1981).

C. **Biologic variations**
1. Biologic variations appear in certain ethnic groups that can have an effect on the pregnancy, the mother, or the newborn.
   a. African Americans and others of Mediterranean descent may have sickle cell disease
   b. Native Americans and Hispanics are susceptible to diabetes mellitus
   c. Jewish populations from Europe (Ashkenazi) carry the traits for Tay-Sachs & Gaucher's diseases
   d. Greek and Southeast Asian women often present with thalassemias, along with women of Arab/Eastern Mediterranean descent.
   e. Amish women may have phenylketonuria (PKU), and infant boys with hemophilia B (Moore, Moos, & Callister, 2009).
2. Differences in pelvic shape and size related to race (see Chapter 10 for further discussion)
3. Differences in infant size related to ethnic influences (see Chapter 17 for further discussion)

D. **Interventions/Outcomes**
Basically, interventions would be directed to any gaps in congruency between the mother/family's expectations of care and that of the nurse, or for any significant biologic variations noted. Most center around the following:
1. Traditional beliefs about hot and cold
   a. Offer warm drinks immediately postpartum.
   b. Offer heat lamps or hot packs rather than sitz baths or ice application to the perineum.
   c. Provide extra blankets for warmth.
   d. Provide a balance between the hot and cold forces by offering medications with warm liquids, if requested by client.
2. Language barrier
   a. Provide and use an interpreter, when necessary; ideally a medically trained interpreter should be available. This person:
      (1) Knows interpreting techniques
      (2) Has a health care background
      (3) Understands patients' rights
      (4) Can help bridge the cultural gap by interpreting nonverbal messages and pass them on to you
      (5) Can give advice concerning the cultural appropriateness of recommendations (Andrews, 2008a)
   b. Use the interpreter appropriately.
      (1) Most women prefer another woman when discussing intimate matters.
      (2) The interpreter should not be a child.
         (a) It is not appropriate for a child to have knowledge of childbearing.
         (b) The child will have unusual power over the parent because of the knowledge gained.
      (3) Refrain from using slang or medical jargon that might be difficult for the interpreter to translate.
   c. Assess the client's ability to read and write before providing written information in the native language.
3. The traditional cultural group's dietary practices (usually related to the hot/cold theory described previously)
   a. Assess what foods the client prefers to eat or not to eat.
   b. Encourage preferred dietary practices if they are not shown to cause harm to the mother or fetus.
   c. Permit and encourage family members to bring foods into the hospital if necessary.
4. Postpartum traditional cultural group's practices
   a. Assess what practices the mother wishes to follow related to:
      (1) Bathing
      (2) Ambulation
      (3) Infant caretaking
      (4) Support persons
      (5) Dietary practices (for mother and infant)

    5. Modify usual hospital practices to accommodate client preferences.
      a. Explain the rationale for early ambulation.
      b. Encourage the mother to move frequently in bed and perhaps to sit by the bedside rather than to completely ambulate.
      c. Provide an opportunity for bathing in bed with warm water, rather than showering.
      d. Encourage family members or the other support person to assume care of the infant.

E. An unknown environment
    1. Encourage family members to remain with the client if so desired.
    2. Explain procedures and reinforce the explanations given by others.
      a. Use terminology that is understood.
      b. Avoid taboo or inappropriate language or terminology.
    3. Include family members in decision making, particularly the expectant father or husband if the woman so wishes.
    4. Incorporate traditional practices as expressed by the client when possible, particularly in regard to activity during labor, position for birth, nonpharmacologic pain management, and support persons.
      a. Perceptions of childbirth pain, pain behaviors, and preferences for pain management are culturally determined and bound (Callister, 2006). Pain may be seen as a normal part of giving birth, or it may be viewed as suffering that requires aggressive pharmacologic management.
      b. Culturally diverse women may use herbs, acupressure, massage, meditation, movement, hydrotherapy, birthing balls, and position changes to increase comfort and decrease pain (Moore, Moos & Callister, 2009).
    5. Avoid practices in conflict with cultural traditions, when possible, especially in regard to modesty requests/requirements of the culture.

F. Anxiety due to culturally unusual expectations for behavior and treatment
    1. Assess the level of anxiety through overt and covert manifestations.
    2. Assess the client's expectations for behavior and treatment.
    3. Incorporate culturally traditional expectations into care
      a. Allow the activity and position of choice during labor and delivery.
      b. Allow the family member(s) of choice to provide support.
      c. Alter Western expectations for activity and hygiene during the postpartum period to allow comfort for the new mother.
      d. Observe mother-infant interactions in the context of cultural expectations.

HEALTH EDUCATION

A. Before education can begin with culturally diverse clients, the assessment just described must be performed to establish a valid database.
    1. Strategies that are based on cultural knowledge are more likely to be successful than those not based on such data.
    2. Unless based on cultural information, nursing interventions might be inappropriate or incomplete, rather than allowing modification to meet the client's cultural needs.

B. Approaches might:
    1. Integrate scientific knowledge and folk practices, if necessary.
    2. Affect the client's behavior.
    3. Result in understanding on the nurse's part about why change cannot occur.

C. Educational strategies
    1. Explain the rationale for a scientific approach to care if it is significantly different from that proposed by the client.
    2. If proposed practices are not harmful to the mother or fetus, allow them to continue.
    3. If proposed practices are harmful, attempt to alter behaviors to include more beneficial ones.
    4. Elicit assistance and support from the established caretaker in the family (e.g., a grandmother or an aunt).
    5. Obtain approval and consent for treatment from the proper person (e.g., the husband or father).

6. Demonstrate how scientific and folk practices can be combined to provide optimal care for the mother and infant.
7. Recognize when compromise is not possible without destroying the family's entire cultural belief system.

CASE STUDIES AND STUDY QUESTIONS

Mrs. G., a Mexican-American, has come to your antepartum clinic for the first time. She is a gravida 3, para 2 (G3, P2) woman and is at 32 weeks' gestation. Through an interpreter she tells you that she is feeling fine, had no problems with her previous pregnancies, and has come for prenatal care only at the urging of the nurse in the well-child clinic where her two children receive immunizations. She believes it is important to balance the hot and cold humors and eats according to the prescriptions for accomplishing this during pregnancy; she avoids "hot" foods, iron preparations, and milk (because of lactose intolerance). She is kept active caring for her family (her children are ages 2 and 5 years) and believes that this will ensure a small infant and an easy delivery; she also believes that sleeping flat on her back protects the fetus from harm.

1. Who is the best person to serve as an interpreter for this woman?
   a. A woman 20 to 30 years old
   b. A man 20 to 30 years old
   c. A young girl in her early teens
   d. A young boy 8 to 10 years old
2. What is an appropriate approach to discussing her possible dietary deficiencies?
   a. Tell her the beliefs in a balance of hot and cold are superstition.
   b. Tell her that it is important that she include milk and an iron preparation in her diet.
   c. Explore with her acceptable alternatives to milk and iron preparations that she can ingest.
   d. Refer her to a nutritionist who will construct a specific diet for her.
3. What is an appropriate question to ask this woman?
   a. "Will your husband be with you during labor and delivery?"
   b. "Who will you want to be with you during labor and delivery?"
   c. "Are you attending any childbirth preparation classes?"
   d. "Do you know that sleeping on your back is actually bad for the infant?"

4. What is a good approach for the nurse in caring for this woman?
   a. Instruct her in the components of a balanced diet.
   b. Tell her the benefits of regular and early prenatal care.
   c. Enroll her and her husband in a childbirth preparation class.
   d. Ensure female care providers as often as possible.

You are assigned to care for Mrs. T., a Vietnamese woman who gave birth 12 hours previously. When you enter the room she is lying in bed with the infant in the bassinet beside her. There is a full bottle in the crib. She has not had a shower, and most of her food remains on her breakfast tray. She has had only the tea and toast. When you exclaim over the infant, she merely turns her head away and does not comment.

5. What is an appropriate comment or question for her regarding her food intake?
   a. "If you don't eat more, you won't have the strength to care for your infant."
   b. "Why didn't you eat your cereal, juice, and fruit?"
   c. "Do you have special food requirements during this time that I could help with or that your family could bring in?"
   d. "Don't you like our food?"
6. What should you assess about her activity and bathing?
   a. Whether there are cultural restrictions on her activity that prohibit her from showering at this time
   b. When she will take a shower
   c. When she will get out of bed and ambulate
   d. Whether she is going to feed the infant soon
7. How would you expect this mother to behave toward her infant?
   a. Expresses great joy about the birth of the infant
   b. Appreciates compliments about the infant by the staff
   c. Willing to take complete charge of caring for the infant

d. Remains distant toward the infant during the first few days, with caretaking done by others

8. Who would you expect to be at her bedside helping her to take care of herself and the infant?
   a. No one
   b. Her mother or grandmother
   c. Her husband
   d. Her neighbors

Mrs. C., a Laotian, her husband, and her mother come into the labor and delivery area. She is a 20-year-old gravida 1, para 0 (G1, P0) at term. When being examined, she frequently pulls the sheet over herself and looks away from her husband, who appears uncomfortable. She is found to be 7 cm dilated, completely effaced, and at 0 station. She sits upright in the bed, only grimacing with contractions. Her mother asks if her daughter may have a cup of hot tea to drink.

9. What are important components of a care plan for this family?
   a. Determine which family member(s) the patient would prefer to support her during labor.
   b. Make sure that the patient has ice chips at the bedside at all times.
   c. Assess the patient frequently for signs and behavior indicative of increasing discomfort.
   d. Provide for as much privacy and modesty as possible.
   e. Insist that the patient lie on one side or the other during the rest of her labor.
      (1) All of the above
      (2) a, c, d
      (3) a, c
      (4) b, c, e

10. Which of the following are essential to providing effective perinatal care to families of different cultures?
    a. Including cultural and family assessments as part of the routine history
    b. Insisting that the family adhere to scientific and medical principles of care at all times
    c. Assessing all culturally different beliefs as harmful
    d. Providing the services of an interpreter if a language barrier exists
    e. Fostering an attitude of respect for alternative healing practices
       (1) a, c, e
       (2) b, c, e
       (3) a, d, e
       (4) All of the above

11. What might prevent culturally diverse families from seeking maternity care in health care institutions in the United States?
    a. The presence of interpreters to assist with language differences
    b. Culturally competent care provided by health care practitioners
    c. Clinics that are easily accessible and in local neighborhoods
    d. Long clinic waits in urban centers that are structured to accommodate clients as a group, not as individuals

12. Applying transcultural concepts to nursing practice includes:
    a. Identifying cultural needs
    b. Understanding the cultural context of the client and family
    c. Using culturally sensitive strategies to meet mutually satisfying goals
    d. All of the above

ANSWERS TO STUDY QUESTIONS

1. a	4. d	7. d	10. 3
2. c	5. c	8. b	11. d
3. b	6. a	9. 2	12. d

REFERENCES

American Academy of Nursing. (1992). AAN expert panel report: Culturally competent health care. *Nursing Outlook, 40*(6), 277–283.

American Academy of Nursing. (1993). *Promoting cultural competence in and through nursing education. Subpanel on Cultural Competence in Nursing Education*. New York: American Academy of Nursing.

Andrews, M. (1989). Culture and nutrition. In J. Boyle, & M. Andrews (Eds.), *Transcultural concepts in nursing care* (pp. 333–355). Glenview, IL: Scott, Foresman/Little, Brown College.

Andrews, M. (1995). Transcultural nursing care. In M. Andrews, & J. Boyle (Eds.), *Transcultural concepts in nursing care* (2nd ed., pp. 49–96). Philadelphia: Lippincott.

Andrews, M. (2003). Culturally competent nursing care. In M. Andrews, & J. Boyle (Eds.), *Transcultural concepts in nursing care* (4th ed., pp. 15–35). Philadelphia: Lippincott Williams & Wilkins.

Andrews, M. (2008a). Culturally competent nursing care. In M. Andrews, & J. Boyle (Eds.), *Transcultural concepts in nursing care* (5th ed., pp. 15–33). Philadelphia: Wolters Kluwer/Lippincott Williams & Wilkins.

Andrews, M. (2008b). The influence of cultural and health belief systems on health care practice. In M. Andrews, & J. Boyle (Eds.), *Transcultural concepts in nursing care* (5th ed., pp. 66–82). Philadelphia: Wolters Kluwer/Lippincott Williams & Wilkins.

Andrews, M., & Boyle, J. (1997). Competence in transcultural nursing care. *American Journal of Nursing, 98*(8), 16AAA–DDD.

Beck, C. (2008). State of the science on postpartum depression: What nurse researchers have contributed. Part 1. *MCN: The American Journal of Maternal Child Nursing, 33*(2), 121–126.

Boyle, J., & Mackey, M. (1999). Pica: Sorting it out. *Journal of Transcultural Nursing, 10*(1), 65–68.

Callister, L. (2006). Pain and celebrating new life: Women giving birth. In A. Lucas (Ed.), *Frontiers in pain research* (pp. 157–176). Happauge, NY: Nova Science Publishers.

Callister, L. (2008). Cesarean birth rates: Global trends. *MCN: The American Journal of Maternal Child Nursing, 33*(2), 124.

Callister, L., & Birkhead, A. (2007). Mexican immigrant childbearing women: Social support and perinatal outcomes. In D. R. Crane, & E. S. Marshall (Eds.), *Families in poverty: An interdisciplinary approach* (pp. 181–197). Thousand Oaks, CA: Sage.

Campanella, L., Korbin., J., & Acheson, L. (1993). Pregnancy and childbirth among the Amish. *Social Science Medicine, 36*(3), 333–342.

Campinha-Bacote, J. (2000). A model of practice to address culturally competent health care in the home. *Home Care Provider, 5*, 213–219.

Campinha-Bacote, J. (2003). *The process of cultural competence in the delivery of healthcare services* (4th ed.). Cincinnati: Transcultural C.A.R.E. Associates.

Carlton, T., Callister, L., & Stoneman, E. (2005). Decision making in laboring women: Ethical issues for perinatal nurses. *Journal of Perinatal and Neonatal Nursing, 19*(2), 145–154.

Chaudron, L., Kitzman, H., Peifer, K., Morrow, S., Perez, L., & Newman, M. (2005). Self-recognition and provider response to maternal depressive symptoms in low-income Hispanic women. *Journal of Women's Health, 14*(4), 331–338.

Choudry, U. (1997). Traditional practices of women from India: Pregnancy, childbirth and newborn care. *Journal of Obstetric, Gynecologic, and Neonatal Nursing, 26*(5), 533–539.

Clark, A. (1978). *Culture, childbearing, health professionals.* Philadelphia: F.A. Davis.

Geron, S. (2002). Cultural competency: How is it measured? Does it make a difference? *Generations, 26*(3), 39–45.

Goldbort, J. (2005). Transcultural analysis of postpartum depression. *MCN: The American Journal of Maternal Child Nursing, 31*(2), 121–126.

Greener, D. (1989). Transcultural nursing care of the childbearing woman and her family. In J. Boyle, & M. Andrews (Eds.), *Transcultural concepts in nursing care* (pp. 95–119). Glenview, IL: Scott, Foresman/Little, Brown College.

Kay, M. (1982). *Anthropology of human birth.* Philadelphia: F.A. Davis.

Lauderdale, J. (2008). Transcultural perspectives in childbearing. In M. Andrews, & J. Boyle (Eds.). *Transcultural concepts in nursing care* (5th ed.). Philadelphia: Lippincott Williams & Wilkins.

Leininger, M., & McFarland, M. (2002). *Transcultural nursing: Concepts, theories, research & practice.* New York: McGraw-Hill.

Lewis, J. (2003). Jewish perspectives on pregnancy and childbearing. *MCN: The American Journal of Maternal Child Nursing, 28*(5), 306–312.

Mattson, S. (1993). Mental health of Southeast Asian refugee women: An overview. *Health Care for Women International, 14*, 155–165.

Mattson, S. (1995). Perinatal care for Southeast Asians in the United States. *Journal of Obstetric, Gynecologic, and Neonatal Nursing, 24*(4), 335–341.

Mattson, S. (2003). Caring for Latino women. *AWHONN Lifelines, 4*(4), 258–260.

Meleis, A. (1999). Culturally competent care. *Journal of Transcultural Nursing, 10*(1), 12.

Meleis, A. (2003). Theoretical consideration of health care for immigrant and minority women. In P. Hill, J. Lipson, & A. Meleis (Eds.), *Caring for women crossculturally* (pp. 1–10). Philadelphia: F.A. Davis.

Meleis, A., & Sorrell, L. (May-June, 1981). Bridging cultures. Arab-American women and their birth experiences. *American Journal of Maternal-Child Nursing, 6*(3), 171–176.

Moore, M., Moos, M. K., & Callister, L. (2009). *Health disparities and cultural competence in the 21st century.* White Plains, NY: March of Dimes.

Office of Minority Health. (1999). Assuring cultural competence in health care: Recommendations for national standards and an outcomes-focused research agenda. Washington, DC: Department of Health & Human Services, U.S. Public Health Service. Available online at www.omhrc.gov/clas/ds.htm.

Posmontier, B., & Horowitz, J. (2004). Postpartum practices and depression prevalences: Technocentric and ethnokinship cultural perspectives. *Journal of Transcultural Nursing, 15*(1), 34–43.

Purnell, L., & Paulanka, B. (2008). *Transcultural health care: A culturally competent approach* (3rd ed.). Philadelphia: F.A. Davis.

Taggart, L., & Mattson, S. (1996). Delay in prenatal care as a result of battering in pregnancy: Cross-cultural implications. *Health Care for Women International, 17*, 25–34.

Tiedje, L. (2000). Returning to our roots: 25 years of maternal/child nursing in the community. *MCN: The American Journal of Maternal Child Nursing, 25*(6), 315–317.

Tripp-Reimer, T., Brink, P., & Saunders, J. (1984). Cultural assessment: Content and process. *Nursing Outlook, 32*(2), 78–82.

Waxler-Morrison, N., Andrews, J., & Richardson, E. (1990). Cross-cultural caring: *A handbook for health professionals in western Canada*. Vancouver, BC: University of British Columbia Press.

Wells, M. (2000). Beyond cultural competence: A model for individual and institutional cultural development. *Journal of Community Health Nursing, 17*(4), 189–199.

Zlot, A., Jackson, D., & Korenbrot, C. (2005). Association of acculturation with cesarean section among Latinas. *Maternal and Child Health Journal, 9*(1), 11–20.

ADDITIONAL RESOURCES

Alexander, G., Mor, J., Kogan, M., Leland, N., & Kieffer, E. (1996). Pregnancy outcomes of U.S.-born and foreign-born Japanese Americans. *American Journal of Public Health, 86*(6), 820–824.

Al-Shahri, M. (2002). Culturally sensitive caring for Saudi patients. *Journal of Transcultural Nursing, 13*(2), 133–138.

American Public Health Association (Maternal/child Health). www.apha.org/ppp/red/index.htm.

Andrews, M., & Boyle, J. (2008). *Transcultural concepts in nursing care* (5th ed.). Philadelphia: Wolters Kluwer/Lippincott Williams & Wilkins.

Berry, A. (1999). Mexican American women's expressions of the meaning of culturally congruent prenatal care. *Journal of Transcultural Nursing, 10*(3), 203–212.

Callister, L., Semenic, S., & Foster, J. (1999). Cultural and spiritual meanings of childbirth: Orthodox Jewish and Mormon women. *Journal of Holistic Nursing, 17*(3), 280–295.

Callister, L., & Vega, R. (1998). Giving birth: Guatemala women's voices. *Journal of Obstetric, Gynecologic and Neonatal Nursing, 27*(3), 289–295.

Center for Cross Cultural Health. www.crosshealth.com.

Choi, E. (1995). A contrast of mothering behaviors in women from Korea and the United States. *Journal of Obstetric, Gynecologic and Neonatal Nursing, 24*(4), 363–369.

Cooper, M., Grywalski, M., Lamp, J., Newhouse, L., & Studlien, R. (2007). Enhancing cultural competence: A model for nurses. *Nursing for Women's Health, 11*(2), 149–159.

Cross Cultural Health Care Program. www.xculture.org.

Darby, S. (2007). Pre-and-perinatal care of Hispanic families: Implications for nurses. *Nursing for Women's Health, 11*(2), 162–169.

Edwards, N., & Boivin, J. (1997). Ethnocultural predictors of postpartum infant-care behaviours among immigrants in Canada. *Ethnicity and Health, 2*(3), 163–176.

Ferguson, B. (2008). Health literacy & health disparities: The role they play in maternal and child health. *Nursing for Women's Health, 12*(4), 287–298.

Hill, P., Lipson, J., & Meleis, A. (2003). *Caring for women cross-culturally*. Philadelphia: F.A. Davis.

Hyman, I., & Dussault, G. (2000). Negative consequences of acculturation on health behaviour, social support and stress among pregnant Southeast Asian immigrant women in Montreal: An exploratory study. *Canadian Journal of Public Health, 91*(5), 357–360.

Klingberg-Allvin, M., Binh, N., Johansson, A., & Berggren, V. (2008). One foot wet and one foot dry: Transition into motherhood among married adolescent women in rural Vietnam. *Journal of Transcultural Nursing, 19*(4), 338–346.

Kridli, S. (2002). Health beliefs and practices among Arab women. *MCN: The American Journal of Maternal Child Nursing, 27*(3), 178–182.

Mattson, S., & Lew, L. (1992). Culturally sensitive prenatal care for Southeast Asians. *Journal of Obstetric, Gynecologic and Neonatal Nursing, 21*(1), 48–54.

Morrow, M., Smith, J., Lai, Y., & Jaswal, D. (2008). Shifting landscapes: Immigrant women and postpartum depression. *Health Care for Women International, 29*, 593–617.

Morgan, M. (1996). Prenatal care of African American women in selected US urban and rural cultural contexts. *Journal of Transcultural Nursing, 7*(2), 3–9.

National Center for Cultural Competence. http://www.guccdc.georgetown.edu/nccc.

National Institutes of Health Office of Research on Minority Health. www.od.nih.gov/ormh.

Office on Women's Health. www.4woman.gov.

Pritham, U., & Sammons, L. (1993). Korean women's attitudes toward pregnancy and prenatal care. *Health Care for Women International, 14*(2), 145–153.

Purnell, L., & Paulanka, B. (2005). *Guide to culturally competent health care*. Philadelphia: F.A. Davis.

Savage, C., Anthony, J., Lee, R., Kappresser, M., & Rose, B. (2007). The culture of pregnancy and infant care in African American women: An ethnographic study. *Journal of Transcultural Nursing, 18*(3), 215–223.

Spector, R. (2004). *Cultural diversity in health and illness* (6th ed.). Upper Saddle River, NJ: Prentice-Hall Health.

Spring, M., Ross, P., Etkin, N., & Deinard, A. (1995). Sociocultural factors in the use of prenatal care by Hmong women. *Minneapolis. American Journal of Public Health, 85*(7), 1015–1017.

Transcultural C.A.R.E. Associates. www.transcultural-care.net.

Weber, S. (1996). Cultural aspects of pain in childbearing women. *Journal of Obstetric, Gynecologic, and Neonatal Nursing, 25*(1), 67–72.

Yosef, A. (2008). Health beliefs, practices and priorities for health care of Arab muslims in the United States. *Journal of Transcultural Nursing, 19*(3), 284–291.

4-1 Quick Reference Guide to Ethnocultural Differences

	Native American	African American	Asian	Hispanic	Arabic Heritage
Pregnancy normal	Yes	Yes	Yes (must maintain balance between yin/yang)	Yes	Yes (but seek care)
Prefer female attendants	Yes	No	Yes	Yes	Yes
Diet	Often have lactose intolerance (especially Eskimos, who are used to high protein and low carbohydrates)	Pica; eat salty (soul) foods; avoid acids; use sassafras tea; are at risk for overeating of fats and carbohydrates	Often are vegetarian; use herbal teas; often have lactose intolerance (tofu is a good alternative)	Are clay eaters; use herbal teas and remedies; use much fat in cooking; do not consider greens to be vegetables (use fish bones for calcium); may not eat eggs; may refuse iron (believe it causes a difficult recovery)	If Moslim, eat no pork or pork products, caffeine, or alcohol
Activity	Should be active	Should continue sexual activity	Remain moderately active; avoid sexual activity in third trimester	Are active; use massage	Have no restrictions
Emotions	Should be happy	Avoid stress	Should be serene, calm, and not sad	Do not quarrel with husband	Have no special needs

■ TABLE 4-2
■ **Intrapartum Variations**

	Native American	African American	Asian	Hispanic	Arabic Heritage
Prefer female attendants	Yes; some want the whole family (Navajo)	Yes (especially mother or grandmother)	Yes	Yes	Yes
Pain	Endure quietly	Usually are taught not to show weakness or call attention to themselves	Should not show pain; shameful to scream; often avoid verbal expression; use no medication (Samoan)	Endure pain with patience, but consider it acceptable to cry out	Are verbally expressive; cry and scream loudly; may refuse medication
Positions	Choose various positions; often use birth chair	Choose various positions	Like to move around, but must stay warm to not lose heat; come to hospital in advanced labor; squatting (Laotian, Hmong)	Use massage; will use birth chair; like to move around and walk; come to hospital in advanced labor	Choose various positions
Food and drink	Have no special needs	Have no special needs	Drink herbal teas	Drink manzanilla tea (makes uterine contractions stronger)	Have no special needs

■ TABLE 4-3
■ ■ **Postpartum Variations**

	Native American	African American	Asian	Hispanic	Arabic Heritage
Hot and cold beliefs	Not applicable	Prevent cold air from entering uterus; wear pad and use abdominal binder	Believe that exposure to cold may cause arthritis or asthma; avoid showers, ice packs, and ice water; use hot blankets; avoid drafts	Believe that exposure to cold may cause sterility; use abdominal binder	Have no special needs
Diet	Drink hot herbal teas	Use sassafras tea; avoid eggplant, okra, tomatoes, cold drinks, and milk (Haitians); avoid chitterlings, liver, and onions (southern African Americans believe that these will affect breast milk)	Drink ginseng tea; eat only "hot" foods (chicken every day, plus other meats and fish for 30 days; may eat warm, dry salty foods with little liquid [Korean, Vietnamese]; avoid fruits and green vegetables)	Eat cold food for 1 to 2 months; corn gruel is good; avoid acidic foods (citrus fruits, vegetables, chili, pork)	Have no special needs
Activity	Have no special needs	See themselves as sick; avoid bathing, washing hair, and heavy work	Need to rest; relatives do all work, including care of the infant; avoid contact with others and going out into the sun	Remain indoors, stay in bed up to 1 month; avoid strenuous work and bathing; avoid sexual contact for 40 days	Expect a lot of visitors; often request pain medications
Purification	Take a ritual bath on the fourth postpartum day (Navajo)	Not applicable	Avoid sexual contact for 3 to 4 months	Take a ritual bath 2 weeks postpartum	Not applicable

■ TABLE 4-4
■ ■ **Variations in Newborn Care**

	Native American	African American	Asian	Hispanic	Arabic Heritage
Breastfeeding	Yes; urban dwellers may use bottle	Yes; urban dwellers may use bottle	Yes	Yes (after milk comes in); consider colostrum bad for the infant; use bottle	Varies
Special clothes	Use cradle boards in urban areas	Use belly bands to prevent hernias	Wear old, ragged clothes (Southeast Asians)	Swaddle tightly; abdominal binder is common (infant is susceptible to "bad air")	Do not plan ahead for the infant, which would tempt the evil eye; often have no layette ready
Activity	Consider infants important to the family; keep infant close and handle often	Not applicable	Keep infant close continually; have no circumcision performed	Believe that the infant is vulnerable to the evil eye (if a stranger admires the infant, believe the stranger should touch the infant to dispel harm); no circumcision performed	Believe that the infant is vulnerable to the evil eye and needs protection
Praise of infant	Not applicable	Not applicable	No; believe that praise will call attention of the gods to the vulnerable newborn	Yes	No; praise mother instead; if do praise the infant, touch wood or mention God's blessing

■ TABLE 4-5
■ ■ Biologic Variations to Consider

	Native American	African American	Asian	Hispanic	Arabic Heritage
Sickle cell trait	Yes	Yes	No	No	Yes
Diabetes	Yes (especially Pima and Papago of Arizona)	No	No	No	No
Abnormal hemoglobin (other than sickle cell)	No	No	Yes (especially Thai and Cambodian)	No	No
Tuberculosis	No	No	Yes (especially recent refugees)	No	No
Glucose-6 phosphate dehydroge-nase deficiency (G6PD)	No	Yes	Yes (especially Chinese, no Filipino, Thai)	No	Yes

5 Physiology of Pregnancy

Linda Bond

OBJECTIVES

1. Describe systemic changes occurring in a woman's body during pregnancy.
2. Describe changes in the uterus, cervix, vagina, and vulva during pregnancy.
3. Identify the presumptive, probable, and positive diagnostic signs and symptoms of pregnancy.
4. Differentiate between normal and abnormal laboratory findings observed during pregnancy.
5. Define optimal nutritional adequacy based on pregnancy outcome indicators.
6. Identify specific changes in nutrient requirements during pregnancy.
7. Examine weight gain recommendations during pregnancy for different women.
8. Design an individualized patient education plan based on data from the history.
9. Detect potential complications of pregnancy based on data from a history, a physical examination, and laboratory test results.
10. Formulate nursing interventions to prevent anticipated problems identified from the nursing assessment.

INTRODUCTION AND BACKGROUND

A. **Conception and 40 weeks' gestation involve numerous maternal physiologic adaptations.**
   1. Regular health care supervision is necessary to ensure that subtle and untoward changes will not go undetected, ensuring a positive outcome for mother, infant, and the entire family. It is necessary for the nurse to be knowledgeable of the physiologic changes of pregnancy to provide competent, high-quality care.
   2. The course of pregnancy and the outcome are directly related to the nutritional status of the mother.
   3. The health care team is responsible for monitoring expected physiologic and psychologic changes and for providing health teaching for greater understanding of the events of pregnancy as well as preparation for parturition and postpregnancy events.
B. **Maternal system changes**
   1. Reproductive system
      a. Uterus
         (1) Size increases to 20 times that of nonpregnant size.
            (a) Hyperplasia and hypertrophy of myometrial cells, including muscle fibers, occur.
            (b) Increases are related to estrogen and progesterone, with mechanical factors of stretching related to the developing fetus.
         (2) Wall thins to 1.5 cm (0.6 inch) or less (changes from almost a solid globe to a hollow vessel).
         (3) Weight increases from 70 to 1100 g (1.8 ounces to 2.2 pounds).
         (4) Volume (capacity) increases from less than 10 mL to 5 L (2 teaspoons to 1 gallon).
         (5) Uterine contractility (Braxton Hicks contractions)
            (a) Irregular, painless contractions due to structural and functional changes in myometrium resulting from estrogen increases in pregnancy
            (b) As pregnancy advances, these contractions become more intense, frequent, and easily felt.
            (c) Braxton Hicks contractions do not typically lead to cervical changes.
         (6) Shape changes from that of an inverted pear to that of a soft globe that enlarges, rising out of the pelvis by the end of the first trimester.

(7) Endometrium is called the decidua after implantation.
  (a) Decidua parietalis: all of the uterine lining that is not in contact with the fetus
  (b) Decidua basalis: uterine lining beneath implantation
  (c) Decidua capsularis: portion of the decidua that surrounds the embryo and the chorionic sac
  b. Cervix
  (1) Softening related to increased vascularity, edema, slight hypertrophy, and hyperplasia (Goodell's sign)
  (2) Cervical glands occupy approximately half of the cervical mass near term.
  (3) Mucus plug (operculum) fills the cervical canal soon after conception.
    (a) Formed from the thick mucus produced by endocervical glands
    (b) Function is to prevent ascending infections
  c. Ovaries and fallopian tubes
  (1) Anovulation results from the suppression of follicle-stimulating hormone (FSH) and luteinizing hormone (LH) related to high levels of estrogen and progesterone.
  (2) Corpus luteum remains active for 6 to 7 weeks into pregnancy, producing progesterone and estrogen to maintain pregnancy; after 6 to 7 weeks' gestation, the placenta will produce the progesterone to maintain pregnancy.
  d. Vagina
  (1) Increased vascularity results in bluish, violet discoloration (Chadwick's sign)
  (2) Hypertrophy and hyperplasia of epithelium and elastic tissues
  (3) Leukorrhea, with an acid pH of 3.5 to 6.0, functions to control the growth of pathogens.
  e. Vulva
  (1) Increased vasculature
  (2) External structures enlarged due to hypertrophy of structures, along with fat deposits
  f. Breasts
  (1) Changes begin soon after conception.
  (2) External changes
    (a) Size increases; weight increases by about 400 g (12 ounces).
    (b) Breasts become nodular.
    (c) Skin appears thinner.
    (d) Blood vessels become more prominent with a twofold increase in blood flow.
    (e) Areola and nipples
      [i] Pigmentation darkens, beginning during the first trimester.
      [ii] Montgomery's tubercles become more prominent.
      [iii] Secondary pinkish areola might develop.
      [iv] Nipples enlarge and become more erect (second trimester).
  (3) Internal changes
    (a) Proliferation of glandular tissue and lactiferous ducts begins in first trimester (influenced by estrogen and progesterone).
    (b) Alveoli begin producing colostrum.
      [i] Pre-colostrum, which is a thin, clear liquid, can be found in acini cells in early second trimester.
      [ii] Colostrum is the creamy, white-to-yellowish pre-milk secreted as early as 16 weeks' gestation.
2. Cardiovascular system
  a. Heart
  (1) Slight enlargement (hypertrophy) (approximately 12%)
  (2) Auscultatory changes
    (a) Exaggerated split heard in S_1 and S_2
    (b) S_2 and S_3 are more obvious.
    (c) Systolic and diastolic murmurs are common.
  (3) Shift in chest contents: heart is displaced upward, forward and to the left in late pregnancy.
  b. Hemodynamic changes
  (1) Heart rate increases about 15 to 20 beats/minute (20% increase).
  (2) Cardiac output increases by 30% to 50% during first two trimesters and then declines to about 20% near term.

(3) Blood volume increases by approximately 1500 mL or 30% to 50% (might be even greater with multiple births) over prepregnancy level.

(4) Stroke volume increases by as much as 30% over prepregnancy level.

(5) Vasodilation occurs because of progesterone.

(6) Arterial blood pressure
   (a) Readings, positional variations (Lowdermilk & Perry, 2007; Walsh, 2001)
      [i] Supine hypotension results from uterine pressure on inferior vena cava (supine hypotensive syndrome).
      [ii] Left lateral recumbent position is optimal for cardiac output and uterine perfusion.
      [iii] Brachial artery pressure is highest when woman is sitting.
   (b) Systolic and diastolic pressures begin to fall in the first trimester; they decrease until midpregnancy and then slowly rise back to the prepregnancy levels.

(7) Venous pressure does not change despite the increase in blood volume.
   (a) Increased vascular capacity influenced by hormonal changes.
   (b) Pressure below the uterus is increased related to compression of the large pelvic veins and those distal to the uterus.
      [i] Venous pooling might occur late in pregnancy after long periods in the upright position.
      [ii] Late in pregnancy the enlarged uterus might also contribute to slowed venous return, pooling, dependent edema, hemorrhoids, and varicose veins in the legs and vulva.

c. Hematologic changes

(1) Red blood cell (RBC) production escalates.
   (a) Total RBC volume increases approximately 33% (450 mL) with iron supplementation.
   (b) Blood iron levels in RBC volume increase only approximately 20% to 30% (250 mL).

(2) White blood cell (WBC) count increases 5000 to 12,000/mm³; might normally increase to 20,000/mm³ during parturition without infection.
   (a) WBCs in pregnant women are less effective in fighting infection and disease than they are in nonpregnant women.
   (b) History and physical examination must confirm diagnosis of infection.

(3) Blood volume expansion is made up of increased volume of plasma and increased numbers of RBCs (plasma volume increases more rapidly than RBC production and causes hemodilution or physiologic anemia of pregnancy).
   (a) Primary function is to offset blood loss at delivery.
   (b) Supplies the hypertrophied vascular system during pregnancy.

(4) Clotting factors increase.
   (a) Plasma fibrin levels increase by approximately 40%.
   (b) Fibrinogen levels increase by approximately 50%.
   (c) Pregnancy is a hypercoagulable state, placing the woman at risk for thrombosis and alterations in coagulation (e.g., disseminated intravascular coagulation).

(5) Hemoglobin and hematocrit decrease (in relation to plasma volume).
   (a) Hemoglobin of less than 10 g/dL indicates anemia.
   (b) Hematocrit lower than 35% indicates anemia.

3. Respiratory system

   a. Respiratory rate and maximal breathing capacity remain unchanged, whereas vital capacity might increase slightly.

   b. Tidal volume increases 30% to 40%; minute ventilatory volume and minute oxygen uptake increase as pregnancy advances, as evidenced by deeper breathing.

   c. Carbon dioxide output increases.

   d. Increased vascularity of the upper respiratory tract is influenced by increased estrogen levels.

   e. Thoracic circumference increases by 5 to 7 cm (2 to 3 inches), and the diaphragm elevates approximately 4 cm (1.5 inches).

   f. Basal metabolic rate increases and oxygen requirement increases by 15% to 20% to supply the uterine-placental unit and increased cardiac activity.

   g. Acid-base balance: arterial blood is slightly more alkaline.

4. Urinary system
    a. Renal structure changes
        (1) Influenced by:
            (a) Hormone effects, particularly the influence of progesterone on smooth muscle
            (b) Uterine pressure
            (c) Alterations in the cardiovascular system, including increased cardiac output and increased blood volume
        (2) Collection system changes (physiologic hydronephrosis)
            (a) Renal pelvis dilates.
            (b) Ureters elongate and become tortuous; the upper one third of the ureters might dilate (particularly the right ureter).
            (c) Urinary stasis or stagnation occurs and increases the danger of pyelonephritis.
        (3) Increased urinary frequency is related to the increasing size of the uterus and its pressure on the bladder.
        (4) Bladder is pulled up into the abdominal cavity by the growing uterus, and the bladder tone is decreased.
    b. Renal function changes
        (1) Changes in kidney function occur to accommodate a heavier workload while maintaining stable electrolyte balance and blood pressure.
            (a) Increased glomerular filtration rate
            (b) Increased renal plasma flow
        (2) Urine output is 25% higher during pregnancy.
        (3) Laboratory values (Cunningham et al., 2005; Walsh, 2001)
            (a) Glucosuria occurs in 20% of pregnant women (might not be abnormal; warrants further evaluation and monitoring).
            (b) Proteinuria is abnormal, except in very concentrated urine or in the first-voided specimen on arising (total urine protein of more than 300 mg in 24 hours is a warning of impaired kidney function and/or pregnancy-induced hypertension).
5. Gastrointestinal system
    a. Mouth and teeth
        (1) Gums become hyperemic, swollen, and soft (friable) and have a tendency to bleed (estrogen influence).
        (2) Saliva becomes more acidic.
            (a) Production remains unchanged.
            (b) Some women experience increased saliva production (ptyalism) due to decreased swallowing associated with nausea and vomiting.
        (3) Teeth remain unchanged.
    b. Gastrointestinal tract
        (1) Smooth muscle relaxation and decreased peristalsis occur related to progesterone influence; this can lead to:
            (a) Decreased motility, resulting in fluids and nutrients remaining in the intestine longer, facilitating greater absorption but also resulting in constipation
            (b) Hemorrhoids: associated with constipation, increased venous pressure, and pressure of the gravid uterus
            (c) Heartburn (pyrosis), slowed gastric emptying, and esophageal regurgitation (reflux)
        (2) Positional changes of organs occur because of uterine enlargement.
            (a) Upward displacement of the stomach
            (b) Colon shifted and compressed
    c. Liver function undergoes insignificant, minor changes.
    d. Gallbladder
        (1) Volume is increased, muscle tone decreased.
        (2) Emptying time is prolonged, which could lead to formation of gallstones.
        (3) Retained bile salts can lead to pruritus
6. Musculoskeletal system
    a. Distention of the abdomen and a shift in the center of gravity can result in lordosis.
    b. Relaxation and increased mobility of joints occur because of the hormones relaxin and progesterone, and lead to a characteristic "waddle gait."

    c. Diastasis recti, a separation of the rectus muscles of the abdominal wall, is associated with the enlarging uterus in some women.

    d. Relaxation and increased mobilitiy of pelvic joints facilitate labor.

  7. Integumentary system

    a. Skin undergoes hyperpigmentation (primarily due to estrogen influence).

      (1) Melasma (also called chloasma) is the blotchy, brownish "mask of pregnancy."

      (2) Linea alba can darken and become linea nigra (abdomen).

      (3) Nipples, areolae, axillae, vulva, and perineum all darken.

    b. Hair: some women may note increased growth.

    c. Stretch marks (striae gravidarum) in the breasts, abdomen, thighs, and inguinal area result from the separation within connective tissue related to the action of adrenocorticosteroids (Blackburn, 2008).

    d. Blood vessels have increased permeability, causing:

      (1) Edema

      (2) Spider nevi or angiomas

      (3) Palmar erythema

    e. Skin disorders and skin problems associated with pregnancy include noninflammatory pruritus and acne vulgaris (especially in the first trimester).

  8. Endocrine system

    a. Pituitary gland (not essential to maintain pregnancy) (Cunningham et al., 2005)

      (1) Anterior lobe: slight increase in size

        (a) FSH and LH production is suppressed.

        (b) Thyrotropin and adrenocorticotropic (ACTH) hormones might increase slightly.

        (c) Human chorionic somatomammotropin (hCS; formerly called human placental lactogen) from the placenta has been suggested to be a growth hormone, responsible for breast development.

        (d) Prolactin production is increased and ensures lactation.

      (2) Posterior lobe: oxytocin production gradually increases as the fetus matures.

        (a) Influences uterine contractibility

        (b) Stimulates milk ejection from breasts (Blackburn, 2008)

    b. Thyroid gland activity and hormone production increase.

      (1) Gland enlarges (related to increased vascularity and growth of glandular tissue).

      (2) Total triiodothyronine (T_3) and thyroxine (T_4) increase in early pregnancy and remain high until term.

      (3) Increases in thyroid hormone levels occur and function to support maternal metabolic changes along with fetal growth and development (Blackburn, 2008).

    c. Parathyroid gland activity increases, and blood levels of parathyroid hormone are elevated to meet the demands for growth of the fetal skeleton.

    d. Adrenal glands: little change in function

    e. Pancreas: insulin production increased throughout pregnancy to compensate for placental hormone insulin antagonism

      (1) Insulin antagonists (hCS, estrogen, progesterone, and adrenal cortisol) decrease tissue sensitivity or the ability to use insulin.

      (2) Normal pancreatic beta cells can meet the increased demand for insulin.

    f. Ovaries

      (1) Estrogen (also from adrenal cortex and later the placenta) is responsible for:

        (a) Enlargement of breasts, uterus, and genitals

        (b) Fat deposit changes

        (c) Alterations in thyroid function and nutrient metabolism

        (d) Changes in sodium and water retention

        (e) Hematologic changes

        (f) Vascular changes

        (g) Stimulation of melanin-stimulating hormones, hyperpigmentation

      (2) Progesterone from the corpus luteum (later, the placenta) is responsible for:

        (a) Facilitating implantation and maintaining the endometrium

        (b) Decreasing uterine contractility

        (c) Development of secretory ducts and the lobular-alveolar system of the breasts

        (d) Fat deposit changes

(e) Reducing smooth muscle tone in renal and gastrointestinal systems

(f) Increasing sensitivity of respiratory system to carbon dioxide

(3) Relaxin from the corpus luteum (later, the placenta) is thought to be responsible for inhibiting uterine contractility and cervical ripening (Blackburn, 2008).

9. Immunologic system

a. Resistance to infection is decreased due to depressed leukocyte function, which can also lead to improvement in certain autoimmune diseases.

b. Immune system tolerates the fetus while continuing to function against microorganisms (Blackburn, 2008; Cunningham et al., 2005).

C. **Pregnancy signs and symptoms**

1. Presumptive evidence of pregnancy

a. Signs

(1) Amenorrhea

(2) Breast changes: increase in size, tenderness

(3) Vaginal mucosa discoloration (Chadwick's sign; significant sign only in primiparous women)

(4) Skin pigmentation changes (melasma/chloasma, linea nigra, and linea alba)

b. Symptoms

(1) Nausea with or without vomiting

(2) Urinary frequency

(3) Fatigue

(4) Perception of fetal movement (quickening)

(5) Maternal perception of pregnancy

2. Probable evidence of pregnancy

a. Signs

(1) Abdominal enlargement and striae

(2) Uterine changes: softening of isthmus (Hegar's sign); cervical softening (Goodell's sign)

(3) Braxton Hicks contractions

(4) Ballottement of the fetus

(5) Endocrine tests positive for human chorionic gonadotropin (hCG) levels

b. Symptoms are the same as presumptive symptoms.

3. Positive evidence of pregnancy

a. Fetal heartbeat (distinct from the heart sounds of the mother) heard by the examiner. Doppler ultrasonography can detect heartbeat as early as 8 weeks.

b. Fetal outline visualized by radiographic studies (Lowdermilk & Perry, 2007)

c. Fetal movements visible and detected by examiner

D. **Nutritional consideration during pregnancy: although attitudes have varied over the years and within cultures about desirable weight gain, much of the scientific body of knowledge allows some general observations.**

1. Prepregnancy weight and weight gain

a. Weight before pregnancy and weight gain during pregnancy are directly related to the birthweight of the infant and the incidence of morbidity and mortality.

b. Prepregnancy weight and height along with stores of micronutrients affect health and size of the newborn (Kaiser & Allen, 2002).

c. Body mass index (BMI) is commonly used to evaluate weight for height.

(1) BMI is expressed as weight/height^2 in which weight is in kilograms (kg) and height is in meters (m).

(2) BMI classifications are used to categorize nutritional status based on prepregnancy measurements (Cesario, 2003).

(a) Underweight: BMI less than 18.5

(b) Healthy/normal weight: BMI 18.6 to 24.9

(c) Overweight: BMI greater than 25 to 29.9

(d) Obese: BMI greater than 30

d. A weight gain of between 11.5 and 16 kg (25 and 35 pounds) is recommended for healthy pregnant women (Reifsnider & Gill, 2000).

(1) Weight gain should be steady throughout the pregnancy and depends on the stage of pregnancy.

(a) Progressive weight gain during pregnancy is essential to ensure normal fetal growth and development and the deposition of maternal stores.

        (b) Recommended weight gain during pregnancy is determined largely by prepregnancy weight for height (Lowdermilk & Perry, 2007).

    (2) Approximately 200 to 450 g/week (0.5 to 1 pound) should be adequate during the second and third trimesters.

  e. Recommended weight gain for overweight women is between 7 and 11.5 kg (15 and 25 pounds), depending on nutritional status and degree of obesity (Cesario, 2003).

    (1) Women must be aware of the adverse effects of maternal malnutrition on infant growth and development.

    (2) All pregnant women should gain at least enough weight to equal the weight of the products of conception.

    (3) Dietary restriction can result in inadequate intake of essential nutrients and in catabolism of fat stores.

        (a) This process augments the production of ketones leading to ketonuria, which has been found to be correlated with preterm labor.

        (b) Long-term effects of mild ketonemia during pregnancy are not known (see Chapter 22 for discussion of endocrine disorders).

    (4) Ideally, obese women should address weight management issues before conception.

  f. If prepregnancy weight is estimated at 10% to 20% below ideal body weight, the mother is considered to have poor nutritional status.

    (1) This might also indicate an inability to attain proper weight or the presence of poor or unusual dietary habits.

    (2) It is recommended that gains for pregnant underweight women be 12.5 to 18 kg (28 to 40 pounds).

    (3) Emphasis should be placed on the quality of food intake.

2. Nutritional needs during pregnancy

  a. Energy and calorie requirements are increased during pregnancy due to deposition of new tissue, increased metabolic expenditure, and increased energy needed to move the pregnant body.

  b. Optimal weight gain from a nutritionally sound diet contributes to a successful pregnancy (Lederman, 2001).

  c. Nutrients needed during pregnancy can be obtained with a diet that provides all essential nutrients, fiber, and energy in adequate amounts.

    (1) Dietary supplementation is justified when there is concern that adequate nutrition or a well-balanced diet is compromised.

        (a) Indicators of nutritional risk include:

           [i] Adolescence

           [ii] Short interval between pregnancies

           [iii] Obesity or low prepregnancy weight

           [iv] Use of alcohol, drugs, or tobacco

           [v] Poor dietary habits

           [vi] Poverty; lack of access to food distribution programs

           [vii] Multiple-gestation pregnancy

           [viii] Medical conditions (e.g., diabetes, heart disease, errors in metabolism)

           [ix] Social conditions (e.g., homelessness, battering)

    (2) Vegetarian diets have many variations; however, almost all contain vegetables, fruits, legumes, nuts, seed, and grains (Lowdermilk & Perry, 2007).

        (a) For strict vegetarians (vegans), vitamin B_{12} supplement or fortified foods are recommended.

        (b) Vitamin B_6, iron, calcium, zinc intake might also be low, so intake must be assessed and supplements added as needed.

    (3) To meet the increased need for iron during the second and third trimesters, a low-dose iron supplement is recommended (60 mg ferrous iron daily).

  d. To meet the energy needs of pregnancy, the recommended dietary allowance (RDA) states that pregnant women need 300 kcal/day over prepregnancy intake.

  e. These additional kilocalories can be adequately met by the following recommended increases:

    (1) Milk intake from 480 mL (2 cups) prepregnancy to the recommended 720 to 960 mL (3 to 4 cups)

    (2) Protein intake by 1 serving

(3) Fruits and vegetables by 2 servings

(4) Breads and cereals by 1 to 2 servings

3. Achieving nutritional adequacy during pregnancy is closely associated with meeting the nutrient requirements based on the RDA.

   a. Protein requirements are increased for the development of new tissue; the RDA for pregnant women includes an additional 10 to 12 g per day for a daily total of 60 g.

   b. Vitamins and mineral requirements are usually increased during pregnancy.

      (1) Folic acid

         (a) Should be increased from 400 to 600 mcg/day to support increase in RBC production, cell division, and deoxyribonucleic acid (DNA) synthesis

         (b) Requirement can be met by an increased intake of leafy green vegetables, citrus fruits, fortified ready-to-eat cereals and other grains.

      (2) B vitamin requirements are increased because of energy metabolism.

         (a) Adequate intake of protein foods and grains should meet this requirement.

         (b) The RDA for the B vitamins is as follows:

            [i]   Riboflavin: 1.4 mg

            [ii] Thiamine: 1.4 mg

            [iii] Pyridoxine (B_6): 1.9 mg

            [iv] Niacin: 18 mg

            [v] B_{12}: 2.6 mcg

      (3) Vitamin C

         (a) The RDA during pregnancy is 70 mg/day or 10 mg/day more than the prepregnancy intake.

         (b) This need is easily met by a minimal increase of foods rich in vitamin C (e.g., citrus fruits, certain melons, peppers, leafy green vegetables).

      (4) Vitamin A

         (a) The RDA is not different during pregnancy.

         (b) Adequate vitamin A can be obtained from consuming, at least every other day, a yellow, orange, or red vegetable or fruit or a leafy green vegetable, and/or fortified butter or margarine.

      (5) Vitamin D

         (a) Essential role in the absorption and metabolism of calcium

         (b) Disorders of calcium metabolism are evident in mother and fetus with a vitamin D deficiency.

         (c) Although there is no increased requirement in pregnancy, women who do not get sunlight exposure or adequate intake of fortified foods rich in vitamin D (milk products, ready-to-eat cereals, fatty fish, and egg yolk) should be given vitamin D supplements (Lowdermilk & Perry, 2007; Penney & Miller, 2008).

      (6) Vitamin K

         (a) Essential for assisting in the normal process of blood clotting.

         (b) Maternal dietary deficiency is rare.

      (7) Calcium

         (a) Requirement remains at 1000 to 1300 mg/day to ensure adequate calcium for changes in bone metabolism during pregnancy and for development of the fetal skeleton and deciduous teeth.

         (b) Phosphorus and vitamin D are also involved in bone and calcium metabolism, and imbalances of either might affect calcium requirements.

      (8) Iron requirements are greatly increased during pregnancy because of increased maternal blood volume and fetal demands.

         (a) The RDA for iron is 30 mg/day.

            [i] It is difficult to get adequate iron intake from food sources during pregnancy; therefore, iron supplements (simple ferrous salts) are prescribed.

            [ii] Food sources include lean red meat, poultry, fish, deep green leafy vegetables, enriched breads and cereals, legumes, liver, soy products, and dried fruits.

         (b) Pica, or consumption of nonfood substances, might displace more nutritious foods and interfere with absorption of nutrients, especially iron.

            [i] Either pica or iron deficiency anemia should lead to the investigation for the other problem.

[ii] Women at highest risk for pica are from rural or inner-city areas, African American, or those who have a family or childhood history of pica (Kaiser & Allen, 2002).

   (9) Sodium

      (a) Is not restricted unless a medical condition so warrants

      (b) No less than 2 to 3 g of sodium should be consumed daily during a normal pregnancy.

   (10) Other requirements can be met by a well-balanced diet and include:

      (a) Vitamin E (10 mg/day)

      (b) Zinc (15 mg/day)

      (c) Iodine (175 fg/day)

4. Nutrition for optimal fetal health

  a. The fetus is dependent on the maternal host for nutrients.

  b. Because the fetus is in a state of growth and development, deprivation of essential nutrients can lead to stunted growth, various birth abnormalities, or spontaneous abortions.

  c. Nutritional knowledge in this area is not yet complete. Human research is based on observation and epidemiologic data (Worthington-Roberts & Williams, 1997).

  d. The following evidence is based on animal studies and may not be conclusive or extensive (Worthington-Roberts & Williams, 1997).

    (1) Riboflavin (vitamin B_2) deficiency has been associated with poor skeletal formation.

    (2) Pyridoxine (vitamin B_6) deficiency has been associated with neuromotor problems.

    (3) Vitamin B_{12} deficiency has been associated with hydrocephalus.

    (4) Folic acid deficiencies are associated with neural tube defects.

    (5) The fetal growth stage known as hyperplasia, the time during the first trimester when the cells are rapidly dividing and multiplying, requires folic acid and vitamin B_{12}, which play a role in the synthesis of nucleic acids and prevention of neural tube defects.

    (6) The next fetal growth stage, known as hypertrophy, occurs during the second and third trimesters of pregnancy when the cells increase in size, and require amino acids and vitamin B_{12} for protein synthesis.

    (7) Iron is essential to maintain the maternal hemoglobin levels, which in turn supply oxygen to the developing fetus.

    (8) Inadequate caloric intake increases the risk of delivering an infant with intrauterine growth restriction (IUGR).

    (9) Excessive caloric intake (preexisting obesity or obesity that develops during pregnancy) increases the likelihood of macrosomia and the associated increases in operative births, birth trauma, and infant mortality.

CLINICAL PRACTICE

A. The goal of clinical practice is to have a healthy pregnancy as the outcome, leading to a successful parturition. Because pregnancy is considered a normal life process, interventions will involve a comprehensive assessment followed by a series of periodic visits to the health care provider to monitor the health of the maternal-fetal unit. Evidence-based protocols (National Guideline Clearinghouse [NGC], 2008) for the delivery of prenatal care provide guidelines for the health care team. The pregnant woman is a central member of the team. When all measurements stay within expected parameters, the most important intervention will be education that will empower the woman to be active in guiding the course of the pregnancy.

B. Assessment (comprehensive general health examination at first prenatal visit)

  1. History

    a. Current pregnancy

      (1) Menstrual history

        (a) Last menstrual period

        (b) Previous menstrual period

        (c) Last normal menstrual period

        (d) Menarche, age of onset

    b. Signs and symptoms (see earlier discussion of pregnancy signs and symptoms)

    c. Risk assessment (at risk for a problem pregnancy)
- (1) Younger than 16 years, older than 35 years (see Chapter 7 for a complete discussion)
- (2) History of induced abortions
- (3) Previous stillbirth or neonatal loss
- (4) Infant born prematurely, large for gestational age (LGA), with isoimmunization, or with congenital anomaly
- (5) History of maternal malignancy, genital tract anomaly, or medical indication for termination of previous pregnancy
- (6) Substance use or abuse: tobacco products, alcohol, or illicit or prescription drugs (see Chapter 25 for a complete discussion)
- (7) Environmental factors: exposure to high levels of noise, radiation, or pollution of air, food, and water
- (8) Occupational hazards: anesthetic gases, lead, or paternal exposure to toxic agents (can transfer to female partner during intercourse; see Chapter 9 for complete discussion of environmental effects)
- (9) Abuse assessment; research suggests that intimate partner violence might increase during pregnancy. Screening should be instituted for women with unusual bruising, injury, or depression (Barash & Weinstein, 2002; see Chapter 18 for a complete discussion).

2. Obstetric and gynecologic history
- **a.** Gravida/para system or gravidity, term, preterm, abortions, living children (G/TPAL) system (system often confusing due to regional variations) (Cunningham et al., 2005)
- **b.** Sexual history, including sexually transmitted infections: syphilis, gonorrhea, herpes genitalia, trichomoniasis, condylomata acuminata (genital human papillomavirus [HPV] infection or genital warts), hepatitis B, chlamydial infection, and human immunodeficiency virus (HIV) infection (see Chapter 20 for a complete discussion)
- **c.** Contraceptive history and use
- **d.** Infertility problems
- **e.** Description of previous pregnancies and their outcomes (length of gestations, type of delivery, and fetal outcome, including birthweight and maternal complications)

3. Cultural assessment including racial or ethnic background (see Chapter 4 for complete discussion)

4. Medical history (elements of this portion of the examination are the same for all instances of history taking)
- **a.** Childhood diseases (especially infectious diseases)
- **b.** Other diseases (e.g., diabetes, asthma, urinary tract infections, varicosities, seizures)
- **c.** Surgery (blood transfusions)
- **d.** Injuries (especially to the pelvic region)
- **e.** Allergies (especially to drugs)
- **f.** Immunizations (especially rubella and chickenpox)
- **g.** Alcohol, caffeine, tobacco, and other drug use, including prescription, over-the-counter, and recreational drugs
- **h.** Exercise patterns
- **i.** Elimination patterns
- **j.** Sleep patterns
- **k.** Any significant stress
- **l.** Relationships with significant others, including potential for abuse

5. Nutrition history
- **a.** Overall factors to consider
  - (1) Parity, in addition to the time intervals between each pregnancy, has an effect on nutrition reserves and the outcome of pregnancy, and it might generate increased nutritional needs.
    - (a) Primigravidas usually gain more weight during pregnancy than multigravidas.
    - (b) Short intervals between pregnancies increase the challenge for nutrient repletion and maintenance of adequate nutrient stores.
    - (c) A woman who had a previous low-birthweight, IUGR, or preterm delivery needs to be identified in subsequent pregnancies for early counseling and assessment.
  - (2) Age is an important consideration.
    - (a) Adolescent pregnancy adds important considerations to clinical assessment.

[i] Pregnant adolescents who, at the time of conception, are less mature gynecologically and undernourished have the greatest risks.

[ii] Infants born to teenagers suffer a higher incidence of prematurity (fewer than 37 weeks), stillbirth, and low birthweight (less than 2500 g).

(b) At the other range of the age spectrum, older women (over 40) might incur more health risks during pregnancy than younger women (this effect is confounded with parity and might be associated with concurrent chronic illnesses; see Chapter 7 for further considerations of age).

(3) Women of very low socioeconomic status are at risk for undernutrition, which leads to inadequate nutrient and energy intake, poor weight gain, and increased pregnancy complications and poor pregnancy outcomes.

(4) A more careful dietary assessment is needed for women with chronic diseases, such as pregnancy-induced hypertension, diabetes, and cardiovascular disease, to prevent nutrition-related complications (see Chapters 19, 22, and 26, respectively, for further discussion).

(5) Ethnic/cultural and religious background may determine which foods are customarily desirable and those that are not consumed.

(6) Allergies might determine the need for dietary substitutions or supplements.

(7) Women with multiple fetuses are advised to consult a dietitian or nutritionist to ensure optimal nutrition and weight gain.

b. A 24-hour recall, a verbal or written recollection of all foods, meals, and snacks (include ice [pagophagia]) eaten within the last 24-hour period can be helpful. NOTE: For women who are vegetarians, taking a 3- to 7-day food history is necessary to get a comprehensive assessment of adequacy of nutrient intake (Penney & Miller, 2008).

(1) Food frequency analysis: the number of times each week a basic food is eaten

(2) Additional factors to be considered

(a) Where food is eaten

(b) How much is eaten

(c) How food is prepared (e.g., fried with a bread coating)

(d) Which foods or odors seem to precipitate discomfort

(e) Which foods are limited and for what reasons

(f) Dietary supplements, vitamin and herbal supplements

(3) Visit www.mypyramid.gov for personalized eating plans for pregnancy and lactation (Figure 5-1 shows the general MyPyramid).

6. Family medical history
   a. Health status of parents and siblings
   b. Family incidence of diabetes, cardiovascular disease, and hypertension
   c. Genetic and congenital diseases, abnormalities, or unexplained stillbirths
   d. Multiple births
7. Father's health history
   a. Current health status, including health problems
   b. Blood type and rhesus (Rh) factor
   c. Family medical history
   d. Alcohol and drug use and abuse
8. Social, family, and emotional history
9. Review of physical systems
   a. General: weight change, fatigue, night sweats, chills, or fever
   b. Skin, hair, and nails
   c. Head, ears, eyes, nose, and throat
   d. Mouth and teeth
   e. Breasts
   f. Respiratory
   g. Cardiovascular
   h. Gastrointestinal
   i. Genitourinary
   j. Musculoskeletal
   k. Neurologic (especially history of seizure activity)
   l. Hematologic

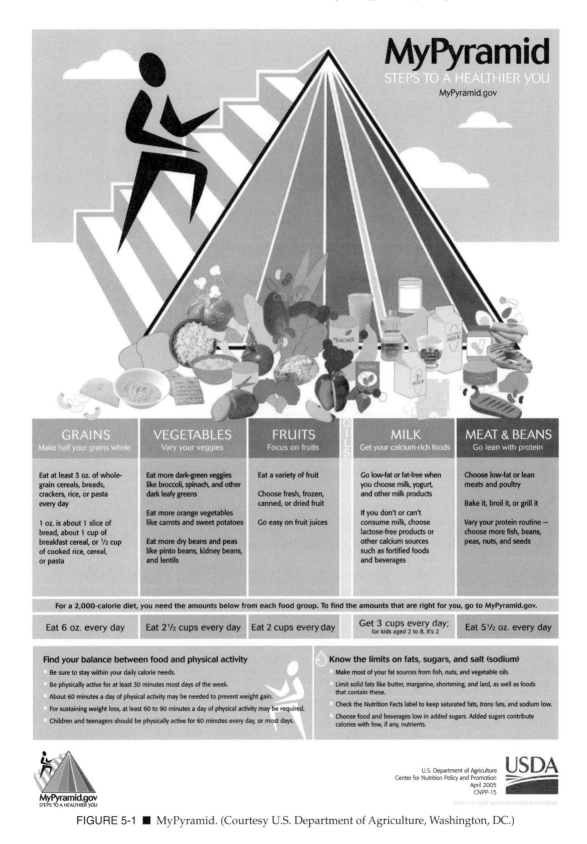

FIGURE 5-1 ■ MyPyramid. (Courtesy U.S. Department of Agriculture, Washington, DC.)

      m. Endocrine

      n. Psychiatric (mental disorders, especially depression)

C. Physical examination

  1. Initial visit

    a. Temperature, pulse, and respiration; blood pressure; height; weight

    b. Breasts (changes consistent with early pregnancy)

    c. Abdomen (changes consistent with pregnancy)

    d. Pelvis (external genitalia, vagina, uterus, cervix, and adnexa) (see Chapter 1 for a complete discussion of anatomy and Chapter 10 for pelvic sizes and shapes)

      (1) Bony pelvis, internal

        (a) Diagonal conjugate measurement: 12.5 cm

        (b) Sacral curve and shape (concave)

        (c) Ischial spines (prominence or bluntness)

        (d) Coccyx (movable)

      (2) Pelvic outlet

        (a) Subpubic arch 4 to 5 cm wide and rounded

        (b) Distance between ischial tuberosities (biischial diameter) more than 11 cm

  2. Calculation of expected delivery date (EDD), expected confinement date (ECD), expected date of birth (EDB)

    a. Nägele's rule: first day of last normal menstrual period – 3 months + 7 days + 1 year (Littleton & Engebretson, 2002)

    b. Ultrasonic examination: measurement of crown-to-rump length; most accurate in first trimester to date the gestation

  3. Physical assessment of nutritional status (Table 5-1)

    a. Blood pressure readings greater than 140/90 mm Hg or an increase of 30 mm Hg systolic or 15 mm Hg diastolic over baseline blood pressure might indicate pregnancy-induced hypertension, if combined with other signs.

    b. Temperature readings greater than 37° C (98.6° F) might indicate infection, which might increase basal metabolic rate and protein requirements

    c. Weight and height; calculation of BMI

    d. Special nutritional consideration/problems

      (1) A well-planned vegetarian diet is considered a healty choice in pregnancy (Penney & Miller, 2008).

        (a) Generally, a vegetarian diet is practiced because of physiologic, philosophic, or religious commitments.

        (b) Ensuring adequate protein and vitamin intake is an important consideration (Mangels, 2000).

        (c) Foods are usually combined to ensure enough protein in the diet (examples: legumes and grains; legumes and seeds; seeds and grains).

          [i] Only animal proteins are complete.

          [ii] By combining particular vegetable proteins, a complete source of essential amino acids can be achieved.

        (d) Vegetarianism classifications are:

          [i] Lacto-ovo: excludes all animal protein but includes eggs and dairy products and all plant foods

          [ii] Lacto: excludes all animal protein and eggs but includes dairy products and all plant foods

          [iii] Vegan: excludes all animal products, including eggs and dairy products; diet consists of plant foods only

      (2) Obesity: research has confirmed that obese pregnant women have a higher incidence of obstetric complications

        (a) These women are at an increased risk for developing pregnancy-induced hypertension, diabetes, wound complications, thromboembolism, urinary tract infections, prolonged labor, and postpartum hemorrhage.

        (b) Obese women are at a greater risk to deliver macrosomic infants.

        (c) Newborns of obese mothers might also become obese infants.

        (d) Weight loss is not recommended during pregnancy; low-carbohydrate or low-calorie diets are ketogenic and can cause glucose deprivation to the fetal brain.

■ TABLE 5-1
■ ■ **Physical Assessment of Nutritional Status**

Signs of Good Nutrition	Signs of Poor Nutrition
GENERAL APPEARANCE	
Alert, responsive, energetic, good endurance	Listless, apathetic, cachectic, easily fatigued, looks tired
MUSCLES	
Well developed, firm, good tone, some fat under skin	Flaccid, poor tone, tender, "wasted" appearance
GASTROINTESTINAL FUNCTION	
Good appetite and digestion, normal regular elimination, no palpable organs or masses	Anorexia, indigestion, constipation or diarrhea, liver or spleen enlargement
CARDIOVASCULAR FUNCTION	
Normal heart rate and rhythm, no murmurs, normal blood pressure for age	Rapid heart rate, enlarged heart, abnormal rhythm, elevated blood pressure
HAIR	
Shiny, lustrous, firm, not easily plucked, healthy scalp	Stringy, dull, brittle, dry, thin and sparse, depigmented, can be easily plucked
SKIN (GENERAL)	
Smooth, slightly moist, good color	Rough, dry, scaly, pale, pigmented, irritated, easily bruised, petechiae
FACE AND NECK	
Skin color uniform, smooth, pink, healthy appearance; no enlargement of thyroid gland; lips not chapped or swollen	Scaly, swollen, skin dark over cheeks and under eyes, lumpiness or flakiness of skin around nose and mouth; thyroid enlarged; lips swollen, angular lesions or fissures at corners of mouth
ORAL CAVITY	
Reddish pink mucous membranes and gums; no swelling or bleeding of gums; tongue healthy pink or deep reddish in appearance, not swollen or smooth, surface papillae present; teeth bright and clean, no cavities, no pain, no discoloration	Gums spongy, bleed easily, inflamed or receding; tongue swollen, scarlet and raw, magenta color, beefy, hyperemic and hypertrophic papillae, atrophic papillae; teeth with unfilled caries, absent teeth, worn surfaces, mottled
EYES	
Bright, clear, shiny, no sores at corners of eyelids, membranes moist and healthy pink color, no prominent blood vessels or mound of tissue (Bitot's spots) on sclera, no fatigue circles beneath	Eye membranes pale, redness of membrane, dryness, signs of infection, redness and fissuring of eyelid corners, dryness of eye membrane, dull appearance of cornea, blue sclerae
EXTREMITIES	
No tenderness, weakness, or swelling; nails firm and pink	Edema, tender calves, tingling, weakness; nails spoon-shaped, brittle
SKELETON	
No malformations	Bowlegs, knock-knees, chest deformity at diaphragm, beaded ribs, prominent scapulas

From Lowdermilk, D.L., & Perry, S.E. (2007). *Maternity & women's health care* (9th ed.). St. Louis: Mosby.

(3) Pica is the compulsive ingestion of nonfood substances that have little or no nutritive value; one suggested reason for pica is that the body is lacking in some essential nutrient (Littleton & Engebretson, 2002).
   (a) The most commonly ingested substances are:
      [i] Dirt
      [ii] Clay
      [iii] Dry laundry starch
      [iv] A variety of other substances have also been known to be eaten, however, such as:
         • Ice
         • Hair
         • Gravel
         • Charcoal
         • Antacid tablets
         • Baking soda
         • Coffee grounds
         • Inner tubes
   (b) Pica is neither a new phenomenon nor one that is solely correlated to a geographic area, race, creed, culture, gender, or socioeconomic status.
   (c) Etiology and medical implications are not well understood, but the practice can lead to:
      [i] Inadequate intake of essential nutrients
      [ii] Intake of substances that might contain toxic compounds
      [iii] Interference with the absorption of certain minerals (e.g., iron)
(4) Lactose intolerance should not hinder a pregnant woman's ingestion of calcium-fortified foods during pregnancy.
   (a) Suggested substitutions for milk or dairy products that are fairly well tolerated are:
      • Calcium-fortified tofu
      • Soy milk
      • Canned salmon with bones
      • Naturally aged hard cheese
      • Milk products (e.g., yogurt, sweet acidophilus milk, buttermilk, chocolate milk, cocoa)
      • Fortified orange juice
      • Commercial products that contain lactase (e.g., Lactaid)
   (b) Although leafy green vegetables are high in calcium, the bioavailability of calcium may be inhibited by phytates.
4. Diagnostic procedures (NGC, 2008)
   a. Pregnancy test (hCG levels in serum or urine) (Cunningham et al., 2005; Walsh, 2001)
      (1) Radioimmunoassay (RIA)
         (a) Based on antibodies against beta subunit hCG, radioimmunoassay is accurate as early as 1 week postovulation.
         (b) Other bioassay tests are prone to false-positive and false-negative results because of cross-reaction with LH.
         (c) Test time 1 to 5 hours, viewed as a disadvantage
      (2) Enzyme-linked immunosorbent assay (ELISA); most popular test
         (a) Monoclonal antibody binds with hCG (levels as low as 5 mIU/mL) in serum
         (b) Positive test indicated by color change in as little as 5 minutes
         (c) Home pregnancy tests (based on ELISA technology) are sensitive and accurate as early as day 1 of the expected menstrual cycle (provided the directions have been carefully followed).
   b. Blood
      (1) Complete blood count with differential smear
      (2) Hemoglobin, 12 to 16 g/dL (less than 11 g/dL might indicate iron deficiency anemia)
      (3) Hematocrit, 38% to 47% (less than 35% may indicate iron deficiency anemia)
      (4) Type and Rh factor
      (5) Antibody screen (Rh, D [Rho], rubeola, varicella, and toxoplasmosis)

(6) Rubella titer more than 1:10 to confirm immunity
(7) Screening for genetic diseases based on family history, ethnic or racial background (e.g., Tay-Sachs disease, thalassemia, sickle cell anemia)
(8) Syphilis tests (serologic test for syphilis or Venereal Disease Research Laboratory [VDRL] test)
(9) Hepatitis B screen
(10) Additional testing might be indicated based on the woman's history: HIV, alpha-fetoprotein (MSAFP), blood lead screening, rubeola, tuberculosis or group B streptococci.

  c. Urinalysis: urine screening for glucose, protein, RBCs, WBCs, and bacteria
    (1) Ketone and glucose: elevated levels might indicate gestational or overt diabetes mellitus; low intake or absorption of ketones might indicate starvation ketosis.
    (2) Protein (albumin): increased levels after 20 weeks in the presence of hypertension might indicate preeclampsia.

  d. Cervical smears
    (1) Papanicolaou
    (2) Gonorrhea culture
    (3) Chlamydia culture
    (4) Herpes simplex (types 1 and 2), if indicated by history or observation

  e. Periodic revisits: normal pregnancy (NGC, 2008; Walker, McCully, & Vest, 2001; Wilkinson, 2000)
    (1) Schedule is usually:
      (a) Monthly until 28 weeks' gestation
      (b) Biweekly from 28 to 36 weeks' gestation
      (c) Weekly from 36 weeks until delivery
      (d) Healthy women might be placed on a reduced number of visits (9 versus the traditional 14) (Walker et al., 2001).
    (2) Interval history: physical symptoms and maternal well-being, including emotional adjustment
    (3) Blood pressure and weight
    (4) Fetal well-being
      (a) Fundal height (Figure 5-2)
        [i] Fundus elevates out of pelvic area and can be palpated just above the symphysis pubis at about 12 weeks.
        [ii] Fundus rises to the level of the umbilicus at about 20 weeks and to the xiphoid process near term.

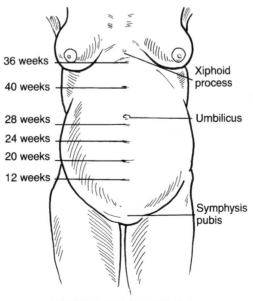

FIGURE 5-2 ■ Fundal height.

- (b) Value of symphysis-fundal height measurement called into question as a valid measure of fetal size and weight (Neilson, 2002)
- (c) Fetal heart rate
- (d) Fetal position determination: Leopold's maneuvers (see Chapter 10 for complete discussion of Leopold's maneuvers)
- (e) Other possible tests: chorionic villus sampling, fetal movements determined by examiner, nonstress test (see Chapter 8 for complete discussion of antepartum fetal testing)
- (f) Ultrasonography considered optional by some providers (Barash & Weinstein, 2002; Bickler & Neilson, 2003; NGC, 2008)
  - [i] Controversy over value of routine screening in second trimester (Barash & Weinstein, 2002)
  - [ii] Routine early screening is related to a decrease in induction rate for postterm infants.
  - [iii] Routine late screening has not been shown to decrease morbidity or mortality.
- (5) Cervical examination if indicated
- (6) Repeated or additional laboratory examinations
  - (a) Maternal serum screening for maternal serum AFP (MSAFP) at 15 to 20 weeks is offered to all women (optional test) (Barron, 2008).
    - [i] Multiple marker (double, triple, or quadruple screen; MSAFP, hCG, and unconjugated estriol) are used to detect Down syndrome and other chromosomal abnormalities (Barash & Weinstein, 2002; Barron, 2008; Cunningham et al., 2005)
    - [ii] High levels of MSAFP associated with neural tube defects; low levels of MSAFP associated with Down syndrome and other chromosomal abnormalities
    - [iii] Positive screening test results call for further diagnostic studies (see Chapter 8 for further discussion)
  - (b) Hemoglobin or hematocrit at 26 to 28 weeks
  - (c) Gestational diabetes screen at 24 to 28 weeks (Barron, 2008)
  - (d) Antibody screen (D [Rho]) at 28 weeks
  - (e) Group B streptococci at 35 to 37 weeks (NGC, 2008)
  - (f) Tests for sexually transmitted infections, if indicated (e.g., gonorrhea)

HEALTH EDUCATION

A. Pregnancy is a normal process that takes a woman and her family on a 280-day journey.
Delivery of evidence-based prenatal education is a primary role for the nurse. Trimester-specific education topics provide the woman the tools she will need to stay healthy and to maintain a normal pregnancy. Successful health teaching demands that the nurse be aware of and apply the principles of teaching and learning. This type of health education can be individualized and will empower the woman to be an active participant in the delivery of prenatal care, but does not substitute for formal childbirth or prenatal education programs.

B. First trimester
  1. Physiologic changes of pregnancy with resulting discomforts
     a. Pain and tingling in breasts
     b. Nausea and vomiting (morning sickness)
     c. Urinary frequency
     d. Fatigue
     e. Mood swings
  2. Warning signs that should be reported
     a. Vaginal bleeding
     b. Abdominal cramping
     c. Severe and prolonged vomiting
  3. Health teaching
     a. Schedule of return visits for routine prenatal care
     b. General hygiene
     c. Comfort measures for trimester-related discomforts
     d. Anticipatory guidance regarding duration of current discomforts

    e. Sexual activity
    f. Safety issues
      (1) Auto safety including proper use of seatbelts
      (2) Avoid getting overtied—schedule rest/relaxation periods.
      (3) Avoid cancerous chemicals in the home and the workplace.
      (4) Select shoes that provide comfort, and good balance and posture
    g. Physical activities, exercise, and rest
      (1) Exercise is safe in uncomplicated pregnancies (Lively, 2002).
      (2) Mild to moderate exercise is encouraged.
      (3) Athletes should avoid sports that carry a risk of abdominal trauma.
      (4) Recommend adequate hydration and nutrition essential for well-being of client and fetus (Dundas & Taylor, 2002)
    h. Nutritional guidance, weight gain, and diet
      (1) Multiple pregnancy
        (a) Theoretically the nutritional needs of a woman carrying more than one fetus should be greater to support extra blood volume and placental/fetal tissue.
        (b) There has been no formal evaluation of needs, however, and specific guidelines have not been developed (Reifsnider & Gill, 2000).
        (c) Total weight gain recommendations are between 18.2 and 20.5 kg (40 and 45 pounds) for twins and 20.5 and 22.7 kg (45 and 50 pounds) for triplets.
        (d) General dietary recommendations include the following:
          [i] Follow all dietary recommendations of nonrisk pregnancy (see earlier).
          [ii] Eat nutrient-dense foods.
          [iii] Increase protein and calcium intake as necessary.
          [iv] Eat small, frequent meals.
      (2) For women who are vegetarians, the assumption of malnutrition is not supported by nutrition research, although supplements may be recommended to meet nutritional needs.
    i. Encourage avoidance of alcohol (leading cause of mental retardation; fetal alcohol syndrome).
    j. Encourage avoidance of self-medication with over-the-counter drugs, herbal remedies, and even vitamins.
    k. Educate on smoking cessation (if indicated).
C. Second trimester
  1. Physiologic changes with resulting discomforts
    a. Enlargement of abdomen
    b. Skin pigmentation
    c. Striae gravidarum
    d. Vascular spiders
    e. Constipation
    f. Heartburn
    g. Leg cramps
    h. Groin pain from round ligament stretching
    i. Leukorrhea
  2. Warning signs that should be reported
    a. Vaginal bleeding
    b. Burning or painful urination
    c. Signs of fever
    d. Reduction in or absence of fetal movements
    e. Nausea and vomiting
    f. Abdominal pain or cramping
    g. Swelling of face or fingers, headaches, visual disturbances, or epigastric pain
  3. Health teaching
    a. Reinforcement and reiteration of previous teaching
    b. Comfort measures specific to trimester-related discomforts
    c. Anticipatory guidance regarding duration of current discomforts
    d. Choices of prenatal education classes
    e. Signs and symptoms of preterm labor

D. **Third trimester**
   1. Physiologic changes with resulting discomforts
      a. Dyspnea
      b. Leg and foot cramps
      c. Constipation
      d. Indigestion, heartburn
      e. Pedal edema
      f. Fatigue
      g. Vaginal discharge
      h. Urinary frequency
      i. Braxton Hicks contractions
   2. Warning signs that should be reported
      a. Visual disturbance
      b. Headache
      c. Hand and facial edema
      d. Fever
      e. Vaginal bleeding
      f. Abdominal pain; uterine contractions
      g. Premature rupture of membranes
      h. Decreased or lack of fetal movement
   3. Health teaching
      a. Signs and symptoms of labor/preterm labor
      b. When to call the health care provider; when to go to the hospital or birthing place
      c. Comfort measures for trimester-related discomforts
      d. Anticipatory guidance regarding duration of present discomforts
      e. Reinforcement and reiteration of previous teaching

CASE STUDIES AND STUDY QUESTIONS

Ms. L. is a 26-year-old who has registered at the clinic for prenatal care. She reports fatigue, nausea, and constipation. Her last normal menstrual period was 8 weeks ago, and the home pregnancy test result was positive. This is her first pregnancy.

1. Presumptive signs of pregnancy include:
   a. Ballottement
   b. Braxton Hicks contractions
   c. Breast changes
   d. Positive pregnancy test results
2. The bluish discoloration of the vagina is known as:
   a. Chadwick's sign
   b. Hegar's sign
   c. Goodell's sign
   d. Braxton's sign
3. A normal physiologic change associated with the first trimester of pregnancy is:
   a. Increased respirations
   b. Increased peristalsis
   c. Increased resistance to infection
   d. Increased cardiac output
4. Health teaching of particular importance at this early stage of pregnancy includes:
   a. Comfort measures for trimester-related discomforts

   b. Choices of prenatal education classes
   c. Signs and symptoms of labor
   d. Infant feeding techniques

Ms. T., at 27 weeks' gestation, comes to the clinic for a routine prenatal visit. This is her fourth pregnancy, and she has four living children (with one set of twins).

5. How would her obstetric history be recorded?
6. Routine laboratory tests that should be repeated at this visit include:
   a. hCG level
   b. Rubella titer
   c. Antibody screen
   d. Complete blood count with differential smear
7. She reports feeling fatigued and is bothered by constipation. These symptoms are related to the hormone:
   a. Estrogen
   b. hCG
   c. Thyroxine
   d. Relaxin
8. Her hemoglobin value is 11.7 g/dL. Which factor explains this finding?
   a. The trimester of pregnancy

b. Hemodilution of pregnancy
c. The presence of iron deficiency anemia
d. Greater-than-expected weight gain

Ms. S., age 16, is a finicky eater. She is very weight conscious and has tried several fad diets in the past. Ms. S. rarely eats breakfast; when she does, it consists of a glass of orange juice and a piece of toast. At noon she usually eats an apple or an orange. After school she is famished and snacks on cookies, soda, and ice cream. Frequently her evening meal consists of pizza, or a milkshake and a hamburger. She has just learned that she is pregnant, and she is horrified that she might become fat. Her medical history includes anemia. Present weight is 50.9 kg (112 pounds) and height is 1.86 m (5 feet, 7 inches) .

9. How much weight should she gain to ensure a healthy pregnancy?
   a. 28 to 40 pounds
   b. 25 to 35 pounds
   c. More than 55 pounds
   d. 15 to 22 pounds

10. The RDA for energy includes an extra _____ kilocalories to support needs associated with the second and third trimesters of pregnancy.
    a. 200
    b. 250
    c. 300
    d. 350

11. When assessing the nutritional status of Ms. S., one of the best methods for obtaining dietary information is to:
    a. Consult with family members
    b. Ask her where she usually eats
    c. Ask her how many meals she eats
    d. Obtain a verbal and written 24-dietary recall

12. Which of the following factors is not a nutritional risk at the onset of pregnancy or during pregnancy?
    a. Low hemoglobin or hematocrit
    b. BMI within 90% to 110% of standard prepregnancy BMI
    c. Inadequate weight gain
    d. Poverty

ADDITIONAL STUDY QUESTIONS

13. The increase in uterine size during pregnancy is primarily the result of which of the following factors?
    a. Growth of the fetus
    b. Formation of new muscle fibers
    c. Increase in blood circulation to the uterus
    d. Stretching of existing muscle fibers
14. The primary source of the hormones estrogen and progesterone during early pregnancy is the:
    a. Placenta
    b. Anterior lobe of the pituitary gland
    c. Corpus luteum
    d. Adrenal cortex
15. The expected height of the fundus at 20 weeks' gestation is:
    a. At the xiphoid process

    b. At the umbilicus
    c. Halfway between the symphysis pubis and umbilicus
    d. At the symphysis pubis
16. A pregnant woman should immediately report which of the following symptoms to her health care provider?
    a. Leg cramps
    b. Abdominal pain
    c. Dyspnea
    d. Heartburn
17. Normal physiologic responses to pregnancy include:
    a. Increased cardiac output
    b. Increased peristalsis
    c. Increased respirations
    d. Increased blood pressure

ANSWERS TO STUDY QUESTIONS

1. c
2. a
3. d
4. a
5. G4, P3

6. c
7. d
8. b
9. a
10. c

11. d
12. b
13. d
14. c
15. b

16. b
17. a

REFERENCES

Barash, J. H., & Weinstein, L. C. (2002). Preconception and prenatal care. *Primary Care Clinical Office Practice, 29,* 519–542.

Barron, M. L. (2008). Antenatal care. In K. R. Simpson, & P. A. Creehan (Eds.), *AWHONN perinatal nursing* (pp. 88–124). Phildelphia: Wolters Kluwer/ Lippincott Williams & Wilkins.

Bickler, L., & Neilson, J. P. (2003). Routine Doppler ultrasound in pregnancy. In *The Cochrane Library* (Vol 1). Oxford: Update Software.

Blackburn, S. T. (2008). Physiologic changes of pregnancy. In K. R. Simpson, & P. A. Creehan (Eds.), *AWHONN perinatal nursing* (pp. 59–77). Phildelphia: Wolters Kluwer/Lippincott Williams & Wilkins.

Cesario, S. K. (2003). Obesity in pregnancy: What every nurse should know. *AWHONN Lifelines, 7,* 119–125.

Cunningham, F. G., Leveno, K. J., Bloom, S., Hauth, J. C., Gilstrap, L., & Wenstrom, K. D. (2005). *Williams obstetrics* (22nd ed.). New York: McGraw-Hill.

Dundas, M. L., & Taylor, S. (2002). Perinatal factors, motivation, and attitudes concerning pregnancy affect dietary intake. *Topics in Clinical Nutrition, 17,* 71–79.

Kaiser, L. L., & Allen, L. (2002). Position of the American Dietetic Association: Nutrition and lifestyle for a healthy pregnancy outcome. *Journal of the American Dietetic Association, 102*(10), 1479–1490.

Lederman, S. A. (2001). Pregnancy weight gain and postpartum loss: Avoiding obesity while optimizing the growth and development of the fetus. *Journal of the American Medical Women's Association, 56*(2), 53–58.

Littleton, L. Y., & Engebretson, J. C. (2002). *Maternal, neonatal, and women's health nursing.* Albany, NY: Delmar-Thompson Learning.

Lively, M. W. (2002). Sport participation and pregnancy. *Athletic Therapy Today, 7,* 11–15.

Lowdermilk, D. L., & Perry, S. E. (2007). *Maternity & women's health care* (9th ed.). St. Louis: Mosby.

Mangels, R. (2000). *Protein in the vegan diet.* The Vegetarian Resource Group. Available at www.vrg.org/ nutrition/protein.htm. Accessed March 11, 2003.

National Guideline Clearinghouse (NGC). (August 2008). Routine prenatal care (NGC 006704). Available at www.guideline.gov/summary. Accessed February 10, 2009.

Neilson, J. P. (2002). Symphysis-fundal height measurement in pregnancy. In *The Cochrane Library* (Vol 4). Oxford: Update Software.

Penney, D. S., & Miller, K. G. (2008). Nutritional counseling for vegetarians during pregnancy and lactation. *Journal of Midwifery & Women's Health, 53*(1), 37–44.

Reifsnider, E., & Gill, S. L. (2000). Nutrition for the childbearing years. *Journal of Obstetric, Gynecologic, and Neonatal Nursing, 29*(1), 43–55.

Walker, D. S., McCully, L., & Vest, V. (2001). Evidence-based prenatal care visits: When less is more. *Journal of Midwifery and Women's Health, 46*(3), 146–151.

Walsh, L. V. (2001). *Midwifery: Community-based care during the childbearing years.* Philadelphia: Saunders.

Wilkinson, L. D. (2000). Care and counseling by trimester. *Family Practice Recertification, 22,* 61–76.

Worthington-Roberts, B. S., & Williams, S. R. (1997). *Nutrition in pregnancy and lactation* (6th ed.). Boston: McGraw-Hill.

6 Psychology of Pregnancy

Catherine R. Coverston

OBJECTIVES

1. Describe two stages of family development pertinent to pregnancy.
2. List the developmental tasks of pregnancy.
3. List the general concepts in Rubin's tasks of pregnancy.
4. Discuss two psychosocial findings in normal pregnancy.
5. Discuss strategies to minimize self-concept disturbances during pregnancy.
6. Discuss risks related to eating disorders during pregnancy.
7. Discuss the effects of increased technology on a woman's psychologic experience of pregnancy.
8. Describe three needs of fathers during labor and delivery.
9. Identify two reactions of fathers to pregnancy.
10. Describe changes in sexual feelings, fears,and behaviors in pregnancy.
11. Discuss the concept of developmental crises in pregnancy.
12. Describe how to assist families in developing a birth plan and selecting childbirth education.
13. Enumerate maternal behaviors exhibited during pregnancy validation.
14. Describe maternal behaviors exhibited during fetal embodiment.
15. Differentiate maternal behaviors seen during fetal distinction.
16. List the most common maternal behaviors observed in role transition.
17. Identify maternal behaviors indicative of Rubin's task of safe passage in the last trimester of pregnancy.
18. Describe issues seen in the last trimester involving acceptance of the child by others.

INTRODUCTION

Pregnancy is a time of increased susceptibility to psychologic stress for expectant mothers and fathers. Pregnancy and childbearing are developmental phases in family life often characterized by ambivalence and conflicting emotions, as expectant parents face significant role and lifestyle changes.

CLINICAL PRACTICE

A. Assessment
  1. History
    a. Family background
      (1) Economic status
      (2) Marital status
      (3) Age
      (4) Support system
      (5) Self-esteem
      (6) Role models
      (7) Culture (see Bibliography)
      (8) Religion/spirituality
      (9) Stability of living conditions
    b. Obstetric experience
      (1) Previous pregnancies
      (2) Prior pregnancy outcomes

      (3) Pregnancy experiences of extended family and friends
      (4) Previous experience with infants and neonates
      (5) Unresolved grief or anger related to previous experiences
  c. Current pregnancy
      (1) Wanted or unwanted
      (2) Planned or unplanned
      (3) Mother's health: healthy or unhealthy before and during this pregnancy
      (4) The woman's and partner's learning capabilities and/or limitations
      (5) Whether the woman has healthy or unhealthy personal relationships
      (6) The status of her pregnancy: low risk or high risk (Lutz & May, 2007; Sittner, DeFrain, & Judson, 2005)

2. Duvall's (1985) stages of family development
  a. Married couple beginning a family
      (1) Attainment of a satisfying relationship
      (2) The dyad is the easiest and first relationship of family development.
  b. Expectant family: role preparation
      (1) Reorganization of the household for the infant
      (2) Development of new patterns of making and spending money
      (3) Realignment of tasks and responsibilities
      (4) Adaptation of sexual relationship to the pregnancy
      (5) Reorientation of relationships with relatives
      (6) Adaptation of relationships with friends and associates
      (7) Increase in knowledge about pregnancy, birth, and parenting
      (8) Adaptation to accelerated emotional changes
  c. Childbearing family (from the first birth to the time when the last child attains the age of 30 months)
      (1) Adjust to a changing relationship (i.e., dyad to triad).
      (2) Encourage the development of the new infant.
      (3) Introduce each new infant to the existing siblings (Duvall, 1985).

3. Psychosocial findings
  a. Thoughts and desires
      (1) Food cravings might occur during pregnancy.
      (2) Sexual behaviors, desires, and thoughts vary throughout pregnancy.
        (a) Might decrease in late pregnancy for some
        (b) Might remain unchanged for others
      (3) Dream life is very active in pregnancy.
      (4) Fatigue, especially during the first and third trimesters, might influence desires and thoughts.
  b. Mood swings
      (1) Ambivalence about becoming a mother appears in early pregnancy in most women.
      (2) Irritability may increase throughout pregnancy and peak in the ninth month, as fatigue increases.
      (3) Increased sensitivity might exist throughout the entire pregnancy.
      (4) A sense of vulnerability tends to peak during the seventh month.
      (5) The woman might experience frustration with her own indecisiveness throughout the pregnancy.
      (6) Normal fears might exist (e.g., about the health of the infant and about her ability to give birth safely). Extreme fear of birth (i.e., requests cesarean to avoid vaginal birth) may be accompanied by other psychosocial problems (Nerum, Halverson, Sorlie, & Oian, 2006).

4. Pregnancy as a developmental (maturational) crisis
  a. Danger of increased psychologic vulnerability at this time
  b. Increased opportunity for personal growth
  c. Increased susceptibility to stress because of potential changes in areas such as work, housing needs, and access to care
  d. Alteration in role and identity for each parent and for each member of the family

5. Developmental tasks of pregnancy are progressive over time.
  a. Pregnancy validation

        (1) Most women have an initial ambivalence about being pregnant.

        (2) Many women experience fantasies and dreams about themselves and how pregnancy will change their lives.

   b. Fetal embodiment

        (1) The woman incorporates the fetus into her body image.

        (2) She becomes dependent on her partner or on significant others.

        (3) She is typically introspective and calm.

   c. Fetal distinction

        (1) The woman conceptualizes her fetus as a separate individual.

        (2) She accepts her new body image and might characterize it as being full of life.

        (3) She typically becomes more dependent on her mother or feels closer to her mother at this time.

   d. Role transition

        (1) She prepares to separate from and give up the physical, symbiotic attachment with her fetus.

        (2) She becomes anxious about impending labor and delivery.

        (3) She exhibits "nesting" behaviors or a need to get all the supplies needed for the infant (preterm labor is a major disruption of the need to nest).

        (4) She becomes impatient with her awkward body and is anxious for pregnancy to end; she states frequently that she is tired of being pregnant.

        (5) She feels prepared to mother the infant.

6. Rubin's (1984) tasks of pregnancy occur concurrently with each other.

   a. General principles

        (1) Pregnancy progressively becomes a part of the woman's total identity.

        (2) The woman is able to share little of her sensory experience with others, making her feel unique.

        (3) The woman's focus turns progressively inward as the pregnancy advances.

        (4) The woman generally becomes overly sensitive.

        (5) She seeks the company of other women, especially other pregnant women.

        (6) The absence of a female support system during pregnancy is an index of a high-risk pregnancy.

   b. "Binding-in" is acceptance of pregnancy and incorporating the reality of pregnancy into her self-concept.

        (1) First trimester: she accepts the idea of pregnancy, but not of the child

        (2) Second trimester: there is a dramatic change, with the sensation of fetal movement (quickening); she becomes aware of the child as a separate entity within her

        (3) Third trimester: she wants the child and is tired of being pregnant

   c. Acceptance of the child

        (1) First trimester: acceptance of the pregnancy by herself and others

        (2) Acceptance of the child by others is the keystone of a successful adjustment to pregnancy

        (3) Second trimester: the family needs to relate to the infant (e.g., as a son or brother)

        (4) Third trimester: the critical issue is the unconditional acceptance of the child; conditional acceptance implies rejection

   d. Reordering of relationships and learning to give of herself

        (1) First trimester: examines what needs to be given up

            (a) Trade-offs for having the infant

            (b) Might grieve the loss of a carefree life

        (2) Second trimester: identifies with the child

        (3) Third trimester: has decreased confidence in her ability to become a good mother to her child

   e. Safe passage: Rubin (1984) suggested this task usually receives most of the woman's attention

        (1) First trimester: focuses on herself, not on her infant

        (2) Second trimester: develops an attachment of great value to her infant

        (3) Third trimester: has concern for herself and her infant as a unit

            (a) At the seventh month she is in a state of high vulnerability.

            (b) She sees labor and delivery as deliverance and as a hope, not as a threat.

7. Expectant fathers: less is known about men's transition to parenthood (Halle, Dowd, Fowler, Rissel, Hennessy et al., 2008).
    a. Psychosocial findings during pregnancy
        (1) Couvade: some men actually experience symptoms of pregnancy
            (a) Weight gain
            (b) Nausea
            (c) Other common physical symptoms of pregnancy
        (2) Expectant fathers vary widely in their reactions to pregnancy as well as to the psychologic and physical changes in the woman.
            (a) Some enjoy the role of nurturer.
            (b) Some experience alienation, which might lead to extramarital affairs.
            (c) Some view the pregnancy as a proof of masculinity and assume a dominant role.
            (d) Some believe pregnancy has no meaning and brings no responsibility to the mother or child.
    b. Paternal tasks of pregnancy
        (1) First trimester: announcement phase
            (a) Must cope with ambivalence about becoming a father
            (b) Strives to accept the biologic fact of pregnancy
            (c) Attempts to take on the expectant father role
        (2) Second trimester: moratorium phase
            (a) Often has a delay of "binding-in" to the pregnancy compared with the woman
            (b) Accepts the woman's changing body
            (c) Accepts the reality of the fetus, particularly when fetal movement is felt
            (d) Adapts to the changes in their sexual relationship
                [i] Frequently has fears about harming the fetus during sexual intercourse
                [ii] Might experience a potential rivalry with a male obstetrician
            (e) Experiences confusion when dealing with the woman's intense introspection
            (f) Fantasizes about the father-child relationship (not as an infant but as an older child—playing ball, for example)
        (3) Third trimester: focusing phase
            (a) Negotiates what his role will be during labor and delivery
            (b) Prepares for the reality of parenthood
            (c) Might change his self-concept and image (e.g., might shave his beard and buy new clothes).
            (d) Engages in preparing the nursery
            (e) Copes with fears about the mutilation or the death of his partner and child
    c. Fathers at labor and birth
        (1) Benefits
            (a) Might dispel his feelings of alienation
            (b) Might increase his sense of significance and importance
            (c) Might increase his sense of control
            (d) Might increase his appreciation for his laboring woman/partner
            (e) Might develop a closer attachment to his newborn earlier in the father-child relationship
        (2) Roles of fathers during labor and birth
            (a) The father as a *labor coach* is very involved and needs a high level of control.
            (b) A father as a *teammate* needs less control but provides emotional and physical support.
            (c) A father as a *witness* is there as a companion, providing support, but looks to others for instruction and support; needs very little control.
        (3) There is a need for sensitivity to a father's unfamiliarity with such things as:
            (a) Unfamiliar sights; for example:
                [i] His wife/girlfriend in pain and grimacing
                [ii] Bulging perineum
                [iii] Blood and fluids
                [iv] Others touching his partner in intimate ways
            (b) Unfamiliar sounds; for example:
                [i] Moans, grunts
                [ii] Hospital noises

        (c) Unfamiliar smells; for example:
           [i] Vaginal discharge, amniotic fluid
           [ii] Cleaning solutions and medications
        (d) The father has his own needs to meet.
           [i] Fatigue
           [ii] Hunger
           [iii] Fears and concerns
    (4) Other considerations about expectant fathers at labor and birth
        (a) Some cultures bar men from labor and birth (e.g., certain Middle Eastern cultures).
        (b) Some men do not want to be present for labor and/or birth.
        (c) Some women do not want the father to see them "like that."

8. Other family members' psychosocial reactions to pregnancy and childbirth
  a. Expectant siblings
    (1) Reaction to pregnancy is age dependent.
    (2) Siblings might express excitement and anticipation.
    (3) Siblings might verbalize negative reactions.
    (4) Siblings might be unaware or noncommittal.
    (5) Siblings present at birth need a caretaker whose major focus is meeting the needs of the sibling (i.e., involvement or withdrawal from the process).
    (6) Siblings might exhibit ambivalent reactions to a newborn in the home.
        (a) Show affection and excitement
        (b) Might vacillate, with regressive behavior, anger, or both
  b. Expectant grandparents
    (1) Often express excitement and anticipation
    (2) Might express resentment (e.g., "I'm too young to be someone's grandmother!")
    (3) Might verbalize anger if the pregnancy was unplanned or if the mother is a teenager or is unwed
    (4) Often express anxiety about the health and well-being of the expectant mother and fetus
    (5) Might be concerned about the expectant parents' age, income, and emotional stability

9. Single expectant mother's psychosocial needs
  a. Reason for single status needs to be assessed to better understand the meaning of pregnancy
    (1) Single by choice: pregnancy might have been by artificial insemination
    (2) Single by accident: becoming a widow after conception or pregnant through rape
    (3) Single by divorce or separation after conception
    (4) Single and pregnant by a casual acquaintance (unplanned or planned)
  b. Presence or absence of strong support persons can significantly influence the woman's adaptation to pregnancy.
  c. Future plans for the child are an important factor influencing the mother's psychologic needs (i.e., is she planning to keep and raise the child or planning to place the child for adoption? Is she a surrogate parent?).

10. Ethnocultural considerations
  a. In the United States, there are mixed cultural messages about behavior during pregnancy and birth.
  b. Technologic culture is dominant in U.S. health care.
    (1) Use of technology creates a potential to increase stress and anxiety in the pregnant woman (Kornelsen, 2005).
        (a) Moral and ethical dilemmas frequently are associated with diagnostic tests.
        (b) The woman's interpersonal and emotional needs and feelings might be missed or ignored in favor of technologic information.
    (2) There is an increased chance of caregivers' shifting their focus from the woman to the equipment.
    (3) "Tentative pregnancy" is the concept of inability or unwillingness to fully accept or embrace one's pregnancy until all prenatal diagnostic test results have been received.

    (4) Technology might prevent women from viewing pregnancy with the "ignorant bliss" of earlier generations.

    (5) The woman might feel that she must trust technology more than herself.

  c. General principles regarding pregnancy among varying cultures may or may not apply to individuals.

    (1) Pregnancy is considered to be normal, not a state of illness in many cultures (e.g., some Native American tribes, most Latin cultures).

    (2) Women of some cultures might only seek care if they believe there is something wrong or for technology, such as ultrasound.

    (3) Pregnancy often has many rigid taboos (e.g., some African nations).

    (4) Pregnancy might be viewed as only woman's work (e.g., Middle Eastern cultures).

    (5) Yin/yang: everything in nature is balanced; for example, hot/cold (e.g., Korean cultures).

    (6) Some cultures stress pregnancy behaviors that are protective, whereas others do not (avoidance of substance abuse, improved diet).

    (7) Protective behaviors might be compromised as immigrants become more acculturated and give up protective behaviors (e.g., use of tobacco, less healthy food such as fast food).

11. Psychosocial alterations affecting perinatal adaptation and outcomes

  a. Postpartum mood disorders

  b. Eating disorders

    (1) Three types in the *Diagnostic and Statistical Manual of Mental Disorders,* 4th edition *(DSM-IV)*

      (a) Anorexia nervosa

        [i] Intentional loss of body weight 15% below recommended weight

          • Body image distortion and amenorrhea are common.

          • Preoccupation with weight and eating

        [ii] Achieved by severe food restriction, exercise, fasting, as well as purging through vomiting, laxative and diuretic abuse, and diet pills

        [iii] Affects about 0.3% to 1% of the population

        [iv] Very difficult to treat; often chronic and concurrent with other psychiatric disorders

      (b) Bulimia nervosa

        [i] Binge eating with purging; excessive exercise

        [ii] Usually normal weight

        [iii] Undue focus on body image

      (c) Eating disorders not otherwise specified

        [i] Do not meet criteria for anorexia or bulimia but might binge eat

        [ii] Pregnancy might push a woman into full-blown anorexia or bulimia.

    (2) Effects on pregnancy

      (a) Anorexia nervosa

        [i] Fertility: contrary to popular belief, women with anorexia do not seem to have decreased fertility, even with amenorrhea.

        [ii] Complications (Bansil et al, 2008)

          • Higher miscarriage, cesarean, and induction rates

          • Low infant birthweight

          • Higher incidence of congenital malformation

      (b) Bulimia nervosa

        [i] Symptoms increase in pregnancy.

        [ii] Might smoke or restrict eating to control weight

        [iii] Complications

          • Higher miscarriage rate

          • Hypertension more common

      (c) Complications associated with all eating disorders

        [i] Infant

          • Low-birthweight infants

          • Low Apgar scores

          • Higher occurrence of breech presentation

- Higher incidence of cleft palate
- Higher incidence of stillbirth

[ii] Mother

- Higher incidence of bleeding during pregnancy
- Delay in wound healing
- Complications are no more prevalent in women with eating disorders than in any other pregnancy if normal pregnancy weight gain is maintained.

(3) Detection of eating disorders

(a) Evaluate feelings about being weighed.

(b) Evaluate history of amenorrhea, unexplained pregnancy loss, or infants with difficulties.

(c) Evaluate for history of sexual or physical abuse and other psychiatric disorders.

(d) Determine if cosmetic surgery has been obtained to alter the body.

(e) Evaluate history, which is likely to indicate many past weight gains and losses.

(f) Evaluate exercise and caffeine patterns, food allergies or phobias, restrictions such as vegetarianism.

(g) Look for failure to gain weight in two consecutive visits during the second trimester.

c. Grief and loss in the perinatal period

(1) Grief and loss might be triggered by several events related to pregnancy.

(a) Spontaneous abortion

[i] Loss of various roles and privileges associated with pregnancy

[ii] Loss of trust in one's body; feelings of inadequacy as a woman

[iii] Might feel guilt if she had been ambivalent about the pregnancy

[iv] Father of the infant might not have the same sense of the reality of the pregnancy as the mother.

[v] The lack of any "rituals" related to spontaneous abortion might leave the woman feeling alone and unsupported.

[vi] Each member of a couple or family will likely grieve differently and might be perceived as unsupportive or unfeeling by the others.

(b) Relinquishing child for adoption

(c) Loss of the perfect child

[i] Preterm or ill child

[ii] Child of a gender other than that wanted

[iii] Child with congenital anomalies

d. Parental reaction

(1) Parents will likely experience a grief response that includes shock, denial, depression, equilibrium, and acceptance and reorganization of the family

(2) Might separate from the preterm or ill child, which can delay attachment

(3) Might anticipate grief of potential loss of the infant

(4) Might acknowledge failure to produce a healthy infant

(5) Might change ways of relating to the infant in face of the threat of disability or death

(6) Might strive to learn to live with the special needs of their infant

12. Childbirth preparation education: the goal of childbirth education is to assist individuals and family members to make informed decisions about pregnancy and birth based on knowledge of their options and choices; the goal is operationalized via the provision of specific information about the components of a healthy pregnancy and the process of labor and birth; necessary tools and skills to deal with pregnancy, labor, and birth are acquired.

a. Basic underlying principles of childbirth education

(1) Partner or support person participation is important.

(2) Relaxation and breathing strategies can be learned and practiced as a conditioned response to the stimulus of a uterine contraction.

(3) Relaxation and breathing patterns are aids to cope with labor pain and enhance labor effectiveness.

(4) Knowledge of choices, options, and alternatives can empower a laboring woman and her support person.

(5) Confidence in one's ability to accomplish unmedicated birth is the most important predictor of success.

    b. Various approaches are available; the two most common are:

      (1) Lamaze

        (a) Active relaxation strategies and breathing techniques to deal with pain of labor (e.g., touch, imagery, music, hydrotherapy)

        (b) Basic breathing awareness and breathing strategies

      (2) Bradley

        (a) Diaphragmatic breathing (i.e., from the abdomen) is believed to be most efficient for relaxation during labor.

        (b) Women are taught to become aware of their own breathing to determine the rate and depth of breath to take in labor.

      (3) Others

        (a) Many childbirth educators have taken what they believe are the best of several approaches and created a hybrid approach.

        (b) Many childbirth educators will tailor a program that is right for the couple.

      (4) Women and their partners should be encouraged to broadly explore the many options available for childbirth through books, articles, classes, and electronic media presentations.

      (5) Women who are unable to attend prenatal classes due to bedrest or other situations might find an educator willing to work with them individually.

C. Interventions/Outcomes

    1. Disturbed body image due to body changes, eating disorders

    2. Taking on new roles; changes in roles related to pregnancy

    3. Low self-esteem related to pregnancy complications, changes in body image, and roles

      a. Interventions

        (1) Use effective listening and nonjudgmental communication skills.

        (2) Encourage woman to seek early and continual prenatal care.

        (3) Provide resources—books, magazines, electronic media, and support groups—to assist in role changes of pregnant woman to a new mother.

        (4) Encourage participation in childbirth and childcare classes.

        (5) Encourage family to provide material symbols of role changes.

          (a) Maternity clothes

          (b) Infant equipment

        (6) Explain normal, expected emotional ramifications of pregnancy and role changes.

        (7) Help couple to set realistic goals and expectations for themselves.

        (8) Explore expectations for labor through:

          (a) Birth plans (Deering, Zaret, McGaha, & Satin, 2007; Lothian, 2006)

          (b) Choice of support persons

          (c) Options and opportunities for decision making to increase self-esteem

        (9) Offer realistic concepts of early parent-infant attachment process.

          (a) Provide early infant contact.

          (b) Explain normal newborn behaviors.

      (10) Evaluate weight gain and other possible signs of eating disorders.

      b. Outcomes

        (1) Woman has received prenatal care.

        (2) Couple has attended childbirth and/or child care classes.

        (3) Woman exhibits acceptance of role (e.g., can be concerned about being a good mother but not ambivalent about becoming a mother).

        (4) Woman gains appropriate weight in the pregnancy.

        (5) Woman has determined how she will feed her child (by breast or bottle).

        (6) Couple has chosen possibilities for the infant's name.

        (7) Couple has prepared the home for the infant.

        (8) Couple negotiates options and desires for labor and birth.

        (9) Parents demonstrate an active interest in the newborn at birth.

    4. Changes in libido during pregnancy

      a. Interventions

        (1) Explain wide variety of normal sexual feelings and behaviors.

          (a) Couple might enjoy sexual activity more because there is:

            [i] No fear of pregnancy

            [ii] No need for contraceptive use (which may have disrupted spontaneity)

[iii] Increased pelvic congestion with fulminating orgasm (some women experience their first orgasm during pregnancy)

[iv] Increased vaginal lubrication

[v] Perception of the pregnancy as very sensuous

(b) Couple might have decreased desires and responses because of:

[i] Negative body image (might be experienced by the man, the woman, or both)

[ii] A belief in myths about harming the fetus by intercourse

[iii] Physical symptoms such as fatigue and nausea might influence desire and response.

[iv] Psychologic restriction some couples feel toward sexual intercourse during pregnancy

[v] Taboos some cultural and social groups have against sexual intercourse during pregnancy

(2) Determine and fulfill informational needs.

(a) There are many ways of expressing affection and intimacy beyond intercourse alone (e.g., kissing, massage, and romantic dinner).

(b) Positions for intercourse might need to change as the uterus grows (e.g., to side-lying or female superior).

(c) Masturbation or manual stimulation might cause a more intense orgasm than intercourse (needs to be avoided if intercourse is contraindicated for preterm labor risk).

(d) Provide accurate information about the safety of intercourse throughout a normal pregnancy.

(e) Pregnancy is a time of vulnerability, and couples need to be encouraged to be sensitive to each other's needs for affection and intimacy.

(f) Orgasm causes harmless contractions and does not cause any problems in normal pregnancy.

(g) Blowing into the vagina is contraindicated because of the potential of causing an air embolus.

(3) Contraindications to intercourse

(a) Ruptured membranes: contraindicated because of potential for infection

(b) Incompetent cervix: contraindicated because of potential to cause preterm labor

(c) Spotting or bleeding: contraindicated, especially with a placenta previa

(d) Preterm labor history in current pregnancy: contraindicated because of potential to start premature labor

b. Outcomes

(1) Comfort for open dialogue with health care provider about sexual concerns is established.

(2) Couple maintains intimacy during pregnancy.

(3) Couple can discuss satisfaction with options for expressing affection.

5. Stressors of pregnancy or loss

a. Interventions

(1) Offer anticipatory guidance about normal developmental stressors of pregnancy, such as:

(a) Ambivalence during early pregnancy

(b) Vulnerability

(c) Impatience, irritability

(d) Active dream/fantasy life

(2) Encourage couple to ask questions.

(3) Help couple appreciate the normal and universal nature of the emotional changes in pregnancy and identify areas of stress.

(4) Acknowledge ethical dilemmas and emotional stress of prenatal diagnostic testing procedures.

(5) Discuss common phases through which men progress during pregnancy.

(a) Announcement phase: when diagnosis is made

(b) Moratorium phase: occurring during early pregnancy, when there is often little overt interest on the expectant father's part

(c) Focusing phase: related to new role as father, which occurs during late pregnancy (Deave & Johnson, 2008).

      (6) Provide encouragement that couple's adaptive coping strategies are effective; help the couple alter them if the strategies are not working (Figueiredo, Field, Diego, Hernandez-Reif, Deeds, & Ascencio, 2008).

      (7) Help couple to identify and use support systems.

  b. Outcomes

      (1) Couple can verbalize feelings and concerns to each other and to the health care provider.

      (2) Couple discusses available support systems and uses them (family, friends, and other expectant families).

      (3) Couple attends childbirth and/or childcare classes together.

      (4) Couple demonstrates mutual support.

      (5) Couple seeks help with emotional concerns about prenatal testing (Griffiths & Kuppermann, 2008; Lobel, Dias, & Myer, 2005; Sun, Hsia, & Sheu, 2008; Wright, 2008).

6. Fear of the unknown

  a. Interventions

      (1) Offer individual education and information and encourage attendance at childbirth classes and parenting classes.

      (2) Explain all procedures and rationales before implementing them, and keep parents informed of progress.

      (3) Help couple verbalize fears and determine the level of anxiety (from mild anxiety to panic).

      (4) If anxiety is related to a specific maternal or fetal complication, refer the couple to an appropriate resource.

      (5) Avoid overburdening couple with too much information at one time.

      (6) Assist family to develop a realistic birth plan focusing on concerns and to gain a sense of control.

         (a) Primigravida: help to focus on alternatives and to transform dreams and fantasies into choices.

         (b) Multigravida: assess what went well in the last labor and birth and what she would like to change this time.

  b. Outcomes

      (1) Couple develops a realistic birth plan with several different, appropriate alternatives and options.

      (2) Couple seeks appropriate resources for specific problems.

      (3) Couple can verbalize fears to health care providers and to each other.

      (4) Couple demonstrates a calmer demeanor with relaxed voices and body language.

      (5) Couple states a feeling of less anxiety and fearfulness.

7. Enhanced family coping due to opportunity for growth and mastery

  a. Interventions

      (1) Offer couple the necessary information for decision making.

      (2) Encourage couple to make decisions based on realistic alternatives.

      (3) Praise couple each time they demonstrate effective coping (e.g., a birth plan, breathing in synchrony, and mutual support).

      (4) If couple is not coping effectively, actively help them regain control.

      (5) Offer oneself as role model to demonstrate skills the couple can learn (e.g., relaxation strategies, breathing techniques).

      (6) Help couple envision changes in plans (e.g., undergoing an unplanned epidural or cesarean birth procedure) as an appropriate coping mechanism within context of a particular situation and not as a failure.

  b. Outcomes

      (1) Couple verbalizes a sense of pride of accomplishment.

      (2) Couple discusses resources and support systems used during pregnancy and childbirth.

      (3) Couple seeks to understand any events during labor and birth that were unclear or misinterpreted and to put them into an appropriate context.

      (4) Couple expresses realistic uncertainties about infant care while expressing confidence in learning.

8. Lack of knowledge and skills about parenting
    a. Interventions
        (1) Help couple develop realistic expectations of themselves as parents.
            (a) Primigravida: help shift the focus from the common myth of blissful newborn parenting to a realistic view of initial sleep deprivation and disorganization
            (b) Multigravida: help identify how a new infant will change the present family constellation and assess family plans to incorporate the new infant into the family's daily life
        (2) Offer hands-on demonstration or return demonstration opportunities for infant care (e.g., bathing or cord care) to increase practical parenting skills.
        (3) Give parents community resources to solicit assistance and support, as needed.
        (4) Send parents home from hospital with written materials to reinforce hospital staff teaching about infant care and parenting.
    b. Outcomes
        (1) Couple demonstrates basic infant care skills with beginning confidence.
        (2) Couple verbalizes a plan for meeting early parenting demands.
        (3) Couple identifies appropriate resources to offer assistance.
9. Coping with mood disorders, eating disorders, or loss
    a. Interventions
        (1) Assess frequently.
        (2) Provide motivational stimulation for health-directed behavior.
        (3) Use praise to affirm weight gain, coping abilities, and adjustment.
        (4) Provide consultation with appropriate health care providers.
        (5) Provide support group information and encouragement.
        (6) Evaluate grief response of father and mother of ill or preterm infants separately as well as together.
    b. Evaluation
        (1) Women with eating disorders will gain adequate weight during pregnancy and transit through the postpartum period without additional difficulties.
        (2) Women with mood disorders will demonstrate appropriate care of self and infant.
        (3) Couples experiencing loss of the perfect child will experience an appropriate adjustment.
10. Grief due to the birth of an ill, preterm, or congenitally anomalous newborn
    a. Interventions
        (1) Provide information and support.
        (2) Allow parents to participate in care as much as they desire and as is possible.
        (3) Encourage couple to talk about their feelings and concerns.
    b. Outcomes
        (1) Couple will verbalize their feelings and concerns; ask appropriate questions.
        (2) Couple will verbalize realistic expectations.
11. Dysfunctional grieving due to stillbirth, ill or preterm newborn, loss of perfect child, loss of pregnancy, or loss of desired labor or birth experience
    a. Interventions
        (1) Provide information and support.
        (2) Allow venting of feelings and concerns.
        (3) Encourage parental participation in care.
        (4) Assess parental grief responses; provide validation of their experience and feelings.
        (5) Provide "tokens" of stillborn or expired infant with pictures, hair clippings, handprints and footprints, etc.
        (6) Maintain continuity in caregivers as possible.
        (7) Refer to support groups.
    b. Outcomes
        (1) Couple will demonstrate individual and family progress in the grieving process.
        (2) Parents of ill or preterm infants will participate in infant care.

HEALTH EDUCATION

A. **Early pregnancy**
   1. Developmental tasks of pregnancy
      a. Mother: acceptance of pregnancy integration into her self-system
      b. Father: announcement and realization of the pregnancy
      c. Couple: realignment of relationships and roles
   2. Psychosocial changes of pregnancy
      a. Ambivalence about pregnancy
      b. Introversion
      c. Passivity and difficulty with decision making
      d. Sexual and emotional changes (Foux, 2008)
      e. Changing self-image
      f. Ethical dilemmas of prenatal testing (Ekberg, 2007)
B. **Second trimester**
   1. Developmental tasks of pregnancy (Brotherson, 2007).
      a. Mother: binding-in to the pregnancy, ensuring safe passage, and differentiating the fetus from herself
      b. Father: anticipation of adapting to the role of fatherhood
      c. Couple: realignment of roles and division of tasks
   2. Psychosocial changes
      a. Active dream and fantasy life
      b. Concerns with body image
      c. Nesting behaviors
      d. Sexual behavior adjustment
      e. Expanding to a variety of methods of expressing affection and intimacy
C. **Third trimester**
   1. Developmental tasks of pregnancy
      a. Mother: separating herself from the pregnancy and the fetus; trying various caregiving methods
      b. Father: role adaptation; preparation for labor and birth
      c. Couple: preparation of the nursery
   2. Psychosocial changes
      a. Dislikes being pregnant but loves the child
      b. Although anxious about childbirth, the mother also sees labor and delivery as a deliverance.
      c. The couple experiments with various mothering or fathering roles.
      d. Mother is introspective.
D. **Evaluation**
   1. Couple can verbalize the educational content.
   2. Couple seeks assistance and support with psychologic concerns.
   3. Couple demonstrates insight into psychologic processes (e.g., increasing introspection and isolation during labor).

CASE STUDY AND STUDY QUESTIONS

Mrs. L. is a 30-year-old primigravida and the last of her friends to become pregnant. Although she and her husband wanted a child, they had not expected it to happen so quickly after stopping birth control pills. She confided to the nurse that she was not sure she really wanted to be pregnant. When her ultrasound and alpha-fetoprotein tests were normal, she began to really embrace pregnancy. She frequently spent time with her friends and family who had children to learn about their experiences.

Mr. L. was very excited about the pregnancy and had nausea when his wife did and even gained more weight than she did in the first trimester. However, Mrs. L. was experiencing strange dreams and fantasies and was beginning to think she was crazy until her friends told her they had also had strange dreams. Her mother, who is a labor nurse, bought them almost every book about pregnancy and birth that was available at the local bookstore. Some of the ideas the couple read sounded really strange and "far-out." However, as they continued to read, they found ideas that were comfortable for them. Mr. L. was enthusiastic about learning to be a good support person for Mrs. L., but wanted Mrs. L. to have the most say about the experience because it was she who would actually experience labor. They learned that the hospital in which they would deliver had a very high induction and epidural rate, and wished that they had known more before they chose their care provider and hospital. They were concerned about their ability to accomplish their dreams of an unmedicated birth in such an environment. Their childbirth educator helped them to develop a birth plan and coached them in assertiveness techniques while encouraging them to explore alternatives just in case not all went according to the ideal. They arrived in the labor suite feeling confident and able.

1. When a woman desires to have a child and learns that she is pregnant, her emotions might include:
   a. Ambivalence
   b. Joy
   c. Surprise
   d. All of the above
2. Men whose partners are pregnant sometimes experience sympathetic feelings and symptoms called:
   a. Pseudopregnancy
   b. Male pregnancy
   c. Couvade
   d. Pseudogestation
3. Pregnant women who tell the nurse about strange dreams should be:
   a. Referred to a psychiatrist
   b. Assured that such dreams are common and normal in pregnancy
   c. Offered a psychosocial interpretation
   d. Told to ignore them
4. The concept of developing a birth plan:
   a. Should upset nurses who are the real experts about labor and birth
   b. Is illegal in some states
   c. Is acceptable only in home births
   d. Increases a couple's sense of control and mastery
5. Many Native American women do not seek prenatal care because:

a. They see tribal healers instead
b. They remain in bed throughout pregnancy
c. They believe that pregnancy is normal, and it is therefore unnecessary to see a physician
d. None of the above
6. The critical third-trimester issue in acceptance of the child is that:
   a. The nursery is ready
   b. The family describes the fetus as a real person
   c. Acceptance is unconditional
   d. The father is concerned about the infant's well-being
7. Nesting behaviors are disrupted by:
   a. Baby showers
   b. Preterm labor
   c. Father's business plans
   d. Anxiety about labor
8. Two third-trimester developmental tasks of expectant fathers include:
   a. His changing image and negotiation of his role during labor and delivery
   b. Taking on the expectant father role and preparing the nursery
   c. Preparing for parenthood and accepting the woman's changing body
   d. Dealing with the woman's introspection and accepting the biologic fact of pregnancy
9. A common principle found among many ethnic cultures is that:
   a. Pregnant women are sick
   b. Everything in nature is balanced (e.g., yin/yang)
   c. A pregnant woman must wear a gold necklace in labor
   d. A pregnant woman's mother must be barred from the birth
10. If expectant parents tell the labor nurse that they have taken childbirth classes, have chosen a possible name for their infant, have decided to breastfeed, and have prepared their home for the newborn, the nurse can surmise they are successfully coping with changes in:
    a. The expectant couple role
    b. Self-concept as a couple
    c. The developmental stressors of pregnancy
    d. Anxiety

ANSWERS TO STUDY QUESTIONS

1. d
2. c
3. b
4. d

5. c
6. c
7. b
8. a

9. b
10. b

REFERENCES

Bansil, P., Kulina, E. V., Whiteman, M. K., Kourtis, A. P., Posner, S. F., Johnson, C. H., & Jamieson, D. J. (2008). Eating disorders among delivery hospitalizations; prevalence and outcomes. *Journal of Women's Health, 17*(9), 1523–1528.

Brotherson, S. E. (2007). From partners to parents: Couples and the transition to parenthood. *International Journal of Childbirth Education, 22*(2), 7–12.

Deave, T., & Johnson, D. (2008). The transition to parenthood: What does it mean for fathers? *Journal of Advanced Nursing, 6*(3), 399–420.

Deering, S. H., Zaret, J., McGaha, K., & Satin, A. J. (2007). Patients presenting with birth plans: A case-control study of delivery outcomes. *Journal of Reproductive Medicine, 52*(10), 884–887.

Duvall, E. (1985). *Marriage and family development.* New York: Harper & Row.

Ekberg, M. (2007). Maximizing the benefits and minimizing the risks associated with prenatal genetic testing. *Health, Risk & Society, 9*(1), 67–81.

Figueiredo, B., Field, T., Diego, M., Hernandez-Reif, M., Deeds, O., & Ascencio, A. (2008). Partner relationships during the transition to parenthood. *Journal of Reproductive and Infant Psychology, 26*(2), 99–107.

Foux, E. (2008). Sex education in pregnancy: Does it exist? A literature review. *Sexual and Relationship Therapy, 23*(3), 271–277.

Griffiths, C., & Kuppermann, M. (2008). Perceptions of prenatal testing for birth defects among rural Latinas. *Maternal and Child Health Journal, 12*(1), 34–42.

Halle, C., Dowd, T., Fowler, C., Rissel, K., Hennessy, K., et al. (2008). Supporting fathers in the transition to parenthood. *Contemporary Nurse: A Journal for the Australian Nursing Profession, 31*(1), 57–70.

Kornelsen, J. (2005). Essences and imperatives: An investigation of technology in childbirth. *Social Science and Medicine, 61*(7), 1495–1504.

Lobel, M., Dias, L., & Meyer, B. A. (2005). Distress associated with prenatal screening for fetal abnormality. *Journal of Behavioral Medicine, 28*(1), 65–76.

Lothian, J. (2006). Birth plans: The good, the bad, and the future. *JOGNN: Journal of Obstetric, Gynecologic, & Neonatal Nursing, 35*(2), 295–303.

Lutz, K., & May, K. A. (2007). The impact of high-risk pregnancy on the transition to parenthood. *Journal of Childbirth Education, 22*(3), 20–22.

Nerum, H., Halverson, L., Sorlie, T., & Oian, P. (2006). Maternal request for cesarean section due to fear of birth: Can it be changed through crisis-oriented counseling? *Issues in Perinatal Care, 33*(3),221–228.

Rubin, R. (1984). *Maternal identity and the maternal experience.* New York: Springer.

Sittner, B. J., DeFrain, J., & Judson, D. B. (2005). Effects of high-risk pregnancies on families. *The American Journal of Maternal Child Nursing, 30*(2), 121–126.

Sun, J., Hsia, P., & Sheu, S. (2008). Women of advanced maternal age undergoing amniocentesis: A period of uncertainty. *Journal of Clinical Nursing, 17*(21), 2829–2837.

Wright, J. A. (2008). Prenatal and postnatal diagnosis of infant disability: Breaking the news to mothers. *Journal of Perinatal Education, 17*(3), 27–32.

BIBLIOGRAPHY

Ahmed, S., Hewison, J., Green, J. M., Cuckle, H. S., Hirst, J., & Thornton, J. G. (2008). Decisions about testing and termination of pregnancy for different fetal conditions: A qualitative study of European white and Pakistani mothers of affected children. *Journal of Genetic Counseling, 17*(6), 560–572.

American Psychiatric Association (2000). *Diagnostic and statistical manual of mental disorders* (4th ed.). Arlington, VA: American Psychiatric Association.

Bronte-Tinkew, J., Carrano, J., Horowitz, A., & Kinukawa, A. (2008). Involvement among resident fathers and links to infant cognitive outcomes. *Journal of Family Issues, 29*(9), 1144–1211.

Dallas, C. (2004). Family matters: How mothers of adolescent parents experience adolescent pregnancy and parenting. *Public Health Nursing, 21*(4), 347–353.

Essex, H. N., & Pickett, K. E. (2008). Mothers without companionship during childbirth: An analysis with the millennium cohort study. *Birth: Issues in Perinatal Care, 35*(4), 266–276.

Fleuriet, K. J. (2009). Problems in the Latina paradox: measuring social support for pregnant immigrant women from Mexico. *Anthropology and Medicine, 16*(1), 49–59.

Paul, T. A. (2008). Prevalence of posttraumatic stress symptoms after childbirth: Does ethnicity have an impact? *Journal of Perinatal Education, 17*(3), 17–26.

Waller, M. R., & Bitler, M. P. (2008). The link between couples' pregnancy intentions and behavior: Does it matter who is asked? *Perspectives on Sexual and Reproductive Health, 40*(4), 194–201.

Wilson, E. K. (2008). Acculturation and changes in the likelihood of pregnancy and feelings about pregnancy among women of Mexican origin. *Women and Health, 47*(1), 45–64.

MATERNAL-FETAL WELL-BEING

 7 Age-Related Concerns

Connie Sampson von Köhler

OBJECTIVES

1. Identify the risks of childbearing that are related to adolescents.
2. Identify the risks of childbearing that are related to advanced maternal age.
3. Distinguish between the risks that can be attributed solely to biologic age factors and the risks that can be attributed to sociocultural and economic factors.
4. Select interventions that correspond to the developmental level of a pregnant adolescent.
5. Design and implement health education that reflects a sensitivity to the specialized needs of younger expectant parents and older expectant parents

INTRODUCTION

Pregnancy that occurs at the two age extremes (younger than 19 and older than 35 years) of a woman's childbearing years places the expectant mother and the fetus at risk for age-related complications. The maternal mortality risk for adolescents younger than 17 years has been reported to be twice that of adult pregnant women (Klein, 2005). However, the increased risks of age extremes might be related more to sociocultural and economic factors than to the biologic factors of age. Many of these risks can be minimized through the use of current technology, education, and consistent prenatal care. Certainly, preexisting biologic conditions might require management by a high-risk team, regardless of the age of the woman (Suplee, Dawley, & Bloch, 2007).

Pregnancy in women 35 years and older who deliver in settings in which current technology is available might be at no higher risk for an adverse outcome than pregnancy in younger women. The trend toward technology to treat infertility has led to the possibility of childbirth in women of any age (Suplee, Dawley, & Bloch, 2007). Using surrogacy or egg donors, women well into the menopausal years can have children.

Each year more than 750,000 adolescents become pregnant in the United States (American College of Obstetricians and Gynecologists [ACOG], 2007a). For the first time in 15 years, the teen birth rate rose in 2006 by 3%. This followed a 14-year downward trend in which teen births steadily fell 34% from the 1991 peak (Hamilton, Martin, & Ventura, 2007). In 2007 the birth rate among teens 15 to 19 years old was 45.2% (Hamiton, Martin & Ventura, 2007). The United States continues to have the highest teen pregnancy rate among all developed countries (ACOG, 2007b). Once an adolescent has had an infant, she is at increased risk for another teen pregnancy (Ladewig, London, & Davidson, 2010). Approximately 25% of adolescents giving birth had a previous birth (Klein, 2005). With early and thorough prenatal care, adolescents older than the age of 15 years experience no greater risks than those of the general pregnant population (Ladewig, London, & Davidson, 2010). Although the incidence of certain complications might be higher because of age extremes, the diagnoses, interventions, and evaluations remain relatively unchanged from those for the general pregnant population with the same complications.

CLINICAL PRACTICE

Adolescence

A. **Assessment**
  1. History (specifics to add related to the adolescent's age)
     a. Age at menarche
        (1) Several of the first menstrual cycles are anovulatory and irregular, making gestational dating difficult.

(2) Long bone growth is incomplete until approximately 2 years after menarche, and the pelvis does not reach adult size until 1 to 3 years after menarche; there is an increased risk of cephalopelvic disproportion (CPD) among young adolescents because of lack of pelvic maturity (Davidson, London, & Ladewig, 2008).

b. Number of sexual partners

(1) Having multiple sexual partners increases the risk of concurrent sexually transmitted diseases; adolescents will frequently have serial monogamous relationships (i.e., one short-term monogamous relationship that is followed by another, and then another).

(2) Each year young adults who are 15 to 24 years old account for 48% of all newly reported cases of sexually transmitted diseases in the United States (Guttmacher Institute, 2006).

c. Knowledge about how conception occurs

d. Planned or unplanned pregnancy: more than 90% of teens described their pregnancies as unintended (Klein, 2005)

e. Previous pregnancies

(1) Term or preterm

(2) Spontaneous abortions

(3) Therapeutic abortions

f. Contraceptive use: although statistics indicate an increased use of condoms among the adolescent population, adolescents are still inconsistent contraceptive users (Ladewig, London, & Davidson, 2010). The majority of sexually active teens (74% of females and 82% of males) used contraceptives the first time they had sex (Guttmacher Institute, 2006) and 62.8% reported using a condom during their last sexual intercourse (Ladewig, London, & Davidson, 2010).

(1) Type

(2) Frequency of use

(3) Last time used

(4) Non-use

g. Dietary intake

(1) Is frequently inadequate in adolescents; there is a high incidence of pregnancy-related, iron deficiency anemia in pregnant adolescents who are younger than 17 (Davidson, London, & Ladewig, 2008)

(2) Caloric restriction can occur when the pregnant adolescent attempts to "not get fat," to control abdominal protrusion, or to deny the pregnancy to herself and others (Davidson, London, & Ladewig, 2008).

(3) Overeating might occur to mask the body's changes of pregnancy.

(4) Overweight and obesity prior to pregnancy: 17.4% of the adolesent population is overweight (National Center for Health Statistics, 2006). There are significant health risks and implications for prepregnant maternal obesity for mother and child (Stothard, Tennant, Bell, & Rankin, 2009)

(5) The incidence of eating disorders might be high among adolescents as a group (Ladewig, London, & Davidson, 2010).

(6) Good maternal weight gain during an adolescent pregnancy improves fetal growth and reduces mortality (Ladewig, London, & Davidson, 2010).

(a) Young pregnant adolescents should strive for a weight gain at the upper end of the range for an adult pregnant woman.

(b) Young pregnant adolescents should consume as much as 50 kcal/kg of nutrition per day, if active.

h. Prenatal care

(1) Some adolescents have no prenatal care, might not have known they were pregnant, deny their pregnancy, or are confused about available prenatal services (Corbett, 2007).

(2) Prenatal care is frequently started in middle to late pregnancy (ACOG, 2007b; Ladewig, London, & Davidson, 2010).

(3) Sporadic prenatal care and missed appointments are prevalent.

(4) Adolescents who lack adequate and early prenatal care have an increased incidence of pregnancy complications and tend to give birth to low-birthweight babies (ACOG, 2007b). Among this age group, prenatal care is the critical factor that has the most influence on the pregnancy outcome (Ladewig, London, & Davidson, 2010).

    i. Risk taking behaviors

        (1) Adolescents between the ages of 15 and 19 have a high incidence of sexually transmitted infections (STIs) including genital herpes, gonorrhea, syphilis, and chlamydia (Ladewig, London, & Davidson, 2010).

        (2) Alcohol, tobacco, and illicit drug use

        (3) Tattooing and piercing

    j. Social support system plays an important part in transitioning the teen to the role of mother (Logsdon & Koniak-Griffin, 2005).

        (1) Financial

            (a) Having a child at an early age is a strong predictor that the the adolescent's children will live in poverty.

            (b) Adolescent mothers tend to fail at establishing a stable family at such a young age (Ladewig, London, & Davidson, 2010).

        (2) Emotional: father of child

            (a) An adolescent father is usually not prepared (maturational or psychologic) to deal with the consequences of pregnancy.

            (b) Studies indicate that between 16% to 37% of pregnant adolescents experience domestic violence (Ladewig, London, & Davidson, 2010).

        (3) Marital status; majority of adolescent marriages end in divorce

        (4) Parents' awareness of and attitude toward their teenage daughter's pregnancy

    k. Attendance at prenatal classes

2. Developmental assessment

    a. The overall developmental tasks of an adolescent are:

        (1) Acceptance of and comfort with one's body image

        (2) Internalization of a sexual identity and role

        (3) Development of a personal value system

        (4) Development of a sense of productivity

        (5) Identification of a life's work

        (6) Achievement of a sense of independence

        (7) Development of an adult identity

    b. The early-adolescent girl (younger than 15 years)

        (1) Is a concrete thinker

        (2) Usually has some degree of discomfort with normal body changes and body image

        (3) Usually has only a minimal ability to foresee the consequences of her behavior and see herself in the future

        (4) Usually has an external locus of control

    c. The middle-adolescent girl (15 to 17 years)

        (1) Is prone to experimentation and challenges

            (a) Drugs and alcohol

            (b) Tattoos and piercings

            (c) Sex

            (d) Feeling invulnerable

        (2) Seeks independence and frequently turns to her peer group for support, information, and advice; pregnancy at this age can force a parental dependency and interfere with her striving for independence (Ladewig, London, & Davidson, 2010)

        (3) Is capable of formal operational thought and abstract thinking, but might have difficulty anticipating the long-term implications of her actions

    d. The late-adolescent girl (17 to 19 years)

        (1) Is developing individuality

        (2) Is capable of thinking abstractly and anticipating consequences

        (3) Is capable of problem solving and decision making

        (4) Can picture herself in control

3. Physical findings (specifics related to the adolescent girl's age)

    a. Bone growth is still incomplete in early adolescence.

        (1) If pregnancy occurs before bone growth is complete, it can interfere with or arrest further bone growth.

            (a) The first 4 years after menarche carry the highest risk (Ladewig, London, & Davidson, 2010).

(b) An increase of estrogen during this time, caused by pregnancy, can lead to the early closure of the epiphysis.

(2) Pelvic bones have not reached adult female dimensions: the incidence of cephalopelvic disproportion, leading to cesarean section, is increased (Davidson, London, & Ladewig, 2008).

b. Signs of hypertensive disorders in pregnancy; preeclampsia is primarily a disease of first pregnancies and maternal age extremes (Peters, 2008). (See Chapter 19 for a complete discussion of hypertensive disorders in pregnancy.)

c. Signs of intrauterine growth restriction

(1) Morbidity in babies of adolescents might be attributed to two common causes: prematurity and low birthweight (Klein, 2005).

(2) Adolescents have a higher incidence of low-birthweight infants, especially very young girls ages 14 or younger (Klein, 2005).

(3) Fundal height and gestational age discrepancy might be noted.

(4) Inadequate nutritional status might be evidenced by low weight gain; nutritional needs include:

(a) Additional amounts of protein, iron, and calcium needed to support the adolescent's growth and fetal development (Ladewig, London & Davidson, 2010).

(b) Folic acid supplementation (Ladewig, London, & Davidson, 2010)

(5) Signs of infection (see Chapter 20 for a complete discussion of intrauterine infection and Chapter 17 for a discussion of congenital infections of the neonate)

B. Interventions/Outcomes

1. Delayed growth and development due to adolescent pregnancy

a. Interventions

(1) Adapt the nutritional requirements of pregnancy to the individual adolescent's likes, cultural influences, economic resources, and peer-group habits.

(a) Instruct the adolescent about how to make the most nutritious selections from fast-food menus without attracting peer attention.

(b) Instruct the adolescent about how to select and plan for healthy snacks when she is away from home and at home.

(2) Adapt all interventions to correspond with the adolescent's developmental level.

(a) Help her develop and use decision-making skills that are appropriate to her developmental level; because teens tend to be self-centered, consider ways to motivate her to participate in health care and health education.

(b) Help her develop and use problem-solving skills that are appropriate to her developmental level; focus on those areas that are of most concern to her (Davidson, London, & Ladewig, 2008).

(c) Actively involve her in her own care.

[i] Have her listen to fetal heart tones.

[ii] Have her place her hands on palpable fetal parts in late pregnancy and help her to visualize the fetal position.

[iii] Help her see how good nutrition benefits her skin and hair texture and how it prevents her from gaining excess weight.

b. Outcomes

(1) Pregnant adolescent will be able to select and consume a nutritious diet without feeling conspicuous among her peers.

(2) Pregnant adolescent will show an active involvement in her own care.

(3) Pregnant adolescent will seek information and make decisions that are appropriate for her developmental level.

2. The adolescent's denial of pregnancy

a. Interventions

(1) Develop a trusting relationship with the adolescent (King-Jones, 2008).

(a) Listen attentively.

(b) Maintain a nonjudgmental approach.

(c) Avoid sounding like a parent to the adolescent (i.e., avoid using the word "should," giving unwanted advice, making decisions for her).

(d) Recognize the unique problems of the adolescent as they relate to her individual situation.

(e) Determine her individual strengths, and compliment her on these strengths.

(2) Assist her in developing and using decision-making and problem-solving skills related to her developmental level.

(a) Encourage her to include her family as a resource, if appropriate, in decision making and problem solving.

(b) If inappropriate to include her family in the decision-making process, encourage the adolescent to communicate to her family the thoughts and resources she used to arrive at her decisions.

(c) Support and encourage her well-thought-out decisions; praise her abilities and her approximations toward thoughtful decisions.

(3) Seek involvement of the adolescent's mother, older sister, or other close female relative, if appropriate.

b. Outcomes

(1) Pregnant adolescent will develop a trusting relationship with the nurse.

(2) Pregnant adolescent will be able to include her parents or another relative in the problem-solving process, if at all possible, and seek the support of her family, if appropriate.

3. Poor eating habits and inadequate nutritional balance

a. Interventions

(1) Adapt nutritional requirements of pregnancy to the individual adolescent's likes, cultural influences, economic resources, and peer-group habits.

(2) Instruct adolescent about how to make the most nutritious selections from fast-food menus without attracting peer attention.

(3) Instruct adolescent about how to select and plan for healthy snacks when she is both away from home and at home.

(4) Describe to her how good nutrition benefits her skin and hair texture and how it prevents her from gaining excess weight.

b. Outcome: pregnant adolescent will select and consume all nutrients necessary for continued individual growth and fetal development

4. Inconsistant and/or late prenatal care

a. Interventions

(1) Give specific information about the effect or purpose of each procedure that is conducted during a prenatal visit.

(a) Explanations must be appropriate to the adolescent's developmental level.

(b) Provide attractive drawings of the fetus at the current gestational stage, and inform the client of the appearance and capabilities of the fetus at every visit.

(c) Adolescents have a tendency to be egocentric.

[i] Effects of maternal health and habits on the fetus might not be regarded as important by the adolescent.

[ii] Emphasize the effects of health maintenance on her own well-being (see previous discussion under alteration in growth and development).

(2) Adapt prenatal instructions to the adolescent's lifestyle as much as possible.

b. Outcomes

(1) Adolescent will seek prenatal care within the first trimester of her pregnancy.

(2) Adolescent will receive consistent prenatal care throughout her pregnancy.

(3) Pregnant adolescent will demonstrate an adequate knowledge of the value of prenatal care and demonstrate compliance with instructions.

Advanced Maternal Age

In 2007 the U.S. birth rates for women in the age range of 35 to 39 years was 47.5%; in the age range of 40 to 44 years 9.5%, and in the age range of 45 to 49 years, 6%. This trend has shown an increase over previous years (Hamilton, Martin, & Ventura, 2007). Clearly, pregnancy at or beyond what was commonly thought of as the far end of a woman's reproductive age has become more prevalent. With implementation of infertility technologies, the boundaries of reproductive age have been challenged.

A. Assessment

1. History

a. Conception problems: in the average woman, declining fertility begins at ages 37 to 38. Fertility rates are 26% to 46% lower in women ages 35 to 39 and as much as 95% lower between ages 40 and 45 (Speroff & Fritz, 2005). The chances of pregnancy decrease with age whether assisted or unassisted (Suplee, Dawley, & Bloch, 2007).

(1) Any tests, treatments, or procedures that were used to facilitate conception
    (a) Diagnostic tests
        [i] Ovarian function
        [ii] Semen analysis
        [iii] Uterine assessment
        [iv] Hormonal function tests
        [v] Endometrial assessment
        [vi] Tubal patency assessment
    (b) Treatments/procedures
        [i] Fertility drugs to induce ovulation
        [ii] Artificial insemination
    (c) Assisted reproductive technologies (ART) (Speroff & Fritz, 2005)
        [i] In vitro fertilization (IVF): oocyte fertilized in the laboratory; resulting embryo transferred to uterus
        [ii] Gamete intrafallopian transfer (GIFT): gametes (oocyte and sperm) transferred to fallopian tubes; zygote intrafallopian transfer (ZIFT) or tubal embryo transfer (TET) via laparoscopy (Speroff & Fritz, 2005)
        [iii] Intracytoplasmic sperm injection (ICSI): one sperm injected into the cytoplasm of the oocyte
          • Microsurgical epididymal sperm aspiration (MESA)
          • Testicular sperm extraction (TESE)
        [iv] Assisted hatching: hole made in zona pellucida with microinjection needle or laser to enhance embryo hatching (used with frozen embryos)
        [v] Donor oocytes: oocytes retrieved from donor, inseminated, and resulting embryo transferred to recipient using IVF
        [vi] Gestational carrier: IVF with resulting embryos transferred to the uterus of another woman who will carry the pregnancy
        [vii] Embryo cryopreservation: pregnancy can be achieved by using previously frozen embryos from IVF, GIFT, or ZIFT
        [viii] Embryo donation: previously cryopreserved embryos are donated to be transferred to the uterus of a recipient woman who has been prepared for implantation with estrogen and progesterone
(2) Duration of the conception problem
(3) Gynecologic conditions predisposing to fertility problems
    (a) Uterine fibroids
    (b) Endometriosis
    (c) Pelvic inflammatory disease (PID)

b. Previous pregnancies (parity)
    (1) Problems conceiving
    (2) Complications during the pregnancy
c. Planned or unplanned pregnancy
d. Occupation or career
    (1) Women older than 35 years might have advanced in their careers to a level of high responsibility and high stress (Suplee, Dawley, & Bloch, 2007). They:
        (a) Frequently are college educated
        (b) Frequently have high achievement needs
        (c) Usually have a deep psychologic investment in their careers
    (2) Career women older than 35 years might have difficulty balancing a career with the physical and psychologic demands of pregnancy.
    (3) Women older than 35 years might have difficulty with or feel an increased ambivalence about changing their roles.
        (a) During the postpartum period, women must make decisions about whether to return to work and, if they plan to, when they will return.
        (b) They must make decisions about obtaining adequate child care if they will return to work and must deal with the feelings of combining motherhood and a career.

    e. Comorbidities are more common (38% to 50%) in women older than 35 years and might affect the pregnancy (e.g., diabetes, hypertension, obesity, cancer, decreased cardiovascular reserve, lupus, or multiple sclerosis) (Bravemen, 2006; Luke & Brown, 2007; Suplee, Dawley, & Bloch, 2007).

2. Physical assessment (specific to advanced maternal age)

    a. Genetic testing (see Chapter 2 for a complete discussion of genetics.)

        (1) Incidence of chromosomal abnormalities increases with age.

        (2) Quad marker screen: maternal serum alpha-fetoprotein (MS-AFP) detection of chromosomal abnormalities

        (3) Chorionic villus sampling or amniocentesis is performed for the detection of chromosomal abnormalities.

        (4) Ultrasound; alternative and possible complementary screen for Down syndrome; first-trimester fetal nuchal translucency, second-trimester genetic sonogram (Benacerraf, 2005)

    b. Signs of diabetes (see Chapter 22 for a complete discussion of diabetes in pregnancy)

        (1) Incidence of gestational diabetes is increased in women older than 35 years (Luke & Brown, 2007; Suplee, Dawley, & Bloch, 2007).

        (2) Blood glucose tolerance screening may be performed earlier than the routine screening.

    c. Signs of hypertension (see Chapter 19 for a complete discussion of hypertensive disorders in pregnancy). Incidence of hypertensive disorders in pregnancy (preeclampsia) are increased in women older than 35 years (Luke & Brown, 2007; Peters, 2008).

    d. Fundal height and due-date discrepancy

        (1) Women older than 35 years are at higher risk for low-birthweight term infants, preterm delivery prior to 32 weeks, and very-low-birthweight infants (Luke & Brown, 2007).

        (2) There is an increased incidence of multiple gestation in women older than 35 years.

    e. Women of advanced maternal age have an increased risk of stillbirth (Huang, Sauve, Birkett, Fergusson, & van Walraven, 2008).

    f. Vaginal bleeding: there is an increased incidence of gestational bleeding in women older than 35 years (see Chapter 21 on hemorrhagic disorders in pregnancy for a complete discussion of bleeding during pregnancy).

        (1) Increased incidence of abruptio placentae (Luke & Brown, 2007)

        (2) Increased incidence of placenta previa (Luke & Brown, 2007)

        (3) Increased incidence of trophoblastic disease, particularly in women who are older than 40 years; possibly related to defects in oocyte function (Altman, Bentley, Murray, & Bentley, 2008).

    g. For pregnant women older than age 35, and particularly those who have had infertility treatment/assisted reproduction, there is an increased incidence of cesarean section, elective and emergency as well as prolonged and dysfuntional labor (Luke & Brown, 2007).

B. Interventions/Outcomes

1. Anxiety due to possible complications of pregnancy

    a. Interventions

        (1) Treat the pregnancy as normal unless specific complications are identified.

        (2) Reassure client that good nutrition, health habits, and consistent prenatal care significantly reduce the risks associated with advanced maternal age.

        (3) Stress importance of consistent prenatal care to detect any complications early, when treatment is most effective.

        (4) Review danger signs in pregnancy, and rehearse the appropriate responses to them so that the client feels confident about what to do.

    b. Outcomes

        (1) Client of an advanced maternal age will feel that her pregnancy is normal, unless specific complications are identified.

        (2) Pregnant client of an advanced maternal age who has identified risks and complications will feel confident in the care and treatment she receives to minimize her risks and complications.

        (3) Client of an advanced maternal age will seek and receive early prenatal care.

2. Anxiety due to possible chromosomal abnormality in the fetus

    a. Interventions

        (1) Encourage genetic counseling to identify risks, and discuss implications of testing to enhance decision making.

    (2) Decision to undergo genetic screening might be related to beliefs and attitudes about abortion; therefore, the nurse must respect the client's decision.

    (3) Support client and encourage her to ventilate her anxiety during days of waiting for genetic screening results.

  b. Outcomes

    (1) Pregnant client of an advanced maternal age will make an informed choice about whether she will undergo genetic studies and will feel confident about her decision.

    (2) Pregnant client of an advanced maternal age and her partner will understand what is taking place on a technical level during the waiting period after amniocentesis for a chromosomal study and will verbalize their frustration and anxiety associated with delayed results.

 3. Parenting related to late childbearing

  a. Interventions

    (1) Encourage expectant parents' attendance at parenting classes before the infant's birth.

    (2) Identify and promote individual strengths and the advantages related to late childbearing.

     (a) Financial security has usually been achieved.

     (b) Education has usually been completed.

     (c) Expectant mother usually is secure in a career or occupation.

     (d) Marriage or relationship has had opportunity to stabilize.

     (e) Woman has had a child-free period for personal development before childbearing.

     (f) Personal maturity will generally result in mothers who are more accepting and feel less conflict in their parenting role.

    (3) Anticipate the informational needs of older couples.

     (a) Handling feelings of social isolation that might occur because peers have children who are already teenagers

     (b) Coping with increased energy required to care for newborn and developing strategies to meet the added energy demands

      [i] Getting help in the house, if finances permit

      [ii] Sharing care of newborn with partner

      [iii] Planning naps

      [iv] Preparing and eating simple, nutritious meals

  b. Outcomes

    (1) Pregnant client of an advanced maternal age and her partner will feel confident in their ability to parent their newborn.

    (2) Expectant couple of an advanced age will develop a plan to meet the high-energy demands of newborn care and tailor it to their individual lifestyle.

HEALTH EDUCATION

A. **Adolescence**

 1. Preparation for childbirth classes focused on pregnant adolescents' special concerns

  a. Lack of knowledge about conception and pregnancy, as well as labor and delivery

  b. Alteration in body image issues

  c. Isolation from peer groups

  d. Alteration in education and career goals and plans

 2. Female anatomy and physiology: before, during, and after pregnancy

 3. Conception and contraception

 4. Information about pregnancy alternatives to assist in decision making

  a. Abortion

  b. Adoption: public and private

  c. Single parenting

 5. Parenting classes for adolescents

  a. Child development

  b. Child safety

  c. Discipline

  d. Childcare arrangements

6. Setting realistic short-term and long-term goals
   a. Returning to school or continuing educational plans
   b. Career or life plans
   c. Adequate child care
   d. Financial considerations
   e. Social relationships

B. Advanced maternal age
   1. Preparation for childbirth and parenting skill classes developed to accommodate the special concerns and needs of older expectant parents
   2. Alteration in lifestyles and habits to adapt to a child
   3. Combining career and quality parenting

CASE STUDIES AND STUDY QUESTIONS

Ms. C. is a 14½-year-old high school student, gravida 1, para 0 (G1, P0). Her last menstrual period was approximately 5 months ago, as best she remembers. She has had unprotected intercourse sporadically during the past year. She has had three sexual partners since she became sexually active and one steady boyfriend for the past 6 months. She states that her parents are unaware that she is sexually active and would never suspect that she might be pregnant. In fact, she is surprised that her pregnancy test result is positive and stated that she "doesn't do it that often." She says that her periods have always been irregular since the beginning (menarche was at age 12). Skipping a few months was not unusual, and she did not think much about it. She states that recently it has been difficult to control her weight, that she has had to be stringent about what she eats, and that some days she does not eat at all, just to stay at her present weight. She complains that despite all this effort, her clothes are uncomfortably tight and she feels fat. She denies tobacco or other drug use and states that she drinks beer only at parties. She has come to the clinic for birth control. The results of a physical examination are as follows: blood pressure, 118/60; height, 162.6 cm (5 feet, 4 inches); weight 52.6 kg (116 pounds) (prepregnant weight, 52.6 kg); urine, trace protein, no sugar; fundal height, 14 cm; ultrasound test results, intrauterine pregnancy at 16 weeks' gestation.

1. Ms. C. states that she cannot believe she is pregnant and that maybe a mistake has been made in the tests. This remark is not unusual because, appropriate to her age, she:
   a. Has the ability to foresee the consequences of her behavior but will not admit it to herself or to anybody else
   b. Is a concrete thinker and has difficulty believing something she cannot see, such as a 16-week pregnancy
   c. Really does know she is pregnant because she is capable of thinking abstractly but cannot deal with the thought of her parents finding out that she is sexually active and now pregnant

2. From the physical findings and her history, she is at greatest risk for and already showing signs of:
   a. Intrauterine growth restriction
   b. Preeclampsia
   c. Gestational diabetes
   d. Sexually transmitted disease because of her multiple sexual partners

3. She proudly states that she has not gained any weight but complains that her clothes are fitting tighter and that she feels fat. The most appropriate intervention would be to:
   a. Reinforce the fact that she is pregnant and needs to eat more to support her own growth and the growth of her fetus.
   b. Tell her not to worry about gaining weight, and explain to her that after she has had the child she will return to her normal weight.
   c. Review her food intake during the past 24 hours, determine her likes and dislikes, and adapt a nutritious diet to her needs.
   d. Encourage her to wear looser clothing so that she will not feel so constricted.

Ms. C. explains that it was difficult for her to get to the clinic. She had to make an excuse to her mother and had to get an older friend to give her a ride. When given the schedule for prenatal clinic visits, she states that the appointments are too frequent and, in her opinion, nothing much is done at each visit. She says she will come as often as she can, but she does not know how often that will be.

4. Her anticipated missed appointments represent the largest problem in the management of adolescent pregnancy, which is:
    a. An adolescent seeks independence; however, the clinic represents authority and has rules.
    b. The pregnant adolescent pictures herself in control and resents being told what she has to do.
    c. Late and inconsistent prenatal care is the cause of most of the complications associated with adolescent pregnancy.

Mrs. M., 42, is an accountant with a prestigious firm in a large metropolitan area. She typically works long hours and must travel on occasion. She enjoys the responsibilities of her career as well as the authority of her position. She has been married to her husband, 43, for 10 years. They had always planned to have a family, but Mrs. M. wanted time to develop her career. She is now pregnant for the first time. She has a history of uterine fibroids, one of which measures 3 cm. Physical findings are as follows: blood pressure, 130/82; height, 167.6 cm (5 feet, 6 inches); weight, 64.9 kg (143 pounds), prepregnant weight, 59 kg (130 pounds); urine, no protein/no sugar; fundal height, 26 cm; ultrasound results show an intrauterine pregnancy at 25 weeks' gestation and marginal placenta previa.

At 16½ weeks' gestation, Mr. and Mrs. M. elected to have amniocentesis performed for genetic testing. They had to wait nearly 2 weeks (10 business days) for the results, making Mrs. M. 18½ weeks into gestation before any information was available.

5. Mr. and Mrs. M. were undecided about what their actions would be if the fetus had chromosomal abnormalities. An important intervention with them would be:
    a. To assist them in clarifying and deciding what their decision is before getting the results so that their emotions will not confuse their decision
    b. To encourage them to talk about their anxieties and concerns about the upcoming results and to delay their final decision making until the results are known

    c. To have them put their worry about the test results aside because there is nothing that they can do about it during the waiting period, and they will just make themselves more anxious by worrying

6. Because of the marginal placenta previa, Mrs. M. is instructed to immediately report any vaginal bleeding, no matter how slight. There is a possibility that the birth will have to be by cesarean section. She cries and wonders aloud why she just cannot be normal, like any other pregnant woman. She states she feels so out of control. The best intervention for her is one based on the concept that:
    a. This is a normal feeling for all pregnant mothers, and she will just have to work through it psychologically.
    b. Because of her age, her fears are heightened related to the fact that she might not have another chance to have a child.
    c. She is exaggerating her situation and creating her own anxiety.
    d. Her career and lifestyle have elements of personal control in them to which she has become accustomed; feeling out of control is distressing for her.

7. Pregnant women older than 35 years have a higher incidence of all of the following except:
    a. Neural tube defects
    b. Gestational diabetes
    c. Multiple gestation
    d. Preeclampsia

8. Women older than 35 years have a higher incidence of gestational bleeding related to:
    a. An incompetent cervix
    b. Clotting abnormalities
    c. Abruptio placentae
    d. Anemia

ANSWERS TO STUDY QUESTIONS

1. b
2. a
3. c
4. c

5. b
6. d
7. a
8. c

REFERENCES

Altman, A. D., Bentley, B., Murray, S., & Bently, J. R. (2008). Maternal age-related rates of gestional trophoblastic disease. *Obstetrics & Gynecology, 112*(2), 244–250.

American College of Obstetricians and Gynecologists. (2007a). *Adolescent facts: Pregnancy and STDs.* Available at www.acog.org/departments/adolescent Health Care.htm. Accessed February 15, 2009.

American College of Obstetricians and Gynecologists. (2007b). *Strategies for adolescent pregnancy prevention.* Available at www.acog.org/department/adolescent HealthCare.htm. Accessed February 15, 2009.

Benacerraf, B. R. (2005). The role of the second trimester genetic sonogram in screening for fetal Down syndrome. *Seminars in Perinatology, 29,* 386–394.

Braveman, F. R. (2006). Pregnancy in patients of advanced maternal age. *Anesthesiology Clinics, 24*(3), 637–646.

Corbett, R. W. (2007). Nursing care during pregnancy. In D. L. Lowdermilk, & S. E. Perry (Eds.), *Maternity & women's health care* (9th ed., pp. 380–427). St. Louis: Mosby.

Davidson, M., London, M., & Ladewig, P. (2008). *Olds' maternal-newborn nursing & women's health across the lifespan* (8th ed.). Upper Saddle River, NJ: Pearson Prentice-Hall.

Guttmacher Institute (2006). *Facts on American teens' sexual and reproductive health.* Available at www.gutmacher.org/pubs/fb_ATSRH.html. Accessed February 15, 2009.

Hamilton, B., Martin, J., & Ventura, S. (2007). Births: Preliminary data for 2007. *National Vital Statistics Report, 57*(12). Available at www.cdc.gov/nchs/data/nvsr/nvsr57_12_tables.pdf. Accessed November, 2009.

Huang, L., Sauve, R., Birkett, N., Fergusson, D., & van Walraven, C. (2008). Maternal age and risk of stillbirth: A systematic review. *Canadian Medical Association Journal, 178*(2), 165–172.

King-Jones, T. (2008). Pregnant adolescents: Perils and pearls of communication. *Nursing for Women's Health, 12*(2), 114–119.

Klein, J. (2005). Adolescent pregnancy: Current trends and issues. *Pediatrics, 116*(1), 281–286.

Ladewig, P., London, M., & Davidson, M. (2010). *Contemporary maternal-newborn nursing care* (7th ed.). Upper Saddle River, NJ: Pearson Education, Inc.

Logsdon, M. C., & Koniak-Griffin, D. (2005). Social support in postpartum adolescents: Guidelines for nursing assessments and interventions. *Journal of Obstetric, Gynecologic, and Neonatal Nursing, 34,* 761–768.

Luke, B., & Brown, M. B. (2007). Elevated risks of pregnancy complications and adverse outcomes with increasing maternal age. *Human Reproduction, 22*(5), 1264–1272.

National Center for Health Statistics. (2006). *Prevalence of overweight among children and adolescents: United States, 2003-2004.* Available at www.cdc.gov/nchs/products/pubs/pubd/hestats/overweight/overwght_child_03.htm. Accessed Feb 15, 2009.

Peters, R. M. (2008). High blood pressure in pregnancy. *Nursing for Women's Health, 12*(5), 410–422.

Speroff, L., & Fritz, M. A. (2005). *Clinical gynecologic endocrinology and infertility* (7th ed., pp. 1013–1067, 1215–1275). Philadelphia: Lippincott Williams & Wilkins .

Stothard, K. J., Tennant, P., Bell, R., & Rankin, J. (2009). Maternal overweight and obesity and the risk of congenital anomalies. *JAMA, 301*(6), 636–650.

Suplee, P. D., Dawley, K., & Bloch, J. R. (2007). Tailoring peripartum nursing care for women of advanced maternal age. *Journal of Obstetric, Gynecologic, and Neonatal Nursing, 36,* 616–623.

8 Antepartum Fetal Assessment

Keiko L. Torgersen

OBJECTIVES

1. Describe the various fetal diagnostic tests performed to evaluate fetal development and well-being.
2. Explain the risks and benefits of the various fetal diagnostic tests.
3. Identify high-risk pregnancy conditions that require fetal surveillance, and discuss appropriate tests for each condition.
4. List the steps in performing each test.
5. Explain the sensitivity of testing parameters for fetal well-being.
6. Describe client needs for high-risk pregnant clients undergoing a fetal diagnostic testing program and the interventions that might be helpful.

INTRODUCTION

Antepartum fetal assessment is an area of increasing importance today, especially as technology has grown and more studies have presented evidence-based information. It is no longer acceptable to take a "wait and see" stance when problems appear during pregnancy. Antepartum fetal assessment can be considered a twofold assessment. The first antepartum assessments occur early in pregnancy often prior to the 20th week of gestation, and generally consist of a variety of diagnostic tests to determine fetal viability, dating of the pregnancy, and/or abnormal fetal development. See Chapter 3 for additional information on fetal development. The second antepartum assessments occur later in pregnancy, after the 20th week of gestation and generally consist of a variety of diagnostic tests to determine fetal well-being or assess for fetal abnormalities. Overall, antepartum fetal assessment is based on biochemical assessment, placental grading, fetal heart rate monitoring, ultrasound biometry, amniotic fluid assessment, Doppler blood flow studies of fetal and uteroplacental circulation, and an evaluation of biophysical fetal parameters. After a pregnancy has been validated, a number of diagnostic tests may be performed to assess the viability, stability, and dating of the pregancy. As the fetus matures in utero, it begins to demonstrate a variety of fetal behaviors. If a fetus demonstrates reassuring behaviors (normal baseline fetal heart rate [FHR], normal FHR variability, presence of accelerations, and absence of decelerations, along with the presence of fetal breathing movements, fetal movements, normal amniotic fluid), the fetus is deemed "healthy" and management is usually conservative. However, in the absence of these reassuring fetal behaviors, additional fetal surveillance and/or preparation for delivery may be indicated.

"Fetal behavior is an excellent diagnostic tool for evaluation of fetal well-being" (Curran & Torgersen, 2006, p. 262). Fetal behavior can be defined as any observable action or reaction to an external stimulus by the fetus (Andonotopo, Stanojevic, Kurjak, Azumendi, & Carrera, 2004; Harman, 2009). Normal fetal behavior can be equated to a normal healthy fetus. Functional development of the fetal brain begins as early as 8 to 10 weeks' gestation, also known as the late embryonic period. With the institution of three-dimensional (3D) and 4D ultrasound, fetal behavior has become more easily tracked in utero. Between 9 and 12 weeks' gestation, fetal movements are characterized by brisk positional and postural changes. Between 13 and 16 weeks' gestation, the changes of position become more prolonged and include flexion and extension of the fetal limbs. Fetuses between 17 and 20 weeks' gestation make slow flexion and extension movements of the trunk, sometimes accompanied by movement of a single limb. By the time the fetus reaches 18 to 20 weeks' gestation, he/she performs slow, supple, and harmonious movements with isolated leg movements (Andonotopo et al, 2004; Harman, 2009; Kurjak et al, 2005).

During the 9 months of gestation, fetal activities constantly expand, which correlates precisely with the development of fetal structures and the maturation of the fetal central nervous system (Morokuma et al 2004). The organization of behavioral states during the last weeks of pregnancy demonstrates that the connection between the fetal cerebral cortex and the fetal periphery is established (Blackburn, 2007). In addition, this organization demonstrates that the fetal cerebral cortex takes control over fetal activity. As a result, the fetus possesses the ability to perceive and process external signals (Harman, 2009; Morokuma et al, 2004).

The majority of fetal deaths occur prior to the onset of labor. These deaths can be attributed to uteroplacental insufficiency, a state of poor perfusion at the maternal-fetal interface. Therefore, antenatal testing needs to include fetal and placental evaluations (Curran & Torgersen, 2006). In every pregnancy, basic fetal assessment is conducted at every prenatal visit by assessing for fundal height, presence of fetal movement, and auscultation of the fetal heart rate. "Antenatal testing is not routine" (Curran & Torgersen, 2006, p. 262). Assessing a fetus during the antenatal period should be used to help identify the "at risk" fetus, one that is at risk for disrupted fetal oxygenation. In the high-risk pregnancy, in which the risk of fetal morbidity and mortality can increase, fetal assessment becomes more specialized. The information gleaned from these tests and procedures helps the perinatal provider identify the risk, whether high or low, and manage the pregnancy better by weighing the risks of delivery versus the benefits of the fetus remaining in the uterine environment. In essence, antenatal testing gives the perinatal provider a way to see how the fetus is tolerating living in the intrauterine environment and how the placenta is functioning.

The American Academy of Pediatrics (AAP) and American College of Obstetricians and Gynecologists (ACOG) (AAP & ACOG, 2007; ACOG, 1999) list some of the more common high-risk conditions of pregnancy that include (but are not limited to) the following:

1. Maternal conditions
   a. Hypertensive disorders
   b. Antiphospholipid antibody syndrome
   c. Poorly controlled hyperthyroidism
   d. Hemoglobinopathies (hemoglobin SS, SC, or S-thalassemia)
   e. Cyanotic heart disease
   f. Systemic lupus erythematosus
   g. Chronic renal disease
   h. Type 1 diabetes mellitus
   i. Pulmonary disease (i.e., uncontrolled asthma)
2. Pregnancy-related conditions
   a. Hypertensive disorders of pregnancy (preeclampsia, superimposed preeclampsia)
   c. Hydramnios (oligohydramnios or polyhydramnios)
   d. Postterm pregnancy
   e. Type 2 diabetes or gestational diabetes
   f. Preterm premature rupture of membranes
   g. Third-trimester bleeding
3. Fetal conditions
   a. Intrauterine growth restriction
   b. Rh isoimmunization (moderate to severe)
   c. Multiple gestation (especially with significant growth discordance)
   d. Decreased fetal movement
   e. Fetal infections
   f. Unexplained or recurrent fetal demise
4. Genetic assessment: may be done for clients of certain ethnic origins or with a personal or family history of genetic defect.

Although there is no optimum gestational age to begin antenatal testing, most fetal surveillance for at-risk clients begins about 32 to 34 or 36 weeks' gestation but may begin as early as 26 to 28 weeks with some high-risk conditions (ACOG, 1999; Society of Obstetricians & Gynaecologists of Canada [SOGC], 2007). For genetic concerns, assessment can begin as early as the first trimester.

In summary, there are two goals of antepartum testing: (1) to identify fetuses that are at risk for permanent injury or death due to disrupted oxygenation, and (2) to identify fetuses that are "healthy," thus preventing the use of unnecessary intervention (ACOG, 1999; Curran & Torgersen, 2006; Tucker, Miller, & Miller, 2009).

Fetal Behavioral States

In assessing the fetus during the antenatal period, it is important to consider the behavioral states of the fetus. Four behavioral states have been identified (Druzin, Smith, Gabbe, & Reid, 2007; Harman, 2009; Richardson & Gagnon, 2009).

1. State 1F (fetal)—characterized by quiescence (i.e., occasional brief gross body movements); eye movements are absent; FHR is stable with narrow oscillation bandwith
2. State 2F—characterized by frequent gross body movements, eye movements are present continually; FHR has a wider oscillation bandwidth; frequent FHR accelerations with fetal body movements
3. State 3F—characterized by zero gross body movements; eye movements are present continually; FHR stable with wider oscillation bandwidth than state 1F
4. State 4F—characterized by frequent and vigorous gross body movements; eye movements are present continually; FHR unstable with large and prolonged acceleration
5. Non–rapid eye movement (NREM; quiet sleep) and rapid eye movement (REM; active sleep) compare directly with states 1F and 2F (Richardson & Gagnon, 2009).

Fetal Growth and Development

It is important for the nurse to understand fetal growth and development. This understanding will greatly assist in his or her role during myriad antenatal assessments (see Chapter 3 for more detailed information on fetal growth and development).

A. **The normal length of gestation for full fetal development is 280 days (40 weeks) from the first day of the mother's last menstrual period (LMP) or 266 days (38 weeks) from actual conception; because the conception date is usually not known, the delivery date given to the mother is the estimated date of confinement (EDC), with a range of plus or minus 2 weeks to account for variations in time of ovulation from LMP.**

B. **With unknown LMP, an estimation of gestational age (EGA) can be determined by estimating fetal size; one method is to measure the distance from the upper aspect of the maternal symphysis pubis to the top of the uterus (fundal height).**

1. Given a normal uterus, normal amniotic fluid volume, and a nondiabetic singleton gestation, a 20-week fetus usually causes a fundal height of 20 cm, with a normal growth rate of 1 cm per week until 36 weeks, after which engagement of the presenting part may occur.
2. If a discrepancy is found in the size-for-dates estimate, ultrasonography can be performed, preferably in the first or second trimester, a time that demonstrates the most steady growth rates.
   a. First trimester
      (1) The gestational sac can be measured and visualized during the first 13 weeks; measurements provide an estimated gestational age with plus or minus 9 days' accuracy (Robinson, 1980).
      (2) Crown-rump length (CRL) also can be evaluated and has been accurate in 95% of cases within plus or minus 4.7 days (Box 8-1).

BOX 8-1
MENSTRUAL AGES PER CROWN-RUMP LENGTH

1. 6.1 Weeks: 0.4 cm
2. 7.2 Weeks: 1 cm
3. 8.0 Weeks: 1.6 cm
4. 9.2 Weeks: 2.5 cm
5. 9.9 Weeks: 3 cm
6. 10.9 Weeks: 4 cm
7. 12.1 Weeks: 5.5 cm
8. 13.2 Weeks: 7 cm
9. 14.0 Weeks: 8 cm

    b. Second trimester
      (1) Biparietal diameter is among the most accurate second trimester measurement for determining gestational age providing a 95% accuracy within 10 to 14 days (Brookside Associates, 2008). After 30 weeks a significant difference to the altered growth rates may be found in the small-for-gestational-age (SGA), average-for-gestational-age (AGA), and large-for-gestational-age (LGA) fetuses seen in the graphs demonstrating intrauterine growth curves of weight, head growth, and length developed by Lubchenko in 1963 (Robinson, 1980).
      (2) Femur length
      (3) Ratios between fetal head and abdominal circumference
  3. Human intrauterine growth charts are clinically useful in assessing adequate serial fetal growth; the normal fetus grows from a weight of 2 to 4 g (0.1 to 0.12 ounce) and less than 2 to 3 cm (1 inch) at the onset of the fetal period (the beginning of the ninth week), up to an average weight of 3000 to 3600 g (6 pounds, 10 ounces to 7 pounds, 15 ounces) and a length of 48 to 53 cm (19 to 21 inches) at term.

C. Fetal organ growth is not synchronous; fetal systems grow in staggered periods.
  1. Because all body organ systems are present at least in rudimentary form by the end of the embryonic stage (8 weeks), the fetal period involves tissue and organ specialization and growth accompanied by changes in body proportions.
  2. Depending on their level of development, the systems have a varying degree of susceptibility to malformations caused by environmental agents and maternal conditions.
  3. The fetal heart is usually large enough at 18 to 20 weeks' gestation to be audible with a DeLee stethoscope or 12 to 14 weeks' gestation with a Doppler ultrasound. This finding is another confirmation of gestational age.

D. Viability can be defined in terms of ability or capacity of a product of conception to survive for a finite time in a defined environment. Viability by law is defined as when a baby can survive for an indefinite period outside the womb with natural or artificial life-support measures. The upper limit of fetal viability is 36 weeks' gestation plus 6 days (Behrman & Butler, 2007). **The lower limit of viability is determined by fetal organ development and the current advancements in high-risk obstetric and neonatal care** (Behrman & Butler, 2007).
  1. Although infants born at 22 weeks' gestation have been known to survive, most authorities believe that 23 weeks is the time of earliest survival.
  2. Some systems are more immediately critical than others for survival; the respiratory system is critical because gas exchange must occur even if assisted ventilation is used.
    a. Pulmonary maturity generally is not achieved until approximately 37 weeks' gestation.
    b. Surfactant—the substance that prevents the collapse of the alveoli—increases significantly at the 34th week; the absence of surfactant contributes to respiratory distress, a common condition of prematurity. Surfactant is stored in lamellar bodies, discharged into the alveoli, and carried into the amniotic cavity and pulmonary fluid (Leung & Lai, 2008).
    c. Phospholipids make up most of surfactant, the most common being lecithin and the second most common being phosphatidylglycerol (PG).
    d. The presence of lecithin increases significantly at about the 35th week of gestation.
    e. PG appears at 35 weeks' gestation and increases rapidly between 37 and 40 weeks.

Fetal Response to Hypoxemia

In the presence of hypoxemia, the fetus uses a variety of compensatory mechanisms (Curran & Torgersen, 2006). One of the first compensatory mechanisms is to increase its oxygen supply. The fetus can do this in several ways: increase the baseline FHR, increase the hemoglobin concentration, improve cardiac contractions, and/or increase fetal oxygen extraction (Armour, 2004; Curran & Torgersen, 2006; Harman, 2009). A second compensatory mechanism the fetus uses is to control its oxygen resources by redistributing cardiac output; shunting blood to support the vital organs such as heart, lungs, brain, adrenals, and placenta; and shunting blood/oxygen away from fetal periphery or nonvital organs (i.e., stomach, colon). This redistribution is increased two- to threefold and is known as "brain sparing"—essentially keeping the brain oxygenated and alive while limiting oxygen supply to the peripheral organs and limbs (Blackburn, 2007; Curran & Torgersen, 2006). The result is decreased fetal movement while maintaining a normal pH, normal neurologic function, and normal cardiac efficacy (Blackburn; Curran & Torgersen). The final mechanism the fetus uses is to decrease oxygen consumption by decreasing FHR accelerations (or reactivity), decreasing fetal movement, and/or decreasing FHR variability (Blackburn; Curran & Torgersen; Harman, 2009). Once the compensatory mechanisms are used, the hypoxemic situation needs to be resolved (i.e., eliminate or decrease decelerations or provide supplemental oxygen to the mother, or stopping uterine activity), or the compensatory mechanisms will become depleted. Once depleted, the fetus begins to demonstrate signs of metabolic acidemia as evidenced by an increase in lactic acid in the bloodstream, cardiac dysfunction, and a progressive acidosis. If the metabolic acidemia is not corrected, permanent fetal injury can occur because lactic acid is a potent acid and severe asphyxia can cause swelling in the brain and eventually rupture the cells (Myers, Beard, & Adamson, 1969). Antepartal testing of the fetus provides a way to assess fetal oxygenation, intrauterine environment, and placental function (Blackburn; Curran & Torgersen).

CLINICAL PRACTICE

Role of the Nurse

For each test, the role of the nurse will vary. For some tests the nurse will provide direct assistance to the physician, certified nurse-midwife, or nurse practitioner. In others, the nurse conducts the test him- or herself, interprets the test, and reports the findings to the health care provider. In all cases, the nurse must be able to explain the procedure to the client, as well as to understand the results so that these may be either interpreted and reinforced to the client, providing appropriate nursing interventions or education when required. Regardless of the antenatal test performed, there is always a risk for maternal or fetal injury. The nurse must be knowledgeable in specific high-risk pregnancy conditions, their associated treatment options, and fetal diagnostic tests and surveillance regimens.

Biochemical Assessments

Often during the first or second trimester, a pregnant woman may have her blood drawn to assess fetal status. Additionally, ultrasonography can be used to further assist the provider in identifying a fetus or a woman at risk for problems during the pregnancy.

A. **Alpha-fetoprotein**
   1. Protein produced by the fetus. Its presence can identify fetuses that may be at risk for problems during the pregnancy.
   2. However, high levels do not always indicate a problem. They can be indicative of normal and abnormal conditions such as the following:
      a. A fetus with a neural tube defect of the brain or spinal cord
      b. A baby with a birth defect of the abdominal wall
      c. Multiple pregnancy (more than one fetus)
      d. Pregnancy complications, to include miscarriage, discordant growth or death of the fetus, and placental abruption
   3. If blood tests detect an abnormal alpha-fetoprotein level in a pregnant woman, an ultrasound is usually done to:
      a. Confirm the length (in time) of the pregnancy.
      b. Determine if there is more than one fetus present.
      c. Determine fetal status (fetal death; discordant growth).
      d. Detect the presence of birth defects (visual inspection and/or chromosomal studies).
   4. Amniotic fluid can also be assessed for acetylcholinesterase. The presence of acetylcholinesterase, when combined with a high alpha-fetoprotein, is indicative of an increased risk of a neural tube defect.
   5. The presence of alpha-fetoprotein, with or without acetylcholinesterase, indicates a neural tube defect and other abnormalities located in the esophagus (i.e., esophageal atresia) and the abdominal wall (i.e., gastroschisis).

B. **Triple and quad screening**
   1. Triple and quad screening is usually done around 15 to 20 weeks' gestation.
   2. This screening assesses estriol and beta-human chorionic gonadotropin (hCG) levels in addition to alpha-fetoprotein and inhibin A.
   3. Triple screening includes alpha-fetoprotein, estriol, and beta-hCG.

4. Quad screening includes alpha-fetoprotein, estriol, beta-hCG, and inhibin A.
5. If these levels are elevated it could indicate an increased risk of chromosomal abnormalities (i.e., Down syndrome). Quad screening results are "positive" (abnormal) in as much as 80% of Down syndrome cases (Dungan & Elias, 2003).

C. **Delta OD 450**
   1. Some pregnancies can be complicated by alloimmunization when the mother's ABO and/or Rh is different from the fetus's. This mismatch of blood can lead to a variety of complications from jaundice to fetal death secondary to severe fetal anemia. Essentially, this mismatch leads to a breakdown of red blood cells (RBCs) through hemolysis. This hemolysis causes an accumulation of bilirubin (a byproduct of RBC breakdown). The higher the bilirubin level, the more severe the hemolysis. If diagnosed early in pregnancy, and treated with lifesaving blood transfusion via the umbilical cord, 90% of these fetuses can survive (Oepkes et al, 2006)
   2. Dr. Liley, in 1961, was the first to propose using a sample of amniotic fluid to measure the deviation of optical density at 450 nm, commonly referred to as (delta OD 450). This measurement would be used to predict life-threatening fetal anemia in the third trimester (Sikkel, et al, 2002).
   3. This test was initially used solely in the first trimester. However, when intrauterine transfusion, via percutaneous umbilical cord sampling (PUBS), became a relatively safe procedure as early as 18 weeks, the procedure was also used in the second trimester to predict fetal anemia (Figure 8-1) (Oepkes et al, 2006).
   4. However, amniocentesis is not without its problems, which include risk of membrane rupture, infection, worsening sensitization, and fetal loss. Some have suggested the use of Doppler ultrasound to achieve the same results as the delta OD 450 (Oepkes et al, 2006).
   5. Following a number of studies conducted between 2002 and 2006, it has been determined that Doppler measurement of the peak velocity of systolic blood flow in the middle cerebral artery can safely replace invasive testing in the management of Rh-alloimmunized pregnancies. (Oepkes et al, 2006; Sikkel et al, 2002).

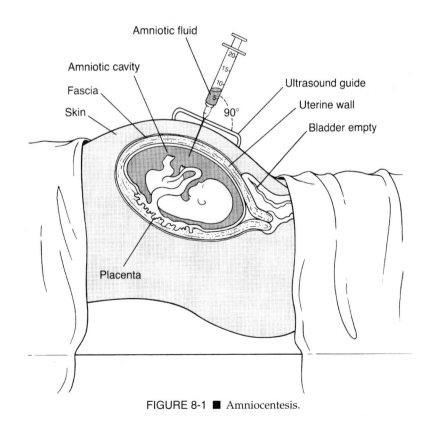

FIGURE 8-1 ■ Amniocentesis.

Biophysical Assessment

A. Ultrasonography
1. With the advent of imaging via ultrasound, tissue can be assessed in either static or real time; a wide variety of information can be gathered pertinent to maternal and fetal issues in low- and high-risk pregnancies.
2. Ultrasonography is a method of tissue imaging based on graphic analysis of the spectral characteristics of reflected high-frequency sound waves (Sonek & Nicolaides, 1998).
3. Equipment
    a. Transducer
    (1) Most scanning in obstetrics is done with 3.5- and 5-MHz transducers.
    (2) The transducer contains crystals that emit ultrasound wave energy; it also receives the reflected sound energy as echoes.
    b. Signal display (B-scan)
    (1) Reflected sound waves are converted first into electrical signals then into a spot on the oscilloscope.
    (2) The intensity (brightness) of the spot varies directly with the strength of the echo, which can be amplified by the gain controls.
4. Safety concerns: dosage levels
    a. The ratio between emitting and receiving time with diagnostic ultrasonography is only 1:1000.
    (1) Total exposure time during 24 hours is less than 84 seconds.
    (2) Therefore a fetus that is 8 cm from the source receives an average of 0.01 to 0.03 mW per square centimeter (mW/cm^2), which is only 0.01% of the maximal safe level of 100 mW/cm^2.
    b. More than 25 years of follow-up by the American College of Radiology have shown no adverse effects of diagnostic ultrasonography.
5. Routes
    a. Abdominal and vaginal ultrasound can be used.
    b. Advantages of vaginal ultrasound include the following:
    (1) Earlier visualization of the products of conception
    (2) Increased detail
    (3) Better evaluation of extrauterine pregnancies or masses (Predanic, Chervenak, & Reece, 2007)
6. Assessment: obstetric ultrasound can assess the following (Torgersen, 2005)
    a. First trimester
    (1) Gestational dating and/or confirmation of pregnancy
    (2) Diagnosis of ectopic pregnancy
    (3) Placental evaluation and localization
    (4) Diagnosis of multiple gestation
    (5) Guidance tool for obstetric tests such as chorionic villus sampling (CVS)
    b. Second and third trimesters
    (1) Fetal presentation and position
    (2) Placental evaluation for abnormalities associated with bleeding (i.e., placenta previa)
    (3) Confirmation of fetal viability
    (4) Evaluation of amniotic fluid volume or fetal well-being (i.e., biophysical profile [BPP])
    (5) Survey of fetal anatomy for gross anomalies
    (6) Guidance tool for obstetric tests (i.e., PUBS or amniocentesis)
7. Physical findings
    a. Gestational dating and confirmation of pregnancy
    (1) Because clients in some clinic populations have questionable menstrual histories, a more accurate method for determining EDC than that based on LMP was needed.
    (2) This is especially true in high-risk pregnancies in which the fetal maturity estimate weighs heavily in the risk-benefit decision in planning a delivery.
    (3) In 1985, Queenan developed the scoring system given in Table 8-1 to identify a term fetus.
    (4) Using measurements of various parts of fetal anatomy according to the trimester, Sabbagha (1978) and others developed equations and reference tables for serial size and age determinations.

■ TABLE 8-1
■ ■ **Fetal Maturity Scoring***

Traits of Parameter	Maturity
Biparietal diameter (BPD)	>9 cm
Placental grading	II-III
Amniotic fluid volume (AFV)	Normal to crowding

*See the related findings discussions for explanation of each parameter.

    (5) Fundal height measurement to assess uterine size provides a subjective assessment; however, ultrasound provides a more precise determination of gestational age. Gestational age assessment is accurate to 3 to 4 days when completed between 14 and 22 weeks' gestation (Abuhamad, 2007).

    (6) Three-dimensional (3D) ultrasound can offer improved assessment of fetal growth and fetal weight (Torgersen, 2005).

b. Diagnosis of ectopic pregnancy

    (1) Normally a fertilized egg travels down the fallopian tube, leaves the tube, and implants in the lining of the uterus. However, in about 1.9% of reported pregnancies, the fertilized egg implants in the fallopian tube.

    (2) Endovaginal ultrasound can be used to detect an intrauterine pregnancy. However, if unable to detect an intrauterine pregnancy with the endovaginal ultrasound, serum hCG levels are assessed. When serum hCG levels reach 1100 to 1500 mIU/mL, it can strongly suggest an abnormal gestation or ectopic pregnancy (Lozeau & Potter, 2005).

c. Placental evaluation

    (1) Grading criteria: In 1979, Grannum, Berkowitz, and Hobbins reported on a method of categorizing maturation into grades 0 to III.

       (a) This method was based on the identification and distribution of calcium deposits within the placenta and the increasing delineations with maturity, as in the appearance of the basal and chorionic plate of placenta and the placental substance (Figure 8-2).

       (b) Clinical implications (Grannum, Berkowitz, & Hobbins, 1979; Schuler-Maloney & Lee, 2004)

          [i] Grade 0
- Straight, smooth, dense, unbroken chorionic plate
- No distinct echogenic areas within the placental parenchyma
- Smooth transition of the basal plate
- Indicative of immature placenta; seen in the first and second trimesters of pregnancy

          [ii] Grade I
- Well-defined unbroken chorionic plate with undulations
- Multiple echogenic areas in the parenchyma
- No changes in the basal plate
- Seen as early as 30 to 32 weeks' gestation; associated with about 67.7% fetal lung maturity

          [iii] Grade II
- Deeper, more numerous indentations of the chorionic plate
- Larger and more numerous echogenic areas that appear to be contiguous with the chorionic plate indentations
- Larger and more dense linear echogenic areas parallel to the basal plate
- Associated with 87.5% fetal lung maturity

          [iv] Grade III
- Indentations of the chorionic plate extend to the basal layer with central echo-free areas.
- Adjacent dense irregular echogenic areas up to 2 cm

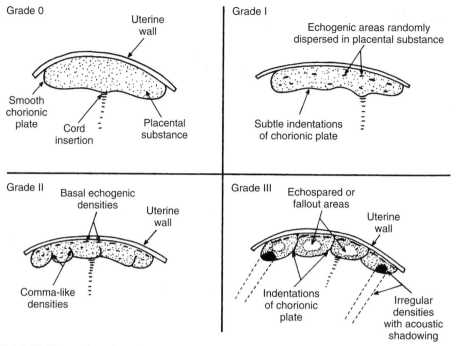

FIGURE 8-2 ■ Placental grading. (From Grannum, P., Berkowitz, R., & Hobbins, J. [1979]. The ultrasonic changes in the maturing placenta and the relation to pulmonic maturity. *American Journal of Obstetrics and Gynecology, 133*[8], 916.)

- Basal plate echogenic areas are larger, more dense, and more confluent than those in the parenchyma
- Placentas more than 36 weeks' gestation or presence of hypertension or growth-restricted fetus; this grade was associated in one study with 100% fetal lung maturity (Grannum et al, 1979) and in another with 93% lung maturity (Harman, Manning, Stearns, & Morrison, 1982).
- Placenta of more than 42 weeks' gestation; this grade has 40% incidence of villous changes, which can reduce blood flow leading to fetal hypoxia (e.g., increased calcification, intervillous thrombosis, perivillous fibrin [Eden, 1990]).

(2) Placental position

(a) In the presence of vaginal bleeding episodes, diagnostic ultrasonography is used to screen for low-lying placenta or placenta previa (implantation partially or completely over the cervical os).

(b) *Placental migration* is a term widely used to describe a placenta that appears to be "low-lying" in the first trimester and then is resolved by the third trimester. However, the term *migration* is a misnomer because the placenta does not move. Instead, it grows toward a better blood supply at the fundus (referred to as trophotorpism). This leaves the distal portions of the placenta to atrophy. Therefore, as the uterus continues to grow so does the lower uterine segment, giving it the appearance that the "low-lying" placenta "migrated" up to a more fundal position (Hull & Resnick, 2009).

d. Multiple gestation

(1) Risk of discordant growth: Multiple pregnancies can be high risk, especially if monozygotic.

(a) Two fetuses compete for nutrition from the same placenta.

(b) The cords can become entangled in utero (monoamniotic).

(2) Mode of delivery planning

(a) The third-trimester presentation of twin fetuses determines the mode of delivery; if vertex-vertex, many practitioners consider a vaginal birth to be safe.

(b) If the first twin is vertex, some may do an external cephalic version (ECV) of the second transverse twin after the first has been born vaginally.

(c) Cesarean birth is the preferred delivery method for all other presentations.

(3) Clinical implication: Serial ultrasonic antepartum assessment of multiple pregnancies for fetal weight and growth discordance should start at approximately 18 weeks, with assessment occurring every 3 to 4 weeks. In the presence of fetal growth discordance or growth restriction of more than 20%, ultrasonic assessment should increase to every 2 weeks. Additionally, Doppler velocimetry may be used to further evaluate fetal well-being in multiple gestations (Malone & D'Alton, 2009).

e. Guidance tool for obstetric tests such as CVS

(1) CVS is a screening test taken during early pregnancy in which a small piece of placental tissue (chorionic villi) is removed from the uterus. The placental tissue is sent to the lab to assess for genetic defects.

(2) CVS can be done through the cervix or through the abdomen. Ultrasound is used to find the safest approach to gather the chorionic villi specimen and to guide the medical provider to the right location.

(3) Initially an abdominal ultrasound is performed to assess the position of the uterus, evaluate the size of the gestational sac, and assess the position of the placenta within the uterus (Figure 8-3).

(4) If done via the cervix (transcervical), a thin plastic tube is inserted through the vagina and the cervix to reach the placenta. The ultrasound is used to help guide the plastic tube to the appropriate area. Then a small sample of chorionic villi tissue is removed.

(5) If done via the abdomen (transabdominal), a needle is inserted through the abdomen and uterus and into the placenta. The ultrasound is used to help guide the needle to the appropriate area. Then a small sample of chorionic villi tissue is removed.

f. Fetal presentation and position

(1) Vertex: Malpresentations have a much higher incidence of morbidity associated with vaginal birth than do cephalic presentations; identifying the fetal presentation in labor accurately is crucial; visualization by ultrasonography of the fetal skull outline at the maternal pelvic brim is a reassuring finding.

(2) Breech: Breech presentation in the last trimester may be manipulated into a vertex presentation by an external cephalic version (ECV) procedure; antepartum assessment

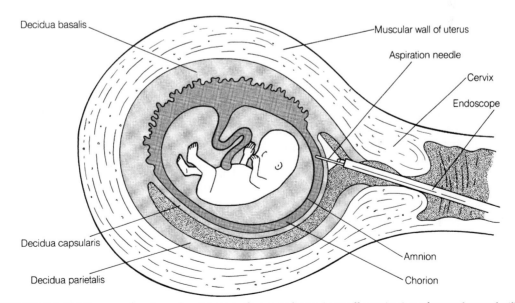

FIGURE 8-3 ■ Diagram of an 8-week pregnancy shows endoscopic needle aspiration of extraplacental villi. (From Rodeck, C.H., & Morsman, J.M. [1983]. First trimester biopsy. In M.A. Ferguson-Smith [Ed.]. *Early prenatal diagnosis* [p. 338]. Edinburgh: Churchill Livingstone.)

of presentation can also be of value in enabling a timely intervention to avoid a malpresentation at delivery.

    (3) Transverse: Just as with breech presentation, transverse presentation in the last trimester may be manipulated into a vertex presentation by an ECV, and ultrasound evaluation can provide timely intervention to avoid a malpresentation at delivery.

    (4) The position of the fetus plays an important role in determining the course of labor. It also plays an important part in whether the fetus will fit through the maternal pelvis (see Chapter 10 for additional information on fetal positions).

        (a) The most common position for birth is with the fetus's head positioned down, facing the mother's back, with the fetal chin tucked to its chest. This position allows the back of the head (smallest diameter) to enter the pelvis. Most fetuses settle into this position between 32 and 36 weeks' gestation.

        (b) Occasionally the fetus is positioned with the head down as it should be, but it is facing the mother's abdomen. This position is referred to as occiput posterior and can increase the chance of painful and prolonged delivery because the softer part of the fetal head is presenting first, trying to dilate the cervix.

g. Placental evaluation for abnormalities associated with bleeding. See Chapter 21 for additional information on hemorrhagic disorders.

    (1) Although the majority of women presenting with second- or third-trimester vaginal bleeding may experience minimal blood loss, it is still a situation that needs immediate evaluation. Ultrasound is a useful tool to assess the degree and potential cause of vaginal bleeding (Hertzberg, 2007).

    (2) Bleeding in the second and third trimesters can be attributed to a variety of conditions including, but not limited to, placenta previa, abruptio placentae (placenta separates from the uterine lining), placenta cretas (placenta invades into the uterine lining and/or the uterine musculature), uterine rupture (uterus develops a hole in the uterine musculature with the fetus/fetal parts extruding into the peritoneal cavity), or vasa previa (placental or umbilical cord blood vessels are trapped between the fetus and the opening to the birth canal) (Hertzberg, 2007).

h. Confirmation of fetal viability

    (1) Fetal life can be confirmed by the visualization of the heart's beating and of fetal movements.

    (2) Real-time ultrasonography provides a fast and effective method of assessing intrauterine fetal demise (Merz, 2007).

i. Evaluation of amniotic fluid volume or fetal well-being

    (1) Amniotic fluid

        (a) Most researchers agree that less than 500 mL (or amniotic fluid index [AFI] <5 cm) of amniotic fluid at term is considered oligohydramnios, or decreased fluid, and more than 2000 ml (or AFI ≥25 cm) is considered polyhydramnios (Beall & Ross, 2009; Brace & Wolf, 1989).

        (b) AFI

            [i] The AFI is an index developed by Rutherford, Phelan, Smith, and Jacobs (1987) in which the depths of amniotic fluid measured in all four quadrants surrounding the maternal umbilicus are totaled. The depths are described in centimeters.

            [ii] Interpretation currently recommended is based on findings of an increased perinatal morbidity (low Apgar scores, meconium staining, fetal distress) in pregnancies with lower-than-normal measurements at term (Richards, 2007).
               • Normal: 10 to 24 cm
               • Low normal: 5 to 9.9 cm

    (2) Fetal well-being: It is important to be able to assess the fetus during the course of pregnancy, especially in light of underlying maternal medical or obstetric problems (i.e., hypertensive disorders; diabetes mellitus) that can have an effect on the fetus. Ultrasound can be used alone or is often combined with other assessment tools to determine the status of fetal well-being. Assessment tools using ultrasonography include the biophysical profile, modified biophysical profile, 3D or 4D ultrasound, and Doppler velocimetry. Further descriptions of these assessment tools are described under Ancillary Antenatal Tests (see section B, following).

j. Survey of fetal anatomy for gross anomalies: Congenital anomalies and follow-up directed (level-2) scans. See Chapter 2 for further information on genetics and Chapter 17 for further information on congenital abnormalities.
  (1) Incidence
    (a) Based on 2007 Centers for Disease Control and Prevention (CDC) data (CDC, 2007), approximately 1% to 2% of live-born infants have a major anomaly.
    (b) At least 500 known developmental anomalies have been discovered.
    (c) Between 6% and 11% of all stillbirths and neonatal deaths are the result of aneuploid fetuses; morbidity as the result of chromosomal defects accounts for another 0.65% of newborns (ACOG, 2007a).
    (d) Testing, using integrated tests from the first and second trimesters, has a 92% to 96% detection rate and a 5% false-positive rate for Down syndrome (Barclay, 2008).
    (e) The recognition of an anomaly may influence the location and method of delivery so that neonatal outcome may be optimized (CDC, 2007).
    (f) Nuchal lucency has been added to the screening tests for Down syndrome, done between 11 and 14 weeks' gestation; congenital anomalies and heart disease, along with Down syndrome, have been associated with the increase in size of the normal clear area posterior to the fetal neck (ACOG, 2007a; Dungan & Elias, 2003).
  (2) Directed scans are performed as a thorough examination of a client suspected of carrying a physiologically or anatomically defective fetus, based on her history, clinical evaluation, or previous ultrasonography.
  (3) Management of anomalies depends on consideration of variables such as:
    (a) Expected prognosis for the lesion
    (b) Demonstration of progressive pathophysiology
    (c) Availability of treatment modalities, if any
    (d) Fetal age at the time of diagnosis
k. Guidance tool for obstetric tests, such as amniocentesis and PUBS
  (1) Amniocentesis for determination of fetal lung maturity (AAP & ACOG, 2007)
    (a) Lecithin/sphingomyelin (L/S) ratio: The chance of lung maturity is 98% if the concentration of lecithin is twice that of sphingomyelin in lung surfactant secreted by the fetus into the amniotic fluid (L/S ratio greater than 2:1) in the nondiabetic client.
      [i] Lecithin is key to the formation and stablization of the active surface layer that prevents the pulmonary alveoli from collapsing (Schuler-Maloney & Lee, 2004).
      [ii] Sphingomyelin is a membrane lipid present in amniotic fluid. It is not related to fetal lung maturity (Schuler-Maloney & Lee, 2004).
      [iii] L/S ratio 1:1: before 32 to 34 weeks' gestation
      [iv] L/S ratio 2:1: as early as 35 weeks' gestation
      [v] In the presence of maternal diabetes, fetal acidosis, or fetal sepsis, the L/S ratio can be favorable, yet still result in an infant with respiratory distress syndrome (Mercer, 2009; Schuler-Maloney & Lee, 2004). See Chapter 22 for further discussion on testing in diabetic women.
    (b) Phosphatidylglycerol (PG)
      [i] PG is one of the last pulmonary phospholipids to be evident in amniotic fluid, usually appearing after 35 weeks' gestation.
      [ii] PG is highly predictive of fetal lung maturity in diabetic clients, or in specimens contaminated with blood or vaginal fluids.
      [iii] In addition to the L/S ratio, the presence of PG is required for definitive maturity assessment.
    (c) Lamellar body count (LBC)
      [i] Lamellar bodies are surfactant-containing particles secreted by type II pneumocytes. Lamellar bodies carry surfactant, are the same size as platelets, and can be counted via the same laboratory equipment that performs a platelet count (e.g., Coulter counter). They are found in the amniotic fluid. The number of lamellar bodies increases with the onset of functional fetal lung maturity (Mercer, 2009).
      [ii] The test requires 1 mL of amniotic fluid and takes less than 15 minutes to complete (Greenspoon, Rosen, Roll, & Dubin, 1995).
      [iii] An LBC ≥50,000/μL is highly predictive of pulmonary maturity (Mercer, 2009).

(d) An LBC ≤15,000/μL is highly predictive of pulmonary immaturity (Mercer, 2009).

(e) The following can interfere with LBC results:

[i] Meconium; LBC not recommended with meconium (Mercer, 2009)

[ii] Vaginal bleeding. If vaginal bleeding is present, a hematocrit should be performed. If the hematocrit is more than 1%, notify the primary health care provider because an elevated hematocrit will falsely elevate LBC results (Mercer, 2009).

[iii] Vaginal mucus can disrupt the counters leading to a decreased count (Mercer, 2009).

[iv] Hydramnios: Severe oligohydramnios can falsely increase the LBC (indicating lungs are mature), whereas polyhydramnios can falsely decrease the LBC (indicating the lungs are immature) (Mercer, 2009).

(2) PUBS (Dungas & Elias, 2003)

(a) Used after ultrasound has detected an anomaly in the fetus

(b) Used when a rapid chromosome analysis is needed, especially if analysis is needed toward the end of the pregnancy. Results are usually available within 48 hours, depending on the laboratory process.

(c) The procedure is conducted much like an amniocentesis; under ultrasonography, the provider inserts a needle through the abdominal wall. However, instead of the needle staying in a pool of amniotic fluid, it is guided to insertion into the umbilical cord (Figure 8-4).

(d) A sample of the fetal blood is then withdrawn and sent to the laboratory for analysis.

(e) Loss of pregnancy with this procedure is approximately 1 in 100 pregnancies.

(f) Clients, and their fetuses, undergoing amniocentesis and PUBS are not without risk. For example, there is risk for maternal-fetal injury and risk for infection. Clients should be provided with a simple, clear explanation of each procedure that includes the purpose of the test, the frequency of the test, the risks, the benefits, and complications of the procedure.

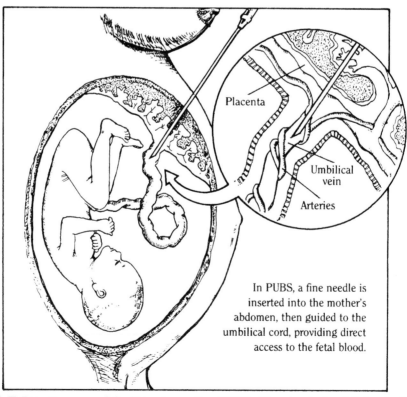

Placenta

Umbilical vein

Arteries

In PUBS, a fine needle is inserted into the mother's abdomen, then guided to the umbilical cord, providing direct access to the fetal blood.

FIGURE 8-4 ■ Percutaneous umbilical blood sampling (PUBS). (Drawing by Jonel Sofian for Pennsylvania Hospital, Philadelphia.)

Interventions

A. Allow the client to vent her frustrations with the discomfort, time-consuming demands, and limitations imposed by this high-risk pregnancy and fetal surveillance program.

B. Assist the client in setting realistic goals for progress in her pregnancy so that she experiences a sense of accomplishment.
   1. Each day in utero is beneficial to the normal development of her fetus.
   2. The fetus has improved chances for survival as long as the testing remains reassuring.
   3. Compliance with treatment and testing regimens is beneficial to the fetus.

C. Nursing actions
   1. Use sterile technique to prevent chorioamnionitis.
   2. Position client properly (in lateral or wedged position) to avoid supine hypotension during fetal monitoring tests.
   3. Administer local anesthesia when starting an IV, as permitted by the institutional protocol.
   4. Use comforting measures such as touch during difficult procedures.
   5. Explain procedures step by step.
   6. Encourage the client's significant other to be with her if she requests it during procedures.
   7. Have terbutaline, 0.25 mg, available for subcutaneous (or IV) injection for uterine contractions, should they occur.
   8. Schedule testing appointments at the client's convenience when possible.
   9. Follow up when the client does not keep an appointment. Reinforce the value of testing.

Ancillary Antenatal Tests

Fetal Movement Counting (FMC)
A. Introduction

As early as 8 to 9 weeks gestation, the fetus begins to move, to kick, and to stretch; however, maternal perception of her fetus moving is often delayed until 16 to 20 weeks' gestation (ACOG, 1999; Curran & Torgersen, 2006). In all pregnancies, fetal movement is a sign of fetal well-being. In high-risk pregnancies the fetus may be at an increased risk for altered perfusion, that is, a redistribution of the fetal cardiac output. Fetal movement (FM) is an inexpensive and noninvasive method of screening that is often taught to high-risk pregnant women (Grant, Elbourne, Valentin, & Alexander, 1989; Harman, 2009). In low-risk pregnancies, perception of FM is discussed at every prenatal visit, and women are told to inform their health care provider or to call/go to Labor and Delivery if there is a decrease in FM or if no FM is felt. FMC is also referred to as fetal kick counting or kick counts (ACOG, 1999; Atterbury, Mikkelsen, & Santa-Donato, 2003; Curran & Torgersen, 2006).

B. Assessment
   1. History: physiologic basis
      a. Decreased activity in a previously active fetus may reflect disturbance of placental function and may be a clue to impending demise (Sadovsky, 1985a). A sudden total cessation of fetal movement is definitely alarming and may signify a premortem event and not just a "warning" of impending fetal compromise (Harman, 2009).
      b. Many variables, such as gestational age, diurnal rhythm, fetal behavior states, medications, tobacco or fetal malformation, can affect FM and should be considered when evaluating decreased fetal movement (Curran & Torgersen, 2006)
   2. Physical findings
      a. The literature proposes a variety of ways to perform FMC. However, the literature does not define an optimum, or ideal, number of movements or the time duration for counting those movements (AAP & ACOG, 2007; ACOG, 1999; Armour, 2004; Barron, 2008; Curran & Torgersen, 2006; Harman, 2009; Littleton & Engebretson, 2005). As a result, any of the protocols identified in the literature are considered to be acceptable (ACOG, 1999). A recent Cochran Database Review of four trials consisting of 71,370 women compared the available methods of FM assessment and found that there were "no advantages" to any specific method but that there was more compliance with women using the Cardiff count-to-10 method (Mangesi & Hofmeyr, 2007). Whatever method is used, it is important for the institutional policies to be standardized to include the same instructions given to the mother regardless of where the mother is seen—clinic or Labor and Delivery (Curran & Torgersen, 2006).

    b. According to Sadovsky (1990), the mean daily FM recording (DFMR) rises from about 200 in the 20th week to a maximum of 575 in the 32nd week of gestation and then decreases gradually thereafter until delivery, with a mean of 282 daily FMs. Even with increasing gestational age, the fetus never stops moving.

    c. Interpretation is complicated for a variety of reasons: every pregnancy has its own rhythm, a woman's perception is subjective, and confusion and inconsistent instructions may be given to the woman; physician noncompliance in doing fetal assessment or updating their knowledge; waiting to report the decrease for the next prenatal visit versus the day the decrease occurs; or total reliance on the nonstress test (NST) to rule out fetal compromise (Harman, 2009; Sadovsky, 1990). However, when compared with an FM-sensing device, there was an 80% to 90% correlation with maternal perception of FM (Grant et al, 1989; Moore & Piacquadio, 1989; Sadovsky, 1990).

    d. Fetuses have a diurnal rhythm. They have been found to move more in the late evening between the hours of 1900 (7 P.M.) and 2300 (11 P.M.) (Gilbert, 2007).

3. The mother is asked to count distinctive FMs for up to 2 hours. Once the 10th FM is reached, the count is stopped and the test is considered reassuring (AAP & ACOG, 2007; ACOG 1999; Barron, 2008; Freeman, Garite, & Nageotte, 2003).

    a. An alternative method is to have the mother count the FMs for 1 hour three times per week. If the count equals or exceeds the mother's established baseline count, the test is considered reassuring (ACOG, 1999).

    b. Another accepted abbreviated method of FMC has the mother assessing 3 FMs in 30 minutes. If needed, the mother can assess an additional 30 minutes for a total time of 60 minutes.

    c. If the mother feels fewer than 10 FMs or if she perceives that the FMs are less than the previous day, she is instructed to call her primary health care provider and/or perinatal nursing unit to be evaluated. Adjunct fetal assessment may be required (NST or BPP) (AAP & ACOG, 2007).

    d. If the mother does not perceive any fetal movement in a 10-hour period, she should be instructed to notify her primary health care provider and/or perinatal nursing unit for further evaluation (Armour, 2004).

4. Although FM is considered a reassuring sign, the lack of FM should not be interpreted as ominous due to the variety of factors that influence fetal behavior (as discussed previously) (Barron, 2008). Any report by the mother that she perceives decreased fetal movement should be assessed. The woman can be instructed to lie down in a quiet environment, have something to eat, rest, and focus on her fetus's movement for 1 hour. If she perceives 4 FMs in that hour, the test is considered reassuring; however, if there are fewer than 4 FMs in 2 hours, the woman should contact her primary health care provider and/or the perinatal nursing unit (Barron, 2008; Curran & Torgersen, 2006).

Nonstress Test (NST)

A. Introduction

  1. The NST was first introduced to the perinatal community in the 1970s. It is considered to be one of the most common methods of perinatal screening and continues to be the cornerstone for today's fetal surveillance (Barron, 2008; Malcus, 2004).

    a. Definition: The NST assesses the FHR externally when there is no stress (i.e., contractions) or stimulus to the fetus and evaluates the FHR in the absence of regular uterine contractions to determine fetal oxygenation and cardiac or neurologic function (Curran & Torgersen, 2006).

    b. Rationale

      (1) In the healthy fetus with an intact central nervous system (CNS), 92% of gross fetal body movements are associated with fetal heart accelerations (Richardson & Gagnon, 2009). An FHR acceleration in response to movement is indicative of an intact CNS and a normal fetal pH (Armour, 2004; Atterbury et al, 2003; Volpe, 2008).

      (2) Loss of reactivity can be caused by fetal sleep, CNS depression, and acidosis (ACOG, 1999; Barron, 2008; Tucker et al, 2009).

      (3) The NST is a quick test to perform and has no known side effects (ACOG, 1999). An NST carries a low false-negative rate of <1% meaning that the incidence of fetal death within 1 week of the NST is <1% (ACOG, 1999; Armour, 2004; Gilbert, 2007; Tucker et al, 2009)

B. **Indications** (ACOG, 1999; Armour, 2004; Atterbury et al, 2003; Barron, 2008; Curran & Torgersen, 2006; Gilbert, 2007; Tucker et al, 2009)
   1. Hypertensive disorders of pregnancy
   2. Postterm gestation (>42 weeks' gestation)
   3. Hydramnios (polyhydramnios or oligohydramnios)
   4. Diabetes mellitus (type 1 or type 2)
   5. Prior stillbirth or intrauterine fetal demise (IUFD)
   6. Chronic maternal disease (asthma, autoimmune disease)
   7. Multiple gestation
   8. Trauma and/or bleeding
   9. Client complaint: decreased or no fetal movement.
C. **Interventions** (ACOG, 1999; Armour, 2004; Atterbury et al, 2003; Barron, 2008; Curran & Torgersen, 2006; Gilbert, 2007; Tucker et al, 2009)
   1. Explain the procedure to the client.
   2. Have the client void prior to her procedure. Have the client position herself in a semi-Fowler's or lateral position.
   3. Perform Leopold's maneuvers to determine the fetal position and proper placement of the external fetal heart ultrasound transducer (U/S) and tocodynamometer (toco).
   4. Apply the external U/S and toco on the maternal abdomen.
   5. Obtain baseline maternal vital signs and continue to assess per the institutional policy.
   6. Run a 20-minute fetal tracing; testing time may be extended to 40 minutes to accommodate the fetal sleep-wake cycle.
   7. If after the first 20 minutes of tracing there is no reactivity (i.e., no accelerations), acoustic stimulation may be applied (refer to vibroacoustic stimulation, in the following section). An FHR acceleration in response to vibroacoustic stimulation is highly predictive of a normal pH (Edersheim, Hutson, Druzin, & Kogut, 1987; Tucker et al, 2009).
   8. Interpret the NST and document the results; report the results to the primary health care provider.
   9. Document primary health care provider notification.
D. **Interpretation** (ACOG, 1999; Armour, 2004; Atterbury et al, 2003; Curran & Torgersen, 2006; Gilbert, 2007; Tucker et al, 2009)
   1. Reactive (normal/reassuring)
      a. Term fetus: two or more FHR accelerations with a peak amplitude of at least 15 beats per minute above the baseline lasting for ≥15 seconds (from beginning to end of acceleration) within a 20-minute period. Other reassuring features of the FHR include moderate variability and the absence of decelerations.
      b. Preterm fetus: two or more FHR accelerations with a peak amplitude of at least 10 beats per minute above the baseline lasting for more than 10 seconds (from beginning to end of acceleration) within a 20-minute period; testing time can be increased to 60 to 90 minutes.
      c. The accelerations can occur with or without maternal perception of FM.
      d. For fetuses >30 weeks' gestation, an FHR greater than 160 beats per minute is considered tachycardia. Accelerations that occur as the result of acoustic stimulation are considered reassuring (AAP & ACOG, 2007). When vibroacoustic stimulation is used for fetuses >26 weeks' gestation, accelerations will occur, thus producing a reactive NST (Baird & Ruth, 2002; Curran & Torgersen, 2006)
   2. Nonreactive (negative; no accelerations; National Institute of Child Health & Development [NICHD] Category II or Category III FHR tracings) (AAP & ACOG, 2007; Armour, 2004; Atterbury et al, 2003; Curran & Torgersen, 2006; Macones, Hankins, Spong, Hauth, & Moore, 2008)
      a. Term: no accelerations or accelerations that do not meet the "reactive" criteria, as defined previously, in a 40-minute period; even one acceleration is considered inadequate
      b. Preterm: no accelerations or accelerations that do not meet the "reactive" criteria, as defined previously, in a maximum testing time of 90 minutes
      c. If variable decelerations are present, an assessment of amniotic fluid is warranted (ACOG, 1999).
      d. FHR decelerations persisting for ≥1 minute are associated with increased risk of cesarean delivery for Category II or Category III FHR patterns and fetal demise (ACOG, 1999; Macones et al, 2008; Tucker et al, 2009; Volpe, 2008).

    e. Variable decelerations are seen in approximately 50% to 75% of the NSTs performed, especially in the preterm fetus (ACOG, 1999). If variable decelerations are present and they are nonrepetitive and <30 seconds in duration, the fetus is considered to not be compromised and there is little, if no, need for intervention (ACOG, 1999; Atterbury et al, 2003)

    f. Minimal or absent variablity

    g. FHR baseline may be within the normal range (110 to 160 beats per minute) or outside of the normal range

E. Testing regimen/management

    1. Once or twice weekly (ACOG, 1999; Gilbert, 2007) because reactive results are associated with fetal survival for 1 week or more in 99% of the cases (Armour, 2004; Barron, 2008; Parer, 1999)

    2. Twice weekly regimen is considered in some of the higher risk conditions.

        a. Postterm pregnancy (>42 weeks' gestation)

        b. IUGR

        c. Type 1 diabetes

        d. Hypertensive disorders of pregnancy

    3. Testing can occur more frequently depending on the maternal and/or fetal condition (Curran & Torgersen, 2006).

    4. In the presence of any Category II FHR patterns (Macones et al , 2008) further evaluation can be completed with a contraction stress test (CST), oxytocin challenge test (OCT), or biophysical profile (BPP).

    5. Once a fetus has achieved a reactive NST, regardless of gestational age, the fetus should continue to have a reactive NST, as long as there is no evidence of fetal compromise (Curran & Torgersen, 2006).

Vibroacoustic Stimulation

A. Introduction

    1. Vibroacoustic stimulation (VST) is also known as fetal vibroacoustic stimulation (FAST) or vibroacoustic stimulation (VAS) (Curran & Torgersen, 2006). In the event of a nonreactive NST, VST can be effective in eliciting a change in fetal behavior, fetal startle movements, and increased FHR variability (Curran & Torgersen, 2006; Harman, 2009).

    2. VST is used for a number of reasons

        a. Shortening the fetal testing time during an NST

        b. Decreasing the incidence of a false nonreactive NST, or

        c. Eliminating the need for retesting in the antenatal period (Baird & Ruth, 2002; Curran & Torgersen, 2006; Ohel, Birkenfield, Rabinowitz, & Sadovsky, 1987)

    3. If a fetus is in behavioral state 1F, the acoustic stimulation can induce fetal body movements, change in fetal posture, increase in FHR and FHR variability comparable with behavioral state 2F (Harman, 2009). If the fetus is already in a 2F behavioral state, the acoustic stimulation can induce an exaggerated fetal response comparable to behavioral state 4F, such as increased frequency of FMs, FHR increase (can induce tachycardia), and exaggerated FHR variability. In addition, the acoustic stimulation in the 2F behavioral state has produced decelerations (Harman, 2009; Sherer, Menashe, & Sadovsky, 1988).

B. Mechanism of action

    1. It is still unclear whether the response from the fetus results from the vibrations coupled with the auditory sound or if the vibrations alone elicit the fetal response. The vibration sense of the fetus is fully developed by 22 to 24 weeks and the auditory capability of the fetus is fully developed by 26 to 28 weeks (Blackburn, 2007; Harman 2009). In light of this, it is acceptable to use VST on fetuses >26 weeks' gestation.

    2. Despite some concern about the use of sound on the fetus, studies have shown that the sound elicited from an acoustic stimulation device is 83 decibels at 1 meter air, which is less than that of a hair dryer (Druzin et al, 2007). Additionally, there have been no adverse effects, neurologic or auditory, found in fetuses exposed to VST (Tan & Smyth, 2001).

    3. The VST may shorten the NST testing time by 10 to 20 minutes (Harman, 2009; Mardin, McDuffie, Allen, & Abitz, 1997; Saracoglu, Gol, Sahin, Turkkani, & Oztopcu, 1999).

    4. Preterm fetuses may require more sound to elicit a response (Kisilevsky, Pang, & Hains, 2000).

    5. Inaccuracies can occur in the high-risk population (Harman, 2009). Fetal responsiveness has been found to be decreased in fetuses that were considered to be "abnormal" (Vindla,

James, & Sahota, 1999), fetuses with exposure to cocaine early in gestation (Gingras & O'Donnell, 1998), fetuses of hypertensive mothers (Warner, Hanes, & Kisilevsky, 2002), fetuses of mothers with depression (Allister, Lester, Carr, & Liu, 2000), and fetuses with severe IUGR treated with magnesium, antenatal steroids, or beta-sympathomimetic drugs for preterm labor (Gagnon, Hunse, Carmichael, & Patrick, 1989; Rotmensch, Celentano, Liberati, Sadan, & Glezerman, 1999; Sherer, 1994).

C. **Indications** (ACOG, 1999; Atterbury et al, 2003; Baird & Ruth, 2002; Harman, 2009; Simpson, 2008)
  1. Nonreactive NST
  2. If 10 to 20 minutes of zero accelerations (reactivity) during an NST

D. **Interventions** (ACOG, 1999; Atterbury et al, 2003; Baird & Ruth, 2002; Curran & Torgersen, 2006; Harman, 2009; Simpson, 2008)
  1. The VST device (i.e., artificial larynx) is attached to the fetal monitor and elicits a mark—either a line, arrow, or musical note on the fetal tracing paper at the time of stimulation.
  2. Explain the procedure to the patient.
  3. Position the patient in a semi-Fowler's or lateral position.
  4. Perform Leopold's maneuvers to find the fetal head position. The proper placement for the VST is near the fetal head.
  5. Place the VST on the maternal abdomen near the fetal head.
  6. Press and hold the button down on the VST to create a stimulus for 1 to 2 seconds for the first time. If there is no fetal response, the stimulus may be repeated every 1 minute up to three times to achieve longer durations of time, not to exceed 3 seconds for each stimulus. The maximum time of application is 9 seconds (three applications that equal a total of 9 seconds). Once a fetal response (i.e., accelerations) is achieved, additional stimuli are not required.
  7. The VST should not be used during a vaginal exam, during uterine contractions, or in the presence of FHR decelerations.
  8. After three applications and accelerations, notify the primary health care provider and prepare for additional antenatal testing (i.e., CST or BPP).
  9. Interpret the test results; notify the primary health care provider of the results.
  10. Document the test results and primary health care provider notification.

E. **Interpretation** (ACOG, 1999; Atterbury et al, 2003; Baird & Ruth, 2002; Curran & Torgersen, 2006; Simpson, 2008)
  1. Reactive VST
    a. Two or more accelerations within a 10-minute period
    b. Accelerations meet gestational age and NICHD definitions.
  2. Nonreactive VST
    a. Inability to fulfill the reactive criteria within 10 minutes of starting the VST
    b. The test should be continued for 40 minutes before it is classified as nonreactive

F. **Management** (ACOG, 1999; Baird & Ruth, 2002; Atterbury et al, 2003; Curran & Torgersen, 2006; Tucker et al, 2009)
  1. If, in response to the vibroacoustic stimulation, the fetus elicits a prolonged acceleration or tachycardia, there is no need to elicit any additional accelerations. However, the FHR should return to the previously established FHR baseline (the FHR baseline before the VST), before discharging the client home.
  2. In low-risk pregnancies, VST has some usefulness, that being to assess the fetus that may be in a 1F behavioral state and not reacting to an NST along with shortening the NST testing time. However, in light of the high false-negative rate of VST and the safety concerns of using the VST, it is not recommended for use in the routine testing of high-risk pregnancies (Harman, 2009).
  3. VST is not to be used on a fetus demonstrating fetal bradycardia (Simpson, 2008; Tucker et al, 2009).

Biophysical Profile (BPP) (Also Biophysical Profile Score (BPS)) (Harman, 2009)

A. **Introduction**
  1. The BPP was first introduced in 1980 by Dr. F. Manning (Manning, Platt, & Sipos, 1980) as a form of intrauterine Apgar score. Since then, there have been two modifications to Dr. Manning's original research. The first modification came in 1987 when Dr. Manning added the NST when any of the other parameters was abnormal (Manning, Morrison, & Lange,

1987). The second modification came in 1993, when he reported a change in the amniotic fluid parameter from 1-cm pocket to a 2-cm pocket (Manning, 1995). (See Table 8-2.)

2. The BPP provides an indication of fetal well-being when there is an increased risk for altered fetal oxygenation. The BPP uses ultrasound with electronic fetal monitoring to assess five different CNS reflex activities that are sensitive to hypoxia (Curran & Torgersen, 2006). These five parameters include:
    a. NST (this can be eliminated only if the other four parameters are normal) (ACOG, 1999; Harman, 2009)
    b. Fetal breathing movements
    c. Gross body movements
    d. Fetal tone
    e. Qualitative amniotic fluid volume

B. Mechanism of action
1. Perfusion to the uterus and across the placenta affects the delivery of fluids, nutrients, electrolytes, and oxygen; fetal hypoxemia and acidosis trigger a redistribution of cardiac output to the vital organs (brain, heart, adrenals, placenta) and away from those not essential to fetal life (lung, kidney, gut) (Manning, 1999).
2. The following relationships have been made with the BPP:
    a. Neonatal morbidity is increased as BPP score drops.
    b. Low Apgar score is associated with low BPP score.
    c. Cord pH shows an inverse relationship.
        (1) Normal BPP: pH of 7.28
        (2) Equivocal score: pH of 7.19
        (3) Abnormal score: pH of 6.99 (Vintzileos, Gaffney, Salinger, Campbell, & Nochemison, 1987)
3. Fetal tone is initiated at 7.5 to 8.5 weeks' gestation and disappears when the fetal pH is <7.0 (Curran & Torgersen, 2006; Gilbert, 2007).
4. Fetal movement begins at about 9 weeks' gestation and disappears when the fetal pH is 7.10 to 7.20 (Curran & Torgersen, 2006; Gilbert, 2007).
5. Fetal breathing begins at 20 to 21 weeks' gestation and disappears at a fetal pH <7.0 (Curran & Torgersen, 2006; Gilbert, 2007).
    a. Variables influencing fetal breathing movements are as follows (Richardson & Gagnon, 2009)
        (1) Increased fetal breathing movements (FBMs)
            (a) Increased glucose concentration
            (b) Smoking
            (c) Chronic caffeine consumption (acute has no effect)
            (d) Tocolytics
        (2) Decreased FBM
            (a) Ethanol alcohol (ETOH)
            (b) Chronic methadone use
6. A reactive FHR baseline begins to function at about 26 to 28 weeks' gestation and is abolished when the fetal pH is <7.19 (Curran & Torgersen, 2006; Gilbert, 2007).
7. Amniotic fluid volume (AFV) or index (AFI) is considered to be an important marker of chronic asphyxia; the lower the AFV/AFI, the greater the incidence of a nonreactive NST (Gilbert, 2007).
    a. Measuring AFI is key to assessing placental function.
    b. Interpretation
        (1) Normal: 10 to 24 cm
        (2) Low normal: 5.1 to 9.9 cm
        (3) Oligohydramnios: ≤5 cm
        (4) Polyhydramnios: ≥24
    c. Severe oligohydramnios
        (1) AFI ≤1 cm
        (2) Associated with 47-fold increase in perinatal mortality when compared to clients with normal fluid volumes (Tarsa & Moore, 2005)
        (3) Delivery is the preferred intervention as decreased amniotic fluid is associated with decreased placental perfusion and can result in meconium staining in the postterm pregnancy (ACOG, 1999; Tarsa & Moore, 2005)

(4) The resulting oligohydramnios may be a reflex induced by hypoxia, causing blood to be shunted away from the lung and kidney, thereby decreasing fetal urine output, which leads to a drop in amniotic fluid volume.

(5) Oligohydramnios may also be related to a decrease in fluid perfusion across the placenta to the fetus.

8. As asphyxia evolves, the first fetal biophysical activities to develop are the last to disappear (i.e., there is a resulting loss of fetal breathing movements, fetal movement, fetal tone, and fetal heart rate reactivity while maintaining normal amniotic fluid volume).

9. Vintzileos et al (1991) further assessed cord gases and determined that fetal breathing movements and FHR accelerations associated with movement seem to be the most sensitive of the variables affected, with fetal tone being the least sensitive.

10. A number of factors can affect the BPP/BPS

   a. Drugs

   (1) Sedatives or drugs with sedative side effects: decreased activity of all parameters assessed; should not totally stop or abolish the parameters (Harman, 2009)

   (2) Drugs with excitatory effects (beta-sympathomimetics): FBMs are continuous with "picket fence" pattern (Harman, 2009, p. 369)

   (3) Street drugs (cocaine, methamphetamine): FM is rigid, jerky, furious, or bizarre (Harman, 2009; Shieh & Kravitz, 2002).

   (4) Indomethacin: oligohydramnios (Harman, 2009)

   b. Maternal cigarette smoking: can totally stop or attenuate fetal breathing movements; can have no effect on fetal breathing movements; can decrease FM (Harman, 2009)

   c. Maternal hyperglycemia: sustained fetal breathing movements, fetal acidosis, decrease of FM, fetal tone, or FHR variability (Harman, 2009)

   d. Maternal hypoglycemia: abnormal quantity (less) of all behaviors with normal AFI (Harman, 2009).

C. **Indications** (ACOG, 1999; Armour, 2004; Atterbury et al, 2003; Curran & Torgersen, 2006; Gilbert, 2007; Harman, 2009; Manning et al, 1980; Menihan & Kopel, 2007)

   1. Nonreactive NST
   2. Positive CST/OCT
   3. Preterm fetal assessment

D. **Interventions** (ACOG, 1999; Armour, 2004; Atterbury et al, 2003; Curran & Torgersen, 2006; Gilbert, 2007; Harman, 2009; Manning et al, 1980; Menihan & Kopel, 2007; Tucker et al, 2009)

   1. A BPP is performed by a provider or ultrasound technician who is credentialed in obstetric ultrasound or limited obstetric ultrasound.
   2. The procedure takes 30 minutes from start to finish.
   3. Explain the procedure to the mother.
   4. Have the mother void prior to the procedure.
   5. Place the mother in a semi-Fowler's or wedged supine position.
   6. Ultrasonic gel or lotion is applied to the mother's abdomen.
   7. BPP is interpreted by the provider/sonographer and reported to the mother. The interpretation results should be documented in the client's medical record.

E. **Interpretation/management** (Table 8-2)(ACOG, 1999; Armour, 2004; Atterbury et al, 2003; Curran & Torgersen, 2006; Gilbert, 2007; Harman, 2009; Manning et al, 1980; Menihan & Kopel, 2007; Tucker et al, 2009)

   1. The BPP has been used in similar fashion to the Apgar score, with the evaluation of the five criteria having a total possible score of 10. (Refer to Table 8-2 for BPP point assignment.) Essentially, a score of 2 points is awarded for each criterion met and a score of 0 is awarded for each criterion not met.

   a. Normal: 8 to 10

   (1) Minimal risk of acute or chronic asphyxia; predicted perinatal mortality = <1/1000 (Harman, 2009)

   (2) If oligohydramnios is the reason for the BPP score of 8, futher evaluation is warranted (ACOG, 1999; Armour, 2004; Harman, 2009). Predicted perinatal mortality with 8/10— oligohydramnios = 89/1000 (Blackburn, 2007; Harman, 2009).

   (3) Repeat in 3 to 4 days (Gilbert, 2007).

   (4) High-risk pregnancy: repeat twice/week if >42 weeks' gestation or diabetic (ACOG, 1999).

■ TABLE 8-2
■ ■ **Biophysical Profile**

	POINTS	
Criteria	None	Present
Reactive nonstress test (≥2 accelerations associated with FM in 30 minutes)	0	2
Fetal breathing movements (at least one episode of 30 seconds or more in 30 minutes)	0	2
Gross body movements (at least 3 discrete body/limb movements in 30 minutes)	0	2
Fetal tone (at least 1 episode of active extension with return to flexion of fetal limbs or trunk; opening and closing of hand = normal tone)	0	2
Qualitative AFV (at least 1 pocket of AF that measures at least 2 cm in two perpendicular planes)	0	2

AFV, Amniotic fluid volume; *FM,* fetal movement.

      b. Equivocal: 6—suspected chronic asphyxia
          (1) BPP can be repeated (ACOG, 1999; Gilbert, 2007; Harman, 2009), the testing time can be extended (Harman, 2009), or additional ancillary tests can be added (Harman, 2009; Simpson, 2008).
          (2) If initial score 6/10 and repeat is 10/10, manage as if BPP 10/10 (Harman, 2009).
          (3) Mature fetus with repeat score of 6 indicative of delivery (Gilbert, 2007).
          (4) Immature fetus with repeat score of 6—repeat test in 24 hours (Gilbert, 2007). If repeat score is same or worse, recommendation is for steroids and planned delivery for 48 hours after last steroid administration (Curran & Torgersen, 2006).
          (5) If 6/10 and AFI normal, predictive perinatal mortality 61/1000 depending on progression (Blackburn, 2007; Harman, 2009)
      c. Abnormal: ≤4—strong suspicion of chronic asphyxia; score of 0 or 2 = immediate delivery (Curran & Torgersen, 2006)
          (1) If 4/10, predicted perinatal morbidity = 91/1000. Delivery is the recommended management with continuous fetal monitoring (Blackburn, 2007; Harman, 2009)
          (2) If 2/10, predicted perinatal morbidity = 125/1000 and cesarean delivery for fetal indications is recommended management (Harman, 2009)
          (3) If 0/10, predicted perinatal morbidity = 600/1000. If fetus is viable, immediate cesarean delivery is indicated (Harman, 2009)
  2. McKenna et al (2003) suggest using ultrasound between 30 and 32 weeks' gestation in the low-risk population to identify a high-risk fetus and again between 36 and 37 weeks in the event that borderline IUGR has been identified.
  3. A negative predictive value at greater than 99.9% is reported for a "negative" BPP (ACOG, 1999; Harman, 2009).

Modified BPP
A. Introduction
  1. The modified BPP is considered to be less invasive, less expensive, and less time consuming than the CST (Blackburn, 2007; Curran & Torgersen, 2006).
  2. AAP/ACOG (2007) indicates that the predictive value of the modified BPP to be as good as other biophysical fetal surveillance tests. Armour (2004) and Freeman et al, (2003) reported that the modified BPP had lower false-negative results and required fewer interventions when it was used as an alternative test to the BPP instead of using the CST.
  3. Modified BPP combines the NST and AFI assessment (ACOG, 1999; Curran & Torgersen, 2006; Harman, 2009; Simpson, 2008).
    a. NST—short-term (acute) indicator of fetal well-being
    b. AFI—long-term (chronic) indicator of placental function and fetal well-being
  4. Same predicitive results as weekly CST (Clark, Sabey, & Jolley, 1989)

B. **Indications—same as for NST**
C. **Interventions** (ACOG, 1999; Freeman et al, 2003; Gilbert, 2007; Harman, 2009; Tucker et al, 2009)
  1. NST performed as previously described
  2. AFI performed as follows (Curran & Torgersen, 2006):
     a. Explain procedure to mother.
     b. Have the mother void prior to the procedure.
     c. Place the mother in a semi-Fowler's or wedged supine position.
     d. Ultrasonic gel or lotion is applied to the mother's abdomen.
     e. The uterus is visually divided into four quadrants using the maternal umbilicus as the center point. Using the ultrasound transducer, the sonographer will view each quadrant individually for the largest pocket of amniotic fluid. The pocket is to be free of umbilical cord and small fetal body parts.
     f. The four numbers are added up for a total AFI and is reported/recorded in centimeters.
     g. Modified BPP is interpreted by the provider/sonographer and reported to the mother. The interpretation results should be documented in the client's medical record.
D. **Interpretation**
  1. AFI as indicated previously
  2. Modified BPP
     a. Normal (both criteria must be met): reactive NST *and* AFI >5 cm
     b. Abnormal
        (1) Reactive NST and AFI <5 cm
        (2) Nonreactive NST and AFI >5 cm
        (3) Nonreactive NST and AFI <5 cm
E. **Management**
  1. AFI
     a. Decreased
        (1) If fetus is term or postterm = delivery
        (2) If AFI is zero = further ultrasound testing to rule out anomalies and assess for rupture of membranes
     b. Low-normal
        (1) Assess gestational age of fetus
        (2) AFI <10 should be evaluated for IUGR.
        (3) Should be evaluated every 3 to 4 days if all other findings are normal
     c. Normal: reassuring; no need for further treatment
     d. Increased (polyhydramnios)
        (1) Serial AFI measurements can be initiated.
        (2) Thorough ultrasound examination to rule out fetal or placental abnormalities
  2. Modified BPP
     a. Normal = no further testing required
     b. Abnormal = needs further evaluation if BPP score is ≤8

Doppler Ultrasound (Doppler Velocimetry) Blood Flow Assessment
A. **Introduction**
  1. One of the major new advances in perinatal medicine, developed in the 1970s, is the ability to study blood flow noninvasively in the fetus and placenta, as well as heart motion. With the advanced technology of color coding, more in-depth assessment is possible. More commonly, in a fetus, the umbilical vessels are assessed. However, vessels such as the aorta and cerebral blood flow can also be examined. The maternal uterine circulation can also be evaluated (Trudinger, 1999). The assessment of the growth-restricted fetus has been advanced with the use of Doppler blood flow assessment (AAP & ACOG, 2007; ACOG, 1999).
  2. The most common vessels measured are the uterine, umbilical, and middle cerebral arteries (Armour, 2004; Callen, 2000; Woo, 2001). Doppler velocimetry has evolved over the last 30 years to become a comprehensive multivessel assessment of the fetal and maternal circulatory systems (Harman, 2009).
  3. The Doppler principle
     a. When an ultrasound wave is directed at an acute angle to a moving target, as with blood flowing through a vessel, the frequency of the echoes is altered in response to the systolic and diastolic components of the cardiac cycle (Trudinger, 1999).

b. This change, called the Doppler shift, indicates forward movement of blood within the vessel; Doppler shifts can be analyzed and displayed as velocity waveforms (Figure 8-5).

c. Physical findings

  (1) Visual representation of the blood flow can be calculated at the time of the procedure by dividing the systolic (S) peak by the end-diastolic (D) component (Blackburn, 2007; Harman, 2009; Trudinger, 1999; Woo, 2004). Essentially, Doppler velocimetry uses systolic/diastolic flow ratios and resistance indices to estimate the blood flow in the fetal, umbilical, and uterine vessels (Blackburn, 2007; Tucker et al, 2009).

  (2) The normal S/D ratio declines from 2.8 to 2.2 between midpregnancy and term.

   (a) When uteroplacental perfusion is reduced, either by narrowing of the vessels, underdevelopment of the vessels, partial or complete blockage of the vessels, lesions in the placenta or abnormal placental pathology, diastolic flow decreases, stops or reverses, resulting in an elevated S/D ratio.

   (b) Elevations greater than 3 are abnormal.

   (c) The higher the S/D ratio, the lower the diastolic flow, leading to fetal growth restriction.

   (d) Reversed flow velocities lead to the most unfavorable fetal outcome (Karsdorp et al, 1994), 70% blockage of placental arteries (Woo, 2004) and birthweight below the 10th percentile in 84% of cases studied have been associated with a 5% to 10%

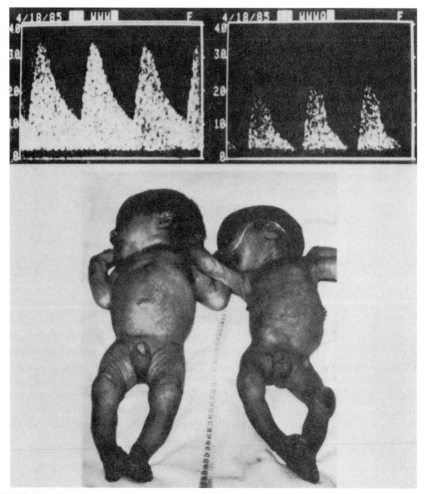

FIGURE 8-5 ■ Doppler ultrasound comparison of N1 twin to twin with intrauterine growth restriction (IUGR). (From Schulman, H. [1990]. Doppler ultrasound. In R. Eden & F. Boehm [Eds.]. *Assessment and care of the fetus: Physiological, clinical and medicolegal principles* [p. 402]. Norwalk, CT: Appleton & Lange.)

incidence of fetal anomalies (Farrine, Kelly, Ryan, Morrow, & Ritchie, 1995). If the flow is reversed, the waveform will be upside down (inverted) (Woo, 2004).

    (e) Color flow mapping shows the blood flow through the fetal and maternal vessels with a different color representing a different directional flow of the blood (Harman, 2009; Woo, 2004).

B. Clinical significance (Divon, Girz, Lieblich, & Langer, 1989; Harman, 2009; Hecher, Campbell, Doyle, Harrington, & Nicolaides, 1995)

The use of this technology has shown significant improvement in perinatal outcomes in pregnancies complicated by IUGR (Harman, 2009; Alfirevic & Neilson, 1995). However, in conditions beyond the growth-restricted fetus, Doppler velocimetry is not a useful screening tool to determine fetal compromise and is not recommended in the general obstetric population (Harman, 2009; Tucker et al, 2009). The clinical significances listed below relate to the growth-restricted fetus.

    1. Umbilical artery

        a. Absent end-diastolic velocity (AEDV)

            (1) Considered to be not stable

            (2) Will progress to reverse end-diastolic velocity (REDV)

            (3) Many fetuses with AEDV also have brain blood flow that is altered with increased diastolic velocities (brain sparing) (Harman, 2009).

            (4) Indicative of immediate delivery regardless of fetal age (not compatible with term pregnancy) (Harman, 2009)

        b. REDV

            (1) Very unstable situation

            (2) Can be indicative of acute vascular accidents such as placental abruption or fetal-maternal hemorrhage (Pattinson, Norman, Kirsten, & Odendaal, 1995).

            (3) Delivery as soon as possible is indicated (Harman, 2009; Pattinson et al, 1995)

    2. Fetal middle cerebral artery (MCA)

        a. If fetus is IUGR and fetal compensatory mechanisms are initiated, MCA diastolic velocities increase.

        b. If fetus has REDV and fetal hypoxemia, cardiac decompensation can occur.

        c. In the event of fetal anemia, MCA can increase. It is considered to be a better predictor of moderate to severe fetal anemia than the traditional use of amniocentesis to determine the delta OD 450 (Dukler, Oepkes, Seaward, Windrim, & Ryan, 2003; Mari et al, 2007).

        d. Increased velocimetries in the MCA indicates need for further antepartum testing (Harman, 2009); multivessel Doppler and BPP are indicated on a frequent basis (Baschat & Harman, 2001).

    3. Fetal vein

        a. According to Harman (2009), the ability to predict fetal outcome is incomplete without the use of venous Doppler.

        b. Elevated resistance in the ductus venosus coupled with the depresson of the alpha-wave is indicative of a threefold increase in major neonatal complications (Harman, 2009).

    4. Maternal uterine artery

        a. Often used in the assessment of maternal hypertensive disease, especially if the mother is being treated with multiple antihypertensive agents

        b. Monitoring the uterine artery, especially in the third trimester, has not been established because as much as two thirds of preeclamptic mothers have normal uterine artery Doppler tracings (Harman, 2009).

C. Summary

    1. Umbilical artery Doppler tracings provide key information regarding the placentation and placental vascular resistance.

    2. If the umbilical artery Doppler tracings worsen, a multivessel approach is highly recommended (Harman, 2009). The multivessel approach includes monitoring the systemic arterial (MCA) and venous (precordial veins) Doppler waveforms to provide a direct assessment of fetal circulation (Harman, 2009).

Three-Dimensional (3D) View, Planes, or 4D Ultrasonography

A. Introduction

    1. Developed due to the limitations of 2D ultrasonography that include the inability to visualize complex facial movements or fine architecture and branching of placental stem vessels, and difficulty in interpretation of umbilical vessels to the chorionic plate (Curran & Torgersen, 2006)

2. 3D and 4D ultrasounds are transabdominal ultrasounds. A 3D ultrasound exam takes thousands of images at once. These are stored and shaded to make a 3D image, which looks more lifelike. A 4D image is similar to a 3D image, but it also shows movement and provides a 360-degree assessment (ACOG, 2006).
3. Advantages of 3D ultrasounds (ACOG, 2004; Stanojevic, Hafner, & Kurjak, 2002; Woo, 2004)
    a. Improved assessment of complex fetal anatomic structures
    b. Decreased time of fetal exposure to ultrasound beam (15 to 30 minutes/2D vs. 2 to 5 minutes/3D)
    c. Identification of placental anastomoses
    d. Volumetric measuring of fetal organs
    e. Spatial presentation of blood flow information
    f. 3D examination of the fetal skeleton
    g. Easily conducted
    h. Economical—it is cheaper than x-ray, magnetic resonance imaging (MRI), or computed tomography (CT)
4. Limitations of 3D ultrasounds (ACOG, 2004; Stanojevic et al, 2002; Woo, 2004)
    a. FM and/or maternal movement can degrade the image quality.
    b. Surface view can be difficult to see due to oligohydramnios and superimposed fetal structures.
    c. Inability to observe facial movement
    d. Inability of real-time observation
    e. Limited to the competency of the sonographer/health care provider
5. Advantages of 4D ultrasounds
    a. Able to evaluate fetal brain morphology and neonatal brain lesions (i.e., identification of presence, type, and extent) (Stanojevic et al, 2002)
    b. Real-time observation
    c. Spatial imaging of fetal structures, especially the face (Curran & Torgersen, 2006)
    d. Strengthens parental bond with unborn fetus (Kurjak et al, 2002, 2004; Woo, 2004)
6. Disadvantages of 4D ultrasound
    a. Due to real-time assessment can only measure quality of expressions, not quality
    b. Limited experienced sonographers administering the exam (i.e., mall shops)
B. **Indications** (Curran & Torgersen, 2006; Kurjak et al, 2002, 2004; Woo, 2004)
    1. Diagnosis/confirmation of early pregnancy
    2. Diagnosis of:
        a. Fetal malformations
        b. Uterine or pelvic abnormalities during pregnancy
        c. Hypoxic ischemic brain injury
        d. Inflammatory disorders of the brain and secondary complications
    3. Determination of:
        a. Gestational age and assessment of fetal size
        b. Hydramnios (polyhydramnios or oligohydramnios)
        c. Fetal presentation
        d. Vaginal bleeding in early pregnancy
        e. Ventriculomegaly and hydrocephaly
        f. Congenital brain defects
    4. Confirmation of:
        a. Fetal well-being via BPP
        b. Intrauterine death
        c. Fetal presentation
    5. Grading intracranial hemorrhage
    6. Assessing multiple gestation
C. **Interventions** (Curran & Torgersen, 2006; Kurjak et al, 2002; Kurjak, et al 2004; Woo, 2004)
    1. Explain the procedure to the mother.
    2. Have the mother void before the procedure.
    3. Place the mother in a low semi-Fowler's position.
    4. Apply ultrasonic gel or lotion to the mother's abdomen.
    5. Assist the sonographer or health care provider as he/she uses the transducer to scan the abdomen.

6. Doppler velocimetry studies are performed on a segment of the artery closest to the placenta.
7. The tests are interpreted by the sonographer/health care provider, reported to the client, and documented in the mother's medical record.

Contraction Stress Test (CST)

A. **Introduction** (Blackburn, 2007; Curran & Torgersen, 2006; Harman, 2009; Tucker et al, 2009)
   1. CSTs are antepartum surveillance tests that assess the ability of the fetus to maintain a normal FHR in response to uterine contractions.
   2. A CST can be achieved by either stimulating the endogenous release of oxytocin via nipple stimulation (CST) or by an exogenous titrated dose of oxytocin administered via intravenous infusion (OCT).
   3. A fetus that is healthy can tolerate short periods of decreased oxygen during the "normal" stress of uterine contractions. However, if a fetus is compromised (e.g., maternal diabetes, severe preeclampsia, IUGR, etc.) the fetus may not be able to tolerate the lack of oxygen availability caused by normal uterine contractions. As a result, the fetus can develop fetal hypoxemia, which in turn leads to the FHR pattern of late decelerations (ACOG, 1999).
   4. Late decelerations associated with uterine contractions have been associated with an increased rate of fetal death, fetal growth restriction, lower 5-minute Apgar scores, cesarean section, and the need for neonatal resuscitation due to neonatal depression (Harman, 2009; Huddleston, 2002; Kubli, Hon, Khazin, & Takemura, 1969).
   5. A CST is found to be more sensitive to fetal oxygen reserves than an NST. A CST has a <1% false-negative rate (ACOG, 1999).

B. **Indications**
   1. Nonreactive NST
   2. Nonreactive VST

C. **Contraindications (relative)—associated with conditions that have an increased risk of preterm labor, bleeding that is related to pregnancy, or uterine rupture** (ACOG, 1999; Atterbury et al, 2003; Baird & Ruth, 2002; Curran & Torgersen, 2006; Littleton & Engebretson, 2005)
   1. Patients at high risk for preterm labor
   2. Preterm labor
   3. History of uterine surgery or classical cesarean delivery
   4. Known placenta previa
   5. Third-trimester bleeding
   6. Incompetent cervix
   7. Multiple gestation

D. **Interventions** (Curran & Torgersen, 2006; Harman, 2009; Tucker et al, 2009)
   1. Setting is either outpatient (nipple stimulation) or inpatient (OCT)
   2. Explain the procedure to the mother.
   3. Have the mother void prior to the procedure.
   4. Place mother in a semi-Fowler's or lateral position.
   5. Perform Leopold's maneuvers to determine fetal position.
   6. Place external U/S and toco on the maternal abdomen.
   7. Obtain and assess an initial set of maternal vital signs; continue to monitor maternal vital signs in accordance with institutional policy; otherwise, monitor maternal BP and pulse every 30 to 45 minutes.
   8. Run a 10-minute fetal tracing; obtain a baseline FHR and uterine activity tracing.
   9. If three or more spontaneous uterine contractions are obtained, lasting a minimum of 40 seconds, for 10 minutes, testing can be deferred.
      a. The goal of CST is to obtain three or more contractions lasting 40 seconds each in a 10-minute period.
      b. If uterine contractions are present but do not meet the required timing in a 10-minute period, nipple stimulation or oxytocin administration can be started.

Nipple Stimulation (CST) (Curran & Torgersen, 2006)

   1. Before the test, apply warm packs to the breasts for approximately 10 minutes as this helps to improve relaxation and circulation.
   2. Instruct the mother to brush her palm across one nipple or roll her nipple using the palmar surface of the index finger and thumb.

    a. The mother can perform the nipple stimulation through her clothes or skin-to-skin.

    b. If skin-to-skin method is used, give mother some mineral oil to use on her fingers to ease the stimulation.

3. The nipple stimulation occurs in four cycles of 2 minutes on and 2 to 5 minutes off (one cycle = 2 minutes on and 2 to 5 minutes off).

    a. "Stimulate the nipples until contractions begin or 2 minutes have passed" (Curran & Torgersen, 2006, p. 274).

    b. If a uterine contraction begins during the stimulation, the mother is instructed to *stop* the stimulation. She can begin the nipple stimulation when the uterine contraction stops.

    c. If there are no uterine contractions after 4 cycles, 2 different methods can be used

        (1) Allow the mother to rest for 5 to 10 minutes. After the rest, begin *bilateral continuous* stimulation for 5 to 10 minutes, stopping when uterine contractions begin. The mother can resume the stimulation when the uterine contractions stop.

        (2) Allow the mother to rest for 5 to 10 minutes. After the rest, begin stimulation again, *alternating* nipples, stopping when uterine contractions begin. The mother can resume the stimulation when the uterine contractions stop.

4. The stimulation should stop when:

    a. Three or more uterine contractions lasting $\geq$40 seconds each, within a 10-minute period occur.

    b. Late decelerations occur.

    c. Unsuccessful nipple stimulation occurs (i.e., two rounds of four cycles without uterine contractions).

5. If the nipple stimulation test is unsuccessful, a titrated intravenous (IV) oxytocin infusion can be initiated (i.e., OCT).

Oxytocin Administration. Oxytocin administration should be done in a facility capable of an emergency response in the presence of tachysystole resulting in fetal bradycardia (Harman, 2009).

1. Ensure that informed consent has been obtained prior to administration of oxytocin.

2. Start mainline IV with 5% dextrose in lactated Ringer's (D_5LR) or lactated Ringer's (LR) (per institutional policy) and infuse at 125 mL/hr or as directed by institutional policy.

3. Piggyback the secondary IV infusion of oxytocin, via continuous infusion pump, into mainline IV. Begin titration of oxytocin at 0.5 to 2 milliunits/min or per institutional policy (AAP & ACOG, 2007; ACOG 1999; Armour, 2004; Atterbury et al, 2003; Curran & Torgersen, 2006; Harman, 2009).

4. Increase the dosage of oxytocin infusion by 0.5 to 2 milliunits/min at 15- to 30-minute intervals (or per institutional policy). If started at 0.5 milliunit/min, the dosage can be doubled until it reaches 4 milliunits/minute, then increased by 2 milliunits/min (ACOG, 1999; Gilbert, 2007). With either method, oxytocin is increased until there are three or more uterine contractions of $\geq$40 seconds' duration each for a 10-minute period (AAP & ACOG, 2007; ACOG, 1999, Armour, 2004; Atterbury et al, 2003; Menihan & Kopel, 2007).

5. Oxytocin infusion is discontinued when:

    a. Three or more spontaneous uterine contractions, lasting >40 seconds each within a 10-minute period occur.

    b. Maximum dose of 16 milliunits/min has been achieved (Gilbert, 2007).

    c. Late decelerations are present.

    d. Tachysystole occurs.

    e. Prolonged bradycardia is seen.

6. After the oxytocin infusion has been discontinued, continue to monitor the FHR and uterine contractions until they have returned to the prestimulation (baseline) state.

7. Interpret the test results.

8. Report the results to the primary health care provider.

9. Document test results and provider notification.

E. Interpretation (AAP & ACOG, 2007; ACOG, 1999; Armour, 2004; Atterbury et al, 2003; Blackburn, 2009; Curran & Torgersen, 2006; Freeman et al, 2003; Gilbert, 2007; Harman, 2009; Menihan & Kopel, 2007)

  1. Negative

    a. 10-minute strip with minimum of three uterine contractions $\geq$40 seconds' duration, *each without late or variable decelerations*

    b. Usually associated with moderate variability

2. Positive
    a. Late decelerations with ≥50% of uterine contractions, even if there are fewer than three uterine contractions in 10 minutes
    b. Usually associated with absent or minimal variability
    c. Associated with increased incidence of:
        (1) IUGR
        (2) Low 5-minute Apgar scores
        (3) Meconium-stained amniotic fluid
        (4) Intrauterine fetal distress
        (5) Late decelerations in labor
        (6) Intrauterine death (Druzin et al , 2007; Harman, 2009)
3. Equivocal/suspicious
    a. Intermittent late decelerations (late decelerations with <50% of uterine contractions)
    b. Significant (severe) variable decelerations
4. Equivocal/tachysystole
    a. Late decelerations occuring with uterine contractions that are more than five contractions in 10 minutes, averaged over 30 minutes (Macones et al, 2008) *or*
    b. Late decelerations occuring with uterine contractions that are more frequent than every 2 minutes (AAP & ACOG, 2007; ACOG, 1999) *or*
    c. Late decelerations occuring with uterine contractions lasting >90 seconds (AAP & ACOG, 2007; ACOG, 1999)
5. Unsatisfactory or equivocal/unsatisfactory
    a. Fewer than three uterine contractions within a 10-minute period
    b. Poor quality FHR data tracing that is perceived as uninterpretable or indeterminate
F. **Management** (AAP & ACOG, 2007; ACOG, 1999; Armour, 2004; Atterbury et al, 2003; Freeman et al, 2003; Gilbert, 2007; Menihan & Kopel, 2007)
    1. Reassuring—indicative of a fetus that is likely to survive labor should labor occur within 1 week of the test
    2. The test can be repeated weekly, especially with a "negative" test, unless there is some change in the mother's medical or obstetric condition such as:
        a. Deterioration in maternal diabetic control
        b. Decreased FM
        c. Worsening maternal hypertension
        d. Worsening maternal renal, cardiac, or respiratory status
    3. Management of the equivocal/suspicious test can be challenging. The test can be repeated in 24 hours or immediately followed by further assessment with BPP (ACOG, 1999; Armour 2004). If BPP is a reliable alternative to the CST/OCT, especially in the presence of a high-risk pregnancy, the BPP should be the tool chosen to assess the fetus versus the CST/OCT (Blackburn, 2007; Harman, 2009).
    4. Any result other than a "negative" test needs further evaluation. The entire clinical situation needs to be considered to include the fetal gestational age, fetal maturity, maternal condition, and/or results of additional fetal assessment tools (Curran & Torgersen, 2006; Harman, 2009).
    5. Any CST/OCT that elicits variable decelerations needs sonographic examination to assess oligohydramnios (Curran & Torgersen, 2006; Harman, 2009).
    6. Timing and mode of delivery for a "positive" CST/OCT is determined by the primary health care provider. Transfer of the client to a tertiary care facility with advanced neonatal support (i.e., neonatal intensive care unit [NICU]) may be warranted depending on the maternal condition, fetal gestational age, and/or fetal maturity.
        a. Even if a 10-minute window of three contractions occurs in which no decelerations occur, if a contraction is associated with a late deceleration elsewhere in the tracing, Freeman and Lagrew (1990) believe this should be considered a suspicious test result.
        b. The perinatal mortality rate with this criterion for a negative result was 0 to 2.2 per 1000 compared with 10 per 1000 when the window interpretation was used. ACOG (1999) reports the negative predictive value at greater than 99.9%.
        c. Contraindications to performing a test include the following (ACOG, 1999):
            (1) Clients at high risk for preterm labor
            (2) Presence of premature rupture of membranes (PROM)
            (3) History of uterine surgery
            (4) Diagnosis of placenta previa

HEALTH EDUCATION

A. Several client education issues have already been addressed during the description of the various tests; therefore, these sections are provided for a complete review of this topic.

B. Because certain high-risk pregnancy conditions are preventable and relate to lifestyle choices that are hazardous to the fetus, counseling during some testing sessions can assist clients in making better choices.

1. Obtain prenatal care within the first trimester.
   a. Prenatal care increases the accuracy of gestational age assessment.
   b. It allows more timely intervention in true cases of postterm pregnancies.
   c. It improves determination of inadequate fetal growth for a given fetal age.
2. Avoid alcohol, illegal drugs, caffeine, and over-the-counter drugs during pregnancy, especially during the first trimester, to prevent teratogenic effects. Some prescription medications may have negative effects on the growing fetus. The woman's provider will assess prescription medications to determine their appropriateness for pregnancy. If deemed inappropriate the prescription will be modified to accommodate the pregnancy.
3. Normal fetal growth can result if smoking is stopped early in the pregnancy.
4. Maintain a good diet with proper nutrition (ACOG, 2007b; U.S. Department of Health and Human Services, [USDHHS] 2006). See Chapter 5 for a complete discussion of nutrition in pregnancy.
   a. A healthy diet is low in fat, sugar, and cholesterol and high in vegetables, fruits, and grains.
   b. A healthy diet should also include proteins, carbohydrates, vitamins, minerals, and fat. Depending on the woman's diet, the provider may prescribe prenatal vitamins to ensure the correct amount of nutrients are ingested during pregnancy.
   c. Iron, folic acid, protein, and calcium are essential for fetal growth. Iron and folic acid are needed to generate the additional red blood cells (RBCs) (thus, oxygen-carrying capability) during pregnancy. Protein is needed to assist with RBC production and building fetal tissues and muscles. Calcium is needed to build fetal bones and teeth.
5. Abuse, whether physical, sexual, or emotional, needs to be assessed throughout the pregnancy, especially as the fetus begins to be visible on the pregnant woman's body. The pregnant woman should have access to information and education on abuse to include contact information for support agencies (ACOG, 2007b). See Chapter 18 for a complete discussion of intimate partner violence in pregnancy.

CASE STUDIES AND STUDY QUESTIONS

Ms. J. is a 37-year-old gravida 1, para 0 (G1, P0) woman whose last menstrual period was March 17. Her first prenatal visit was on July 3, at which time her fundal height was 22 cm. Fetal heart rate was audible by Doppler ultrasonography but not by DeLee stethoscope, and she has not yet felt fetal movement. Select from among the following items those that apply to Ms. J. or the issue addressed.

1. High-risk factor(s)
   a. Fetal cardiac anomaly
   b. Advanced maternal age
   c. Size greater than dates
   d. IUGR
   e. Decreased fetal movement
2. Differential diagnoses for size greater than dates
   a. Oligohydramnios
   b. Polyhydramnios

   c. Twins
   d. Uterine fibroids
   e. Inaccurate date of LMP
   f. Pregnancy-induced hypertension
3. Diagnostic testing options
   a. CST
   b. Amniocentesis for genetics
   c. NST
   d. Ultrasonography for dating
4. Risk of miscarriage because of amniocentesis
   a. Less than 1%
   b. 10%
   c. 5%
   d. 8%

Ms. S. is a 30-year-old G3 P2002 woman at 43 weeks' gestation (by poor dates) with late prenatal care. Her obstetric ultrasonography at 42½ weeks showed a grade III placenta and biparietal diameter of 9.2 cm. She has complained of decreased FM since the previous night. Her next scheduled office visit is in 3 days. Select from among the following items those that apply to Ms. S. or the issue addressed.

5. High-risk factor(s)
   a. Preterm labor
   b. Postdate pregnancy
   c. Abruptio placentae
   d. Decreased fetal movement
   e. Grand multipara
6. Possible diagnoses
   a. Postterm pregnancy
   b. Term pregnancy
   c. Placenta previa
   d. Inaccurate maternal perception of fetal movement
   e. Uterine dystocia
   f. Fetal distress
   g. Preterm pregnancy
7. Diagnostic testing options
   a. Amniocentesis for L/S ratio
   b. NST
   c. CST
   d. AFI
   e. Biophysical profile
8. Is it true or false that Ms. S. is at no additional risk if she waits until her next scheduled office visit to be evaluated?
9. Is it true or false that all clients should be induced for postterm pregnancy at 42 weeks by dates, regardless of the accuracy of their EGA dating method, fetal surveillance results, or evidence of fetal maturity?

Ms. G. is a 25-year-old G2, P1001 woman at 32 weeks' gestation. Her prenatal blood pressures have ranged from 116 to 130/68 to 74. At her current prenatal visit her blood pressure was 160/104 and her urine dipstick was 2+ for protein. In addition, her fundal height is 30 cm. Select from among the following items those that apply to Ms. G. or the issue addressed.

10. High-risk factor(s)
    a. Preeclampsia
    b. Rh sensitization
    c. Maternal anemia
    d. IUGR

Ms. L. is a 25-year-old G4, P3 woman at 34 weeks' gestation (by good dates) who has a history of drug abuse and smoking. Fetal serial ultrasound

tests show poor interval growth, with a current biparietal diameter (BPD) of 7.8 cm and femur length of 6 cm, both consistent with 30 weeks' gestation. Select from among the following items those that apply to Ms. L. or the issue addressed.

11. High-risk factor(s)
    a. Preeclampsia
    b. Diabetes
    c. IUGR
    d. Multiple pregnancy
    e. Substance abuse
12. Diagnostic testing for IUGR pregnancy and treatment planning
    a. Cervical culture
    b. Biophysical profile
    c. Amniocentesis for lung profile
    d. Maternal urine toxicology screen
    e. Maternal glucose testing
    f. NST and AFI (modified BPP)
13. Is it true or false that if Ms. L. were to stop smoking now, her fetus would have an improved blood supply and would gain weight more rapidly?

M., a 35-year-old G5, P3012 woman, is at 33 weeks' gestation and has experienced a 7-pound weight gain in the last 4 weeks, has an elevated diastolic BP of 104, and has 2+ protein in her urine. The physician has required her to quit work and maintain bedrest at home.

14. Because of the potential for uteroplacental insufficiency associated with preeclampsia, M. may have the following parameters evaluated in the home:
    a. AFI
    b. BPP
    c. CST
    d. NST
    e. Fetal movement
15. Two weeks later, she experiences spontaneous rupture of the membranes. She continues to leak amniotic fluid daily, and the AFI has just decreased by 50% at 36 weeks' gestation. To determine fetal maturity, which of the following tests might be performed?
    a. L/S ratio
    b. delta OD 450
    c. AFP
    d. LBC
    e. PG

ANSWERS TO STUDY QUESTIONS

1. b, c	6. a, b, d, f	11. c, e
2. b, c, d, e	7. a, b, c, d, e	12. b, c, d, f
3. b, d	8. False	13. True
4. a	9. False	14. d, e
5. b, d	10. a, d	15. a, d, e

BIBLIOGRAPHY

Abuhamad, A. (2007). Uterine size less than dates: A clinical dilemma. In E. I. Bluth, C. B. Benson, P. W. Ralls, & M. J. Siegel (Eds.), *Ultrasound: A practical approach to clinical problems* (2nd ed., pp. 342–346). New York: Thieme Publishers.

ACOG. (1999). *Antepartum fetal surveillance. Practice Bulletin No. 9.* Washington, DC: ACOG.

ACOG. (2004). *Guidelines for diagnostic imaging during pregnancy. (ACOG Committee Opinion, Number 299.* Washington, DC: ACOG, September 2004.

ACOG. (2006). *Ultrasounds. ACOG educational pamphlet.* Washington, DC: ACOG.

ACOG. (2007a). *Screening for fetal chromosomal abnormalities. Practice Bulletin No. 77.* Washington, DC: ACOG.

ACOG. (2007b). *You and your baby: Prenatal care, labor and delivery, and postpartum care.* Washington, DC: ACOG Educational Pamphlet Author.

Alfirevic, Z., & Neilson, J. P. (1995). Doppler ultrasonography in high-risk pregnancies: Systematic review with meta-analysis. *American Journal of Obstetrics and Gynecology, 172*(5), 1379–1387.

Allister, L., Lester, B. M., Carr, S., & Liu, J. (2000). The effects of maternal depression on fetal heart rate response to vibroacoustic stimulation. *Developmental Neuropsychology, 20,* 639–651.

American Academy of Pediatrics (AAP) & American College of Obstetricians and Gynecologists (ACOG). (2007). *Guidelines for perinatal care* (6th ed., pp. 83–137). Washington, DC: AAP/ACOG.

Andonotopo, W., Stanojevic, M., Kurjak, A., Azumendi, G., & Carrera, J. M. (2004). Assessment of fetal behavior and general movements by four-dimensional sonography. *Ultrasound. Review of Obstetrics and Gynecology, 4,*103-114.

Armour, K. (2004). Antepartum maternal-fetal assessment. *AWHONN Lifelines, 8,* 232–240.

Association of Women's Health Obstetrics and Neonatal Nurses (AWHONN). (2008). *Fetal assessment: Clinical position statement* Washington, DC: AWHONN.

Atterbury, J., Mikkelsen, G., & Santa-Donato, A. (2003). Antepartum fetal surveillance. In N. Feinstein, K. Torgersen, & J. Atterbury (Eds.), *Fetal monitoring principles and practices* (3rd ed., pp. 261–288). Dubuque, IA: Kendall-Hunt Publications.

Baird, S. M., & Ruth, D. J. (2002). Electronic fetal monitoring of the preterm fetus. *Journal of Perinatal & Neonatal Nursing, 16*(1), 12–24.

Barclay, L. (2008). *New guidelines recommend universal prenatal screening for Down Syndrome.* Medscape Medical News, online journal released January 2008. http://cme.medscape.com.

Barkai, G., Reichman, B., Modan, M., Goldman, B., Serr, D., & Mashiach, S. (1988). The influence of abnormal pregnancies on fluorescence polarization of amniotic fluid lipids. *Obstetrics and Gynecology, 67*(4), 566–568.

Barron, M. L. (2008). Antenatal care. In K. R. Simpson, & P. A. Creehan (Eds.), *AWHONN perinatal nursing* (3rd ed., pp. 88–124). Philadelphia: Lippincott Williams & Wilkins.

Baschat, A. A., & Harman, C. R. (2001). Antenatal assessment of the growth restricted fetus. *Current Opinions in Obstetrics and Gynecology, 13*(2), 161–168.

Beall, M. H., & Ross, M. G. (2009). Amniotic fluid dynamics. In R. Creasy, R. Resnick, J. Iams, C. J. Lockwood, & T. R. Moore (Eds.), *Creasy & Resnik's maternal-fetal medicine: Principles and practice* (6th ed., pp. 47–54). Philadelphia: Saunders.

Behrman, R. E., & Butler, A. S. (2007). *Preterm birth: Causes, consequences, and prevention. Committee on Understanding Premature Birth and Assuring Healthy Outcomes; Institute of Medicine (U.S.).* Washington, DC: National Academies Press.

Blackburn, S. T. (2007). Fetal assessment. In *Maternal, fetal, and neonatal physiology: A clinical perspective* (3rd ed., pp. 173–192). Philadelphia: Saunders.

Boehm, F., Salyer, S., Shah, D., & Waughn, W. (1986). Improved outcome of twice weekly nonstress testing. *Obstetrics and Gynecology, 67*(4), 566–568.

Brace, R. A., & Wolf, E. J. (1989). Normal amniotic fluid volume changes throughout pregnancy. *American Journal of Obstetrics and Gynecology, 161*, 382–388.

Brookside Associates (2008). OB/GYN 101: *Second and third trimester*. Retrieved from www.brooksidepress. org/Products/OBGYN_101/MyDocuments4/ Ultrasound/2nd_and_3rd_Trimester_Ultrasound_ Scanning.htm. Accessed May 4, 2009.

Callen, P. (2000). Amniotic fluid: Its role in fetal health and disease. In P. Callen (Ed.), *Ultrasonography in obstetrics and gynecology* (4th ed., pp. 638–659). Philadelphia: Saunders.

Centers for Disease Control and Prevention (CDC). (2007). *National Vital Statistics Report*, Vol. 1, No. 55. Accessed from www.cdc.gov/nchs/data/nsvr. May 11, 2009.

Clark, S., Sabey, P., & Jolley, K. (1989). Nonstress testing with acoustic stimulation and amniotic fluid volume assessment: 5973 tests without unexpected fetal death. *Journal of Obstetrics & Gynecology, 160*(3), 694–697.

Curran, C., & Torgersen, K. (2006). Fetal antepartal testing: Techniques & implications. In C. Curran, & K. Torgersen (Eds.), *abcdEFM The Textbook: Electronic Fetal Monitoring* (pp. 261–294). Virginia Beach, VA: Colley Avenue Copies & Graphics Publishers.

D'Amore, L. (2006). *Antenatal fetal assessment, Clinical Practice Guideline Review* (No. 6). Association of Midwives.

Divon, M. Y., Girz, B. A., Lieblich, R., & Langer, O. (1989). Clinical management of the fetus with markedly diminished umbilical artery end-diastolic flow. *American Journal of Obstetrics and Gynecology, 161*(6), 1523–1527.

Druzin, M. L., Smith, J. F., Gabbe, S. G., & Reid, K. L. (2007). Antepartum fetal evaluation. In S. G. Gabbe, J. R. Niebyl, & J. L. Simpson (Eds.), *Obstetrics: Normal and problem pregnancies* (5th ed., pp. 313–352). Philadelphia: Churchill Livingstone.

DuBose, T. J. (1997). Assessment of fetal age and size. In M. C. Berman, & H. L. Cohen (Eds.), *Diagnostic medical sonography: A guide to clinical practice* (2nd ed., pp. 359–398). Philadelphia: Lippincott Williams & Wilkins.

Dukler, D., Oepkes, D., Seaward, G., Windrim, R., & Ryan, G. (2003). Noninvasive tests to predict fetal anemia: A study comparing Doppler and ultrasound test to predict fetal anemia. *American Journal of Obstetrics and Gynecology, 188*(5), 1310–1314.

Dungan, J. S., & Elias, S. (2003). Antenatal screening tools. In M. H. Beers, A. J. Fletcher, T. V. Jones, & R. Porter (Eds.), *The Merck manual of medical information* (2nd ed., pp. 1432–1434). Whitehouse Station, NJ: Merck Research Labs.

Eden, R. (1990). Postdate pregnancy. In R. Eden, & F. Boehm (Eds.), *Assessment and care of the fetus: Physiological, clinical and medicolegal principles* (pp. 767–778). Norwalk, CT: Appleton & Lange.

Edersheim, T. G., Hutson, J. M., Druzin, M. L., & Kogut, E. A. (1987). Fetal heart rate response to vibratory acoustic stimulation predicts fetal pH in labor. *American Journal of Obstetrics and Gynecology, 157*(6), 1557–1560.

Farrine, D., Kelly, E., Ryan, A., Morrow, R., & Ritchie, J. (1995). Absent and reversed umbilical artery and diastolic velocity in Doppler ultrasound. In J. Copel, & K. Reed (Eds.), *Doppler ultrasound in obstetrics and gynecology* (pp. 187–188). New York: Raven.

Freeman, R. (2008). Antepartum testing in clients with hypertensive disorders in pregnancy. *Seminars in Perinatology, 32*(4), 271–273.

Freeman, R. K., Garite, T. J., & Nageotte, M. J. (2003). *Fetal heart rate monitoring* (3rd ed.). Philadelphia: Lippincott Williams & Wilkins.

Freeman, R., & Lagrew, D. (1990). The contraction stress test. In R. Eden, & F. Boehm (Eds.), *Assessment & care of the fetus: Physiological, clinical, and medicolegal principles* (pp. 351–363). Norwalk, CT: Appleton & Lange.

Gagnon, R., Hunse, C., Carmichael, L., Fellows, F., & Patrick, J. (1987). External vibroacoustic stimulation near term: Fetal heart rate and heart rate variability responses. *American Journal of Obstetrics and Gynecology, 156*(2), 323–327.

Gagnon, R., Hunse, C., Carmichael, L., & Patrick, J. (1989). Vibratory acoustic stimulation in 25- to 32-week, small-for-gestational age fetus. *American Journal of Obstetrics and Gynecology, 150*, 172–175.

Gardner, R. J. M., & Sutherland, G. R. (1996). Prenatal diagnostic procedures. In *Chromosome abnormalities and genetic counseling* (2nd ed.). New York: Oxford University Press, Oxford monographs on medical genetics, No 29.

Garite, T., & Freeman, R. (1986). Fetal maturity cascade: A rapid and cost effective method for fetal lung maturity testing. *Obstetrics and Gynecology, 67*(4), 619–622.

Gilbert, E. S. (2007). Assessment of fetal well-being. In *Manual of high risk pregnancy & delivery* (4th ed., pp. 43–86). St. Louis: Mosby.

Gingras, J., & O'Donnell, K. J. (1998). State control in the substance-exposed fetus. I. The fetal neurobehavioral profile: An assessment of fetal state, arousal, and regulatory competency. In J. A. Harvey, & B. E. Kosofsky (Eds.), *Cocaine: Effects on the development of the brain: Annals of the New York Academy of Science* (Vol. 846, pp. 262–276). New York: Academy of Science.

Grannum, P. A., Berkowitz, R. L., & Hobbins, J. C. (1979). The ultrasonic changes in the maturing placenta and their relation to fetal pulmonic maturity. *American Journal of Obstetrics and Gynecology, 133*(8), 915–922.

Grant, A., Elbourne, D., Valentin, L., & Alexander, S. (1989). Routine formal fetal movement counting and risk of antepartum late death in normally formed singletons. *Lancet, 2*(8659), 345–349.

Greenspoon, J. S., Rosen, D. J., Roll, K., & Dubin, S. B. (1995). Evaluation of lamellar body number density as the initial assessment in a fetal lung maturity test cascade. *Journal of Reproductive Medicine, 40*(4), 260–266.

Haddow, J. E., Palomaki, G. E., Knight, G. J., Cunningham, G. C., Lustig, L. S., & Boyd, P. A. (1994). Reducing the need for amniocentesis in women 35 years of age or older with serum markers for screening. *New England Journal of Medicine, 330*(1), 114–118.

Harman, C. R. (2009). Assessment of fetal health. In R. Creasy, R. Resnick, J. Iams, C. J. Lockwood, & T. R. Moore (Eds.), *Creasy & Resnik's maternal-fetal medicine: Principles and practice* (6th ed., pp. 361–395). Philadelphia: Saunders.

Harman, C., Manning, F., Stearns, E., & Morrison, I. (1982). The correlation of ultrasonic placental grading and fetal pulmonary maturation in five hundred sixty-three pregnancies. *American Journal of Obstetrics and Gynecology, 143*(8), 941–943.

Hecher, K., Campbell, S., Doyle, P., Harrington, K., & Nicolaides, K. (1995). Assessment of fetal compromise by Doppler ultrasound investigation of the fetal circulation. *Circulation, 91*(1), 129–138.

Henry, G., & Miller, W. (1992). Early amniocentesis. *Journal of Reproductive Medicine, 37*(5), 396–402.

Hertzberg, B. S. (2007). Second- and third-trimester bleeding. In E. I. Bluth, C. B. Benson, P. W. Ralls, & M. J. Siegel (Eds.), *Ultrasound: A practical approach to clinical problems* (2nd ed., pp. 296–306). New York: Thieme Publishers.

Hobbins, J. C., Grannum, P. A., Berkowitz, R. L., Silverman, R., & Mahoney, M. J. (1979). Ultrasound in the diagnosis of congenital anomalies. *American Journal of Obstetrics and Gynecology, 134*(3), 331–345.

Huddleston, J. F. (2002). Continued utility of the contraction stress test? *Clinical Obstetrics and Gynecology, 45*(4), 1005–1014.

Hull, A. D., & Resnick, R. (2009). Placenta previa, placenta accreta, abruptio placentae, and vasa previa. In R. K. Creasy, R. Resnick, J. D. Iams, C. J. Lockwood, & T. R. Moore (Eds.). *Creasy & Resnick's maternal-fetal medicine: Principles and practice* (6th ed., pp. 725–737). Philadelphia: Saunders.

Karsdorp, V. H., van Vugt, J. M., van Geijn, H. P., Kostense, P. J., Arduini, D., Montenegro, N., & Todros, T. (1994). Clinical significance of absent or reversed end diastolic velocity waveforms in umbilical artery. *Lancet, 344*(8938), 1664–1668.

Kisilevsky, B. S., Pang, L., & Hains, S. M. (2000). Maturation of human fetal responses to airborne sound in low- and high-risk fetuses. *Early Human Development, 58*(3), 179–195.

Kubli, F. W., Hon, E. H., Khazin, A. F., & Takemura, H. (1969). Observations on heart rate and pH in the human fetus during labor. *American Journal of Obstetrics and Gynecology, 104*(8), 1190–1206.

Kurjak, A., Stanojevic, M., Andonotopo, W., Salihagic-Kadie, J., Carrera, J., & Azumendi, G. (2004). The potential of four-dimensional (4D) ultrasonography in the assessment of fetal awareness. *Journal of Perinatal Medicine, 32*(4), 46–53.

Kurjak, A., Stanojevic, M., Andonotopo, W., Scazzocchio-Duenas, E., Azumendi, G., & Carrera, J. M. (2005). Fetal behavior assessed in all three trimesters of normal pregnancy by four-dimensional ultrasonography. *Croatian Medical Journal, 46*(5), 772–780.

Kurjak, A., Vecek, N., Hafner, T., Bozek, T., Funduk-Kurjak, B., & Ujevic, B. (2002). Prenatal diagnosis: What does four-dimensional ultrasound add? *Journal of Perinatal Medicine, 30*, 57–62.

Leung, S. W., & Lai, J. C. K. (2008). Protein and cell signaling with biomaterials: Influence of surfactants. In G. E. Wnek, & G. L. Bowlin (Eds.), *Encyclopedia of biomaterial and biomedical engineering* (pp. 2337). New York: Informa Health Care.

Littleton, L. Y., & Engebretson, J. (2005). Fetal development and well-being. In L. Y. Littleton, & J. Engebretson (Eds.), *Maternity nursing care* (3rd ed., pp. 441–442). Clifton Park, NY: Thomson Delmar Learning.

Lozeau, A. M., & Potter, B. (2005). Diagnosis and management of ectopic pregnancy. *American Family Physician, 72*(9), 1707–1714.

Macones, G. A., Hankins, G. D. V., Spong, C. Y., Hauth, J., & Moore, T. (2008). The 2008 National Institute of Child Health and Human Development Workshop report on electronic fetal monitoring. *Obstetrics & Gynecology, 112*(3), 661–666.

Malcus, P. (2004). *Antenatal fetal surveillance. Current Opinion in Obstetrics and Gynecology.* (Vol 16, pp. 123-128). Philadelphia: Lippincott Williams & Wilkins .

Malone, F. D., & D'Alton, M. E. (2009). Multiple gestation: Clinical characteristics and management. In R. K. Creasy, R. Resnick, J. D. Iams, C. J. Lockwood, & T. R. Moore (Eds.), *Creasy & Resnick's maternal-fetal medicine: Principles and practice* (6th ed., pp. 453–476). Philadelphia: Saunders.

Mangesi, L., & Hofmeyr, G. J. (2007). Fetal movement counting for assessment of fetal wellbeing. *The Cochrane Database of Systematic Reviews*, Issue 1; CD004909.

Manning, F. A. (1995). Fetal biophysical profile scoring. In F. A. Manning (Ed.), *Fetal medicine: principles and practice* (pp. 124). Norwalk, CT: Appleton and Lange.

Manning, F. (1999). Fetal assessment by evaluation of biophysical variables. In R. Creasy, & R. Resnick (Eds.), *Maternal-fetal medicine* (4th ed., pp. 319–330). Philadelphia: Saunders.

Manning, F. A., Lange, I. R., Morrison, I., & Harman, C. R. (1983). Determination of fetal health: Methods for antepartum and intrapartum fetal assessment. *Current Problems in Obstetrics and Gynecology, 7*(3), 733–737.

Manning, F. A., Morrison, M., & Lange, I. (1987). Fetal biophysical profile scoring: Selective use of the nonstress test. *American Journal of Obstetricians and Gynecologists, 156,* 709–712.

Manning, F., Morrison, I., Lange, I., Harman, C., & Chamberlain, P. (1985). Fetal assessment based on fetal biophysical profile scoring: Experience in 12,620 referred high-risk pregnancies. *American Journal of Obstetrics and Gynecology, 151*(3), 343–350.

Manning, F., Platt, L., & Sipos, L. (1980). Antepartum fetal evaluation: Development of a fetal biophysical profile. *American Journal of Obstetrics and Gynecology, 136*(6), 787–795.

Mardin, D. M., McDuffie, R. S., Allen, R., & Abitz, D. (1997). A randomized controlled trial of a new fetal acoustic stimulation test for fetal well-being. *American Journal of Obstetrics and Gynecology, 176*(6), 1386–1388.

Mari, G., Hanif, F., Kruger, M., Cosmi, E., Santolaya-Forgas, J., & Treadwell, M. C. (2007). Middle cerebral artery peak systolic velocity: A new Doppler parameter in the assessment of growth-restricted fetuses, *Ultrasound in Obstetrics and Gynecology, 29*(3), 310–316.

McKenna, D., Tharmaratnam, R. A., Mahsud, S., Baile, C., Harper, A., & Dornan, J. (2003). A randomized trial using ultrasound to identify the high risk fetus in a low risk population. *Obstetrics and Gynecology, 4*(101), 626–632.

Menihan, C. A., & Kopel, E. (2007). Antepartum fetal assessment. In C. A. Menihan, & E. Kopel (Eds.), *Electronic fetal monitoring: Concepts and applications* (2nd ed., pp. 69–78). Philadelphia: Lippincott Williams & Wilkins.

Mercer, B. M. (2009). Assessment and induction of fetal pulmonary maturity. In R. K. Creasey, R. Resnick, J. D. Iams, C. J. Lockwood, & T. R. Moore (Eds.), *Creasy & Resnick's maternal-fetal medicine: Principles and practice* (6th ed., pp. 419–431). Philadelphia: Saunders.

Merz, E. (2007). Intrauterine death. In E. Merz (Ed.), *Ultrasound in obstetrics and gynecology* (2nd ed., pp. 200–202). New York: Thieme Publishers.

Moore, T. R., & Piacquadio, K. (1989). A prospective evaluation of fetal movement screening to reduce the incidence of antepartum fetal death. *American Journal of Obstetrics and Gynecology, 60*(5 Pt 1), 1075–1080.

Morokuma, S., Fukushima, K., Kawai, N., Tomonaga, M., Satoh, S., & Nakano, H. (2004). Fetal habituation correlates with functional brain development. *Behavioural Brain Research, 153,* 63–459.

Myers, R., Beard, R., & Adamson, K. (1969). Brain swelling in the newborn rhesus monkey following prolonged partial asphyxia. *Neurology, 19*(10), 1012–1018.

Oepkes, D., Seaward, M. B., Vandenbussche, F. P., Windrim, R., Kingdom, J., Beyene, J., Kanhai, H. H., Ohlsson, A., & Ryan, G. (2006). Doppler ultrasonography vs. amniocentesis to predict fetal anemia. *New England Journal of Medicine, 355,* 156–164.

Ohel, G., Birkenfield, A., Rabinowitz, R., & Sadovsky, E. (1987). Fetal response to vibratory acoustic stimulation in periods of low heart rate reactivity and low activity. *American Journal of Obstetrics and Gynecology, 154*(3), 619–621.

Parer, J. (1999). Fetal heart rate. In R. Creasy, & R. Resnick (Eds.), *Maternal-fetal medicine* (4th ed., pp. 270–299). Philadelphia: Saunders.

Paspulati, R. M., Bhatt, S., & Nour, S. G. (2004). Sonographic evaluation of first trimester bleeding. *Radiology Clinics of North America, 42*(2), 297–314.

Pattinson, R. C., Norman, K., Kirsten., G., & Odendaal, H. J. (1995). Relationship between the fetal heart rate pattern and perinatal mortality in fetuses with absent end-diastolic velocities of the umbilical artery: A case-controlled study. *American Journal of Perinatology, 12*(4), 286–289.

Predanic, M., Chervenak, F. A., & Reece, E. A. (2007). Basic principles of ultrasound. In E. A. Reece, & J. C. Hobbins (Eds.), *Clinical obstetrics: The fetus and the mother* (3rd ed., pp. 117–120). Hoboken, NJ: Wiley-Blackwell.

Queenan, J. (1985). *Management of high-risk pregnancy* (2nd ed.). Oradell, NJ: Medical Economics.

Richards, D. S. (2007). Ultrasound for pregnancy dating, growth, and the diagnosis of fetal malformations. In S. Gabbe, J. Neibyl, & J. Simpson (Eds.), *Obstetrics: Normal and problem pregnancies* (5th ed., pp. 251–296). New York: Churchill Livingstone.

Richardson, B. S., & Gagnon, R. (2009). Fetal breathing and body movements. In R. K. Creasy, & R. Resnick (Eds.), *Maternal-fetal medicine* (5th ed., pp. 171–179). Philadelphia: Saunders.

Robinson, H. (1980). Ultrasound measurements in the evaluation of the normal early pregnancy. In R. Sanders, & A. James (Eds.), *The principles and practice of ultrasonography in obstetrics and gynecology* (pp. 121–130). New York: Appleton-Century-Crofts.

Rotmensch, S., Celentano, C., Liberati, M., Sadan, O., & Glezerman, M. (1999). The effect of antenatal steroid adminstration on the fetal response to vibroacoustic stimulation. *Acta Obstetricia et Gynaecologica Scandinavica, 78,* 847–851.

Rutherford, S., Phelan, J., Smith, C., & Jacobs, N. (1987). The four-quadrant assessment of amniotic fluid volume: An adjunct to antepartum fetal heart rate testing. *Obstetrics and Gynecology, 70*(3), 353–356.

Sabbagha, R. (1978). Standardization of sonar cephalometry and gestational age. *Obstetrics and Gynecology, 52*(4), 402–409.

Sadovsky, E. (1985a). Fetal movements. In J. Queenan (Ed.), *Management of high-risk pregnancy* (2nd ed., pp. 183–193). Oradell, NJ: Medical Economics.

Sadovsky, E. (1990). Fetal movements. In R. Eden, & F. Boehm (Eds.), *Assessment and care of the fetus: Physiological, clinical, and medicolegal principles* (pp. 341–349). Norwalk, CT: Appleton & Lange.

Saracoglu, F., Gol, K., Sahin, I., Turkkani, B., & Oztopcu, C. (1999). The predictive value of fetal acoustic stimulation. *Journal of Perinatology, 19*(2), 103–105.

Schuler-Maloney, D., & Lee, S. (2004). Clinical definitions. In D. Schuler-Maloney, & S. Lee (Eds.), *The placenta: To know me is to love me* (pp. 143–145). Des Moines, IA: DSM PathWorks, Inc.

Schulman, H. (1990). Doppler ultrasound. In R. Eden, & F. Boehm (Eds.), *Assessment and care of the fetus: Physiological, clinical and medicolegal principles* (pp. 397–407). Norwalk, CT: Appleton & Lange.

Sherer, D. M. (1994). Blunted fetal response to vibroacoustic stimulation associated with maternal intravenous magnesium sulfate therapy. *American Journal of Perinatology, 11*(6), 401–403.

Sherer, D. M., Menashe, M., & Sadovsky, E. (1988). Severe fetal bradycardia caused by external vibratory acoustic stimulation. *American Journal of Obstetrics and Gynecology, 159*(2), 334–335.

Shieh, C., & Kravitz, M. (2002). Maternal-fetal attachment in pregnant women who use illicit drugs. *Journal of Obstetric, Gynecologic, and Neonatal Nursing, 31*(2), 156–164.

Sikkel, E., Vandenbussche, F., Oepkes, D., Meerman, R., Le Cessie, S., & Kanhai, H. (2002). Amniotic fluid [Delta] OD 450 values accurately predict severe fetal anemia in d-alloimmunization. *Obstetrics & Gynecology, 100*(1), 51–57.

Simpson, K. R. (2008). Fetal assessment during labor. In K. R. Simpson, & P. A. Creehan (Eds.), *AWHONN perinatal nursing* (3rd ed., pp. 431–432). Philadelphia: Lippincott Williams & Wilkins.

Society of Obstetricians & Gynaecologists of Canada (SOGC). (2007). *Clinical Practice Guideline: Fetal health surveillance*. Ottawa, Ontario, Canada: Antepartum and intrapartum guidelines. Author.

Sonek, J., & Nicolaides, K. (1998). The ultrasound examination. In N. Gleicher (Ed.), *Principles and practice of medical therapy in pregnancy* (3rd ed., pp. 48–70). Stamford, CT: Appleton & Lange.

Stanojevic, M., Hafner, T., & Kurjak, A. (2002). Three-dimensional ultrasound—A useful imaging technique in the assessment of the neonatal brain. *Journal of Perinatal Medicine, 30*(1), 74–83.

Tan, K., & Smyth, R. (2001). Fetal vibroacoustic stimulation for facilitation of tests of fetal well being. *Cochrane Database of Systematic Reviews, CD002963*, #1, 2001.

Tarsa, M., & Moore, T. R. (2005). Oligohydramnios. In J. T. Queenan, J. C. Hobbins, & C. Y. Spong (Eds.), *Protocols for high risk pregnancies* (4th ed., pp. 428–433). Hoboken, NJ: Wiley-Blackwell.

Torgersen, K. L. (2005). Maternal and fetal health. In S. M. Nettina (Ed.), *Lippincott manual for nursing practice* (8th ed., pp. 1174–1199). Philadelphia: Lippincott Williams & Wilkins.

Trudinger, B. (1999). Doppler ultrasound assessment of blood flow. In R. K. Creasy, & R. Resnick (Eds.), *Maternal-fetal medicine* (4th ed., pp. 216–229). Philadelphia: Saunders.

Tucker, S. M., Miller, L. A., & Miller, D. A. (2009). Antepartal fetal assessment. In *Mosby's pocket guide to fetal monitoring: A multidisciplinary approach* (6th ed., pp. 191–209). Mosby: St. Louis.

U.S. Department of Health and Human Resources. (2006). *What to eat while pregnant*. Found at: www.womenshealth.gov/pregnancy/pregnancy/eat.cfm. Accessed May 19, 2009.

Vindla, S., James, D., & Sahota, D. (1999). Comparison of unstimulated and stimulated behavior in human fetuses with congenital abnormalities. *Fetal Diagnostic Therapies, 14*(3), 156–165.

Vintzileos, A., Fleming, A., Scorza, W., Wolf, E., Balducci, J., Campbell, W., & Rodis, J. F. (1991). Relationship between fetal biophysical activities and umbilical cord blood gas values. *American Journal of Obstetrics and Gynecology, 165*(3), 707–713.

Vintzileos, A., Gaffney, S., Salinger, I., Campbell, W., & Nochemison, D. (1987). The relationship between fetal biophysical profile and cord pH in patients undergoing cesarean section before the onset of labor. *Obstetrics and Gynecology, 70*(2), 196–201.

Volpe, J. J. (2008). Hypoxic ischemic encephalopathy intrapartum assessment. In J. J. Volpe (Ed.), *Neurology of the newborn* (5th ed., pp. 325–346). Philadelphia: Saunders.

Warner, J., Hanes, S. M., & Kisilevsky, B. S. (2002). An exploratory study of fetal behavior at 33 and 36 weeks gestational age in hypertensive women. *Developmental Psychobiology, 41*, 156–168.

Woletz, P. S. (1997). The use of ultrasound in the first trimester. In M. C. Berman, & H. L. Cohen (Eds.), *Diagnostic medical sonography: A guide to clinical practice* (2nd ed., pp. 211–232). Philadelphia: Lippincott Williams & Wilkins.

Woo, J. (2001). *A short history of the development of ultrasound in obstetrics and gynecology*, Parts 1, 2, and 3. Internet document available at www.ob-ultrasound.net/history3. Accessed February 15, 2009.

Woo, J. (2004). *What are obstetric ultrasound scans? Obstetric Ultrasound*. Internet document available at www.ob-ultrasound.net/omeasure.html. Accessed February 20, 2009.

9 Environmental Hazards

Beverly Bowers

OBJECTIVES

1. Assess childbearing families for potential exposure to environmental hazards.
2. Discuss elements of the prenatal occupational and environmental history to assess maternal or paternal risk factors.
3. Identify potential risks of environmental hazard exposure to the fetus.
4. Provide support and information to prenatal patients who have had exposure to environmental risks.
5. Identify community resources for health education or referrals relevant to environmental hazards.
6. Educate women of childbearing age regarding potential environmental hazards and how to protect against or minimize exposure.

INTRODUCTION

A. **Scope of the problem**
   1. There are more than 29,000,000 commercially available chemicals and more than 240,000 regulated chemical substances in use in the environment today (Chemical Abstracts Service, 2009).
   2. More than 84,000 chemical substances are used in the work environment with more than 2000 more added each year.
   3. Although the majority of these chemicals are safe and contribute to our daily lives, only a small proportion (<5%) of these chemicals have even been tested for toxic effects on humans (March of Dimes, 2009).
   4. Exposure to environmental hazards can occur in the home, at work, or in recreational settings.
   5. Environmental hazardous agents are found in the air, water, soil, food, and in household and personal care products.
   6. All pregnancies are exposed to potential environmental toxins; physical, biological or chemical substances that are harmful.
   7. All pregnancies have a 2% to 4% risk that the fetus will be affected with a major congenital defect (Fisher, Rose, & Carey, 2008).
   8. About 5% of congenital defects are caused by exposure to environmental agents (Fisher et al, 2008).
B. **Definition of terms**
   1. Toxic agent: a physical, biological, or chemical substance that is harmful. Toxins can target specific organs or tissues or can have a systemic effect on the entire body (Arble, 2004).
   2. Reproductive toxin: a substance or agent that can cause adverse effects on the reproductive system of males or females. The effects of toxic agents may target the reproductive organs, the adrenals, or the thyroid.
   3. Fetotoxin: a chemical substance that can poison or cause degenerative effects in a fetus.
   4. Teratogen: an agent that acts directly on replicating cells of the developing zygote, embryo, or fetus causing irreversible abnormal development or defects (Arble, 2004).
   5. Mutagen: a chemical or physical agent (such as ionizing radiation or hyperthermia) that is genotoxic (capable of inducing changes to deoxyribonucleic acid [DNA]). Germ cell mutagens affect the sperm or ova, causing inheritable effects. If other types of cells are affected, altered cell growth or cell death can result. Harm occurs during early stages of cell division of the zygote.

6. Carcinogen: a substance or condition that increases the incidence of cancer
7. Xenobiotic: a chemical substance, not inherent to the body, which is introduced into the body. Some xenobiotics are beneficial, such as folic acid supplements, but others can be toxic, such as lead.
8. Developmental toxicity: adverse effects observed in the embryo, fetus, or newborn
9. Embryolethality: failure to conceive or spontaneous abortion or stillbirth
10. Embryotoxicity: growth restriction or delayed growth of specific organ systems
11. Endocrine disruptor: a chemical capable of interfering with the proper functioning of estrogen, androgen, and thyroid hormones in humans and animals possibly resulting in alteration in sex ratios or fetal sex development and/or growth
12. Reproductive risk: likelihood that an adverse reproductive outcome will result from a given exposure

OVERVIEW OF PRINCIPLES OF TOXICOLOGY

A. **Toxicology is the study of how chemical, physical, or biological agents adversely affect living organisms and the ecosystem, and how these effects can be prevented or mitigated.**
B. **Dosage: the amount of a chemical administered to an individual measured in mg/kg body weight at one time or over a period of time**
   1. Dose toxicity is dependent on the chemical's properties; amount, duration, and timing of dose; route of exposure; absorption; metabolism; excretion; presence of other chemicals (antagonizers or potentiaters); and gender and age (fetus is at increased risk).
   2. Effects of exposure to a toxic agent are dose dependent.
C. **Duration of exposure**
   1. Acute: a single brief exposure to a substance
   2. Subacute: exposure of up to 14 days
   3. Subchronic: exposure lasts up to 90 days
   4. Chronic: exposure lasts more than 90 days
D. **Routes of exposure to toxins (exposure may involve more than one route)**
   1. Inhalation: Toxin is inhaled and passes directly to bloodstream, resulting in increased bioavailability of the agent (Greim & Snyder, 2008).
      a. Air pollution
         (1) Agents
            (a) Carbon monoxide
            (b) Carbon dioxide
            (c) Nitrogen dioxide
            (d) Sulfur dioxide
            (e) Particulate matter (PM) with aerodynamic diameter <2.5 µm
            (f) Fumes which may or may not have an odor
            (g) Indoor air quality
            (h) Secondhand smoke
            (i) Substance abuse
         (2) Associated with intrauterine growth restriction and prematurity (Slama et al, 2008)
         (3) Maternal and paternal exposures possibly important
      b. Ingestion: Toxin is taken in orally. Agent undergoes a process of absorption by the intestinal mucosa and is metabolized by the liver (first-pass effect) decreasing the bioavailability of the agent to the systemic circulation (Greim & Snyder, 2008).
         (1) Contaminated food products
         (2) Contaminated water
         (3) Recreational substance use
         (4) Medications (prescribed, over-the counter, or herbal remedies)
   2. Dermal contact (absorbed through direct contact with skin)
      a. Chemicals
      b. Personal products
   3. Direct effect
      a. Radiation (ionizing or nonionizing)
      b. Temperature extremes (heat or cold)
      c. Noise

    4. Other exposure modalities

      a. Parenteral (direct introduction of chemical into bloodstream)

      b. Ergonomics and workplace requirements

        (1) Prolonged standing

        (2) Shift work

        (3) Working long hours

      c. Exposure to occupational-related disease that could affect pregnancy outcomes

        (1) Health care workers and daycare workers

          (a) Human immunodeficiency virus (HIV)

          (b) Cytomegalovirus (CMV)

      d. Exposure to rodents

        (1) Risk for lymphocytic choriomeningitis virus (LCMV)

          (a) Fetal illness or death

          (b) Developmental problems

          (c) Hydrocephalus

E. Dose-response relationship

    1. The response to a toxin changes as the dose increases.

    2. "The right dose differentiates a poison from a remedy" (Paracelsus)

      a. No observable effect level (NOEL)

      b. Highest exposure level that produces no measurable effect

      c. Effective dose

        (1) The amount of substance required for a therapeutic beneficial effect

        (2) Might be the desired effect if the agent is a pharmaceutical substance

      d. Threshold

        (1) Dosage at which a toxic effect is first encountered

        (2) Occurs at point where body's ability to detoxify the substance or repair toxic injury is exceeded

        (3) There is individual variation in threshold dose from very susceptible to tolerant.

F. The target organ for the same chemical can change based on route of entry.

    1. Ingested substances

      a. Absorbed by intestines and directly detoxified by the liver

    2. Inhaled substances

      a. Enter the bloodstream via respiration and can distribute to body cells before being detoxified by the liver.

OVERVIEW OF PRINCIPLES OF TERATOLOGY

A. Timing of exposure

    1. Susceptibility varies with the developmental stage at the time of exposure.

      a. Pre-embryonic stage

        (1) First 2 weeks after conception

        (2) Period of rapid cell division and differentiation

        (3) Mesoderm, endoderm, and ectoderm differentiated

        (4) Gastrulation and cardiac looping begin.

        (5) Effects of exposure during this time

          (a) Pregnancy loss

          (b) Birth defects

      b. Embryonic stage

        (1) Organogenesis (3 to 8 weeks after conception)

        (2) Period of rapid cell growth and differentiation into essential organs

        (3) Main external features develop.

        (4) Embryo is most susceptible to damage during this period.

        (5) Effects of exposure during this time (Polifka & Friedman, 2002)

          (a) Growth retardation

          (b) CNS dysfunction evident later in life

          (c) Pregnancy loss

          (d) Major anatomic anomalies

            [i] Neural tube defects or cleft lip

    c. Fetal stage

      (1) From 9 weeks until birth

      (2) All organ systems and external structures are present.

      (3) Period of growth and development

      (4) Period of maximum brain growth and myelination begins at 20 weeks.

      (5) Effects of exposure during this time

        (a) Altered fetal growth

        (b) Low birthweight

        (c) Alterations in structural function

        (d) Altered neurologic development

B. Dose of the agent

  1. Factors that affect dosage

    a. Maternal pharmacokinetics

    b. Placental exchange

    c. Fetal and placental metabolism of substance

    d. Fetal distribution of substance

    e. Presence of tissue specific receptors in fetus

    f. These factors explain the variation of outcomes in pregnancies with similar exposures.

  2. Threshold levels exist.

    a. Agent can be taken safely in lower dosages but can cause birth defects at dosages that exceed threshold levels.

      (1) With low dose, no effect may occur.

      (2) With intermediate dose, malformation may result.

      (3) With high dose, death of embryo may occur.

C. Duration of exposure to agent

  1. Continual exposure to agents can affect structural and functional fetal development.

D. Other considerations

  1. Determining and quantifying exposures is difficult.

  2. Causal relationships between exposure and negative outcomes are difficult to confirm.

  3. Exposure to more than one agent at a time may have occurred.

  4. Exposure to pharmaceutical agents

    a. The benefits of treatment must be weighed against the potential risks.

Reproductive Risks of Environmental Toxins

A. Exposure to environmental toxins has reproductive implications for the mother, the father, and the fetus.

B. Exposure to environmental toxins by either parent prior to conception or by mother or fetus during early development can put the embryo or developing fetus at risk for adverse developmental or genetic outcomes (Silbergeld & Patrick, 2005).

C. For some toxins, the residual reproductive effects can last for several years after exposure.

D. Reproductive outcomes

  1. Reduced fertility

    a. Males

      (1) Decreased sperm count

      (2) Quality of sperm

    b. Females

      (1) Menstrual irregularities

      (2) Early menopause

  2. Pregnancy loss

    a. Increased preimplantation loss

    b. Spontaneous abortions

      (1) 15% to 20% of known pregnancies end in spontaneous abortion (Fisher et al, 2008).

    c. Fetal demise

    d. Neonatal deaths

  3. Altered gestational lengths (preterm or late preterm)

  4. Low birthweight or growth restriction

5. Genetic changes
   a. Gene mutation
      (1) Change in DNA sequence within the gene
   b. Chromosomal aberration
      (1) Changes in chromosome structure
   c. Aneuploidy/polyploidy
      (1) Increase or decrease in the number of chromosomes
      (2) Examples include trisomy 21, Turner's syndrome, or Klinefelter's syndrome.
      (3) Can cause embryonic death
6. Congenital malformations
   a. All pregnancies have a 2% to 4% background risk that the fetus will be born with a major congenital malformation (Fisher et al, 2008).
7. Altered secondary sex ratio (proportion of male births)
   a. May be influenced by endocrine disruptors such as diethylstilbestrol (DES) (Wise et al, 2007)
8. Conditions that develop later in child's life
   a. Developmental effects (Rice & Barone, 2000)
      (1) Transient or persistent deficits
      (2) Developmental delays
   b. Behavioral disorders
   c. Chronic diseases
   d. Malignancies
9. Intergenerational effects may continue across future generations if germ cell line affected.

Environmental Hazards in the Workplace

A. **Background**
   1. Approximately 39 million women of childbearing age between ages 16 and 44 are employed in the civilian workforce accounting for about 46% of the workforce (U.S. Department of Labor, 2008).
   2. The workplace has been designed predominantly for men.
   3. The National Institute of Occupational Safety and Health (NIOSH, 1999) reports that more than 5000 chemicals have possible reproductive toxicity.
   4. Occupational exposures affect the reproductive health of male and female workers.
   5. Inaccurate and incomplete exposure data during gestation make determining reproductive risk difficult.
   6. Occupational and nonoccupational exposures are difficult to separate.
      a. Age, lifestyle factors, social class, nutrition, and occupational exposures have been associated with various reproductive outcomes.
      b. Results of studies to support relationships between occupational exposures and outcomes, specifically birth defects, are not convincing (Thulstrup & Bonde, 2006)
B. **Common occupationally related environmental hazards**
   1. Chemical agents
      a. Antineoplastic drugs (Connor & McDiarmid, 2006)
         (1) Use
            (a) Drugs used for treatment for cancer
            (b) Combination therapy of antineoplastic drugs more common
            (c) Antineoplastic drugs are also used to treat conditions other than cancer.
         (2) At-risk populations
            (a) Health care workers and pharmacists are at increased risk.
               [i] Prepare and handle antineoplastic drugs
               [ii] Handle contaminated excreta of patients taking antineoplastic drugs while providing care
               [iii] Unsafe handling of antineoplastic drugs
                  • Lack of use of personal protective equipment or other safeguards
            (b) Workers where drugs are produced
         (3) Classes of antineoplastic drugs
            (a) Alkylating agents: nitrogen mustard, nitrosoureas

   (b) Antimetabolites
    [i] 5-fluorouracil (disrupts folic acid metabolism)
    [ii] Methotrexate
   (c) Mitotic spindle inhibitors
    [i] Vinca alkaloids: vincristine and vinblastine
   (d) Epipodophylotoxins: teniposide and etoposide
   (e) Antitumor antibiotics: bleomycin, daunorubicin, doxorubicin
   (f) Hormones
    [i] Antiandrogenic agents
    [ii] Antiestrogenic agents
   (g) Miscellaneous drugs: L-asparaginase
   (h) All classes of antineoplastic drugs are mutagenic and carcinogenic.
    [i] Many are FDA pregnancy Category D and five are Category X.
  (4) Exposure
   (a) Inhalation of droplets or particles during preparation
   (b) Dermal exposure during preparation or cleanup
   (c) Ingestion
    [i] Accidental hand-to-mouth exposure
    [ii] Contamination of food or drink in workplace
  (5) Effects
   (a) Fetal loss
    [i] Congenital malformations (two-fold increase if exposed during first trimester)
    [ii] Low birthweight
    [iii] Infertility
 b. Colorants
  (1) Use
   (a) Permanent hair dyes, nail polish, and furniture paints or fabric dyes
    [i] Some hair colorants contain lead acetate as possible agent.
  (2) At-risk populations
   (a) Cosmetologists
   (b) Leather workers
   (c) Auto mechanics who handle corroded parts
  (3) Route of exposure
   (a) Absorbed through skin or scalp at work or during hobbies
  (4) Effects
   (a) Animal studies show linkage to birth defects, whereas human studies are inconclusive.
   (b) Implicated as teratogen with nearly double the risk of gastroschisis in the exposed fetus
   (c) Recommended to avoid usage of colorants during first trimester of pregnancy
 c. Ethylene oxide (Center for the Evaluation of Risks to Human Reproduction [CERHR], 2002)
  (1) Use
   (a) Production of ethylene glycol for antifreeze, polyester fibers and films, and detergents
   (b) Sterilization of equipment and supplies in health care facilities
   (c) Fumigant in the manufacture of medical products and foodstuffs
  (2) At-risk populations
   (a) Operators of sterilization equipment for medical or dental supplies and equipment
  (3) Route of exposure
   (a) Inhalation
   (b) Skin contact
   (c) Exposure during all stages of cell division is important.
  (4) Effects
   (a) Reproductive problems (males and females)
   (b) A teratogen and genotoxin
   (c) Adverse reproductive outcomes (Gresie-Brusen, Kielkowski, Baker, Channa, & Rees, 2006)
    [i] Spontaneous abortion
    [ii] Birth defects

d. Nanoparticles
  (1) Use
    (a) Engineered particles of extremely small size (1 to 1000 nanometers) with unique optical, chemical and magnetic properties that differ from their related chemical compound
    (b) Used in suntan lotion, cosmetics, clothing, cleaning materials, medicines, and food
    (c) Emerging applications for nanoparticles are under development.
  (2) At-risk populations
    (a) Nanotechnology research and development workers
    (b) Chemical and pharmaceutical workers
    (c) Workers who handle powders related to paint, pigments, and concrete
    (d) Welders
  (3) Exposure
    (a) Inhalation is the most frequent route in humans.
    (b) Dermal exposure
    (c) Ingestion
  (4) Effects
    (a) Nanoparticles are small enough to penetrate the body at the molecular level.
    (b) They bypass the body's usual defense mechanisms.
    (c) Reproductive effects are unknown.
      [i] Nanoparticles cross the blood-testes barrier.
      [ii] Deposit in testes and have potential for adverse effects on sperm (McAuliffe & Perry, 2007)
      [iii] More research is needed to determine safety and reproductive effects of this emerging technology (U.S. Department of Health and Human Services [USDHHS], 2009).
e. Organic solvents
  (1) Description
    (a) Chemicals with high volatility and high vapor pressure that are lipid soluble, used to dissolve oil, resins, and rubber
      [i] Aliphatic hydrocarbons (mineral spirits, varnish, kerosene)
      [ii] Aromatic hydrocarbons (benzene, toluene, xylene)
      [iii] Halogenated/chlorinated hydrocarbons (carbon tetrachloride, trichloroethylene, tetrachloroethylene [also known as perchloroethylene, or perc])
        • Also used as pesticides
      [iv] Aliphatic alcohols (methanol)
      [v] Glycols (ethylene glycol)
      [vi] Glycol ethers (methoxyethanol)
  (2) Uses
    (a) Spot removers, aerosol sprays, paints
    (b) Chemical laboratories
    (c) Auto work, gasoline
    (d) Furniture stripping, glues
    (e) Fixative in medical care
    (f) Nail polish and polish remover
    (g) Floor and tile cleaner
  (3) At-risk populations
    (a) Workers in manufacturing and industry jobs
    (b) Nail salon workers
    (c) Painters
    (d) Dry cleaners
    (e) Medical laboratories workers
    (f) Funeral service workers
    (g) Abusers of solvents such as paint sniffers
    (h) Chemical manufacturers of inks and plastics
  (4) Exposure
    (a) Inhalation of vapor; one of the most common types of workplace exposures

(b) Ingestion
[i] Some organic solvents are contaminants in drinking water.
(c) Skin or eye contact
(5) Effects
(a) Women exposed to organic solvents in work or hobbies have an increased risk for infants born with gastroschisis (Torfs, Katz, Bateson, Lam, & Curry, 1996).
(b) Increased risk for intrauterine growth restriction (IUGR) and small-for-gestational-age (SGA) infant (Ahmed & Jaakkola, 2007)
(c) Carcinogen
[i] Exposure is important during any stage
(d) Neurodevelopmental toxicity (Laslo-Baker et al, 2004)
(e) Color blindness
(f) Congenital solvent exposure syndrome may exist (Bowling, Gaudette, & Pergament, 2006).
(g) Specific agents
[i] Benzene
• May act as a teratogen and carcinogen
• Decreased fertility in women
• Irregular periods and smaller ovaries
• Effects on fetus are not known
[ii] Propylene and glycol
• May act as teratogens
• Reported to double the risk of gastroschisis in the exposed fetus
f. Pesticides (Frazier, 2007)
(1) Use
(a) Control of unwanted pests or vegetation in crops
(b) Classification of pesticides
[i] Organophosphates
[ii] Carbamates
[iii] Pyrethroids
[iv] Herbicides
[v] Fungicides
[vi] Fumigants
[vii] Organochlorines
(2) At-risk populations
(a) Farm workers
(b) Greenhouse workers
(3) Exposure
(a) Inhalation
(b) Ingestion of contaminated food or water
[i] Passes to breast milk
(c) Dermal exposure
(d) Exposure at any stage of pregnancy may be important.
(4) Effects
(a) Alterations in male fertility
[i] Altered sperm count, sperm motility or morphology
[ii] Decreased male fertility (Roeleveld & Bretveld, 2008)
(b) Endocrine disruptors
[i] Deficit of male children
[ii] Fetal growth restriction
(c) Spontaneous abortion
(d) Birth defects
[i] Limb defects
[ii] Musculoskeletal defects
(e) Altered neurobehavioral development of the fetus
(f) Carcinogenic
[i] Some links to childhood leukemia reported

   g. Phthalates (Gray, 2000; Khattak et al, 1999)
- (1) Use
  - (a) Chemicals used to soften plastic
  - (b) Found in many personal care products and medical supplies
  - (c) Plastic products including water bottles, food wrap
  - (d) Found in polymers coating some medications (Hernández-Diáz, Mitchell, Kelley, Calafat, & Hauser, 2009)
- (2) At risk populations
  - (a) Nearly 100% of population has been exposed.
  - (b) Women of reproductive age have high levels of exposure.
- (3) Exposure
  - (a) Inhalation
  - (b) Ingestion
  - (c) Dermal exposure
  - (d) Crosses placenta
  - (e) Found in breast milk
  - (f) Agents associated with reproductive health effects
    - [i] Diethylhexyl phthalate (DEHP)
    - [ii] Dibutyl phthalate (DBP)
    - [iii] Butyl benzyl phthalate (BBP)
- (4) Effects
  - (a) Developmental effects
  - (b) Reproductive toxin; endocrine disruptors
    - [i] Can cause changes to genitals of developing male fetus
    - [ii] Shorter anogenital index
    - [iii] Cryptorchidism
    - [iv] Smaller penis
    - [v] Increased risk for testicular tumors in adulthood
    - [vi] Decreased sperm count

   h. Polychlorinated biphenyls (PCBs)
- (1) Use
  - (a) A group of 290 synthetic organic compounds
  - (b) Used to manufacture dielectric capacitors and transformers
  - (c) Found in heat-exchange fluid and hydraulic fluid
  - (d) Production of PCBs in the United States was banned in 1977.
- (2) At-risk populations
  - (a) Capacitor manufacturing workers
  - (b) Women who consume moderate to high amounts of contaminated fish
- (3) Exposure
  - (a) Inhalation
    - [i] Fire or leaks from older buildings
    - [ii] Landfills where not disposed of properly
  - (b) Ingestion
    - [i] Consumption of contaminated fish
    - [ii] Contaminated well water
  - (c) Crosses placental barrier
  - (d) Found in breast milk
- (4) Effects
  - (a) Preterm delivery and induced abortion (Tsukimori et al, 2008)
  - (b) Spontaneous abortion
  - (c) Low birthweight
  - (d) Low intelligence quotient (IQ) scores in the child
  - (e) Possibly at least 2-year lag in reading comprehension
  - (f) Immunotoxic effect
  - (g) Exposure during fetal development poses increased risk for health effects.

   i. Toxic metals (heavy metals)
- (1) Arsenic
  - (a) Use

[i]   Naturally found in soil and minerals.

[ii]   Used in the production of various alloys to improve characteristics such as corrosion resistance, to improve machinability, and to increase annealing temperatures

[iii]   Wood preservation

[iv]   Production of lead acid batteries, semiconductors, and light-emitting diodes

(b) At-risk populations

   [i]   Smelter workers

   [ii]   Ceramic artists

   [iii]   Painters

(c) Exposure

   [i]   Ingestion of food or water

   [ii]   Inhalation

   [iii]   Crosses placenta and found in fetal tissues

   [iv]   Passes to breast milk

(d) Effects

   [i]   Spontaneous abortion

   [ii]   Low birthweight

   [iii]   Fetal loss

   [iv]   Studies of fetal effects of inhaled arsenic are inconclusive

(2) Lead

(a) Use

   [i]   Production of gasoline, batteries, paints, ink, ceramics, pottery, ammunition, and textiles

- Workplace exposures occur with smelting
- Lead fishing weights or ammunition
- Hobbies with use of lead solder; stained glass
- Lead acetate found in some hair colorants

   [ii]   At-risk populations

- Occupational exposures by woman or others living in the home
- Ingestion of clay, plaster, or paint chips (pica) either on purpose or by accident
- Live in an older home where renovations are occurring or with water pipes made of lead or with lead solder
- Use traditional or folk remedies or cosmetics that are homemade or not sold in regular stores.
  - *Greza* and *azarcon*—used by some Hispanic women as a morning sickness remedy.
  - *Bint al zahab (dhahab)*—a lead oxide compound that is burned by some Arabic women (Silbergeld & Patrick, 2005)

   [iii]   Women with hobbies that expose them to lead (stained glass making, oil paints, ceramic glazes)

   [iv]   Eat or drink from noncommercial pottery or leaded crystal

(b) Exposure

   [i]   Inhalation of dust

   [ii]   Ingestion of contaminated food or water

   [iii]   Skin contact (especially nonintact skin)

(c) Effects

   [i]   Increased testicular risks

   [ii]   Premature birth

   [iii]   Low birthweight (Cleveland, Minter, Cobb, Scott, and German, 2008)

   [iv]   Early fetal death

   [v]   Neurodevelopmental effects

- Most pronounced with exposure in the first trimester
- Cognitive defects in child associated with perinatal lead exposure (Chetty, et al, 2001).

(3) Mercury

(a) Three forms of mercury

   [i]   Metallic

   [ii]   Organic (combines with carbon) and salts

[iii] Methylmercury
- A form of organic mercury converted by microorganisms (bacteria, phyto-plankton and fungi) and other natural processes
- Found in freshwater and saltwater fish and marine mammals
- Shark and swordfish have highest levels.

(b) Uses
[i] Production of chlorine gas, used to extract gold from other minerals
[ii] Found in mercury thermometers, barometers, and dental amalgam fillings (50% mercury)
[iii] Red tattoo dye
[iv] Antibacterials (mercurochrome) and preservatives (thimerosal)

(c) At-risk populations
[i] Chloralkali plant workers
[ii] Thermometer factory workers
[iii] Dental clinic workers
[iv] Mercury mine and refinery workers

(d) Exposure
[i] Inhalation
- Inhalation of metallic mercury increases dose
- If inhaled, 80% of metallic mercury is absorbed
[ii] Ingestion of contaminated water and food (especially certain seafood)

(e) Effects
[i] Metallic mercury
- Fetus is more at risk for central nervous system (CNS) damage during critical periods of development.
[ii] Inorganic mercury
- Passes to breast milk
- Does not cross placenta easily
[iii] Methylmercury (Myers & Davidson, 2000)
- Passes to fetus in higher concentrations than the maternal concentration
  o Goes to fetal brain
- Fetus is more at risk for CNS damage during critical periods of development.
  o Passed in breast milk
[iv] Effects of all mercury products
- Decreased fertility
- Spontaneous abortions
- Low birthweight
- Developmental disabilities or mild retardation
  o Seizures
  o Blindness
  o Cerebral palsy

j. Waste anesthetic gases
(1) Use
(a) Gases used for general anesthesia
[i] Nitrous oxide
[ii] Halothane
[iii] Enflurane
(2) At-risk populations
(a) Health care workers who work around anesthesia gases
(b) Dentists
(c) Laboratory personnel
(d) Veterinarians
(3) Exposure
(a) Inhalation
[i] Gases can cross the placental barrier.
[ii] Exposure may occur at any stage, including before pregnancy.
(4) Effects
(a) Carcinogenic, teratogenic, and mutagenic

    (b) Embryotoxicity

    (c) Reduced male fertility

    (d) Early fetal death

    (e) Altered sex ratio

    (f) Late fetal death

    (g) Low birthweight

    (h) Birth defects

2. Ergonomic factors: physical and psychological aspects of the work environment

  a. Physiologic changes during pregnancy that may affect work

    (1) Increased risk of ligament strain due to decreased elasticity

    (2) Spine is more curved, change in center of gravity, with increased risk of back strain

    (3) Reaching distance increases due to increased abdominal girth

    (4) Increased strain on back muscles when lifting

    (5) Edema in joints

      (a) Increased risk of carpal tunnel syndrome

    (6) Impeded blood return from legs

  b. Ergonomic tasks and associated risks during pregnancy

    (1) Heavy physical work

      (a) There is great variation in women's tolerance of strenuous exertion, such as lifting, pulling, pushing, or climbing, based on physical fitness and strength, load handled, and the environment (Figá-Talamanca, 2006).

        [i] Risks

          • Spontaneous abortion

          • Preterm labor

          • Low birthweight

    (2) Awkward postures

      (a) Increased risk of muscle strain

      (b) Increased mechanical load (bending and lifting)

      (c) Increased risk of spontaneous abortion

    (3) Repetitive work

      (a) Risk of injury to ligaments, carpal tunnel syndrome

    (4) Prolonged standing

      (a) Increased risk of spontaneous abortion (for women with previous history of spontaneous abortion)

      (b) Fetal growth restriction

    (5) Prolonged sitting at a desk

      (a) Increased risk of blood clots

    (6) Other ergonomic-associated risks

      (a) Lack of rest

      (b) Worker fatigue

      (c) Irregular work hours

        [i] Slight risk of decreased fertility

        [ii] Slight risk of spontaneous abortion

      (d) Combined factors may increase risks.

        [i] Working long hours, lengthy periods of standing, and night work have been associated, in some studies, with increased risk for preterm delivery (Mozurkewich, Luke, Avni, & Wolf, 2000).

  c. Ergonomic environmental risks

    (1) Ionizing radiation

      (a) Source

        [i] Occurs naturally

          • Natural internal sources inside human body (accounts for about 10% of radiation dose in the United States)

          • Radon, cosmic, and terrestrial radiation account for about 82% of radiation dose in the United States (Agency for Toxic Substances and Disease Registry [ATSDR], 1999).

        [ii] Found in industrially produced radioactive materials

          • Medical radiation accounts for 15% of radiation dose exposure

- Production and testing of nuclear weapons account for 1% of exposure (ATSDR, 1999).
  - [iii] Used diagnostically and therapeutically in the health care industry (alpha, beta, gamma, and x-rays)
    - Exposures to x-rays and gamma rays are usually well controlled and with proper protection do not pose a major threat.
    - High-dose techniques—computed tomography (CT) and interventional radiology—require radiation protection.
    - Exposure from alpha rays: ingestion or inhalation—do not penetrate skin easily
    - Gamma rays—can pass through body
  - (b) At-risk populations
    - [i] Female flight personnel and pregnant frequent flyers exposure to cosmic radiation may exceed recommended radiation exposure (Geeze, 1998).
    - [ii] Nuclear workers
  - (c) Route of exposure
    - [i] Inhalation
    - [ii] Consumption of plants or animals that ingest contaminated food or water
    - [iii] Most exposure is from naturally occurring radiation such as radon.
  - (d) Exposure risks
    - [i] Mutagen at any stage of pregnancy
    - [ii] Teratogen during early weeks of pregnancy (differentiation)
  - (e) Recommended limits for radiation doses
    - [i] Current federal and state regulations limit radiation workers' doses to 0.05 Sv/year (5 rem/year).
    - [ii] The limit for the unborn child of a female radiation worker is 0.005 Sv (0.5 rem) per 9-month gestation period (ATSDR, 1999).
    - [iii] A dose to a pregnant woman should not exceed 1.5 rad during pregnancy. High doses of ionizing radiation may lead to:
      - Spontaneous abortion
      - Late fetal death
      - Neonatal death
      - Low birthweight
      - Microcephaly or mental retardation (especially with excessive exposure during first 8 weeks' gestation)
      - Childhood mortality
    - [iv] Low doses of ionizing radiation may lead to:
      - Altered sex ratio
      - Childhood malignancies: solid tumors and leukemia
      - Childhood mortality
    - [v] Nonionizing radiation sources
      - Ultraviolet radiation
      - Microwaves
      - Ultrasound
    - [vi] No reproductive data are available to support concern for exposure to nonionizing radiation.
- (2) Noise: sound transmits to the fetus, but the effects on the fetus are inconclusive.
  - (a) Source
    - [i] Loud noise is common in manufacturing processes, heavy-equipment operation, rock concerts, or the airline industry.
  - (b) Exposure risk
    - [i] Exposure to more than 85 dB associated with low birthweight of infant
      - 80 dB equivalent to subway, heavy city traffic, or factory noise.
      - Noise levels greater than 85 dB usually interfere with communication.
      - 90 dB equivalent to truck traffic, noisy home appliances, shop tools, lawnmowers
    - [ii] Prolonged exposure to loud noise (for more than 8 hours increases risk)
      - Prematurity and IUGR
      - An increase in the child's risk of high-frequency hearing loss (American Academy of Pediatrics [AAP], 1997)

(3) Temperature extremes
  (a) Hyperthermia
    [i] Source
      • Exposure to high temperatures in hot tubs, Jacuzzis, workplace, or from febrile illness (Andersen et al, 2002)
    [ii] At-risk populations
      • Outdoor workers
      • Military personnel
      • Recreational users of hot tubs, saunas, or Jacuzzis (Li, Janevic, Odouli, & Liu, 2001)
      • History of prolonged febrile illness in early pregnancy (Graham, Edwards & Edwards, 1998)
    [iii] Exposure risks
      • Increased risk of abortions and birth defects (Graham et al, 1998)
      • Hyperthermia increases the body's core temperature, and prolonged high temperature may affect the CNS of the fetus (Araujo, 1997).
      • Hyperthermia is considered a suspected teratogen with greatest harm caused during early differentiation.
      • Exposure at all stages of pregnancy can carry risk.
      • Some experts conclude that hyperthermia causes no reproductive hazard.
      • Neural tube defects such as spina bifida, encephalocele, and anencephaly are associated with hyperthermia (Graham et al, 1998).
      • Exposure to hot tubs and Jacuzzis early in pregnancy may increase the risk of birth defects by two to three times.
      • Pregnant women should be advised to avoid hot tub or Jacuzzi temperature of 38° C (100° F) or higher (Pergament, Schectman, & Rochanayon, 1997).
  (b) Hypothermia
    [i] Source
      • Work with deep freezers
      • Outdoor winter seasonal work or recreation
      • Medically induced hypothermia
    [ii] At-risk populations
      • Outdoor workers; construction, park rangers
      • Women who work in meat-packing plants
      • Women undergoing medically induced hypothermia during surgical procedures
    [iii] Exposure risk
      • Fetal bradycardia (Stange & Halldin, 1983)
      • Possible miscarriage
(4) Secondhand smoke (environmental tobacco smoke and passive smoking)
  (a) Background:
    [i] Approximately 30% of all reproductive-age women in the United States smoke during pregnancy (Talbot, 2008).
    [ii] In 2005 only 10.7% of women smoked during pregnancy.
    [iii] American Indian/Native Alaskan women have highest rate of smoking during pregnancy (17.8%) (American Lung Association, 2008)
    [iv] Cigarette smoke contains more than 4000 chemicals, of which more than 250 are known to be toxic and 69 are known carcinogens.
      • Toxic effects of most of these chemicals have not been studied.
    [v] Components of cigarette smoke
      • Mainstream smoke (inhaled directly by smoker)
      • Sidestream smoke emitted from a smoldering cigarette
      • Some compounds in sidestream smoke are emitted at 10 times the concentration as mainstream smoke.
    [vi] Secondhand smoke, also known as environmental tobacco smoke (ETS), includes sidestream smoke and exhaled smoke of smokers.
      • Inhaled passively by the smoker and nonsmokers

[vii] At-risk populations
- Exposure occurs at workplace, home, or recreational settings.
- Bartenders and casino workers have increased risk of exposure.

[viii] Exposure risks
- Reproductive effects of secondhand smoke in females target uterus, ovary, oviducts (Talbot, 2008)
  - Reduced fertility with acceleration of oocyte loss
  - Conception delay
  - Premature menopause
  - Increased risk for ectopic pregnancy
  - Increased risk of prematurity
- Affects uterine artery contractility, placental growth, and attachment and amniotic fluid
- Evidence suggests that maternal exposure to secondhand smoke during pregnancy adversely affects the unborn child.
  - Cigarette smoke targets the placenta, umbilical cord, and embryo/fetus (Talbot, 2008).
  - Measurable concentrations of cotinine (a biomarker of nicotine uptake in nonsmokers) have been found in the hair of infants born to mothers exposed to secondhand smoke (Joad, 2000).
  - Evidence is conclusive to infer relationship between secondhand smoke and sudden infant death syndrome (SIDS) (USDHHS, 2006).
  - Evidence is suggestive of causal link between environmental tobacco smoke and preterm delivery and small reductions in birthweight (USDHHS, 2006).
  - Suggestive but not sufficient evidence to infer causal relationship between secondhand smoke exposure during prenatal and postnatal periods and leukemia, childhood cancer, lymphoma, or childhood brain tumors (USDHHS, 2006).

Pharmaceuticals

A. Introduction
1. Pharmaceuticals are chemical substances with medicinal properties; they include prescribed drugs, over-the-counter drugs, and herbal therapies that are taken as part of a treatment regimen or to provide relief of symptoms.
2. Drugs that are absorbed systemically or are known to be potentially harmful to the fetus are required by the U.S. Food and Drug Administration (FDA) (2009) to be categorized according to one of five pregnancy categories as follows (the letter signifies the level of risk to the fetus):
   a. Category A: drugs that have failed to pose a demonstrated risk to the fetus in controlled studies in pregnant women
   b. Category B: drugs that have not posed a demonstrated fetal risk in animals but for which no controlled studies in pregnant women have been conducted
   c. Category C: drugs that have revealed adverse effects on the fetus in animal studies, but no controlled studies in women have been conducted
      (1) Also includes drugs for which no animal or human well-controlled studies are available
      (2) Note that most drugs are in this category due to lack of available studies.
   d. Category D: drugs for which positive evidence of human fetal risk exists, but the benefits might outweigh the risk if no safer effective drugs are available
   e. Category X: drugs with animal and human studies that have demonstrated positive evidence of fetal abnormalities
      (1) These drugs are contraindicated in women who are or may become pregnant.
3. The FDA pregnancy risk category system is undergoing revision.
   a. The current system falsely implies that drugs at higher levels such as D or X are more dangerous than lower levels (Category A, B, or C).
   b. The assigned category is actually based only on the presence of research studies to support data.
   c. The proposed new system will provide more detailed information related to the areas of fertility, fetal effects, pregnancy, and lactation (FDA, 2009).

4. Many women take some sort of pharmaceutical while pregnant.
   a. In studies of U.S. prescription practices for pregnant women, 56% to 65% of pregnant women were prescribed a drug during pregnancy (Andrade et al, 2004; Riley et al, 2005).
   b. At least half of all pregnant women were prescribed medications of FDA category C, D, or X for which there is no established safety during pregnancy or evidence in animal or human studies of fetal risk (Andrade et al, 2004).
   c. Many women take a prescribed drug during the preconceptual period and may be unaware when they become pregnant, increasing early trimester exposure.
   d. Prescriptions for potentially harmful drugs decrease during the first trimester (Malm, Martikainen, Klaukka, & Neuvoven, 2004).
   e. Most commonly prescribed therapeutic drug classes during pregnancy (Andrade et al, 2004; Riley et al, 2005)
      (1) Antibiotics
      (2) Respiratory drugs; asthma drugs
      (3) Opioid and nonopioid analgesics
      (4) Gastrointestinal drugs; antiemetics
   f. Most commonly dispensed Category D drugs (excluding ovulation stimulants, fertility drugs, contraceptive hormones, estrogens, and progesterones)
      (1) Atenolol
      (2) Secobarbital
      (3) Doxycycline
      (4) Lorazepam
      (5) Clonazepam
   g. Most commonly dispensed Category X drugs (excluding ovulation stimulants, fertility drugs, contraceptive hormones, estrogens, and progesterones)
      (1) Temazepam
      (2) Flurazepam
      (3) Testosterone
      (4) Misoprostol
      (5) Triazolam
5. Approximately 30 drugs are known to be teratogenic in humans.
6. No safe dose has been established for many pharmaceuticals during pregnancy.
7. Some drugs are prescribed during pregnancy specifically for fetal pharmacotherapy, to treat or prevent a problem with the fetus (Blackburn, 2008).
   a. Preconceptual folic acid to prevent neural tube defects
   b. Antenatal corticosteroids to accelerate maturation of fetal lungs, for treatment of congenital lupus, or to treat female fetuses at risk for congenital adrenal hyperplasia
   c. Treatment of inherited metabolic disorders
   d. Treatment of fetal cardiac arryhthmias or heart failure
   e. Prevention of Rh sensitization with antenatal recombinant human (Rh) immune globulin
8. Results of studies related to safety of some pharmaceuticals are unequivocal; therefore, caution is advised.
9. Many women self-medicate with herbal therapies.
10. Availability of drugs on the internet, sometimes without a prescription, can make it easier for women to self-medicate with a possible harmful drug when pregnant.
11. Dose and method of administration must also be considered in evaluating risk.
12. Evaluation of each drug taken must be based on its potential effect as a carcinogen, mutagen, or teratogen.
13. For drugs with known pregnancy risks, implementation of risk management programs such as iPLEDGE with isotretinoin have been demonstrated to be an effective way to mitigate the risks (Honein, Lindstrom, & Kweder, 2007).
    a. Drug distribution system that requires registration of patients, health care provider, distributors, and wholesalers
    b. Links real-time pregnancy testing to dispensing of medication
14. Pregnancy registries around the world collect and organize information related to outcomes of various drugs taken during pregnancy and are a resource for health care providers, nurses, and pregnant women (Karceski, 2008).

Assessment for Exposure to Environmental Hazards

A. **Assess exposure history of males and females.**
   1. Identify current or past exposures.
   2. Reduce or eliminate current exposures.
   3. Reduce adverse health effects.
B. **Reproductive health assessment**
   1. Discuss obstetric history.
      a. Infertility
      b. Previous pregnancy loss
      c. Health of current children
         (1) Birth defects
         (2) Developmental delay
         (3) Learning or behavior problems
   2. Identify any potential toxins or agents to which parents may be exposed on an ongoing basis.
      a. Solvents
      b. Dust
      c. Fumes
      d. Pesticides
      e. Other chemicals
      f. Radiation
      g. Loud noise
   3. Assess possible signs of illness after previous exposure to a chemical or pesticide
   4. Assess whether symptoms improve when parent is away from work or the home
   5. Establish time of exposure.
      a. Preconceptual
      b. Stage during pregnancy
      c. For accuracy, pinpoint gestational age in weeks and days (e.g., 10 week and 3 days).
   6. Establish exposure levels in the workplace.
   7. Establish duration of exposure.
      a. Acute: seconds to minutes
      b. Chronic: over months or years
   8. Establish route of exposure (inhalation, ingestion, direct skin contact, direct effect, other)
   9. Evaluate precautions taken to control exposure.
      a. Use of personal protective equipment (PPE) in the workplace
      b. Evaluate whether a uniform is worn, or if either parent wears work clothes to and from work.
      c. Potential for exposure to contaminated clothing of other family members
      d. Hygienic procedures after work (bathing)
      e. Laundry procedures (NIOSH, 1999)
   10. History of occupational or home exposure
      a. Type of work
         (1) Current work
         (2) Past work
         (3) Longest job held
         (4) Military service
      b. Hobbies
         (1) Gardening
         (2) Fishing or hunting
            (a) Ask if they eat fish or game that is caught or hunted
         (3) Stained glass
         (4) Ceramics
      c. Pets
      d. Ergonomic risks of work
         (1) Noise, lifting, prolonged standing or sitting
   11. Identify sociocultural practices that might increase pregnancy risks.
      a. History of pica increases risk of ingestion of heavy metals.
      b. Use of votives or cosmetics that contain lead-based products

12. Home/neighborhood location
    a. Air quality
    b. Water concerns: lead pipes, well water
    c. Located near landfill
    d. Located near factories
    e. Located near farms (risk of contaminated water runoff)
    f. Age of home
    g. Recent remodeling
    h. Lead paint
    i. Type of heating
    j. Storage of any chemicals
    k. Pesticide use in the home
13. Review use of pharmaceuticals taken preconceptually and during pregnancy
    a. Prescribed
    b. Over-the counter
    c. Nonprescription or borrowed
    d. Recreational
    e. Herbal therapies
14. Establish patient's level of exposure through review of records when possible.
    a. Review biologic samples when appropriate.
       (1) Urine screening to determine levels of organic solvents and pesticides
       (2) Blood samples to determine lead or other toxic metal levels
    b. Establish level of exposure through environmental monitoring of workplace.
    c. Consider an ergonomic assessment of workplace to evaluate risk.
    d. Dosimeter to monitor noise level
    e. Coordinate with occupational health nurse if available.
    f. Gather material safety data sheets (MSDSs).

Nursing Interventions and Outcomes for Environmental Hazards

A. **Introduction: Most nurse-patient encounters related to environmental hazards occur after the exposure happens. Key interventions focus on minimizing physical and psychological effects of the exposure, providing patient education, referral, and support after the exposure.**
B. **Patient Education**
   1. Encourage preconceptual counseling for couples considering pregnancy.
      a. Discuss potential environmental or occupational hazards of both parents with health care provider.
      b. Advise health care provider of any medications currently taking and discuss need to change medications.
      c. Advise of potential reproductive dangers of pharmaceuticals, whether prescribed or over-the-counter.
      d. Ensure the prepregnant woman is up-to-date on immunizations prior to pregnancy.
         (1) Some vaccines are teratogens.
      e. Outcomes
         (1) Parents will seek a preconceptual counseling visit with health care provider.
         (2) Parents can identify potential risks of environmental hazards in the home and workplace.
         (3) Patient informs health care provider of medications used.
         (4) Maternal medications are adjusted prior to conception to avoid use of potential teratogens.
         (5) Maternal immunizations are updated prior to seeking conception.
         (6) Exposure to environmental hazards is avoided or minimized preconceptually by both parents.
   2. Teach males and females of reproductive age the risks of occupational and environmental exposures.
      a. Sources of reproductive toxins at work and in the home
      b. Potential reproductive outcomes of exposure
      c. Explain role of the occupational health nurse as a consultant for males and females of reproductive age related to identification of environmental hazards in the workplace.

■ BOX 9-1
■ **RESOURCES FOR ENVIRONMENTAL HAZARDS**

The following resources may provide useful information on environmental hazards:

- Agency for Toxic Substances & Disease Registry: www.atsdr.cdc.gov
- Association of Occupational & Environmental Clinics: www.aoec.org
- Environmental Protection Agency: www.epa.gov
- Material safety data sheets: www.hazard.com/msds
- Occupational Safety & Health Administration: www.osha.gov
- March of Dimes: www.marchofdimes.com
- Local health department, environmental agency, poison control center
- National Society of Genetic Counselors: www.nsgc.org/
- American Lung Association: www.lungusa.org
- State teratogen registries
- U.S. Food and Drug Administration: www.fda.gov
- Teratogen Information System (TERIS): www.depts.washington.edu/terisweb/teris
- Reprotox: www.reprotox.org
- Organization of Teratology Information Specialists: www.otispregnancy.org/hm

    d. Provide reliable resources about environmental hazards in the workplace and home (i.e., internet websites, material safety data sheets) (Box 9-1).

    e. Outcomes

        (1) Males and females of reproductive age are able to identify environmental hazards in the workplace and home that may affect fertility, pregnancy, and health of developing fetus.

        (2) Patients can discuss the role of the occupational health nurse as a resource in the workplace.

        (3) Patients can identify resources for further information on specific environmental hazards.

3. Teach strategies to minimize exposure to toxic work-related or environmental hazards during pregnancy

    a. Advise patient to evaluate environmental hazards she is exposed to and discuss strategies to avoid them as much as possible.

    b. Reinforce use of personal protective equipment.

    c. Avoid contamination from the workplace to home.

        (1) Wear a uniform that is only used for work.

        (2) Change clothes between work and home if possible.

        (3) Use safe laundering practices.

        (4) Practice good personal hygiene after work.

    d. Outcomes

        (1) Patient is able to identify potential hazards in the workplace.

        (2) Patient uses appropriate personal protective equipment if working in an at-risk environment.

        (3) Both parents implement practices to minimize contamination from workplace to home.

4. Teach ways to minimize duration and dosage of an actual toxic environmental or work related exposure during preconceptual period and throughout critical periods of pregnancy.

    a. Physically remove self from exposed area if inhalation risk occurs.

    b. Immediately remove contaminated clothing if skin exposure occurs.

    c. Perform decontamination procedures based on type of exposure.

    d. Outcomes

        (1) Duration and dosage of the exposure event are minimized.

        (2) Appropriate decontamination procedures are applied in a timely manner.

5. Teach woman how to minimize ergonomic risks during pregnancy.
   a. Teach about the normal body changes in pregnancy that affect work (i.e., changes in center of gravity, lordosis that can affect back strain).
   b. Use of proper body mechanics for turning, lifting, pushing, pulling, or during prolonged standing required during pregnancy to prevent back strain.
   c. Identify alternatives for work practices that involve heavy lifting (get help or use other lifting aids).
   d. Avoid awkward postures during pregnancy such as crawling on stomach.
   e. Use ergonomic keyboards to reduce risks of carpal tunnel.
   f. Alternate work activities during the day if possible to avoid prolonged sitting or standing.
   g. Follow precautions and use protective equipment if working in areas with exposure to ionizing radiation.
   h. If prolonged exposure to loud noise, seek breaks away from areas of exposure to areas of quiet.
   i. Outcomes
      (1) Woman uses proper body mechanics during work performance for lifting, turning, pushing, pulling, or if prolonged standing is required as evidenced by absence of back strain or injury during pregnancy.
      (2) Patient can identify alternative ways to accomplish work requirements to protect self during pregnancy if exposed to environmental hazards.
      (3) Ergonomic risks are minimized during pregnancy as evidenced by absence of maternal injury and normal fetal growth and development.
6. Teach importance of avoiding temperature extremes during pregnancy (hypothermia or hyperthermia).
   a. Teach about normal range of body temperature (36.4° to 37.1° C [97.5° to 98.8° F]).
   b. Provide information about the possible dangers to fetus of prolonged exposure to heat or cold during pregnancy.
   c. Teach signs of hyperthermia (high body temperature, cessation of sweating, headache, dizziness, faintness, nausea, rapid respirations, and rapid heart rate).
   d. Advise use of Jacuzzis or hot tubs only at temperatures of less than 38° C (100° F) for short intervals (10 minutes at a time) while pregnant.
   e. Discourage strenuous physical activities and exercise that might increase body temperature when climate is hot or humid.
   f. Encourage patient to drink fluids to maintain adequate hydration, even if not thirsty.
   g. Discuss ways to minimize effects of hyperthermia.
      (1) Move to cooler environment.
      (2) Use other cooling measures (cold compresses, ice pack, or fan).
      (3) Take in extra liquids for hydration.
      (4) Seek medical attention if temperature exceeds 38° C (101° F) with signs of hyperthermia.
   h. Teach signs of hypothermia (drowsiness, confusion, slow speech, shivering, slow heartbeat, slow respirations, cold pale skin, blue fingers and toes)
   i. Discuss ways to minimize effects of hypothermia.
      (1) Wear layers of clothing if at risk for cold exposure.
      (2) Move to a warm environment.
      (3) Add extra clothing or blankets
      (4) Drink warm fluids.
      (5) Seek medical attention if symptoms of hypothermia occur.
   j. Outcomes
      (1) Patient is able to identify signs and symptoms of hypothermia and hyperthermia.
      (2) Patient is able to discuss ways to minimize exposure to temperature extremes in the workplace and environment.
      (3) Maternal core body temperature maintained within a normal range of 36.4° to 37.1° C (97.5° to 98.8° F)
7. Minimize exposure to active and passive smoking during pregnancy.
   a. Teach patient about risks of active and passive smoking on the developing fetus
   b. Advise patient to maintain a smoke-free environment during pregnancy
   c. Inform of laws and legislation that provide smoke-free environments.

    d. Encourage patient to be assertive in not allowing smoking in environments she can control.

    e. Advise patient of increased risk of respiratory problems, ear infections, SIDS, and childhood cancers in infants and children exposed to secondhand smoke.

    f. Outcomes

      (1) Patient protects self and fetus from exposure to secondhand smoke.

      (2) Patient avoids smoke-polluted environments.

      (3) Patient selects nonsmoking areas in public places.

      (4) Patient restricts smoking in personal environments at home and work.

      (5) Patient is knowledgeable of the health risks associated with active and passive smoking for self, fetus, and newborn.

      (6) Patient informs employer of potential dangers of exposure to secondhand smoke during pregnancy if working in an at-risk environment and demands a smoke-free environment.

      (7) Patient makes plan to create smoke-free home environment for self and infant.

8. Teach woman about risks of pharmaceutical use during pregnancy (prescribed, over-the-counter, and herbal therapies).

    a. Advise patient to inform health care provider of plans for pregnancy to discuss implications of prescribed drugs.

    b. Instruct preconceptual and pregnant women not to take any type of pharmaceutical or herbal therapy without consulting their health care practitioner.

    c. Instruct women who are considering pregnancy never to restart a drug previously prescribed without consulting their health care practitioner.

    d. Instruct women never to take borrowed medications that were prescribed for others.

    e. Instruct patient to read all pharmaceutical labels and adhere to their precautions.

    f. Outcomes

      (1) Patient obtains information about potentially hazardous pharmaceuticals.

      (2) Patient discontinues all drugs not approved by health care provider.

      (3) Patient follows through on all referrals.

    g. Exposure to environmental and workplace hazards by the mother is minimized during pregnancy as evidenced by maintenance of pregnancy and normal pattern of fetal growth and development during each trimester.

C. **Referrals**

  1. Occupational health nurse

    a. Occupational health nurses employed by the specific industry will be knowledgeable of identified reproductive and pregnancy risk issues in the workplace.

    b. Evaluates the need for possible work reassignment during preconceptual period and/or early embryonic period if needed (Cannon, Schmidt, Cambardella, & Browne, 2000)

    c. Instructs those at risk of occupational exposures about where to locate and how to read the MSDSs for chemical agents to which they have potential to be exposed

    d. Ensures that safety manuals in the workplace have policies and procedures to address issues related to workplace environmental hazards

      (1) Approved chemicals and their use

      (2) Methods of exposure

      (3) Risk reduction methods

      (4) Proper methods of disposal of hazardous substances

      (5) Requirements for personal protective equipment

      (6) Procedures to follow when exposures occur

  2. Health care provider: Refer for further evaluation of pregnancy and fetus post exposure.

    a. Evaluate risk to pregnancy post exposure according to type of agent, developmental stage of pregnancy, dose and duration of exposure, health of the mother prior to and after exposure, type of protection used to control exposure, and fetal status post exposure.

  3. Genetic counseling: refer if exposed to a known teratogen during critical stages of pregnancy

  4. Other agencies: refer to appropriate agencies for further information about the potential hazard or to report exposure

    a. Refer a pregnant woman exposed to potentially hazardous pharmaceuticals preconceptually or during first trimester of pregnancy to teratogen registries, the March of Dimes, and other agencies who are interested in collecting data to generate or support hypotheses about the link between the use of pharmaceuticals and pregnancy outcome.

5. Outcomes
   a. Patient will follow through with referrals.
   b. Patient will participate in or support research on the correlation between pharmaceutical use and pregnancy outcomes.

D. **Provide support to parents if exposure to environmental hazard occurs.**
   1. Listen to patient's expression of anxiety or fear.
   2. Provide emotional support.
   3. Provide factual information to provide a realistic perspective to pregnant women concerned about potentially hazardous exposures to environmental toxins or pharmaceuticals.
   4. Provide resources to parents for accurate information of risks.
   5. Provide reassurance that not every exposure results in a negative outcome; many uncertainties exist.
   6. Refer for genetic or psychological counseling as needed.
   7. Assist in finding a support system or support group.
   8. Assist with making decisions related to work based on severity of past exposure or probability of continued exposure (Drozdowsky & Whittaker, 1999).
      a. Reduce exposure to environmental hazard.
      b. Transfer to a different job.
      c. Take compensated or uncompensated leave.
      d. Terminate current job.
   9. Outcomes
      a. Patient is able to express her anxiety or fear related to possible hazardous environmental exposure.
      b. Patient is able to identify sources of accurate information related to the hazardous environmental exposure.
      c. Patient will follow up with appointments for referrals for genetic or psychological counseling.
      d. Patient is able to identify sources of support available after a hazardous environmental exposure.
      e. Patient is able to make decisions related to job if potential for further exposures exists during pregnancy.

CASE STUDIES AND STUDY QUESTIONS

Occupational Hazards

Mrs. T. is a 24-year-old woman who has been employed full-time as a dental assistant for the past 3 years. Her work involves standing about 75% of the time. She has just learned that she is 6 weeks pregnant. This is her first pregnancy. Her husband is employed by a company that produces chemicals used as pesticides. They planned this pregnancy but did not seek preconceptual care. Mrs. T. also is a member of a local spa and attends aerobic exercise classes three times per week.

1. When taking the occupational history on Mrs. T., which of the following areas need further assessment? (Choose all that apply.)
   a. Why they did not seek preconceptual counseling
   b. Does Mrs. T. use a sauna or hot tub at the spa?
   c. Types of chemicals with which Mr. T. works
   d. Potential ergonomic or chemical exposures for Mrs. T.

2. What would you include in health education for Mrs. T.? (Choose all that apply.)
   a. Importance of reviewing MSDSs on each chemical to which she and her husband are exposed
   b. Importance of using recommended protective equipment
   c. Importance of informing her employer of the pregnancy
   d. Importance of taking 5- to 10-minute activity breaks every hour to avoid prolonged standing and sitting
      (1) a, b
      (2) a, b, d
      (3) a, c
      (4) All of the above

3. What recommendations would you make regarding her recreational activities?
   a. Aerobic class activities should be evaluated to determine level of safety.
   b. Advise her to discontinue aerobic classes because they are too strenuous.

c. Advise her to continue aerobic classes because they do not pose a potential health threat.

d. Recommend that she discuss her pregnancy with her aerobics instructor.

Pharmaceuticals

Mrs. C., 33 years old, is 8 weeks pregnant with her third child. During the intake interview she reports that since she became pregnant, she has taken aspirin for headaches and antihistamines for allergy symptoms. She also uses antacids occasionally. She reports that she takes herbal teas for relaxation.

4. Which drugs that she is using would concern you? (Choose all that apply.)
   a. Antacids
   b. Aspirin
   c. Antihistamines
   d. Herbal teas
5. Which would you recommend during her pregnancy? (Choose all that apply.)
   a. The drugs she is taking are safe during pregnancy because they are not Category D or X.
   b. She should not take any medications or herbal therapies during pregnancy without discussing them with her health care provider first.
   c. Herbal teas are a good way to relax during pregnancy.
   d. The teratogenic effects of many drugs and herbal therapies are not known.

Temperature Extremes

Mrs. D. is a pregnant 31-year-old mother of three children. She and her husband live in a large home in an affluent neighborhood. They have a swimming pool and hot tub. They enjoy relaxing in the hot tub nightly before retiring. She also reports that she likes to exercise outside several times a week. Her favorite activities are jogging and bike riding.

6. Which recommendation will help her control her exposure to high temperatures? (Choose all that apply.)
   a. Stop using the hot tub.
   b. Use the hot tub for only 10 minutes at a time with the temperature less than 38° C (100° F)
   c. Sit with only her legs or feet dangling in the hot water.
   d. Suggest that she take an evening walk with her husband instead of using the hot tub.

Secondhand Smoke

Ms. R. is a 22-year-old single woman, pregnant with her second child, who works for a metropolitan newspaper in the newsroom, where smoking is permitted. Ms R. quit smoking when she first discovered she was pregnant with this child. Ms. R. usually dates every Friday and Saturday evening. She especially enjoys dancing at a local bar. She does not permit smoking in her home or car.

7. Which response to her work situation would you support?
   a. Quit her job and find one in a smoke-free workplace.
   b. Discuss with her employer the potential dangers of secondhand smoke to the fetus and request a separate office that would be smoke free.
   c. Use a fan to vent the smoke away from her.
   d. Request a transfer to a different department immediately.
8. What health teaching would you include related to her social life?
   a. Suggest that she stop dating because of potential dangers to fetus.
   b. Advise her to avoid dancing because finding a dance floor free of smoke is impossible.
   c. Encourage her to discuss her concern regarding effects of passive smoking with her date and consider alternatives that would be safe.
   d. Do nothing because the dangers of secondhand smoke to the fetus have not been well documented.

Workplace Exposures

Ms. S. is a 19-year-old gravida 3, para 0 woman who is 8 weeks pregnant and being seen for her intake appointment at the prenatal clinic. She reports that she works in a furniture factory in the wood finishing department. She states that her job involves use of aerosol spray paints and varnishes and that she does a moderate amount of heavy lifting. She denies taking any medications prior to pregnancy and reports she is a nonsmoker and denies drinking alcoholic beverages. She is very excited but cautious about this pregnancy as she lost two other pregnancies at about 8 weeks' gestation. She affirms that there is an employee health nurse at her workplace.

9. What information is needed by the nurse during the intake interview related to exposure to environmental hazards? (Choose all that apply.)

a. Gather more information about the circumstances and outcomes of her two past pregnancies that did not go to term.

b. Get a complete list of the types of paint products or chemicals she works with.

c. Ask whether personal protective equipment is available and if she uses it while on the job.

d. Ask whether she contacted the employee health nurse prior to getting pregnant.

10. Ms. S. reports that she is supposed to wear a respirator at work but does not always use it. What health teaching or referral would be most appropriate for Ms. S.? (Choose all that apply.)

a. Inform her that working with paints and solvents can increase the risk of birth defects and she should protect herself.

b. Refer her to the employee health nurse to develop a plan for avoidance of workplace hazards during pregnancy.

c. Teach her about the importance of protecting herself and her fetus from workplace environmental hazards by using personal protective equipment.

d. Notify her employer that she is pregnant and that she must use the personal protective equipment.

ANSWERS TO STUDY QUESTIONS

1. b, c, d	6. b, c
2. 4	7. b
3. a	8. c
4. b, d	9. a, b, c
5. b, d	10. b, c

REFERENCES

Agency for Toxic Substances and Disease Registry (ATSDR). (1999).Toxicological profile for ionizing radiation. Atlanta: U.S. Department of Health and Human Services, Department of Public Health. Retrieved April 1, 2009, from www.atsdr.cdc.gov/toxprofiles/phs149.html.

Ahmed, P., & Jaakkola, J. (2007). Exposure to organic solvents and adverse pregnancy outcomes. *Human Reproduction, 22*(10), 2751–2757.

American Academy of Pediatrics, Committee on Environmental Health. (1997). Noise: A hazard for the fetus and newborn. *Pediatrics, 100,* 724–727.

American Lung Association. (2008). Smoking and women fact sheet. Retrieved March 6, 2009, from American Lung Association website: www.lungusa.org/site/c.dvLUK9O0E/b.33572/k.9D28/Smoking_and_Women_Fact_Sheet.htm

Andersen, A., Vastrup, P., Wohlfhart, J., Andersen, P., Olsen, J., & Melbye, M. (2002). Fever in pregnancy and risk of fetal death: A cohort study, *Lancet, 360*(9345), 1552–1556.

Andrade, S. E., Gurwitz, J., Davis, R., Chan, K., Finkelstein, J., Fortman, K., McPhillips, H., Raebel, M., Roblin, D., Smith, D., Yood, M., Morse, A., & Platt, R. (2004). Prescription drug use in pregnancy. *American Journal of Obstetrics and Gynecology, 191,* 398–407.

Araujo, D. (1997). Expecting questions about exercise and pregnancy? *The Physician and Sportsmedicine, 27*(8), 51.

Arble, J. (2004). Toxicology primer: Understanding workplace hazards and protecting worker health. *AAOHN Journal, 52*(6), 25.

Blackburn, S. (2008). Fetal pharmacotherapy. *Journal of Perinatal and Neonatal Nursing, 22*(4), 264–266.

Bowling, L., Gaudette, M., & Pergament, E. (2006). Organic solvents during pregnancy: An update on occupational exposure. Illinois Teratogen Information Service Newsletter, *13*(1), 1–5. Retrieved March 14, 2009, from www.fetal-exposure.org.

Cannon, R., Schmidt, J., Cambardella, B., & Browne, S. (2000). High risk pregnancy in the workplace: Influencing positive outcomes. *AAOHN Journal, 48*(9), 435–448.

Center for the Evaluation of Risks to Human Reproduction (CERHR). (2002). *NTP-CERHR expert panel report on the reproductive and developmental toxicity of ethylene glycol, National Toxicology Program.* Washington, DC: U.S. Department of Health and Human Services. Retrieved on February 12, 2009, from cerhr.niehs.nih.gov/chemicals/egpg/ethylene/EG_Report_Final.pdf.

Chemical Abstracts Service. (2009). Registry number and substance counts. Retrieved on February 12, 2009, from www.cas.org/cgi-bin/cas/regreport.pl.

Chetty, C. S., Reddy, G. R., Murthy, K. S., Johnson, J., Sajwan, K., & Desaiah, D. (2001). Perinatal lead exposure alters the expression of neuronal nitric oxide synthase in rat brain. *International Journal of Toxicology, 20*(3), 113–120.

Cleveland, L., Minter, M., Cobb, K., Scott, A., & German, V. (2008). Lead hazards for pregnant women and children: Part 2: More still can be done to reduce the chance of exposure to lead in at-risk populations. *American Journal of Nursing, 108*(11), 40–47.

Connor, T., & McDiarmid, M. (2006). Preventing occupational exposure to antineoplastic drugs in health care settings. *CA: A Cancer Journal for Clinicians, 56,* 354–365.

Drozdowsky, S., & Whittaker, S. (1999). Workplace hazards to reproduction and development: A resource for workers, employers, health care providers, and health & safety personnel. Safety and Health Assessment and Research for Prevention (SHARP), Technical Report Number 21-3-1999. Retrieved March 14, 2009, from www.lni.wa.gov/ Safety/Research/files/repro_dev.pdf.

Figá-Talamanca, I. (2006). Occupational risk factors and reproductive health of women. *Occupation Medicine, 56,* 521–531.

Fisher, B., Rose, N., & Carey, J. (2008). Principles and practice of teratology for the obstetrician. *Clinical Obstetrics and Gynecology, 51*(1), 106–118.

Frazier, L. (2007). Reproductive disorders associated with pesticide exposure. *Journal of Agromedicine, 12*(1), 27–37.

Geeze, D. S. (1998). Pregnancy and in-flight cosmic radiation. Aerospace Medical Association. *Aviation Space and Environmental Medicine, 69*(11), 1061–1064.

Graham, J., Edwards, M., & Edwards, M. (1998). Teratogen update: Gestational effects of maternal hyperthermia due to febrile illnesses and resultant patterns of defects in humans. *Teratology, 58,* 209–221.

Gray, L. E. (2000). Perinatal exposure to the phthalates DEHP, BBP, and DINP, but not DEP, DMP, or DOTP, alters sexual differentiation of the male rat. *Toxicology Sciences, 58*(2), 357–365.

Greim, H., & Snyder, R. (2008). *Toxicology and risk assessment: A comprehensive introduction.* Wiltshire: Anthony Rowe, Ltd.

Gresie-Brusen, D., Kielkowski, D., Baker, A., Channa, K., & Rees, D. (2006). Occupational exposure to ethylene oxide during pregnancy and association with adverse reproductive outcomes. *International Archives of Occupational and Environmental Health, 80*(7), 559–565.

Hernández-Diáz, S., Mitchell, A., Kelley, K., Calafat, A., & Hauser, R. (2009). Medications as a potential source of exposure to phthalates in the U.S. population. *Environmental Health Perspectives, 117*(2), 185–189.

Honein, M., Lindstrom, J., & Kweder, S. (2007). Can we ensure the safe use of known human teratogens? The iPLEDGE test case. *Drug Safety, 30*(1), 5–15.

Joad, J. (2000). Smoking and pediatric respiratory health. *Clinics in Chest Medicine, 21*(1), 37–46.

Karceski, S. (2008). Epilepsy and pregnancy: Are seizure medications safe? *Neurology, 71*(14), e32–e33.

Khattak, S., K-Moghtader, G., McMartin, K., Barrera, M., Kennedy, D., & Koren, G. (1999). Pregnancy outcome following gestational exposure to organic solvents: A prospective controlled study. *Journal of the American Medical Association, 282*(11), 1033.

Laslo-Baker, D., Barrera, M., Knittel-Keren, D., Kozer, E., Wolpin, J., Khattak, S., Hackman, R., Rovet, J., & Koren, G. (2004). Childhood neurodevelopmental outcome and maternal occupational exposure to solvents. *Archives of Pediatric Adolescent Medicine, 158,* 951–956.

Li, D. K., Janevic, R., Odouli, R., & Liu, L. (2001). Use of hot tub or Jacuzzi during pregnancy and the risk of spontaneous abortion (SAB). *Journal of Pediatric and Perinatal Epidemiology, 15,* A20.

Malm, H., Martikainen, J., Klaukka, T., & Neuvoven, P. (2004). Prescription of hazardous drugs during pregnancy. *Drug Safety, 27*(12), 899–908.

March of Dimes. (2009). Environmental risks and pregnancy. Retrieved February 16, 2009, from www. marchofdimes.com/855_9146.asp.

McAuliffe, M., & Perry, M. (2007). Are nanoparticles potential male reproductive toxicants? A literature review. *Nanotoxicology, 1*(3), 204–210.

Mozurkewich, E., Luke, B., Avni, M., & Wolf, F. (2000). Working conditions and adverse pregnancy outcome: A meta-analysis. *Obstetrics and Gynecology, 95*(4), 623–635.

Myers, D., & Davidson, P. (2000). Does methylmercury have a role in causing developmental disabilities in children? *Environmental Health Perspectives, 108*(3), 413–420.

National Institute for Occupational Safety and Health (NIOSH). (1999). The effects of workplace hazards on female reproductive health. USDHHS Publication No. 99–104. Retrieved March 14, 2009, from www.cdc.gov/NIOSH/docs/99-104/default.html.

Pergament, E., Schechtman, A., & Rochanayon, A. (1997). Hyperthermia and pregnancy. Risk Newsletter. Retrieved February 24, 2009, from www.fetal-exposure.org/HYPERTH.html.

Polifka, J., & Friedman, J. M. (2002). Medical genetics: Clinical teratology in the age of genomics. *Canadian Medical Association Journal, 167*(3), 265–273.

Rice, D., & Barone, S. (2000). Critical periods of vulnerability for the developing nervous system: Evidence from humans and animal models. *Environmental Health Perspectives, 108*(Suppl 3), 511–533.

Riley, E., Fuentes-Afflick, E., Jackson, R., Escobar, G., Brawarsky, P., Schreiber, M., & Haasm, J. (2005). Correlates of prescription drug use during pregnancy. *Journal of Women's Health, 14*(5), 401–409.

Roeleveld, N., & Bretveld, R. (2008). The impact of pesticides on male fertility. *Current Opinion in Obstetrics and Gynecology, 20*(3), 229–233.

Silbergeld, E., & Patrick, T. (2005). Environmental exposures, toxicologic mechanisms and adverse pregnancy outcomes. *American Journal of Obstetrics and Gynecology*, *192*, S11–S21.

Slama, R., Darrow, L., Parker, J., Woodruff, T., Strickland, M., Nieuwenhuijsen, M., Gliniani, S., Hoggatt, K., Kannan, S., Hurley, F., Kalinka, J., Sram, R., Brauer, M., Wilhelm, M., Heinrich, J., & Ritz, B. (2008). Meeting report: Atmospheric pollution and human reproduction. *Environmental Health Perspective*, *116*(6), 791–798.

Stange, K., & Halldin, M. (1983). Hypothermia and pregnancy. *Anesthesiology*, *58*, 460–461.

Talbot, P. (2008). In vitro assessment of reproductive toxicity of tobacco smoke and its constituents. *Birth Defects Research (Part C)*, *84*, 61–72.

Thulstrup, A., & Bonde, J. (2006). Maternal occupational exposure and risk of specific birth defects. *Occupational Medicine*, *56*(8), 532–543.

Torfs, C., Katz, E., Bateson, T., Lam, P., & Curry, C. (1996). Maternal medications and environmental exposures as a risk for gastroschisis. *Teratology*, *54*, 84–92.

Tsukimori, K., Tokunaga, K., Shibata, S., Uchi, H., Nakayama, D., Ishimaru, T., Nakano, H., Wake, N., Yoshimura, T., & Furue, M. (2008). Long-term effects of polychlorinated biphenyls and dioxins on pregnancy outcomes in women affected by the Yusho incident. *Environmental Health Perspectives*, *116*(5), 626–630.

U.S. Department of Labor. (December, 2008). *Employment status of the civilian noninstitutional population by sex and age, 2007 annual averages. Women in the labor force*. Washington DC: A data book. Current Population Survey, U.S. Bureau of Labor Statistics.

U.S. Department of Health and Human Services (USDHHS). (2006). The health consequences of involuntary exposure to tobacco smoke: A report of the Surgeon General. Public Health Service, Office of the Surgeon General, Rockville, MD. Retrieved on March 14, 2009, from www.surgeongeneral.gov/library/secondhandsmoke/report/citation.pdf.

U.S. Department of Health and Human Services (USDHHS), Centers for Disease Control and Prevention (CDC), and National Institute for Occupational Safety and Health (NIOSH). (March 2009). Approaches to safe nanotechnology: Managing the health and safety concerns associated with engineered nanomaterials. USDHHS-NIOSH Publication 2009-125. Retrieved April 16, 2009, from NIOSH website: www.cdc.gov/niosh/docs/2009-125/pdfs/2009-125.pdf.

U.S. Food and Drug Administration (FDA). (2009). Pregnancy and lactation labeling. Center for Drug Evaluation and Research. Retrieved February 12, 2009, from www.fda.gov/cder/regulatory/pregnancy_labeling/default.htm.

Wise, L., Palmer, J., Hatch, E., Troisi, R., Titus-Ernstoff, L., Herbst, A., Kaufman, R., Noller, L., & Hoover, R. (2007). Secondary sex ratio among women exposed to diethylstilbestrol in utero. *Environmental Health Perspectives*, *115*(9), 1314–1319.

INTRAPARTUM PERIOD

10 Essential Forces and Factors in Labor

Gail M. Turley

OBJECTIVES

1. List the forces affecting labor.
2. Identify the possible causes of the onset of labor.
3. Discuss the oxytocin release theory of labor onset.
4. Discuss the fetal prostaglandin theory of labor onset.
5. Describe the amount of uterine activity required to effect cervical changes.
6. Differentiate between muscle contraction and muscle retraction, and discuss the significance of both to the progress of labor.
7. List the techniques used for assessing uterine activity and uterine efficiency.
8. Differentiate between true labor and false labor, using information gathered by history and physical examination.
9. Identify the basic pelvic shapes.
10. Recognize adequate pelvic dimensions.
11. Describe methods for assessing pelvic capacity.
12. Compare and contrast the anticipated progress of labor for each of the four pelvic shapes.
13. Identify and discuss maternal conditions that may alter or influence pelvic capacity.
14. Analyze the relation between maternal posture and the pelvic passage.
15. Define fetal lie, attitude, presentation, presenting part, position, and station.
16. List the mechanisms of spontaneous vaginal delivery.
17. Discuss the significance of breech presentation or transverse lie to the progress of labor.
18. Recognize fetal variables that may interfere with the progress of labor.
19. Discuss the significance of fetal malpositioning to the course and outcome of labor.
20. Describe the characteristic emotions associated with labor.
21. Identify variables that determine a couple's expectations for the labor and birth experience.
22. Distinguish between adaptive coping and maladaptive coping during labor.
23. Describe the nursing actions that maximize the forces of labor.
24. Predict when a woman is at risk for a difficult labor as the result of an alteration in one of the forces of labor.

INTRODUCTION

Traditionally, four essential forces or powers have been identified as the determinants of labor outcome (Biancuzzo, 1993). These "4 P's," which are interrelated, are:
1. Power: The uterine muscle provides the power of labor, and the onset and establishment of a satisfactory contraction pattern is a readily recognized force of labor.
2. Passage: The bony boundaries of the pelvis define the labor passage, and its shape and configuration determine the ease with which the infant is expelled from the uterus.
3. Passenger: The infant, or passenger, is an active participant in the labor process as it moves and turns to accommodate to the maternal pelvis.
4. Psyche: A woman's psyche, or emotional system, determines her total response to labor and influences physiologic and psychologic functioning.

CLINICAL PRACTICE

A. Power of labor
1. History
   a. Onset of contractions
      (1) Maternal factor theories
         (a) The uterus is stretched to threshold point, leading to synthesis and release of prostaglandin.
         (b) The pressure on the cervix and its nerve plexus reaches threshold point.
         (c) Oxytocin stimulation theory (Gay, 1978)
            [i] Exogenous oxytocin is known to stimulate myometrial contractions, but no evidence clearly documents its role in the onset of labor.
            [ii] Progesterone inhibits myometrial response throughout pregnancy.
            [iii] Estrogen at term enhances myometrial sensitivity to oxytocin.
            [iv] A surge of oxytocin may be released by stretching of the cervix at term (Ferguson's reflex), but studies do not agree about this possibility.
         (d) Progesterone withdrawal theory
            [i] In animals, a decrease in progesterone is followed by evacuation of the uterus.
            [ii] In humans, no firm evidence documents that progesterone is decreased at term.
            [iii] Many researchers, however, support the view that an altered progesterone-estrogen ratio leads to increased myometrial contractility.
      (2) Fetal factor theories
         (a) Placental aging and deterioration trigger initiation of contractions.
         (b) Fetal cortisol theory (Gay, 1978)
            [i] It is reasoned that normal fetal adrenal glands produce a steroid, cortisol, which stimulates the onset of labor
            [ii] It is recognized that anencephaly causes adrenal dysfunction secondary to pituitary dysfunction
            [iii] Empirically, anencephalic fetuses tend to have prolonged gestations
         (c) Prostaglandin synthesis theory (Gay, 1978)
            [i] Prostaglandins are known to stimulate uterine contractions at any gestational age
            [ii] Prostaglandin is present in increased quantities in blood and amniotic fluid during labor
            [iii] Prostaglandin production requires the precursor arachidonic acid
            [iv] Esterified arachidonic acid is stored in fetal membranes
            [v] It is postulated that free arachidonic acid is released at term and is then converted by agents in the uterine decidua to prostaglandin
   b. Physiology of contractions (Cunningham et al, 2005)
      (1) Myometrium
         (a) Uterine muscle is controlled by involuntary innervation.
         (b) Alpha-receptors stimulate uterine contractions.
         (c) Beta-receptors stimulate uterine relaxation.
         (d) Norepinephrine and epinephrine stimulate alpha- and beta-receptors.
            [i] When progesterone is present, beta-receptors are stimulated.
            [ii] When estrogen is present, alpha-receptors are stimulated.
      (2) Contraction: the shortening of a muscle in response to a stimulus, with return to its original length (Figure 10-1)
         (a) Increment: building up; the longest phase of a contraction
         (b) Acme: peak
         (c) Decrement: letting up
      (3) Retraction: the shortening of a muscle in response to a stimulus, without return to its original length; muscle becomes fixed at a relatively shorter length, but no increase in baseline tension occurs after the contraction (also known as brachystasis)
         (a) With each uterine contraction, the upper segment of the uterus becomes shorter and thicker, and the lower segment of the uterus becomes longer, thinner, and more distended

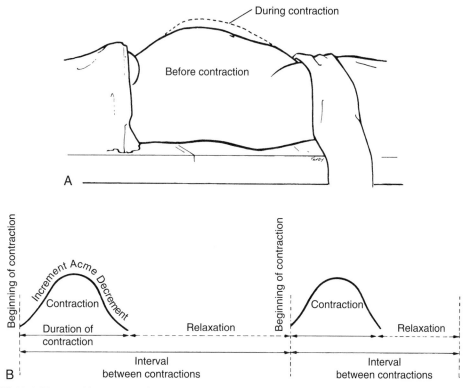

FIGURE 10-1 ■ Wavelike pattern of contractile activity. (From Lowdermilk, D.L., & Perry, S.E. [2007]. *Maternity & women's health care* [9th ed.]. St. Louis: Mosby.)

(b) The division between the contractile upper segment of the uterus and the passive lower uterine segment is the physiologic retraction ring.

(c) Longitudinal traction on the cervix by the upper portion of the uterus as it contracts and retracts leads to cervical effacement and dilation.

(d) The shortening and thickening of the upper uterine segment lead to fetal descent.

(4) Tonus: the degree of pressure exerted by the uterine musculature as measured by intrauterine pressure

  (a) Tonus is measured in millimeters of mercury (mm Hg), which is also called torr.

  (b) Normal baseline tonus between contractions is 8 to 12 mm Hg.

  (c) Pressure at peak of a contraction ranges from 35 to 75 mm Hg.

(5) Intensity: the rise in intrauterine pressure above baseline brought about by a contraction

  (a) Intensity is measured as the difference between peak pressure and baseline pressure.

  (b) Normally, 30 to 50 mm Hg intensity is necessary for effective labor.

(6) Pacemaker: the site of electrical activity responsible for triggering a uterine contraction

  (a) Pacemakers are generally located in the fundus of the uterus (fundal dominance).

    [i] Previously thought that specialized cells existed that acted as pacemakers

    [ii] Current thinking is that the cells responsible for initiating electrical stimuli are not different from surrounding myometrial cells.

    [iii] Fundal dominance occurs because the fundus contains a greater number of myometrial cells than other areas of the uterus

  (b) The wave of the contraction begins in the fundus then proceeds downward to the rest of the uterus (descending gradient).

    [i] The duration of the contraction diminishes progressively as the wave moves away from the fundus; therefore, during any contraction, the upper portion of the uterus is contracted for a longer time.

[ii] The intensity of the contraction diminishes from top to bottom, so that the upper segment contracts more strongly than the lower segment.

[iii] If the duration and intensity of the contraction were constant throughout, effacement and dilation could not occur.

(c) Asymmetry results when the uterine halves function independently, leading to ineffective contractions with minimal dilation.

(d) Ectopic pacemakers (i.e., pacemakers located outside the uterine fundus) result in spasmodic myometrial contractions, which are disorganized and colicky, and rarely effective in producing dilation (see Chapter 11 for a complete discussion of dysfunctional labor).

c. False labor

(1) Discomfort is perceived, but cervical changes do not occur.

(2) Discomfort is usually perceived more in lower abdomen than in back.

(3) Discomfort may be caused by uterine contractions, intestinal or bladder spasm, or abdominal wall muscle tension.

(4) Despite perceived discomfort, the uterus is often relaxed, although mild contractions may be palpated.

(5) Contractions are irregular and short in duration.

(6) The interval between contractions is long and irregular, and it does not decrease as discomfort continues.

(7) The intensity does not increase with time.

(8) Contractions are easily interrupted by medication and activity, such as walking.

(9) There is an absence of cervical bloody show.

(10) False labor is mentally and physically tiring for the patient.

d. True labor

(1) By definition, true labor is the onset of contractions that leads to progressive cervical effacement and dilation.

(2) Discomfort is perceived in both front and back.

(3) Hardening of the uterus is palpable.

(4) Contractions occur at regular intervals, usually beginning 20 to 30 minutes apart, lasting 10 to 20 seconds, and of mild intensity.

(5) Frequency, duration, and intensity increase as contractions continue.

(6) Medication does not easily disrupt true labor.

(7) Walking increases the intensity.

(8) Presenting part descends.

(9) Bulging of the membranes may occur.

(10) Bloody show is present.

2. Physical examination

a. Contraction strength

(1) Myometrial activity

(a) Myometrial activity is solely responsible for effacement and dilation of the first stage of labor.

(b) Uterine contractions create increased intrauterine pressure, which exerts tension on cervix and pressure on the descending fetus.

(c) Myometrial effectiveness is improved by good uterine blood flow.

[i] Lateral positions avoid the vena caval syndrome.

[ii] Walking and activity increase circulating blood to the uterus.

[iii] Relaxation and sense of well-being mitigate fight-or-flight response, avoiding diminished blood flow to the uterus.

(2) Expulsive activity

(a) During the second stage of labor, involuntary and voluntary forces are present.

(b) Involuntary myometrial activity continues to create increased intrauterine pressure, which exerts pressure against the fetus.

(c) Full dilation causes involuntary reflex desire to bear down, which increases intraabdominal pressure, thereby increasing intrauterine pressure (Roberts, Goldstein, Gruener, Maggio, & Mendez-Bauer, 1987).

(d) Voluntary efforts to bear down increase intraabdominal pressure, thereby increasing intrauterine pressure.

       (e) Positions that flex the legs on the abdomen increase intraabdominal pressure, thereby increasing intrauterine pressure.
- **b.** Contraction frequency
  - (1) Contraction frequency is measured from the beginning of one contraction to the beginning of the next contraction.
  - (2) Typical frequency of contractions during active labor is two to five contractions per 10 minutes.
- **c.** Contraction duration
  - (1) Contraction duration is measured from the beginning of the increment to the end of the decrement.
  - (2) Typical duration of contractions during active labor is 30 to 90 seconds.
- **3.** Diagnostic studies and techniques
  - **a.** Manual palpation of contractions
    - (1) Judge indentability of the uterine wall and assign a rating of mild, moderate, or strong.
      - (a) Mild: Uterine wall easily indented.
      - (b) Moderate: Uterine wall demonstrates resistance to pressure, though some indentation occurs.
      - (c) Strong: Uterine wall cannot be indented.
  - **b.** External monitoring of contractions: tocotransducer
    - (1) The tocotransducer reflects increased intraabdominal pressure.
    - (2) Placement of the tocotransducer influences the accuracy of information.
    - (3) Intraabdominal pressure does not directly correlate with intrauterine pressure; therefore, it does not measure the actual intensity of contractions.
    - (4) No known risks have been found of using the tocotransducer, but some women feel confined and uncomfortable.
  - **c.** Internal monitoring of contractions: intrauterine pressure catheter
    - (1) Allows direct measurement of intrauterine pressure
    - (2) Provides accurate measurement of actual intensity of uterine contraction
    - (3) Associated risks
      - (a) Introduction of infection into uterine cavity
      - (b) Uterine rupture caused by traumatic insertion (see Chapter 12 for complete discussion of contraction monitoring)
  - **d.** Montevideo units
    - (1) Developed by Calderyo-Barcia to measure and quantify uterine work
    - (2) Calculated by multiplying the frequency of contractions (as expressed by the number of contractions in 10 minutes) by their intensity
    - (3) Expressed as mm Hg per 10 minutes
    - (4) Example
      - (a) The patient is contracting every 3 minutes; therefore, three contractions occur in 10 minutes
      - (b) The intensity of the contraction at its peak is 35 mm Hg.
      - (c) Three contractions per 10 minutes x 35 mm Hg per contraction = 105 mm Hg per 10 minutes

B. Labor passage
- **1.** History
  - **a.** Musculoskeletal deformities and diseases
    - (1) A contracted pelvis may lead to disproportion between the pelvis and the fetus.
    - (2) Uterine neoplasms (e.g., fibromyomas, ovarian cysts) may block the birth canal, impeding the passage.
    - (3) Bicornuate uterus
      - (a) May lead to abortion, premature labor, or premature rupture of membranes
      - (b) Has been implicated in incompetent cervix
      - (c) May be causative factor of breech or transverse lie
      - (d) Vaginal delivery is possible but may be accompanied by uterine inertia or obstruction of descent.
    - (4) Maternal dwarfism
      - (a) Defined as a height of less than 1473 cm (4 feet, 10 inches) at maturity
      - (b) Pelvic dimensions may be favorable if dwarfism is proportionate.

(5) Kyphoscoliosis

(a) If the thoracic area is involved, little or no reduction of pelvic capacity occurs.

(b) If the dorsolumbar or lumbosacral area is involved, marked pelvic deformity is common.

(6) Bony disease of femurs or acetabula may result in abnormal pressures on the pelvis during development, leading to pelvic asymmetry and reduced pelvic capacity.

(7) Nutritional deficiencies and diseases (e.g., rickets) may contribute to bony deformities of the pelvic passage.

b. Pelvic trauma or injury may lead to asymmetry and reduced capacity.

c. Cervical trauma or injury:

(1) Includes accidental insults as well as those resulting from surgical procedures (e.g., dilation and curettage [D&C], cone biopsy, uterine aspiration)

(2) May result in loss of cervical integrity with resultant incompetence

(3) May result in cervical scarring and adhesions, with resultant failure to dilate

(4) Cervical abnormalities are frequently found among women exposed in utero to diethylstilbestrol (DES).

2. Physical examination

a. Pelvic shapes (Figure 10-2) (Cunningham et al, 2005)

(1) Rigid classification is not possible.

(a) Name assigned is based on classification of inlet.

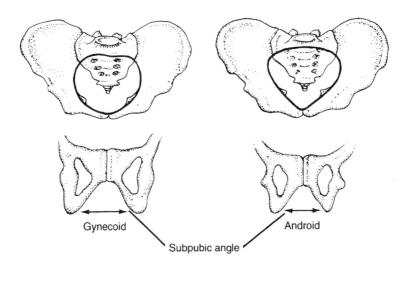

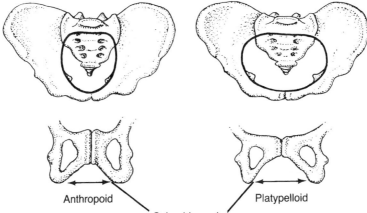

FIGURE 10-2 ■ Caldwell-Moloy classification of pelvis. (From Sloane, E. [2002]. *Biology of women* [4th ed.]. Albany, NY: Delmar.)

(b) Nonconforming characteristics are then described.

(c) Shape and size of pelvis influence fetal position and attitude.

(2) Gynecoid: normal female

(a) Uterine function is good.

(b) Early and complete internal rotation occurs.

(c) Labor prognosis is good.

(d) This shape offers the optimal diameters in all three planes of the pelvis.

(e) Approximate incidence is 50%.

(3) Android: male

(a) Posterior segments are reduced in all the pelvic planes.

(b) Deep transverse arrest is common.

(c) Failure of rotation is common.

(d) Labor prognosis is poor.

(e) Approximate incidence is 20%, but it occurs more frequently among white women (30%) than nonwhite women (15%).

(4) Anthropoid: apelike

(a) Reduced transverse measurements are compensated by large anteroposterior diameters.

(b) Prognosis is generally more favorable than android or platypelloid.

(c) This shape may deliver occiput posterior.

(d) Approximate incidence is 25%, but it occurs more frequently among nonwhite women (50%) than white women (25%).

(5) Platypelloid: flat female

(a) Arrest at inlet is common.

(b) Labor prognosis is poor.

(c) Approximate incidence is 5%.

b. Pelvic dimension

(1) The measurements that define the obstetric capacity of the pelvis

(2) Important measurements

(a) Obstetric conjugate of the inlet (Figure 10-3)

[i] Is the shortest diameter through which the infant must pass

[ii] Extends from the middle of the sacral promontory to the posterior superior margin of the symphysis pubis

[iii] Can be approximated by manually measuring the diagonal conjugate, extending from the subpubic angle to the middle of the sacral promontory, then subtracting 15 cm (0.6 inch)

[iv] Adequate measurement: 11 cm (4.4 inches)

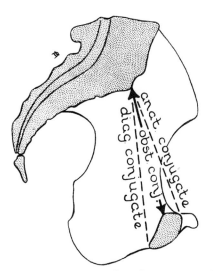

FIGURE 10-3 ■ Obstetric conjugate. (From Oxorn, H. [1986]. *Oxorn-Foote human labor and birth* [5th ed., p. 29]. New York: Appleton & Lange.)

(b) Transverse diameter between the ischial spines
[i] The spines form the lateral boundaries of the pelvic cavity plane of least dimension (Figure 10-4).
[ii] Adequate measurement: 10.5 cm (4.2 inches)

(c) Subpubic angle (see Figure 10-2)
[i] Forms the apex of the anterior triangle of the pelvic outlet
[ii] Adequate measurement: 90 degrees or more

(d) Bituberous diameter
[i] Transverse diameter of the pelvic outlet
[ii] Adequate measurement: 11 cm (4.4 inches)

(e) Posterior sagittal diameters (Figure 10-5)
[i] Extend from the intersection of the transverse and anteroposterior diameters to the posterior limit of the latter
[ii] Represent the back portion of the anteroposterior diameters
• Inlet: 4.5 cm (1.8 inches)
• Cavity: 4.5 to 5 cm (1.8 to 2 inches)
• Outlet: 9 cm (3.6 inches)

(f) Curve and length of the sacrum
[i] The sacrum forms the curved canal of the pelvic cavity.

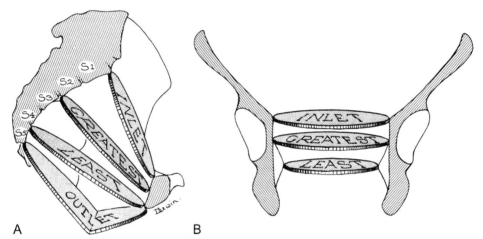

FIGURE 10-4 ■ Pelvic cavity planes. (From Oxorn, H. [1986]. *Oxorn-Foote human labor and birth* [5th ed., p. 27]. New York: Appleton & Lange.)

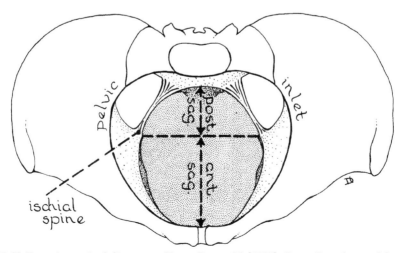

FIGURE 10-5 ■ Posterior sagittal diameters. (From Oxorn, H. [1986]. *Oxorn-Foote human labor and birth* [5th ed., p. 29]. New York: Appleton & Lange.)

        [ii] Posterior wall should be deep and concave.

        [iii] Sacrum should measure 10 to 15 cm (4 to 6 inches).

(3) Maternal posture influences pelvic size and contours (Fenwick & Simkin, 1987; Roberts, 1980a,b).

    (a) There is no correct position; each offers advantages and disadvantages.

    (b) Walking and changing positions effect changes in pelvic joints, facilitating descent and rotation.

    (c) Horizontal postures

        [i] Contribute to vena caval syndrome

- Decreased placental blood flow can lead to fetal compromise.
- Decreased uterine blood flow can lead to uterine muscle hypoxia (Mayberry et al, 2000).
  - Decreased strength of uterine contractions
  - Increased pain perception

        [ii] Decrease the ability of the patient to push voluntarily

        [iii] Require expulsive forces to work against gravity

        [iv] Foster dependency and passivity of patient; mirror is required for patient to see birth

        [v] Provide for ease of attendant

        [vi] Associated with increased incidence of interventions

- Instrument-assisted delivery
- Episiotomy

        [vi] Positions

- Dorsal or supine
  - Legs may be extended or knees flexed.
  - Pelvic angle is 30 degrees, which directs the fetal head away from the pelvic inlet.
  - Probably best reserved for rare instances when delivery difficulties anticipated
  - Lithotomy: patient legs are in stirrups
  - Semi-Fowler's: head of bed is elevated
- Lateral (Lehrman, 1985)
  - Relaxation of the pelvic muscles facilitates descent and rotation of the presenting part.
  - Avoids vena caval syndrome
  - Left side-lying may offer increased control of pushing efforts (Roberts & Woolley, 1996).
  - Lateral Sims', with mother lying on the side where the fetal spine is positioned, may enhance rotation from occiput posterior to occiput anterior (Ridley, 2007).
  - Lateral positions associated with increased likelihood of intact perineum (Shorten, Donsante, & Shorten, 2002)
  - Requires a support person to hold the anterior leg
  - May impede interaction with the attendant or infant because the delivery occurs at the woman's back

    (d) Upright postures

        [i] Avoid vena caval syndrome

        [ii] Abdominal muscles work in synchrony with uterine contractions, maximizing expulsive forces; associated with a shortened second stage (Gennaro, Mayberry, & Kafulafula, 2007; Liu, 1989).

        [iii] Abdominal wall relaxes, allowing the fundus to fall forward because of the force of gravity and straightening the longitudinal axis of the birth canal (Shermer & Raines, 1997).

- Fetus is well aligned with the angle of the pelvis.
- Effect of gravity is maximized.
- Fetal descent is enhanced.

        [iv] Pelvic angle is 90 to 120 degrees, directing the fetal head to enter the pelvis in the anterior position and enhancing application of the fetal head against the cervix.

[v] Uterine contractions are more efficient.
  • Gravity increases pressure to the cervix by 10 to 35 mm Hg.
  • Contractions may be less frequent but of greater amplitude.
[vi] Fosters participation of patient in the birth process
  • Increases patient's perception of control
  • Facilitates interactions with care providers
  • May reduce anxiety
[vii] Technically more difficult for some attendants
[viii] Associated with fetal and newborn well-being
  • Decreased incidence of abnormal fetal heart patterns
  • Decreased incidence of acidosis at birth
  • Decreased incidence of Apgar score less than 7
[ix] Epidural anesthesia is not an absolute contraindication to upright postures (Gilder, Mayberry, Gennaro, & Clemmens, 2002; Mayberry, Strange, Suplee, & Gennaro, 2003).
  • Determined by agent used as well as dosing regimen
  • Requires sufficient leg strength to support maternal weight
[x] Positions
  • Squatting
    ○ Enlarges the pelvic outlet by approximately 28%
    ○ Increases the efficiency and effectiveness of expulsive forces (Golay, Vedam, & Sorger, 1993; Romond & Baker, 1985)
    ○ Often cited as best position for second stage of labor (Roberts & Woolley, 1996)
    ○ Efficacy of position requires less forceful pushing and may be less tiring.
    ○ Induces a slight separation of the lower symphysis pubis, resulting in an enlarged outlet
    ○ Thighs are flexed and abducted, creating leverage on the innominate bones, thereby opening the bony outlet (McKay, 1984).
    ○ Without the pressure of a bed, the sacrum and coccyx are easily pushed back by the descending fetus, thereby enlarging the outlet.
    ○ Pressure of the thighs on the abdomen increases intraabdominal pressure.
    ○ Pressure is evenly distributed to the perineum, reducing the need for episiotomy.
    ○ Reduces visibility of perineum for the attendant
    ○ Often used in non-Western cultures, though not customary in Western societies (McKay, 1984)
    ○ Decreased muscle strength and joint flexibility can be fatiguing and uncomfortable.
    ○ Use of squatting bar provides opportunities for rest.
    ○ Playing tug-of-war with support person simulates squatting while minimizing stress on thighs.
  • Sitting
    ○ Increases the pelvic diameters but not as much as squatting
    ○ May increase edema of perineum and perineal blood loss
    ○ Continuous pressure on lower buttocks leads to venous congestion and dependent edema.
      — More pronounced when using a molded birthing chair, which inhibits position changes and weight shifts
    ○ Patient can unintentionally slide into a semirecumbent posture if she relies too much on back support.
  • Standing
    ○ Is tiring for the patient
    ○ Requires the assistance of two attendants or support persons
(e) Kneeling postures (hands-knees)
  [i] May facilitate rotation of fetus from posterior to anterior position (Biancuzzo, 1993; Stremler et al, 2005)

                    [ii] Coccyx is freely mobile, maximizing pelvic diameter
                    [iii] Are tiring for the patient
                    [iv] May reduce participation in birth process and interaction with the infant
                          because the woman may be using her arms and hands to support herself
        c. Cervical changes
            (1) Effacement
                (a) Shortening of the cervix
                (b) Passive reduction in the length of the cervical canal from 2 cm (0.8 inch) to a
                    paper-thin orifice
                (c) Internal os disappears as cervical canal is drawn up into the lower uterine
                    segment
                (d) In nulliparas, effacement generally begins before the onset of labor.
                (e) In multiparas, effacement may not begin until labor ensues.
            (2) Dilation (Figure 10-6)
                (a) Opening of the external os
                (b) Caused by two forces
                    [i] Pressure of the presenting part
                    [ii] Contraction and retraction of the uterine muscle
    3. Diagnostic studies and techniques
        a. Vaginal examination to assess cervical changes
            (1) Effacement
                (a) 0%: Cervical canal is 2 cm (0.8 inch) long.
                (b) 50%: Cervical canal is 1 cm (0.4 inch) long.
                (c) 100%: Cervical canal is obliterated.
            (2) Dilation
                (a) 0 cm: External os is closed.
                (b) 10 cm (4 inches): External os is fully dilated and will permit passage of the fetus.
        b. Manual determination of pelvic capacity
            (1) Measurement of the diagonal conjugate permits calculation or estimation of the
                obstetric conjugate.
            (2) Engagement of the presenting part signals adequacy of the inlet but does not predict
                adequacy of the midpelvis or the pelvic outlet.

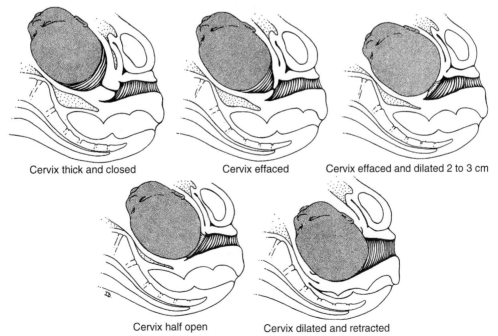

Cervix thick and closed   Cervix effaced   Cervix effaced and dilated 2 to 3 cm

Cervix half open   Cervix dilated and retracted

FIGURE 10-6 ■ Dilation of the cervix. (From Oxorn, H. [1986]. *Oxorn-Foote human labor and birth* [5th ed., p.
119]. New York: Appleton & Lange.)

C. Passenger
  1. History
    a. Previous pregnancies
       (1) Birthweight of previous children
       (2) Malpresentation or disproportion encountered during previous labors
    b. Current pregnancy: unusual perceptions by the patient that suggest a large infant or atypical positioning
  2. Physical examination (Cunningham et al, 2005)
    a. Fetal lie: relation of the long axis of the fetus to the long axis of the mother
       (1) Longitudinal lie: The long axes of the fetus and of the mother are parallel.
       (2) Transverse or oblique lie: The long axis of the fetus is perpendicular to the long axis of the mother.
    b. Fetal attitude: the relation of fetal parts to one another
       (1) Flexion: the typical fetal attitude in utero
       (2) Extension: tends to present larger fetal diameters
    c. Presentation: determined by the pole of the fetus that first enters the pelvic inlet
       (1) Cephalic: head first (95% of term deliveries)
       (2) Breech: pelvis first (3% of term deliveries)
       (3) Shoulder: shoulder first (2% of term deliveries)
    d. Presenting part: the specific fetal structure lying nearest to the cervix
       (1) Determined by the attitude of the fetus
       (2) Each presenting part has an identified denominator that is used to describe the fetal position in the pelvis.
       (3) Cephalic presentations (Figure 10-7)
           (a) Vertex (denominator is occiput)
               [i] Flexion
                   • Normal fetal position, with infant's chin resting on the chest
                   • Presents optimal fetal dimensions during labor
                   • At term, the position of 95% of fetuses
               [ii] No flexion and no extension
                   • Known as a military attitude
                   • Presents slightly larger diameters than full flexion
                   • Usually converts to flexion or full extension
                   • Prognosis for labor and delivery generally favorable
           (b) Frontum or brow (denominator is frontum)
               [i] Partial extension
               [ii] Incidence less than 1%
               [iii] May be related to fetal anomaly
               [iv] May be associated with polyhydramnios or a small fetus
               [v] Presents relatively larger fetal diameters to pelvis
               [vi] Spontaneous delivery possible if pelvis is large, contractions are adequate, and infant is small
               [vii] Delivery expedited by conversion to vertex or face presentation
           (c) Face (denominator is mentum-chin)
               [i] Full extension
               [ii] Incidence less than 1%
               [iii] More frequent in multiparas
               [iv] May be secondary to fetal factors that cause hyperextension, such as enlarged thyroid or multiple nuchal cords
               [v] Fetal diameters essentially the same as with a vertex presentation
               [vi] Vaginal delivery possible only if mentum is anterior
       (4) Breech presentations (denominator is sacrum) (Figure 10-8)
           (a) Complete breech: flexion at hips, flexion at knees
           (b) Frank breech: flexion at hips, extension at knees
           (c) Footling breech: extension at one or both hips, extension at one or both knees
           (d) Kneeling breech: extension at hips, flexion at knees
           (e) Passage of meconium may occur secondary to pressure changes and does not necessarily indicate fetal stress or distress.

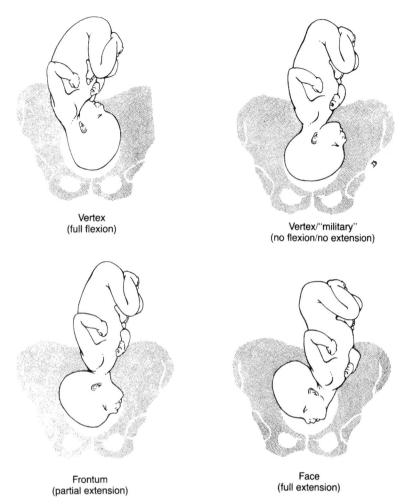

Vertex
(full flexion)

Vertex/"military"
(no flexion/no extension)

Frontum
(partial extension)

Face
(full extension)

FIGURE 10-7 ■ Cephalic presentations. (From Oxorn, H. [1986]. *Oxorn-Foote human labor and birth* [5th ed., p. 55]. New York: Appleton & Lange.)

(f) Associated with prematurity, placenta previa, multiparity, pelvic abnormality, and some congenital anomalies, such as hydrocephaly
(g) Associated with increased fetal mortality and morbidity
   [i] Prematurity
   [ii] Malformations
   [iii] Asphyxia caused by prolonged compression of cord, prolapse of cord, or trauma to after-coming head, which does not have the opportunity to undergo molding
   [iv] Injury to brain and skull, resulting in minute hemorrhages or fractures
   [v] Trauma of manipulation during delivery may lead to cervical fractures, brachial plexus paralysis, liver rupture, or spinal cord traction/injury.
(h) Associated with protracted and dysfunctional labor
(i) Maternal positioning may facilitate conversion to cephalic presentation (Founds, 2005; Smith, Crowther, Wilkinson, Pridmore, & Robinson, 1999).
   [i] Scientific evidence weak
     • Few controlled studies
     • Most evidence derived from noncontrolled studies or anecdotal reports
     • Study results may have been confounded by noncompliance of participants.
   [ii] Elkins procedure: knee-chest position for 15 minutes every 2 hours while awake for 5 days

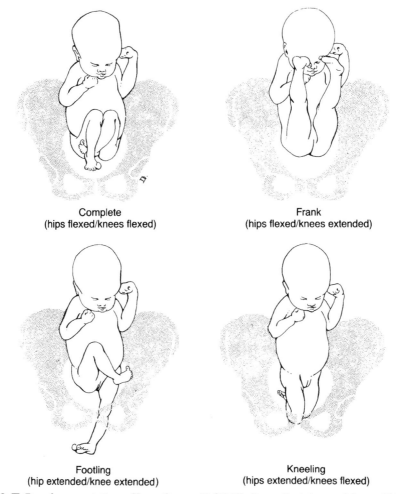

Complete
(hips flexed/knees flexed)

Frank
(hips flexed/knees extended)

Footling
(hip extended/knee extended)

Kneeling
(hips extended/knees flexed)

FIGURE 10-8 ■ Breech presentations. (From Oxorn, H. [1986]. *Oxorn-Foote human labor and birth* [5th ed., p. 57]. New York: Appleton & Lange.)

        [iii] Modified Elkins procedure: knee-chest position with a full bladder for 15 minutes three times a day for 7 days

        [iv] Indian procedure: supine with head down, hips elevated on pillows, knees bent, feet flat for 10 minutes twice daily, for 4 to 6 weeks beginning at 30 weeks' gestation

  (5) Transverse presentation (Figure 10-9)

     (a) Shoulder is the usual presenting part (denominator is scapula)

     (b) May be caused by anything that prevents descent of the head or the breech into the lower pelvis

        [i] Placenta previa

        [ii] Neoplasm

        [iii] Anomalies of the lower uterine segment

        [iv] Multiple gestation

        [v] Fetal anomalies

     (c) Associated with multigravidas, possibly secondary to increased relaxation of uterine and abdominal muscles

     (d) Vaginal delivery impossible without injury to mother and fetus

  (6) Compound presentation

     (a) The infant assumes a unique posture, usually with the arm or the hand presenting alongside the presenting part

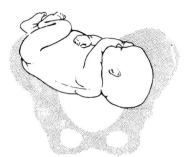

FIGURE 10-9 ■ Transverse presentation. (From Oxorn, H. [1986]. *Oxorn-Foote human labor and birth* [5th ed., p. 57]. New York: Appleton & Lange.)

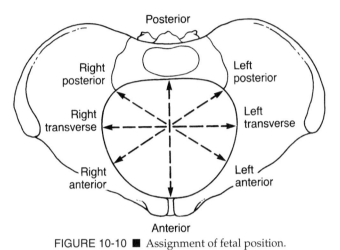

FIGURE 10-10 ■ Assignment of fetal position.

      (b) Presents increased fetal diameters
      (c) May interfere with the cardinal movements of labor
  e. Fetal position: the relation of the denominator to the maternal pelvis
    (1) In practice, eight points are demarcated.
    (2) The denominator is assigned right or left, depending on which side of the maternal pelvis it is in.
    (3) The denominator is assigned anterior, posterior, or transverse according to maternal front, back, or side (Figure 10-10).
    (4) The occiput anterior position is most facilitative of vaginal delivery.
    (5) The occiput transverse position typically requires rotation to anterior or posterior position for delivery.
    (6) The occiput posterior position presents slightly larger diameters to pelvis.
      (a) May slow progress of descent
      (b) Usually converts to anterior position during descent for delivery
      (c) An increased degree of internal rotation is required to align occiput beneath the maternal symphysis.
      (d) Typically causes increased back pain during labor
      (e) Associated with higher rates of cesarean delivery (Ridley, 2007)
  f. Fetal station: the relation of the presenting part to an imaginary line drawn between the ischial spines
    (1) Designations
      (a) The ischial spines are 0 station.
      (b) Above the spines is a negative value.
      (c) Below the spines is a positive value.
    (2) Engagement: when the widest diameter of the presenting part has passed the inlet
      (a) Usually corresponds to a 0 station

(b) Depth of the pelvis and amount of caput succedaneum that is present influence the actual station at engagement.

(c) In primigravidas

[i] Often occurs before labor

[ii] When the fetus is unengaged at the outset of labor, disproportion is suggested.

(d) Engagement may occur any time in multigravidas.

(3) Floating: when the presenting part is entirely out of the pelvis and freely movable in the inlet

(4) Synclitism: when the biparietal diameter (BPD) of the fetal head is parallel to the planes of the maternal pelvis (Figure 10-11)

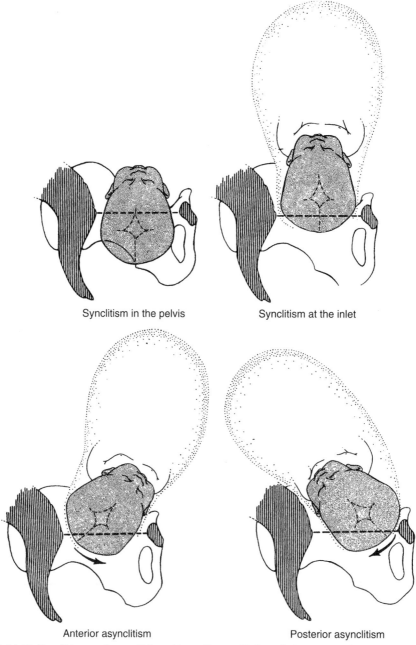

Synclitism in the pelvis   Synclitism at the inlet

Anterior asynclitism   Posterior asynclitism

FIGURE 10-11 ■ Synclitism and asynclitism. (From Oxorn, H. [1986]. *Oxorn-Foote human labor and birth* [5th ed., p. 71]. New York: Appleton & Lange.)

(5) Asynclitism: when the biparietal diameter is not parallel to the maternal pelvis (i.e., the fetal head appears tilted); may lead to a disproportion or delayed descent (see Figure 10-11)

g. Fetal size

(1) Size alone is less significant than the relation between fetal size and pelvic dimensions.

(2) Macrosomia

(a) Generally defined as birthweight more than 4500 g (9 pounds, 15 ounces) (American College of Obstetricians and Gynecologists [ACOG], 2000)

(b) Incidence is between 0.5% and 1.8%.

(c) Associated variables

[i] Family history

[ii] Multiparity

[iii] Advanced maternal age

[iv] Excessive maternal weight gain

[v] Maternal diabetes

[vi] Postterm gestation

[vii] Male fetus

[viii] Father of infant at least 10 years older than mother

(d) Associated complications

[i] Prolonged second stage of labor

[ii] Shoulder dystocia (Camune & Brucker, 2007)

[iii] Maternal genital tract injury

[iv] Postpartum hemorrhage related to atony

[v] Separation of pubic symphysis

[vi] Birth trauma

• Skull fracture

• Brachial plexus damage

• Clavicle fracture

• Asphyxia or depression (see Chapter 17 for risks associated with gestational age and birthweight)

(3) Microsomia

(a) Typically occurs in the preterm gestation but may be associated with intrauterine growth restriction

(b) Is associated with shortened second stage of labor

(c) May be possible to deliver the infant through an incompletely dilated cervix, predisposing to entrapment of the placenta or after-coming fetal parts and cervical lacerations or injury

(4) Fetal anomalies influencing fetal size

(a) Hydrocephalus

(b) Thyroid hypertrophy

(c) Abdominal distention secondary to kidney disease

(d) Omphalocele

(e) Myelocele

h. Fetal skull

(1) The most important structure because it is the largest and least compressible

(2) Landmarks (Oxorn, 1986)

(a) Cranial bones

[i] At birth, they are thin, poorly ossified, and easily compressible.

[ii] Occipital: located posteriorly

[iii] Parietal (two): located laterally

[iv] Temporal (two): located anteriorly

[v] Frontal (two): located anteriorly

(b) Sutures

[i] The membranous tissue between the bones

[ii] Sagittal: lies between the parietal bones, in an anteroposterior direction

[iii] Lambdoidal: separates the occipital bone from the two parietal bones, and runs in a transverse direction

[iv] Coronal: separates the parietal bones from the frontal bones and runs in a transverse direction

[v] Frontal: lies between the frontal bones and is a continuation of the sagittal suture
  (c) Fontanelles
      [i] The intersections of the sutures
      [ii] Anterior (bregma)
          • Junction of the sagittal, frontal, and coronal sutures
          • Diamond shaped, 3 × 2 cm (1 × 1 inch)
      [iii] Posterior (lambda)
          • Junction of the sagittal and lambdoidal sutures
          • Triangular shaped, 1 × 2 cm (0.5 × 1 inch)
  (3) Molding
      (a) The ability of the fetal head to change shape to accommodate the maternal pelvis
      (b) Accomplished because of the lack of fusion of the cranial bones
      (c) May decrease dimensions by 0.5 to 1 cm (0.2 to 0.4 inch)
  (4) Caput succedaneum
      (a) Soft-tissue edema caused by cervical pressure against the presenting head
      (b) If severe, may obscure the suture lines, making determination of fetal position difficult
      (c) May make determination of fetal station difficult
i. Cardinal movements (Cunningham et al, 2005)
  (1) The manner in which the infant moves and rotates to accommodate to the maternal pelvis
  (2) Although often conceptualized as separate and sequential, the movements more typically are concurrent.
  (3) Engagement and descent
      (a) In nulliparas, engagement usually precedes the onset of labor, with additional descent occurring during labor.
      (b) In multiparas, engagement and descent may not occur before labor.
      (c) Absence of descent in a primigravida may signal disproportion or malpresentation.
      (d) The fetal head typically enters the pelvis with the sagittal suture aligned in the transverse diameter.
      (e) Responsible for lightening, the subjective sensation felt by the mother as the fetus settles into the lower uterine segment; more commonly perceived by primigravidas.
  (4) Flexion
      (a) Relative flexion is the natural posture of the fetus and is enhanced as the descending part encounters pelvic resistance.
      (b) Flexion achieves the smallest fetal diameters presenting to the maternal pelvic dimensions.
  (5) Internal rotation
      (a) Aligns the long axis of the fetal head with the long axis of the maternal pelvis
      (b) The sagittal suture aligns in the anteroposterior diameter.
      (c) Occurs mainly during the second stage of labor
  (6) Extension
      (a) Resistance of the pelvic floor causes the presenting part to pivot beneath the symphysis pubis.
      (b) Delivery is accomplished through extension of the head beneath the symphysis pubis.
  (7) Restitution
      (a) The sagittal suture returns to an oblique diameter.
      (b) The oblique position realigns the sagittal suture with the fetal trunk axis.
  (8) External rotation
      (a) Continuation of restitution, with the sagittal suture moving to a transverse diameter and the shoulders aligning in the anteroposterior diameter
      (b) The sagittal suture maintains alignment with the fetal trunk as the trunk navigates through the pelvis.
  (9) Expulsion: After the delivery of the presenting part, the trunk typically follows easily.

3. Diagnostic studies and techniques
   a. Leopold's maneuvers (Figure 10-12) (Olds, London, Ladewig, & Davidson, 2003)
      (1) Inspection and palpation of the maternal abdomen to determine the fetal position, station, and size
      (2) When performed by experienced clinicians, the maneuver is effective as a screening assessment for malpresentation (Lydon-Rochell, Albers, Gotwocia, Craig, & Qualls, 1993).
      (3) First maneuver: What is in the fundus?
         (a) Clinician stands at the patient's side and palpates the fundus.
         (b) The head feels hard and smooth.
         (c) The breech feels more irregular.
      (4) Second maneuver: Where is the back?
         (a) Clinician faces the patient and places hands on the sides of her abdomen.

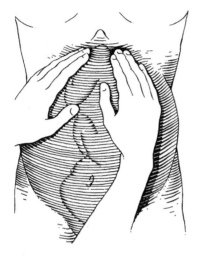

1. What is in the fundus?

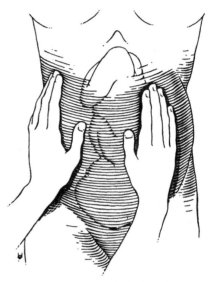

2. Where is the back?

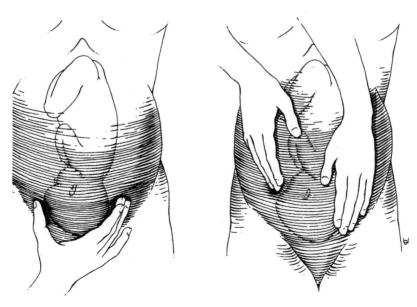

3. What is the presenting part?   4. Where is the cephalic prominence?

FIGURE 10-12 ■ Leopold's maneuvers. (From Oxorn, H. [1986]. *Oxorn-Foote human labor and birth* [5th ed., pp. 77-79]. New York: Appleton & Lange.)

      (b) The back feels firm and smooth.
      (c) The small parts feel irregular.
   (5) Third maneuver: What is the presenting part?
      (a) Clinician moves hands down the sides of the abdomen to grasp the lower uterine
          segment.
      (b) The breech feels soft and irregular.
      (c) The head feels globular and firm.
   (6) Fourth maneuver: Where is the cephalic prominence?
      (a) Clinician faces the patient's feet and slides hands down the sides of the uterus to
          locate the side of greater resistance; this is the prominence.
   b. Vaginal examination (Figure 10-13)
      (1) Determine presentation
         (a) Cephalic
         (b) Breech
         (c) Shoulder
      (2) Determine station.
         (a) Presenting part at level of ischial spines: 0 station
         (b) Presenting part above level of ischial spines: −1, −2, −3 station
         (c) Presenting part below level of ischial spines: +1, +2, +3 station
      (3) Determine position.
         (a) Denominator located by palpating sutures, facial features, or anatomic
             landmarks
         (b) Denominator defined in relation to the maternal pelvis (see Figure 10-10)
   c. Ultrasonography (see Chapter 8 for complete discussion of antepartum testing)
      (1) Size
         (a) BPD is measured with accuracy beginning at 13 weeks.
         (b) BPD is predictive of fetal age and fetal weight.
      (2) Presentation: Contents in lower pelvis are identified.
      (3) Morphology
         (a) Anencephaly is demonstrated by lack of cerebral formation.
         (b) Hydrocephaly is suggested if BPD is greater than 11 cm (4.4 inches).
         (c) Microcephaly may be suspected but can be difficult to diagnose.
         (d) Anatomic structural defects may be recognizable.

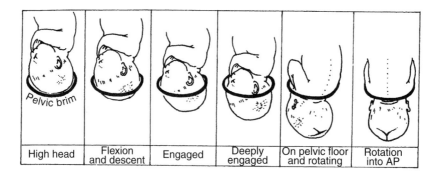

| High head | Flexion and descent | Engaged | Deeply engaged | On pelvic floor and rotating | Rotation into AP |

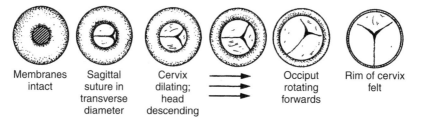

| Membranes intact | Sagittal suture in transverse diameter | Cervix dilating; head descending | | Occiput rotating forwards | Rim of cervix felt |

FIGURE 10-13 ■ Fetal head progressing through pelvis and changes in cervix. (From Fraser, D.M., & Cooper, M.A. [2003]. *Myles textbook for midwives* [14th ed., p. 448]. Edinburgh: Churchill Livingstone.)

D. Psyche
1. History
    a. Previous birth experiences
        (1) Complications of pregnancy, labor, and birth that occurred in previous pregnancies
        (2) Birth outcome of previous pregnancies
        (3) The degree to which the patient's personal expectations for birth were achieved in previous pregnancies
    b. Current pregnancy experience
        (1) Planned versus unplanned pregnancy
            (a) A planned pregnancy imparts increased feelings of acceptance.
            (b) An unplanned pregnancy may be accompanied by anger and rejection.
        (2) Patient age
            (a) Adolescent women must complete the developmental tasks of adolescence as well as pregnancy.
            (b) Mature women are more accustomed to being in control of their lives and may be easily frustrated by the loss of control during pregnancy and birth (Winslow, 1987).
        (3) Difficulty in conceiving
            (a) Relative infertility may result in increased anxiety about the well-being of a premium pregnancy.
            (b) Technology to assist conception and maintenance of the pregnancy may reduce a patient's sense of involvement and control.
        (4) Pregnancy discomforts may increase the patient's anticipation of discomfort and difficulty during labor and birth.
        (5) High-risk pregnancy
            (a) The patient may experience increased anxiety and fears about her own well-being and the well-being of the fetus.
            (b) The need for technology may interfere with the patient's expectations for a natural birth.
        (6) Completion of the developmental tasks of pregnancy: failure to complete the developmental tasks of pregnancy may result in increased fears and anxiety about the birth experience.
    c. Cultural considerations (Clark, 1978) (see Chapter 4 for a complete discussion of cultural considerations of childbearing)
        (1) One of the most important factors influencing women's perception of chilbirth (Callister, 1995)
        (2) Establishes values and beliefs about sickness and health.
            (a) Pregnancy as physiologic process, a wellness experience
            (b) Pregnancy as a state of illness, a time of vulnerability
        (3) Defines the childbirth experience.
            (a) Shameful versus joyful experience
            (b) Intimate experience versus social event
            (c) Superstitions about pregnancy and birth
            (d) Prescribed behaviors and taboos influencing activities, food, and drink
        (4) Defines kinship structure and relationships.
            (a) Interaction between the couple
            (b) Parent-infant interactions
            (c) Role expectations of mother, father, and grandparents, for example
            (d) Involvement of support persons
            (e) Intergenerational behaviors
        (5) Defines pain
            (a) Identifies the meaning and context of pain
            (b) Determines the acceptable response to pain (perceived pain is not always expressed as pain)
        (6) Determines the significance of touch
            (a) Soothing versus intruding
            (b) May be viewed as a symbol of intimacy
    d. Expectations for birth experience
        (1) Childbirth can be viewed as either a meaningful or a stressful event.

(2) Goals can be realistic and attainable or too idealistic and in conflict with reality, thus leading to disappointment.

(3) Acceptable behavior for self and others is defined by cultural as well as other influences.

(4) Labor may be viewed as a test.

e. Preparation for birth

   (1) Type of childbirth preparation

   (2) Familiarity with the institution and its policies and procedures

   (3) Type of relaxation techniques learned and practiced

f. Support system

   (1) The presence and support of valued companions during birth are invaluable to most women (Price, Noseworthy, & Thornton, 2007).

      (a) The woman's spouse or partner is the most frequently chosen labor companion

         [i] The anticipated or unplanned separation from spouse or partner may be a source of anxiety (Chiota, Goolkasian, & Ladewig, 1976).

      (b) The woman's mother and other female relatives often provide additional support.

         [i] Young grandmothers may not be prepared to assume the grandparent role and thus may subconsciously withhold support.

         [ii] Grandparents may have misinformation and misperceptions and may need knowledge of current practices (Horn & Manion, 1985).

   (2) The support of a trained labor attendant supplements and enhances familial support (Simkin, 2002).

      (a) Types of attendants

         [i] Doula

           • From the Greek, meaning in service of or woman's servant (Perez & Herrick, 1998)

           • Provides continuous physical and emotional support (Campbell, Lake, Falk, & Backstrand, 2006)

           • Does not assess maternal or fetal well-being

           • Does not intervene to ensure safe outcome for mother or baby

           • Relationship with patient often begins before labor.

           • May serve as a bridge between patient and caregivers (Gilliland, 2002)

         [ii] Professional nurse

           • Provides physical and emotional support, though not always on a continual basis

           • Critical factor in the achievement of improved birth outcomes (Association of Women's Health, Obstetric and Neonatal Nurses [AWHONN], 2000)

           • Assesses maternal and fetal well-being

           • Intervenes to ensure safe outcome for mother and baby

         [iii] Roles should be complementary, not adversarial (Ballen & Fulcher, 2006).

      (b) Supportive activities (Gale, Fothergill-Bourbonnais, & Chamberlain, 2001; Hodnett, 1996; Mackey & Lock, 1989; Manogin, Bechtel, & Rami, 2000; Miltner, 2000)

         [i] Emotional support

           • Sustaining physical presence ("keeping company") (Heffron, 2006)

           • Words of encouragement, reassurance, and praise

         [ii] Physical support

           • Comfort measures and pain relief

           • Hygiene

           • Reassuring touch/massage

           • Application of heat or cold

           • Calm environment (lighting, sounds, temperature)

           • Therapeutic music (Browning, 2000; Zwelling, Johnson, & Allen, 2006)

              ○ Anxiolytic music

              ○ Causes reduction or absence of anxiety

              ○ Typically characterized by no extremes of rhythm, melody, or dynamics

              ○ Selections chosen by patient are best.

- Aromatherapy (Zwelling et al, 2006)
  - ○ Therapeutic use of plant-derived essentials oils
  - ○ Promotes physical and psychological well-being, enhances relaxation, influences perception of pain
  - ○ May be interally applied or inhaled
  - ○ Limited research studying its use during labor
- [iii] Information and advice
  - Provide information regarding progress of labor.
  - Interpret medical language and jargon.
- [iv] Advocacy
  - Support decisions.
  - Ensure that others respect patient's decisions.
  - Manage visitors.
- [v] Support of partner
  - Role model therapeutic interactions
  - Assist to meet own self-care needs (e.g., nutrition, hygiene)
- (c) Caring modalities (Hottenstein, 2005)
  - [i] Auditory
    - Music
    - Words of praise and encouragement
    - Quiet whispers to help patient focus
  - [ii] Visual
    - Internal visualization or imagery
    - External focal point or object
    - Quiet, calming decor
  - [iii] Olfactory
    - Aromatherapy
  - [iv] Tactile
    - Intentional touch
      - — May include acupressure and reflexology
  - [v] Kinesthetic
    - Swaying or pelvic rocking
    - Rocking chair
  - [vi] Caring consciousness
- (d) Measurable effects on birth outcome (AWHONN, 2000; Kennell, Klaus, McGrath, Robertson, & Hinckley, 1991; Sauls, 2002; Zhang, Bernasko, Leybovich, Fahs, & Hatch, 1996)
  - [i] Reduced likelihood of needing pharmacologic pain relief
  - [ii] Shorter duration of labor
  - [iii] Reduced likelihood of operative vaginal delivery, cesarean delivery, and oxytocin augmentation
  - [iv] Increased likelihood that infant's 5-minute Apgar score is greater than 7
  - [v] Increased likelihood of patient satisfaction with birth experience
  - [vi] Increased likelihood of exclusive breastfeeding
  - [vii] Increased likelihood of longer duration of breastfeeding
  - [viii] Increased likelihood that patient demonstrates positive mother-infant behaviors at birth
- (3) Religious values and spiritual faith also provide a supportive structure.
2. Psychosocial responses
   a. Emotions of labor (Clark & Affonso, 1979)
      (1) Latent phase
         (a) Is excited
         (b) Is ready for anything
         (c) Experiences anxiety and fear
      (2) Active phase
         (a) Has decreased energy
         (b) Experiences fatigue
         (c) Turns attention to internal sensations
         (d) Feels serious

    (3) Transition
        (a) Is discouraged
        (b) Is irritable or nasty
        (c) Is panicky and overwhelmed by fears of death
        (d) Is impatient
        (e) Feels out of control
    (4) Second stage
        (a) Is focused
        (b) Has increased energy, though is still fatigued
        (c) May subconsciously "hold back," resulting in decreased pushing efforts (McKay & Barrows, 1991)
        (d) Is gratified that she can actively participate to bring about birth
    (5) Immediate postpartum period
        (a) Experiences joy and relief
           [i] Is able to see and hold baby
           [ii] Is eager to share the news with others
        (b) Begins grief work
           [i] Experiences loss of valued object (the pregnancy)
           [ii] Experiences loss of valued status (as a pregnant woman)
           [iii] May feel sense of failure at not achieving own expectations for labor and birth
           [iv] Experiences loss of some aspect of self
               • Altered body image
               • Changed self-esteem
               • Changed self-concept
               • Loss of former role
        (c) Fatigue: finally able to sleep after hours of work
  b. Psychologic reactions to labor
    (1) Anxiety
        (a) Anxiety is defined as an uneasiness in response to a vague, nonspecific threat.
        (b) At mild to moderate levels, anxiety is an effective stimulant to action.
        (c) Excessive anxiety interferes with labor.
        (d) Somatic cues
           [i] Muscular pain and stiffness (especially in neck and back)
           [ii] Chest pain or tightness
           [iii] Nausea
           [iv] Flushing
           [v] Numbness in hands and face
        (e) Behavioral cues
           [i] Crying, tearfulness
           [ii] Tremulous voice
           [iii] Inability to focus or concentrate
           [iv] Jitteriness
        (f) Physiologic cues
           [i] Elevated blood pressure
           [ii] Elevated heart rate
           [iii] Dilated pupils
           [iv] Diarrhea
    (2) Fear
        (a) Fear is defined as a painful, uneasy feeling in response to an identifiable threat
        (b) Possible intrapartum threats
           [i] Labor is an unknown despite the best of preparations.
           [ii] Maternal or fetal injury during labor and birth
           [iii] Pain
           [iv] Institutional procedures (e.g., IVs, fetal monitor)
           [v] Impending irreversible lifestyle changes created by the birth of a baby
        (c) Fear causes peripheral vasoconstriction that may decrease uterine blood flow, decreasing uterine contractility.
        (d) Fear typically enhances pain perception, leading to increased fear.

    (3) Loss of control and sense of helplessness
        (a) For many women, childbirth is their first hospitalization.
        (b) Personal belongings and clothing are removed.
        (c) Routine procedures are unfamiliar and intimidating.
        (d) Most patients recognize that at some point in the labor process, they must depend on others for assistance.
    (4) Feelings of aloneness or abandonment
        (a) Removal from familiar home environment
        (b) Restriction of support system
        (c) Changing patterns of communication
            [i] Increased reliance on nonverbal messages
                • Vision
                • Touch
                • Facial expression
                • Body movements
                • Vocal quality
            [ii] When verbal and nonverbal messages are out of synchrony, nonverbal communications are usually more accurate.
            [iii] As labor progresses, most women turn inward, which may lead to distorted message reception.
        (d) Isolation may decrease reality orientation, leading to increased anxiety and fear.
    (5) Fatigue and weariness
        (a) Etiologic factors
            [i] Sleep deprivation
            [ii] Sensory overload
            [iii] Generalized fatigue, which is common in late pregnancy
            [iv] Energy expended during labor
        (b) Fatigue generally leads to reduced energy and inability to focus and concentrate.
        (c) Fatigue may decrease myometrial activity.
  c. Personality styles
    (1) There is no one correct style, and a patient may demonstrate aspects of each.
    (2) Controlling
        (a) The patient seeks the opportunity to have influence in the decisions regarding her care.
        (b) The patient explores the options and alternatives in a given situation.
        (c) The patient relies on her knowledge base and relaxation skills.
        (d) The patient's belief that she will succeed is affirmed.
        (e) Inability to participate in decision making leads to conflict.
    (3) Optimistic
        (a) The patient freely releases the surge of energy that is generated by her emotions and feelings.
        (b) The patient smiles, laughs, cries, and demonstrates increased activity levels.
        (c) The patient accepts the expertise and assistance of those around her.
        (d) The patient demonstrates basic trust in the outcome.
    (4) Fatalistic
        (a) The patient focuses on her perceived loss of control.
        (b) The patient avoids choosing options and participating in decision making.
        (c) The patient becomes preoccupied with details.
        (d) The patient has a heightened perception of danger, leading to increased fears.
        (e) The patient displays hostility, aggression, and withdrawal.
        (f) The patient demonstrates generalized distrust in the outcome and therefore views her own actions and those of others as meaningless.
  d. Behaviors
    (1) Effective coping
        (a) Rhythmic activity during contractions (rocking, swaying, self-stroking)
        (b) Attention-focusing activity during contractions
            [i] Tactile: touch, massage, stroking
            [ii] Auditory: music, murmuring, verbal encouragement (Browning, 2000)

        [iii] Visual: partner's face, designated picture or object
        [iv] Kinesthetic: rocking, swaying, tapping
        [v] Mental: counting breaths, reciting verse, visualizing a favorite scene
        [vi] Vocalization: moaning, counting, chanting
   (c) Ritual
        [i] Repetition of the same rhythmic and attention-focusing activities during each contraction
        [ii] May include use of introspective self-talk
  (2) Ineffective coping
   (a) Random or uncoordinated activity during contractions (wincing, writhing)
   (b) Unfocused or panicked activity during contractions
   (c) Absence of a consistent reaction to each contraction

INTERVENTIONS

A. Power of labor
  1. Facilitate the establishment of an effective uterine contraction pattern.
    a. Therapeutic
      (1) Encourage the patient to walk about as much as possible.
      (2) When the patient is in bed, assist her to assume adaptive postures and positions.
        (a) Lateral position with the head of the bed slightly elevated, using pillows and other supports
        (b) Frequent position changes
        (c) Positions of comfort
    b. Diagnostic
      (1) Assess contraction frequency, duration, and intensity.
        (a) Every hour during early labor
        (b) Every 30 minutes during active labor
  2. Minimize the risk of infection related to the use of an intrauterine pressure catheter (IUPC).
    a. Therapeutic
      (1) Use aseptic technique when assembling the pressure catheter.
      (2) Maintain asepsis during insertion of the pressure catheter.
      (3) Use aseptic technique during vaginal examinations.
      (4) Limit vaginal examinations to those necessary for clinical decision making.
    b. Diagnostic
      (1) Every 2 to 4 hours, or as indicated by the stage of labor and the patient's clinical status, obtain temperature.
      (2) As appropriate to the patient's stage of labor and clinical status, assess fetal heart rate.
      (3) On an ongoing basis, assess characteristics of amniotic fluid.
      (4) On an ongoing basis, assess for uterine tenderness.
      (5) On an ongoing basis, monitor laboratory results.
B. Labor passage
  1. Facilitate the achievement of maximum pelvic capacity.
    a. Therapeutic
      (1) Help the patient assume adaptive positions.
        (a) Upright
        (b) Squatting
        (c) Sitting
        (d) Modified knee-chest
      (2) Encourage the patient to change position frequently.
      (3) Reassure the patient that absolute pelvic measurements are less important than the relation between the pelvis and the infant.
    b. Diagnostic
      (1) As appropriate to the patient's stage of labor and clinical status, perform a vaginal examination to assess cervical effacement and dilation.
      (2) As appropriate to the patient's stage of labor and clinical status, assess fetal descent.

C. **Passenger**
   1. Facilitate achievement of the fetal cardinal movements.
      a. Therapeutic
         (1) Assist the patient to assume adaptive positions that foster fetal descent and rotation.
            (a) Upright
            (b) Squatting
            (c) Sitting
            (d) Modified knee-chest
         (2) Encourage the patient to change position frequently.
      b. Diagnostic
         (1) As appropriate to the patient's stage of labor and clinical status, assess fetal position and descent.
   2. Minimize the likelihood of injury (fetal trauma, uterine trauma, cervical trauma, fetal distress, or asphyxia) related to malpresentation.
      a. Therapeutic
         (1) Report breech, transverse, and compound presentations promptly to the physician or nurse-midwife.
         (2) Report arrest of the cardinal movements to the physician or nurse-midwife.
         (3) Prepare the patient for cesarean delivery as directed by the physician.
      b. Diagnostic
         (1) At the outset of labor perform Leopold's maneuvers and a vaginal examination to determine fetal lie and presentation.
         (2) As appropriate to the patient's stage of labor and clinical status, perform a vaginal examination to assess fetal presentation and station.
         (3) As appropriate to the patient's stage of labor and clinical status, assess fetal heart rate.
         (4) On an ongoing basis, assess for uterine tenderness.

D. **Psyche**
   1. Minimize anxiety and fear associated with labor.
      a. Therapeutic
         (1) Orient the patient to her surroundings .
         (2) Familiarize the patient with the usual routine and procedures, and explain all procedures and interventions to the patient.
         (3) Provide the patient with factual information about the baby's condition.
            (a) Fetal heart rate
            (b) Information regarding size and morphology gained from ultrasound examination
         (4) Inform the patient of her status and progress, offering reassurance when everything is normal.
         (5) Reassure the patient that cephalopelvic disproportion is not necessarily caused by fetal abnormalities.
         (6) Encourage the patient to avoid engaging in unrealistic fantasies about the baby.
         (7) Provide a quiet, restful environment with minimal stimulation.
         (8) Remain with the patient as much as possible.
         (9) Be direct and specific in communicating with the patient, offering her a limited number of options.
         (10) Speak and behave calmly.
         (11) Do not communicate one's own problems and concerns to the patient.
         (12) Encourage the patient to remain focused on now and to avoid a past or future orientation.
      b. Diagnostic
         (1) Every 4 hours or as appropriate for the stage of labor, obtain blood pressure, pulse, and respirations.
         (2) On an ongoing basis, evaluate the patient's concerns and expectations.
         (3) On an ongoing basis, determine the patient's understanding of what is happening.
         (4) On an ongoing basis, evaluate the patient's ability to focus and concentrate.
         (5) On an ongoing basis, evaluate the patient's ability to respond to messages.
         (6) On an ongoing basis, determine the synchrony between the patient's verbal and nonverbal communications.

2. Maximize the patient's coping skills.
    a. Therapeutic
        (1) Reinforce or teach relaxation techniques.
        (2) Encourage the use of rhythmic and focused behaviors.
        (3) Control the environment to minimize sensory overload and intrusion.
            (a) Eliminate unnecessary lights and noises.
            (b) Remove unnecessary equipment and supplies from the bedside.
            (c) Avoid unnecessary conversation at the bedside.
            (d) Provide a single source of sensory input.
                [i] Music through earphones (in some patients, using earphones may contribute to isolation from their support system and health care providers)
                [ii] A focus point
        (4) Keep the patient informed about her condition and her progress, explaining all procedures and interventions.
        (5) Assist the patient in identifying her strengths, and praise her for her demonstration of adaptive coping skills.
        (6) Acknowledge the patient's feelings of discouragement, then refocus her toward adaptive behaviors.
        (7) Provide physical comfort measures.
            (a) Cool cloth
            (b) Mouthwash
            (c) Back rub
            (d) Sponge bath
            (e) Pillows
        (8) Remain with the patient as much as possible.
        (9) Identify things within the patient's control and encourage her to be involved.
        (10) Establish effective communication with the patient.
            (a) Be direct, using a *take charge* style.
            (b) Exude calm confidence.
            (c) Maintain eye contact.
            (d) Speak calmly, quietly, and slowly to the patient.
            (e) Create a pacing rhythm.
            (f) Develop a contraction ritual.
            (g) Respond to verbal and nonverbal communication.
            (h) Communicate with the patient in her own communication mode.
                [i] Return eye contact.
                [ii] Return touch.
            (i) During active labor, use direct questions ("Does this cool cloth help?") because open-ended questions become difficult for the patient to answer ("How can I help?").
        (11) Include support persons of the patient's choosing, and support the support person.
            (a) Provide nourishment.
            (b) Provide episodic relief from responsibility.
            (c) Provide praise and encouragement.
        (12) Discuss with the patient her expectations and values and integrate them into the labor experience as much as possible.
    b. Diagnostic
        (1) On an ongoing basis, evaluate the patient's use of relaxation techniques and coping behaviors.
        (2) On an ongoing basis, evaluate the patient's patterns of communication.
        (3) On an ongoing basis, evaluate the patient's ability to receive and use information that is provided.
        (4) On an ongoing basis, evaluate the patient's degree of satisfaction with the experience.
        (5) On an ongoing basis, determine the patient's reaction to the environment.
        (6) On an ongoing basis, determine the patient's problem-solving abilities.
3. Maximize the patient's knowledge and understanding about the birthing process.
    a. Therapeutic

(1) Explain the principles of labor and birth as related to the patient's specific circumstances.

(2) Explain all procedures.

(3) Encourage the patient to ask questions and answer questions honestly and promptly.

(4) Identify changes in the patient's status that might be misunderstood, and offer anticipatory education.

    b. Diagnostic

      (1) On an ongoing basis, determine the patient's level of comprehension.

HEALTH EDUCATION

A. Optimizing labor power

  1. Encourage normal activity and exercise patterns throughout pregnancy.

    a. Women with generally well-toned musculature tend to have more efficient uterine contractions.

    b. Good abdominal musculature assists during the second stage of labor.

    c. Women who exercise are generally more aware of their bodies and can more effectively control pushing efforts.

  2. Instruct the patient in exercises specific to pregnancy and childbearing.

    a. Kegel exercise to tone perineal floor

    b. Pelvic tilt to tone abdominal muscles and relieve backache (Figure 10-14)

    c. Adductor stretching to tone thighs (tailor sitting)

  3. Instruct the patient in intrapartum activities that strengthen uterine effort.

    a. Walk and remain active as long as possible.

    b. Lateral positions and an elevated head of the bed improve regularity and intensity of contractions.

    c. Avoid supine hypotension, which leads to decreased uterine blood flow and decreased muscle strength.

B. Maximizing labor passage

  1. Instruct the patient in postures that increase pelvic capacity.

  2. Instruct support person in techniques to achieve alternative postures.

  3. Encourage the patient to change positions frequently during labor.

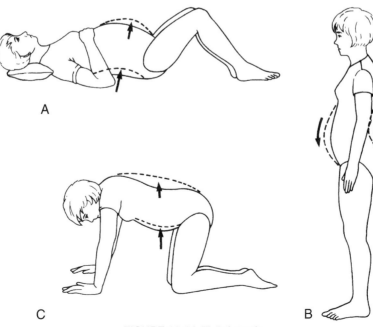

FIGURE 10-14 ■ Pelvic tilt.

    a. Provides dynamic pelvic capacity, which facilitates fetal passage
    b. Avoids excessive stress and tension on a single muscle group

C. Emotional preparation for birth
    1. Encourage attendance at childbirth preparation classes.
    2. Support self-study efforts, such as books and videos.
    3. Encourage rehearsal of coping behaviors and relaxation techniques.
    4. Encourage guidance and support of family members.

CASE STUDIES AND STUDY QUESTIONS

Primigravida in Early Labor

Mrs. W. is a 37-year-old, gravida 1 (G1) woman who began experiencing irregular contractions late Tuesday afternoon. Throughout Tuesday evening, she and her husband diligently timed each contraction. They were very excited that labor had begun. They were equally excited that the baby's arrival had waited until the end of the academic year. She had recently been promoted to associate professor and took great pride in personally reviewing all of her students' papers before issuing final grades.

Near midnight, the contractions were 3 to 4 minutes apart, lasting 45 to 50 seconds. Her discomfort was increasing, although she remained able to focus on the relaxation breathing techniques she had learned. Her husband was becoming tired, but he remained excited and eager to time each new contraction. When her membranes ruptured at 12:30 AM, she phoned her physician, confident that her baby would be born soon.

Mr. and Mrs. W. arrived in labor and delivery at 1:10 AM Wednesday. On arrival she provided the nurse with a detailed summary of the previous 8 hours. She also shared with the nurse her goals for the birth experience, which included being permitted to breastfeed immediately after birth and going home as soon as possible. She was obviously uncomfortable with contractions, but she used her breathing techniques well.

The nurse escorted the couple to a labor-delivery-recovery (LDR) room, oriented them to the hospital environment, and assisted Mrs. W. in changing into a hospital gown. Her initial assessment findings included:
- Maternal vital signs within normal limits (WNL)
- Fetal heart rate of 136 bpm
- Contractions every 4 to 5 minutes, lasting 45 to 50 seconds, and of moderate intensity
- Cervix 100% effaced and 3 to 4 cm dilated
- Baby at 0 station, in the right-occipitoanterior (ROA) position

When the nurse informed Mr. and Mrs. W. of her findings, Mrs. W. was obviously distressed and disappointed. "How can I be only 3 cm? I've been in labor for hours. I should be almost finished by now." As she spoke, she became increasingly agitated, and each new contraction heightened her frustration. She became restless and had difficulty implementing her breathing techniques.

1. What factor is most responsible for Mrs. W.'s reaction to the nurses' information?
   a. Maternal age
   b. The frequency and duration of her contractions
   c. Unrealistic expectations
   d. Her unfamiliarity with the hospital environment

2. How should the nurse respond to her?
   a. Remind her that first babies usually take 18 to 24 hours.
   b. Assist her in resuming the relaxation techniques she had been using on admission.
   c. Inform her that the physician will be contacted to obtain something to help her relax.
   d. Obtain additional information about her birth plan.

3. How can the nurse assist her to cope adaptively with her labor and birth?
   a. Provide her with information and encouragement.
   b. Leave her and her husband alone as much as possible.
   c. Share with Mrs. W. her own birth experience.
   d. Teach her how to time her contractions.

4. What immediate intervention does Mr. W. require?
   a. Provision of scrub attire
   b. Information about the early discharge procedure
   c. Instruction about how to time contractions
   d. Information about how best to support his wife

Primigravida, Multiple Gestation

Mr. and Mrs. C., a couple in their mid-20s, were thrilled when they first learned that Mrs. C. was pregnant. They had been married for more than a year, and Mrs. C. had quit her job at the local bookstore shortly after their marriage in anticipation of raising a family. Both individuals came from large families, and they hoped to continue the tradition. Despite their desire for children and plans for a large family, they were shocked when the physician informed them that they were expecting twins.

As the shock faded, Mrs. C. began to revel in the specialness of her pregnancy and enjoyed the extra attention that her friends and family paid her. She was unprepared, however, for the increased discomfort she experienced. Her physician reassured her that both fetuses were healthy and that everything was normal. Nonetheless, with each new sensation, she worried that something was wrong.

At 37 weeks' gestation, she began having contractions. She telephoned her physician immediately and went to the hospital.

On admission to labor and delivery, she was quiet and reserved. She told the nurse that her contractions had begun 2 hours earlier. Her husband drove a delivery truck, and the company was trying to contact him to meet her at the hospital. She had tried to telephone her mother but was unable to reach her at home. The nurse also learned that Mr. and Mrs. C. had not attended childbirth-preparation classes. According to Mrs. C., "My husband's schedule is very unpredictable, and I couldn't go alone. Besides, most of the time I didn't have the energy to do much of anything."

The nurse's assessment revealed:
- Blood pressure 144/86, pulse 88, respirations 20
- Fetal heart rate 124 bpm in right lower quadrant (RLQ) and 136 bpm in right upper quadrant (RUQ)
- Contractions every 10 minutes, lasting 20 seconds, and of mild intensity
- Cervix 0% effaced and 4 cm dilated
- Fetus A presented vertex, at 0 station; fetus B also was vertex

5. What factors should the nurse consider as contributing to Mrs. C.'s anxiety level?
   a. Her lack of attendance at childbirth preparation classes
   b. Multiple gestation
   c. Maternal age
   d. Inadequate support system
      (1) a, c
      (2) a, b, d
      (3) a, c, d
      (4) All of the above
6. What should the nurse do first to minimize Mrs. C.'s anxiety?
   a. Notify the physician, and obtain an order for medication.

b. Instruct her in childbirth-preparation information.
   c. Permit her to listen to the fetal hearts, and reassure her that the fetuses are doing well.
   d. Remain with her.
7. What is the significance of fetus A's station?
   a. Suggestive of pelvic adequacy
   b. Indicative of malpresentation
   c. Suggestive of a short labor
   d. Indicative of the need to prepare for a cesarean delivery
8. What actions can the nurse take to increase the likelihood of a vaginal delivery?
   a. Encourage Mrs. C. to walk around during the early stage of labor.
   b. When Mrs. C. is in bed, keep the head of the bed slightly elevated.
   c. Assist Mrs. C. in assuming upright positions.
   d. Assist Mrs. C. with relaxation breathing techniques.
      (1) a, c
      (2) b, c, d
      (3) b, d
      (4) All of the above
9. At the outset of her labor, what information would best assist Mrs. C. in coping adaptively?
   a. An explanation of the procedures she should expect
   b. A discussion of the anatomy and physiology of labor
   c. A description of the institution's policies about support persons' attendance at cesarean birth
   d. Instruction in relaxation techniques
      (1) a, c
      (2) a, b, d
      (3) a, c, d
      (4) All of the above

Multigravida, Active Labor

Mrs. A. is a 34-year-old, 41-week-gestation, gravida 3, para 2 (G3, P2) woman who arrived in labor and delivery on Friday at 10:20 AM. She states that when she awoke she noticed some pelvic heaviness, but that she ignored it as she got her 9-year-old and 6-year-old children off to school. Once the house was quiet, she became aware that she was contracting regularly, though she describes the contractions as mild and cramplike. Because her previous labors were quick (first pregnancy, 11 hours; second pregnancy, 4 hours), she went right to the hospital without notifying her physician or husband: "The last time, it was over almost before it had begun." Throughout the admission process, she remained calm. When the nurse was finished, she remarked, "Well, I guess I should call my husband if I expect him to get here in time."Admission assessment includes:

- Maternal vital signs within normal limits
- Fetal heart rate 148 bpm RLQ
- Contractions every 5 to 6 minutes, 30 to 45 seconds, and of mild to moderate intensity
- Cervix 70% effaced and 2 cm dilated
- Fetal position in right occipitoposterior (ROP), at a –1 station

10. What additional findings would reassure the nurse that Mrs. A. was in true labor?
    a. The presence of a bloody show
    b. Bulging membranes
    c. A progressive increase in the length of time between contractions
    d. A progressive increase in the duration of contractions
       (1) a, c
       (2) a, c, d
       (3) a, b, d
       (4) All of the above

11. What is the significance of the baby's station and position?
    a. Of little significance at this time
    b. Suggestive of cephalopelvic disproportion
    c. Suggestive of a prolonged labor
    d. Indicative of the need to prepare for cesarean delivery

12. What additional assessments would be helpful to the nurse in planning care for the patient?
    a. The gestational age and birth weight of Mrs. A.'s previous deliveries
    b. The time and amount of Mrs. A.'s last oral intake
    c. Mrs. A.'s preparation for this birth experience
    d. Mrs. A.'s expectations about pain management
       (1) a, c
       (2) a, b, d
       (3) a, c, d
       (4) All of the above

13. Which cardinal movement is most affected when a baby is occipitoposterior ?
    a. Flexion
    b. Internal rotation
    c. Extension
    d. External rotation

14. Which factors may contribute to the baby's presenting occipitoposterior?
    a. Maternal pelvic shape
    b. Maternal age
    c. Fetal size
    d. Postmaturity
       (1) a, c
       (2) b, c, d
       (3) b, d
       (4) All of the above

ADDITIONAL STUDY QUESTIONS

15. What is characteristic of the powers of the first stage of labor?
    a. Controlled by the involuntary nervous system
    b. Responsible for cervical effacement and dilation
    c. Responsive to nursing interventions
    d. Quantified by calculating frequency times intensity
       (1) a, c
       (2) a, b, d
       (3) a, c, d
       (4) All of the above

16. True or false: Women should be encouraged to go through labor in an upright position because this is the most facilitative posture for childbirth.

17. What describes the birth of a macrosomic baby?
    a. The infant is at increased risk of birth trauma.
    b. Prolonged labor is likely.
    c. The mother is at increased risk of birth trauma.

    d. Postpartum hemorrhage is likely.
       (1) a, c
       (2) a, b, d
       (3) a, c, d
       (4) All of the above

18. What is characteristic of the anxiety and fear experienced during labor?
    a. Results in an elevated blood pressure and pulse rate
    b. Results in an improved ability to concentrate
    c. Results in increased pain perception
    d. May prolong labor
       (1) a, c
       (2) a, b, d
       (3) a, c, d
       (4) All of the above

19. What nursing intervention is indicated to reduce sensory overload?
    a. Keep the room's lighting subdued.
    b. Speak quietly and calmly to the patient and her support person.
    c. Provide music in the room.

d. Avoid doing a procedure during a contraction.
  (1) a, c
  (2) a, b, d

(3) a, c, d
(4) All of the above

ANSWERS TO STUDY QUESTIONS

1. c	6. d	11. c	16. True
2. b	7. a	12. 3	17. 4
3. a	8. 4	13. b	18. 3
4. d	9. 2	14. 1	19. 2
5. 2	10. 3	15. 4	

REFERENCES

American College of Obstetricians and Gynecologists (2000). *Fetal macrosomia: Practice bulletin no. 22.* Washington, DC: Author.

Association of Women's Health, Obstetric and Neonatal Nurses (AWHONN). (2000). *Professional nursing support of laboring women: Position statement.* Washington, DC: Author.

Ballen, L., & Fulcher, A. (2006). Nurses and doulas: Complementary roles to provide optimal maternity care. *Journal of Obstetric, Gynecologic, and Neonatal Nursing, 35*(2), 304–311.

Biancuzzo, M. (1993). Six myths of maternal posture during labor. *MCN The American Journal of Maternal Child Nursing, 18*(5), 264–269.

Browning, C. A. (2000). Using music during childbirth. *Birth, 27*(4), 272–276.

Callister, L. C. (1995). Cultural meanings of childbirth. *Journal of Obstetric, Gynecologic, and Neonatal Nursing, 24*(4), 327–331.

Campbell, D., Lake, M., Falk, M., & Backstrand, J. (2006). A randomized controlled trial of continuous support in labor by a lay doula. *Journal of Gynecologic & Neonatal Nursing, 35*(4), 456–464.

Camune, B., & Brucker, M. (2007). An overview of shoulder dystocia—The nurse's role. *Nursing for Women's Health, 11*(5), 488–498.

Chiota, B. J., Goolkasian, P., & Ladewig, P. (1976). Effects of separation from spouse on pregnancy, labor and delivery, and the postpartum period. *Journal of Obstetric, Gynecologic, and Neonatal Nursing, 5*(1), 21–23.

Clark, A. (1978). *Culture, childbearing, health professionals.* Philadelphia: F.A. Davis.

Clark, A., & Affonso, D. (Eds.). (1979). *Childbearing: A nursing perspective* (2nd ed.). Philadelphia: F.A. Davis.

Cunningham, F., Leveno, K., Bloom, S., Gilstrap, L., Hauth, J., & Wenstrom, K. (2005). *Williams obstetrics* (22nd ed.). New York: McGraw-Hill.

Fenwick, L., & Simkin, P. (1987). Maternal positioning to prevent or alleviate dystocia in labor. *Clinical Obstetrics and Gynecology, 30*(1), 83–89.

Founds, S. (2005). Maternal posture for cephalic version of breech presentation: A review of the evidence. *Birth, 32*(2), 137–144.

Gale, J., Fothergill-Bourbonnais, F., & Chamberlain, M. (2001). Measuring nursing support during childbirth. *MCN: The American Journal of Maternal Child Nursing, 26*(5), 264–271.

Gay, J. (1978). Theories regarding endocrine contributions to the onset of labor. *Journal of Obstetric, Gynecologic, and Neonatal Nursing, 7*(5), 42–47.

Gennaro, S., Mayberry, L., & Kafulafula, U. (2007). The evidence supporting nursing management of labor. *Journal of Obstetric, Gynecologic, and Neonatal Nursing, 36*(6), 598–604.

Gilder, K., Mayberry, L. J., Gennaro, S., & Clemmens, D. (2002). Maternal positioning in labor with epidural analgesia—Results from a multi-site survey. *AWHONN Lifelines, 6*(1), 40–45.

Gilliland, A. L. (2002). Beyond holding hands: The modern role of the professional doula. *Journal of Obstetric, Gynecologic, and Neonatal Nursing, 31*(6), 762–769.

Golay, J., Vedam, S., & Sorger, L. (1993). The squatting position for the second stage of labor: Effects on labor and on maternal and fetal well-being. *Birth, 20*(2), 73–78.

Heffron, C. (2006). The honor of your presence. *AWHONN Lifelines, 10*(6), 532–533.

Hodnett, E. (1996). Nursing support of the laboring woman. *Journal of Obstetric, Gynecologic, and Neonatal Nursing, 25*(3), 257–264.

Horn, M., & Manion, J. (1985). Creative grandparenting: Bonding the generations. *Journal of Obstetric, Gynecologic, and Neonatal Nursing, 14*(3), 233–236.

Hottenstein, S. (2005). Continuous labor support. *AWHONN Lifelines, 9*(3), 242–247.

Kennell, J., Klaus, M., McGrath, S., Robertson, S., & Hinckley, C. (1991). Continuous emotional support during labor in a U.S. hospital: A randomized controlled trial. *Journal of the American Medical Association, 265*(17), 2197–2201.

Lehrman, E. (1985). Birth in the left lateral position: An alternative to the traditional delivery position. *Journal of Nurse-Midwifery, 30*(4), 193–197.

Liu, Y. C. (1989). The effects of the upright position during childbirth. *Image, 21*(1), 14–18.

Lydon-Rochelle, M., Albers, L., Gotwocia, J., Craig, E., & Qualls, C. (1993). Accuracy of Leopold maneuvers in screening for malpresentation: A prospective study. *Birth, 20*(3), 132–135.

Mackey, M. C., & Lock, S. E. (1989). Women's expectations of the labor and delivery nurse. *Journal of Obstetric, Gynecologic, and Neonatal Nursing, 18*(6), 505–512.

Manogin, T. W., Bechtel, G. A., & Rami, J. S. (2000). Caring behaviors by nurses: Women's perceptions during childbirth. *Journal of Obstetric, Gynecologic, and Neonatal Nursing, 29*(2), 153–157.

Mayberry, L. J., Strange, L. B., Suplee, P. D., & Gennaro, S. (2003). Use of upright positioning with epidural analgesia—findings from an observational study. *MCN The American Journal of Maternal Child Nursing, 28*(3), 152–159.

Mayberry, L. J., Wood, S. H., Strange, L. B., Flee, L., Heisler, D., & Neilson-Smith, K. (2000). Managing second-stage labor—Exploring the variables during the second stage. *AWHONN Lifelines, 3*(6), 28–34.

McKay, S. (1984). Squatting: An alternative position for the second stage of labor. *MCN The American Journal of Maternal Child Nursing, 9*(3), 181–183.

McKay, S., & Barrows, T. (1991). Holding back: Maternal readiness to give birth. *MCN The American Journal of Maternal Child Nursing, 16*(5), 251–254.

Miltner, R. S. (2000). Identifying labor support actions of intrapartum nurses. *Journal of Obstetric, Gynecologic, and Neonatal Nursing, 29*(5), 491–499.

Olds, S., London, M., Ladewig, P., & Davidson, M. (2003). *Maternal-newborn nursing and women's health care* (7th ed.). Princeton, NJ: Prentice-Hall.

Oxorn, H. (1986). *Oxorn-Foote human labor and birth* (5th ed.). New York: Appleton-Century-Crofts.

Perez, P. G., & Herrick, L. M. (1998). Doulas: Exploring their roles with parents, hospitals, and nurses. *AWHONN Lifelines, 2*(2), 54–55.

Price, S., Noseworthy, J., & Thornton, J. (2007). Women's experience with social presence during childbirth. *MCN The American Journal of Maternal Child Nursing, 32*(3), 184–191.

Ridley, R. (2007). Diagnosis and intervention for occiput posterior malposition. *Journal of Obstetric, Gynecologic, and Neonatal Nursing, 36*(2), 135–143.

Roberts, J. (1980). Alternative positions for childbirth. Part I: First stage of labor. *Journal of Nurse-Midwifery, 25*(4), 11–18.

Roberts, J. (1980). Alternative positions for childbirth. Part II: Second stage of labor. *Journal of Nurse-Midwifery, 25*(5), 13–19.

Roberts, J., & Woolley, D. (1996). A second look at the second stage of labor. *Journal of Obstetric, Gynecologic, and Neonatal Nursing, 25*(5), 415–423.

Roberts, J. E., Goldstein, S. A., Gruener, J. S., Maggio, M., & Mendez-Bauer, C. (1987). A descriptive analysis of involuntary bearing-down efforts during the expulsive phase of labor. *Journal of Obstetric, Gynecologic, and Neonatal Nursing, 16*(1), 48–55.

Romond, J., & Baker, I. (1985). Squatting in childbirth. *Journal of Obstetric, Gynecologic, and Neonatal Nursing, 14*(5), 406–411.

Sauls, D. J. (2002). Effects of labor support on mothers, babies, and birth outcomes. *Journal of Obstetrics, Gynecologic, and Neonatal Nursing, 31*(6), 733–741.

Shermer, R. H., & Raines, D. A. (1997). Positioning during the second stage of labor: Moving back to basics. *Journal of Obstetric, Gynecologic, and Neonatal Nursing, 26*(6), 727–734.

Shorten, A., Donsante, J., & Shorten, B. (2002). Birth position, accoucheur, and perineal outcomes: Informing women about choices for vaginal birth. *Birth, 29*(1), 18–27.

Simkin, P. (2002). Supportive care during labor: A guide for busy nurses. *Journal of Obstetrics, Gynecologic, and Neonatal Nursing, 31*(6), 721–732.

Smith, C., Crowther, C., Wilkinson, C., Pridmore, B., & Robinson, J. (1999). Knee-chest postural management for breech at term: A randomized controlled trial. *Birth, 26*(2), 71–75.

Stremler, R., Hodnett, E., Petryshen, P., Stevens, B., Weston, J., & Willan, A. (2005). Randomized controlled trial of hands-and-knees positioning for occipitoposterior position in labor. *Birth, 32*(4), 243–252.

Winslow, W. (1987). First pregnancy after 35: What's the experience? *MCN The American Journal of Maternal Child Nursing, 12*(2), 92–96.

Zhang, J., Bernasko, J. W., Leybovich, E., Fahs, M., & Hatch, M. (1996). Continuous labor support from labor attendant for primiparous women: A meta-analysis. *Obstetrics and Gynecology, 88*(4 Pt 2), 739–744.

Zwelling, E., Johnson, K., & Allen, J. (2006). How to implement complementary therapies for laboring women. *MCN The American Journal of Maternal Child Nursing, 31*(6), 364–370.

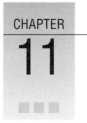

11 Normal Childbirth

Makeba B. Felton

OBJECTIVES

1. Determine the potential for alteration in health status during the intrapartum period.
2. Recognize the signs and symptoms of labor.
3. Identify phases of the first stage of labor.
4. Describe the normal physiologic changes occurring in all four stages of labor.
5. Discuss methods of pain relief used during labor.
6. Use nursing interventions that reflect knowledge of standards of care, while using evidence-based nursing practice.
7. Accurately record documentation of nursing care.
8. Identify variables that may alter the course of labor and delivery.
9. Modify the nursing plan of care to changes in patient status.
10. Recognize the variables that influence the normal progress of labor.
11. Practice the concept of family-centered care during the intrapartum period.

INTRODUCTION

A. The intrapartum period of pregnancy or labor begins with the first stage's uterine contractions and the progressive dilation of the cervix.
B. From complete dilation of the cervix to the infant's delivery is the second stage of labor.
C. The third stage of labor is completed with the expulsion of the placenta and membranes.
D. The fourth stage of labor is the first hour postpartum.

CLINICAL PRACTICE

Premonitory Signs

A. Assessment
   1. History
      a. Lightening
         (1) On the average, lightening occurs 10 days before onset of labor in a primigravida.
         (2) Increased pressure of presenting part leads to:
            (a) Urinary frequency
            (b) Backache and leg pain
            (c) Increased vaginal discharge
            (d) Dependent edema
            (e) Lower abdominal pressure or discomfort
         (3) Lightening results in easier respirations.
      b. Increased mucus-like vaginal discharge
      c. Braxton Hicks contractions
         (1) Called false labor
         (2) Walking lessens discomfort.
         (3) Is usually irregular
         (4) No progressive shortening of interval between contractions
         (5) No changes in cervix

    d. Vaginal show
- (1) Late sign: occurs after the beginning of cervical changes and increased pressure of presenting part
- (2) Blood-tinged cervical mucus

    e. Spontaneous rupture of amniotic sac: leakage of clear or cloudy amniotic fluid

    f. Burst of energy due to increased epinephrine release caused by decreased progesterone release
- (1) Often 24 to 48 hours before labor onset

    g. Gastrointestinal (GI) symptoms
- (1) Diarrhea
- (2) Indigestion
- (3) Nausea and vomiting

    h. Sleep disturbances
- (1) Change in sleep pattern
- (2) Restlessness

2. Physical findings

    a. Lightening
- (1) The uterus and presenting part descend into pelvis.
- (2) Occurrence is determined by abdominal and pelvic examination.

    b. Braxton Hicks contractions
- (1) Uterus not easily indented with palpation
- (2) Irregular uterine contractions
- (3) No changes in cervix

    c. Cervical changes
- (1) Ripening and softening of cervix resulting from hormonal changes
- (2) Effacement: thinning of the cervix
- (3) Dilation: opening of the cervix

    d. Spontaneous rupture of the amniotic sac
- (1) Increased risk of infection; barrier is now open
- (2) There is danger of cord prolapse.

    e. Burst of energy
- (1) Weight loss: patient may experience a 2- to 3-pound weight loss 24 to 48 hours before onset of labor.
- (2) Increased vaginal discharge

3. Psychosocial

    a. Burst of energy may result in nesting urge.

4. Diagnostic procedures

    a. Spontaneous rupture of amniotic sac
- (1) Visible pooling of fluid is observed.
- (2) pH is tested with Nitrazine strip.
- (3) Sterile speculum examination is performed to obtain specimen for microscopic ferning pattern.
- (4) Other testing to assess presence of amniotic fluid, such as Amnisure®

    b. Vaginal examination for cervical status

B. Interventions

1. Offer support to patient and family.

    a. Listen attentively to concerns.
- (1) Allow verbalization of feelings.
- (2) Provide information and support.
- (3) Reinforce and encourage use of prenatal education.
- (4) Provide an awareness of changes as labor begins.
- (5) Give clear, concise explanations, and repeat as necessary.
- (6) Review, demonstrate, and implement anxiety-reduction techniques.
- (7) Provide for the presence of a support person.
- (8) Explain all nursing activities.
- (9) Answer questions presented.

    b. Assist with pain management.
- (1) Discuss pain-relief methods.

   c. Assist with prevention of infection.
       (1) Monitor the patient's temperature every 2 hours for elevation.
       (2) Observe for foul-smelling vaginal discharge or amniotic fluid.
       (3) Educate the patient about the need for perineal cleanliness.
            (a) Handwashing after voiding or defecation
            (b) Cleansing of perineal area from front to back
       (4) Administer antibiotics as indicated.
       (5) Implement Standard Precautions with emphasis on strict handwashing.

First Stage of Labor: Dilation

A. **Assessment**
   1. Physical findings
       a. Cardiovascular changes
           (1) Cardiac output increases.
           (2) Slight pulse changes: may increase to more than 100 beats per minute as a result of exhaustion or dehydration.
           (3) Blood pressure (BP) changes very little.
                (a) Increases are noted if monitored during a contraction.
                (b) Hypotension may occur: vena caval syndrome or supine hypotension resulting from pressure of pregnant uterus on inferior vena cava
       b. Hematologic changes
           (1) White blood cell (WBC) count increases up to $20,000/mm^3$ with strenuous labor.
       c. GI changes
           (1) Motility and absorption are decreased.
           (2) Gastric emptying time is decreased.
           (3) Nausea and vomiting are common.
           (4) Dry lips and mouth occur, resulting from mouth breathing and dehydration.
       d. Renal changes
           (1) The tendency to concentrate urine results in specific gravity greater than 1.025.
           (2) Pressure of full bladder may not be felt due to anesthesia; however, without anesthesia, pressure is increased.
                (a) Requires frequent assessment, and often catheterization
                (b) Can impede labor and fetal descent
           (3) Pressure of presenting part on urethra may require catheterization to empty the urinary bladder.
           (4) Proteinuria
                (a) Caused by increased metabolic activity
                (b) May be sign of gestational hypertension (formerly pregnancy-induced hypertension [PIH])
       e. Respiratory changes
           (1) Exhalation of more CO_2
           (2) Hyperventilation
                (a) Tingling and numbness of hands and feet
                (b) Dizziness
B. **Phases of labor: latent phase**
   1. Patient history
       a. Identification of patient
           (1) Date and time of arrival
           (2) Reason for admission
           (3) Time physician notified and time seen
           (4) Last food intake
       b. Prenatal history (prenatal record)
           (1) Estimated date of confinement (EDC)
           (2) Pregnancies, births, abortions, and living children
           (3) Allergies
           (4) Medications taken during pregnancy (frequency; time and date of last dose)

      (a) Medical conditions
         [i] Pregnancy induced
         [ii] Chronic
      (b) Acute illness during pregnancy: recent exposures and present infections
  (5) Results of laboratory work done during pregnancy (see Chapters 5 and 8 for discussion and interpretation of pregnancy laboratory tests)
      (a) Complete blood count (CBC) to include hemoglobin and hematocrit (H&H)
      (b) Blood type and Rh factor
      (c) Urinalysis
      (d) Venereal Disease Research Laboratory (VDRL)/serologic testing (syphilis screening)
      (e) Gonorrhea (GC)
      (f) Rubella titer
      (g) Papanicolaou smear
  (6) Special tests
      (a) Glucose screen
      (b) Sickle cell screen
      (c) Ultrasonography
      (d) Genetic studies: chorionic villus sampling (CVS), amniocentesis, percutaneous umbilical blood sampling (PUBS)
      (e) Lecithin/sphingomyelin (L/S) ratio, phosphatidylglycerol (PG)
      (f) Maternal serum alpha-fetoprotein (MS-AFP)
      (g) Human immunodeficiency virus (HIV) titer
      (h) Hepatitis B surface antigen (HbsAg) titer for hepatitis screening
      (i) Rh antibody screen
      (j) Nonstress test (NST), oxytocin challenge test (OCT), or contraction stress test (CST)
      (k) Biophysical profile (BPP)
  (7) Childbirth preparation
      (a) Birth plan
      (b) Support system
      (c) Previous experience and coping skills
      (d) Cultural influences
c. Physical findings
  (1) Vital signs: BP, temperature, pulse, respirations, fetal heart rate (FHR), and fetal activity
  (2) Contraction status
      (a) Onset of contractions
      (b) Present contraction status
         [i] Frequency of contractions; contractions may be irregular and may occur every 5 to 10 minutes.
         [ii] Duration: 30 to 45 seconds
         [iii] Intensity
            • Mild by palpation
            • 5 to 40 mm Hg by intrauterine pressure catheter (IUPC)
      (c) Vaginal examination if no abnormal vaginal bleeding
         [i] Cervix location (posterior, moving to anterior)
         [ii] Dilation: 0 to 3 cm; effacement: 0% to 40%
         [iii] Fetal presentation, position, and station
         [iv] Status of membranes
      (d) Vaginal discharge
         [i] Amniotic fluid
             • Time of rupture
             • Color, amount, and odor
         [ii] Bloody show
             • Onset and amount
             • Characteristics
      (e) Abdominal examination
         [i] Fundal height
         [ii] Leopold's maneuvers to determine fetal position and lie

            [iii] Scars, ridges, or masses
        (f) Chest examination
            [i] Heart and lung sounds
        (g) Deep tendon reflexes
            [i] Patellar or brachial reflexes
            [ii] Clonus
    d. Psychosocial findings
        (1) Emotional status
            (a) Confident, low anxiety level
                [i] Excited, talkative
                [ii] Anticipatory, apprehensive
        (2) Support systems
        (3) Fears and concerns
        (4) Nonverbal clues (restlessness, muscle tension, frowning)
    e. Diagnostic procedures
        (1) Urine screen
            (a) Specific gravity; protein, glucose
        (2) Routine blood screen
            (a) CBC (especially H&H)
            (b) Serologic testing
            (c) Blood type and Rh factor
            (d) Obtain other labs from prenatal clinic if available.
C. Phases of labor: active phase
  1. Patient history
    a. Contraction pattern
    b. Hydration status
        (1) Last oral intake
        (2) Current dietary status
        (3) Any nausea or vomiting
    c. Vaginal assessment
        (1) Vaginal bleeding
        (2) Loss of fluid (rupture of membrane [ROM])
  2. Physical findings
    a. Contraction pattern evaluated (by electronic fetal monitoring [EFM] or by palpation) every
        30 minutes or more frequently, if indicated
        (1) Frequency: every 2 to 5 minutes
        (2) Duration: 45 to 60 seconds
        (3) Intensity
            (a) Moderate to strong by palpation
            (b) 50 to 70 mm Hg by IUPC
    b. Vaginal examination
        (1) Dilation: 4 to 7 cm; effacement: 40% to 80%; station: −2 to 0
        (2) Presenting part and position
        (3) Status of membranes
            (a) Intact
            (b) If ruptured:
                [i] Time of rupture
                [ii] Color, amount, and odor of fluid
                [iii] Consistency of fluid
        (4) Progression of labor: suggested dilation rate
            (a) 1.2 cm/hr for primipara
            (b) 1.5 cm/hr for multipara
        (5) Cervix location: anterior
    c. Intake and output (I&O)
        (1) Monitor intake and output hourly
            (a) Insert catheter if indicated
            (b) Hydration status, intravenous fluid intake (IVF)
            (c) Nausea and vomiting

3. Psychosocial findings
   a. Absorbed in serious work of labor
   b. Intense and quieter
   c. Increased dependency
   d. Wavering self-confidence
D. **Phases of labor: transition phase**
   1. Patient history
      a. Childbirth preparation is important.
      b. Time for relaxation between contractions decreases.
   2. Physical findings
      a. Dilation 8 to 10 cm; effacement 80% to 100%; station −1 to +1
      b. Contractions
         (1) Frequency: every 2 to 3 minutes
         (2) Duration: 60 to 90 seconds
         (3) Intensity
             (a) Strong by palpation
             (b) 70 to 90 mm Hg by IUPC
         (4) Strong urge to push if station is low
         (5) Backache
         (6) Nausea and vomiting
         (7) Trembling limbs
         (8) Vaginal discharge: bloody show increases
         (9) Intake and output (I&O)
             (a) Monitor oral and IV intake.
             (b) If patient does not have catheter at this point, monitor frequently for urge to void.
   2. Psychosocial findings
      a. Supportive needs increase, but client is agitated and irritable.
      b. Patient is increasingly discouraged because of fatigue and may want to give up.
      c. Patient's coping ability decreases because she feels overwhelmed.
      d. Patient relaxation is almost impossible.
E. **Pain management during first stage of labor**
   1. Goal: Change perception through relaxation to decrease tension and medication to increase pain threshold.
   2. Pain receptors are stimulated by uterine contractions that result in:
      a. Myometrial anoxia
      b. Cervical stretching or dilation
      c. Distention of lower uterine segment and pelvic floor
      d. Pressure on pelvic nerves
      e. Traction on supporting and nearby structures
   3. Pain perception may be affected by:
      a. Experience
      b. Cultural expectations and support system
      c. Fatigue, anemia
      d. Fear, anxiety, and emotional stress
      e. Environment
      f. Pain anticipation
   4. Medications
      a. Barbiturates (phenobarbital [Nembutal], secobarbital [Seconal])
         (1) Provide sedation or sleep
         (2) Reduce tension and fear
      b. Tranquilizers (hydroxyzine [Vistaril] and promethazine [Phenergan])
         (1) Various agents with such added effects as antianxiety and/or antiemetic
         (2) Provide muscle relaxation
         (3) May potentiate narcotics
      c. Narcotics (meperidine [Demerol], morphine, butorphanol [Stadol], nalbuphine [Nubain], fentanyl [Sublimaze], sufentanil)
         (1) Increase pain threshold: Patient's ability to tolerate or cope with discomfort increases.
         (2) May increase or decrease uterine activity

(3) May cause drowsiness

(4) Have narcotic antagonist available: naloxone (Narcan)

(5) Administer during uterine contraction to minimize fetal effect.

   d. Regional anesthesia

    (1) Paracervical block (NOTE: This anesthesia is rarely used anymore and is described here only for historic purposes.)

      (a) Local anesthesia is injected transvaginally lateral to cervix at dilation of 4 to 6 cm.

      (b) Lower uterine segment, cervix, and upper vagina are affected.

      (c) Effect on fetus is transient bradycardia.

    (2) Epidural or caudal

      (a) Local anesthesia is injected into epidural or caudal space.

      (b) Nerves leaving the spinal cord are blocked.

      (c) Entire pelvis and lower extremities are affected so that the patient perceives touch but not pain.

      (d) Monitor for urinary retention.

      (e) Fetal effect: Uterine blood flow is decreased if maternal hypotension occurs, leading to potential fetal distress.

      (f) Keep antidote on hand (naloxone).

    (3) Nonpharmacologic methods

      (a) Transcutaneous electrical nerve stimulation (TENS)

        [i] Electrodes are placed on either side of patient's lower spine.

        [ii] Patient provides electrical stimulation during contractions.

        [iii] TENS provides alternate sensation to decrease perception of pain from contractions.

      (b) Touch

        [i] Acupressure: increases endorphin release and reduces sensation.

        [ii] Cutaneous stimulation: effleurage provides an alternative sensation.

        [iii] Massage and counterpressure

        [iv] Hot or cold application

      (c) Therapeutic touch and healing touch

      (d) Relaxation techniques

        [i] Biofeedback

        [ii] Visual imagery

        [iii] Controlled breathing patterns

        [iv] Shower or Jacuzzi

        [v] Movement, position changes, and ambulation

F. Interventions

  1. Assist with positioning during labor.

    a. Discourage supine position to prevent supine hypotension or vena caval syndrome.

    b. Use pillows to assist with positioning.

    c. Encourage frequent position changes.

  2. Monitor vital signs

    a. Assess BP between contractions for an accurate reading.

    b. Monitor BP, pulse, and respirations every 30 to 60 minutes.

    c. Observe for vital signs that may indicate bleeding (e.g., elevated pulse, decreased BP).

    d. Monitor temperature every 4 hours (every 2 hours after ROM) for elevation, which may indicate dehydration.

  3. Maintain an accurate I&O record.

    a. Encourage adequate intake of oral fluids.

    b. Monitor IV fluid intake.

    c. Encourage bladder elimination every 2 hours.

    d. Catheterize patient as indicated.

  4. Actively integrate patient and family in laboring process.

    a. Orient the patient to her environment.

    b. Call the patient by her name.

    c. Encourage verbalization of feelings, listening attentively.

    d. Respect the patient's privacy.

    e. Provide information about routine procedures to patient and her family.

      f. Encourage participation by support persons.

      g. Encourage expression of feelings.

      h. Reinforce previously learned coping methods.

      i. Present new methods of coping with the situation.

      j. Encourage rest between contractions in active phase and transition.

   5. Implement pain management regimen.

      a. Minimize environmental stimuli.

      b. Assess level of comfort before and after pain management intervention, throughout all stages of labor.

      c. Offer comfort measures, including pharmacologic and nonpharmacologic methods of pain relief (see previous section for discussion of options).

      d. Offer and explain analgesia or anesthesia, if indicated and desired.

      e. Assist with pain management regimen as needed.

      f. Encourage rest in latent phase and promote relaxation.

   6. Monitor fetal well-being during labor.

      a. Monitor FHR for signs of distress caused by decreased uteroplacental perfusion (see Chapter 12 for further discussion of fetal assessment in labor)

         (1) May be done continuously with EFM.

         (2) Monitor every 15 minutes if not on EFM.

   7. Monitor I&O

      a. Encourage voiding every 2 hours; catheterize as indicated.

      b. Test urine for specific gravity (normal is 1.010 to 1.025).

      c. Administer oral or IV fluids as indicated.

      d. Observe for obvious vaginal bleeding.

   8. Assess membrane status.

      a. Document time of ROM and characteristics of amniotic fluid.

      b. Monitor temperature every 2 hours after ROM.

      c. Monitor laboratory data as indicated, to include WBC count.

      d. Perform vaginal examinations only when necessary.

      e. Ensure aseptic technique during procedures.

      f. Observe FHR for tachycardia, often an early indication of maternal infection.

Second Stage of Labor: Infant Expulsion

A. Assessment

   1. Physical findings

      a. Vaginal examination

         (1) Dilation: 10 cm (complete cervical dilation); effacement 100%; station 0 to +2

      b. Contractions

         (1) Frequency: every 2 to 3 minutes

         (2) Duration: 60 to 90 seconds

         (3) intensity

            (a) Strong by palpation

            (b) 80 to 100 mm Hg by IUPC

      c. Diaphoresis

      d. Methods to facilitate fetal descent

         (1) Laboring down

            (a) Second stage rest period for patients with epidural

            (b) Begin pushing when the urge is felt

         (2) The urge-to-push method, in which the mother bears down as she feels the urge and in a manner that feels right to her

            (a) Most women make three to five brief (4- to 6-second) pushes with each contraction.

            (b) Most pushes are accompanied by the release of air.

         (3) Provide caution in using the traditional method of pushing, and avoid instructing the patient to hold her breath; bear down as in a Valsalva maneuver; and push

            (a) Pushing in this fashion leads to prolonged second stage of labor and fetal effects such as lower Apgar scores and abnormal cord blood levels (Yildirim, 2008).

        (4) The open-glottis method in which air is released during pushing so that no intrathoracic pressure builds up, is recommended as a method with fewer maternal and fetal effects.

    e. Signs of descent of presenting part

        (1) Bulging of perineum occurs, as vaginal introitus opens.

        (2) Rectal changes occur.

            (a) Passing of flatus or stool

            (b) Rectal mucosa exposed

        (3) The presenting part is visible (crowning).

        (4) Burning or stretching sensation is felt in the perineal area.

        (5) Urine may be expressed during pushing.

B. Anesthesia during delivery

  1. Continuation of caudal or epidural anesthesia

  2. Integration of pudendal anesthesia

    a. Definition: a transvaginal block of the pudendal nerve near ischial spines

    b. Affects vaginal and perineal area and has little or no fetal effect

    c. Perineal body is injected with local anesthesia.

    d. Performed just before delivery at site of episiotomy

  3. Saddle block: low spinal anesthesia

    a. Definition: Local anesthesia is introduced into the subarachnoid space.

    b. Motor and sensory nerves are blocked.

    c. Effect on fetus is decreased blood flow with maternal hypotension secondary to peripheral vasodilation.

C. Episiotomy: incision into the perineum to provide more space for delivery of presenting part

  1. Indications

    a. To prevent tearing

    b. To prevent undue stretching of bladder and rectal supports

    c. To reduce time and stress of second stage

    d. To allow for ease in manipulation with a forceps, suction, or breech delivery

  2. Types

    a. Median or midline

        (1) Advantages: heals quickly; easily repaired; less discomfort; less dyspareunia

        (2) Disadvantage: Extension can involve rectal area.

    b. Mediolateral: 45-degree angle to left or right

        (1) Advantages: used for large infant; has no rectal involvement

        (2) Disadvantages: heals slowly; is more painful; causes greater blood loss

D. Laceration: injury to soft tissue in perineal area as a result of truamatic birth, generally when the fetal head is being delivered

  1. Classifications

    a. First degree: involves perineal skin and vaginal mucous membrane

    b. Second degree: involves skin and mucous membrane plus fascia of perineal body

    c. Third degree: involves skin, mucous membrane, and muscle of perineal body; extends into rectal sphincter

    d. Fourth degree: extends into rectal mucosa to expose the lumen of the rectum

E. Psychosocial

  1. Patient is less irritable and agitated.

  2. Patient is more cooperative.

  3. Trying to maintain modesty often not a priority with patient

  4. Patient may doze off between contractions.

  5. Patient is intent on work of pushing.

F. Delivery methods

  1. Controlled vaginal vertex delivery

    a. Maintain gentle pressure on presenting part.

    b. Provide perineal support.

    c. Support fetal head as it is delivered.

    d. Check for nuchal cord.

    e. Suction infant's mouth, then nose.

    f. Deliver anterior shoulder under symphysis.

g. Deliver posterior shoulder over coccyx.
h. Rest of infant delivers easily.
i. Note time of delivery, the point at which the entire infant body is free of the mother
2. Vaginal-assisted delivery: involves the use of forceps or vacuum suction to assist in vaginal delivery
  a. Indications
    (1) Maternal
      (a) Progress of second stage stops as the result of inadequate contraction strength, poor pushing efforts, excessive infant size, or nonvertex fetal position.
      (b) Maternal condition that warrants a shortened second stage (e.g., cardiac problems)
      (c) Extreme fatigue of mother after prolonged labor, particularly second stage
    (2) Fetal
      (a) Preterm infant (potential for cranial damage with prolonged pushing)
      (b) Distress that warrants a shortened second stage
  b. Prerequisites
    (1) No cephalopelvic disproportion (CPD) is present.
    (2) Head is engaged.
    (3) Membranes are ruptured.
    (4) Cervix is completely dilated.
    (5) Bladder is empty.
  c. Types of assisted deliveries
    (1) Low/outlet forceps: used when the head is visible at the perineum
    (2) Midforceps
      (a) Head is at the ischial spines.
      (b) Often needed for rotation to anteroposterior position
    (3) Vacuum
      (a) Head is visible.
      (b) Silastic suction cup is applied to presenting part and gentle traction is exerted while the mother pushes.
  d. After any assisted delivery, the infant should be examined thoroughly for possible injuries.
    (1) Bruising
    (2) Cephalhematoma (collection of blood under the skull bones, so does not cross suture lines) (NOTE: area of edema of scalp at location of Silastic cup is usual with vacuum extractions)
    (3) Facial nerve damage
  e. Use of forceps or vacuum may predispose the client to lacerations of the vagina or perineum.
G. **Interventions**
1. Monitor vital signs and oxygenation status.
  a. Closely monitor vital signs after analgesia or anesthesia.
  b. Monitor pulse oximetry as indicated.
  c. Administer oxygen as indicated
2. Assist with pain management during fetal expulsion.
  a. Assess level of comfort of client.
  b. Encourage, support, and guide patient and labor coach related to second stage of labor.
  c. Encourage rest periods between pushing contractions.
  d. Provide comfort measures; facilitate optimal breathing techniques.
  e. Offer other nonpharmacologic options to include TENS, massage, hydrotherapy, etc.
  f. Assist with pharmacologic techniques.
    (1) Provide information on analgesia and/or anesthesia as necessary.
    (2) Answer patient's questions regarding therapeutic options.
    (3) Administer analgesia and/or anesthesia as indicated.
    (4) Monitor response to pain relief method used.
    (5) Maintain patient safety.
      (a) Put side rails up after analgesia or anesthesia has been administered
3. Monitor the patient's I&O.
  a. Encourage emptying of bladder and catheterize distended bladder if the patient is unable to void.
  b. Maintain adequate fluid intake.

4. Assist with expulsion of fetus
   a. Encourage side-lying or pillow-propped position because dorsal recumbent position occludes the inferior vena cava.
   b. Encourage upright rather than recumbent position for pushing.
   c. Encourage gentle pushing efforts to allow for gradual stretching of tissue.
   d. Discourage Valsalva maneuvers while pushing.
   e. Encourage open-glottis pushing.
   f. Avoid precipitous or uncontrolled delivery when possible.
   g. Position the patient to facilitate perineal floor relaxation and increased pelvic diameters (see Chapter 10 for a complete discussion of optimal positions for expulsion).
   h. Provide mirror to observe progress of pushing.
5. Monitor patient for signs and symptoms of infection.
   a. Document and intervene when deviations from norm occur.
   b. Use clean or aseptic technique as appropriate.
   c. Using institution's designated solutions, cleanse perineal area before delivery.

Third Stage of Labor: Placental Expulsion

A. **Assessment**
   1. Physical findings
      a. Signs of separation of placenta
         (1) Gush of blood occurs.
         (2) Cord lengthens at vaginal opening.
         (3) Fundus rises in abdomen.
         (4) Uterine shape changes from flat to firm and globular as placenta drops into lower uterine segment
      b. Types of placental delivery
         (1) Spontaneous
             (a) Schultz's mechanism: Fetal side delivers first.
             (b) Duncan's mechanism: Maternal side delivers first.
         (2) Manual extraction: Delivery attendant assists with placental separation and removal.
      c. Placental abnormalities (Figure 11-1)
         (1) Battledore: Cord is inserted at or near the placental margin, rather than in the center.
         (2) Circumvallate: The fetal surface of the placenta is exposed through a ring of chorion and amnion opening around the umbilical cord.
         (3) Succenturiate: One or more accessory lobes of fetal villi have developed.
             (a) Only the membranes support the vessels from the major to the minor lobe, increasing the risk of retention of the minor lobe during the third stage.
             (b) Blood loss may also occur if these vessels are nicked during intrauterine procedures.
         (4) Velamentous insertion of cord: Fetal vessels separate in the membranes before reaching the placenta.
             (a) If bleeding is visible, it should be tested for fetal hemoglobin by means of Kleihauer-Betke or Apt test to determine if fetal or maternal blood
             (b) Fetus may become hypovolemic.
             (c) Fetus is most vulnerable during labor and delivery.
             (d) Condition is more common with:
                 [i] Multiple gestation
                 [ii] Placental anomalies (Olds, London, & Ladewig, 1996)
         (5) Vasa previa: associated with velamentous insertion of the cord
             (a) The umbilical vessels in the membranes cross the region of the internal os and present ahead of the fetus.
             (b) Potential danger to the fetus is considerable if rupture of the membranes is accompanied by rupture of a fetal vessel.
             (c) In severe cases, vasa previa can lead to exsanguination of the fetus (Perry, Hockenberry, Lowdermilk, & Wilson, 2010).

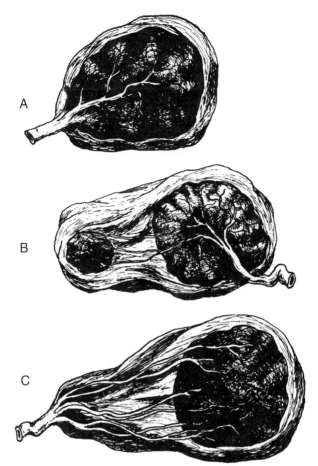

FIGURE 11-1 ■ Placental variations. **A,** Battledore placenta. **B,** Placenta succenturiate. **C,** Velamentous insertion of the umbilical cord. (From Lowdermilk, D.L., & Perry, S.E. [2007]. *Maternity & women's health care* [9th ed.]. St. Louis: Mosby.)

      (d) Vasa previa may be diagnosed by:
         [i] Vaginal examination
         [ii] Amnioscopy
         [iii] Palpation of a vessel pulsating synchronously with the FHR in the membranes in front of the fetus
         [iv] Cesarean delivery may be indicated if the health care provider believes the risk of hemorrhage to be great.

B. Interventions
    1. Facilitate bonding of infant and mother.
      a. Provide early infant contact as soon as possible: Place the infant on the mother's abdomen after delivery if not contraindicated.
      b. Encourage touching and holding of the infant, including skin-to-skin contact.
    2. Explain procedures to patient and family.
      a. Explain process of placental delivery to patient and labor coach.
      b. Offer reassurance of fetal well-being.
        (1) Explain any procedures for routine stimulation or resuscitation of the infant to allay anxiety.
    3. Monitor for and prevent bleeding during immediate postpartum period.
      a. Monitor vaginal bleeding with delivery of the placenta.
      b. Monitor firmness of the uterus, and massage if indicated.
      c. Administer oxytocin (Pitocin) as indicated.
      d. Monitor vital signs for indications of bleeding.

Fourth Stage of Labor: Immediate Postpartum Period

A. **Assessment**
   1. Physical findings
      a. Vital signs
         (1) BP is taken every 15 minutes.
            (a) Transient changes are secondary to decreased blood volume after delivery.
            (b) Excitement may elevate BP.
            (c) Low reading is often a late sign of blood loss.
         (2) Pulse is checked every 15 minutes.
            (a) Bradycardia may occur to compensate for decreased vascular bed and decreased intraabdominal pressure.
            (b) Tachycardia may indicate an increase in blood loss or a temperature elevation.
         (3) Temperature: Slight elevation is normal (37.8° C [100° F]) as the result of dehydration and the fatigue of labor.
      b. Fundal assessment every 15 minutes
         (1) Fundus is firm and well contracted.
         (2) Fundus is 2 cm below the level of the umbilicus immediately after delivery of placenta (Lowdermilk & Perry, 2007).
         (3) Fundus rises slowly to the level of umbilicus during the first hour after placental delivery.
      c. Lochia assessment every 15 minutes
         (1) Nature of flow: intermittent, trickle, continuous
         (2) Amount of flow
            (a) Hemorrhage
               [i] Weigh peripads or Chux (1 g = 1 mL)
               [ii] Greater than 500 mL indicates postpartum hemorrhage in a vaginal delivery (see Chapter 28 for further discussion of postpartum hemorrhage).
               [iii] Saturated peripad in less than 1 hour (see Chapter 13 for more details regarding lochial flow and evaluation)
         (3) Character and odor of flow
      d. Perineal assessment
         (1) Episiotomy and/or laceration assessment
            (a) Intact: edges approximated
            (b) Minimal pain or discomfort
            (c) No hematomas, redness, or edema
            (d) Ice to episiotomy/laceration site for first 24 hours, then heat
            (e) Episiotomy/laceration site is clean and dry
   2. Psychosocial
      a. Attachment process begins.
      b. Mother inspects the newborn.
      c. Mother wants to cuddle the infant and begin breastfeeding.
      d. Rubin's phases of maternal postpartum adjustment
         (1) Taking-in: first 24 hours; excited and talkative; reliving birth experience; focus is primarily on self and one's personal needs
         (2) Taking-hold: days 2 and 3; eager to learn; baby blues might settle in; focus is primarily on taking care of baby
         (3) Letting-go: day 4 on; eager to incorporate other family members into care and life of infant; focus is on relationships at this point (Lowdermilk & Perry, 2007; see Chapter 13 for further discussion)

B. **Interventions**
   1. Facilitate maternal-infant bonding.
      a. Provide for early infant contact, to include skin-to-skin contact.
      b. Encourage familial involvement in infant's care.
      c. Assist with early breastfeeding.
      d. Postpone eye prophylaxis if indicated.
   2. Educate patient and family on fetal well-being.
      a. Call attention to quiet, alert state of infant.
      b. Provide information about infant's ability to see and hear.

3. Monitor I&O.
    a. Encourage emptying of the bladder, catheterize distended bladder if the patient is unable to void.
    b. Monitor fundal height for indication of bladder distention.
    c. Administer IV and oral fluids as indicated.
4. Monitor for signs of excessive bleeding.
    a. Monitor pad count.
    b. Monitor vital signs for signs of bleeding.
    c. Monitor fundal height and firmness.
5. Monitor and assess level of comfort.
    a. Assist with nonpharmacologic methods of relief (as discussed previously).
    b. Assist with pharmacologic methods of relief.
        (1) Provide medication as ordered.
        (2) Monitor for effectiveness and side effects of medication.
6. Monitor for and prevent maternal and neonatal infection.
    a. Use clean or aseptic technique, as appropriate.
    b. Clean the perineal area from front to back.
    c. Inspect the perineal area for indications of infection.
    d. Emphasize good handwashing technique to patient.
    e. Monitor client's vital signs for indications of infection.

Variables Influencing Labor and Delivery

Induction or Augmentation
Initiation or augmentation of uterine contractions will often accomplish delivery.
A. **Assessment**
    1. History
        a. Relative indications for induction or augmentation
            (1) Maternal
                (a) Medical complications such as diabetes or gestational hypertension
                (b) Slowed progress of labor
                (c) History of precipitate labor
                (d) Chorioamnionitis
            (2) Fetal
                (a) Intrauterine growth restriction (IUGR)
                (b) Prolonged ROM
                (c) Postdates gestation
                (d) Rh sensitization
                (e) Fetal death
        b. Relative contraindications for induction or augmentation
            (1) Maternal
                (a) Previous classical uterine incision
                (b) Placenta previa
                (c) Grand multipara
                (d) Overdistended uterus
                (e) Active genital herpes
            (2) Fetal
                (a) Cephalosporin disproportion (CPD)
                (b) Severe fetal distress
                (c) Fetal malposition
                (d) Fetal immaturity
    2. Physical findings
        a. Bishop score measures physiologic readiness of cervix (Table 11-1)
            (1) Dilation
            (2) Effacement
            (3) Station
            (4) Cervical consistency
            (5) Cervical position

3. Diagnostic findings
   a. Maternal readiness
      (1) Informed consent
      (2) Bishop score of 5 to 7 indicates probable induction success.
   b. Fetal readiness
      (1) Gestational age established by early ultrasound test or measurement of appropriate parameters
      (2) Acceptable lecithin/sphingomyelin (L/S) ratio (usually 2:1 or higher)
      (3) Presence of phosphotidylglycerol (PG) in amniotic fluid (see Chapter 8 for a complete discussion)
4. Methods of induction or augmentation
   a. Mechanical
      (1) Amniotomy: Artifically rupture membranes in an attempt to stimulate onset of labor.
         (a) Potential complications: infection; prolapsed cord
   b. Chemical
      (1) Prostaglandin E (PGE)
         (a) Used as suppository or gel to ripen cervix to improve the Bishop score
         (b) Side effects: nausea, vomiting and diarrhea, and/or fever

■ TABLE 11-1
■ ■ Bishop Score

PARAMETER	POINTS ASSIGNED			
	0	**1**	**2**	**3**
Position of Cervix	Posterior (towards the back)	Midposition	Anterior (towards the front)	---
Consistency	Firm	Medium	Soft	---
Effacement (%)	0-30	40-50	60-70	>80
Dilation (cm)	Closed/0	1-2	3-4	>5
Baby's Station	−3	−2	−1 to 0	+1, +2
+ Cervical Sensations	None	Slight	Strong and frequent	Coordinated with some or all toning contractions
+ Yoni (vaginal) Secretions	No increase	Increased mucus	Increase with bloody mucus	---
+ Toning Contractions	None to slight	Mild	Strong, sporadic, frequent	Almost regular, visible on abdominal observation

+ All items with a plus sign are added by Anne Frye, *Holistic midwifery volume II*, and have been proven helpful from a midwifery-model perspective. All others are original components of the Bishop Score.

Modifiers:
Add 1 point to score for:
1. Preeclampsia
2. Each prior vaginal delivery
Subtract 1 point from score for:
1. Postdates pregnancy
2. Nulliparity (Never having borne children)
3. Premature or prolonged rupture of membranes

Total Score=sum of all points for each parameter. The meaning of the score:
7 or less: Do **not** attempt induction without ripening the cervix first.
9 or more: Favorable to attempt induction
12 or more: She is quite ready for labor or in early labor; a little encouragement should get her going.

Sources: Modified from Romney S et al, editors: *Gynecology and obstetrics: The health care of women, ed 2,* New York, 1981, McGraw-Hill. *Holistic Midwifery volume II,* Anne Frye, Labrys Press, http://www.mothercare.ca/bishop.htm, www.cdc.gov/, Jennifer A. McFarland, My Birth By Design, http://www.mybirthbydesign.com/, Jennifer@MyBirthByDesign.com, 312-805-5280, 856-740-4858

(2) Oxytocin (Pitocin): synthetic hormone used to initiate uterine contractions
    (a) Given intravenously (diluted in an isotonic electrolyte solution) in secondary line with an infusion pump
    (b) Side effects
       [i] Tetanic contractions
       [ii] Maternal hypotension
       [iii] Antidiuretic effect
       [iv] Neonatal hyperbilirubinemia has been reported (Perry et al, 2010)
(3) Other methods of induction
    (a) Membrane stripping
    (b) Nipple stimulation (Lowdermilk & Perry, 2007)

B. Interventions

1. Offer reassurance to patient and family.
   a. Present procedure with clear explanations.
2. Monitor fetal well-being
   a. Maintain frequent presence, with continuous EFM for fetus and maternal contractions.
   b. Reassure the patient of fetal status and progress of labor.
3. Monitor and assess level of comfort.
   a. Anticipate that the patient will feel the pain from contractions sooner than with naturally occurring labor.
   b. Provide pharmacologic and nonpharmacologic methods of pain control as indicated by patient.
4. Monitor I&O strictly for imbalances.
   a. Maintain an accurate record of the amount of oxytocin administered.
   b. Observe for signs of water intoxication; discontinue oxytocin if indicated.
      (1) Altered consciousness
      (2) Assess respiratory status for shortness of breath and/or presence of crackles.
      (3) Edema
5. Administer oxytocin (Pitocin) if indicated.
   a. Review institution's written policy or protocol for medication use; a suggested oxytocin protocol follows:
      (1) Dilute 10 units of oxytocin in 1000 mL of lactated Ringer's solution or other physiologic electrolyte solution so that each mL contains 10 mU of oxytocin
      (2) Administer by means of infusion pump as secondary line, connected as close as possible to the primary IV site.
      (3) Initial dose is usually 0.5 to 1 mU/min
      (4) Dose may be gradually increased in increments of 1 to 2 mU/min every 30 to 60 minutes.
      (5) Once the desired frequency of contractions is reached (usually every 3 minutes), the rate may be maintained (a client seldom requires more than 20 to 40 mU/min).
      (6) Nurse-patient ratio should be 1:1 or 1:2.
   b. During administration, accurate monitoring is required for:
      (1) Uterine contractions: frequency, duration, and intensity
      (2) Uterine resting tone
      (3) FHR response to contractions
      (4) Maternal vital signs
      (5) Maternal I&O
   c. Discontinue oxytocin infusion:
      (1) With a tetanic contraction (one lasting longer than 90 seconds)
      (2) With uterine tachysystole (contractions occurring less than 2 minutes apart)
      (3) With elevated uterine resting tone
      (4) With nonreassuring FHR patterns (see Chapter 12 for complete discussion of FHR patterns)
6. Administer prostaglandin if indicated. Review institution's written policy or protocol for medication use; a suggested prostaglandin protocol follows:
   a. In all patients an IV should be started and continuous EFM begun.
   b. Supine or nearly side-lying bed rest for 1 to 2 hours after cervical ripening agent with vital signs
   c. Continuous FHR and contraction monitoring for 1 to 4 hours

  d. Oxytocin may be initiated no sooner than 4 hours before or after the last misoprostol dose (if this drug is being used).
  e. If uterine tachysystole occurs, notify health care provider.
  f. If FHR indicates fetal compromise, institute measures to remove the tablet and improve fetal oxygenation (Murray, 1996).

Dysfunctional Labor

A. Assessment
  1. History
     a. Abnormal progress of labor (some overlapping exists between classifications)
     b. Nulliparous women are more subject to certain conditions that occur in early labor, such as:
        (1) Hypertonic uterine dysfunction
        (2) Primary inertia
        (3) Prolonged latent phase
     c. Multiparous women more often demonstrate problems that occur in the active phase, such as:
        (1) Hypotonic uterine dysfunction
        (2) Secondary inertia
        (3) Protraction or arrest of the active phase
     d. Altered Friedman curve (Figure 11-2)
        (1) Friedman demonstrated a normal labor pattern by plotting, on a graph, cervical dilation and degree of descent against lapsed time.
     e. Categories of delayed progression according to his terminology:
        (1) Prolonged latent phase
        (2) Protraction disorders
        (3) Arrest disorders
  2. Physical findings
     a. Hypertonia (primary inertia)
        (1) Uncoordinated uterine activity: no normal resting phase
        (2) More than one uterine pacemaker sending signals
        (3) Frequent contractions
        (4) Occurs in latent phase (protracted latent phase)
        (5) Painful because of uterine anoxia
        (6) Management with therapeutic rest (Lowdermilk & Perry, 2007)
     b. Hypotonia (secondary inertia)
        (1) Ineffective tightening and pressure
           (a) Infrequent contractions that are insufficient in dilating the cervix
           (b) Poor contraction intensity
           (c) Occurs in active phase (protracted active phase)
           (d) Management with labor augmentation (Lowdermilk & Perry, 2007)

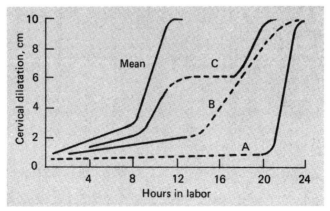

FIGURE 11-2 ■ Abnormal Friedman curve. (From Friedman, E. [1965]. In J.P. Greenhill [Ed.], *Obstetrics* [13th ed.]. Philadelphia: Saunders.)

   c. Precipitate labor
     (1) Labor of less than 3 hours
     (2) Low maternal tissue resistance
     (3) Often rapid transit of fetus through birth canal
     (4) More common in women older than 35 and younger than 20 years (Lowdermilk & Perry, 2007)
     (5) Previous history is good indicator of subsequent precipitous deliveries.
  3. Diagnostic findings
    a. Pathologic retraction ring (Bandl's ring) (Figure 11-3)
     (1) A normal physiologic retraction ring develops at the junction of the active upper and passive lower segments of the uterus.
     (2) A pathologic ring is an exaggeration of this physiologic ring; it grips the fetus, preventing descent.
     (3) Labor is arrested at this point.
     (4) The uterus above the ring becomes thicker, and the lower segment thins out and ruptures unless the obstruction is relieved.
     (5) Tocolytic drugs to relax the uterus are often used.
     (6) If drug therapy is not successful, delivery must be made by cesarean birth.
    b. Fetus in occiput posterior position
     (1) A larger diameter presents to the pelvis.
     (2) The degree of flexion is altered.
     (3) Cervical dilation and fetal descent are slowed.
B. Interventions
  1. Monitor and document progress of labor.
    a. Assess patient tolerance to labor.
    b. Document contractions, patient's response, and coping ability.
    c. Perform vaginal examinations to determine cervical dilation and fetal descent.
    d. Communicate deviations from normal to health care provider.
    e. Explain unknown or unplanned situations in an easily understood manner.
    f. Identify how this situation may alter birth plan and assist patient with making adjustments.
    g. Maintain a positive attitude about ability to cope.
    h. Reassure the patient as to the status of the fetus.
  2. Educate patient on deviations from normal laboring process.
    a. Assess patient's knowledge of alterations in labor process.
    b. Encourage questions and expression of feelings.
    c. Provide factual information about dysfunctional labor.
    d. Explain expected treatment and outcome.
  3. Monitor and assess level of comfort.
    a. Offer pharmacologic and nonpharmacologic methods of pain control.
  4. Monitor for and prevent maternal and neonatal infection.
    a. Monitor and document vital signs and FHR for indications of infection.
    b. Maintain good aseptic technique.

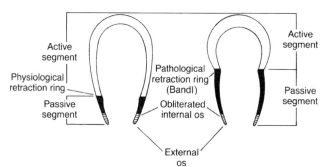

FIGURE 11-3 ■ Bandl's ring. *Left,* normal second stage; right, abnormal second stage—dystocia. (Redrawn from Cunningham, G., MacDonald, P., & Gant, N. [1988]. *Williams obstetrics* [18th ed., p. 214]. Norwalk, CT: Appleton & Lange.)

    c. Minimize vaginal examinations, using sterile technique when indicated.

    d. Maintain good perineal hygiene.

    e. Monitor characteristics and odor of amniotic fluid.

    f. Administer antibiotics as indicated.

    g. Assess labs as indicated, including WBC count.

Cesarean Birth

Delivery is through incision in abdominal and uterine walls.

A. Assessment

  1. History

    a. Previous uterine surgery

    b. Fetal conditions (see following)

    c. Maternal condition (e.g., hemorrhage, cardiac disease, hypertension)

  2. Physical findings

    a. Indications for cesarean birth

      (1) Fetal

        (a) Fetal distress, disease, or anomaly

        (b) Umbilical cord prolapse

        (c) Fetal malposition or malpresentation

        (d) Fetal macrosomia

        (e) CPD

      (2) Maternal

        (a) Multiple gestation

        (b) Active herpes genitalia

        (c) Maternal positive HIV status

        (d) Placental abnormality (e.g., placenta previa or abruptio placentae)

    b. Vaginal birth after cesarean (VBAC)

      (1) Decision making

        (a) Nonrepeating condition

        (b) Desire to avoid cesarean birth

        (c) Ability to perform emergency cesarean birth, if indicated

        (d) Benefits mother by shortening recovery time

      (2) Risks

        (a) Possibility of uterine rupture, particularly when previous type of uterine scar is unknown

        (b) Need for close monitoring during labor

  3. Psychosocial

    a. Relief after long labor with failure to progress

    b. Fear if fetus or mother is stressed

    c. Helplessness if birth plan is altered

    d. Disappointment if vaginal delivery is not achieved

  4. Diagnostic findings

    a. Preoperative CBC, urinalysis; blood typed and crossmatched

    b. Fetal lung maturity and gestational age if elective

    c. Ultrasonography for fetal position and placental placement

  5. Anesthesia (see Chapter 24 for complete discussion of anesthesia and surgery during pregnancy)

    a. General

      (1) General anesthesia usually is used only in emergency situations or when regional anesthesia is contraindicated.

      (2) General anesthesia leads to CNS depression of patient and fetus.

      (3) Patient must be NPO.

      (4) Nonparticulate antacids may be administered prior to surgery.

      (5) Because of the resulting hypoxia in the infant, it is recommended that induction time to birth be less than 8 minutes.

      (6) Patient is not awake during the delivery.

    b. Regional

      (1) Spinal

(a) Local anesthesia is injected into the subarachnoid space.
(b) Motor and sensory block ensues.
(c) Spinal anesthesia has the potential for causing severe headaches during recovery period.
(d) Patient may remain awake.
(2) Epidural
(a) Local anesthesia is injected into epidural space.
(b) Sensory block of entire pelvis and legs ensues.
(c) Epidural block has the potential for hypotensive episode if the mother is not well hydrated first.
(d) If hypotension occurs, fetus may suffer distress.
(e) Patient may remain awake.

B. Interventions
1. Keep patient informed of variations in normal laboring process.
    a. Assist patient with appropriate coping techniques.
    b. Encourage active participation in decision making.
    c. Encourage verbalization of feelings about a cesarean birth rather than a vaginal delivery.
    d. Provide clear explanations of all proposed treatment options.
    e. Facilitate involvement of support person.
    f. Reassure patient about infant if surgery is performed for fetal distress.
    g. Provide positive reassurance.
2. Educate patient on surgical process.
    a. Provide factual information about cesarean birth and verify informed consent obtained.
    b. Explain expected procedures.
        (1) Anesthesia preparation
            (a) IV fluid
            (b) Patient takes nothing by mouth.
            (c) Nonparticulate antacid administered if general anesthesia planned, as indicated
        (2) Foley catheter insertion
        (3) Skin preparation
    c. Encourage questions and verbalization of situation.
3. Monitor and assess level of comfort.
    a. Assess level of pain every 2 to 4 hours, and more often if indicated.
    b. Use nonpharmacologic and pharmacologic methods of relief as appropriate.
    c. Assess effectiveness of pain management intervention.
4. Monitor I&O and hydration status.
5. Observe and document blood loss.
    a. Monitor hematocrit and hemoglobin levels to assess blood loss.
    b. Monitor vital signs for indications of blood loss and/or impending shock.
6. Monitor for signs and symptoms of infection, to include vital signs and skin assessment.
7. Monitor for and prevent maternal and neonatal infection.
    a. Maintain good sterile technique during:
        (1) Vaginal examinations
        (2) Catheterization
    b. Provide preoperative skin preparation.
    c. Administer antibiotics as indicated.

HEALTH EDUCATION

A. Intrapartum health education should provide the following:
1. Information about the process of labor
2. Clear explanations about the procedures (risk versus benefits) performed during the process of labor and delivery
3. Information about the available pain relief methods, including pharmacologic and nonpharmacologic methods
4. Methods of involvement and participation during the intrapartum period
5. Preoperative teaching for cesarean birth
6. Information about variables that may alter or influence a birth plan

CASE STUDY AND STUDY QUESTIONS

Mrs. V., a 24-year-old gravida 2, para 1 (G2, P1) woman is admitted to labor and delivery at 39 weeks' gestation. A vaginal examination indicates her cervix is 80% effaced and 3 cm dilated. The presenting vertex is at –1 station. The amniotic sac is not palpated, and Mrs. V. says she thinks it has ruptured.

1. What should the nurse ask about the amniotic sac?
    a. The time the membranes ruptured
    b. The color and amount of fluid, if observed
    c. The presence of back pain
    d. The presence of bloody show
2. During this early phase of labor, how often should the FHR be evaluated?
    a. Every 5 minutes
    b. At least every 15 minutes
    c. At least every 30 minutes
    d. At least every hour
3. To promote comfort, she is encouraged to assume certain positions while in labor and to avoid others. Which position should not be used during labor?
    a. Lateral position
    b. Squatting position
    c. Standing position
    d. Supine position
4. As her labor progresses to 5 cm, she becomes increasingly uncomfortable and requests an epidural anesthetic. After this is in place, the nurse should be particularly alert to:
    a. Possible hypertensive rebound
    b. Possible hypotensive episode
    c. Increased thirst
    d. Signs of water intoxication

When she is comfortable from the epidural, it is observed that her contractions have spaced out to a frequency of every 5 to 6 minutes and are only mild to palpation. An oxytocin infusion is started to augment her labor.

5. What would be the most likely classification for the dysfunctional labor?
    a. Pathologic retraction ring
    b. Hypertonic labor
    c. Protracted active phase
    d. Prolonged latent phase
6. All of the following are possible side effects of oxytocin administration except:
    a. Fetal hyperglycemia
    b. Fetal hyperbilirubinemia
    c. Uterine tachysystole
    d. Water intoxication

7. When should the oxytocin infusion be discontinued?
    a. When the client is comfortable with her contractions
    b. When signs of fetal distress are observed on the fetal monitor
    c. When the contractions are 3 minutes apart
    d. When the client is ready to push
8. On assessment, Mrs. V. is found to be completely dilated and effaced and at a +1 station. Which finding suggests transition to the second stage of labor?
    a. Decreased urge to push
    b. Decreased bloody show
    c. FHR accelerations
    d. Bulging of the perineum

Because of the epidural anesthetic, she is not able to push effectively. She pushes the infant to a +3 station but cannot bring it under the symphysis to effect delivery. It is decided to assist her by use of a vacuum extractor.

9. Prerequisites for use of the vacuum are:
    a. Membranes intact
    b. Presenting part engaged
    c. Cervix completely dilated
    d. Documentation of gestational age
    e. Empty bladder
       (1) a, b, c
       (2) b, d, e
       (3) b, c, e
       (4) c, e
10. After this procedure, the infant should be carefully examined for:
    a. Brachial plexus injury
    b. Respiratory distress
    c. Facial bruising
    d. Cephalhematoma
11. Which structures are involved when an episiotomy is performed?
    a. Vaginal mucosa
    b. Levator ani muscle
    c. Glans clitoris
    d. Cardinal ligament
    e. Fourchette
12. Which signs would indicate that delivery is imminent?
    a. The mother has the desire to defecate.
    b. An increase in frequency, duration, and intensity of uterine contractions
    c. The mother begins to bear down spontaneously with uterine contractions.
    d. Bulging of the perineum occurs.

e. There is an increase in the amount of blood-stained mucus flowing from the vagina.
  (1) d
  (2) a, c, d
  (3) b, d, e
  (4) b
  (5) All of the above
13. A nurse caring for a mother and infant in the fourth stage of labor would:
  a. Keep the mother warm and out of drafts.
  b. Massage the uterus every 15 minutes, or more often, if needed.
  c. Massage the uterus continuously.
  d. Check maternal vital signs every 15 minutes.
  e. Administer oxytocin as ordered.
    (1) a, b, d
    (2) b, d, e
    (3) c, d
    (4) b, d
    (5) a, d, e
14. Identify and match the most important risks of the various methods of obstetric anesthesia.
  a. General anesthesia
  b. Regional conduction anesthesia
  c. Paracervical block
    (1) Fetal bradycardia
    (2) Aspiration of stomach contents
    (3) Maternal hypotension
15. Match each term or phrase with the definition that best fits it.
  a. Enlargement of the external os to 10 cm in diameter
  b. Maximum shortening of the cervical canal
  c. A condition caused by failure of the uterine muscle to stay contracted after delivery
  d. Surgical incision of the perineum during the second stage of labor
  e. Settling of the infant's head into the brim of the pelvis
    (1) Uterine atony
    (2) Complete dilation
    (3) Lightening
    (4) Complete effacement
    (5) Episiotomy

ANSWERS TO STUDY QUESTIONS

1. a	5. c	9. 3	13. 2
2. c	6. a	10. d	14. (a) 2, (b) 3, (c) 1
3. d	7. b	11. a	15. (a) 2, (b) 4, (c) 1,
4. b	8. d	12. 5	(d) 5, (e) 3

BIBLIOGRAPHY

Callister, L. C., & Hobbins-Garbett, D. (2000). Cochrane pregnancy and childbirth database: Resource for evidence-based practice. *Journal of Obstetric, Gynecologic, and Neonatal Nursing, 29*(2), 123–128.

Clayworth, S. (2000). The nurse's role during oxytocin administration. *MCN The American Journal of Maternal Child Nursing, 25*(2), 80–85.

Davies, B. L., & Hodnett, E. (2002). Labor support: Nurses' self-efficacy and views about factors influencing implementation. *Journal of Obstetric, Gynecologic, and Neonatal Nursing, 31*(1), 48–56.

Faucher, M. A., & Brucker, M. C. (2000). Intrapartum pain: Pharmacologic management. *Journal of Obstetric, Gynecologic, and Neonatal Nursing, 29*(2), 169–180.

Gagnon, A. J., & Waghorn, K. (1999). One-to-one nurse labor support of nulliparous women stimulated with oxytocin. *Journal of Obstetric, Gynecologic, and Neonatal Nursing, 28*(4), 371–376.

Gale, J., Fothergill-Bourbonnais, F., & Chamberlain, M. (2001). Measuring nursing support during childbirth. *MCN The American Journal of Maternal Child Nursing, 26*(5), 264–271.

Gilder, K., Mayberry, L. J., Gennaro, S., & Clemmens, D. (2002). Maternal positioning in labor with epidural analgesia: Results from a multi-site survey. *AWHONN Lifelines, 6*(1), 40–45.

Kardong-Edgren, S. (2001). Using evidence-based practice to improve intrapartum care. *Journal of Obstetric, Gynecologic, and Neonatal Nursing, 30*(4), 371–375.

Lowdermilk, D. L., & Perry, S. E. (2007). *Maternity & women's health care* (9th ed.). St Louis: Mosby.

Mayberry, L. J., Wood, S. H., Strange, L. B., Lee, L., Heisler, D. R., & Neilsen-Smith, K. (2000). Managing second-stage labor: Exploring the variables during the second stage. *AWHONN Lifelines*, *3*(6), 28–34.

McCartney, P. R. (1998). Caring for women with epidurals using the "laboring down" technique. *MCN The American Journal of Maternal Child Nursing*, *23*(5), 274.

McRae-Bergeron, C. E., Andrews, C. M., & Lupe, P. J. (1998). The effect of epidural analgesia on the second stage of labor. *Journal of the American Association of Nurse Anesthetists*, *66*(2), 177–182.

Minato, J. F. (2000). Is it time to push? Examining rest in second-stage labor. *AWHONN Lifelines*, *4*(6), 20–23.

Murray, M. (1996). *Advanced fetal monitoring: Maternal/ fetal challenges for the caregiver*. Albuquerque, NM: Learning Resources International, Inc.

Olds, S., London, M., & Ladewig, M. (1996). *Maternal-newborn nursing: A family-centered approach* (5th ed.). Redwood City, CA: Addison-Wesley.

Perry, S., Hockenberry, M., Lowdermilk, D., & Wilson, D. (2010). *Maternal child nursing care* (4th ed.). St Louis: Mosby.

Ruchala, P. L., Metheny, N., Essenpreis, H., & Borcherding, K. (2002). Current practice in oxytocin dilution and fluid administration for inducting of labor. *Journal of Obstetric, Gynecologic, and Neonatal Nursing*, *31*(5), 545–550.

Searing, K. A. (2001). Induction vs. post-date pregnancies: Exploring the controversy of who's really at risk? *AWHONN Lifelines*, *5*(2), 44–48.

Simpson, K. R., & Knox, G. E. (2001). Fundal pressure during the second stage of labor: Clinical perspectives and risk management issues. *MCN The American Journal of Maternal Child Nursing*, *26*(2), 64–71.

Sprague, A., & Trèpanier, M. J. (1999). Charting in record time: Setting guidelines for documenting FHR enhances care for laboring women. *AWHONN Lifelines*, *3*(4), 35–40.

Wilson, C. (2000). The nurse's role in misoprostol induction: A proposed protocol. *Journal of Obstetric, Gynecologic, and Neonatal Nursing*, *29*(6), 574–583.

Yildirim, G. (2008). Effects of pushing techniques on mother and fetus: A randomized study. *The Cochrane Central Register of Controlled Trials*, *35*(1), 25–30.

Intrapartum Fetal Assessment

Keiko L. Torgersen

OBJECTIVES

1. Identify techniques and methods of fetal assessment.
2. Identify baseline (BL) features, including rate, rhythm, and variability.
3. Identify, interpret, and discuss probable causes of periodic patterns of variable, late, and early decelerations and accelerations.
4. Identify, interpret, and discuss probable causes of episodic patterns of variable and prolonged decelerations and accelerations.
5. Identify, interpret, and discuss probable causes of arrhythmic and dysrhythmic fetal heart rate (FHR) patterns.
6. Assess probable fetal status.
7. Discuss strategies to document FHR events accurately and completely for the patient record.
8. Reiterate the critical values of fetal blood gases and pH, and relate these to fetal outcome.
9. State appropriate physiologic interventions for deceleration patterns and altered variability in relation to fetal outcome.

INTRODUCTION

Intrapartum fetal assessment is essential to providing critical information regarding fetal well-being and the fetal response to labor. FHR and uterine activity (UA) data can be collected by nonelectronic or electronic methods. Regardless of the method chosen to assess fetal status, the nurse is accountable for knowing and responding to auditory and electronically obtained data (Curran & Torgersen, 2006; Harmon, 2009). Nonelectronic assessment uses auscultation and palpation to assess the FHR and UA. Electronic assessment or electronic fetal monitoring (EFM) uses electronic techniques, such as tocodynamometer, ultrasound, fetal scalp electrode (FSE), or intrauterine pressure catheter (IUPC) to monitor FHR and UA. The technique provides a permanent record that can be observed and discussed instantaneously or retrospectively by professional care providers. Events that cannot be heard or measured by auscultation, such as variability, are available through EFM. Therefore, EFM is another tool available to the care provider to easily provide information that would otherwise consume many hours of care and yield less complete data. The ability to monitor using short- or long-distance telemetry influences nursing care management and patient comfort and may aid consultation and transport practices. Although there are few confirmatory data that show that the use of EFM has significantly improved outcomes, it is still used in the labor and delivery arena (Simpson, 2008a). The reader should also be aware of research in progress to refine or augment interpretation of fetal status and probable outcomes. Such methods that may become available include oxicardiotocograph, computer analysis of fetal electrocardiogram, near-infrared spectroscopy for high-risk pregnancies, lactate measurement as a replacement for pH fetal blood sampling, ST-segment analysis, and artificial intelligence to assess all fetal data and clinical events. Today, proper interpretation of FHR patterns may be the best method to reliably determine fetal status.

In 1995-1996 the Eunice Kennedy Shriver National Institute of Child Health and Development (NICHD) pulled together EFM experts to discuss EFM terminology. In 1997 this group of experts published new EFM definitions that were based not only on clinical data, but also on laboratory, manufacturing, and published research. These definitions were "reaffirmed and updated at the 2008 meeting" (Lyndon, O'Brien-Abel, and Simpson, 2009, p. 104). One goal of these definitions was to allow the predictive value of fetal monitoring to be assessed more meaningfully. Another was to allow evidence-based clinical management of intrapartum fetal compromise (Macones, Hankins, Spong,

Hauth, & Moore, 2008). In December 2004, the Society of Obstetricians and Gynecologists in Canada (SOGC) adopted the NICHD nomenclature as their standard in the interpretation of FHR tracings. In May 2005, the American College of Obstetricians and Gynecologists (ACOG) and the Association for Women's Health, Obstetric, and Neonatal Nurses (AWHONN) followed suit and also adopted the NICHD nomenclature to be used in the interpretation of FHR tracings. The language used in this chapter is consistent with the most recently understood interpretations of EFM tracings in general use and is consistent with AWHONN's current Fetal Heart Monitoring Program, revised in 2006, 2008, and 2009 to coincide with the NICHD. The reader must recognize that although the NICHD committee agreed to the FHR that was definitely evident of a fetus that was well oxygenated and agreed to the FHR that definitely needed immediate intervention, there was not consensus on FHR patterns that fell between those two extremes (Parer & Ikeda, 2007).

Regardless of the practice setting, the terminology, or even the areas of non-consensus, the process of interpreting a FHR monitoring tracing includes (a) examining the tracing for trends of FHR and UA parameters and (b) answering the question, "At the present time, what is the likely status of this fetus?" (Curran & Torgersen, 2006; Lyndon et al, 2009; Macones et al, 2008). Nurses using EFM should know the capabilities, benefits, limitations, and troubleshooting of the assessment modalities used.

CLINICAL PRACTICE

Methods of FHR Assessment

A. **Nonelectronic methods of FHR assessment**
   1. Auscultation (Curran & Torgersen, 2006; Feinstein, Sprague, & Trepanier, 2008)
      a. Fetoscope
         (1) Detects FHR baseline (BL)
         (2) Detects FHR rhythm
         (3) Verifies presence of an irregular rhythm (i.e., dysrhythmia)
         (4) Detects increases and decreases from FHR BL
         (5) Clarifies halving or doubling on the EFM tracing
         (6) Differentiates fetal and maternal heart rates, eliminating errors related to fetal demise and EFM equipment errors
      b. Doptone
         (1) Detects FHR BL
         (2) Detects FHR rhythm
         (3) Detects increases and decreases from FHR BL
      c. Benefits (Feinstein et al, 2008)
         (1) Outcomes are comparable to those with EFM based on current randomized clinical trials (RCTs).
         (2) Lower cesarean birth rates have been associated more with auscultation than EFM in some RCTs.
         (3) Noninvasive
         (4) Promotes the "high-touch, low-tech" approach to care
         (5) Widespread application is possible.
         (6) Patients have increased freedom of movement and ambulation.
         (7) Allows for FHR assessment during water immersion
         (8) Equipment costs less than EFM.
      d. Limitations (Curran & Torgersen, 2006; Feinstein et al, 2008)
         (1) May limit ability to hear FHR resulting from maternal obesity, increased amniotic fluid volume, and maternal or fetal movement
         (2) Uterine tension disrupts assessment.
         (3) Certain FHR characteristics associated with EFM cannot be detected (e.g., variability, types of decelerations).
         (4) Some women may believe that auscultation is more intrusive or disruptive.
         (5) Is not automatically documented on paper; therefore, cannot go back and review tracing
         (6) Creates a potential need to increase or realign staff to meet 1:1 nurse/patient ratio
         (7) Requires education, practice, and skill in auditory assessment

e. Documentation
   (1) Numerical BL rate
   (2) Rhythm
   (3) Increases and decreases (abrupt or gradual) in BL rate
   (4) Timing related to contraction
   (5) Frequency for intermittent auscultation (IA) (ACOG, 2005; AWHONN, 2008; SOGC, 2007). NOTE: These guidelines may change as new data are presented. This information is a guideline and not suggestive of or dictating an exclusive procedure or plan of action. The individual patient and her clinical situation must always be considered to ensure an individualized plan of care.
       (a) AWHONN: auscultation and EFM
           [i] Low risk: every 15 to 30 minutes during active phase, every 5 to 15 minutes during second stage
           [ii] High risk: every 15 minutes during active phase, every 5 minutes during second stage
       (b) SOGC
           [i] Low risk: Latent phase. Regularly after rupture of the membranes or other clinically significant change. (NOTE: These patients are usually at home during this time. However, if they are in the hospital, this is one recommended way to perform IA. There is just not enough evidence to recommend optimal frequency time for latent phase of labor [SOGC, 2007]).
           [ii] Low risk: Auscultate every 15 to 30 minutes in active labor, every 15 minutes in second stage then every 5 minutes once pushing has started.
           [iii] EFM: every 15 minutes during the active phase of labor, at least every 5 minutes during the second stage of labor
2. Palpation
   a. Detects relative uterine resting tone (Harmon, 2009)
   b. Detects relative frequency, duration, and relative strength of uterine contractions (Harmon, 2009).
   c. Benefits (Curran & Torgersen, 2006; Harmon, 2009; Simpson, 2008a)
       (1) Noninvasive; allows for hands-on assessment or care of patient
       (2) Widely used; not limited by access to equipment
       (3) Patient has increased freedom of movement and ambulation
       (4) Allows for touch therapy that may be reassuring to some patients
       (5) Easy to use
       (6) Inexpensive when compared to additional devices such as an IUPC
       (7) Nurse-to-patient interaction is increased
   d. Limitations (Curran & Torgersen, 2006; Harmon, 2009; Simpson, 2008a)
       (1) Actual intrauterine pressures cannot be detected.
       (2) Certain conditions may limit ability to palpate contractions (e.g., maternal size, large amount of adipose tissue).
       (3) Subjective assessment; varies from examiner to examiner
       (4) No permanent record is provided.
       (5) Potential for the mother not to tolerate palpation during labor

B. **Electronic methods of FHR assessment**
   1. Doppler ultrasound for FHR assessment
      a. Detects FHR BL rate, accelerations, decelerations, and variability of the FHR
      b. Benefits (Curran & Torgersen, 2006; Harmon, 2009; Simpson, 2008a)
          (1) Is noninvasive; easy to use
          (2) Rupture of membranes or cervical dilation is not required.
          (3) Creates a permanent record via hard copy, electronic disks, or microfilm process
          (4) Can be observed from many locations when visual screens are used as a central display or as a bedside monitor to track all patients
          (5) Can use in the intrapartum and antepartum arena.
          (6) Can be used with telemetry allowing for monitoring during ambulation
      c. Limitations (Curran & Torgersen, 2006; Moffatt & Feinstein, 2003; Simpson, 2008a)
          (1) Signal transmissions may be influenced by maternal obesity, occiput posterior fetal position, anterior placenta, and fetal movement (e.g., weak, absent, or false signal).

(2) Maternal movement may be restricted.

(3) Maternal and fetal movement may interfere with continuous record.

(4) Artifact may artificially increase variability.

(5) Monitor may half- or double-count, especially if FHR tachycardia or bradycardia is present.

(6) May detect maternal aorta movement and trace as FHR, especially if fetus is small

(7) May detect maternal heart rate as FHR at random or in the event of fetal demise

(8) Artifact may artificially change variability.

2. FSE for FHR assessment

    a. Detects FHR BL rate, variability, accelerations, and decelerations

    b. Detects FHR dysrhythmias

    c. Benefits (Harmon, 2009; Simpson, 2008a)

        (1) Provides continuous detection of FHR

        (2) Accurately detects variability

        (3) Maternal position change does not alter assessment ability or tracing quality.

        (4) Provides a permanent record

        (5) Can be observed from many locations when visual screens are used

    d. Limitations (Harmon, 2009; Simpson, 2008a)

        (1) The procedure is invasive.

        (2) Rupture of membranes, cervical dilation, and accessible or appropriate fetal presenting part are required.

        (3) Moist environment is required for detection of FHR.

        (4) Potential small risk of infection, fetal hemorrhage, or fetal injury is presented.

        (5) May not be accurate when fetal demise occurs; maternal heart rate may be detected and traced.

        (6) Fetal dysrhythmias may not be evident if logic or electrocardiogram (ECG) button is turned on or engaged.

        (7) Electronic interference and artifact may occur.

3. Tocodynamometer (tocotransducer) for UA assessment

    a. Detects relative uterine resting tone

    b. Detects relative frequency and duration of uterine contractions

    c. Benefits (Curran & Torgersen, 2006; Harmon, 2009; Simpson, 2008a)

        (1) Is noninvasive

        (2) Is easily placed

        (3) Ruptured membranes or cervical dilation is not required.

        (4) Creates a tracing via hard copy, electronic disks, or microfilm process for future assessment and for permanent medical record

        (5) Can be used in antepartum and intrapartum arena

        (6) Can be used with telemetry providing for monitoring during ambulation

    d. Limitations (Curran & Torgersen, 2006; Harmon, 2009; Simpson, 2008a)

        (1) Subjective assessment

        (2) Cannot detect uterine contraction intensity and resting tone

        (3) May be unable to accurately detect exact uterine contraction frequency and duration in some conditions (e.g., maternal obesity or preterm labor)

        (4) Location sensitive; placement may lead to false information.

        (5) Sensitive to maternal or fetal motion that may be superimposed on the waveform

        (6) Transducer presence or position may be uncomfortable for mother.

        (7) Maternal movement and ambulation during labor may be limited.

        (8) May need frequent readjustments secondary to maternal and fetal movement.

4. IUPC for UA assessment

    a. Detects actual uterine resting tone and frequency, duration, and strength of uterine contractions

    b. Access for amniotic fluid testing (e.g., amniotic fluid sampling)

    c. Allows for amnioinfusion

    d. Benefits (Curran & Torgersen, 2006; Harmon, 2009; Simpson, 2008a)

        (1) Objective; accurate assessment of uterine contraction frequency, duration, intensity, and resting tone

        (2) Correlation of timing of FHR changes with UA is more accurate.

(3) Provides a tracing via hard copy, electronic disks, or microfilm process for future assessment and for permanent medical record

(4) Provides means for aspiration of amniotic fluid to assess for chorioamnionitis

(5) Provides means for amnioinfusion as intervention for oligohydramnios or thick meconium-stained amniotic fluid

(6) Solid-tipped IUPC is easily zeroed/rezeroed to atmospheric pressure.

(7) Solid-tipped IUPC design avoids pressure artifacts that may be caused by a catheter containing air, that becomes kinked, or becomes lodged against the uterine wall, as may occur with fluid-filled IUPC.

(8) Can be used to calculate Montevideo units during oxytocin infusion

(9) Assists in interpretation of late versus variable decelerations

e. Limitations (Curran & Torgersen, 2006; Moffatt & Feinstein, 2003; Simpson, 2008a)

(1) General

(a) Rupture of membranes (ROM) or adequate cervical dilation required.

(b) An invasive procedure

(c) Maternal ambulation may be limited during labor.

(d) Increased risk of uterine perforation (rupture), placental abruption or perforation, infection, or umbilical cord prolapse.

(e) IUPC reading may be different between fluid-filled and sensor-tipped catheters.

(f) May be contraindicated with infections in which ROM is discouraged to prevent maternal-fetal transmission (e.g., group B-streptococci, genital herpes, human immunodeficiency virus [HIV]).

(g) May be contraindicated in presence of vaginal bleeding

(2) Fluid-filled IUPC

(a) Catheter tip may become wedged against uterine wall or fetal part; might prevent production of pressure data or produce distorted or truncated waveform.

(b) Catheter tip may affect pressures, especially as related to external pressure transducer.

(c) Catheter may become obstructed with meconium, vernix, or blood.

(d) Pressure readings may be lower than solid-tipped IUPC transducer.

(e) Air may dissipate or pass through balloon at tip; may change pressure waveform or provide inaccurate pressure data (solid-tipped IUPC with pressure balloon).

(3) Solid-tipped IUPC

(a) Pressure readings, including uterine resting tone, may be higher than fluid- or air-filled IUPCs.

(b) Larger tip may require further dilation for insertion when compared to fluid- or air-filled IUPCs.

(c) Possibility of extraovular placement (between chorionic membrane and endometrial lining)

FETAL FACTORS INFLUENCING THE FHR

A. **Parasympathetic nervous system**
1. Slows FHR and variability
2. Provides variability; greatest influence on short-term variability (STV)
3. Is of vagal origin
4. Increases with increasing gestational age
5. Effect on FHR may be exaggerated during hypoxemia.
6. Blocking (e.g., with atropine) produces increased FHR and loss of variability

B. **Sympathetic nervous system**
1. Increases FHR and cardiac output
2. Some influence on long-term variability (LTV) in conjunction with parasympathetic nervous system.
3. Influences epinephrine and norepinephrine (epinephrine secreted in significantly smaller amounts than norepinephrine)
4. Effect on FHR may be stimulated during hypoxemia.
5. Blocking the sympathetic system, as with maternal medication, produces decrease in the BL FHR.

C. **Baroreceptors**
   1. Located in carotid artery and aortic arch
   2. Respond rapidly to fetal blood pressure (BP) changes; transfer information to sympathetic and parasympathetic systems
   3. An increase in fetal BP produces decrease in the FHR, which decreases fetal cardiac output and BP
   4. Decreases in fetal BP result in sympathetic stimulation to increase FHR.
D. **Chemoreceptors** (Nageotte & Gilstrap, 2009; O'Brien-Abel, 2009; Simpson, 2008a)
   1. Located in aortic arch and carotid artery
   2. Consists of peripheral receptors in the central nervous system (CNS)
   3. Responds to fetal oxygen or carbon dioxide changes and in pH levels of blood and cerebrospinal fluid; transfers information to sympathetic and parasympathetic nervous systems
   4. Least-understood factor influencing FHR
   5. Stimulation caused by mild increases in carbon dioxide or mild decreases in oxygen produces an increase in fetal BP and FHR; more severe changes can produce bradycardia.
E. **CNS**
   1. Responsible for variations in FHR and variability in response to fetal sleep state and body movements; in fetal sleep cycles of 20 to 40 minutes, variability and reactivity decrease
   2. In alert states, FHR variability and reactivity increase.
   3. Integrative center for central and peripheral neural influences that produces variability and net increase or decrease in BL FHR
F. **Hormonal influences**
   1. Catecholamines facilitate hemodynamic changes in response to hypoxemia and adaptational changes in neonate at birth (Lagercrantz & Slotkin, 1986; Parer, 1976, 1999).
   2. Epinephrine increases FHR and blood flow to skeletal muscle.
   3. Norepinephrine
      a. Associated with initial increase in FHR (Lagercrantz & Slotkin, 1986; Parer, 1999)
      b. Increases blood flow to vital organs and away from nonvital organs
      c. Hemodynamic changes elevate BP and may cause parasympathetic response resulting in decreased FHR (norepinephrine cannot overcome this parasympathetic response).
      d. Secreted in greater amounts than found in resting adult.
   4. Vasopressin
      a. Secreted by pituitary; increases during hypoxemia and hemorrhage
      b. Helps regulate BP
      c. Produces rise in BP by increasing peripheral vascular resistance and decreasing FHR
      d. Decreases blood flow to nonvital organs
   5. Renin-angiotension system
      a. Renin secreted by kidneys; increases in response to hemorrhage
      b. Angiotension II
         (1) Secreted by kidneys; increases in response to hemorrhage and hypovolemia.
         (2) Causes vasoconstriction of peripheral vascular bed resulting in maintenance of systemic arterial BP and umbilical-placental blood flow.
         (3) Increased level produces marked increase in BP with initial decrease in FHR followed by increase to higher than previous FHR; produces increased cardiac output and blood flow to heart.
         (4) Decreases renal blood flow

BASELINE CHARACTERISTICS

Baseline Fetal Heart Rate

The FHR BL is assessed by determining the mean FHR rounded to increments of 5 beats per minute (bpm) during a 10-minute window. Additionally, there needs to be 2 minutes of interpretable data to determine FHR BL. The 2 minutes do not necessarily have to be contiguous—they may be 2 consecutive minutes or two 1-minute segments (Curran & Torgersen, 2006; Macones et al, 2008; Nageotte & Gilstrap, 2009; Simpson, 2008a; Tucker, Miller, & Miller, 2009). Normal FHR BL ranges from 110 to 160 bpm; it is assessed when mother has no uterine contraction and excludes accelerations, decelerations, and periods of marked variability (>25 bpm). If a FHR BL cannot be determined (i.e., not enough data to interpret, marked variability present so cannot determine BL, sinusoidal pattern, etc.), the BL is interpreted as "indeterminate" (Figure 12-1).

A. Tachycardia (FHR >160 bpm for ≥10 minutes)

    1. History: possible causes (Curran & Torgersen, 2006; Nageotte & Gilstrap, 2009; Simpson, 2008a; Tucker et al, 2009)

        a. Maternal causes

           (1) Fever

           (2) Infection

           (3) Dehydration

           (4) Hyperthermia

           (5) Hyperthyroidism

           (6) Endogenous adrenaline or anxiety

           (7) Medication or drug response

               (a) Parasympathetics (Hydroxyzine [Visteril/Atarax], atropine, and phenothiazines)

               (b) Ketamine

               (c) Beta-sympathomimetic drugs (Terbutaline; Ritodrine)

               (d) Sympathomimetic bronchodilators used in asthma patients (albuterol)

               (e) Epinephrine

               (f) Selected positive inotropes (e.g., dobutamine, positive chronotropic drugs)

               (g) Over-the-counter medications (e.g., decongestants, appetite suppressants, stimulants or caffeine)

           (8) Illicit drugs (cocaine; methamphetamines)

           (9) Anemia

           (10) Nicotine, if inhaled (if inhaled by smoking, may increase the FHR; if absorbed through nicotine patch, may decrease FHR) (Lyndon et al, 2009; Muller, Antunes, Behle, Teixeira, & Zielinsky, 2002; Oncken et al, 1997; Oncken, Kranzler, O'Malley, Gendreau, & Campbell, 2002)

        b. Fetal causes (Lyndon et al, 2009; Simpson, 2008a)

           (1) Infection

           (2) Activity or stimulation

           (3) Compensatory effort following acute hypoxemia

           (4) Chronic hypoxemia

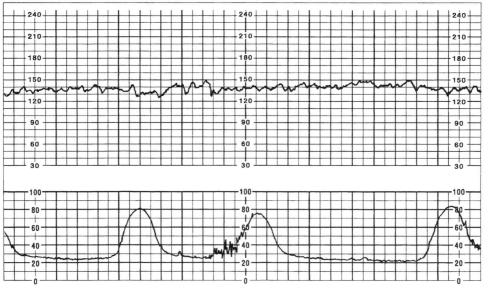

FIGURE 12-1 ■ Normal baseline FHR and moderate variability.

(5) Fetal hyperthyroidism

(6) Fetal tachyarrhythmias (e.g., SVT, atrial fibrillation, atrial flutter)

(7) Prematurity

(8) Congenital abnormalities

(9) Cardiac abnormalities or heart failure

(10) Anemia

2. Physical findings (Figure 12-2)

   a. Persistent FHR greater than 160 bpm for duration of a minimum of 10 minutes with no maximum (days or weeks are possible); if persists at greater than 200 to 220 bpm for extended period, can result in fetal hydrops or fetal demise (Curran & Torgersen, 2006; Lyndon et al, 2009).

   b. Decreased variability common as rate increases, especially at rates greater than 180 bpm (Barnes, 2009; Torgersen, 2003)

   c. Tachyarrhythmias (FHR >240 bpm, i.e., SVT) and ventricular arrhythmias more frequent

   d. Tachycardia with moderate variability and in the absence of FHR decelerations rarely denotes fetal acidemia (Krebs, Petres, Dunn, Jordaan, & Segreti, 1979; Nageotte & Gilstrap, 2009).

3. Related physiology

   a. Increased sympathetic tone

   b. Decreased parasympathetic tone

   c. Persistently high rate associated with fetal hydrops or fetal demise (e.g., SVT, atrial flutter, atrial fibrillation)

4. Interventions—tachycardia

   a. Monitor maternal vital signs, specifically temperature and pulse.

   b. Increase or initiate hydration with intravenous fluids as needed.

   c. Initiate interventions to decrease maternal temperature, if elevated (e.g., antipyretics).

   d. Assess for possible tachyarrhythmias or dysrhythmias; administer appropriate medications to lower FHR (e.g., cardiac agents for SVT, tocolytic agents or discontinuation of uterine-stimulating agents to enhance placental blood flow).

   e. Perform scalp stimulation for tachyarrhythmias or dysrhythmias.

      (1) Vagal stimulation may lower tachycardic FHR.

      (2) FHR accelerations following scalp stimulation usually rule out an acidotic fetus.

      (3) Fetal scalp stimulation is not appropriate in the presence of decelerations or bradycardia.

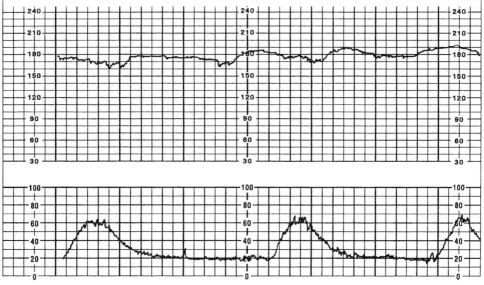

FIGURE 12-2 ■ Tachycardia resulting from maternal fever.

    f. Reduce anxiety, offer explanations, provide comfort measures, and assist with breathing and relaxation techniques (Simpson, 2009).

    g. Change or maintain maternal position that optimizes uteroplacental perfusion (e.g., side lying, walking).

    h. Administer oxygen (10 to 12 L/min via rebreather face mask) as needed.

    i. Assess for use of illicit and legal drugs and alcohol.

    j. If auscultating, intervene as needed and consider application of EFM to further assess FHR, variability, and periodic and episodic changes.

B. **Bradycardia (FHR <110 bpm for ≥10 minutes)** (Figure 12-3) (Curran & Torgersen, 2006; Nageotte & Gilstrap, 2009; Simpson, 2008a; Tucker et al, 2009)

    1. History: possible causes

        a. Maternal causes

            (1) Mother lying in supine position

            (2) Hypotension

        b. Anesthetic agents (e.g., epidural, spinal, pudendal, paracervical)

        c. Adrenergic-receptor blocking agents (e.g., propranolol)

        d. Connective tissue disease (e.g., systemic lupus erythematosus) (Hohn & Stanton, 2002; Tucker et al, 2009)

        e. Prolonged maternal hypoglycemia

        f. Conditions that cause acute maternal cardiopulmonary compromise (e.g., pulmonary embolus, anaphylactoid syndrome of pregnancy [formally amniotic fluid embolism], trauma, uterine rupture)

        g. Fetal causes

            (1) Mature parasympathetic nervous system

            (2) Acute hypoxemia

            (3) Hypothermia

            (4) Umbilical cord occlusion

            (5) Congenital complete heart block (CCHB)

            (6) Cardiac structural defect (resulting from maternal cytomegalovirus infection)

            (7) Sjögren's antibodies

            (8) Excessive parasympathetic nervous system tone (i.e., vagal stimulation) resulting from chronic head compression in a vertex presentation, occiput posterior, or transverse position; FHR usually does not decrease to less than 90 to 100 bpm in this situation (Lyndon et al, 2009; Simpson, 2008a)

            (9) Late or profound hypoxemia

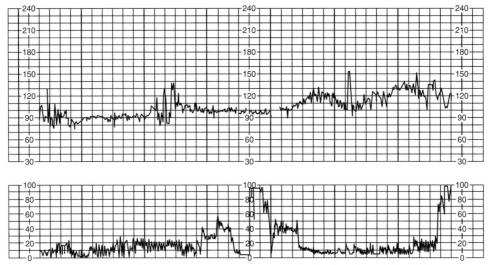

FIGURE 12-3 ■ Bradycardia. (From Lyndon A, Ali L., Barnes J., Cypher R. [2009]. *Fetal heart monitoring: Principles and practices* [4th ed.]. Dubuque, IA: Kendall-Hunt Publications.)

2. Physical findings
   a. FHR less than 110 bpm for duration of 10 minutes
   b. Bradycardia accompanied by adequate variability may be normal (fetal dependent).
   c. Prolonged deceleration resulting in change in FHR BL to bradycardia can be due to a sudden drop in oxygenation (as occurs with abruptio placentae), a decrease or occlusion in umbilical blood flow (cord prolapse or uterine rupture), or a decrease in uterine blood flow (significant maternal hypotension). This type of pattern can be indicative of fetal hypoxemia and may require immediate intervention (Nageotte & Gilstrap, 2009).
   d. Moderate variability less likely if FHR persists at rate less than 90 bpm for more than 10 minutes; if variability and accelerations present, is considered benign or reassuring and not associated with acidemia (Freeman, Garite, & Nageotte, 2003; Simpson, 2008a).
   e. Bradycardia accompanied by loss of variability and late decelerations may indicate current or impending fetal hypoxia (NICHD, 1997).
3. Related physiology
   a. Excessive parasympathetic nervous system tone
   b. Rate of approximately 60 to 70 bpm in second trimester and 50 to 60 bpm at term without variability may indicate CCHB (Eronen, Heikkila, & Teramo, 2001).
   c. Bradycardia may be related to maternal hypotension secondary to supine hypotension, hypovolemia, vasodilation following epidural anesthesia, or maternal catecholamine production.
   d. The lower the FHR, the lower the fetal cardiac output (Curran & Torgersen, 2006; Lyndon et al, 2009; Nageotte & Gilstrap, 2009).
   e. Bradycardia less than 60 bpm or associated with decreased variability requires immediate attention and collaborative management (Curran & Torgersen, 2006; Lyndon et al, 2009; Nageotte & Gilstrap, 2009).
   f. Rate must be differentiated from maternal rate (use real-time ultrasound or palpate maternal apical pulse and compare to FHR).
   g. Rate must be differentiated from prolonged deceleration (prolonged deceleration duration is more than 2 minutes but less than 10 minutes; if deceleration is more than 10 minutes, bradycardia occurs).
4. Interventions—bradycardia
   a. Assess maternal vital signs, specifically BP.
   b. Validate FHR versus maternal HR.
   c. Evaluate fetal movement.
   d. Perform vaginal examination for possible cord prolapse; if prolapse evident, elevate fetal presenting part off of cord.
   e. NOTE: Scalp stimulation has been noted as an intervention for bradycardia. In a nonreassuring FHR (bradycardia or prolonged decelerations without variability or accelerations), scalp stimulation is not recommended. Scalp stimulation in this instance will elicit a vagal response that overrides the sympathetic response and results in a further drop in the FHR (Curran & Torgersen, 2006; Harvey, 1987; Tucker et al, 2009).
   f. Accurately document FHR findings and interventions.

Variability

Variability is defined as "the fluctuations in the FHR over time" and "is present when there are irregular fluctuations in the baseline FHR (Lyndon et al, 2009, p. 109)."These fluctuations are irregular in amplitude and frequency and are visually quantitated as the amplitude of the peak-to-trough in beats per minute" (Curran & Torgersen, 2006, p. 156). The two branches of the autonomic nervous system (parasympathetic and sympathetic) have opposite effects on the FHR. The parasympathetic nervous system slows the FHR, and the sympathetic nervous system speeds the FHR. This continual push-and-pull effect produces the moment-to-moment change in the FHR that is called variability. Variability is interpreted as a single combined term (NICHD, 1997); however, it is important to understand the different types of variability, specifically LTV and STV. These two types provide the visual tracing that is recorded on the EFM.

A. **History of variability**
   1. Described as normal irregularity of cardiac rhythm
   2. Influenced by fetal oxygenation status, cardiac output regulation, fetal behavior during fetal sleep-wake states, humoral regulation, and drug effects (Freeman et al, 2003; Martin, 1982;

Parer, 1997). Also influenced by alcohol and illicit drugs that can cause fetal neurologic damage thus affecting variability: morphine (Kopecky et al, 2000), methadone (Anyaegbunam, Tran, Jadali, Randolph, & Mikhail, 1997), anomalies, and previous insults damaging the fetal brain (Wadhwa, Sandman, & Garite, 2001)

3. Impulse transmission to the FHR is influenced by CNS oxygenation.
4. Adequate oxygenation and a mature and functioning autonomic nervous system contribute to production of variability (Lyndon et al, 2009).
5. Minimal variability may be associated with preterm fetus (less than 28 to 32 weeks' gestation), alteration in the function of the nervous system, inadequate oxygenation, or any combination (Lyndon et al, 2009).
6. Minimal variability without associated decelerations is almost always unrelated to fetal acidemia (Parer & Livingston, 1990).
7. Moderate variability, even in the presence of decelerations, has a 98% association with an umbilical pH >7.15 or an Apgar score ≥7 at 5 minutes (Parer, King, Flanders, Fox, & Kilpatrick, 2006).
8. NICHD nomenclature describes and communicates variability as one unit (versus LTV and STV); however, it is still important to understand the physiology of LTV and STV.
   a. FHR BL variability is determined in a 10-minute window, excluding accelerations and decelerations. Variability is described in four categories (Macones et al, 2008):
      (1) Absent variability: amplitude range undetectable (Figure 12-4)
      (2) Minimal variability: amplitude range > undetectable and ≤5 bpm (Figure 12-5)
      (3) Moderate variability: amplitude range 6 to 25 bpm (see Figure 12-1)
      (4) Marked variability: amplitude range >25 bpm (Figure 12-6)

B. Sinusoidal pattern
1. Defined as "having a visually apparent, smooth, sine wave-line undulating pattern in FHR baseline with a cycle frequency of three to five per minute that persist for ≥20 minutes" (Macones et al, 2008, p. 662)
2. In the presence of a true sinusoidal pattern the BL rate is usually within 110 to 160 bpm, frequency of two to five cycles, and amplitude undulations 5 to 15 bpm above and below the baseline (Simpson, 2008b).
3. A sinusoidal-like pattern can be seen following the administration of some drugs (i.e., Stadol, Fentanyl) and will resolve once the drug has been excreted (Curran & Torgersen, 2006; Simpson, 2008b). However, this pattern differs from the true sinusoidal pattern in that there are fewer and less uniform oscillations, periods of moderate variability and the presence of acceleration patterns (Curran & Torgersen, 2006; Simpson, 2008b) (Figure 12-7).
4. Sinusoidal characteristics (Figure 12-8)

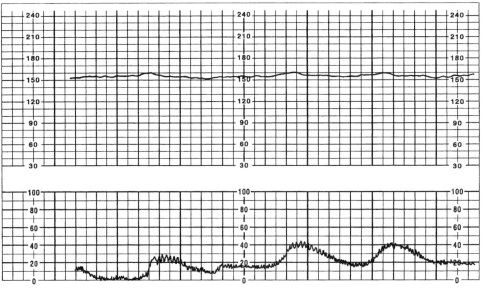

FIGURE 12-4 ■ Absent variability.

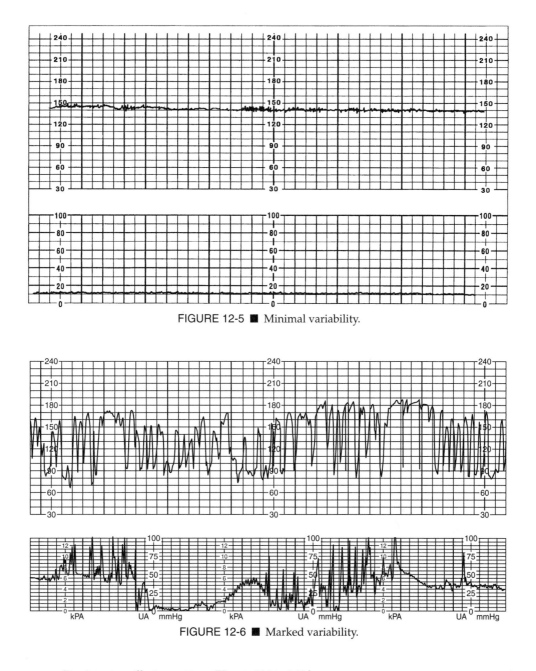

FIGURE 12-5 ■ Minimal variability.

FIGURE 12-6 ■ Marked variability.

    a. Persistent oscillating pattern; BL rate 110 to 160 bpm
    b. Amplitude of undulations usually 5 to 15 bpm greater than and less than BL rate
    c. Frequency of undulation usually two to five cycles per minute
    d. Absent variability
    e. No accelerations present even in response to fetal stimulation or fetal movement
    f. Associated with:
        (1) Severe fetal anemia (Rh isoimmunization; abruptio placentae; fetal-maternal hemorrhage; severe fetal acidosis) (Nageotte & Gilstrap, 2009; Simpson, 2008b; Tucker et al, 2009)
        (2) Unknown causes
  5. Interventions
    a. Kleihauer-Betke test
    b. Expeditious delivery
    c. Intrauterine blood transfusion to fetus via cordocentesis (requires tertiary care facility and skilled staff)

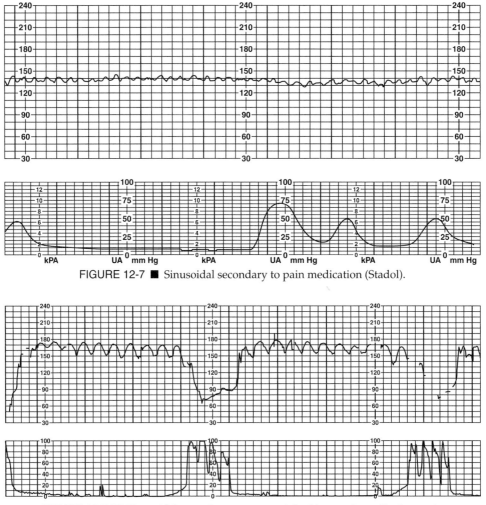

FIGURE 12-7 ■ Sinusoidal secondary to pain medication (Stadol).

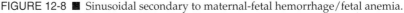

FIGURE 12-8 ■ Sinusoidal secondary to maternal-fetal hemorrhage/fetal anemia.

Fetal Heart Rate Patterns

Fetal heart rate patterns are described as periodic (associated with uterine contractions) or episodic (not associated with uterine contractions) (Macones et al, 2008). Periodic and episodic patterns can be distinguished by the waveform, whether abrupt or gradual, and are described by the NICHD as such. Additionally, the FHR patterns can also be described as recurrent, repetitive or intermittent (Curran & Torgersen, 2006; Macones et al, 2008). These terms are defined below:

1. Gradual: From the onset to the nadir (lowest part of the deceleration) is ≥30 seconds in duration.
2. Abrupt: From the onset to the peak or nadir is <30 seconds in duration.
3. Recurrent: If FHR patterns (periodic or episodic) occur with >50% of the uterine contractions in any 20-minute segment.
4. Repetitive: Periodic or episodic FHR patterns that occur with every uterine contraction (i.e., 100% of time) (Curran & Torgersen, 2006; NICHD, 1997).
5. Intermittent: Periodic or episodic FHR patterns that occur with <50% of the uterine contractions (Curran & Torgersen, 2006; Macones et al, 2008; NICHD, 1997).

PERIODIC PATTERNS

Periodic patterns are FHR patterns that have a direct relation to uterine contractions. Periodic patterns include accelerations and early, variable, and late decelerations.

Accelerations

A. Probable causes
   1. Repetitive fetal stimulation or movement
   2. Direct sympathetic stimulation
   3. Mild umbilical cord compression stimulating fetal compensatory acceleration
B. Physical findings (Figure 12-9)
   1. Pattern characteristics (Curran & Torgersen, 2006; Macones et al, 2008; NICHD, 1997; Parer & Ikeda, 2007; Simpson, 2008b)
      a. Term fetus: visually abrupt FHR increase defined as from the onset of acceleration to the peak of the acceleration in <30 seconds; the peak must be ≥15 beats above the BL FHR and must last a minimum of ≥15 seconds from onset to return
      b. Preterm fetus <32 weeks' gestation: visually abrupt (from onset to peak in <30 seconds) FHR increase from the onset of acceleration to the peak of the acceleration in <30 seconds; the peak acceleration defined as ≥10 beats above the BL FHR for a duration of ≥10 seconds
      c. Prolonged acceleration: acceleration (as described above) lasting ≥2 minutes but <10 minutes
      d. Variability is usually present.
      e. Accelerations are considered to be benign patterns, indicate fetal well-being (well oxygenated), and require no interventions.
      f. Shoulders: physiologic increase in the FHR before or after a variable deceleration secondary to an occlusion of the umbilical vein; increase in rate generally <20 bpm and lasting <20 seconds (Curran & Torgersen, 2006; Lyndon et al, 2009).
      g. Overshoot: smooth, blunt, and prolonged acceleration following a late or variable deceleration; lasts more than 60 to 120 seconds with increase in rate 10 to 20 bpm; has no variability, no abruptness, and returns to BL FHR gradually; if repetitive with absent variability may require fetal intrauterine resuscitation (Curran & Torgersen, 2006; Lyndon et al, 2009)
   2. Clinical findings
      a. When associated with fetal activity or stimuli that meet established criteria, accelerations are called reactivity.
         (1) Observed in an active fetus or a fetus stimulated tactilely, by fetal scalp stimulation, or by vibroacoustic stimulation
         (2) Fetal reactivity is expected by 28 to 30 weeks' gestation; once fetus demonstrates reactivity, should continue through gestation.
      b. When associated with variable decelerations, they are called shoulders or overshoots.

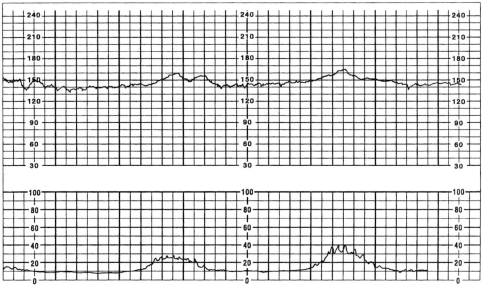

FIGURE 12-9 ■ Acceleration with UC (periodic).

Variable Decelerations

A. Probable causes
1. Decreased umbilical cord perfusion
2. Umbilical cord compression
3. Baroreceptor stimulation with vagal response; depth of deceleration depends on fetal baroreceptor stimulation; depth is reflex mediated and not related to degree of fetal hypoxia or fetal acid-base status (Curran & Torgersen, 2006; Freeman et al, 2003; Lyndon et al, 2009)
4. Hypoxia and hypercarbic states
5. Associated with clinical observation of nuchal cord, body cord entanglement, prolapsed cord, short cord, decreased amniotic fluid, second-stage descent of fetus, true knot of cord, and decreased Wharton's jelly
6. Acceleration that precedes or follows deceleration is a physiologic compensatory response to hypoxemia (oxygen deprivation).

B. Physical findings
1. Pattern characteristics (Curran & Torgersen, 2006; Macones et al, 2008; NICHD, 1997; Parer & Ikeda, 2007; Simpson, 2008b)
   a. Visually apparent abrupt (from onset to beginning of nadir <30 seconds) decrease in the FHR below the baseline
   b. Decrease in FHR is ≥15 bpm, lasting ≥15 seconds, and <2 minutes.
   c. When periodic (associated with uterine contractions), onset, depth, and duration will vary with successive uterine contractions (Macones et al, 2008; NICHD, 1997) (Figures 12-10 and 12-11).
   d. Shoulders and overshoots may be present with variable decelerations (see definition as previously noted).

C. Interventions
1. Change maternal position to left or right lateral, upright, hands and knees, or knee-chest, whichever position relieves the FHR pattern.
   a. Helps to relieve pressure on umbilical cord
   b. Avoids supine hypotension and maximizes uteroplacental and umbilical blood flow
2. Administer oxygen if variable decelerations are recurrent, BL FHR is increasing or decreasing, and variability is absent, or if overshoots are present; oxygen administered via rebreather face mask at 10 to 12 L/min.
3. Perform vaginal examination to assess for prolapsed cord or imminent delivery; if prolapsed cord, elevate fetal presenting part off of umbilical cord.

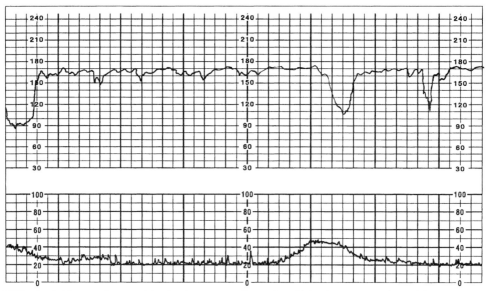

FIGURE 12-10 ■ Periodic variable decelerations tolerated well by fetus as evidenced by recovery and moderate variability.

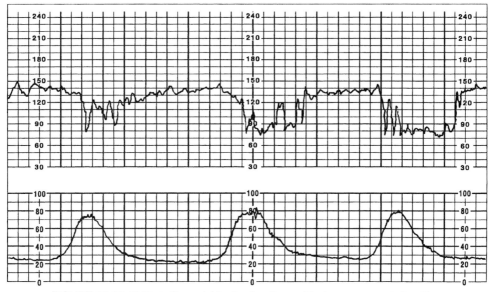

FIGURE 12-11 ■ Periodic variable deceleration, with slow recovery to baseline.

4. Perform amnioinfusion according to institutional protocol.
    a. Increases cushion effect for the umbilical cord
    b. Relieves or lessens variable decelerations when effective
    c. Dilutes thick, particulate meconium, if it is present
    d. Sample protocol (also refer to own institutional guidelines)
        (1) Most protocols recommend initial bolus of 800 mL; follow bolus with maintenance infusion to replace lost amniotic fluid (ACOG, 2005; Simpson, 2009).
        (2) Some protocols recommend titration of fluid bolus at 15 to 20 mL/min until deceleration resolves, followed by an additional 250 mL.
        (3) Warming of solution is not required for full-term fetuses; appropriate for preterm or growth-restricted fetuses; keep temperature between 34° and 37° C (93° and 96° F) (Simpson, 2009).
        (4) Infusion may be discontinued when variables are abolished, the meconium is diluted, 800 mL is infused, or the amniotic fluid index (AFI) is used to determine infusion amounts.
        (5) Maintenance fluid is 120 to 180 mL/hr (Simpson, 2009).
        (6) Amnioinfusion should reach therapeutic result or increase the AFI in approximately 30 minutes (ACOG, 2005; Snell, 1993).
        (7) It is important to monitor maternal vital signs, FHR and variability, resolution of decelerations, and uterine tone.
    e. Discontinue oxytocin or other uterotonics; obtain order for and administer tocolytics (terbutaline) if UA continues.
    f. Assess for accelerations.
    g. Perform scalp stimulation if baseline is normal range and decelerations are not recurrent. Do not perform scalp stimulation during deceleration.
    h. Instruct mother to alter her breathing or pushing technique.
    i. Communicate findings to primary care provider, and document events on the patient's record.
        (1) Note trends and recurrency of deceleration pattern.
        (2) Recovery time: If slow, note the recovery time in seconds.
        (3) Note BL rate and variability.
        (4) Document in trends; use hospital-approved abbreviations (see examples in Box 12-1).
    j. Plan for expedited delivery if unresolved despite interventions.
    k. If auscultating and abrupt decreases in the FHR are heard, change maternal position and reauscultate; consider placing EFM to assess FHR variability and possible deceleration pattern.

■ BOX 12-1
■ **ABBREVIATIONS FOR CHARTING ELECTRONIC FETAL MONITORING**

EFM	Electronic fetal monitoring
FHM	Fetal heart monitoring
FM	Fetal movement
FMC	Fetal movement counting
FHR	Fetal heart rate or rhythm
US	Ultrasonography (external)
TOCO	Tocodynamometer (external)
SE	Spiral electrode (internal)
FSE	Fetal spiral electrode (internal)
IUPC	Intrauterine pressure catheter (internal)
UC	Uterine contraction
UA	Uterine activity
RT	Resting tone
Palp	Palpated/via palpation
Mod	Moderate
MVU	Montevideo units
BL	Baseline (refers to FHR and sometimes to baseline tonus)
bpm	Beats per minute
Var	Variability absent
Var min	Variability minimal
Var +/mod	Variability moderate
Var mark	Variability marked
Late decel	Late deceleration pattern
Early decel	Early deceleration pattern
Var decel	Variable deceleration pattern
Prolonged decel	Deceleration more than 2 minutes but less than 10 minutes

Late Decelerations

A. **Probable causes**
   1. Fetal response to transient alterations in oxygen transport produced or attenuated by uterine contractions (Lyndon et al, 2009), leading to decreased uteroplacental blood flow related to one of the following:
      a. Uteroplacental insufficiency or diminished placental function that alters maternal-fetal gas exchange; associated with decreased variability, fetal myocardial depression, and fetal acidosis
         (1) Hypertension as a result of gestational or chronic hypertension; medications (illicit drugs such as amphetamines or cocaine)
         (2) Placental changes such as postmaturity; premature aging (calcification or necrosis); old or new abruptio placentae sites, placenta previa; or placental malformation
         (3) Uterine tachysystole or hypertonus with or without oxytocin, misoprostol, or prostaglandin administration
         (4) Increased association with other high-risk pregnancy conditions such as chronic maternal diseases (diabetes and collagen disease); maternal smoking; poor maternal nutrition; multiple gestation (usually monochorionic); or maternal anemia
         (5) Cardiopulmonary disease that may decrease maternal arterial hemoglobin or oxygen saturation

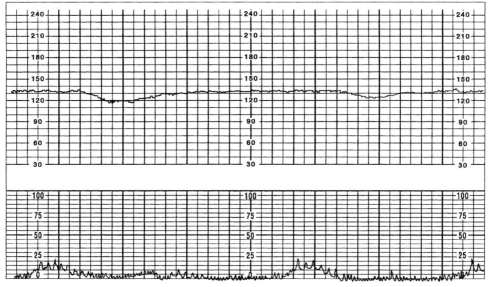

FIGURE 12-12 ■ Late decelerations with external ultrasound, ↓ minimal variability.

    b. Impeded maternal blood flow to placenta or diminished maternal arterial oxygen
saturation; associated with normal pH and variability for at least the first 30 minutes of
blood flow impedance; also called reflex late decelerations (Curran & Torgersen, 2006;
Nageotte & Gilstrap, 2009) resulting from:
        (1) Maternal hypotension from
           (a) Supine hypotension
           (b) Trauma or blood loss
           (c) Regional anesthesia
           (d) Drug use
        (2) Maternal hyperventilation or hypoventilation

NOTE: Although the term *reflex late deceleration* is not a part of the NICHD definitions, it is supported
by recent research and is felt to be neurogenic in origin (Nageotte & Gilstrap, 2009). A reflex late
deceleration occurs due to a fetal physiologic response to uteroplacental insufficiency that occurs
without fetal acidemia. In response to the uterine contraction a well-oxygenated fetus may experience a transient decrease in oxygen availability. This action mobilizes the chemoreceptor response to
the hypoxemia resulting in the deceleration that has a nadir past the peak of the contraction. Once
the contraction resolves, the fetus returns to a normoxic state. Throughout this deceleration the variability is moderate (normal) and there is no evidence of significant acidemia (Curran & Torgersen,
2006; Simpson, 2008b).

B. Physical findings (Figures 12-12 to 12-14)
    1. Visually apparent gradual (from onset to nadir) decrease to the nadir with a subsequent
gradual return to the FHR BL
    2. Deceleration is delayed in timing (can be as much as 20 to 30 seconds).
    3. In most cases, the onset, nadir, and recovery occur after the beginning, peak, and ending of the
contraction, respectively.
    4. Late decelerations with minimal or absent variability can be due to fetal asphyxia (Nageotte &
Gilstrap, 2009; Simpson, 2008b).
    5. Late decelerations accompanied by absent variability may occur over time due to prolonged
periods of variable decelerations, bradycardia, tachycardia, or other periodic patterns.
Such patterns that occur recurrently and over long periods can deplete oxygen reserves
and interrupt or totally stop normal fetal oxygenation (Curran & Torgersen, 2006; Simpson,
2008b).

C. Interventions
    1. Position the patient in lateral left or right position to:
        a. Maximize uteroplacental blood flow.
        b. Avoid supine hypotension effect.

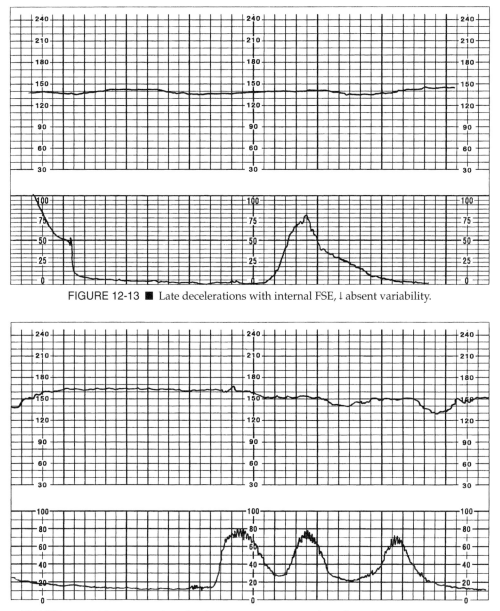

FIGURE 12-13 ■ Late decelerations with internal FSE, ↓ absent variability.

FIGURE 12-14 ■ Recurrent late decelerations, occurring with tripling of uterine contractions.

2. Discontinue oxytocin or other uterotonic medications.
3. Assess hydration; initiate or increase intravenous fluids.
   a. Corrects hypotension
   b. Increases volume to maximize uteroplacental blood flow
4. Administer oxygen via nonrebreather face mask at 10 to 12 L/min to maximize fetal oxygenation.
5. Palpate uterine resting tone to ensure uterine relaxation; consider or request order for tocolytic medication.
6. Communicate the irreversibility or worsening pattern of late decelerations to the appropriate personnel and care providers to include anesthesia and neonatal resuscitation team.
   a. The likelihood of hypoxia, acidosis, and asphyxia increases as duration of the late deceleration pattern increases.
   b. Variability usually reflects fetal status.
   c. Plan for expedited delivery and possible neonatal resuscitation.

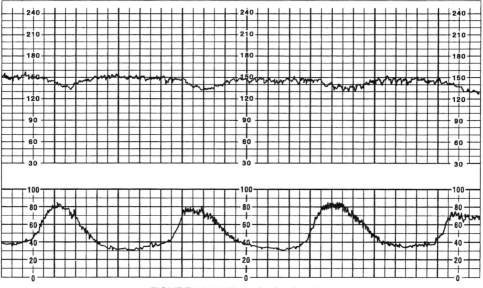

FIGURE 12-15 ■ Early deceleration.

Early Decelerations

A. **Probable causes**
   1. Head compression that results in vagal response
   2. Vagal stimulation via pushing against cervix; compression of head during pushing; forceps or vacuum application
   3. Considered to be benign, requiring no intervention (Curran & Torgersen, 2006; Cypher, Adelsperger, and Torgersen, 2003; Simpson, 2008b; Tucker et al, 2009).
   4. Factors associated with early decelerations include cephalopelvic disproportion (CPD), unengaged presenting part, or persistent occiput posterior presentation.
B. **Physical findings: pattern characteristics** (Figure 12-15)
   1. Visually apparent gradual (≥30 seconds) decrease in FHR with subsequent gradual (≥30 seconds) increase return to FHR BL; nadir coincides with peak of uterine contraction
   2. In most cases the onset, nadir, and recovery of the deceleration coincide with the beginning, peak, and ending of the contraction, respectively.
   3. Are usually associated with moderate variability
   4. Occur more frequently with primigravidas; occurs more often in early active labor, usually between 4 and 7 cm and may also be seen between 8 and 10 cm secondary to head compression
   5. Can be confused with or not identified as late decelerations
C. **Interventions**
   1. Assess progress of labor and perform vaginal examination to assess for dilation, fetal position, and station (descent).
   2. Assess for variability and fetal response to stimulation (scalp stimulation, abdominal, or vibroacoustic stimulation).

Episodic Patterns

Episodic patterns are FHR patterns that do not have a direct relation to uterine contractions. Episodic patterns include accelerations, variable decelerations, and prolonged decelerations.

Accelerations

A. **Probable causes**
   1. Environmental stimuli (e.g., vibroacoustic stimulation)
   2. Fetal movement

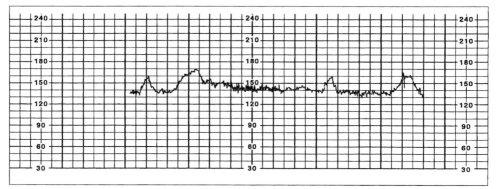

FIGURE 12-16 ■ Accelerations with fetal movement (episodic).

3. Actions or events that may stimulate sympathetic nervous system (e.g., scalp stimulation, occiput posterior presentation, application of FSE)
B. **Physical findings** (Figure 12-16) (Curran & Torgersen, 2006; Macones et al, 2008; Nageotte & Gilstrap, 2009; NICHD, 1997; Simpson, 2008b; Tucker et al, 2009)
   1. Pattern characteristics
      a. Term fetus: visually abrupt FHR increase defined as from the onset of acceleration to the peak of the acceleration in <30 seconds; the peak must be ≥15 beats above the BL FHR and must last a minimum of ≥15 seconds from onset to return
      b. Preterm fetus <32 weeks' gestation: visually abrupt (from onset to peak in <30 seconds) FHR increase from the onset of acceleration to the peak of the acceleration in <30 seconds; the peak acceleration defined as ≥10 beats above the BL FHR for a duration of ≥10 seconds
      c. Prolonged acceleration: acceleration (as described above) lasting ≥2 minutes but <10 minutes
      d. Variability is usually present.
      e. Accelerations are considered to be benign patterns, indicate fetal well-being (well oxygenated), and require no interventions.
   2. Clinical findings
      a. Associated with fetal activity or stimuli, not uterine contractions; accelerations are called reactivity
         (1) Observed in an active fetus or a fetus stimulated tactilely, by fetal scalp stimulation, or by vibroacoustic stimulation
         (2) Fetal reactivity is expected by 28 to 30 weeks' gestation; once fetus demonstrates reactivity, it should continue through gestation.

Variable Decelerations

A. **Probable causes, physical findings, and interventions—same as periodic variable decelerations (see earlier section)** (Figure 12-17)

Prolonged Decelerations

A. **Probable causes**
   1. Any mechanism that has been previously identified for other decelerations (e.g., cord compression, head compression, uteroplacental insufficiency (Curran & Torgersen, 2006)
   2. Profound changes in fetal environment (e.g., abruptio placentae, uterine tachysystole, cord accidents, terminal fetal conditions, maternal death)
   3. Hypotension associated with drug responses or maternal positioning (e.g., sympathetic blockade with anesthesia, paracervical block)
   4. Vagal stimulation with vaginal examination; Valsalva maneuver
   5. Cord impingement, cord prolapse, or cord compression for substantial periods; oligohydramnios with decreased Wharton's jelly allowing for possible cord compression
   6. Uterine rupture
   7. Maternal seizures, status asthmaticus, or maternal cardiorespiratory collapse

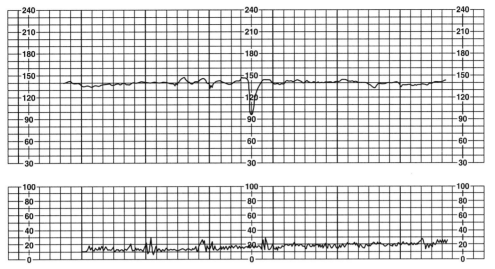

FIGURE 12-17 ■ Episodic variable deceleration. (From Feinstein, N.F., Torgersen, K.L., & Atterbury, J.L. [Eds.]. [2003]. *Fetal heart monitoring: Principles and practices* [3rd ed.]. Dubuque, IA: Kendall-Hunt Publications.)

    8. Rapid fetal descent
    9. Procedures (e.g., vaginal examination, application of internal fetal monitoring devices)
B. Physical findings (Figure 12-18)
    1. Visually apparent decrease in FHR from the baseline that is ≥15 bpm, lasting ≥2 minutes but <10 minutes
    2. A decrease lasting longer than 10 minutes is considered a BL change.
        a. In the absence of tachysystole, numerical intrauterine pressure catheter values are not a diagnostic aid.
        b. Tachysystole is usually defined as more than five uterine contractions in 10 minutes, averaged over a 30-minute window (Macones et al, 2008).
C. Interventions
    1. Change maternal position to left or right lateral, upright, hands and knees or knee-chest—whichever position relieves the FHR pattern.
        a. Helps relieve pressure on umbilical cord
        b. Avoids supine hypotension and maximizes uteroplacental and umbilical blood flow
    2. Perform vaginal examination to assess for prolapsed cord or imminent delivery; if prolapsed cord, elevate fetal presenting part off of umbilical cord.
    3. Discontinue oxytocin or other uterotonics; obtain order for and administer tocolytics (terbutaline) if uterine activity continues.
    4. Assess hydration; initiate or increase intravenous (IV) fluids.
    5. Evaluate presenting part to rule out breech presentation.
    6. Perform vaginal examination to assess for prolapsed cord or imminent delivery; if prolapsed cord, elevate presenting part off of cord.
    7. Administer oxygen via nonrebreather face mask at 10 to 12 L/min.
    8. Communicate findings to primary care provider; document events on the patient's record.
        a. Note the duration and depth of the prolonged deceleration.
        b. Recovery time: If slow, note the recovery time in seconds.
        c. Note BL rate and variability.
    9. Plan for expedited delivery if unresolved despite interventions.
    10. If auscultating and abrupt decreases in the FHR are heard, change maternal position and reauscultate; consider placing EFM to assess FHR variability and possible deceleration pattern.

Uterine Activity

A. Introduction (see Chapter 10 for additional discussion)
    1. Ultimate definition of adequate labor is based on cervical effacement and dilation and fetal descent (Norwitz, Robinson, & Repke, 2007).

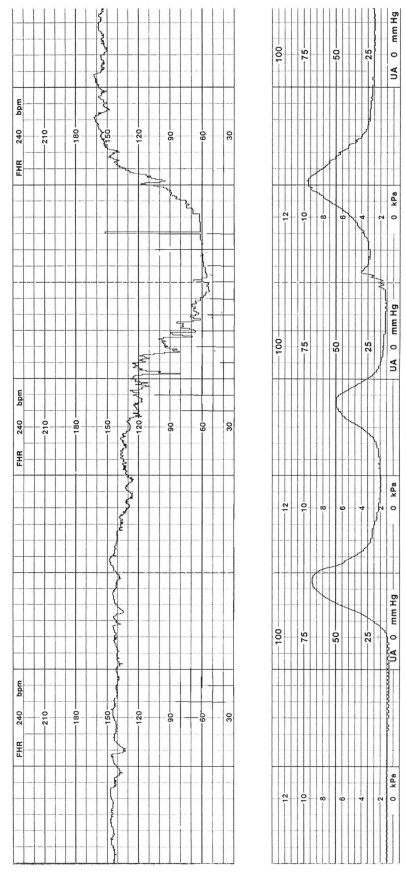

FIGURE 12-18 ■ Prolonged deceleration.

2. Assess three P's of labor to ensure adequacy: power (uterine contractions), passenger (fetus), and passage (pelvis).
3. Montevideo units (MVUs): quantitative measurement of uterine contractions over a 10-minute period
   a. Subtract resting tone of uterus from the peak pressure of the uterine contraction (in mm Hg) for each contraction in the 10-minute period.
   b. Calculated numbers are then added together.
   c. Ranges from 95 to 395 MVUs; average range for adequate labor is 180 to 250 MVUs.
4. Dysfunctional contractions physiologically described as subnormal (or hypotonic, hypertonic, or abnormal) (see Chapter 11 for a complete discussion)
5. Factors affecting labor (UA) that can be changed:
   a. Hydration
   b. Maternal psychological status and anxiety
   c. Intensity and duration of uterine contractions
   d. Maternal positioning and pushing efforts
   e. Drugs or medications taken by or given to mother

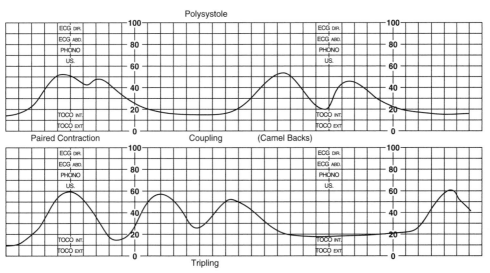

FIGURE 12-19 ■ Uterine contractions with coupling.

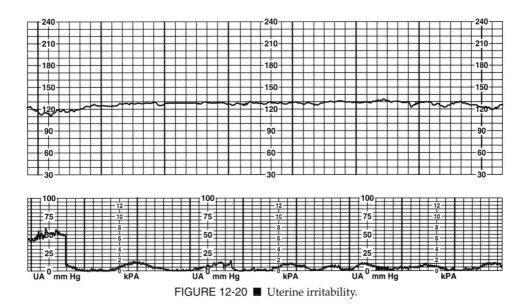

FIGURE 12-20 ■ Uterine irritability.

B. Assessment (Figures 12-19 and 12-20)
1. Frequency: beginning of one contraction to beginning of next contraction; described in minutes
2. Duration: time from beginning of contraction to the end of contraction; measured in seconds or minutes
3. Intensity: strength of uterine contraction; measured externally via palpation (mild, moderate, or strong) or internally with IUPC; IUPC annotated as mm Hg or MVUs.
4. Resting tone: also referred to as BL resting tone; pressure in uterus between uterine contractions; measured externally by palpation (soft or firm) or internally with IUPC in mm Hg
5. Cervical changes as appropriate
   a. Presence of factors affecting uterine contractions
   b. Changes in UA in response to interventions
6. Uterine contractions are quantified as the number of contractions in a 10-minute window averaged over 30 minutes (Macones et al, 2008; NICHD, 1997). The following terminology is used when describing UA:
   a. Normal: ≤5 contractions in 10 minutes, averaged over a 30-minute window
   b. Tachysystole: >5 contractions in 10 minutes, averaged over a 30-minute window
   c. Characteristics of uterine contractions
      (1) "Tachysystole should always be qualified as to the presence or absence of associated FHR decelerations" (Macones et al , 2008).
      (2) Tachysystole is applicable to spontaneous and stimulated (i.e., oxytocin) labor.
      (3) Hyperstimulation and hypercontractility are not defined and the terminology should be abandoned (Macones et al, 2008).

Interpretation of FHR Patterns

A. Three-tier categorization system
1. There are several categorization systems in the recent literature. For example, Parer and Ikeda (2007) described a five-tier system categorized by color. In addition to ACOG, the SOGC and the Royal College of Obstetricians and Gynaecologists (United Kingdom) describe three-tier systems. In collaboration with the NICHD and the Society of Maternal-Fetal Medicine, ACOG adopted a three-tier categorization system.
2. General management principles were agreed upon; however, specific management algorithms (i.e., interventions) were not, as they were determined to be a "function of professional specialty entities" (Macones et al, 2008, p. 664).
3. The categories evaluate the fetus at that specific point in time; FHR patterns can and will change over time.
4. An FHR pattern can move between the categories depending on the clinical situation and the interventions used.
5. Categories
   a. Category I: normal
      (1) Strongly predictive of normal acid-base status at the time of observation
      (2) May be followed routinely
      (3) No specific action/intervention required
      (4) Includes all of the following:
         (a) FHR BL 110 to 160 bpm
         (b) FHR BL variability moderate
         (c) No late or variable deceleration
         (d) Present or absent early decelerations
         (e) Present or absent accelerations
   b. Category II: indeterminate
      (1) Not predictive of abnormal fetal acid-base status; no adequate evidence at present to classify as Category I or Category III
      (2) Requires evaluation and continued surveillance and reevaluation
      (3) Must consider the entire clinical picture
      (4) Includes any of the following:
         (a) Bradycardia not accompanied by absent FHR BL variability
         (b) Tachycardia

(c) Minimal FHR BL variability

(d) Absent FHR BL variability not accompanied by recurrent decelerations

(e) Marked FHR BL variability

(f) Absence of induced accelerations after fetal stimulation

(g) Recurrent variable decelerations accompanied by minimal or moderate baseline variability

(h) Prolonged deceleration

(i) Recurrent late decelerations with moderate FHR BL variability

(j) Variable decelerations with other characteristics, such as slow return to baseline, overshoots, or shoulders

  c. Category III: abnormal

    (1) Predictive of abnormal fetal acid-base status at the specific time of observation

    (2) Requires prompt evaluation

    (3) Includes either:

      (a) Absent FHR BL variability and any of the following:

        [i] Recurrent late decelerations

        [ii] Recurrent variable decelerations

        [iii] Bradycardia

      (b) Sinusoidal pattern

    (4) Interventions can include, but are not limited to:

      (a) Maternal oxygen via nonrebreather face mask at 10 to 12 L/min

      (b) Maternal position change to left or right lateral, knee-chest, or hands and knees, whichever position returns fetus to Category I or Category II status

      (c) Discontinue oxytocin or other uterotonic agent.

      (d) Correct maternal hypotension.

B. Fetal arrhythmias and dysrhythmias

  1. History

    a. Fetal arrhythmias and dysrhythmias have been studied for years. Approximately 1% to 3% of all pregnancies exhibit fetal arrhythmic patterns (Strasburger, Cheulkar, & Wichman, 2007), whereas about 2% to 14% of all pregnancies exhibit fetal dysrhythmic patterns (Chan, Woo, Ghosh, Tang, & Lam, 1990; Copel, Buyon, & Kleinman, 1995; DeVore, Siassi, & Platt, 1984; Southall et al, 1979). Of these, 90% are benign, requiring little or no intervention; however, 10% are potentially life threatening (Bianchi, Crombleholme, & D'Alton, 2000; Drose, 1998).

    b. Terms *dysrhythmia* and *arrhythmia* often used interchangeably; however, they are defined as two distinct patterns.

      (1) Arrhythmia: FHR with irregular rhythm or FHR outside the normal BL FHR; describes sporadic, irregular beats; associated with variability of the R-R intervals; on ECG, shows normal P wave occurring in normal association with each QRS complex (Sklansky, 2009; Torgersen, 2003)

      (2) Dysrhythmia: fetal heart rhythm associated with disordered impulse formation, impulse conduction, or a combination of both (Barnes, 2009; Buttino, Cusick, & Gleicher, 1998; Cabaniss, 1993); on ECG, shows early P waves, or bizarre-looking QRS complexes, or both

    c. Despite the distinctive differences in definition, most dysrhythmic patterns are referred to as "arrhythmias" in most of the maternal-fetal literature. To maintain consistency with the literature, the term *arrhythmia* will be used. According to Barnes (2009), arrhythmias fall into two broad categories.

    d. The two categories of arrhythmias are associated with:

      (1) R-R interval variations: normal P wave with normal occurring QRS complex

      (2) Disordered impulse conduction, disordered impulse formation or a combination of the two: abnormal P-QRS relationship, early or absent P waves, and/or bizarre-appearing QRS complexes (Barnes, 2009)

    e. Arrhythmias derive their names from the anatomic site of variant impulse formation, conduction, or both (Barnes, 2009; Curran & Torgersen, 2006).

  2. Physical findings

    a. A pattern irregularity is audible by auscultation and usually by ultrasound and electrode methods; pattern irregularity can be observed with internal EFM using FSE.

b. Causes (Barnes, 2009; Jaeggi & Nii; 2005; Strasburger et al, 2007)

(1) Conduction system defects

(2) Cardiomyopathy

(3) Cardiac tumors

(4) Cardiac structural disease

(5) Maternal collagen disease

(6) Infections such as cytomegalovirus or coxsackievirus type B

(7) Most return to normal sinus rhythm shortly after birth.

(8) Diagnosis may be aided by Doppler velocimetry, fetal echocardiogram (EchoCG), fetal magnetocardiography, M-mode EchoCG, or pulsed Doppler EchoCG (Barnes, 2009).

c. Fetal arrhythmias are characterized by normal P waves and normal P-QRS relationship; alteration in rhythm

(1) Sinus node variants

   (a) Sinus bradycardia (see Figure 12-3)

      [i] FHR <110 bpm lasting for >10 minutes; from standpoint of arrhythmia, some describe as FHR <100 bpm (Barnes, 2009; Crosson & Brenner, 1999; Shaffer & Wiggins, 1998; Sharland, 2001; Strasburger, 2000; Strasburger et al, 2007)

      [ii] Normal P-QRS complex

      [iii] Most common cause is head compression; less frequent causes are hypothermia (Simpson, 2008b), hypoxia (Strasburger et al, 2007), placental insufficiency (Kleinman, Nehgme, & Copel, 2004), and response to drugs such as beta-blocking agents.

      [iv] Persistent rates of <100 bpm are considered unusual and associated with intrauterine growth restriction (IUGR) (Strasburger et al, 2007), increased vagal tone (Simpson, 2008b), maternal beta-blocker therapy, prolonged QT syndrome or severe hydrops (Allan, Crawford, Anderson, & Tynan, 1984; Ferrer, 1998; Meijboom et al, 1994; Shaffer & Wiggins, 1998; Sharland, 2001; Strasburger et al, 2007; Southall et al, 1979).

   (b) Sinus tachycardia (see Figure 12-2)

      [i] FHR >160 bpm lasting >10 minutes; from standpoint of arrhythmia, some describe as FHR >180 bpm (Crosson & Brenner, 1999; Shaffer & Wiggins, 1998; Sharland, 2001; Strasburger, 2000); does not usually exceed 200 to 210 bpm (Jaeggi & Nii, 2005).

      [ii] Normal P-QRS complex

      [iii] Most common cause: continuous fetal activity, maternal fever, or certain medications such as beta-sympathomimetic drugs (Terbutaline or Ritodrine) or parasympatholytic medications (atropine, hydralazine [Apresoline], or hydroxyzine hydrochloride [Atarax]; other causes are fetal compensatory response to hypoxia secondary to baroreceptor or chemoreceptor stimulation (Barnes, 2009; Shaffer & Wiggins, 1998), acidosis, myocarditis, maternal drug ingestion, and hormone or catecholamine transfer (Jaeggi & Nii, 2005; Mucklow, 1986; Pickoff, 2004; Strasburger et al, 2007)

   (c) Marked sinus arrhythmia (Figure 12-21)

      [i] FHR pattern shows changes as much as 120 bpm within 5-second intervals.

      [ii] Unless repetitive, no significant change in fetal oxygenation is noted.

      [iii] Most common cause is parasympathetic response to fetal hypoxemia (Cabaniss, 1993); often seen with increased UA; commonly associated with bradycardia and seen preceding prolonged or nonreassuring variable decelerations (Simpson, 2008b)

d. Fetal arrhythmias characterized by early or absent P waves and/or bizarre-appearing QRS complex

(1) Supraventricular—pattern originates above the ventricles

   (a) Premature atrial contraction (PAC) (Figure 12-22)—associated with redundancy or an aneurysm of the foraminal flap (Fyfe, Meyer, & Case, 1988; Stewart & Wladimiroff, 1988) and maternal use of caffeine, cigarettes, or alcohol (Nyberg & Emerson, 1990; Strasburger, 2000); premature P wave followed by narrow, normal-appearing QRS complex; EFM tracing shows vertical spikes above and below the BL FHR; upper line is premature beat (often more than 180 bpm); lower line is partial (incomplete) compensatory pause and is short distance from FHR BL; middle line is FHR. PACs typically resolve spontaneously around 2 to 3 weeks after diagnosis. PACs do not represent any risk to the fetus and do not require treatment (Sklansky, 2009).

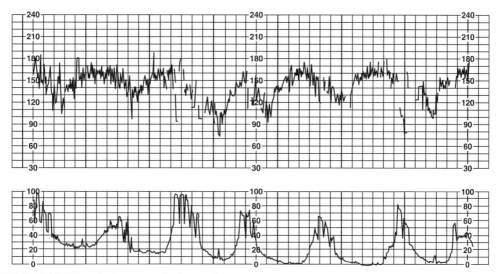

FIGURE 12-21 ■ Marked sinus arrhythmia. (From Feinstein, N.F., Torgersen, K.L., & Atterbury, J.L. [Eds.]. [2003]. *Fetal heart monitoring: Principles and practices* [3rd ed.]. Dubuque, IA: Kendall-Hunt Publications.)

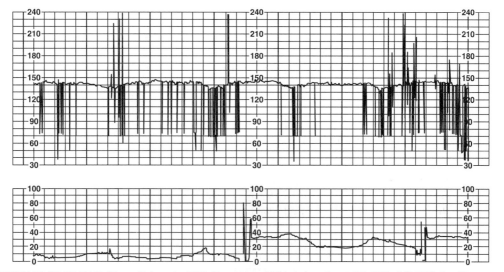

FIGURE 12-22 ■ PAC. (From Feinstein, N.F., Torgersen, K.L., & Atterbury, J.L. [Eds.]. [2003]. *Fetal heart monitoring: Principles and practices* [3rd ed.]. Dubuque, IA: Kendall-Hunt Publications.)

[i] PAC with bigeminy (Figure 12-23)
- PAC occurs with every other beat (e.g., normal beat followed by one premature beat [PAC]).
- Most frequent type of intrapartum fetal dysrhythmia (Cabaniss, 1993; Strasburger, 2000)
- EFM tracing shows two horizontal parallel lines; upper line is the rate between normal and premature beats; lower line is partial (incomplete) compensatory pause; BL FHR obscured.

[ii] PAC with trigeminy (Figure 12-24)
- PAC occurs every third beat (e.g., two normal beats followed by one premature beat [PAC]).
- EFM tracing shows vertical spikes with long upward strokes and short downward strokes (Barnes, 2009; Cabaniss, 1993); upward stroke is premature beat; downward stroke is partial (incomplete) compensatory pause; FHR BL seen intermittently

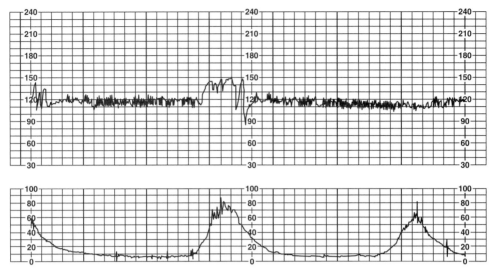

FIGURE 12-23 ■ PAC with bigeminy. (From Feinstein, N.F., Torgersen, K.L., & Atterbury, J.L. [Eds.]. [2003]. *Fetal heart monitoring: Principles and practices* [3rd ed.]. Dubuque, IA: Kendall-Hunt Publications.)

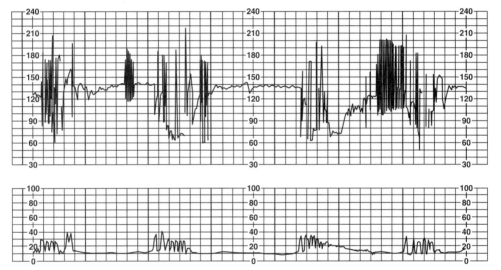

FIGURE 12-24 ■ PAC with trigeminy. (From Feinstein, N.F., Torgersen, K.L., & Atterbury, J.L. [Eds.]. [2003]. *Fetal heart monitoring: Principles and practices* [3rd ed.]. Dubuque, IA: Kendall-Hunt Publications.)

    [iii] PAC with bigeminy and trigeminy
- Bigeminal pattern will dominate.
    - EFM tracing will show uninterrupted parallel vertical lines with FHR BL obscured (Cabaniss, 1993; Strasburger, 2000).

    [iv] Nonconducted PAC (Figure 12-25)
- Premature beat too premature to conduct through atrioventricular (AV) junction
- EFM tracing shows upper line as FHR BL; lower line is the pause produced by nonconducted premature beat; FHR BL is visible.
- Because of slow ventricular rate produced, it may be difficult to differentiate nonconducted PAC from complete heart block (Sharland, 2001).

  (b) SVT: usually presents after 15 weeks, gestation; most commonly seen at 30 to 32 weeks' gestation (Figure 12-26) (Cuneo & Strasburger, 2000; Strasburger et al, 2007).

    [i] Sustained, rapid, regular rate in excess of 210 bpm; rate usually 240 to 260 bpm (Barnes, 2009; Strasburger et al, 2007). SVT of 240 to 280 bpm occurs more frequently in fetuses with normal cardiac structure than in fetuses with congenital heart disease (Sklansky, 2009).

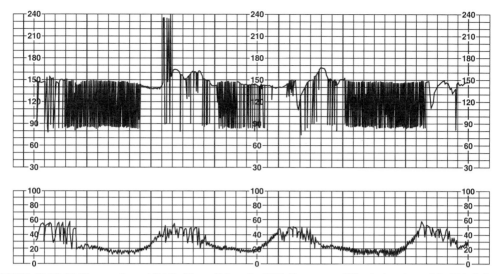

FIGURE 12-25 ■ Nonconducted PAC. (From Feinstein, N.F., Torgersen, K.L., & Atterbury, J.L. [Eds.]. [2003]. *Fetal heart monitoring: Principles and practices* [3rd ed.]. Dubuque, IA: Kendall-Hunt Publications.)

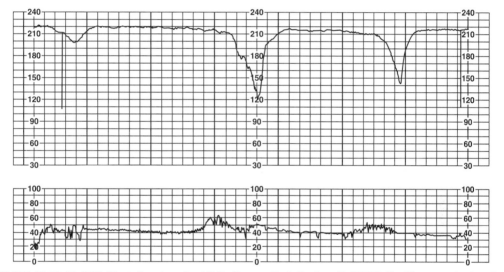

FIGURE 12-26 ■ SVT. (From Lyndon, A., Ali, L., Barnes, J., & Cypher, R. [2009]. *Fetal heart monitoring: Principles and practices* [4th ed.]. Dubuque, IA: Kendall-Hunt Publications.)

      [ii]   May occur suddenly or in waves or spasms (paroxysmal) or may be continuous.
     [iii]   ECG: fixed R-to-R interval with P waves preceding each QRS complex
     [iv]   May contribute to increased birthweight, heavier placenta and neonatal diuresis of a few days' duration (often related to hydrops fetalis) (Crosson & Brenner, 1999); also associated with beta-mimetic therapy (Terbutaline or Ritodrine) (Cabaniss, 1993)
     [v]   Can come directly from atria without relying on ventricles to sustain tachycardic rate (primary atrial tachycardia); if occurs, fetus usually manifests Wolff-Parkinson-White syndrome (Crosson & Brenner, 1999; Sklansky, 2009)
  (c) Atrial flutter (Figure 12-27)
     [i]   Incidence low; associated with high fetal mortality because of difficulty in controlling the pattern and its association with congenital cardiac anomalies (Kleinman et al, 2004; Shaffer & Wiggins, 1998; Sklansky, 2009; Strasburger, 2000)
     [ii]   Rates range from 400 to 500 bpm for fetus and 300 to 360 bpm for neonate.
     [iii]   ECG: regularly recurring sawtoothed atrial activity instead of normal P wave; EFM may half count the FHR

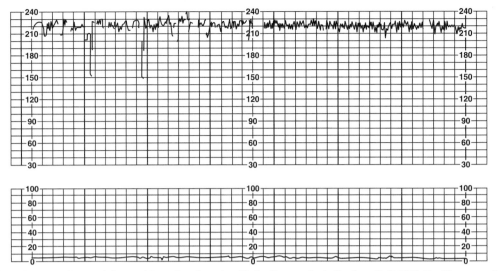

FIGURE 12-27 ■ Atrial flutter. (From Lyndon, A., Ali, L., Barnes, J., & Cypher, R. [2009]. *Fetal heart monitoring: Principles and practices* [4th ed.]. Dubuque, IA: Kendall-Hunt Publications.)

- [iv] Associated with reentrant SVT, atrial septal defect, hypoplastic left heart syndrome; Ebstein's malformation of the tricuspid valve, cardiomyopathy; although very rare, is associated with familial rickets and dislocated hip (Ferrer, 1998; Kleinman et al, 1983; Shenker, 1979; Sklansky, 2009).
- (d) Atrial fibrillation
  - [i] More rare than atrial flutter (Kleinman et al, 2004; Strasburger, 2000)
  - [ii] Associated with fetomaternal hemorrhage, neonatal Wolff-Parkinson-White syndrome, and cardiac structural abnormalities
  - [iii] In antepartum period, variable degree of AV block causes ventricular rate to vary from 60 to 200 bpm.
  - [iv] ECG: low-amplitude irregular atrial activity with complexes of various sizes (Cabaniss, 1993; Torgersen, 2003)
- (2) Ventricular—ventricular in origin; result of premature electrical discharge below the AV junction; considered benign; tend to disappear in late labor or soon after birth; require no treatment in utero or postnatally; if present, mother should avoid cardiac stimulants (Strasburger, 2000)
  - (a) Premature ventricular contraction (PVC) (Figure 12-28)—extremely rare in the fetus (Strasburger, 2000); associated with cardiomyopathy, long QT syndrome, complete AV block with rates <55 bpm, hydrops fetalis, myocarditis, digitalis toxicity, cocaine use, hyperkalemia resulting from hyperemesis (rare in pregnancy), structural cardiac anomalies, or unknown reasons (Allan et al, 1984; Cabaniss, 1993; Ferrer, 1998; Silverman et al, 1985; Southall et al, 1979); frequency may be increased by maternal use of caffeine, nicotine, or alcohol (Cabaniss, 1993).
    - [i] PVC with bigeminy (Barnes, 2009) (Figure 12-29)
      - Will show no middle line
      - FHR or variability obscured
    - [ii] PVC with trigeminy (Barnes, 2009) (Figure 12-30)
      - Top line: premature beat
      - Bottom line: full compensatory pause
      - Middle line: FHR; because of only every third beat being seen, middle line does not represent true beat-to-beat variability (Cabaniss, 1993).
      - Upward and downward strokes are of unequal distance from FHR BL, with upward stroke appearing longer than downward stroke (Torgersen, 2003).
    - [iii] PVC with bigeminy and trigeminy (Barnes, 2009) (Figure 12-31)—BL FHR can appear as uninterrupted line; gives appearance of dotted line between PVCs.
    - [iv] FHR baseline may be obscured (Barnes, 2009).

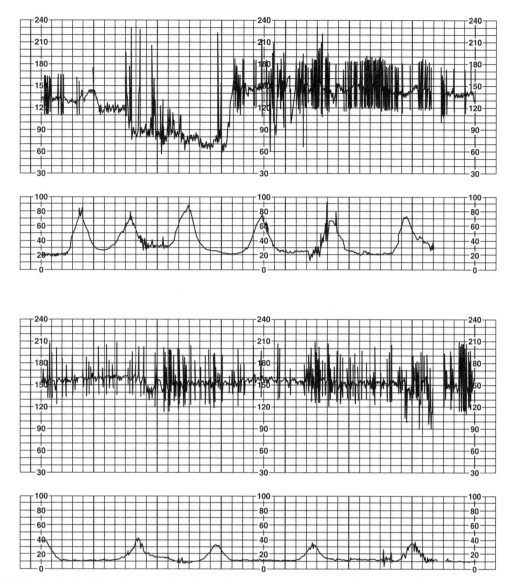

FIGURE 12-28 ■ PVC. (From Lyndon, A., Ali, L., Barnes, J., & Cypher, R. [2009]. *Fetal heart monitoring: Principles and practices* [4th ed.]. Dubuque, IA: Kendall-Hunt Publications.)

    (b) Ventricular tachycardia
        [i]   Rare fetal abnormality; usually a fatal arrhythmia (Sklansky, 2009)
        [ii] Associated with tumors (i.e., rhabdomyosarcoma), structural cardiac disease (i.e., cardiac myopathy, ventricular hypertrophy), prolonged QT interval (Hofbeck, Ulmer, Beinder, Sieber, & Singer, 1997), fetal distress, or fetal acidosis (Sklansky, 2009)
        [iii] FHR varies between 180 and 300 bpm (Sklansky, 2009).
        [iv] Lower rates (180 to 220 bpm) can be treated with lidocaine (administered directly into the umbilical vein) or with propranolol, mexiletine, sotalol, or amiodarone (given orally to mother). However, prognosis is still guarded (Kleinman et al, 2004; Shaffer & Wiggins, 1998; Sklansky, 2009; Strasburger, 2000).
        [v] Important to distinguish between ventricular tachycardia and SVT as digoxin (treatment for SVT) is contraindicated in ventricular tachycardia (Sklansky, 2009)
    (3) Atrioventricular (also referred to as a bradyarrhythmia [Barnes, 2009])—results from AV conduction defect. The type of AV block is described by the degree of the AV block (i.e., first-degree AV block). Impulse conduction through the AV node is abnormal in all

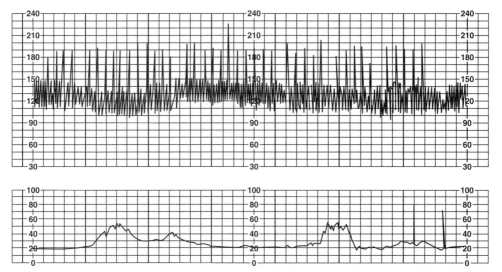

FIGURE 12-29 ■ PVC with bigeminy. (From Feinstein, N.F., Torgersen, K.L., & Atterbury, J.L. [Eds.]. [2003]. *Fetal heart monitoring: Principles and practices* [3rd ed.]. Dubuque, IA: Kendall-Hunt Publications.)

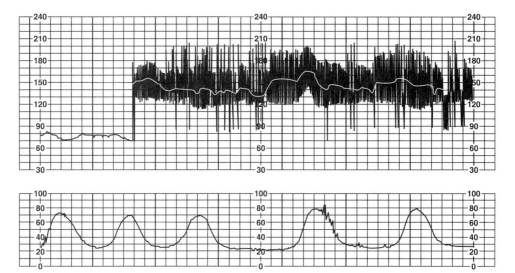

FIGURE 12-30 ■ PVC with trigeminy. (From Feinstein, N.F., Torgersen, K.L., & Atterbury, J.L. [Eds.]. [2003]. *Fetal heart monitoring: Principles and practices* [3rd ed.]. Dubuque, IA: Kendall-Hunt Publications.)

degrees of AV block (Barnes, 2009). First-degree AV block is difficult to recognize in the fetus because the FHR is within the normal BL range. Pathophysiology is difficult to ascertain but it can be due to structural abnormalities (Cabaniss, 1993; Kleinman et al, 2004; Sklansky, 2009). Intermittent failure to conduct an electrical impulse through the AV node can result in second-degree heart block. Second-degree heart block (Mobitz type I; Wenckebach) is not seen in the fetus. However, second-degree heart block (Mobitz type II) can be seen in the fetus but it is difficult to diagnose in the fetus because the atrial and ventricular rates often appear as the same rate (Strasburger et al, 2007)

(a) Second-degree heart block may be associated with:

    [i] Rapid atrial rate resulting from SVT, atrial flutter, or atrial fibrillation (Barnes, 2009; Strasburger et al, 2007)

    [ii] Maternal collagen vascular disease and cardiac structural defects (Crosson & Brenner, 1999; Kleinman et al, 2004; Sklansky, 2009; Strasburger, 2000)

(b) Complete (third degree) heart block (CHB): FHR 40 to 70 bpm (Sklansky, 2009) (Figure 12-32)

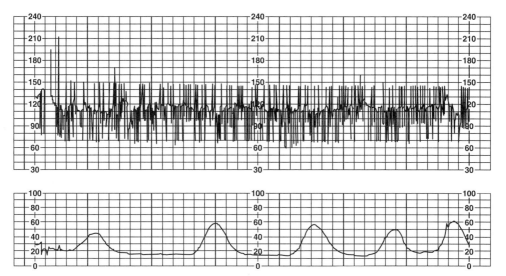

FIGURE 12-31 ■ PVC with bigeminy and trigeminy. (From Feinstein, N.F., Torgersen, K.L., & Atterbury, J.L. [Eds.]. [2003]. *Fetal heart monitoring: Principles and practices* [3rd ed.]. Dubuque, IA: Kendall-Hunt Publications.)

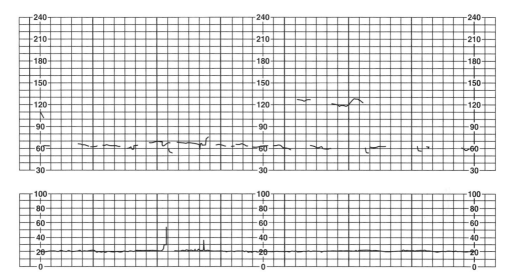

FIGURE 12-32 ■ Third-degree (complete) heart block. (From Lyndon, A., Ali, L., Barnes, J., & Cypher, R. [2009]. *Fetal heart monitoring: Principles and practices* [4th ed.]. Dubuque, IA: Kendall-Hunt Publications.)

[i] Caused by maternal anti-SSA or B antibodies or congenital heart disease (Sklanksy, 2009; Torgersen, 2003); associated with fetal cytomegalovirus infection and antiphospholipid antibody syndrome (Kleinman et al, 2004; Sklansky, 2009; Strasburger, 2000).

[ii] Two categories: (1) CHB associated with complex congenital heart disease (CCHB) or (2) CHB secondary to autoimmune disease-producing autoantibodies that destroy fetal cardiac conductive tissue (Freidman, Zervoudakis, & Buyon, 1998; Horsfall, Venables, Taylor, & Maini, 1991; Litsey, Noonan, O'Connor, Cottrill, & Mitchell, 1985; Kleinman et al, 2004; Moodley et al, 1986; Schmidt, Ulmer, Silverman, Kleinman, & Copel, 1991; Sklansky, 2009; Tanel & Rhodes, 2001; Taylor, Scott, Gerlis, Esscher, & Scott, 1986)

[iii] Fetuses with CHB will have an atrial rate that remains the same but the atrial contractions are not conducted through the AV node to the ventricles (Sklansky, 2009).

[iv] In 50% of fetuses CHB occurs as a result of structural heart disease, a prognosis with a high rate of fetal demise (Sklansky, 2009).

[v] The other 50% result from damage to the AV node by the maternal anti-Ro and/or anti-La antibodies; prognosis is better as fetuses do well in utero (Sklansky, 2009).

[vi] Early treatment for at-risk fetuses (with dexamethasone) may improve fetal cardiac function and prevent the development of CHB, yet this remains a controversial issue (Hornberger & Collins, 2008; Jaeggi et al, 2004; Rosenthal, Gordon, Simpson, & Sharland, 2005; Sklansky, 2009).

3. Interventions

    a. Arrhythmic patterns resulting in normal P-QRS relationship—interventions are the same as discussed in previous FHR BL section.

    b. Arrhythmic patterns resulting in premature or absent P wave and/or bizarre QRS complex.

    (1) SVT: treatment dependent on whether SVT is sustained or intermittent, gestational age of fetus, presence or absence of fetal hydrops and parental wishes (Jaeggi & Nii, 2005; Larmay & Strasburger, 2004)

    (a) Evaluate maternal hydration status.

    (b) Assess mother for fever or other signs of infection.

    (c) Correct any identifiable underlying etiology.

    (d) Monitor FHR for signs of fetal well-being (i.e., moderate variability).

    (e) If pregnancy near term, observation acceptable if tachycardic episodes are short-lived, and if fetal cardiac failure is not evident. May also deliver infant if term and fetus is without evidence of fetal hydrops (Barnes, 2009).

    (f) If term fetus, with presence of fetal hydrops, intrauterine conversion therapy until SVT is converted. After fetus demonstrates normal sinus rhythm, delivery can occur.

    (g) If preterm, intrauterine conversion therapy recommended along with the status of fetal lung maturity. Delivery before term gestation is dependent on fetal gestational age and presence of fetal cardiac failure. Prenatal drug therapy is dependent on gestational age, presence of cardiac failure, duration of pattern, and parental desires.

    (h) For nonhydropic fetus, treatment drug of choice is digoxin administered to mother intravenously. In the absence of contraindications, treatment with digoxin begins with a digoxin load of 0.5 mg intravenously every 6 to 8 hours. A maternal serum digoxin level and ECG are performed before each dose (Sklansky, 2009). Maternal therapy continues until:

    [i] Fetal tachyarrhythmia occurs less than 25% of the time, and/or fetal hydrops resolves.

    [ii] Therapeutic levels are obtained. Therapeutic digoxin level is 0.8 to 2.0 mcg/mL) (Barnes, 2009; Kleinman & Nehgme, 2004).

    [iii] Maternal toxicity as evidenced by maternal symptoms or maternal ECG evidence of second-degree heart block or CHB

    [iv] Fetal toxicity (tachyarrhythmia gets worse) (Sklansky, 2009)

    (i) After desired effect is achieved, administer digoxin 0.25 to 0.5 mg orally two to four times per day (Sklansky, 2009)

    (j) Required dose for cardioversion may be twice the normal dose than required in the nonpregnant adult patient (Barnes, 2009; Strasburger et al, 2007).

    (k) Frequent monitoring of maternal digoxin levels recommended

    (l) Following adequate digitalization and when fetus converts to normal sinus rhythm, the mother is switched to oral digoxin, which is continued until birth (Kleinman & Nehgme, 2004).

    (m) Hydropic fetus may require a change to a different cardiac medication or the use of additional medications such as adenosine, amiodarone, sotalol, and flecainide (Barnes, 2009; Campbell, Best, Eswaran, & Lowery, 2006; Kleinman & Nehgme, 2004; Larmay & Strasburger, 2004; Torgersen, 2003).

    (n) Intrapartum period—scalp stimulation can convert the pattern to normal sinus rhythm (Curran & Torgersen, 2006).

   c. Sinus bradycardia
- (1) Identify underlying etiology.
- (2) Observation acceptable if moderate variability is present and no underlying pathology identified (Barnes, 2009).

   d. Atrioventricular blocks—treatment is the same for second- and third-degree heart block.
- (1) Steroids, such as dexamethasone or betamethasone (cross into the placenta), are used for patients with high anti-SSA/Ro or anti-SSB/La. These steriods may improve fetal cardiac function or prevent further escalation of the disease in the fetus (Barnes, 2009).
- (2) Beta-sympathomimetics, such as Terbutaline, are used to increase the FHR.
- (3) For FHRs that remain less than 55 bpm, dexamethasone plus a beta-stimulant has been successful (Jaeggi & Nii, 2005).
- (4) Postdelivery, fetal epicardial or endocardial leads are placed for temporary pacing of the neonatal heart (Larmay & Strasburger, 2004). Permanent pacing is required in neonates with structural cardiac disease and in about 50% of patients with isolated atrioventricular block. Strasburger and colleagues (2007) recommend specific criteria for pacemaker application:
  - (a) Symptomatic fetus or neonate
  - (b) Resting heart rate <50 to 55 bpm
  - (c) Presence of wide complex escape rhythms.
- (5) Fetus with documented AV block should be delivered at tertiary center capable of cardiac pacing (Strasburger, 2000).

   e. Atrial flutter or atrial fibrillation
- (1) Treatment for atrial flutter is similar to SVT (use of digoxin).
- (2) Atrial flutter treatment may require additional cardiac agents such as flecainide or procainamide.
- (3) Digoxin may not be successful in treating atrial fibrillation, requiring the use of more potent cardiac medications (Barnes, 2009). If unsuccessful, flecainide, quinidine or procainamide, sotalol, amiodarone, or diltiazem can be used (Kleinman et al, 2004; Schmolling et al, 2000; Shaffer & Wiggins, 1998; Strasburger, 2000; Tanel & Rhodes, 2001; Vautier-Rit et al, 2000).

   f. Ventricular tachycardia
- (1) Treated with amiodarone or sotalol given transplacentally (Jaeggi, et al 2004; Strasburger, 2000)
- (2) If fetus shows evidence of congestive heart failure, lidocaine can be given via the umbilical cord (Cuneo & Strasburger, 2000; Ferrer, 1998; Kleinman et al, 2004; Sklansky, 2009). Intracordal administration of lidocaine is often followed by maternal oral therapy of propranolol, mexiletine, quinidine, procainamide, amiodarone, or sotalol (Kleinman et al, 2004; Sklansky, 2009).

   g. Regardless of the type of arrhythmia or dysrhythmia, pretreatment counseling with parents is recommended.
- (1) Treatment options
- (2) Medication regimens
- (3) Plan for labor and delivery.
- (4) Plan for postdelivery care.

ANCILLARY TOOLS TO ASSESS FETAL WELL-BEING

Fetal Scalp Sampling

Fetal scalp sampling is a test in which a sample of fetal scalp blood is obtained to measure the acid and base levels, mainly the pH and base excess of the fetus. Scalp sampling was widespread in most tertiary centers in the 1980s; however, its use did not significantly decrease the rate of cesarean deliveries. Additionally, the test is technically difficult to perform and has been found to be associated with a high level of false-positive results. Often the test required multiple samples and became a costly investment with little or invalid data. As a result, many facilities looked for better noninvasive ways to assess fetal well-being. Fetal scalp sampling has been replaced with scalp stimulation because it is easier to perform and is a good indicator of fetal well-being (Curran & Torgersen, 2006; Ecker & Parer, 1999; Simpson, 2008b).

Fetal Pulse Oximetry

In May 2000, the U.S. Food and Drug Administration (FDA) approved fetal pulse saturation (FSpo$_2$) as an additional method of assessing fetal oxygen status during labor. The FDA approved FSpo$_2$ to be used as an adjunct to EFM, not as a stand-alone assessment tool. Early RCTs demonstrated that the rate of cesarean sections was significantly decreased with FSpo$_2$; however, the rate of cesarean delivery due to dystocia actually increased. Additionally the overall rate of cesarean section showed no difference between the FHR group and the FHR plus fetal pulse oximetry group. In light of these results, the use of FSpo$_2$ was not endorsed by ACOG or the SOGC (Nageotte & Giltrap, 2009; SOGC, 2002) mainly because of their concern that the use of this technology would escalate the cost of medical care without improving clinical outcome (ACOG, 2005). Therefore, in December 2006, FSpo$_2$ devices were pulled from circulation in the United States and are no longer used in the clinical arena (except in those facilities that continue to conduct research on the technology).

Fetal Scalp Stimulation And Vibroacoustic Stimulation

A. Introduction
1. Fetal scalp stimulation has been studied since the 1980s. It is an alternative assessment tool to fetal scalp blood sampling with comparable results (Curran & Torgersen, 2006; Cypher 2009).
2. Any clinician able to perform cervical exams can perform scalp stimulation.
3. Performed with firm, digital pressure on the fetal head during a vaginal examination.
4. In response to the digital pressure, a well-oxygenated fetus will elicit an acceleration (≥15 bpm, lasting for ≥15 seconds from onset to return to FHR BL).
5. Acceleration indicative of fetal blood pH >7.19 to 7.20 100% of the time (Clark, Gimovsky, & Miller, 1984; Elimian, Figueroa, & Tejani, 1997). The presence of an acceleration is reassuring; however, it does not rule out a previous neurologic insult (Ahn, Korst, Phelan, & Martin, 1998).
6. The absence of an acceleration is not an absolute indication of fetal hypoxemia or acidosis (Curran & Torgersen, 2006; Cypher, 2009).
7. Scalp or vibroacoustic stimulation is not used during a deceleration or in the presence of bradycardia (Curran & Torgersen, 2006; Cypher, 2009; Freeman et al, 2003; Tucker et al, 2009).
8. Prolonged scalp stimulation can elicit a vagal response in the fetus leading to bradycardia and absent variability.
9. Vibroacoustic stimulation can be used in the intrapartum period if the FHR needs evaluation and fetal scalp stimulation cannot be performed. See Chapter 8 for vibroacoustic stimulation procedure.
10. About 50% of fetuses that did not elicit an acceleration to scalp stimulation and vibroacoustic stimulation showed acidemia when a fetal scalp blood sample was obtained at the same time (Freeman et al, 2003).
11. If no acceleratory response by the fetus with scalp stimulation or vibroacoustic stimulation, further testing may be warranted (see Chapter 8).

Umbilical Cord Blood Sampling

A. Introduction
1. Considered the most reliable indication of fetal oxygenation and acid-base condition at birth (Cypher, 2009; Thorp & Rushing, 1999).
2. Finding of normal umbilical blood gas measurement precludes the presence of asphyxia at or immediately before delivery (Gregg & Weiner, 1993); more objective than Apgar score.
3. ACOG (2006) recommends umbilical cord gases in the following situations:
   a. Cesarean delivery for fetal compromise
   b. Severe growth restriction
   c. Low 5-minute Apgar scores
   d. Abnormal FHR tracing
   e. Intrapartum fever
   f. Maternal thyroid disease
   g. Multifetal gestations

B. Assessment

1. Identify normal, respiratory, and metabolic acidemia ranges (Table 12-1).
2. Interpret normal, respiratory, and metabolic acidemia with single-digit values (Table 12-2).
3. Respiratory acidemia: excess carbon dioxide in fetal system
4. Metabolic acidemia: excess lactic acid in fetal system
5. Mixed acidemia: excess carbon dioxide and lactic acid in fetal system
6. Essential criteria to indicate hypoxia proximate to delivery severe enough to be associated with an acute neurologic injury (ACOG & American Academy of Pediatrics [AAP], 2003).
   a. Evidence of metabolic acidosis in fetal umbilical cord arterial blood obtained at delivery
      (1) Umbilical artery pH <7.0
      (2) Umbilical artery base excess <15 mEq/L
   b. Early onset of severe or moderate neonatal encephalopathy in infants born at ≥34 weeks' gestation
   c. Spastic quadraplegic or dyskinetic cerebral palsy
   d. Exclusion of other identifiable etiologies, such as trauma, coagulation disorders, infections, or genetic disorders
   e. All four essential criteria must be met to indicate acute neurologic injury.

C. Interventions

1. Provide optimal intrauterine environment with position, fluids, oxygen, and other treatments and medications, as needed.
2. Explain the necessity for the procedure.

■ TABLE 12-1
■ ■ Normal Ranges of Umbilical Cord Arterial Blood Gas Values

Arterial Measure*	Normal Mean Value Range†	Range (± 2 SD)
pH	7.20-7.29	7.02-7.43
p_{CO_2} (mm Hg)	49.2-56.3	21.5-78.3
Bicarbonate (mEq/L)	22.0-24.1	14.8-29.2
Base deficit (mEq/L)	2.7-8.3	−2.0-16.3
pO_2 (mm Hg)	15.1-23.7	2.0-37.8

*Venous values reflect maternal acid-base status; they are generally higher than arterial values; arterial values reflect fetal acid-base status. Venous values may be normal (due to reflecting maternal acid-base status being normal) despite arterial values reflecting fetal acidemia.
†Represent range of normal mean values reported in a review of studies of umbilical arterial cord blood gases (Thorp & Rushing, 1999).
From Cypher, R. (2003). Assessment of fetal oxygenation and acid-base status. In A. Lyndon, L.U. Ali, J. Barnes, & R. Cypher (Eds.). *Fetal heart monitoring: Principles and practices* (4th ed.). Dubuque, IA: Kendall-Hunt Publications.

■ TABLE 12-2
■ ■ Single-Digit Acid-Base Values

Single-Digit Value Guideline for Initial Assessment of Normal and Abnormal Umbilical Cord Blood Acid-Base Values*

	Normal Values	Metabolic Acidemia	Respiratory Acidemia
pH	≥7.10	<7.10	<7.10
pO_2 (mm Hg)	>20	<20	Variable
pCO_2 (mm Hg)	<60	<60	>60
Bicarbonate (mEq/L)	>22	<22	≥22
Base deficit (mEq/L)	≤12	>12	<12
Base excess (mEq/L)	≥12	<12	>12

*Values are suggested as a guide for evaluating acid-base status.
From AWHONN (2006). AWHONN Intermediate Fetal Monitoring Course. AWHONN Fetal Monitoring Program. Dubuque, IA: Kendall-Hunt Publications; Lyndon, A., Ali, L.U., Barnes J., Cypher R. (2009). *Fetal heart monitoring: Principles and practices* (4th ed.). Dubuque, IA: Kendall-Hunt Publications.

3. Explain the procedure, from patient's perspective, step by step; often resulting from expediency to collect sample, procedure may need to be explained after sample is collected.
4. Provide support by significant other if available.
5. Prepare for and gather umbilical cord blood samples according to protocol; arterial and venous samples should be obtained; if only one sample, it should be the arterial sample.
6. Interpret data, document procedure and data collection in patient's medical record, and communicate findings to primary care provider.
7. Anticipate events and explain the possible treatment options based on results of umbilical cord blood sample.

Documentation

A. **Documentation of FHR and UA patterns**
   1. NICHD identified five components that should be included in the documentation of FHR tracings FHR BL rate.
      a. FHR BL variability
      b. Presence of accelerations
      c. Periodic or episodic decelerations
      d. Changes in trends over time
   2. In addition to the NICHD recommendations, the following should also be documented:
      a. Interventions and outcomes
      b. Notification of the primary care provider
   3. Use hospital-approved nomenclature and abbreviations (see Box 12-1).
   4. Examples of documentation can be found in Boxes 12-2 and 12-3.
   5. Uterine contractions should be documented as to:
      a. Frequency
      b. Duration
      c. Intensity
         (1) Can use mm Hg with IUPC or MVUs
         (2) Palpated as mild, moderate, or strong with external monitoring; also palpated with internal monitoring to validate internal IUPC reading
      d. Resting tone
         (1) Can use mm Hg with IUPC
         (2) Palpated as soft or firm with external monitoring; also palpated with internal monitoring to validate internal IUPC reading

▨ BOX 12-2
▨ **INFORMATION INCLUDED IN DOCUMENTATION**

BL FHR

Variability: absent, minimal, moderate, or marked

Accels: periodic or episodic

Decels: periodic or episodic

Type or shape (describe if uncertain of what to call deceleration)

Depth (nadir)

Duration (of nadir)

Recovery time (duration): timed from end of nadir to when FHR returns to BL

UC pattern to include frequency, duration, intensity, and resting tone: if using IUPC, should also validate information via palpation, especially intensity and resting tone

Interventions

Maternal-fetal responses to interventions

Notification of primary care provider (include understanding from provider regarding report)

Understanding of patient

■ BOX 12-3
■ **DOCUMENTATION EXAMPLES OF EFM EVENTS**

1. BL FHR 135 bpm; reassuring var decel, nadir to 80 bpm, return to BL after decel; var moderate; UC q 3-4 minutes, lasting 50-60 seconds, intensity 50-60 mm Hg/palp mod, and RT 10-15 mm Hg/palp soft between UC. Pt turned to left side. Pt tolerating labor; breathing with contractions, father at bedside. Dr.____ notified of FHR, UC pattern, intervention and maternal-fetal response; he/she verbalized understanding.

2. BL FHR 120 bpm; recurrent late decels; return to BL after decel; absent var; UC q 1-2 minutes, lasting 30-45 seconds, intensity strong by palp, and RT palp firm between uterine contractions. Pt on right side; no change in deceleration pattern, turned to left side; oxygen 10 L/min per rebreather face mask applied to pt; oxytocin infusion d/c'd; Dr. ____ paged to come to L&D now; explained to pt and family that fetus is not tolerating labor; pt and family verbalized understanding.

3. FHR BL 155 bpm var decel with nadir 55 bpm; slow recovery from nadir to new BL 140 bpm; overshoots present var minimal to absent; contraction not seen on external monitor; none palp; none perceived by pt; pt turned to left side; oxygen 10 L/min per nonrebreather face mask applied to pt; IVF D_5LR increased to bolus 500 mL; physician called and told of fetal and uterine status as noted above; physician stated he/she is coming right over and to prepare the patient for emergent delivery.

If any one of the examples above continues as written, the subsequent note would state, pattern continues. Need to chart today as if you had to recall the entire labor and delivery process 2 to 20 years in the future.

B. **Chain of command/collaborative resolution**
1. A communication mechanism established by institutions to facilitate problem resolution (Simpson & Knox, 2003)
2. Should be present in all institutions to resolve conflicts or problems in a timely and effective manner
3. Protects the best interest of the patient, family, and staff
4. In 2004, The Joint Commission of Accreditation of Healthcare Organizations (now called The Joint Commission [TJC]) released a Sentinel Event Alert that identified communication issues as the root cause analysis for 72% of the cases reviewed (JCAHO, 2004).
5. In another study, miscommunication between perinatal team members contributed to 40% of maternal deaths and that 45% of near-miss morbidities were preventable (Geller, Rosenberg, & Cox, 2004).
6. Many facilities have adopted the SBAR form of communication during critical times of patient care. The SBAR technique provides a framework for communication between members of the health care team about a patient's condition.
   a. SBAR is an easy-to-remember concrete mechanism useful for framing any conversation, especially critical ones, requiring a clinician's immediate attention and action. It allows for an easy and focused way to set expectations for what will be communicated and how between members of the team, which is essential for developing teamwork and fostering a *culture of patient safety.*
   b. SBAR was adapted by the U.S. Navy during command operations to ensure clear communication (Institute for Healthcare Improvement [IHI], 2009). SBAR means:
      S—Situation: What is happening at the present time?
      B—Background: What are the circumstances leading up to this situation?
      A—Assessment: What do I think the problem is?
      R—Recommendation: What should we do to correct the problem?

Interventions

A. **Specific pattern interventions (see individual sections for specific pattern interventions)**
B. **Physiologic interventions**
1. Aimed at optimizing oxygenation, promoting uteroplacental perfusion, decreasing umbilical cord stretching or compression and/or decreasing UA (Curran & Torgersen, 2006). Attempts should be made to resuscitate the fetus in the intrauterine environment such as:
   a. Change maternal position to left or right lateral position. This action can improve maternal cardiac output, maximize fetal oxygenation, optimize uteroplacental perfusion, decrease UA, and/or decrease umbilical cord compression (Curran & Torgersen, 2006).

  b. Assess maternal blood pressure, especially in the presence of regional anesthesia. This action can increase maternal mean arterial pressure, which, in turn, increases uteroplacental perfusion (Curran & Torgersen, 2006).

  c. Administer oxygen (10 to 12 L/min) via nonrebreather face mask.

  d. Assess hydration and initiate or increase intravenous fluids. Increasing maternal intravascular volume helps to promote uterine perfusion (Curran & Torgersen, 2006).

  e. Assess maternal hemoglobin and hematocrit; if levels indicate anemia, notify primary care provider for preparation and administration of blood as ordered.

  f. If oxytocin is being administered, the infusion can be discontinued or the dosage decreased, depending on the fetal status (ACOG, 1999; Curran & Torgersen, 2006; Simpson & Knox, 2009).

   (1) Oxytocin-induced tachysystole with reassuring (normal) FHR pattern

    (a) Change maternal position to left or right lateral.

     [i] Give IVF (Ringer's lactate) bolus of 500 mL unless otherwise indicated.

     [ii] If UA has not returned to normal after 10 minutes, **decrease** oxytocin infusion rate by at least half.

     [iii] If UA has not returned to normal after *an additional* 10 minutes, **discontinue** oxytocin infusion until UA is less than 5 uterine contractions in 10 minutes.

    (b) Oxytocin-induced tachysystole with nonreassuring (indeterminate or abnormal) FHR pattern:

     [i] Discontinue oxytocin infusion.

     [ii] Change maternal position to left or right lateral.

     [iii] Give IVF (RL) bolus of 500 mL unless otherwise indicated.

     [iv] Consider oxygen administration at 10 to 12 L/min via nonrebreather face mask if first interventions previously do not resolve the Category II or Category III FHR pattern. Discontinue the oxygen as soon as possible when no longer needed.

     [v] If no response, consider 0.25 mL Terbutaline subcutaneously.

  g. Investigate maternal medication intake and possible use of therapeutic or illicit drugs, alcohol, or tobacco.

  h. Observe for alternating periods of moderate variability and accelerations; determine if the fetus is in a sleep cycle; attempt to awaken fetus only when immediate evaluation is necessary.

  i. Encourage mother to alter her breathing, or pushing patterns, or both.

  j. Communicate findings to primary care provider; document findings.

 2. If the FHR pattern does not improve despite intrauterine resuscitation interventions, the fetus may need to be delivered expeditiously. In addition, preparation should be made for possible infant resuscitation.

Health Education

A. **Use a holistic approach for maternal support and education throughout the pregnancy and prenatal period.**

 1. Assess the patient's family and support system.

 2. Assess the educational level, educational needs, language level, and language needs of the patient.

B. **Use standards of care, as identified by AWHONN and agency or institution protocols and procedures.**

C. **Evaluate patient's previous experiences with fetal assessment.**

D. **Assess patient instruction needs regarding fetal assessment technology and purpose.**

E. **Explain the technique used, its purpose, and the appropriate patient compliance needed.**

F. **Answer questions and explain the data obtained, as appropriate, at the patient's level of understanding.**

 1. Anxiety level and educational needs affect outcome.

 2. Catecholamine release and physiologic stress responses are associated with observable changes in FHR.

CASE STUDIES AND STUDY QUESTIONS

Mrs. S., a 30-year-old gravida 6, para 3 (G6, P3003) woman arrives at the labor and delivery room of a local hospital, which performs approximately 125 to 150 deliveries per month. She states she has undergone one previous cesarean section for fetal distress, has had no prenatal care, and believes that she is due in 2 weeks, which, according to her last menstrual period, appears to be accurate. Her FHR is 145 bpm by Doppler ultrasound; she has intact membranes and is 3 cm dilated, 80% effaced, at −1 station, vertex presentation; BP, 120/80; pulse, 76; respirations, 18; temperature, 36.6° C (97.8°F). EFM was applied via the tocodynamometer and Doppler ultrasound.

1. According to the EFM tracing A (Figure 12-33), the BL FHR is the following:
   a. 140 bpm
   b. 150 bpm
   c. Variability marked
   d. BL indeterminate
2. The periodic pattern of tracing A is:
   a. No periodic pattern is shown
   b. Normal BL tracing
   c. Variable decelerations
   d. Early decelerations
3. The uterine contractions are:
   a. Every 1 to 1½ minutes × 50 seconds
   b. Every 2½ minutes × 50 to 60 seconds
   c. Hypotonic
   d. Tachysystole
4. During tracing B (Figure 12-34), Mrs. S. suddenly says, "I have to push," and "something is wrong." The nurse performs

a vaginal examination and finds that Mrs. S. is 3 cm dilated and notes that her fetal heart tracing (via tocodynamometer and Doppler ultrasound) shows:
   a. A need for more tracing; indeterminate FHR BL
   b. A BL FHR of 160 bpm, variability minimal
   c. An agonal FHR pattern
   d. Second-stage labor with impending delivery
5. Her uterine contraction (tracing C in Figure 12-35) shows:
   a. Uterine contractions every 1½ minutes × 40 to 50 seconds
   b. Uterine contractions every 30 seconds × 30 to 40 seconds
   c. Uterine irritability; requires further assessment via palpation
   d. Uterine hypotonus
6. In tracing C (see Figure 12-35), 9 minutes later, an abrupt change in the FHR occurs; Mrs. S.'s nurse applies oxygen, changes the maternal position, gives a fluid bolus, and applies a fetal spiral electrode. UA is still being monitored via tocodynamometer. In addition, preparations for a cesarean delivery have begun. The primary rationale underlying these interventions is:
   a. Enhance maternal status in preparation for a surgical delivery
   b. Suspicion of an abruptio placentae
   c. Maximize oxygenation and uteroplacental blood flow
   d. To show that, legally, everything possible was done

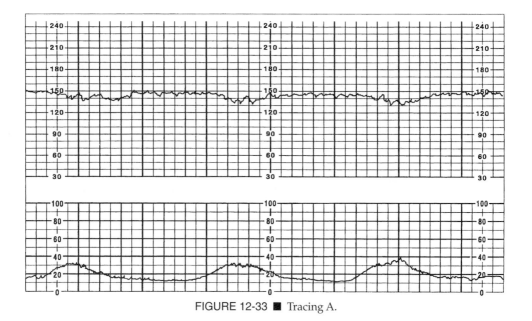

FIGURE 12-33 ■ Tracing A.

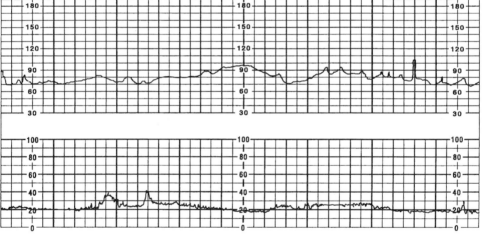

FIGURE 12-34 ■ Tracing B.

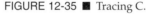

FIGURE 12-35 ■ Tracing C.

7. In tracing D (Figure 12-36), the surgery team is preparing for a cesarean delivery while the physician is en route to the delivery room. The pattern shows a fetus not tolerating labor. This situation means:
   a. The fetus will die no matter what occurs.
   b. The fetus is in immediate need of delivery and expedient interventions may produce a viable newborn that may need resuscitation at delivery.
   c. The fetus will have permanent compromise if it lives.
   d. The fetus will be asphyxiated at birth.

The physician arrived a few minutes after this tracing (see Figure 12-36) had been made and delivered a nonviable fetus that was floating in the abdomen. The entire lower uterine segment had separated from the body of the uterus and the placenta was wedged against this lower segment. The maternal toxicology report was positive for methamphetamines and negative for cocaine.

8. Ms. K., a 27-year-old G1, P0 woman who is 5 days postdates, is admitted in spontaneous labor. Her vital signs at admission

are FHR, 160 bpm; BP, 124/84; pulse, 112; respirations, 20; and temperature, 38.2° C (100.8° F). Her vaginal examination at admission shows a 2- to 3-cm posterior cervix, 50% effacement, –1 station, and light meconium-stained amniotic fluid. At admission, an IV solution of lactated Ringer's was started and opened for a fluid bolus. EFM is being accomplished via tocodynamometer and Doppler ultrasound. Assess tracing E (Figure 12-37), which began 1 hour after admission.

a. Variability moderate, FHR 170 bpm
b. Variability absent, FHR 170 bpm

c. Variability minimal, FHR 170 bpm with prolonged decelerations
d. Variability minimal; FHR 170 bpm initially, then 160 bpm at end of tracing

9. In tracing F (Figure 12-38), an arrow indicates scalp stimulation of the fetus. This fetal response implies:
a. An anomalous fetus
b. A sleeping fetus
c. A nonacidotic fetus
d. An acidotic fetus

Mrs. H. is a 35-year-old G2, P1001 woman who has type 2 gestational diabetes, is at 38 weeks'

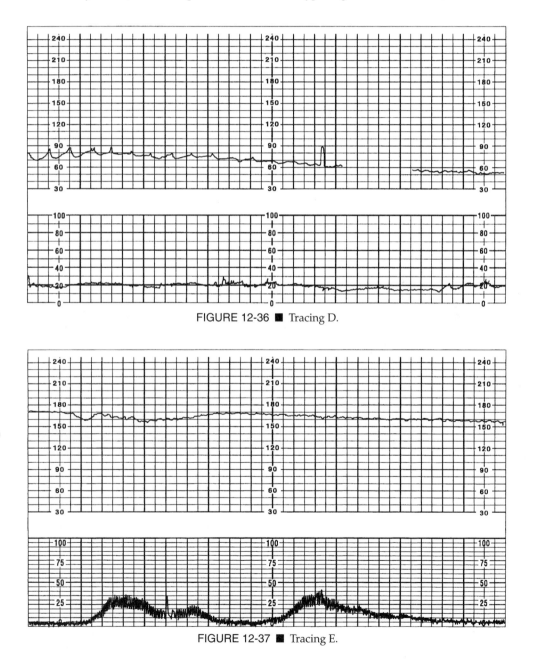

FIGURE 12-36 ■ Tracing D.

FIGURE 12-37 ■ Tracing E.

gestation, and is planning a vaginal birth after cesarean (VBAC). At admission, the FHR is 130 bpm; BP, 158/72; pulse, 80; respirations, 20; and temperature, 36.8° C (98.2° F). Her vaginal examination reveals a thick cervix, ballottable vertex, and intact membranes. EFM is being accomplished via tocodynamometer and Doppler ultrasound.

10. Tracing G (Figure 12-39) began within minutes of her admission to the labor and delivery room. The tracing shows:
    a. Recurrent late decelerations
    b. Variable decelerations
    c. Moderate variability with late decelerations
    d. Diabetic acidosis
11. Interventions for tracing G (see Figure 12-39) that would be expected are:
    a. Change maternal position and administer oxygen (10 to 12 L/min) via nonrebreather face mask to maximize oxygenation and uteroplacental blood flow.
    b. Initiate adequate intravenous fluids and oxytocin augmentation to improve hydration status and adequate labor.

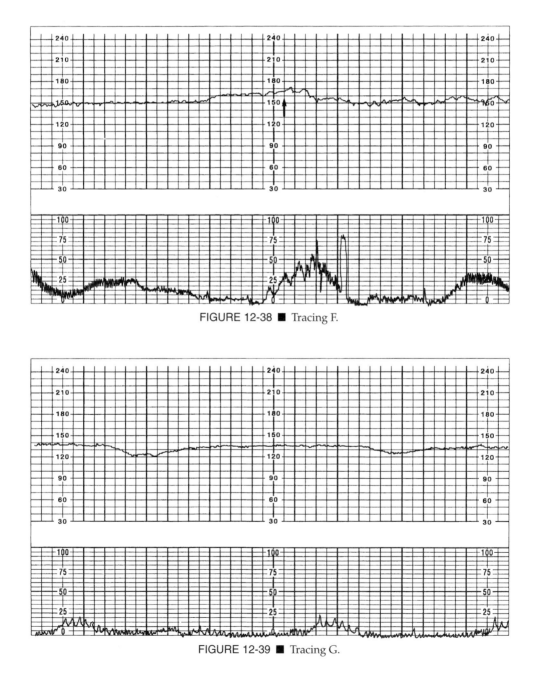

FIGURE 12-38 ■ Tracing F.

FIGURE 12-39 ■ Tracing G.

c. Administer oxygen (10 to 12 L/min) via nonrebreather face mask to maximize oxygenation.

d. Notify anesthesia and prepare for labor epidural anesthesia.

Anesthesia was immediately available, and an epidural was initiated for a cesarean delivery. Mrs. H. was delivered of a male infant weighing 3997 g (8 pounds, 13 ounces). The Apgar score for the infant was 2 and 4 at 1 and 5 minutes, respectively, and umbilical blood gases revealed mixed respiratory and metabolic acidemia.

12. Tracing H (Figure 12-40) represents:
    a. Machine malfunction
    b. Fetal dysrhythmia
    c. Fetal demise
    d. Maternal heart rate

13. Tracing I (Figure 12-41) occurred approximately 1 hour following an amniocentesis while the fetus was undergoing routine observation. Interpretation of the tracing is:
    a. Reactive nonstress test
    b. Marked variability
    c. Machine artifact
    d. Sinusoidal pattern

Tracing J (Figure 12-42) is of a G1, P0 woman who is receiving oxytocin at 4 mU per minute. She is 5 to 6 cm dilated, 90% effaced, and at −1 station. EFM is being accomplished via fetal spiral electrode and tocodynamometer.

14. During the first 2 minutes of the strip, which of the following interpretations can be made?
    a. Variability moderate and fetal reactivity
    b. Variability marked and variable deceleration

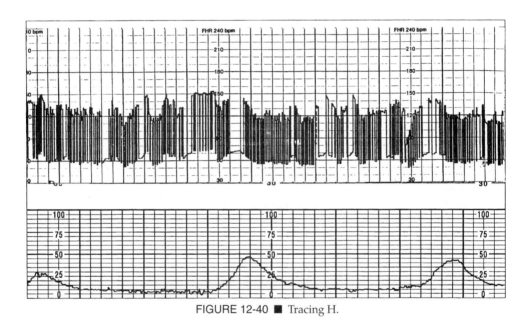

FIGURE 12-40 ■ Tracing H.

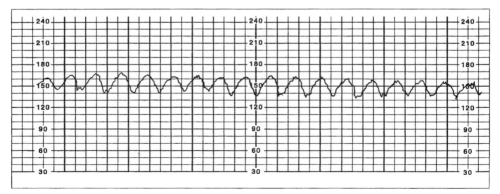

FIGURE 12-41 ■ Tracing I.

c. Fetal atrial fibrillation
d. Fetal SVT (supraventricular tachycardia)

15. In tracing J (see Figure 12-42), during the last 1½ minutes of the strip, the FHR is likely demonstrating:
    a. A prolonged acceleration
    b. Overshoots
    c. Variable decelerations
    d. Compensatory sympathetic response to previous 2 minutes of tracing

Ms. A. is a G1, P0 woman in labor at 6 to 7 cm of dilation, 90% effaced, and −1 station. EFM is accomplished via fetal spiral electrode and toco-dynamometer.

16. Tracing K (Figure 12-43) shows her to have:
    a. Variability moderate; accelerations (reactivity) present
    b. Variability minimal with overshoots
    c. Non–rapid-eye-movement fetal sleep-wake state
    d. Variable decelerations

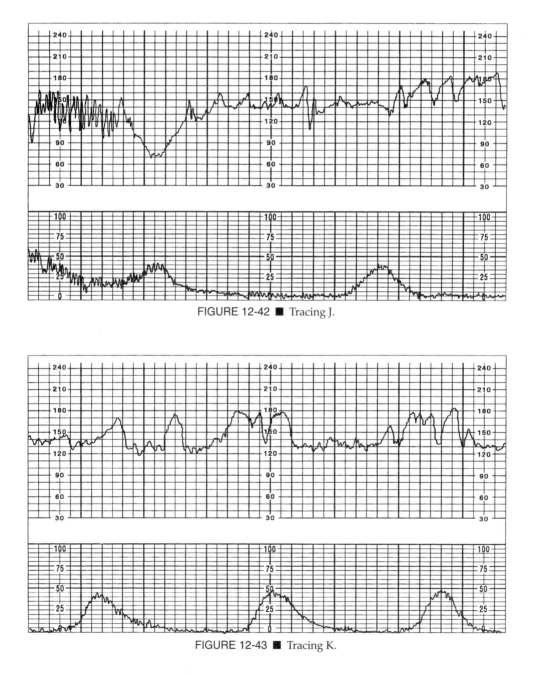

FIGURE 12-42 ■ Tracing J.

FIGURE 12-43 ■ Tracing K.

ANSWERS TO STUDY QUESTIONS

1. b	5. c	9. c	13. d
2. d	6. c	10. a	14. b
3. b	7. b	11. a	15. d
4. a	8. d	12. b	16. a

REFERENCES

Adelsperger, D., & Waymire, V. (2003). Physiological interventions for fetal heart rate patterns. In N. Feinstein, K. L. Torgersen, & J. L. Atterbury (Eds.), *Fetal heart monitoring: Principles and practices* (3rd ed., pp. 159–172). Dubuque, IA: Kendall-Hunt Publications.

Allan, L. D., Crawford, D. C., Anderson, R. H., & Tynan, M. (1984). Evaluation and treatment of fetal arrhythmias. *Clinical Cardiology, 7*(9), 467–473.

American College of Obstetricians and Gynecologists (ACOG). (1999). *Induction of labor (Practice Bulletin No. 10)*. Washington, DC: ACOG.

ACOG. (2005). *Intrapartum fetal heart rate monitoring (Technical Bulletin No. 70)*. Washington, DC: ACOG.

ACOG. (2006). *Umbilical cord blood gas and acid-base analysis (Committee Opinion No. 368)*. Washington, DC: ACOG.

ACOG & American Academy of Pediatrics (AAP). (2003). *Neonatal encephalopathy and cerebral palsy: Defining the pathogenesis and pathophysiology*. Washington, DC: ACOG & AAP.

Ahn, M. O., Korst, L. M., Phelan, J. P., & Martin, G. I. (1998). Does the onset of neonatal seizures correlate with the timing of fetal neurologic injury? *Clinical Pediatrics, 37*(11), 673–676.

Anyaegbunam, A., Tran, T., Jadali, D., Randolph, G., & Mikhail, M. S. (1997). Assessment of fetal well-being in methadone-maintained pregnancies: Abnormal nonstress tests. *Gynecologic and Obstetric Investigations, 43*(1), 25–28.

Association of Women's Health Obstetric, and Neonatal Nurses (AWHONN). (2008). *Fetal heart monitoring (clinical position statement)*. Washington, DC: AWHONN.

AWHONN. (2006). *Intermediate fetal monitoring course. AWHONN Fetal Monitoring Program*. Dubuque, IA: Kendall-Hunt Publications.

Barnes, J. (2009). Fetal arrhythmias. In A. Lyndon, L. Ali, J. Barnes, & R. Cypher (Eds.), *Fetal heart monitoring: Principles and practices* (4th ed., pp. 276–291). Dubuque, IA: Kendall-Hunt Publications.

Bianchi, D., Cromblehome, T., & D'Alton, M. (2000). *Fetology: Diagnosis and management of the fetal patient*. New York: McGraw Hill.

Cabaniss, M. (1993). *Fetal monitoring interpretation*. Philadelphia: Lippincott.

Campbell, J. Q., Best, T. H., Eswaran, H., & Lowery, C. L. (2006). Fetal and maternal magnetocardiography during flecainide therapy for supraventricular tachycardia. *Obstetrics and Gynecology, 108*, 767–771.

Chan, F. Y., Woo, S. K., Ghosh, A., Tang, M., & Lam, C. (1990). Prenatal diagnosis of congenital fetal arrhythmias by simultaneous pulsed Doppler velocimetry of the fetal abdominal aorta and inferior vena cava. *Obstetrics & Gynecology, 76*(2), 200–205.

Clark, S. L., Gimovsky, M. L., & Miller, F. C. (1984). The scalp stimulation test: A clinical alternative to fetal scalp blood sampling. *American Journal of Obstetrics and Gynecology, 148*(3), 274–277.

Copel, J. A., Buyon, J. P., & Kleinman, C. S. (1995). Successful in utero therapy of fetal heart block. *American Journal of Obstetrics and Gynecology, 173*(5), 1384–1390.

Crosson, J. E., & Brenner, J. I. (1999). Fetal arrhythmias. In D. K. James, P. J. Steer, C. P. Weiner, & B. Gonik (Eds.), *High risk pregnancy: Management options* (2nd ed., pp. 371–378). London: Saunders.

Cuneo, B. F., & Strasburger, J. F. (2000). Management strategy for fetal tachycardia. *Obstetrics and Gynecology, 96*(4), 575–581.

Curran, C., & Torgersen, K. (2006). *Abcdefm the textbook: Electronic fetal monitoring* (pp. 115–249). Virginia Beach, VA: Colley Avenue Copies & Graphics Publishers.

Cypher, R. (2009). Assessment of fetal oxygenation and acid-base status. In A. Lyndon, & L. U. Ali (Eds.), *Fetal heart rate monitoring: Principles and practices* (4th ed., pp. 157–176). Dubuque, TA: Kendall-Hunt Publications.

Cypher, R., & Adelsperger, D. (2003). Assessment of fetal oxygenation and acid-base status. In N. Feinstein, K. L. Torgersen, & J. L. Atterbury (Eds.), *Fetal heart monitoring: Principles and practices* (3rd ed., pp. 177–196). Dubuque, IA: Kendall-Hunt Publications.

Cypher, R., Adelsperger, D., & Torgersen, K. L. (2003). Interpretation of the fetal heart rate. In N. Feinstein, K. L. Torgersen, & J. L. Atterbury (Eds.), *Fetal heart monitoring: Principles and practices* (3rd ed., pp. 113–154). Dubuque, IA: Kendall-Hunt Publications.

DeVore, G. R., Siassi, B., & Platt, L. D. (1984). Fetal echocardiography. IV. M-mode assessment of ventricular size and contractility during the second and third trimesters of pregnancy in the normal fetus. *American Journal of Obstetrics and Gynecology, 150*(8), 981–988.

Drose, J. A. (1998). *Fetal echocardiography.* Philadelphia: Saunders.

Ecker, J. L., & Parer, J. T. (1999). Obstetric evaluation of fetal acid-base balance. *Critical Reviews in Clinical Laboratory Sciences, 36*(5), 407–451.

Elimian, A. M., Figueroa, R., & Tejani, N. (1997). Intrapartum assessment of fetal well-being: A comparison of scalp stimulation with scalp blood pH sampling. *Obstetrics and Gynecology, 89*(3), 373–376.

Eronen, M., Heikkila, P., & Teramo, K. (2001). Congenital complete heart block in the fetus: Hemodynamic features, antenatal treatment, and outcome in six cases. *Pediatric Cardiology, 22*(5), 385–392.

Feinstein, N. F., Sprague, A., & Trepanier, M. J. (2008). *Fetal heart rate auscultation* (2nd ed.). Washington, DC: AWHONN.

Ferrer, P. L. (1998). Fetal arrhythmias. In B. J. Deal, G. S. Wolff, & H. Gelband (Eds.), *Current concepts in diagnosis and management of arrhythmias in infants and children* (pp. 17–63). Armonk, NY: Futura.

Freeman, R. K., Garite, T. J., & Nageotte, M. P. (2003). *Fetal heart rate monitoring* (3rd ed.). Philadelphia: Lippincott Williams & Wilkins.

Freidman, D. M., Zervoudakis, I., & Buyon, J. P. (1998). Perinatal monitoring of fetal well-being in the presence of congenital heart block. *American Journal of Perinatology, 15*(12), 669–673.

Fyfe, D. A., Meyer, K. B., & Case, C. L. (1988). Sonographic assessment of fetal cardiac arrhythmias. *Journal of the American College of Cardiology, 12,* 1292–1297.

Geller, S., Rosenberg, B., & Cox, S. (2004). The continuum of maternal morbidity and mortality: Factors associated with severity. *American Journal of Obstetrics and Gynecology, 191,* 939–944.

Gregg, A. R., & Weiner, C. P. (1993). "Normal" umbilical arterial and venous acid-base and blood gas values. *Clinical Obstetrics and Gynecology, 36*(1), 24–32.

Harmon, K. M. (2009). Techniques for fetal heart assessment. In A. Lyndon, & L. U. Ali (Eds.), *Fetal heart monitoring: Principles and practices* (4th ed., pp. 65–100). Dubuque, IA: Kendall-Hunt Publications.

Harvey, C. J. (1987). Fetal scalp stimulation: Enhancing the interpretation of fetal monitor tracings. *Journal of Perinatal Nursing, 1*(1), 13–21.

Hofbeck, M., Ulmer, H., Beinder, E., Sieber, E., & Singer, H. (1997). Prenatal findings in patients with prolonged QT interval in the neonatal period. *Heart, 77,* 98–204.

Hohn, A., & Stanton, R. (2002). The cardiovascular system. In A. Fanaroff, & R. Martin (Eds.), *Neonatal-perinatal medicine: Diseases of the fetus and infant* (7th ed., pp. 883–940). Philadelphia: Mosby.

Hornberger, L. K., & Collins, K. (2008). New insights into fetal atrioventricular block using fetal magnetocardiography. *Journal of the American College of Cardiology, 51,* 85–86.

Horsfall, A. C., Venables, P. J., Taylor, P. V., & Maini, R. N. (1991). Ro and La antigens and maternal anti-La idiotype on the surface of myocardial fibres in congenital heart block. *Journal of Autoimmunity, 4*(1), 165–176.

Institute for Healthcare Improvement (IHI). (2009). *SBAR technique for communication: A situational briefing model.* Found at:www.ihi.org/IHI/Topics/PatientSafety/SafetyGeneral/Tools/SBARTechniqueforCommunicationASituationalBriefingModel.htm. Retrieved March 2, 2009.

Jaeggi, E. T., Fouron, J. C., Silverman, E. D., Ryan, G., Smallhorn, J., & Hornberger, L. K. (2004). Transplacental fetal treatment improves the outcome of prenatally diagnosed complete atrioventricular block without structural heart disease. *Circulation,110,* 1542–1548.

Jaeggi, E. T., & Nii, M. (2005). Fetal brady- and tachyarrhythmias: New and accepted diagnostic and treatment methods. *Seminars in Fetal & Neonatal Medicine, 10,* 504–514.

Joint Commission on Accreditation of Healthcare Organizations (JCAHO). (2004). *Preventing infant death and injury during delivery (Sentinel Event Alert No. 30).* Oak Brook, IL: The Joint Commission.

Kleinman, C. S., Donnerstein, R. L., Jaffe, C. C., DeVore, G. R., Weinstein, E. M., Lynch, D. C., et al. (1983). Fetal echocardiography: A tool for evaluation of in utero cardiac arrhythmias and monitoring of in utero therapy: Analysis of 71 patients. *American Journal of Cardiology, 51*(2), 237–243.

Kleinman, C. S., & Nehgme, R. A. (2004). Cardiac arrhythmias in the human fetus. *Pediatric Cardiology, 25,* 234–251.

Kleinman, C. S., Nehgme, R., & Copel, J. A. (2004). Fetal cardiac arrhythmias: Diagnosis and therapy. In R. K. Creasy, & R. Resnick (Eds.), *Maternal-fetal medicine: Principles and practice* (5th ed., pp. 465–482). Philadelphia: Saunders.

Kopecky, E. A., Ryan, M. L., Barrett, J. F., Seaward, P. G., Ryan, G., Koren, G., et al. (2000). Fetal response to maternally administered morphine. *American Journal of Obstetricians and Gynecologists, 183*(2), 424–430.

Krebs, H. B., Petres, R. E., Dunn, L. J., Jordaan, H. V., & Segreti, A. (1979). Intrapartum fetal heart rate monitoring. I. Classification and prognosis of fetal heart rate patterns. *American Journal of Obstetrics and Gynecology, 140*(4), 435–439.

Lagercrantz, H., & Slotkin, T. A. (1986). The "stress" of being born. *Scientific American, 254*(4), 100–107.

Larmay, H. J., & Strasburger, J. F. (2004). Differential diagnosis and management of the fetus and newborn with an irregular or abnormal heart rate. *Pediatric Clinics of North America, 51,* 1033–1050.

Litsey, S. E., Noonan, J. A., O'Connor, W. N., Cottrill, C. M., & Mitchell, B. (1985). Maternal connective tissue disease and congenital heart block. *British Heart Journal, 60,* 512–515.

Lyndon, A., O'Brien-Abel, N., & Simpson, K. R. (2009). Fetal heart rate interpretation. In A. Lyndon, L. Ali, J. Barnes, & R. Cypher (Eds.), *Fetal heart monitoring: Principles and practices* (4th ed., pp. 101–133). Dubuque, IA: Kendall-Hunt Publications.

Macones, G. A., Hankins, G. D. V., Spong, C., Hauth, J., & Moore, T. (2008). The 2008 National Institute of Child Health and Human Development Workshop Report on Electronic Fetal Monitoring. *Obstetrics & Gynecology, 112*(3), 661–666.

Martin, C. B., Jr. (1982). Physiology and clinical use of fetal heart rate variability. *Clinics in Perinatology, 9*(2), 339–352.

Meijboom, E. J., van Engelen, A. D., van de Beek, E. W., Weijtens, O., Lautenschutz, J. M., & Benatar, A. A. (1994). Fetal arrhythmias. *Current Opinions in Cardiology, 9*(1), 97–102.

Moffatt, F. & Feinstein, N. (2003). Techniques for fetal heart assessment. In N. Feinstein, K. Torgersen, & J. Atterbury (Eds.), *Fetal heart monitoring: Principles and practices* (3rd ed., pp. 77–106). Dubuque, IA: Kendall-Hunt Publications.

Moodley, T. R., Vaughan, J. E., Chuntarpursat, I., Wood, D., Noddeboe, Y., & Schwarting, F. (1986). Congenital heart block detected in utero. A case report. *South African Medical Journal, 70*(7), 433–434.

Mucklow, J. C. (1986). The fate of drugs in pregnancy. *Clinics of Obstetrics and Gynaecology, 13*(2), 161–175.

Muller, J. S., Antunes, M., Behle, I., Teixeira, L., & Zielinsky, P. (2002). Acute effects of maternal smoking on fetal-placental-maternal system hemodynamics. *Arquivos Brasileiros De Cardiologia, 78*(2), 148–155.

Nageotte, M. P., & Gilstrap, L. C. (2009). Intrapartum fetal surveillance. In R. K. Creasy, R. Resnik, J. D. Iams, C. J. Lockwood, & T. R. Moore (Eds.), *Creasy & Resnik's maternal-fetal medicine: Principles and practices* (6th ed., pp. 397–417). Philadelphia: Saunders.

National Institute of Child Health and Development (NICHD). (1997). Electronic fetal heart rate monitoring: Research guidelines for interpretation. *Journal of Obstetric, Gynecologic and Neonatal Nursing, 26*(6), 635–640.

Norwitz, E. R., Robinson, J. N., & Repke, J. T. (2007). Labor and delivery. In S. G. Gabbe, J. L. Simpson, J. R. Niebyl, H. Galan, L. Goetzel, E. Januiaux, & M. Landon (Eds.), *Obstetrics: Normal and problem pregnancies* (5th ed., pp. 353–394). New York: Churchill Livingstone.

Nyberg, D. A., & Emerson, D. S. (1990). Cardiac malformations. In D. A. Nyberg, B. S. Mahony, & D. H. Pretorius (Eds.), *Diagnostic ultrasound of fetal anomalies: Test and atlas* (pp. 300–341). Chicago: Yearbook Medical.

O'Brien-Abel, N. (2009). Physiologic basis for fetal monitoring. In A. Lyndon & L.U. Ali (Eds.), *Fetal heart monitoring: Principles and practices* (4th ed., pp. 21–42). Dubuque, IA: Kendall-Hunt Publications.

Oncken, C. A., Hardardottir, H., Hatsukami, D. K., Lupo, V. R., Rodis, J. F., & Smeltzer, J. S. (1997). Effects of transdermal nicotine or smoking on nicotine concentrations and maternal-fetal hemodynamics. *Obstetrics and Gynecology, 90*(4 Pt 1), 569–574.

Oncken, C. A., Kranzler, H., O'Malley, P., Gendreau, P., & Campbell, W. A. (2002). The effect of cigarette smoking on fetal heart rate characteristics. *Obstetrics and Gynecology, 90*(5 Pt 1), 751–755.

Parer, J. T. (1976). Physiological regulation of the fetal heart rate. *Journal of Obstetric, Gynecologic, and Neonatal Nursing, 5*(Suppl 5), 26s–29s.

Parer, J. T. (1997). *Handbook of fetal heart monitoring* (2nd ed.). Philadelphia: Saunders.

Parer, J. T. (1999). Fetal heart rate. In R. K. Creasy, & R. Resnick (Eds.), *Maternal-fetal medicine* (4th ed., pp. 270–300). Philadelphia: Saunders.

Parer, J. T., & Ikeda, T. (2007). A framework for standardized management of intrapartum fetal heart patterns. *American Journal of Obstetrics & Gynecology, 197*(1), 1–26.

Parer, J. T., & Livingston, E. G. (1990). What is fetal distress? *American Journal of Obstetrics and Gynecology, 162*(6), 1421–1425.

Parer, J. T., King, T., Flanders, S., Fox, M., & Kilpatrick, S. (2006). Fetal acidemia and electronic fetal heart rate patterns: Is there evidence of an association? *Journal of Maternal, Fetal, & Neonatal Medicine, 19*(5), 289–294.

Pickoff, A. S. (2004). Developmental electrophysiology in the fetus and neonate. In R. A. Polin, W. W. Fox, & S. H. Abman (Eds.), *Fetal and neonatal physiology* (3rd ed., pp. 660–690). Philadelphia: Saunders.

Pinsky, W. W., Gillette, P. C., Garson, A., Jr., & McNamara, D. G. (1982). Diagnosis, management, and long-term results of patients with congenital complete atrioventricular block. *Pediatrics, 69*(6), 728–733.

Rosenthal, E., Gordon, P. A., Simpson, J. M., & Sharland, G. K. (2005). Letter regarding article by Jaeggi et al, "Transplacental fetal treatment improves the outcome of prenatally diagnosed complete atrioventricular block without structural heart disease." *Circulation, 111,* 287–288.

Schmidt, K. G., Ulmer, H. E., Silverman, N. H., Kleinman, C. S., & Copel, J. A. (1991). Perinatal outcome of fetal complete atrioventricular block: A multicenter experience. *Journal of the American College of Cardiology, 17*(6), 1360–1366.

Schmolling, J., Renke, K., Richter, O., Pfeiffer, K., Schlebusch, H., & Holler, T. (2000). Digoxin, flecainide, and amiodarone transfer across the placenta and the effects of an elevated umbilical venous pressure on the transfer rate. *Therapeutic Drug Monitor, 22*(5), 582–588.

Shaffer, E. M., & Wiggins, J. W. (1998). Fetal dysrhythmias. In J. A. Drose (Ed.), *Fetal echocardiography* (pp. 279–290). Philadelphia: Saunders.

Sharland, G. (2001). Fetal cardiography. *Seminars in Neonatology, 6*(1), 3–15.

Shenker, L. (1979). Fetal cardiac arrhythmias. *Obstetrics and Gynecologic Survey, 34*(8), 561–572.

Silverman, N. H., Kleinman, C. S., Rudolph, A. M., Copel, J. A., Weinstein, E. M., Enderlein, M. A., et al. (1985). Fetal atrioventricular valve insufficiency associated with nonimmune hydrops: A two-dimensional echocardiographic and pulsed Doppler ultrasound study. *Circulation, 72*(4), 825–832.

Simpson, K. R. (2008a). Labor and birth. In K. R. Simpson, & P. Creehan (Eds.), *Perinatal nursing* (3rd ed., pp. 300–398). Philadelphia: Lippincott.

Simpson, K. R. (2008b). Fetal assessment during labor. In K. R. Simpson, & P. Creehan (Eds.), *Perinatal nursing* (3rd ed., pp. 399–442). Philadelphia: Lippincott.

Simpson, K. R. (2009). Physiological interventions for fetal heart rate patterns. In A. Lyndon, L. U. Ali, J. Barnes, & R. Cypher (Eds.), *Fetal heart monitoring: Principles and practices* (4th ed., pp. 135–156). Dubuque, IA: Kendall-Hunt Publications.

Simpson, K. R., & Knox, G. E. (2003). Communication of fetal heart monitoring information. In N. Feinstein, K. L. Torgersen, & J. L. Atterbury (Eds.), *Fetal heart monitoring: Principles and practices* (3rd ed., pp. 201–232). Dubuque, IA: Kendall-Hunt Publications.

Simpson, K. R., & Knox, G. E. (2009). Oxytocin as a high-alert medication: Implications for perinatal patient safety. *MCN The American Journal of Maternal Child Nursing, 34*(1), 8–15.

Sklansky, M. (2009). Fetal cardiac malformations and arrhythmias: Detection, diagnosis, management, and prognosis. In R.K. Creasy, R. Resnik, J.D. Iams, C.J. Lockwood, & T.R. Moore (Eds.), *Creasy & Resnik's maternal-fetal medicine: Principles and practice* (6th ed., pp. 305–346). Philadelphia: Saunders.

Snell, B. J. (1993). The use of amnioinfusion in nurse-midwifery practice. *Journal of Nurse Midwifery, 38*(2 Suppl), 625–715.

Society of Obstetricians and Gynaecologists of Canada (SOGC). (2002). *SOGC Policy Statement; Fetal Health Surveillance in Labour.* (SOGC Clinical Practice Guidelines No. 1120). Ottawa, Ontario: Canada: SOGC.

Society of Obstetricians and Gynaecologists of Canada (SOGC). (2007). Fetal health surveillance: Antepartum and intrapartum consensus guideline (SOGC Clinical Practice Guidelines No. 197). *Journal of Obstetrics and Gynaecology in Canada, 117,* S3–S32.

Southall, D. P., Arrowsmith, W. A., Oakley, J. R., McEnergy, G., Anderson, R. H., & Shinebourne, E. A. (1979). Prolonged QT interval and cardiac arrhythmias in two neonates: Sudden infant death syndrome in one case. *Archives of Disease in Childhood, 54*(10), 776–779.

Stewart, P. A., & Wladimiroff, J. W. (1988). Fetal atrial arrhythmias associated with redundancy/aneurysm of the foramen ovale. *Journal of Clinical Ultrasound, 16*(9), 643–650.

Strasburger, J. F. (2000). Fetal arrhythmias. *Progress in Pediatric Cardiology, 11*(1), 1–17.

Strasburger, J. F., Cheulkar, B., & Wichman, H. J. (2007). Perinatal arrhythmias: Diagnosis and management. *Clinics in Perinatology, 34,* 627–652.

Tanel, R. E., & Rhodes, L. A. (2001). Fetal and neonatal arrhythmias. *Clinics in Perinatology, 28*(1), 187–207.

Taylor, P. V., Scott, J. S., Gerlis, L. M., Esscher, E., & Scott, O. (1986). Maternal antibodies against fetal cardiac antigens in congenital complete heart block. *New England Journal of Medicine, 315*(11), 667–672.

Thorp, J. A., & Rushing, R. S. (1999). Umbilical cord blood gas analysis. *Obstetrics and Gynecology Clinics of North America, 26*(4), 695–709.

Torgersen, K.L. (2003). Fetal arrhythmias and dysrhythmias. In N. Feinstein, K.L. Torgersen, & J.L. Atterbury (Eds.), *Fetal heart monitoring: Principles and practices* (3rd ed., pp. 289–324). Dubuque, IA: Kendall-Hunt Publications.

Tucker, S. M., Miller, L. A., & Miller, D. A. (2009). *Mosby's pocket guide to fetal monitoring: A multidisciplinary approach* (6th ed., pp. 28–162). St. Louis: Mosby.

Vautier-Rit, S., Dufour, P., Vaksmann, G., Subtil, D., Vaast, P., Valat, A. S., et al. (2000). Fetal arrhythmias: Diagnosis, prognosis, treatment, apropos of 33 cases. *Gynecologic & Obstetric Fertility, 28,* 729–737.

Vlagsma, R., Hallensleben, E., & Meijboom, E. J. (2001). Supraventricular tachycardia and premature atrial contractions in the fetus. *Ned Tijdschr Genneskd, 145*(7), 295–299.

Wadhwa, P. D., Sandman, C. A., & Garite, T. J. (2001). The neurobiology of stress in human pregnancy: Implications for prematurity and development of the fetal central nervous system. *Progress in Brain Research, 133,* 131–142.

Weindling, S. N., Saul, J. P., Triedman, J. K., Burke, R. P., Jonas, R. A., Gamble, W. J., et al. (1994). Staged pacing therapy for congenital complete heart block in premature infants. *American College of Cardiology, 74,* 412–413.

POSTPARTUM PERIOD

Physical and Psychologic Changes

Tamara Whitmer

OBJECTIVES

1. Identify normal physiologic changes in the reproductive system after childbirth.
2. Describe systemic physiologic changes after childbirth.
3. Evaluate common emotional changes in the family in response to childbirth.
4. Recognize normal attachment behaviors in parents and infants.
5. Differentiate between "baby blues" and postpartum depression.
6. Analyze postpartum complications using assessment data.
7. Design individualized patient education based on assessed needs.
8. Develop a discharge teaching plan designed to facilitate competent self-care and assumption of the parenting role.

INTRODUCTION

A. Postpartum period (puerperium)
This period encompasses the time from the delivery of the placenta and membranes to the return of the woman's reproductive system to its prepregnant state.
B. Maternal system changes
   1. Reproductive system
      a. Uterus
         (1) Involution is the retrogressive return to normal condition after pregnancy (Simpson & James, 2005).
            (a) Immediately after delivery
               [i] Weight is approximately 1000 g (2 pounds, 4 ounces).
               [ii] Fundal height is midway between symphysis and umbilicus in midline.
               [iii] Afterpains (uterine contractions) are common, especially for multiparas and breastfeeding mothers.
            (b) At 1 hour postpartum
               [i] Fundal height is at the umbilicus in midline.
               [ii] Consistency is firm and contracted.
            (c) Within 12 hours: uterine muscles relax slightly and uterus returns at the level or 1 cm above the umbilicus.
            (d) At day 2 and after
               [i] Fundal height decreases by 1 cm (0.4 inch)/day and is no longer palpable in the abdomen by day 14 (Simpson & Creehan, 2008).
               [ii] Strong uterine contractions decrease and usually are associated with:
                  • Breastfeeding
                  • Multiparity
                  • Multiple gestation
                  • Conditions producing overdistension of the uterus (e.g., uterine fibroids, polyhydramnios)

(2) Lochia
  (a) Composition
    [i] Endometrial tissue
    [ii] Blood/lymph
    [iii] Bacteria
  (b) Stages
    [i] Rubra (red): 1 to 3 days
      • Scant: less than 2.5 cm (1 inch) on menstrual pad in 1 hour
      • Light: less than 10 cm (4 inches) on menstrual pad in 1 hour
      • Moderate: less than 15 cm (6 inches) on menstrual pad in 1 hour
      • Heavy: saturated menstrual pad in 1 hour
      • Excessive: menstrual pad saturated in 15 minutes
    [ii] Serosa (pink, brown-tinged): 3 to 10 days
    [iii] Alba (yellowish-white): 10 to 14 days but can last 3 to 6 weeks and remain normal
  (c) A danger sign is the reappearance of bright red blood after lochia rubra has stopped.
  (d) Odor is normally that of menstrual flow; foul-smelling lochia might indicate infection.
  (e) Amount might increase temporarily on standing because of pooling in uterus and vagina.
  (f) Amount of lochia might be less after cesarean section, but stages remain unchanged.
  (g) Average amount of lochial discharge varies from 150 to 400 mL (Simpson & James, 2005).
(3) Return of the menstrual cycle
  (a) Nonlactating women
    [i] At 6 to 8 weeks (40% to 45%)
    [ii] At 12 weeks (75%)
    [iii] Within 6 months (100%)
  (b) Lactating women: Some resume menstruation as early as 12 weeks, but some might not resume menstruation for as long as 18 months.
(4) Ovulation: depends on prolactin levels
  (a) For lactating women, 80% of the first few cycles are anovulatory.
  (b) For nonlactating women, 50% of the first few cycles are anovulatory.
  b. Cervical changes (Simpson & Creehan, 2008)
    (1) Cervix is edematous immediately postdelivery.
    (2) Cervix is dilated 2 to 3 cm at 2 to 3 days postdelivery.
    (3) Cervix narrows to 1 cm in diameter by the end of the first week.
    (4) External os widens and appears as a slit.
  c. Vagina
    (1) Rugae reappear in 3 weeks.
    (2) Vagina returns to near prepregnant size at 6 to 8 weeks postdelivery, but will always remain slightly larger.
    (3) Normal mucus production usually returns with ovulation.
  d. Perineum
    (1) Episiotomy is normally without redness, discharge, or edema; most healing takes place within the first 2 weeks.
    (2) Intact perineum might have ecchymosis, edema, or both.
    (3) Lacerations might be present.
      (a) First degree: through skin and structures that are superficial to muscle
      (b) Second degree: extends through perineal muscles (equivalent to a midline episiotomy)
      (c) Third degree: continues through anal sphincter muscle
      (d) Fourth degree: also involves anterior rectal wall
2. Breasts
  a. Changes of pregnancy regress in 1 to 2 weeks' postpartum if mother is not breastfeeding.
  b. Nipples become erect when stimulated.

    c. Breasts increase in vascularity and swell in response to presence of prolactin at the second or third postpartum day (engorgement).

    d. Nonbreastfeeding engorgement subsides in 2 to 3 days (see Chapter 14 for a complete discussion of lactation).

3. Endocrine system

    a. Placental hormones

        (1) Human chorionic gonadotropin (hCG) levels are nonexistent at the end of the first postpartum week.

        (2) Human chorionic somatomammotropin (hCS) (human placental lactogen [hPL]) is undetectable by 24 hours postdelivery.

        (3) Plasma progesterone levels are undetectable by 72 hours postdelivery; production is reestablished with the first menstrual cycle.

        (4) Plasma estrogen levels decrease to 10% of the prenatal value within 3 hours after delivery and reach the lowest levels by day 7.

    b. Pituitary hormones

        (1) Serum prolactin levels rise significantly during the first 2 weeks and rapidly decline to prepregnant levels in the absence of breastfeeding.

        (2) Follicle-stimulating hormone (FSH) and luteinizing hormone (LH) are absent during the first few weeks of the postpartum period.

4. Cardiovascular system

    a. Heart

        (1) Returns to normal position because of shift in diaphragm and abdominal contents

        (2) Cardiac output increases during first and second stages of labor, reaches prelabor values at approximately 1 hour postpartum, and gradually returns to normal within 2 weeks to 3 months (Simpson & James, 2005).

        (3) Cardiac load is increased by 60% to 80% within the first 15 to 20 minutes after birth due to the "autotransfusion" effect, in which 500 mL of blood is redirected to the maternal circulation (Fujitani & Baldisseri, 2005).

    b. Blood volume

        (1) There is an immediate decrease at delivery related to blood loss (normal blood loss at delivery is 200 to 500 mL for a vaginal delivery and 600 to 800 mL for a cesarean delivery).

        (2) Return to normal prepregnant volume takes 1 to 2 weeks (Simpson & Creehan, 2008)

    c. Hematologic changes

        (1) Hematocrit and hemoglobin (Simpson & Creehan, 2008)

           (a) Increase in hematocrit is seen between day 3 and day 7 due to the plasma volume decrease being greater than the loss of red blood cells after birth.

           (b) Returns to prepregnant value in 4 to 8 weeks

           (c) Difficult to determine blood loss during the first 48 hours due to hemodilution. Degree of blood loss is reflected in postpartum hemoglobin levels (500-mL blood loss equals 1- to 1.5-g decrease in hemoglobin levels or 4- to 3-point decrease in hematocrit levels).

           (d) Stabilizes in 2 to 3 days and returns to prepregnant values 4 to 6 weeks postpartum

        (2) White blood cell count

           (a) Might increase to 20,000 to 25,000/mm^3 and returns to normal by the end of the first postpartum week (Blackburn, 2007)

           (b) Increase is primarily in granulocytes (Simpson & Creehan, 2008).

           (c) Might increase without the presence of infection; however, an increase of more than 30% over a 6-hour period is suggestive of infection (see Chapter 28 for further discussion)

    d. Vital signs

        (1) Blood pressure readings immediately postdelivery should be the same as those taken during labor.

           (a) Increased blood pressure might suggest pregnancy-induced hypertension.

           (b) Decreased blood pressure might suggest orthostatic hypotension or uterine hemorrhage.

        (2) Temperature might be slightly elevated in the first 24 hours because of dehydration: 36.2° to 38° C (98° to 100.4° F).

        (3) Pulse rate: Normal range is 40 to 80 beats per minute (bpm).
           (a) Bradycardia (40 to 60 bpm) can be normal during the first 6 to 10 days after birth and is called puerperal bradycardia (Davidson, London, & Wieland-Ladewig, 2008).
           (b) Tachycardia (100 bpm) is abnormal and might indicate uterine hemorrhage or infection.

  5. Respiratory system
    a. Pulmonary function: returns to prepregnant state after the birth of the baby (Simpson & Creehan, 2008)
      (1) Is affected primarily by change in thoracic cage
        (a) Diaphragm descends.
        (b) Organs revert to normal positions.
      (2) Returns to prepregnant levels by 6 to 8 weeks' postpartum
      (3) Respirations are usually in the range of 16 to 24/min.
    b. Acid-base balance returns to prepregnant levels by 3 weeks' postdelivery.
    c. Basal metabolic rate remains elevated for as long as 14 days' postpartum.

  6. Gastrointestinal system
    a. Gastrointestinal motility might remain decreased, leading to constipation and possibly postpartum ileus (Simpson & James, 2005).
    b. Normal bowel elimination resumes at 2 to 3 days postdelivery.
    c. Average weight loss is 5.5 kg (12 pounds) at time of delivery; another 2.3 kg (5 pounds) is lost during the first postpartal week because of diuresis.

  7. Urinary system
    a. Postdelivery edema of bladder, urethra, and urinary meatus is common because of delivery trauma.
      (1) Urinary retention might occur.
      (2) An elevated or laterally displaced uterus (to the right) is a common sign of urinary retention after delivery.
    b. Kidney function
      (1) Mild proteinuria might persist related to catabolism in early postpartum period.
      (2) Diuresis begins within 12 hours postdelivery and continues throughout the first week of the postpartum period.
      (3) Normal function returns by 4 weeks after delivery.

  8. Musculoskeletal system
    a. Abdominal musculature
      (1) Muscles relaxed because of stretching during pregnancy
      (2) Separation of the rectus muscle (diastasis recti), usually 2 to 4 cm (1 to 2.5 inches), can resolve by 6 weeks with gentle exercise.
    b. Joints stabilize again after 6 to 8 weeks postpartum.

  9. Integumentary system
    a. Hyperpigmentation gradually disappears after delivery.
    b. Diaphoresis is common, especially at night, for the first week.
      (1) Can become profuse at times
      (2) Is a mechanism to reduce the fluids retained during pregnancy

  10. Immune system
    a. For women with Rh incompatibility, anti-RhD immunoglobulin is administered within 72 hours after delivery to prevent antibody formation if the mother is nonsensitized.
    b. Blood group incompatibility: ABO incompatibility should be detected early to prevent neonatal complications.
    c. If the rubella titer is 1:18 or less or "equivocal"
      (1) The woman should receive a rubella virus vaccine and instructions to avoid pregnancy for the next 28 days (Centers for Disease Control and Prevention [CDC], 2008a).
      (2) If anti-RhD immunoglobulin and a live virus vacccine, such as measles or rubella, is administered during postpartum, instruct the patient to obtain a postvaccination serology test in 3 months to check immunity (CDC, 2008b).

C. Psychologic changes
  1. Role change is an important psychologic change for the mother.
    a. The mother must relinquish other roles and take on the role of mother.

    b. New mothers typically progress through a series of developmental stages: the rate of progression through these stages is unique to each mother.
- (1) Dependent and taking-in phase of mother (Rubin, 1975)
  - (a) Increase in dependent behavior of mother; wants care for herself
  - (b) Mother asks many questions and talks a great deal about delivery experience.
  - (c) Phase typically lasts 1 to 2 days.
  - (d) Might be the only phase observed by nurse during hospitalization because of a trend toward a shortened inpatient stay for obstetric patients without complications
- (2) Dependent-independent or "taking-hold" phase of mother (Rubin, 1975)
  - (a) Begins to focus on needs of infant
  - (b) Relinquishes pregnant role
  - (c) Takes on maternal role
  - (d) Is interested in learning to care for infant
  - (e) Experiences a period of high fatigue and increased demands by infant
  - (f) Might experience baby blues at 3 to 4 days postpartum during this phase
  - (g) Is typically in this phase 4 to 5 weeks
- (3) Interdependent, or letting-go, phase of mother (Rubin, 1975)
  - (a) Lets go of perception of infant as extension of herself, and views infant as separate
  - (b) Refocuses on relationship with partner
  - (c) Might return to work and relinquish part of child care to other caretakers

2. Attachment
    a. Attachment is the enduring emotional bond between a parent (or parent figure) and an infant (Klaus & Kennell, 1982).
    b. Attachment is essential to the infant's growth and survival.
    c. The mother-infant bond is the basis on which all subsequent attachments are formed and plays a major role in the infant's developing sense of self (Bowlby, 1969).
    d. Besides the mother, infants also attach to the father, siblings, and other significant caregivers.

3. Baby blues
    a. Baby blues or postpartum blues are described as a mild, transient mood disturbance that frequently begins on the third postpartum day and lasts 2 or 3 days.
    b. Approximately 60% to 80% of women experience baby blues during the postpartum period.
    c. The onset of postpartum blues coincides with the normal physiologic drop in estrogen and progesterone, and this, along with fatigue, may be a possible cause of this emotional change.

CLINICAL PRACTICE

Physical Changes

A. Assessment
1. Frequency of postpartum checks according to protocol or as follows:
    a. First hour: every 15 minutes (American Academy of Pediatrics [AAP] & American College of Obstetricians and Gynecologists [ACOG], 1997); second hour: every 30 minutes
    b. First 12 to 24 hours: every 4 hours ("If mother is stable, some institutions defer the 4-hour assessments after the first 12 hours when the mother is sleeping") (Simpson & Creehan, 2008, p. 491)
    c. After 24 hours: every 8 hours
2. Vital signs and blood pressure
3. Breasts
    a. Soft, filling, firm, or engorged
    b. Reddened or painful
    c. Nipples: erectility, possible cracks and redness
4. Uterus
    a. Consistency and tone
    b. Position

  c. Height
  d. Tenderness
5. Cesarean section incision site, if appropriate
  a. Dressing and incision (approximation)
  b. Drainage
  c. Edema, color changes, or both (redness or ecchymosis)
6. Bladder and urinary output
  a. Voiding pattern and amounts voided
  b. Distention
  c. Pain
7. Bowel
  a. Bowel movements
  b. Hemorrhoids
  c. Bowel sounds: auscultate all four quadrants, especially after cesarean section
8. Lochia
  a. Type and amount
  b. Presence of odor
  c. Presence of clots
9. Perineum
  a. Episiotomy, lacerations, and hemorrhoids
  b. Bruising, hematoma, edema, discharge, and loss of approximation
  c. Reddened areas indicative of infection
10. Extremities for thrombophlebitis
  a. Homans' sign (calf pain from passive dorsiflexion of foot)
  b. Check for redness, tenderness, and warmth.
11. Diagnostic studies commonly ordered: complete blood count (CBC), hemoglobin and hematocrit (Hgb/HCT) levels, and urinalysis (UA)
B. **Interventions/Outcomes**
  1. Episiotomy or laceration
    a. Interventions
      (1) Monitor episiotomy for redness, edema, bruising, hematoma, intact sutures, and bleeding.
      (2) Apply ice packs for 2 hours to decrease edema (can be used later for analgesic effect for up to 24 hours).
      (3) Encourage moist heat (sitz bath) after 24 hours.
      (4) Review perineal care with patient
      (5) Pain relief
        (a) Analgesia: oral
        (b) Analgesia: topical
    b. Outcomes: improvement as indicated by:
      (1) Signs that episiotomy is healing; decreased/absent edema
      (2) Signs of infection absent
      (3) Patient reports acceptable control of symptoms.
  2. Urinary retention due to perineal trauma
    a. Interventions
      (1) Check for bladder distention, encourage voiding, and catheterize if indicated.
      (2) Encourage early ambulation.
      (3) Ensure adequate fluid intake.
      (4) Offer warm sitz bath, if needed.
    b. Outcomes: urinary elimination reestablished as indicated by:
      (1) First void within 4 to 8 hours after delivery
      (2) Nondistended bladder
      (3) Voidings more than 200 mL in first two voids
        (a) Less than 150 mL/void suggests retention with overflow; catheterization for residual is suggested (Panayi & Khullar, 2009).
        (b) No complaints of still feeling urge to void immediately after voiding
      (4) No pain or discomfort with voiding

3. Constipation due to perineal discomfort, slowed peristalsis, and/or relaxed abdominal tone
    a. Interventions
        (1) Encourage adequate intake of fluids (2000 to 3000 mL/day) (Simpson & Creehan, 2008).
        (2) Encourage diet high in fiber and roughage.
        (3) Encourage ambulation.
        (4) Administer stool softener, laxative, enema, or suppository if needed.
        (5) Encourage warm sitz baths.
        (6) Apply topical anesthetics.
        (7) Teach methods to avoid constipation and importance of bowel movement within 2 to 3 days (especially important with early discharge practices).
        (8) Acknowledge patient's fear associated with first postdelivery bowel movement.
        (9) Monitor bowel sounds following cesarean section.
    b. Outcomes: bowel elimination reestablished as indicated by:
        (1) Bowel movement (soft, formed stool) by second or third postpartum day
        (2) Return of bowel sounds in cesarean section patient
        (3) Reports of minimal discomfort
4. Pain from episiotomy, hemorrhoids, or cesarean section incision
    a. Interventions
        (1) Inspect condition of perineum.
        (2) Administer cold or hot perineal treatment.
        (3) Administer analgesic medication, as ordered.
        (4) Monitor cesarean section delivery patients for incisional pain.
        (5) Explain cause of pain and how long pain will last.
        (6) Explore various methods of nonpharmaceutical pain relief (e.g., relaxation techniques).
    b. Outcomes
        (1) The patient will report acceptable control of symptoms (Carpenito-Moyet, 2008).
        (2) Communicates need for pain relief in a timely manner

HEALTH EDUCATION

A. **Introduction**
    1. Discharge planning (starting with the admission of the patient) is vital due to shortened in-hospital stays for uncomplicated obstetric care.
    2. Postdischarge follow-up is necessary for the hospital-based nurse to provide.
    3. Communication with community agencies for referral and follow-up of identified problems is essential for the health and welfare of the new family unit.
The teaching plan should include the following components:
B. **Physiologic changes**
    1. Involution of uterus and stages of lochia
    2. Diaphoresis
    3. Weight loss
        a. Usual loss of 4.5 to 5.5 kg (10 to 12 pounds) occurs after delivery.
        b. Additional 2.3- to 3.6-kg (5- to 8-pound) loss occurs from diuresis and involution.
    4. Breast changes occur, whether nursing or not nursing.
    5. Discomforts and measures to provide comfort
        a. Incisional healing (use ice packs, sitz bath, local or topical anesthetic or analgesic)
        b. Afterpains (administer analgesic)
        c. Breast engorgement (provide supportive brassiere or binder, ice packs, or analgesic)
        d. Hemorrhoids (use ice packs, sitz baths, or topical anesthetic; avoid constipation)
C. **Self-care measures**
    1. Personal hygiene, including perineal care
    2. Postpartum exercises, including Kegel exercises
    3. Schedule activities to avoid fatigue.
    4. Diet instructions

5. Special instructions
   a. Breast and nipple care; nursing or nonnursing instructions
   b. Incisional care; post–cesarean section care
6. Smoking cessation, if applicable

D. **Danger signs**
   1. Temperature higher than 38° C (100.4° F)
   2. Excessive vaginal bleeding (two or more pads saturated in 1 hour)
   3. Resumption of bright red bleeding after lochia has already turned brown, especially if accompanied by clots
   4. Vaginal discharge that has a foul odor
   5. Increased swelling, redness, or tenderness of breasts, legs, or incision
   6. Burning sensation on urination, or inability to urinate
   7. Severe headaches, blurred vision
   8. Severe mood swings or thoughts of harming self or infant

Psychologic Changes

A. **Assessment**
   1. Maternal role
      a. History: factors influencing transition to the maternal role
         (1) Condition of mother
            (a) Prolonged labor
            (b) Use of drugs during labor
            (c) Type of delivery (e.g., cesarean birth)
            (d) Other complications at time of delivery
         (2) Condition of infant
            (a) Gestational age
            (b) Admission to neonatal intensive care unit (NICU) for other reasons
            (c) Physical anomalies
         (3) Socioeconomic factors
            (a) Economic resources
            (b) Degree of maternal social support
         (4) Familial factors
            (a) Demands of infant's other siblings
            (b) Quality of maternal relationship with partner
         (5) Maternal age or parity
            (a) Previous experience with maternal role
               [i] Very young mothers might not be informed about infant care.
               [ii] Older mothers might face conflicts related to meeting demands of all family members.
         (6) Role conflict related to career demands: active career women might have difficulty in adjusting to role changes and conflicting demands of infant, family, and job (see Chapter 7 for a complete discussion of age-related concerns).
   2. Postpartum mood disorders (Beck, 2006)
      a. Baby blues
         (1) History: Onset typically occurs on the second or third postpartum day and can last up to 10 days.
         (2) Observable symptoms
            (a) Irritability
            (b) Fatigue
            (c) Crying
            (d) Emotional lability
            (e) Anxiety
      b. Postpartum depression: must have five or more of the following symptoms for at least 2 weeks
         (1) Insomnia or hypersomnia
         (2) Psychomotor agitation or retardation
         (3) Fatigue
         (4) Changes in appetite
         (5) Feelings of worthlessness or guilt

(6) Decreased concentration
(7) Suicidal ideations
   c. Postpartum panic disorder
     (1) Anxiety disorder
     (2) Obsessive-compulsive disorder
   d. Postpartum psychosis (most serious and associated with high rates of suicide and infanticide) (Beck, 2006)
3. Attachment
   a. History: factors influencing attachment
     (1) Maternal factors
       (a) Past experience with one's own mother
       (b) Cultural and ethnic background
       (c) Socioeconomic status
       (d) Wanted versus unwanted status of infant
       (e) Quality of relationship with infant's father
       (f) Degree of paternal support
       (g) Age and maturity level
       (h) Circumstances surrounding delivery
         [i] High-risk versus low-risk delivery
         [ii] Type of delivery
         [iii] Prolonged separation from infant after delivery
         [iv] Labor and/or delivery did not proceed as originally planned
       (i) Physical health
       (j) Intelligence
       (k) Degree to which infant matches expectations
     (2) Infant factors
       (a) Gender
       (b) Appearance/size
       (c) Presence or absence of abnormalities
       (d) Temperament
       (e) Degree of alertness
     (3) Paternal factors
       (a) Age
       (b) Maturity
       (c) Past experiences with infants
       (d) Degree to which infant matches expectations
       (e) Quality of the relationship with infant's mother
       (f) Degree to which father wanted to be and has been included in prenatal and birth experiences
   b. Observable attachment behaviors
     (1) Definition: social signals designed to increase proximity of parent and child
     (2) Observable behaviors in mother toward infant
       (a) Touching
       (b) Holding
       (c) Gazing
       (d) Cuddling
       (e) Kissing
     (3) Behaviors observable in infant
       (a) Signaling behaviors (nondiscriminatory before 8 weeks)
         [i] Crying
         [ii] Smiling
         [iii] Babbling
         [iv] Grasping
         [v] Following with eyes and gazing
       (b) Approach behaviors (require locomotion and are not observed before 6 months of age)
         [i] Clinging
         [ii] Moving toward mother
         [iii] Following mother

    c. Maternal malattachment behaviors
      (1) Prenatally
        (a) Excessive mood swings
        (b) Emotional withdrawal
        (c) Excessive preoccupation with appearance
        (d) Numerous physical complaints
        (e) Failure during last trimester to prepare for infant's birth
      (2) Postnatally
        (a) Negative comments about infant's appearance
        (b) Disappointment about infant's gender
        (c) Failure to look at infant
        (d) Failure to touch or stroke infant
        (e) Failure to respond to infant's signaling behaviors
        (f) Failure to name infant
        (g) Limited handling of infant
        (h) Failure to meet infant's physical needs

B. Interventions/Outcomes
    1. Encouraging maternal bonding/attachment
      a. Interventions
        (1) Meet mother's "taking in" needs; allow mother to express feelings about being a mother.
        (2) Allow and invite mother to participate in infant's care, have infant in room with mother, and encourage skin-to-skin contact with infant, if conditions permit.
        (3) Provide nursing care for infant if mother is too exhausted to participate.
        (4) Provide teaching related to physical caretaking skills.
          (a) Teach mother techniques of infant feeding.
          (b) Demonstrate, encourage, and supervise mother's physical care activities (e.g., diapering and bathing).
          (c) Discuss normal infant rhythm and ways in which infants communicate needs.
        (5) Provide community health follow-up for mother identified to be at risk for failure to assume maternal role; for example, mothers who:
          (a) Are adolescents
          (b) Have inadequate social support
          (c) Fail to demonstrate interest in caring for infant
        (6) Follow up with a phone call 2 days postdischarge for clarification of any of mother's questions.
      b. Outcome: no evidence of impaired parenting at time of discharge
    2. Mood changes
      a. Interventions
        (1) Observe and document alteration in maternal mood.
        (2) Provide supportive environment.
        (3) Provide adequate opportunities for mother to rest and sleep.
        (4) Provide mother with relief from infant care when needed.
        (5) Educate patient's partner or significant other about expected behavior.
        (6) Reassure mother that negative emotions are normal.
        (7) Provide appropriate psychiatric referrals if symptoms have progressed to postpartum depression or psychosis.
      b. Outcome: Patient copes with mood alterations immediately after delivery.
    3. Minimizing barriers to attachment
      a. Interventions
        (1) Provide time for parent-infant interaction as soon after birth as mother's and infant's conditions permit.
        (2) Provide environment that encourages questions and expression of feelings.
        (3) Encourage early and frequent skin-to-skin and eye-to-eye contact between mother and infant (touching, unwrapping, examining infant).
        (4) Allow sufficient time to give information to parents about their infant's condition and to assist them in caretaking.
        (5) Encourage parents to participate in infant's care.

(6) Develop a team approach for support and encouragement of positive parent-infant interactions.

(7) Provide daily information about infant's condition if infant is admitted to the NICU or transferred to another institution.

b. Outcomes

(1) The parent will demonstrate increased attachment behaviors, such as holding infant close, smiling and talking to infant, and seeking eye contact with infant (Carpenito-Moyet, 2008).

(2) Community health follow-up ensured after hospitalization if problems related to parent-infant attachment are observed

HEALTH EDUCATION

A. Psychologic changes
   1. Discuss role changes experienced by all family members.
   2. Discuss plans for maternal reentry into the workforce (if applicable) and provision of criteria for evaluation of daycare centers.
   3. Discuss danger signs of postpartum depression.
B. Care of the newborn
   1. Description of characteristics of a normal newborn
   2. Description of infant-feeding techniques
   3. Demonstration and supervision of physical care of the infant
      a. Bathing
      b. Changing
      c. Holding
      d. Feeding
   4. Discuss normal rhythms and cues of infant related to:
      a. Hunger
      b. Sleep
      c. Socialization
      d. Discomfort
   5. Discuss signs and symptoms of illness.
   6. Discuss balance of maternal and infant needs, as well as those of other household members.
   7. Discuss normal growth and development and appropriate approaches to encourage development.
C. Importance of scheduling a postpartum checkup with health care provider for self and infant
D. Resumption of sexual intercourse may be safely resumed when there is no active bleeding and episiotomy has healed (approximately 3 weeks).
E. Family planning and birth control
   1. Explore her feelings about family planning.
   2. Provide information about various methods.
   3. Discuss methods to use with intercourse before postpartum check (e.g., condoms and foam) (see Chapter 15 for a complete discussion of contraception).

CASE STUDIES AND STUDY QUESTIONS

Ms. B., 15 years of age, delivered her first infant 1 hour ago. It was a normal vaginal delivery. She plans to bottle-feed her infant.

1. What progression can she expect in the stages of the lochia?
   a. Rubra, alba, serosa
   b. Alba, rubra, serosa
   c. Serosa, alba, rubra
   d. Rubra, serosa, alba

2. On examination, where would the uterus normally be located?
   a. At the level of the symphysis pubis
   b. Midway between the umbilicus and symphysis
   c. At the level of the umbilicus
   d. At the level of the xiphoid process

3. She might experience diaphoresis for the first few days of the postpartum period. Diaphoresis occurs because of:

a. An infection in the reproductive tract
b. The restoration of prepregnant body fluid levels
c. The establishment of lactation
d. The toxic side effects of certain pain medications

4. Because she is not breastfeeding, select *all* of the breast changes can she expect during the postpartum period:
   a. The breasts will immediately return to the prepregnant state.
   b. Engorgement might occur for 24 to 36 hours.
   c. Engorgement occurs only with breastfeeding.
   d. The breasts will most likely return to the approximate prepregnant state in 1 to 2 weeks.

5. On her second postpartum day, the nursing assessment indicated the following findings. Which finding is considered abnormal?
   a. Uterus firmly contracted at the level of the umbilicus and shifted to the right
   b. Lochia rubra and a moderate flow without clots
   c. Diaphoretic state
   d. Breast discharge that is clear and yellowish

Ms. S., 31 years of age, delivered her third child by planned cesarean section 3 hours ago. She will breastfeed this infant as she has her other children.

6. Her afterpains are caused by:
   a. Analgesic drugs
   b. Surgical incision into the uterus
   c. Contractions of the uterus
   d. Multiparity

7. Which answer *best* describes the routine postpartum assessment for Ms. S.?
   a. Should be the same as that for any multipara
   b. Should be unnecessary because she already knows what to expect
   c. Should be expanded to include a postoperative check
   d. Should be limited to a postoperative check

Ms. J., a 16-year-old primigravida, gave birth to a 3005-g (6-pound, 10-ounce) infant girl 15 hours ago. She delivered her daughter vaginally with no complications after a 12-hour labor. She is unmarried and has been living with her father since her parents' divorce. She did not receive prenatal care until the last trimester of her pregnancy because she was attempting to conceal her pregnancy from her father. She did not attend childbirth preparation classes. Until delivery, she was ambivalent about keeping her infant. However, she has now decided she wants to keep the child. She has had no previous experience in caring for children and is expressing concern about her ability to care for her child.

8. Which factor predisposes Ms. J. to problems in the area of maternal-infant attachment?
   a. Her marital status
   b. Her lack of prenatal care
   c. Her ambivalence about keeping her infant
   d. Her age
   e. All of the above

9. A plan of care designed to assist her in taking on the maternal role would include:
   a. Allowing her periods of rest when she feels unable to care for her infant
   b. Insisting that she breastfeed her infant on demand
   c. Allowing her to merely observe the nurse as she provides physical care for her infant
   d. Questioning her about whether she is sure she wants to keep her infant

10. During the mother's first contact with her infant, the nurse observes a number of behaviors. Select *all* of the behaviors that are commonly observed during the introductory phase of attachment.
    a. Describing the infant as looking just like her mother
    b. Touching the infant with her fingertips
    c. Examining the infant's fingers and toes
    d. Looking directly at the infant's eyes

11. What is significantly correlated with malattachment?
    a. Cesarean delivery
    b. Multiparity
    c. Child abuse
    d. Age of mother

Ms. C. is a 34-year-old multipara being cared for in the labor delivery postpartum recovery (LDPR) unit. She delivered a 3969-g (8-pound, 12-ounce) boy 10 hours ago. She and her infant are in stable condition after an uncomplicated delivery. Mr. C. has also been present while you are caring for Ms. C.

12. In thinking about your priorities for caring for Ms. C. and her infant, in which stage of the parenting role would you expect her to be?
    a. Taking-in
    b. Taking-hold
    c. Interdependent
    d. Independent-dependent

13. Select all the typical behaviors included during this phase.
    a. Focusing on relationship with partner
    b. Expressing a desire to be cared for physically
    c. Focusing on needs of infant
    d. Reliving the birth experience
14. Ms. C. is very happy about her successful delivery of a healthy infant. On the second day you care for her, she asks you many questions about infant care. Select the important content areas to be included in your discharge teaching plan.
    a. Physical care of infant
    b. Infant-feeding techniques
    c. Ways in which infants communicate needs
    d. Need for proper rest and nutrition for the mother
    e. All of the above

15. After Ms. C.'s discharge from the hospital, you receive a call from her. She is upset and worried. She was so happy when she left the hospital and cannot understand why she is feeling anxious and sad, crying frequently, and having difficulty in sleeping. The most likely explanation for Ms. C.'s behavior is:
    a. Postpartum depression
    b. Marital problems
    c. Baby blues
    d. Exhaustion
16. What would you include in your advice to Ms. C.?
    a. Advise that she seek marital counseling.
    b. Advise that she seek personal counseling.
    c. Advise her that her emotional response is common in the early postpartum period and should be self-limiting.
    d. Advise that she contact her health care provider immediately.

ANSWERS TO STUDY QUESTIONS

1. d	7. c	13. b, d
2. c	8. e	14. e
3. b	9. a	15. c
4. b, d	10. b, c, d	16. c
5. a	11. c	
6. c	12. a	

REFERENCES

Ainsworth, M. D. S., Bleher, M. C., Waters, E., & Wall, S. (1978). *Patterns of attachment.* Hillsdale, NJ: Erlbaum.

American Academy of Pediatrics and American College of Obstetricians and Gynecologists. (1997). *Guidelines for perinatal care* (4th ed.). Elk Grove Village, IL: American Academy of Pediatrics.

Beck, C. T. (2006). Postpartum depression: It isn't just the blues. *American Journal of Nursing, 106*(5), 40–50.

Blackburn, S. T. (2007). *Maternal, fetal, and neonatal physiology: A clinical perspective* (3rd ed.). St. Louis: Saunders.

Bowlby, J. (1959). The nature of the child's tie to his mother. *International Journal of Psychoanalysis, 39,* 350.

Bowlby, J. (1969). *Attachment and loss.* New York: Basic Vol. I. Attachment.

Brazelton, T. B. (1974). The origins of reciprocity: The early mother-infant interaction. In M. Lewis, & L. A. Rosenblum (Eds.), *The effect of the infant on its caregiver.* New York: Wiley.

Carpenito-Moyet, L. J. (2008). *Nursing diagnosis: Application to clinical practice* (12th ed.). Philadelphia: Lippincott Williams & Wilkins.

Centers for Disease Control and Prevention. (2008a). *MMR vaccine—Vaccine information statement.* Available at www.cdc.gov/vaccines/pubs/vis/downloads/vis-mmr.pdf. Retrieved February 27, 2009.

Centers for Disease Control and Prevention. (2008b). *MMR vaccine—Submitted Q&A.* Available at www.cdc.gov/vaccines/vpd-vac/combo-vaccines/mmr/faqs-nipinfo-mmr.htm. Retrieved February 27, 2009.

Cunningham, F. G., Clark, S. L., Gant, N. F., Gilstrap, L. C., Hauth, J. C., Leveno, K. J., & Wenstrom, K. D. (2001). *Williams obstetrics* (21st ed.). Norwalk, CT: Appleton & Lange.

Davidson, M. R., London, M. L., & Wieland-Ladewig, P. A. (2008). *Olds' maternal-newborn nursing & women's health across the lifespan* (8th ed.). Upper Saddle River, NJ: Pearson Education.

Fujitani, S., & Baldisseri, M. R. (2005). Hemodynamic assessment in a pregnant and peripartum patient. *Critical Care Medicine, 33*(10 Suppl), S354–S361.

Kennell, J. H., & Klaus, M. H. (1998). Bonding: Recent observations that alter perinatal care. *Pediatric Review, 19*(1), 4–12.

Klaus, M., & Kennell, J. (1982). *Parent-infant bonding* (2nd ed.). St. Louis: Mosby.

Luegenbiehl, D. (1997). Improving visual estimation of blood volume on peripads. *MCN The American Journal of Maternal Child Nursing, 22*(6), 294–298.

Panayi, D. C., & Khullar, V. (2009). Urogynaecological problems in pregnancy and postpartum sequelae. *Current Opinion in Obstetrics and Gynecology, 21*(1), 97–100.

Rubin, R. (1975). Maternal tasks in pregnancy. *Maternal-Child Nursing Journal, 4*(3), 143–153.

Ruchala, P. (2000). Teaching new mothers: Priorities of nurses and postpartum women. *Journal of Obstetric, Gynecologic, and Neonatal Nursing, 29*(3), 265–273.

Scoggin, J., & Morgan, G. (1997). *Practice guidelines in obstetrics and gynecology*. Philadelphia: Lippincott.

Simpson, K. R., & Creehan, P. A. (Eds.), (2008). *AWHONN's perinatal nursing* (3rd ed). Philadelphia: AWHONN.

Simpson, K. R., & James, D. C. (2005). *Postpartum care: Continuing education for registered nurses and certified nurse midwives*. White Plains, NY: March of Dimes.

Varney, H. (1997). *Varney's midwifery* (3rd ed.). Boston: Jones and Bartlett.

14 Breastfeeding

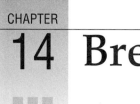

Susan Saffer Orr

OBJECTIVES

1. Identify the two hormones necessary for synthesis of milk and the milk ejection reflex.
2. State two subjective findings that can contribute to a poor initial feeding.
3. Demonstrate criteria for correct positioning of the infant at the breast.
4. List three objective findings that contribute to poor latching-on.
5. List four strategies to decrease breast and nipple pain related to engorgement, plugged ducts, mastitis, or all three.
6. Identify effective swallowing of infant at the breast.
7. Describe two interventions to assist a lactating mother in each of the following special circumstances: infant of a cesarean birth; reluctant or sleepy infant; irritable or fussy infant; infant with physiologic jaundice; preterm or hospitalized infant; multiple-birth infants; or special-needs infant.
8. List three strategies to increase an inadequate milk supply.
9. State nutritional needs of the lactating woman.
10. Identify which infants might benefit from supplemental lactation aids.
11. Participate as a team member in planning care for infants and mothers with special needs in collaboration with a lactation specialist or consultant, physical therapist, occupational therapist, and other health care professionals.
12. Develop a source of referrals for families with special needs.

INTRODUCTION

An understanding of anatomy and physiology of breastfeeding is essential for the nurse who is assisting families during the immediate newborn period. The knowledge the nurse imparts provides the foundation for long-term success with lactation. The nurse has a powerful influence that can positively affect the nursing relationship of the mother-baby couplet. Successful breastfeeding can help prevent hospital readmission of an infant for dehydration or hyperbilirubinemia and can promote infant health. Encouraging frequent and efficient feedings (at least 8 to 10 times in 24 hours) of unlimited length, with the infant correctly positioned and latched on, promotes an adequate supply of breast milk and prevents many common breastfeeding problems.

CLINICAL PRACTICE

A. **Physiology** (Figure 14-1)
   1. Hormonal influences during pregnancy begin in the first trimester related to the following (Ramsey, Kent, & Hartman, 2005):
      a. Ductal sprouting (estrogen)
      b. Ductal branching (estrogen)
      c. Lobular formation (progesterone)
   2. Initiation of milk production (Figure 14-2)
      a. Prolactin level increases (at term, 200 to 400 ng/mL).
      b. Estrogen and progesterone levels decrease after delivery.
      c. Suckling provides continued stimulus for prolactin and oxytocin release.
      d. Prolactin is released from the anterior pituitary and initiates milk production.

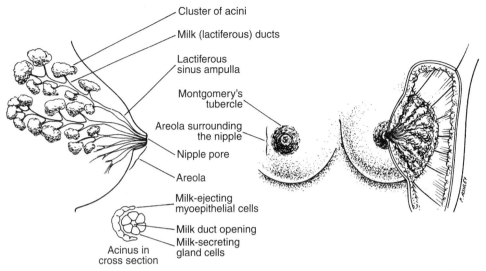

FIGURE 14-1 ■ Anatomy of the breast. (From Burroughs, A. [1992]. *Maternity nursing: An introductory text.* Philadelphia: Saunders.)

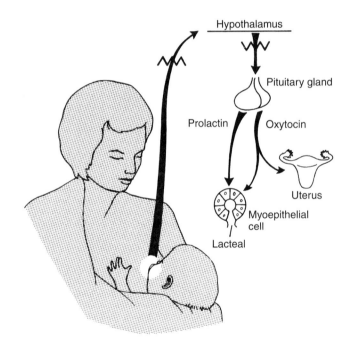

FIGURE 14-2 ■ Hormonal stimulation of milk production and milk ejection. (From Lawrence, R.A. [2005]. *Breastfeeding: A guide for the medical profession* [6th ed.]. Philadelphia: Mosby.)

    (1) Removal of the milk from the breast facilitates continued production of milk.

    (2) Prolactin levels diminish over time in the lactating woman, but they do not return to baseline until 14 days of non-breastfeeding have occurred.

  e. Oxytocin is released from the posterior pituitary and initiates milk ejection (let-down reflex); let-down reflex is triggered by the infant's suckling at the nipple, the mother's emotional response to the infant, or both.

    (1) Alveoli contract and eject milk into the ducts and then into sinuses and out through the nipple.

    (2) There are multiple let-downs during a feeding; many mothers notice only the first one (this is usually not perceptible in the very early weeks of breastfeeding).

(a) The first let-down occurs during the first 1 to 3 minutes of a feeding.

(b) Let-down can also be diminished by stress and anxiety.

(c) Frequency and intensity of let-downs can be variable between feedings and among mothers.

3. Stages of human milk

    a. Lactogenesis I

      (1) Colostrum is available to the infant at delivery and remains available for up to 5 days postpartum.

      (2) Thick and yellow

      (3) The volume varies from 2 to 20 mL per feeding (increased volume in parous women).

      (4) Higher in protein and lower in fat and sugar than mature breast milk

    b. Lactogenesis II

      (1) Onset of copius milk secretion (Anderson, Moore, Hepworth, & Bergmans, 2003; Mannel, Walker, & Martens, 2008)

      (2) Transitional milk: present 2 to 5 days to 2 weeks of postpartum period

        (a) Not as yellow as colostrum

        (b) Protein levels drop as fat, lactose, and calories increase.

      (3) Mature milk: present after transitional milk; whiter and thinner than transitional milk

        (a) Foremilk (a component of mature milk)

          [i] Immediate milk received in feeding

          [ii] Satisfies infant's initial thirst (no normal need to supplement breastfed infant with water)

          [iii] Foremilk is milk that has remained in the breast but has drawn in water and lactose and becomes more dilute.

        (b) Hindmilk (a component of mature milk)

          [i] Later milk received in feeding

          [ii] Higher in fat content (four times higher than foremilk)

          [iii] Satisfies hunger and promotes infant weight gain

          [iv] Milk that has not drawn in the water and the lactose and therefore more concentrated

    c. Lactogenesis III

      (1) Maintenance of lactation is dependent on effective removal of milk from the breast.

      (2) The longer that milk stays in the breast, the slower milk production becomes (Anderson et al, 2003; Mannel et al, 2008).

B. Assessment

1. History

    a. Previous maternal breastfeeding experience

    b. Desire of mother to breastfeed and anticipated duration of breastfeeding

    c. Exposure of mother to breastfeeding education

    d. Cultural influences on mother

    e. Maternal support system

    f. Previous and current maternal infections and sexually transmitted diseases

    g. Any preexisting maternal health condition (such as breast surgery, thyroid dysfunction, polycystic ovary syndrome)

    h. Previous and current maternal use and abuse of tobacco, alcohol, and drugs (illicit, prescription, or over-the-counter)

    i. Difficult labor/delivery, cesarean section, or all

    j. Fetal distress

    k. Preterm infant or multiple births

    l. Hospitalized or special needs infant, or both

    m. Infant with oral motor dysfunction

    n. Infant with poor latching-on

    o. Maternal complaints of pain

      (1) Nipple

      (2) Breast

      (3) Related to incision, episiotomy, or position

2. Physical findings
   a. Inspect nipples for the following changes (when edge of areola is compressed at opposite sides) (Huggins, 2005):
      (1) Protracted: protrude slightly at rest; when stimulated, become erect and are easy for infant to grasp
      (2) Flat: may be more difficult for infant to grasp and are unchanged or retract with compression of areola
      (3) Inverted: are rare; retract at rest as well as when areola is compressed
      (4) Traumatized: are cracked, blistered, fissured, or bleeding; are painful when infant nurses; mother is at greater risk for breast infection (mastitis)
   b. Inspect breast for the following:
      (1) Previous surgery
         (a) Augmentation: patient has the ability to breastfeed as long as milk ducts have not been severed (need to consult with surgeon about specific procedure performed; mother with poor milk production might benefit from supplemental lactation device)
         (b) Reduction: variable lactation success and depends on extent of tissue removed; if nipple has been relocated, ducts usually have been severed (check with surgeon); patient might need supplemental lactation device (Marasco & West, 2005)
         (c) Previous surgery for removal of cysts or lumps: incisions that could disrupt milk ducts
         (d) Single mastectomy: infant can feed from remaining breast
      (2) Size and condition of breast
         (a) Asymmetry of breasts is not uncommon; severe difference in size might indicate reduced milk glands in smaller breast.
         (b) Size of breast not related to ability to produce milk
         (c) Fibrocystic breasts
            [i] Might go into remission during lactation
            [ii] Might improve with decrease in caffeine intake
            [iii] Hand expression of milk might be uncomfortable in fibrocystic breasts, but mechanical pumping is effective.
         (d) Engorgement
            [i] Breasts are tender, swollen, firm, and warm to the touch.
            [ii] Mother might have fever; indicator of inadequate removal of milk from the breast
            [iii] Typically occurs 2 to 4 days postpartum
            [iv] Hand or mechanical expression for a few minutes prior to latch-on will soften the areola and improve latch-on
            [v] Frequent breastfeeding and ice packs might alleviate condition.
            [vi] Prevention is achieved with frequent, effective breastfeeding.
         (e) Plugged duct: blocked milk duct; might have palpable lump and localized tenderness, swelling, and redness in area; warm compresses or shower before frequent breastfeeding might help alleviate condition
         (f) Breast infection or mastitis
            [i] Might be associated with milk stasis and unresolved plugged duct, cracked nipple, or both
            [ii] Mother might have more severe symptoms similar to those of influenza (fever, chills, joint pain, and headache).
            [iii] Stress and fatigue of the mother may increase suceptibility.
            [iv] Usually only one breast with localized redness is involved.
            [v] Heat to the breast before frequent feedings, pumping following feedings, and rest for the mother may alleviate condition.
            [vi] Antibiotic therapy might be required (Huggins, 2005).
   c. Observe maternal positioning of infant; four positions are possible.
      (1) Cradle-hold position
      (2) Cross-cradle hold position
      (3) Football-hold position
      (4) Side-lying position

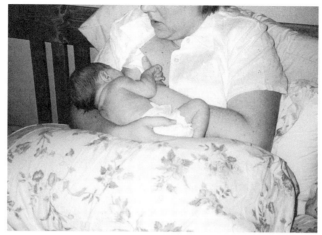

FIGURE 14-3 ■ Cradle-hold position. (Courtesy Susan Saffer Orr, Long Beach, CA.)

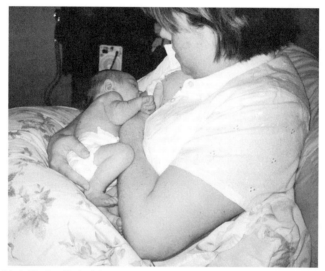

FIGURE 14-4 ■ Cradle-hold position. (Courtesy Susan Saffer Orr, Long Beach, CA.)

    d. Observe suckling infant.
      (1) Check placement of lips, gums, and tongue.
      (2) Listen for infant's swallowing pattern.
      (3) Observe shape of nipple immediately after infant is removed from the breast.
C. Interventions/Outcomes
  1. Positioning the infant
    a. Mother needs to be in a relaxed position as she supports her infant.
      (1) Infant must grasp the breast behind the nipple and keep the nipple drawn to the back of the mouth
      (2) Combination of proper positioning of infant, correct hand position on breast, and correct latching-on prevents or decreases incidence of sore nipples.
      (3) When choosing a position for breastfeeding, first ensure that mother is comfortable and well supported.
      (4) Pillows can be used to further suppport the mother's arm.
        (a) Cradle-hold position (Figures 14-3 and 14-4)
          [i] Infant's head is held in the crook of mother's elbow (lower ear positioned on the bend of mother's elbow).
          [ii] Infant and mother should be tummy to tummy with infant's bottom shoulder tucked in slightly closer to the mother's stomach than the top shoulder.

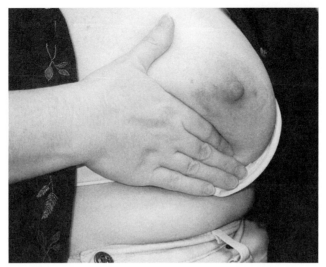

FIGURE 14-5 ■ Hand placement for cradle hold. (Courtesy Susan Saffer Orr, Long Beach, CA.)

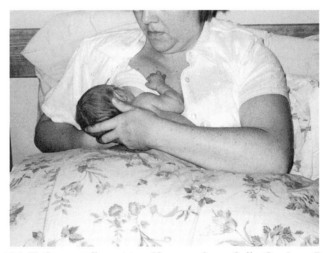

FIGURE 14-6 ■ Cross-cradle position. (Courtesy Susan Saffer Orr, Long Beach, CA.)

      [iii] Grasp infant's bottom with hand, and tuck infant's lower arm next to mother's stomach.

      [iv] Support breast with opposite hand, fingers behind areola, index finger under breast; lift up under breast until nipple is directly in front of infant's mouth; continue to support breast during the early weeks of feeding (Figure 14-5).

      [v] Bring infant to breast with pressure at the infant's upper back; do not push breast into infant; infant's chin should be positioned first and deepest into the breast.

  (b) Cross-cradle hold offers the mother more control over the infant's head position (Figures 14-6 and 14-7).

      [i] Place infant across mother's stomach similar to the cradle hold described previously.

      [ii] Hold the infant with the opposite hand, placing mother's hand at the infant's upper back, supporting the back of his or her neck.

      [iii] The infant's body is held close to mother by tucking her forearm around the infant's bottom and pulling the infant close.

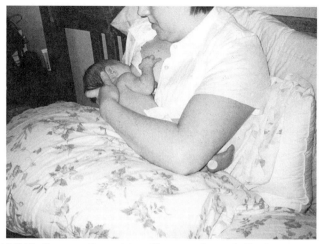

FIGURE 14-7 ■ Cross-cradle position. (Courtesy Susan Saffer Orr, Long Beach, CA.)

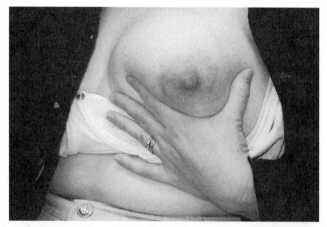

FIGURE 14-8 ■ Hand placement for cross-cradle hold. (Courtesy Susan Saffer Orr, Long Beach, CA.)

[iv] The hand that is supporting the breast is positioned in a "V" shape with the thumb and index finger coming up from the bottom of the breast; the nipple should gently tip toward the infant's mouth (Figure 14-8).

[v] Once the infant has a wide, open mouth, he or she can be brought on to the breast by pressure at the infant's upper back. The infant's chin should be posititioned first and deepest into the breast, resting well behind the nipple.

(c) Football-hold or clutch position offers good control of infant and may be helpful after cesarean birth or with a premature infant (Figure 14-9).

[i] Place infant on pillow at mother's side.

[ii] Have mother support infant's upper back with arm and support infant's neck in hand.

[iii] Have infant's head level with the breast.

[iv] Have mother use opposite hand to support breast, fingers off areola with index finger under breast; palm should remain facing the mother's rib cage; nipple should gently tip down toward infant's mouth (Figure 14-10).

(d) Side-lying position (Figure 14-11)

[i] Mother needs to be well supported in a side-lying position.

[ii] Place infant on side, facing mother's abdomen.

[iii] Have mother support breast with opposite hand.

[iv] Infant should be pulled into breast with pressure at the infant's upper back.

[v] Infant's chin should be positioned deep into breast.

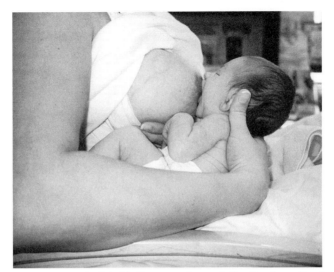

FIGURE 14-9 ■ Football-hold. (Courtesy Susan Saffer Orr, Long Beach, CA.)

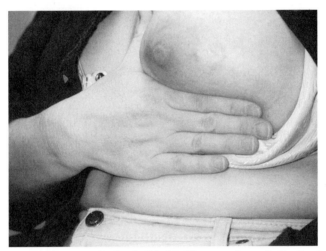

FIGURE 14-10 ■ Hand placement for football-hold. (Courtesy Susan Saffer Orr, Long Beach, CA.)

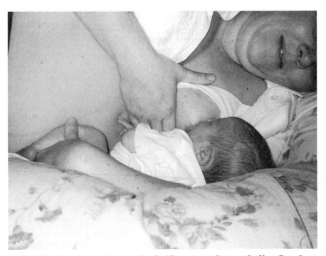

FIGURE 14-11 ■ Side-lying position in bed. (Courtesy Susan Saffer Orr, Long Beach, CA.)

     b. Outcomes

       (1) Mother reports absence of shoulder, neck, or back pain.

       (2) Mother reports absence of nipple pain.

       (3) Nipple protrudes evenly following the feeding and shows no evidence of trauma.

       (4) Mother appears relaxed and verbalizes confidence with positioning infant.

       (5) Infant remains attached to breast.

2. Latching-on problems due to flat or inverted nipples, nipple confusion, or both

     a. Correct placement of the infant's mouth behind the nipple ensures good stimulation for milk supply, promotes good milk transfer to the infant, and decreases or prevents sore nipples.

       (1) Have mother stroke (from superior to inferior in direction) the center of the infant's lip with nipple.

       (2) Allow mouth to open wide, and center breast in mouth.

       (3) Have mother pull infant in close (pull infant in with pressure on infant's upper back or neck), place lower gum well behind nipple with lips flanged; chin is positioned deep into breast.

       (4) Mother can remove infant from breast by breaking the suction: insert a clean finger gently into the corner of infant's mouth, between infant's gums.

     b. Outcomes

       (1) Infant's mouth is opened wide; lips are not tucked or curled.

       (2) Infant's gums are placed behind nipple on areola.

       (3) Tongue is positioned under breast.

       (4) Infant demonstrates burst of suckling.

       (5) Few or no complaints of sore nipples occur.

       (6) Infant does not slip off breast.

     c. Interventions for flat or inverted nipples

       (1) Have patient obtain prenatal breastfeeding education on correct latch-on techniques.

       (2) Have patient place her thumbs on either side of the areola and gently stretch the areola (Hoffman's exercise); thumbs should be rotated around edge of areola to stretch all areas; Hoffman's exercise can be performed several times per day (Amarasena, 2006).

       (3) Have mother apply ice to nipple a few minutes before feeding to increase nipple erection.

       (4) Have mother use breast pump for a few minutes before latch-on to increase nipple protrusion.

       (5) Silicone nipple shields can be used to assist in feeding only if all other interventions have failed and the mother has a good milk supply.

         (a) The mother must be followed closely (best if by a lactation specialist) to ensure that the infant is getting adequate nutrition (Meier et al, 2000).

         (b) A mother who is using a nipple shield may need to pump in addition to breastfeeding to compensate for the reduced stimulation to the breast that occurs when using a nipple shield until her milk supply is well established and infant has demonstrated the ability to transfer adequate amounts of milk.

       (6) Outcomes

         (a) Improved ability of infant to grasp nipple

         (b) Few or no complaints of sore nipples

         (c) Signs of effective breastfeeding observed

     d. Nipple confusion

       (1) Associated with infant having been fed supplements from rubber nipples

       (2) Placement and action of feeding from rubber nipples require the tongue to be up and back

       (3) Infant does not need to use the tongue to hold the artificial nipple in the mouth; when suckling at the breast, the tongue thrusts forward over the lower gum to grasp the nipple and pulls the nipple into the mouth, the lips flange around the areola, and the gums compress the milk sinuses; the tongue then creates a wavelike backward motion to extract milk.

       (4) Have mother avoid using rubber nipples during the first 4 weeks.

       (5) Have mother use a supplemental lactation device if additional fluids are medically necessary.

(6) Place infant skin to skin on mother's chest to identify early feeding cues.

(7) Encourage frequent feedings (every 2 to 3 hours) for practice.

(8) Have mother begin regular pumping to maintain or increase her milk supply if the infant is not breastfeeding adequately.

(9) Outcomes

    (a) Infant accepts breast without pulling away and swallows are heard during the breastfeeding period.

    (b) Milk supply is adequate.

    (c) Infant weight gain is appropriate.

    (d) There is little or no nipple pain.

e. Anxiety with initial feeding due to mother's inexperience

  (1) Evaluate maternal discomfort and institute relief measures (medicate if indicated) for source of pain (incision, episiotomy, or uterus).

  (2) Place infant skin-to-skin on mother's chest as soon as possible after delivery (Anderson et al, 2003).

  (3) Position mother for comfort and provide back, neck, and arm support according to choice of position.

  (4) Initiate correct latching-on and positioning.

  (5) Reassure mother if infant appears disinterested.

    (a) Some newborns are not immediately ready to nurse.

    (b) Encourage her to snuggle, hold, and enjoy her infant instead.

    (c) Skin-to-skin contact in darkened, quiet room may enhance breastfeeding interest in the infant.

  (6) Encourage frequent trials at the breast to enhance practice and confidence.

  (7) Support and encourage mother to verbalize any feelings of disappointment, rejection, or unmet expectations related to initial feeding.

  (8) Educate mother on size of the infant's stomach capacity in the first days of life.

    (a) Infant's stomach holds approximately 5 to 7 mL of fluid on the first day of life and then increases to approximately 22 to 27 mL on the following days.

    (b) It is believed that an infant's stomach does not reach its full capacity until the second week of life (Mohrbacher, 2008).

  (9) Outcomes

    (a) There is an increase in length of time the infant nurses at breast with both breasts being offered; breastfeeding sessions might last 30 to 60 minutes.

    (b) There are frequent feedings; most infants nurse between 8 and 12 times a day during the first month.

    (c) Patient states that she has little or no nipple pain.

    (d) Infant weight gain is appropriate.

    (e) Patient verbalizes confidence; increased breastfeeding skill is observed.

f. Nipple or breast pain because of nipple trauma, engorgement, plugged ducts, mastitis, or all of these conditions

  (1) Sore nipples

    (a) Nipple tenderness is usually associated with breastfeeding incorrectly.

    (b) Contributing factors are:

      [i] Waiting too long between feedings, poor positioning, poor latching-on, or sucking dysfunction

      [ii] Limiting length of feeding times does not prevent sore nipples.

      [iii] Infant thrush might be a cause of nipple soreness if the infant is older than 1 week.

    (c) Inspect nipple tissue for redness, fissures, or blisters.

    (d) Have mother apply ice to nipple immediately before feeding to allow easier grasping of nipple and to produce a numbing effect.

    (e) Application of moist heat to the breast for 10 minutes before feeding encourages milk flow.

    (f) Have mother hand express a few drops of milk before feeding so that infant does not need to nurse as vigorously.

    (g) Have mother pump for 2 to 3 minutes before latching-on to increase nipple protrusion.

(h) Have mother change positions with each feeding so that area of tissue breakdown does not undergo repeated mechanical trauma. The football-hold position may be helpful in encouraging infant to achieve deep latch-on.

(i) Check correct positioning of infant.

(j) Check latching-on and placement of tongue, lips, and gums (tongue under nipple, gums well behind nipple, chin deep into the breast, and lips flared out on the breast).

(k) Correct and prevent engorgement.

(l) Offer patient a mild analgesic 30 to 45 minutes before feeding (if indicated).

(m) Have mother use only cotton breast pads; plastic-lined breast pads retain moisture and paper pads might stick to irritated nipple.

(n) Discontinue use of soap; rinse breast with water.

(o) Have the patient discontinue feeding before she falls asleep.

(p) Do not use lanolin if patient is allergic to wool. Non-lanolin breast creams or hydrogel pads may be soothing to nipples.

(q) Short (10-minute) and more frequent feedings (every 1½ to 2 hours) might be helpful; emphasize importance of active suckling to discourage infant from pacifying at the breast with a sore nipple.

(r) Detach infant by breaking suction with finger.

(s) After feeding, apply a few drops of breast milk to nipple and let dry. Breast milk is very healing unless thrush is noted on the infant's tongue and cheeks. Thrush (yeast infection) appears as a white coating on the tongue or the mucous membranes of the cheeks.

(t) Instruct patient to keep nursing bra flaps down to allow air to reach nipple between feedings (wearing breast shells with multiple holes for good airflow will also keep fabric away from the nipple when bra flaps are closed).

(2) Outcomes

(a) Nipple pain is decreased.

(b) Nipple area decreases in redness, cracking, bleeding, blisters, or fissures.

(3) Pain from engorgement

(a) As breasts start to change from production of colostrum to mature milk, the breasts might swell. A normal fullness is expected in the first days of breastfeeding, but engorgement is generally an exaggerated response related to one of the following: rigid feeding schedules, delayed first feeding, use of supplements, limited time at each feeding, and ineffective infant suckle; the breasts are painful, swollen, and firm and the nipple is difficult for the infant to grasp because of areolar fullness.

[i] Encourage early feedings.

[ii] Encourage frequent feedings: at least every 2 to 3 hours; continue feeding until the infant cannot be persuaded to eat any longer.

[iii] Instruct mother to listen to the infant's swallows (a soft exhalation sound) and promote active swallowing during a feeding; infant should be skin-to-skin with mother to enhance alertness; mother might need to take the infant off the breast, reawake, and relatch several times.

[iv] Discourage or discontinue use of supplements unless medically indicated.

[v] Administer a mild analgesic 30 minutes before feeding, if indicated.

[vi] Instruct mother to apply warm compress to breast (for 10 minutes) or offer a shower before feeding if breast is leaking. Prolonged heat may increase swelling of tissues (Lawrence & Lawrence, 2005).

[vii] Instruct mother in gentle massage of her breast to encourage let-down and soften areolar tissue.

[viii] Encourage and instruct in use of breast pump to soften areolar tissue (CAUTION: excessive pumping can aggravate the problem).

[ix] Apply ice packs to breast for 10 to 15 minutes after feedings.

[x] Instruct patient to wear breast shells between feedings to prevent areolar swelling.

(4) Outcomes

(a) There is decreased pain, swelling, and tenderness within 12 to 24 hours.

(b) Areolar tissue softens, and nipple is easier for infant to grasp.

(c) Swallows can be heard while infant nurses.

(5) Plugged ducts: A decrease in the flow of milk results in a localized obstruction; area might be palpable and reddened.
    (a) Administer a mild analgesic as indicated.
    (b) Apply a warm compress to breast; have mother soak in a warm bath or shower before feeding.
    (c) Have infant feed at involved breast first.
    (d) Position infant's nose or chin in line with palpable lump.
    (e) Ensure frequent feedings (every 2 to 3 hours) and encourage infant to suckle actively as long as possible.
    (f) Avoid supplementary bottles or pacifier use until plug is resolved.
    (g) Suggest pumping, which might be necessary if infant is ill or reluctant to nurse.
    (h) Caution mother to check that her bra is not too tight or to determine if underwires are contributing to the problem.
    (i) Encourage mother to increase fluid intake.
(6) Outcomes
    (a) Decrease in pain, tenderness, and swelling
    (b) Resolution of palpable lump
(7) Mastitis: Reddened and painful area of the breast is accompanied by any or all of the following: fever, symptoms similar to those of influenza, joint pain, headache, and nausea.
    (a) Encourage bedrest for 24 to 48 hours.
    (b) Administer antibiotics as indicated/ordered (usually if starting to resolve within 24 hours).
    (c) Increase fluid intake and ensure adequate nutrition.
    (d) Administer an analgesic as indicated.
    (e) Evaluate hygiene and encourage good handwashing.
    (f) Reassure mother that she can continue breastfeeding.
    (g) Apply warm compress to breast or have mother take warm bath or shower before feeding.
    (h) Encourage frequent feedings (at least every 2 to 3 hours); encourage prolonged active suckling and swallowing in the infant.
    (i) Vary infant's position at the breast.
    (j) Express milk with pump or hand if infant does not empty breast.
(8) Outcomes
    (a) Pain, swelling, and tenderness decrease.
    (b) Fever decreases.
    (c) Inflammation and infection process resolve.

g. Anxiety about ability to breastfeed an infant of a cesarean section, irritable or fussy infant, sleepy or reluctant infant, infant with physiologic jaundice, preterm or hospitalized infant, multiple-birth infants, or special-needs infant.
  (1) Interventions for infant of a cesarean section
    (a) Reassure women who have undergone cesarean sections that they can and do breastfeed as successfully as women who have delivered vaginally.
    (b) Medicate 30 to 45 minutes before feedings to minimize transmission of medication in milk to infant (Hale & Burns, 2002).
    (c) Encourage mobility and self-care for mother.
    (d) Position infant in football-hold to avoid incision discomforts or help mother into side-lying position.
    (e) Encourage night feedings to increase milk supply and decrease engorgement.
    (f) Encourage good nutrition as essential for healing needs.
    (g) Encourage frequent rest periods for mother.
    (h) Encourage mother to obtain help for home responsibilities.
    (i) Allow expressions of any feelings of disappointment.
  (2) Outcomes
    (a) Patient demonstrates ability to latch and feed her infant independently.
    (b) Patient demonstrates increasing competence with self-care and asks for assistance as needed.
    (c) Patient demonstrates knowledge of nutritional needs by diet choices.
    (d) Patient verbalizes confidence with breastfeeding ability.
    (e) Patient has a plan for assistance if needed at discharge.

(3) Interventions for sleepy or reluctant infant: Infant is difficult to awaken, loses interest quickly, and does not feed vigorously.
    (a) Wake infant after 2 to 3 hours during daytime and after 4 to 5 hours at night.
    (b) Encourage at least eight feedings per 24 hours.
    (c) Place infant in skin-to-skin position with mother to increase infant's interest in feeding (Anderson et al, 2003).
    (d) Use arousing techniques: unwrap blankets, undress infant, change diapers, burp frequently; lay sleepy infant down on firm surface, naked, to stretch and arouse for next breast.
    (e) Place drops of sterile water on infant's lips to alert infant.
    (f) Avoid use of rubber nipple and pacifiers.
    (g) Encourage rooming-in so that when infant is awake, mother is available.
    (h) Have mother reduce stimulation to infant, and limit visitors between feedings (overstimulated infants frequently shut down and will not arouse to feed well).
(4) Outcomes
    (a) Interest and time spent at breast increase.
    (b) Infant swallows heard while breastfeeding becomes more frequent.
    (c) Infant weight gain follows expected curve.
    (d) Maternal confidence in meeting infant needs increases.
(5) Interventions for a fussy or irritable infant: Infant might have strong sucking need, might become frantic when beginning feeding, or might want to breastfeed more often than every 2 hours.
    (a) Assess infant's feeding technique to ensure that infant is actively swallowing and nutritional needs are met.
    (b) Use slow, gentle movements.
    (c) Provide a quiet environment (e.g., quiet music, dim lights, rocking chair, cradle).
    (d) Reduce visitors and activity in household.
    (e) Use infant massage and skin-to-skin contact.
    (f) Use soft, cloth infant carriers.
    (g) Follow infant's preference for swaddling.
    (h) Burp infant frequently (might swallow air when fussing).
    (i) Allow infant's nonnutritive sucking needs to be met with sucking of own fingers or pacifier if infant has good weight gain and good latch-on skills.
    (j) Have mother keep diet history (irritable behavior might be associated with an offending food, although this is not as common as once thought); excessive intake of acidic foods bothers some infants.
    (k) Eliminate caffeine and nicotine.
    (l) Avoid using supplements with rubber nipples; this will reinforce impatience and increase the risk of nipple confusion.
    (m) If infant gulps or chokes at breast, have mother pump for 2 to 3 minutes before latch-on to reduce overactive initial let-down; hyperlactation syndrome can be treated in the long term by having the infant nurse on one breast per feeding; reducing the amount of foremilk received on both breasts can reduce fussiness due to fast let-down with increased air swallowing.
    (n) Educate mother on normal infant behavior and normal fussiness.
(6) Outcomes
    (a) Irritability and fussiness decrease.
    (b) Awareness of mother to infant cues increases.
    (c) Mother demonstrates confidence in responding to infant's needs.
(7) Interventions for physiologic jaundice; healthy newborn might show signs of physiologic jaundice (increased bilirubin values, yellowing of the skin, and sclera) on the second or third day of life (see Chapter 17 for complete discussion); bilirubin can be reabsorbed in the intestines; frequent breastfeeding promotes increased bowel movements and decreased reabsorption (Mannel et al, 2008).
    (a) Encourage frequent feedings (every 2 to 3 hours), with a minimum 8 to 10 feedings per day.
    (b) Encourage skin-to-skin contact to enhance infant's interest in nursing.
    (c) Have mother use techniques to arouse infant if he or she is sleepy or uninterested (undress infant, switch positions frequently).

      (d) Discourage use of rubber nipples for supplements (might cause increased nipple confusion, might decrease interest in breastfeeding, and might decrease the number of infant stools); discontinue use of a pacifier, which might reduce infant's willingness to eat. If supplementation is required, consider use of supplemental lactation device. Encourage pumping to maintain or increase milk supply.

      (e) Encourage/consider use of phototherapy in mother's hospital room and/or home phototherapy.

      (f) Encourage mother to verbalize concerns.

  (8) Outcomes

      (a) There is a decrease in bilirubin levels.

      (b) There is an increase in infant's interest in feedings.

  (9) Interventions for breastfeeding a preterm or hospitalized infant

      (a) Can be an overwhelming experience for most parents; the concern about immediate needs, financial costs, and long-term outcomes is of most importance; the immunologic advantages, nutritional components, and digestibility of breast milk are of great value to a preterm or hospitalized infant; preterm infants who receive breast milk tend to have shorter hospital stays (Academy of Breastfeeding Medicine, 2004).

      (b) Encourage and praise patient's decision to breastfeed.

      (c) Provide an electric breast pump while infant is hospitalized (with attachment kit to pump both breasts simultaneously), and instruct in use and cleaning. Begin pumping as soon as possible.

      (d) Have mother use relaxation techniques, use warm compresses, massage breasts, and visualize (or gaze at a picture of) her infant before beginning to pump.

      (e) Provide mother with time to touch infant before pumping: as infant's condition improves and stabilizes, just holding the infant helps with let-down.

      (f) Pump at least 8 to 10 times daily (with a minimum of 10 to 15 minutes for each breast); pump at least once during the night (a pump that can be used on both breasts at once is especially helpful when long-term pumping is necessary) (Hill, Aldag, & Chatterton, 2001).

      (g) Provide mother with written instructions for pumping, milk collection, and storage at discharge.

      (h) Encourage mother to bring pumped milk to the hospital to be used for infant feedings when infant is ready to eat.

      (i) Provide referral for electric pump rental or purchase on discharge.

      (j) Give mother instructions to rest, drink fluids, and maintain adequate nutrition.

      (k) Refer mother to lactation specialist or consultant when necessary for help with immature suck reflex or nipple confusion when infant is put to breast.

      (l) Use supplemental lactation device to increase caloric volume without using rubber nipple (Figure 14-12) (Hill, Ledbetter, & Kavanaugh, 2006).

 (10) Outcomes

      (a) Volume of collected breast milk is increasing.

      (b) Patient expresses increasing confidence and skill when infant is put to breast.

      (c) There is a successful transition of infant to complete breastfeeding.

 (11) Interventions for multiple births

      (a) The patient might have to cope with the challenges of a cesarean section, preterm infants, and providing for long-term follow-up of more than one newborn; breastfeeding can reduce feeding and medical costs and assist in bonding with and meeting the individual needs of each infant.

      (b) Reassure mother that milk supply is determined by milk demand and that the supply adjusts to infant's demands.

      (c) Instruct patient in using "round robin" technique to feed sleepy babies in first weeks (i.e., put one infant to the breast until swallows slow down or stop, then have helper burp and arouse that infant while the mother nurses the other infant; mother continues to switch infants until both are completely fed, changed, and burped, thus making feeding time more efficient).

      (d) Assist patient with positioning of two infants (both in cradle position, legs crossing; both in football position; or one in football position and one in cradle position); breastfeeding infants simultaneously might not be possible in early weeks, but as infants improve latch-on skills, this will become easier.

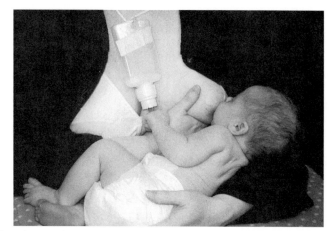

FIGURE 14-12 ■ Supplemental nursing system by Medela, Inc., McHenry, IL. (Courtesy Susan Saffer Orr, Long Beach, CA.)

    (e) Assist patient in anticipatory planning for rest and nutritional needs.
    (f) Provide patient with a referral to a local chapter of Mothers of Twins or Mothers of Multiples.
    (g) Encourage patient to feed infants concurrently to help her get needed rest.
    (h) Provide mother with referral to lactation specialist if breastfeeding problems persist.
  (12) Outcomes
    (a) Patient reports satisfaction with breastfeeding.
    (b) Infant's weight follows growth curve.
  (13) Interventions for a special-needs infant
    (a) When a family's dream of having a so-called perfect infant does not materialize, a period of grieving is appropriate and expected; breastfeeding enhances the bond between mother and child; providing breast milk might increase a mother's ability to nurture and comfort her infant as well as provide ideal nutrition for the infant.
    (b) Encourage and listen to patient's feelings of disappointment, disbelief, and anger.
    (c) Provide flexibility in hospital routine for family support.
    (d) Provide information for support groups specific to disability (e.g., cleft palate, Down syndrome, spina bifida).
    (e) Initiate a collaborative plan, and include a lactation specialist or consultant, occupational therapist, physical therapist, and any other pertinent health care providers to provide consistent, optimal care for specific maternal and infant needs.
    (f) Provide breast pump information as needed for infants with reduced feeding capability (see breastfeeding discussion of preterm infants).
  (14) Outcomes
    (a) Patient has realistic approach to infant's ability to breastfeed and to maternal time and effort needed to explore alternatives (e.g., long-term pumping and/or supplemental nursing device).
    (b) Patient expresses increasing acceptance and understanding of infant's disability.
    (c) Mother expresses increasing confidence and ability with breastfeeding skills.
    (d) Infant demonstrates acceptable growth for condition.
h. Adequate milk supply
  (1) Interventions related to milk supply
    (a) The amount of breast milk produced is related to the demand put on the breast by a suckling infant or to a lesser degree by a breast pump; supply is affected by multiple factors such as inadequate transfer of milk out of the breast by ineffective suckling by the infant, infrequent or shortened feedings, maternal fatigue and/or depression, low thyroid function in the mother, retained placenta, previous surgical history of the breast, or inadequate glandular development of the breast.
    (b) Ensure sufficient stimulation with frequent feedings (every 2 to 3 hours, with a minimum of 10 to 15 minutes of effective suckling/swallowing at each breast).

    (c) Encourage rooming-in.

    (d) Evaluate for any missed or supplemented feedings.

    (e) Wake infant if asleep longer than 3 hours.

    (f) Avoid use of pacifier.

    (g) Use lactation supplemental device if it is medically indicated that infant requires additional calories.

    (h) Evaluate for poor latching-on.

    (i) Listen for infant swallowing, and keep infant aroused at breast.

    (j) Follow feeding with 10 to 15 minutes of pumping with a double electric pump to further increase stimulation to the breast.

    (k) Ensure adequate maternal fluid intake of 1920 mL (2 quarts) daily.

    (l) Evaluate maternal activity level, and encourage rest.

    (m) Consider underlying maternal health condition if poor milk supply continues.

    (n) Refer to lactation specialist.

  (2) Outcomes

    (a) Mother hears consistent infant swallows during breastfeeding.

    (b) Infant younger than 1 month has minimum of one stool per day.

    (c) There are six to eight wet diapers a day.

    (d) Infant has regular patterns of wakefulness, sleep, and feeding.

    (e) Infant's weight loss is not more than 5% to 10% during the first week.

    (f) Infant's weight follows a normal growth curve.

 i. Intake and nutritional demands during lactation

  (1) Interventions

    (a) Nutrition: A wide selection of foods can be offered, according to a mother's individual tastes and preferences.

      [i] Any food, in moderation, can be part of a diet during lactation unless intolerance is noted by the infant.

      [ii] Dairy products, soy, and peanuts have been found to bother some infants.

      [iii] The recommended caloric intake for the size of the mother plus 300 to 500 additional calories are frequently recommended during lactation.

      [iv] It takes an average of 940 calories to produce milk; fat stores from pregnancy help provide some of these additional calories.

      [v] The mother should be encouraged to take adequate liquids to keep her urine pale (drinking more fluids does not increase the milk volume).

      [vi] Servings from all food groups are to be encouraged: protein, three or four; dairy, four to six; fruit, four; grains, four; vegetables, four (Anderson et al, 2003; Mannel et al, 2008).

    (b) Alcohol

      [i] Alcohol passes readily into milk.

      [ii] Even moderate amounts of alcohol might slow brain growth in the infant and inhibit let-down.

      [iii] Occasional intake of one serving of alcohol probably does not constitute considerable danger.

    (c) Drugs and medications

      [i] Several factors affect excretion of maternal medications in breast milk (solubility, route of administration, accumulation of substance, oral bioavailability of medication, duration of use, weight of infant, and amount and number of times infant breastfeeds).

      [ii] For specific prescription and over-the-counter medications see Hale (2008).

    (d) Tobacco

      [i] Smoking 20 cigarettes/day or more might cause nausea and vomiting in the infant and cause decrease in milk supply.

      [ii] Breast milk of smoking mothers has lower level of vitamin C.

      [iii] Any infant exposure to secondhand smoke is detrimental.

      [iv] Parents should not allow smoking when infant is present

    (e) Caffeine

      [i] Might be taken in moderate amounts

[ii] Infants who are frequently colicky, wakeful, or hyperactive might be consuming excessive amounts of caffeine in their breast milk, and maternal consumption of caffeine should be decreased or stopped (Hale, 2008).
- (f) Review dietary choices.
- (g) Provide consultation with a dietitian as needed.
- (h) Offer sample menus.
- (i) Plan menus according to cultural or religious preferences.
- (j) Inform mother of Women, Infants, and Children (WIC) program, a supplemental food and nutritional counseling program for pregnant, postpartum, and lactating mothers with children (pending income and risk qualifications).
- (k) Eliminate foods suspected of aggravating colic, and evaluate effect by keeping a food intake and infant behavior diary.
- (l) Encourage decrease in or elimination of maternal use of tobacco; eliminate infant's exposure to secondhand smoke.
- (m) Discourage moderate to excessive alcohol intake.
- (n) Identify medications that are compatible with breastfeeding.
- (2) Outcomes
  - (a) Mother makes good dietary choices from menu, and maintains an adequate level of fluids.
  - (b) There is an increase in maternal energy levels.
  - (c) There is adequate healing of episiotomy or other incisions.
  - (d) Patient has adequate milk supply.
  - (e) There is a decrease in or elimination of tobacco use.
  - (f) Alcohol intake is limited to one to two servings maximum per week.
  - (g) Mother may continue breastfeeding while taking needed medication.
- j. Role change and sexual identity as a lactating mother
  - (1) Interventions related to sexuality
    - (a) New parents need time to adjust to each other sexually after the birth of their child; time schedules, fatigue, responsibilities, and role changes are all factors that might affect sexual desires and needs.
    - (b) Allow patient to express her concerns and feelings.
    - (c) Use of a water-soluble lubricant might be helpful for decreased vaginal lubrication related to lowered estrogen levels during lactation.
    - (d) Reassure patient that many women notice a let-down reflex during orgasm.
    - (e) Reassure patient that some women find their breasts are very sensitive while lactating; reassure her that an erotic response to breastfeeding can occur and has no particular significance.
    - (f) Reassure her that some women feel overwhelmed by partner's touch after caring for an infant all day.
    - (g) Encourage parents to find time for themselves as a couple.
    - (h) Reaffirm that menstruation might be delayed during lactation, but pregnancy can still occur.
  - (2) Provide patient with information on methods of contraception.
  - (3) Outcomes
    - (a) Parents express realistic expectations for coping with individual sexual needs.
    - (b) Parents have a plan for contraception if an immediate pregnancy is not desired.

HEALTH EDUCATION

A. **The health care provider can offer educational assistance about the following topics through written materials, audiovisual materials, and individual or group instruction.**
   1. Preparation for breastfeeding
      a. Normal physiology
      b. Correction of flat or inverted nipples
      c. Production of milk

    d. Let-down (milk ejection reflex)
    e. Stages of human milk
2. Initial feeding
    a. Correct positioning
    b. Correct latching-on
3. Correction and prevention of common breastfeeding problems
    a. Sore nipples
    b. Engorgement
    c. Plugged ducts
    d. Mastitis
    e. Building and maintaining a milk supply
4. Typical newborn behavior related to feeding in early weeks
5. Resource and referral information available for special situations
    a. Cesarean birth
    b. Irritable or fussy infant
    c. Sleepy or reluctant infant
    d. Infant with physiologic jaundice
    e. Preterm or hospitalized infant
    f. Infants of a multiple birth
    g. Special-needs infant
6. Nutritional guidelines for lactation
7. Sexuality and contraception during lactation

CASE STUDY AND STUDY QUESTIONS

Mrs. M. is a 27-year-old gravida 2, para 1 (G2, P1) woman. She had an uncomplicated spontaneous vaginal delivery at 39 weeks' gestation, and her daughter weighed 3629 g (8 pounds) with Apgar scores of 8 and 9. She had attempted to breastfeed her first daughter, but quit after 2 weeks because of cracked nipples and poor milk supply. She states, "I really want to breastfeed this infant at least 6 months."

1. What additional information is needed to help plan for her care?
    a. Previous breastfeeding experience
    b. Previous use of drugs, tobacco, and alcohol
    c. Maternal support systems
    d. Previous breast surgery
        1. a, b
        2. b, d
        3. c, d
        4. a, d
        5. All of the above
2. On physical examination you observe that Mrs. M.'s nipples are short. What would be helpful to make the nipples easier for the infant to grasp?
    a. Application of ice before feeding
    b. Use of breast shells between feedings
    c. Toughening nipples with washcloth
    d. Use of pump before feeding

    1. a, b, d
    2. a, b, c
    3. b, c, d
3. How soon after delivery should she be encouraged to attempt to breastfeed her daughter?
    a. Immediately after delivery
    b. Between 3 and 6 hours after delivery
    c. Between 6 and 12 hours after delivery
    d. At 12 hours after delivery
4. She expresses concern about how to prevent sore nipples. Which of the following is helpful?
    a. Limiting feedings to 5 minutes at each breast
    b. Checking for correct latching-on
    c. Checking for positioning of infant
    d. Using a supplemental bottle
        1. All of the above
        2. a, b, c
        3. b, c
        4. b, d
5. What initial strategy should be promoted immediately after birth and frequently during the hosptial stay?
6. List three strategies to prevent and decrease engorgement.
7. List four comfort measures to resolve engorgement.
8. List three strategies to increase milk supply.

9. What two breastfeeding aids might be helpful to a mother with a preterm or hospitalized infant?
10. Which of the following are true about a cesarean-section birth mother and breastfeeding?
    a. Usually cannot breastfeed until the fourth postpartum day
    b. Needs help positioning infant during first few days
    c. Might find football-hold position comfortable
    d. Should pump milk while taking pain medication
        1. All of the above
        2. All but a
        3. b, c
        4. a, c
        5. a, c, d

ANSWERS TO STUDY QUESTIONS

1. 5
2. 1
3. a
4. 3
5. Mother-baby skin-to-skin contact
6. Frequent feedings (every 2 to 3 hours); sufficient length feeding; effective suckling of infant; avoidance of supplements
7. Analgesia; warm compresses before feeding if breasts are leaking; hand expression/pumping to soften areolar tissue; frequent feedings (every 2 to 3 hours); sufficient length with effective suckling of infant; avoidance of supplements; application of ice after feeding
8. Frequent feedings (every 2 to 3 hours); sufficient length with effective suckling of infant; additional use of a breast pump following feedings for stimulation to the breast; adequate maternal rest
9. Electric breast pump; supplemental lactation device
10. 3

REFERENCES

Academy of Breastfeeding Medicine (2004). *Transitioning the breastfeeding/breastmilk-fed premature infant from the neonatal intensive care unit to home.* New Rochelle, NY: Academy of Breastfeeding Medicine.

Amarasena, S. (2006). *Sri Lanka Journal of Child Health,* 35: 51–54. Available at www.sljol.info/index.php/SLJCH/article/view/14/14. Accessed January 7, 2009.

Anderson, G.C., Moore, E., Hepworth, J., & Bergmans, N. (2003). *Early skin to skin contact for mothers and their healthy newborn infants.* Available at www.cochrane.org/reviews/en/ab003519.html. Accessed January 7, 2009.

Hale, T. (2008). *Medications and mother's milk* (13th ed.). Amarillo, TX: Pharmasoft Publishing.

Hale, T., & Burns, P. (2002). *Clinical therapy in breastfeeding patients,* Amarillo, TX: Pharmasoft Publishing.

Hill, P. D., Aldag, J. C., & Chatterton, R. T. (2001). Initiation and frequency of pumping and milk production in mothers of non-nursing preterm infants. *Journal of Human Lactation,* 17, 9–13.

Hill, P., Ledbetter, R., & Kavanaugh, K. N. (2006). Breastfeeding patterns of low-birth-weight infants after hospital discharge. *Journal of Obstetric, Gynecologic & Neonatal Nursing,* 26(2), 189–197.

Huggins, K. (2005). *The nursing mother's companion.* Boston: Harvard Common Press.

Lauwers, J., & Breck, S. (2004). *Counseling the nursing mother: A lactation consultant's guide.* (3rd ed.). Boston: Jones and Bartlett.

Lawrence, R. A., & Lawrence, R. M. (2005). *Breastfeeding: A guide for the medical profession* (6th ed.). Philadelphia: Mosby.

Mannel, R., Walker, M., & Martens, P. (Eds). (2008). *Core curriculum for lactation consultant practice (2nd ed.).* Boston: Jones and Bartlett.

Marasco, L., & West, D. (2005). *A breastfeeding mother's guide to making more milk.* New York: McGraw-Hill.

Meier, P., Brown, L., Hurst, N., Spatz, D., Engstrom, J., Borucki, L., & Krouse, A. (2000). Nipple shields for preterm infants: Effect on milk transfer and duration of breast-feeding. *Journal of Human Lactation,* 16(2), 106–114.

Mohrbacher, N. (2008). *Your newborn's stomach.* Available at www.ameda.com/breastfeeding/started/stomach.aspx. Accessed February 2, 2009.

Ramsay, D., Kent, J., Martman, R., & Hartman, P. (2005). Anatomy of the Lactating human breast redefined with ultrasound imaging. *Journal of Anatomy,* 206(6), 525–534.

ADDITIONAL RESOURCES

Academy of Breastfeeding Medicine, 140 Huguenot Street, 3rd floor, New Rochelle, NY 10801; www.bfmed.org.

Breastfeeding and Human Lactation Study Center, University of Rochester School of Medicine and Dentistry, Department of Pediatrics, Box 777, 601 Elmwood Avenue, Rochester, NY 14642; www.us breastfeeding.org.

International Board of Lactation Consultant Examiners (IBLCE), IBLCE International, 6402 Arlington Blvd, Suite 350, Falls Church, VA 22042; www.iblce.org.

International Lactation Consultant Association, 2501 Aerial Center Parkway, Suite 103, Morrisville, NC 27560; www.ilca.org.

La Leche League International, P.O. Box 4079, Schaumburg, IL 60168–4079; www.llli.org.

BREAST PUMPS AND RELATED SUPPLIES

Ameda Inc., 475 Half Day Road, Lincolnshire, IL 60069; 1–866-99-AMEDA. www.ameda.com.

Medela Inc. Breastfeeding U.S., 1101 Corporate Drive, McHenry, IL 60050; 1-800-435-8316; www.medelabr eastfeedingus.com/contact-us.

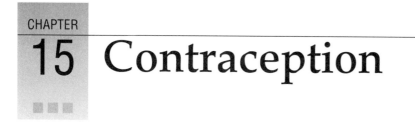

15 Contraception

Denise G. Link

OBJECTIVES

1. Describe the mechanism of action of various methods of birth control.
2. Compare the effectiveness ratings of the various methods of birth control.
3. Construct appropriate questions to use while interviewing a woman about her contraceptive history.
4. Describe the risks and benefits of each method of birth control.
5. Rank the various contraceptives in order of their appropriateness for an individual woman.
6. Explain how postpartum status affects choice of contraception.
7. Identify ethnocultural considerations that can affect the choice of contraception for a woman in postpartum status.
8. Identify social and psychologic considerations that help determine the appropriate choice of a contraceptive method after childbirth.

INTRODUCTION

Helping women and their partners make decisions about contraception is an important role for a nurse who provides care for women and families during the postpartum period. Some contraceptive methods require the participation of the woman's sexual partner, so it may be appropriate to include that person in the discussion. Short hospital stays for women after childbirth means that they and their significant family members might have limited contact with health care providers during the initial days following childbirth. If decisions are not made early in the postpartum period, couples might use contraceptive methods that are inappropriate for the postpartum period and, therefore, ineffective. Nursing practice must include assessment of the couple's contraceptive knowledge, attitudes toward contraception, plans related to future pregnancies, and the need for contraception methods.

CLINICAL PRACTICE

A. **Assessment**
   1. Contraceptive history
      a. Previous contraceptive use
         (1) Identify dissatisfaction with any of the methods.
         (2) Identify satisfaction with any of the methods.
         (3) Identify the method of choice.
         (4) Identify accuracy of knowledge base about methods used and methods rejected.
   2. Reproductive health history
      a. Previous complications associated with contraceptive use including satisfaction or dissatisfaction
      b. Health conditions that affect the choice of contraception
         (1) Hypertension
         (2) Thrombophlebitis
         (3) Diabetes
         (4) Infection
      c. Factors that affect the timing of resumption of sexual intercourse after childbirth
         (1) Operative delivery
         (2) Episiotomy/lacerations

   (3) Infection
   (4) Cultural beliefs and practices
   (5) Hemorrhage
3. Breastfeeding plans
   a. Planned length
   b. Perceived importance
   c. Previous use of contraception while breastfeeding
4. Psychosocial responses regarding contraception
   a. Attitude toward timing of resumption of sexual activities
   b. Religious or cultural views about contraception
      (1) Identify religious or cultural barriers to contraception or to the use of particular contraceptive methods.
      (2) Identify differences in beliefs or values between the woman and her partner.
      (3) Identify conflicts between a desire to avoid conception and religious or cultural values that affect choice.
   c. Attitudes about future pregnancies and their appropriate timing
   d. Motivation to avoid pregnancy
5. Contraceptive knowledge
   a. Postpartum fertility
   b. The use and effectiveness of various methods
   c. Methods of choice
   d. Partner's methods of choice
   e. Recommended physiologic minimum spacing between pregnancies for best outcome
   f. Costs of various methods
   g. Short-term versus long-term contraception
   h. Confidence in methods
B. **Interventions/Outcomes**
   1. Deficient knowledge about postpartum fertility
      a. Interventions
         (1) Explain variations in timing of the return of ovulation and menses during the postpartum period.
         (2) Explain lack of reliable effectiveness of lactation alone to prevent conception during the postpartum period.
         (3) Explain the possibility that pregnancy can occur because ovulation occurs before the resumption of menses.
      b. Outcomes
         (1) Patient states that 4 to 6 weeks after delivery is the usual time for the return of menses in the nonlactating woman.
         (2) Patient explains that breastfeeding on demand (at least six or seven times daily) without supplementing the infant's diet with formula or other food delays the resumption of ovulation and menses for some, but not all, women.
         (3) Patient acknowledges that pregnancy can occur with the first postdelivery ovulation although no menses have occurred.
         (4) Patient states an understanding of the risk of pregnancy during the postpartum period and the need to use effective contraception if pregnancy is not desired.
   2. Deficient knowledge related to proper use of contraceptive method of choice
      a. Interventions (Table 15-1)
         (1) Assess patient's knowledge of all available methods of contraception, including selected method.
         (2) Identify appropriateness and effectiveness of selected method for the postpartum period.
         (3) Describe or review proper use of the method.
         (4) Identify advantages and disadvantages of selected method.
         (5) Determine patient's access to selected method.
         (6) Review signs and symptoms of potential complications of selected method.
         (7) Outline steps the patient should take if complications occur.
         (8) Explain importance of consistent use.
         (9) After teaching, evaluate the patient's understanding of information provided, comfort with use, and confidence in selected method.

■ TABLE 15-1
■ ■ Methods of Contraception

Method	Accidental Pregnancy Rate (Typical Use in First Year)	Postpartum Use	Risks/Disadvantages	Benefits
Abstinence	0%	Is the method of choice for the first 4 to 6 weeks, especially for operative deliveries, complications, and lacerations	Might be unacceptable to patient or partner; might cause relationship problems if there is disagreement	Promotes healing and involution
Vasectomy or male sterilization	0.15%	Has no contraindications	Is permanent; requires minor surgery; risk of surgical complications	No further monitoring required after verification that all sperm in system have been ejaculated
Bilateral tubal ligation or female sterilization	0.5%	Can be performed during cesarean section; can be performed soon after vaginal delivery	Is permanent; risk of surgical complications	Requires no further monitoring
Oral contraceptives (two types: combined pill [estrogen plus progestin] and mini-pill [progestin only])	5% for each type	Might interfere with lactation by decreasing milk supply; if lactating, use mini-pill or wait until lactation is well established	Minor side effects are breast tenderness, nausea, and irregular bleeding (especially with mini-pill); women who weigh more than 155 pounds might have a slightly higher pregnancy rate on lower-dose pills; major risks are rare in women ages 35 and younger who do not smoke, but they may include deep vein thrombosis, liver tumor, cerebrovascular accident (CVA), myocardial infarction (MI), and gallbladder disease; requires regular monitoring by a health care provider	Acceptable for healthy women ages 36 to 50 years who do not smoke; menses are lighter and shorter, and there are fewer cramps; may protect against ovarian and uterine disease
Transdermal contraceptive skin patch	0.88%	Might interfere with lactation by decreasing milk supply; if lactating, wait until lactation is well established	Increased breakthrough bleeding and more breast discomfort in first two cycles than with pills; application site reactions; risk profile similar to combined pills; slightly less effective in women who weigh more than 198 pounds; ethinyl estradiol and norelgestromin	No daily pill required; improved adherence; good skin adhesion in humidity/exercise

Continued

■ TABLE 15-1
■ **Methods of Contraception—cont'd**

Method	Accidental Pregnancy Rate (Typical Use in First Year)	Postpartum Use	Risks/Disadvantages	Benefits
Vaginal ring	0.65%	Might interfere with lactation by decreasing milk supply; if lactating, wait until lactation is well established	Risk profile similar to combined pills; ethinyl estradiol and etonogestrel	Less breakthrough bleeding than with pills; good lipid profile; no fitting required; can be removed for intercourse and replaced within 3 hours
Spermicide with condom (used together)	5%	Has no contraindications	Irritation and allergic reactions are rare; must be inserted/put on just before intercourse; is messy and might decrease sensation	As effective as the pill when used together; available over-the-counter; provides protection against sexually transmitted infections
Diaphragm with spermicide	20%	Decreased levels of estrogen make the vagina thinner and drier than normal and insertion more difficult; must be refitted after a pregnancy; proper fit is not possible until involution is complete	Causes irritation, allergic reactions, and bladder irritation; must be inserted before intercourse and left in place for 6 hours; some positions might dislodge it	Not appropriate during the early postpartum period
Copper-releasing intrauterine device (IUD)	0.7%	Can be placed up to 48 hr after delivery; expulsion rates are higher in the early postpartum period	Might increase menstrual flow and cramps	Once in place, requires little monitoring by the woman; in a suitable candidate, can be placed during first menses after childbirth; approved for up to 10 years of use
Levonorgestrel intrauterine system (LNG-IUS)	0.2%	Can be placed 6 weeks after delivery; contraindicated in women with acute liver disease or tumor; active thrombophlebitis or thromboembolic disorders	Irregular periods for 3 to 6 months after insertion; 20% of women using LNG-IUS will be amenorrheic after 12 months of use	Less cramping and bleeding; once in place, requires little monitoring by the woman; for a suitable candidate, can be placed during first menses after childbirth; approved for up to 5 years of use
Spermicide alone	26%	Might cause irritation because of decreased levels of estrogen	Might cause allergic reactions; messy; inserted just before intercourse	Available over-the-counter

Method	%			
Condoms alone	14%	No contraindications in nonallergic individuals or partners	Irritation and allergic reactions are rare; might break or leak; might decrease sensation	Available over-the-counter; affords some protection against sexually transmitted infections
Female condom	21%	No contraindications	Available over-the-counter	Can be inserted up to 8 hours before intercourse
Natural family planning, fertility awareness, and periodic abstinence	24%	Requires signs and symptoms of hormone fluctuation during normal cycling; this cycling does not occur during the postpartum period, especially during lactation	No risks; requires practice and education from a trained professional; requires self-monitoring and record-keeping as well as varying periods of abstinence	Requires no devices or chemicals; might be acceptable for couples who do not wish to use other methods because of religious or other reasons
Withdrawal	19%	Has no contraindications	Requires interruption of sexual response cycle; fluid with sperm is often released before ejaculation	Requires no devices or chemicals
Progesterone implant	0.05%	Not recommended until lactation is well established; compatible with lactation	Single rod implanted under skin; inserted by health care provider; a change in bleeding pattern is common; risks similar to mini-pill; expensive	Lasts 3 years; little monitoring required after insertion
Depot medroxyprogesterone acetate	0.3%	Not recommended until lactation is well established; compatible with lactation	Requires injection every 3 months; change in bleeding pattern common; risks similar to mini-pill; weight gain averages 5 pounds/year	Progestin only; amenorrhea common; requires no monitoring between injections
EMERGENCY CONTRACEPTION				
High-dose progesterone pills	3.2%	Must be taken within 72 hours of unprotected intercourse	Nausea and vomiting; taken in two doses 12 hours apart	Effective for prevention of unintended pregnancy following unprotected intercourse
Copper-releasing IUD	1.1%	Must be placed within 5 to 7 days of unprotected intercourse	Same as for IUD with routine placement	Effective for prevention of unintended pregnancy following unprotected intercourse

Data from Hatcher, R., Trussell, J., Stewart, F., Kowal, D., Guest, F., Cates, W., & Policar, M. (2008). *Contraceptive technology* (19th ed.). New York: Irvington Publishers.

b. Outcomes
    (1) Patient explains how her method of choice is to be used.
    (2) Patient identifies advantages and disadvantages of her method.
    (3) Patient states how she plans to obtain her method of choice.
    (4) Patient identifies signs and symptoms of complications related to her method of choice.
    (5) Patient states her planned action if problems occur with her method of choice.
    (6) Patient states her understanding of the importance of consistent use of her method of choice to prevent pregnancy.
    (7) Patient states that she feels capable of comfortable use of the selected method.
3. Patient's selection of inappropriate contraceptive method following childbirth
    a. Interventions
        (1) Identify patient's level of commitment to avoiding pregnancy.
        (2) Identify patient's attitude toward contraception and her selected method.
        (3) Identify partner's acceptance of the selected method.
        (4) Review contraceptive methods to assist the patient in selecting an appropriate and perhaps tentative contraceptive method to use following childbirth.
    b. Outcomes
        (1) Patient identifies how highly she values avoiding pregnancy.
        (2) Patient describes how she feels about contraception.
        (3) Patient describes use of her selected method of contraception.
        (4) Patient describes her partner's willingness to accept use of her selected method.
4. Value differences between the woman and her partner about contraceptive choices
    a. Interventions
        (1) Discuss her feelings regarding her partner's anticipated reaction to her contraceptive plans.
        (2) Encourage discussion of contraceptive goals between the patient and her partner.
        (3) Encourage active participation of the partner in contraceptive planning.
        (4) Recognize that conflict regarding contraception between the patient and her partner can lead to increased risk of noncompliance; it can also increase the stress of adjustment during the postpartum period.
    b. Outcomes
        (1) Patient and her partner discuss contraceptive goals with each other.
        (2) Patient's partner discusses his reaction to her contraceptive plans.
        (3) Patient's partner actively participates in decisions regarding contraceptive use.
        (4) Patient and her partner identify any areas of conflict and their potentially negative effects on contraceptive use and family adjustment.

HEALTH EDUCATION

The health education component of family planning is shown in Table 15-1.

CASE STUDIES AND STUDY QUESTIONS

Ms. T., 36, delivered her first child 12 hours ago. She will be discharged after an overnight stay. Her delivery was uncomplicated, and she has no serious health problems except that her social history reveals a habit of smoking two packs of cigarettes per day. She tells you that her partner is anxious to resume sexual relations, and she plans to begin taking birth control pills immediately.

1. What additional information would you need to help her determine whether her plans to use the pill are appropriate?
    a. Her breastfeeding plans
    b. Family history of breast or uterine cancer
    c. The type of pill she used before
    d. Presence of lacerations or episiotomy
2. She tells you that she plans to breastfeed her infant for at least 1 year and that the breastfeeding experience is very important to her. What would be her *best* option in using birth control pills?
    a. Begin taking the same pill she used before pregnancy.
    b. Change to a different brand of birth control pill.
    c. Use an alternative method until lactation is well established.
    d. Use abstinence until lactation is well established.

3. Additional teaching will be planned for her based on your knowledge that:
   a. Her risk of developing serious side effects from birth control pills is greater because she is older than 35, and she smokes.
   b. It is unknown whether she is motivated to avoid an immediate pregnancy.
   c. Her delivery experience makes a minimum 6-week period of abstinence essential to avoid postdelivery complications.
   d. She is unwilling to consider other methods of contraception.
4. Which group of contraceptive methods has the highest typical use effectiveness rates?
   a. Intrauterine device (IUD), fertility awareness, or contraceptive ring
   b. Abstinence, Depo-Provera, or foam and condoms used together
   c. Levonorgestrel IUD, diaphragm, or birth control pills
   d. Condoms, abstinence, or sterilization
5. Which risk is *not* associated with oral contraceptive use?
   a. Clotting disorders
   b. Benign liver tumor
   c. Fibrotic breast cycts
   d. Gallbladder disease
6. Which condition is associated with the copper IUD?
   a. Amenorrhea
   b. Ectopic pregnancy
   c. Increased flow and duration of menses
   d. Clotting disorders
7. Which method of contraception has the *highest* rate of unintended pregnancies during the first year of typical use?
   a. Fertility awareness
   b. Withdrawal
   c. Condoms only
   d. Sterilization
8. Which contraceptive method is available only with a prescription?
   a. Condoms
   b. Spermicide

   c. Contraceptive patch
   d. Natural family planning

Mrs. N., 28, has just delivered her third child without difficulty. She plans a long breastfeeding experience. She states that after a 3- to 4-week period of sexual abstinence, she plans to use a diaphragm that she has had for several years.

9. Which statement is correct?
   a. Contraception is not necessary as long as she breastfeeds because she cannot become pregnant while breastfeeding.
   b. It is appropriate to use the current diaphragm unless it is torn or has obvious holes.
   c. A diaphragm is difficult to use during involution, especially while nursing, because of problems with fit and irritation.
   d. A tubal ligation is a better choice because she already has three children.

Mrs. J., 24, has given birth to her second daughter in 12 months. Jane is crying and tells you that her husband "cannot wait to try again for a boy" and "is glad he does not have to wait any longer for sex." She says she does not feel "like a real woman anymore" because she feels "too tired and sore even to think about making love," and she does not want another baby right away.

10. What should you *not* encourage Mrs. J. to do?
    a. Talk honestly with her partner about her feelings.
    b. Discuss her concerns about family planning with her partner.
    c. Continue to practice abstinence until she feels ready to resume sexual activities.
    d. Sign a consent for bilateral tubal ligation.

ANSWERS TO STUDY QUESTIONS

1. a
2. c
3. a
4. b
5. c

6. c
7. a
8. c
9. c
10. d

BIBLIOGRAPHY

Hatcher, R., Trussell, J., Stewart, F., Kowal, D., Guest, F., Cates, W., & Policar, M. (2008). *Contraceptive technology* (19th ed.). New York: Irvington Publishers.

Lowdermilk, D. L., & Perry, S. (2007). *Maternity & women's health care* (9th ed.). St. Louis: Mosby.

Woods, N. F., & Fogel, C. I. (2008). *Women's health care in advanced practice nursing*. New York, NY: Springer Publishing Co.

THE NEWBORN

16 Transitional Care of the Newborn

Natalie Diane Cheffer and Debra Ann Rannalli

OBJECTIVES

1. Describe the cardiovascular, pulmonary, thermal, and gastrointestinal adaptation of the newborn.
2. Identify indications for instituting neonatal resuscitation.
3. Identify parameters used in the Apgar scoring of a newborn.
4. Describe the importance of maintaining a neutral thermal environment for the newborn, and discuss interventions to achieve a neutral thermal environment.
5. Identify normal physical characteristics of the newborn.
6. Interpret physical and neurologic findings for gestational age classification.
7. Define sensory capabilities of the newborn.
8. Define nutritional needs of the normal newborn, and assess readiness and ability of the newborn to feed orally.
9. Distinguish sleep and wake cycles of the newborn.
10. Devise a health education plan for a particular situation.

INTRODUCTION

Transition from fetus to neonate requires profound physiologic adaptation. Surprisingly, most neonates make this transition without difficulty (Pinheiro, 2009). Key elements in the birth transition are (1) shift from maternally dependent oxygenation to continuous respiration; (2) change from fetal circulation to mature circulation with increase in pulmonary blood flow and loss of left-to-right shunting; (3) commencement of independent glucose homeostasis; (4) independent thermoregulation; and (5) oral feedings (Engle & Boyle, 2005). Close observation of the infant's adaptation to extrauterine life is imperative to identify problems in transition and initiate interventions.

A. **Transition from fetus to neonate**
    1. Respiratory adaptation
        a. Mechanical stimuli: Compression of the fetal chest during vaginal delivery creates negative pressure by which air is drawn into the lung fields as the thorax recoils to its original size when the fetus exits the mother's body. Air fills the alveoli by replacing the lung fluids that have been expelled by chest compression during the vaginal delivery. The remaining lung fluids are removed through reabsorption by the lymphatics. Infant crying creates intrathoracic positive pressure, keeping the alveoli open.
        b. Chemical stimuli: With cessation of placental blood flow, the neonate's lungs must initiate and maintain gas exchange. The stress on the fetus during delivery leads to mild hypoxia, elevated carbon dioxide, and acidosis. Aortic and carotid bodies contain chemoreceptors that stimulate the medulla to trigger respiration. Surfactant, a phospholipid coating the alveolar epithelium, reduces the surface tension of the lung mucosa and allows exhalation without lung collapse.
        c. Thermal stimuli: Sudden chilling of the moist infant after delivery stimulates skin sensory receptors to transmit impulses to the respiratory center.
        d. Sensory stimuli: Normal handling after delivery (e.g., vigorous drying of the newborn) provides strong tactile stimulation to initiate breathing.

2. Cardiovascular adaptation: The neonate's circulatory system undergoes several physiologic changes after birth. The termination of fetal circulation and the transition to newborn circulation involve the closure of the three fetal shunts—the ductus venosus, the foramen ovale, and the ductus arteriosus.
   a. The physiologic changes associated with lung inflation after delivery cause an increase of pressure in the left heart and increase systemic resistance.
   b. With neonatal respiration, oxygenated blood enters the pulmonary musculature. This dilates the pulmonary artery and decreases the pulmonary vascular resistance.
   c. The ductus arteriosus functionally closes by 10 to 15 hours in the full-term infant due to decreasing pressure in the pulmonary vasculature and the increased pressure in the aorta (Blackburn, 2006). This stops the flow of blood through the ductus arteriosus.
   d. Vascular dilation along with the equalization and eventual overriding left atrial pressure forces functional closure of the foramen ovale. The foramen ovale, which acts like a flap valve, closes within minutes after birth with the decreased pulmonary vascular resistance and increased left heart pressure due to termination of placental blood flow (Blackburn, 2006).
3. Thermoregulation
   a. Thermoregulation (a critical component in the physiologic adaptation to extrauterine life) is the means by which the neonate's body temperature is maintained by balancing heat generation and heat loss in a changing environment.
   b. Normal temperature range: Preferred temperatures for term infants are between 36° (96.8° F) and 36.5° C (97.7 F) (axillary) for the first few hours of life. Newborns are at an increased risk of thermoregulatory problems for several reasons (Galligan, 2006; Hackman, 2001).
      (1) The ratio of large body surface to body mass
      (2) Higher metabolic rate with limited stores of metabolic substrates
      (3) Limited subcutaneous fat with poorly developed shivering response
   c. Mechanisms of heat loss
      (1) Convection: Heat is lost to air or fluid around the infant that is cooler than infant's temperature (e.g., air drafts on infant from open door in delivery room).
      (2) Radiation: Heat is lost to solid objects near infant that are cooler than infant's temperature (e.g., windows to the outside not covered by draperies).
      (3) Conduction: Heat is lost to cold surfaces or to objects with which the infant has contact (e.g., x-ray plate or unheated mattress or scale).
      (4) Evaporation: Heat is lost when water evaporates from the infant's skin surface or respiratory tract (e.g., infant not dried immediately after birth).
   d. Newborns attempt to regulate body temperature through flexed fetal positioning, which decreases body surface area; peripheral vasoconstriction; increased metabolic rate; and nonshivering heat production by brown fat metabolism (London, Wieland-Ladewig, Ball, & Bindler, 2007).
   e. Neutral thermal environment (NTE): An NTE is the temperature range in which normal body temperature can be maintained with minimal metabolic demands and oxygen consumption.
      (1) Achieving an NTE
         (a) Incubator: usually single-walled plastic boxes that warm the infant by convection
         (b) Radiant warmers: an open bed with radiant heat panels placed above the infant; convective and evaporative heat losses are increased
         (c) Open crib: Once an infant's temperature is normalized, infant is placed in an open crib with hats and blankets, providing thermal support.
4. Gastrointestinal transition: Feedings initiated as soon as possible after birth help maintain normal metabolism during the transition from fetal to extrauterine life (Heird, 2007). The goal of feeding is to provide adequate nutrition to meet the infant's metabolic requirements and ensure growth.
   a. Infants born beyond 32 to 34 weeks' gestation have adequate suck-and-swallow coordination for oral feedings unless neurologic damage has occurred or the infant is too ill to safely handle feedings.
   b. Feeding newborn infants:
      (1) Breastfeeding: See Chapter 14 for a complete discussion of breastfeeding.
         (a) The best source of nutrition in the first 6 months of life is human milk (Eiger, 2009); provides 20 kcal/ounce (30 mL).
         (b) Should begin as soon as possible after birth, usually within the first hour and continue for at least 12 months (American Academy of Pediatrics [AAP], 2005)

(c) Unless medically contraindicated, alert, healthy infants should have their first feeding in the delivery room. Early breastfeeding in the delivery room has been shown to increase the percentage of mothers who continue breastfeeding at 2 and 4 months postpartum (Schanler, 2009).

(d) Feed every 2 to 3 hours or when infant is awake, alert, and demonstrating behavioral feeding cues (rapid eye movements under the eyelids, sucking movements of the mouth and tongue, hand-to-mouth movements, body movements, small sounds) (Walker, 2007). Each session should last 10 to 15 minutes on each breast. Burp infant between and after each breast.

(e) Do not supplement the breastfed infant with feedings of water, glucose water, or formula, which might actually discourage breastfeeding.

(f) Advantages of breast milk
  [i] Lower incidence and/or severity of a many infectious diseases including diarrhea, respiratory tract infections, otitis media, bacteremia, bacterial meningitis, urinary tract infections, necrotizing enterocolitis (AAP, 2005; Schanler, 2009)
  [ii] Possible protective effect against sudden infant death syndrome (SIDS), type 1 diabetes mellitus, type 2 diabetes mellitus, obesity, hypercholesterolemia, and asthma (AAP, 2005)
  [iii] Economic benefit for the family and society related to reduced health care costs and reduced employee absenteeism for care related to infant illness (Krebs & Primak, 2006)
  [iv] Psychological benefits related to enhanced infant and maternal bonding and attachment

(2) Bottle-feeding
  (a) Commercially prepared formulas are based on cow's milk and have been modified to closely resemble human milk. Provides 20 kcal/ounce (30 mL).
  (b) The first feeding should be initiated in the nursery. Infant should be offered several sips of sterile water before formula to assess for aspiration.
  (c) Bottle-fed infants should be fed 15 to 30 mL of formula every 3 to 4 hours on first day of life increasing to 75 to 90 mL by day 4 or 5.
  (d) Always hold infant during feedings; this provides vital human contact. Bottle-propping can lead to aspiration and middle-ear infections.
  (e) Discard all unused formula left in bottle after feeding.
  (f) Advantages of formula
    [i] Ability to share feedings with partner, family, and friends
    [ii] Lack of physical problems (i.e., sore nipples, nipple confusion, etc.)
  (g) Disadvantages of formula
    [i] Is more costly, especially if purchased in ready-to-serve concentrations
    [ii] Must be prepared if not purchased in ready-to-serve concentration
    [iii] Is more difficult to digest and forms harder curds because of higher casein content

(3) Pacifiers
  (a) Pacifier use is recommended once breastfeeding is well established (approximately 1 month of age) (AAP, 2005).
  (b) Advantage: provides nonnutritive sucking and comfort for a crying infant and may increase arousability of infants during sleep reducing the risk of SIDS (Hunt & Hauck, 2007; Schwartz & Guthrie, 2008)
  (c) Disadvantages: source of bacteria if not cleaned properly, potential for compulsive use, may interfere with normal teeth positioning and eruption and cause alteration in bone growth (Schwartz & Guthrie, 2008)

CLINICAL PRACTICE

A. **Delivery room assessment**
  1. Identify the infant at risk.
    a. Review maternal history and prenatal course.
    b. Assess fetal well-being during labor and delivery.

(1) Apgar scoring
  (a) This scoring system, initially developed by Virginia Apgar in 1952, provides practitioners with a standardized approach for assessing the newborn infant immediately after birth to help identify those infants requiring resuscitation and predict survival in the neonatal period (Stoll, 2007).
  (b) Scoring is done at 1, 5, and sometimes 10 minutes of life; the newborn is given a score from 0 to 2 for each category, based on the elements described in Table 16-1.
(2) Indications for postive pressure ventilation with a tightly fitted face mask using 100% supplemental oxygen (AHA & AAP, 2006)
  (a) Apnea
  (b) Heart rate (HR) absent or less than 100 beats per minute (bpm)
  (c) Central cyanosis
(3) Indications for chest compressions over the lower third of the sternum at a rate of 120/min
  (a) HR absent or remains less than 100 bpm despite adequate assisted ventilation for 30 seconds.
(4) Indications for medication
  (a) HR <60 bpm after a minimum of 30 seconds of adequate ventilation and chest compressions. Administer epinephrine intravenously (IV) at a dose of 0.01 to 0.03 mg/kg.
(5) Indications for endotrachael intubation
  (a) Meconium-stained amniotic fluid
  (b) Ineffectiveness of positive-pressure ventilation with a tightly fitted face mask
  (c) Need for prolonged ventilation (e.g., for an extremely small infant)

B. **Complete newborn assessment**
  1. After stabilization, a thorough and systematic assessment of the newborn is necessary to identify the state of health of the neonate and detect congenital anomalies that might cause problems with extrauterine adaptation. Physical examination of the term infant should be performed with one or both parents in attendance. This fosters discussion with parents about expected physical and behavioral characteristics of their newborn.
  2. Growth parameters
     a. Weight: 2500 to 4000 g (5 pounds, 8 ounces to 8 pounds, 13 ounces)
     b. Length from head to heel: 48 to 53 cm (19 to 21 inches)
     c. Chest circumference: 30.5 to 33 cm (12 to 13 inches)
     d. Head circumference: 33 to 35.5 cm (13 to 14 inches)
  3. Vital signs:
     a. Temperatures should stabilize between 36.4° and 37° C (97.5° and 98.6° F).
     b. Respiratory patterns are irregular, with respiratory rates between 30 to 60 inspirations per minute.
     c. Heart rates are regular, with rates between 110 and 160 bpm depending on the infant's state.
     d. Blood pressure measurements are usually not assessed as part of the newborn examination.

■ TABLE 16-1
■ ■ **Components of Apgar Scoring**

	SCORE		
Sign	**0**	**1**	**2**
Heart rate	Absent	Less than 100 bpm	More than 100 bpm
Respiratory effort	Absent	Weak, irregular	Good, crying
Muscle tone	Flaccid	Some flexion of extremities	Well flexed
Reflex irritability (catheter in nose or slap sole of foot)	No response	Grimace	Cry
Skin color	Blue/pale	Body pink, extremities blue	Completely pink

4. Physical examination
    a. General survey: periods of alertness, symmetric features and movements, easily consolable
    b. Skin: smooth, pink to reddish with possible flaking in areas of major creasing. Vernix caseosa, a cheesy white substance, can be found on the entire body but is more intense between folds. Lanugo, a fine hair, might be seen, especially on the back.
        (1) Benign skin conditions
            (a) Acrocyanosis: cyanosis of hands and feet
            (b) Cutis marmorata: transient mottling, especially when exposed to cool temperatures
            (c) Erythema toxicum: pink papular rash with vesicles on chest, abdomen, back, buttocks, and extermities
            (d) Capillary hemangioma: "stork bite" and "angel kiss" are flat, deep pink areas over eyelids, forehead, or nape of neck in infants with fair skin.
            (e) Mongolian spots: bluish black hyperpigmented areas usually located on the back and buttocks in infants with dark skin
    c. Head
        (1) Molding of the head might occur as the result of the delivery and usually resolves within a few weeks. Bruising is common.
            (a) Caput succedaneum: presents at birth with pitting edema of the scalp crossing suture lines as a result of accumulation of blood or serum above the periosteum (Fuloria & Kreiter, 2002).
            (b) Cephalhematoma: occurs several hours after birth from bleeding between the periosteum and skull, causing swelling that does not cross suture lines; might take several weeks to resolve
    d. Eyes
        (1) Eyelids are usually edematous immediately after birth.
        (2) Color of iris: slate gray, dark blue, or brown
        (3) Pupils reactive to light; red reflex present; focuses on objects and follows to midline
        (4) Mucoid discharge is normal with absence of tears.
        (5) Scleral hemorrhages are possible.
    e. Ears
        (1) Position: Top of pinna is horizontal to outer canthus of eye.
        (2) Pinna is flexible and well formed with cartilage present.
        (3) Loud noise elicits startle reflex.
    f. Nose
        (1) Obligate nose breather.
        (2) Nares are patent with no evidence of choanal atresia.
    g. Mouth
        (1) Intact palate with midline uvula
        (2) Normal frenulum of tongue and lip
        (3) Minimal or absent salivation
        (4) Suck, root, and gag reflexes present
    h. Neck
        (1) Full range of motion without torticollis (asymmetic shortening of the sternocleidomastoid muscle)
        (2) Tonic neck reflex present
        (3) Intact clavicles with no tenderness, swelling, or crepitation
        (4) Absence of webbing
    i. Chest and lungs
        (1) Symmetric, barrel-shaped, with equal anteroposterior and lateral diameters
        (2) Slight subcostal and intercostal retractions are common.
        (3) Breast enlargement and engorgement in either sex with possible physiologic galactorrhea; resolves within several weeks
        (4) Bilateral bronchial breath sounds; fine crackles and transient hoarseness are normal (Colyar, 2003)
    j. Cardiac
        (1) Apex or point of maximal impulse (PMI) at left third or fourth intercostal space
        (2) Significant and persistent murmurs should be evaluated to rule out underlying structural abnormalities (Gaylord & Yetman, 2009).

    k. Abdomen
        (1) Mildly protuberant
        (2) Liver normally palpable 1 to 3 cm below costal margin in the midclavicular line
        (3) Kidneys: 1 to 2 cm above and to both sides of umbilicus and felt with deep palpation
        (4) Bowel sounds present, but might be hypoactive on first day of life
        (5) Three vessels in cord
    l. Genitals
        (1) Female: labia and clitoris edematous; hymenal tag often present; labia majora larger than labia minora; urethral meatus located below clitoris; vaginal discharge whitish or blood-tinged
        (2) Male: scrotum large, edematous, and pendulous; testes palpable; urethral opening at tip of glans penis; foreskin tightly adhered (phimosis)
    m. Extremities
        (1) Symmetric
        (2) Full range of motion
        (3) All 10 fingers and toes present without webbing
        (4) Brachial and femoral pulses present and equal
        (5) Pink nail beds or acrocyanosis
        (6) Creases on anterior two thirds of sole
        (7) Scarf sign present
        (8) Normal hip abduction without clicks
    n. Back
        (1) Spine intact without openings, masses, curves, dimples, or hairy tufts
        (2) Patent anal opening
        (3) Even gluteal folds
        (4) Trunk incurvation reflex present
    o. Neurologic
        (1) Posture: general flexed position similar to that maintained in utero
        (2) Tone: extremities have brisk recoil to flexion; infant able to hold head erect momentarily while sitting
        (3) Tremors or jitteriness: Momentary quivering or tremors might occur as a result of immature nervous system.
        (4) Newborn reflexes: Table 16-2
  5. Behavioral state system: reflects the infant's ability to respond to the environment (VandenBerg, 2007)
    a. Identifying infant's behavioral state is helpful in determining the infant's ability to perceive stimuli and interact with others. The Brazelton Neonatal Assessment Scale (BNAS) is a well-known tool for assessment of full-term neonatal states. The behavioral states described by Brazelton (1999) are as follows:

■ **TABLE 16-2**
■ ■ **Newborn Reflexes**

Name of Reflex	Expected Response
Sucking	Strong sucking movements of mouth can be elicited and might occur during sleep
Swallow	Follows sucking, usually at pauses, and can be seen at the neck
Rooting	When cheek is touched or stroked, infant turns head toward stroked side and opens mouth to receive nipple.
Moro (startle)	Moro (startle): general body response to sudden stimulus that is a combination of full extension and abduction of limbs
Babinski	Upward stroking of sole and across ball of foot causes great toes to hyperextend and foot to dorsiflex.
Palmar and plantar grasps	Touching palms of hands and feet causes flexion of fingers or toes.

(1) Sleep states
  (a) Deep sleep: sleep without movement except for sudden, jerky movements; hard to awaken from this state
  (b) Light sleep: eyes closed with some eye movement seen under lids, active body movements; sucking might be present
  (c) Drowsy: transition state as infant moves from sleep to awake or awake to asleep. Eyes open or closed, lids usually heavy; active body movements with occasional fussing
(2) Awake states
  (a) Quiet alert: alert with eyes open; attentive to close objects; little body movement; good opportunity for newborn to interact with parents (VandenBerg, 2007)
  (b) Active alert: inactivity with mild, agitated vocalizations. An organized term infant may be able to return to a quiet alert state or calm sleep state by calming him- or herself by sucking on the hands (VandenBerg, 2007).
  (c) Crying: eyes tightly closed at times with crying, thrashing, and movements of head and extremities
(3) State organization
  (a) After the delivery, newborns have a period of alertness lasting for a variable amount of time. Infants begin to demonstrate increasing ability to regulate state control as they transition more smoothly between states and develop a more predictible sleep-wake pattern (VandenBerg, 2007).
  (b) Newborns will usually sleep between 16 to 18 hours in a 24-hour period.
  (c) Crying in the newborn period is usually not specific to the type of discomfort. The newborn tends to cry in response to hunger, pain, or disturbing stimuli. During the neonatal period, crying is an important behavior for organizing the day and reducing disturbance in the central nervous system (CNS) (Brazelton, 1999).
  (d) An *organized* newborn can maintain breathing, digestion, smooth movements, tone, and posture and at the same time manage the sleep-wake state. In addition, the *organized* newborn demonstrates self-calming behavior (VandenBerg, 2007). Newborn infants may need help with state self-regulation especially to ensure adequate nutritional intake. Skin-to-skin contact with the mother may help the sleepy, fussy, or closed-down infant begin to self-regulate to a state optimal for feeding (Walker, 2007).

6. Sensory capabilities
   a. Hearing: well-developed at birth; responds to noise
   b. Vision: focuses on close-up objects (e.g., the mother's face when at breast); tracks with eyes to midline or beyond
   c. Taste: distinguishes between sweet and sour at 3 days of age
   d. Smell: distinguishes between mother's breasts and breast milk and those of another by fifth day of age and frequently sooner
   e. Touch: sensitive to pain, usually responds to tactile stimuli

7. Gestational age assessment (see Chapter 17 for a discussion of gestational age significance/risks)
   a. Reliable assessment of gestational age is based on neurologic development and physical characteristics found by direct examination of the infant.
   b. Classification of infant allows clinician to anticipate clinical problems and apply early diagnostic testing.
   c. Classifications: infant's weight and weeks of gestation are classified as follows:
      (1) Appropriate for gestational age (AGA): characterizes approximately 80% of the neonatal population
      (2) Small for gestational age (SGA): less than 2500 g (5 pounds, 8 ounces) for term neonate due to less growth in utero than expected; associated risks include hypoglycemia, asphyxia, respiratory distress syndrome, meconium aspiration, intrauterine infection, and hyperbilirubinemia
      (3) Large for gestational age (LGA): more than 4000 g (8 pounds, 13 ounces) for term neonate due to accelerated growth for length of gestation; associated risks include birth trauma, hypoglycemia, hypocalcemia, hyperbilirubinemia, meconium aspiration, intrauterine infection, and polycythemia.

      d. Assessing for gestational age (see Chapter 8 for a complete discussion of antepartum fetal assessment)

         (1) Guides are frequently used in the nursery to determine neuromuscular and physical maturity. Table 16-2, Table 16-3, and Box 16-1 are commonly used.

         (2) A guide is frequently used to assess neurologic characteristics and maturity (see Box 16-1).

C. Transitional nursing care interventions/outcomes: Delivery room and nursery interventions have been combined in this section. See Figure 16-1 for sequential steps for resuscitative interventions in the delivery room and Table 16-4 for medications used during resuscitation.

  1. Temperature regulation

      a. Interventions

         (1) Close door to delivery rooms and nursery and place radiant warmer away from traffic patterns and air drafts.

         (2) Upon delivery, dry infant thoroughly and quickly; remove wet linens and place the naked infant prone on the mother's bare chest. Cover infant across the back with a warm blanket. Skin-to-skin (STS) contact between the mother and baby at birth keeps the baby warmer. Evidence suggests that this technique is an alternative to traditional rewarming interventions for full-term, low-risk infants that promotes mother-infant attachment (Beal, 2005; Galligan, 2006; Moore, Anderson, & Bergman, 2007).

         (3) Check infant's temperature every 15 to 20 minutes until stable, then every 4 to 8 hours.

         (4) In the nursery, prewarm incubators and radiant warmers.

         (5) Initial bath is recommended only after the newborn's temperature and vital signs have stabilized (2 to 4 hours after birth) (Association of Women's Health, Obstetric and Neonatal Nurses [AWHONN], 2001).

         (6) During the bath, wash one area at a time; dry it, keeping the infant covered at all times. Place hat on infant's head to decrease heat loss (Gaylord & Yetman, 2009). Dress infant in shirt, diaper, and hat or cap.

         (7) Wrap in double blanket until infant can maintain temperature without second blanket (usually about 24 hours) until stable.

         (8) To warm infant, set incubator temperature at 1.5° C (2.6° F) higher than infant's temperature until infant's temperature begins to stabilize.

         (9) Use warming devices, such as heat lamps, sparingly and for only 15-minute intervals to prevent overwarming the infant.

      b. Outcomes

         (1) Skin temperature is 36.4° to 37° C (97.6° to 98.6° F).

         (2) Temperature stabilizes within 4 hours.

  2. Respiratory distress/difficulty

      a. Interventions

         (1) Upon delivery, position infant's head in "sniff" position or slight extension.

         (2) Suction mouth, then the nose.

         (3) Assess respiratory effort and heart rate (HR).

         (4) Provide tactile stimulation (slap foot, flick heel with finger, or rub back).

         (5) Provide positive-pressure ventilation using a bag and mask with 100% oxygen for apnea, HR absent or less than 100 bpm, or central cyanosis.

      b. Outcomes

         (1) Spontanous breathing with good respiratory effort and infant has lusty cry

         (2) Fluid in airways has been removed to allow for normal breathing.

         (3) HR is greater than 100 bpm.

         (4) Skin color is normal with or without acrocyanosis.

         (5) Improved muscle tone

  3. Cardiopulmonary compromise

      a. Interventions

         (1) Assess respiratory rate and HR.

         (2) Begin positive-pressure ventilation using a bag and mask with 100% oxygen if HR absent or less than 100 bpm, or central cyanosis.

         (3) Begin chest compressions if HR absent or remains less than 60 bpm despite adequate assisted ventilation for 30 seconds. The two-thumb technique is recommended in newborn infants (American Heart Association [AHA] & AAP, 2006).

■ TABLE 16-3
■ ■ **Scoring System of External Physical Characteristics***

External Sign	SCORE†				
	0	1	2	3	4
Edema	Obvious edema of hands and feet; pitting over tibia	No obvious edema of hands and feet; pitting over tibia	No edema		
Skin texture	Very thin, gelatinous	Thin and smooth	Smooth; medium thickness; rash or superficial peeling	Slight thickening; superficial cracking and peeling; especially of hands and feet	Thick and parchment-like; superficial or deep cracking
Skin color	Dark red	Uniformly pink	Pale pink; variable over body	Pale; only pink over ears, lips, palms, or soles	
Skin opacity (trunk)	Numerous veins and venules clearly seen, especially over abdomen	Veins and tributaries seen	A few large vessels clearly seen over abdomen	A few large vessels seen indistinctly over abdomen	No blood vessels seen
Lanugo (over back)	No lanugo	Abundant; long and thick over whole back	Hair thinning, especially over lower back	Small amount of lanugo and bald areas	At least half of back devoid of lanugo
Plantar creases	No skin creases	Faint red marks over anterior half of sole	Definite red marks over > anterior half; indentations over > anterior third	Indentations over > anterior third	Definite deep indentations over > anterior third
Nipple formation	Nipple barely visible; no areola	Nipple well defined; areola smooth and flat, diameter <0.75 cm	Areola stippled, edge not raised diameter <0.75 cm	Areola stippled, edge raised, diameter >0.75 cm	
Breast size	No breast tissue palpable	Breast tissue on one or both sides, <0.5 cm	Breast tissue on both sides, one or both 0.5 to 1 cm	Breast tissue on both sides, one or both >1 cm	
Ear form	Pinna flat and shapeless; little or no incurving of edge	Incurving of part of edge of pinna	Partial incurving of whole of upper pinna	Well-defined incurving of whole of upper pinna	
Ear firmness	Pinna soft, easily folded, no recoil	Pinna soft, easily folded, slow recoil	Cartilage to edge of pinna but soft in places, ready recoil	Pinna firm, cartilage to edge, instant recoil	
Genitals: male	Neither testis in scrotum	At least one testis high in scrotum	At least one testis down		
Genitals: female (with hips half abducted)	Labia majora widely separated; labia minora protruding	Labia majora almost cover labia minor	Labia majora completely cover labia minora		

*To be used in conjunction with Box 16-1.
†If score differs on two sides, take the mean.
Adapted from Dubowitz, L., Dubowitz, V., & Goldberg, C. (1970). Clinical assessment of gestational age in the newborn infant. *Journal of Pediatrics*, 77, 1–10.

■ BOX 16-1
■ **TECHNIQUES OF NEUROLOGIC ASSESSMENT***

POSTURE

With the infant supine and quiet, score as follows:

Arms and legs extended = 0
Slight or moderate flexion of hips and knees = 1
Moderate to strong flexion of hips and knees = 2
Legs flexed and abducted, arms slightly flexed = 3
Full flexion of arms and legs = 4

SQUARE WINDOW

Flex the hand at the wrist. Exert pressure sufficient to get as much flexion as possible. The angle between the hypothenar eminence and the anterior aspect of the forearm is measured and scored. Do not rotate the wrist.

ANKLE DORSIFLEXION

Flex the foot at the ankle with sufficient pressure to get maximum change. The angle between the dorsum of the foot and the anterior aspect of the leg is measured and scored.

ARM RECOIL

With the infant supine, fully flex the forearm for 5 seconds, then fully extend by pulling the hands and release. Score the reaction as follows:

Remain extended or random movements = 0
Incomplete or partial flexion = 1
Brisk return to full flexion = 2

LEG RECOIL

With the infant supine, the hips and knees are fully flexed for 5 seconds, then extended by traction on the feet and released. Score the reaction as follows:

No response or slight flexion = 0
Partial flexion = 1
Full flexion (less than 90 degrees at knees and hips) = 2

POPLITEAL ANGLE

With the infant supine and the pelvis flat on the examining surface, the leg is flexed on the thigh and the thigh fully flexed with the use of one hand. With the other hand the leg is then extended and the angle attained scored.

HEEL-TO-EAR MANEUVER

With the infant supine, hold the infant's foot with one hand and move it as near to the head as possible without forcing it. Keep the pelvis flat on the examining surface. Score.

SCARF SIGN

With the infant supine, take the infant's hand and draw it across the neck and as far across the opposite shoulder as possible. Assistance to the elbow is permissible by lifting it across the body. Score according to the location of the elbow:

Elbow reaches the opposite anterior axillary line = 0
Elbow between opposite anterior axillary line and midline of thorax = 1
Elbow at midline of thorax = 2
Elbow does not reach midline of thorax = 3

HEAD LAG

With the infant supine, grasp each forearm just proximal to the wrist and pull gently to bring the infant to a sitting position. Score according to the relationship of the head to the trunk during the maneuver.

No evidence of head support = 0
Some evidence of head support = 1
Maintains head in the same anteroposterior plane as the body = 2
Tends to hold the head forward = 3

VENTRAL SUSPENSION

With the infant prone and the chest resting on the examiner's palm, lift the infant off the examining surface and score.

*To be used in conjunction with Table 16-3.
If score differs on two sides, take the mean. Adapted from Dubowitz, L., Dubowitz, V., & Goldberg, C. (1970). Clinical assessment of gestational age in the newborn infant. *Journal of Pediatrics, 77,* 1–10.

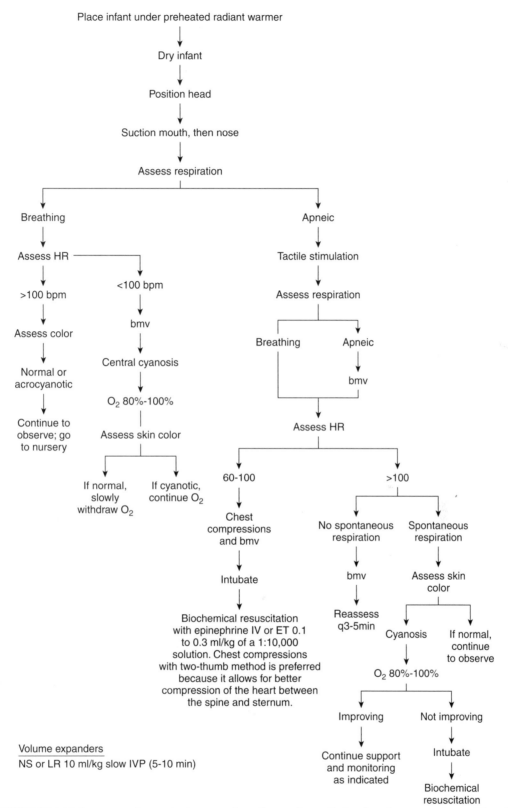

FIGURE 16-1 ■ Summary of resuscitation steps. *bmv,* Bag mask ventilation; *bpm,* beats per minute; *ET,* endotracheal tube; *HR,* heart rate; *IV,* intravenous; *IVP,* intravenous pressure; *LR,* lactated Ringer's; *NS,* normal saline.

TABLE 16-4

Medications for Neonatal Resuscitation

Medication	Concentration to Administer	Preparation	Dosage/Route	Weight:	Total Dose/Neonate		Rate/Precautions
Epinephrine	1:10,000	1 mL	0.1–0.3 mL/kg IV	Weight: 1 kg 2 kg 3 kg 4 kg	Total mL: 0.1–0.3 mL 0.2–0.6 mL 0.3–0.9 mL 0.4–1.2 mL		Give rapidly
Volume expanders	O-negative CBC Whole blood Normal saline Ringer's lactate	40 mL 40 mL	10 mL/kg IV	Weight: 1 kg 2 kg 3 kg 4 kg	Total mL: 10 mL 20 mL 30 mL 40 mL		Give over 5-10 minutes
Sodium bicarbonate	0.5 mEq/mL (4.2% solution)	Two 10-mL prefilled syringes	2 mEq/kg IV	Weight: 1 kg 2 kg 3 kg 4 kg	Total Dose: 2 mEq 4 mEq 6 mEq 8 mEq	Total mL: 4 mL 8 mL 12 mL 16 mL	Give slowly, over a rate of no more than 1 mEq/kg/min Give only if infant is being effectively ventilated
Naloxone hydrochloride	0.4 mg/mL 1.0 mg/mL	1 mL 1 mL	0.1 mg/kg 25 mL/kg IV, IM 0.1 mg/kg 1 mL/kg IV, IM	Weight: 1 kg 2 kg 3 kg 4 kg 1 kg 2 kg 3 kg 4 kg	Total Dose: 0.1 mg 0.2 mg 0.3 mg 0.4 mg 0.1 mg 0.2 mg 0.3 mg 0.4 mg	Total mL: 0.25 mL 0.50 mL 0.75 mL 1.00 mL 0.1 mL 0.2 mL 0.3 mL 0.4 mL	Only recommended for continued respiratory depression and history of maternal narcotic administration within the past 4 hours
Dopamine		$\dfrac{\text{Weight} \times \text{Desired dose}}{6 \times (\text{kg}) \times \text{µg/kg/min}} \bigg/ \text{Desired fluid(mL/n)}$ = $\dfrac{\text{mg of dopamine}}{\text{per 100 mL of solution}}$	Begin at 5 mcg/kg/ min (may increase to 20 mcg/kg/min if necessary) IV	Weight: 1 kg 2 kg 3 kg 4 kg	Total mg/min: 5-20 mcg/min 10-40 mcg/min 15-60 mcg/min 20-80 mcg/min		Give as a continuous infusion using an infusion pump. Monitor heart rate and blood pressure closely. Seek consultation.

CBC, Complete blood count; IM, intramuscular; IV, intravenous. Data from the American Academy of Pediatrics 2006. American Heart Association. 2005 American Heart Association guidelines for cardiopulmonary resuscitation and emergency cardiovascular care of pediatric and neonatal patients: Neonatal resuscitation guidelines. Pediatrics 117(5), e1029-e1038.

          (4) Obtain IV access and administer epinephrine IV at a dose of 0.01 to 0.03 mg/kg if the heart rate remains lower than 60 bpm after a minimum of 30 seconds of adequate ventilation and chest compressions. There is a lack of evidence to support use of endotracheal epinephrine (AHA & AAP, 2006).

      b. Outcomes

          (1) Improvement in cardiac output will be evidenced by the following:

              (a) HR improving and more than 100 bpm

              (b) Skin color improving to within normal limits

  4. Prevention of infection

    a. Interventions

        (1) After temperature stabilization, bathe the infant with warm water to reduce the incidence of skin colonization with pathogenic bacteria (Stoll, 2007). Removal of all vernix is not necessary because it may offer antibacterial protection (AWHONN, 2001).

        (2) Be certain that traces of maternal blood have been removed from infant's skin surface before injections or invasive procedures.

        (3) Clean injection sites with alcohol and friction before injections.

        (4) Clean and observe any scalp monitoring sites for abscesses, redness, or drainage.

        (5) Eye care: Regardless of route of delivery, universal prophylaxis of all newborns with 1% silver nitrate drops, 0.5% erythromycin, or tetracycline is recommended (AAP, 2007; Stoll, 2007).

        (6) Umbilical cord care: Topical antibiotic therapy such as triple dye or bacitracin can be applied to the umbilical cord after the bath to prevent bacterial colonization; however, there is no evidence that applying sprays, creams, or powders is any better than keeping the baby's cord clean and dry at birth (Zupan, Garner, & Omari, 2004). To aid by in cord separation, air-drying by tucking the diaper below the cord is recommended (Lin, Tinkle, & Janniger, 2005).

        (7) Check circumcision site with every diaper change, and remove petroleum jelly–covered gauze after 4 hours. Clean site with water only for 3 to 4 days (AWHONN, 2001).

    b. Outcomes

        (1) Infant has minimal exposure to pathogens.

        (2) Temperature of infant remains within normal limits.

        (3) Signs of infection are absent at any areas where skin integrity has been disturbed.

        (4) Eyes remain free of any purulent drainage.

        (5) Circumcision site remains free of swelling, excess redness, or excess drainage.

  5. Prevent hemorrhagic disease in the newborn or vitamin K–deficiency bleeding (VKDB).

    a. Intervention

        (1) Vitamin K is administered intramuscularly within 1 hour of birth (AAP, 2006).

    b. Outcome

        (1) Signs of early and classic VKDB are absent

  6. Glucose screening

    a. Intervention

        (1) There is no evidence that supports routine measurement of glucose in healthy term neonates (Bloomfield, Dinolfo, & Kokotos, 2009).

        (2) Glucose screening should be performed on any infant with symptoms attributable to hypoglycemia such as jitteriness, irritability, lethargy, hypotonia, poor feeding, diaphoresis, vomiting, apnea, or temperature instabilities (Bloomfield et al, 2009).

        (3) A blood glucose of level of less than 47mg/dL at 4 to 6 hourse of age is accepted as being appropriate for intervention (Canadian Paediatric Society, 2004).

    b. Outcome: Infant will maintain normal blood glucose levels.

HEALTH EDUCATION

Health education centers on the preparation of parents for care of their newborn infant. Educational topics include general newborn care, nutrition, safety, and community resources to aid the family.

A. Delivery room care

  1. Providing family-centered developmental care has become the standard of care for the newborn infant. Whether an infant transitions to extrauterine life smoothly or requires resuscitative efforts, the goal of care must be integration of the child into the family unit (McGrath, 2006). This can only be done when the family is involved in the clinical decision making during the delivery and the entire postpartum stay.

2. It is important to discuss the normal course of events of birth and care of the newborn infant with parents before delivery so that they are not alarmed by normal delivery room events.

3. If there is a need for more in-depth resuscitation, provide parents with information as soon as possible.

B. **General newborn care**
  1. How to bathe while conserving heat and providing for safety
  2. How to take a temperature
  3. How to use bulb syringe
  4. How to diaper
  5. How to care for circumcision site: ordinary cleaning of the diaper area and inspection for bleeding, swelling, or decreased urine output; petroleum jelly gauze applied during the procedure removed after 4 hours
  6. How to clean genitalia
     a. Girls: separating the labia and cleaning from front to back
     b. Boys: wiping under scrotum and penis
  7. How to care for umbilical cord: keeping clean and dry; folding diaper underneath cord
  8. How to detect signs of illness and when to contact the physician or pediatric nurse practitioner

C. **Newborn safety**
  1. Place on his or her back to sleep.
  2. Never leave a newborn unattended on changing table or bed.
  3. Learn first aid for choking.
  4. Always use a car seat in the back seat; must be rear-facing until the infant is 1 year of age and 20 pounds.
  5. Avoid bottle propping.
  6. Wash hands before handling newborn; avoid exposure to others and to illness.
  7. Never leave infant alone in bathtub.
  8. Never shake an infant; shaking can cause severe brain damage.

D. **Newborn nutrition**
  1. Preparation and storage of formulas; collection and storage of breast milk
  2. Cleaning of bottles and nipples
  3. Reasons to avoid honey and corn syrup
  4. Feeding schedules versus on-demand feedings
  5. Expected amounts of intake
  6. Color, consistency, and frequency of stools
  7. Initial weight loss and subsequent gain

E. **Community resources**
  1. Local chapters of La Leche League or other lactation support groups
  2. Home health supply companies (e.g., for breast pumps)
  3. Referrals to local county and state agencies for such concerns as medical insurance, nutritional support (Women, Infants, and Children [WIC]), parenting classes, and early child development and education

F. **Pediatric health maintenance and follow-up**
  1. First health care provider visit should be 48 to 72 hours after discharge (Hernandez & Thilo, 2005).
  2. Schedule and teach importance of immunizations (generally first hepatitis B vaccine given in nursery).

CASE STUDY AND STUDY QUESTIONS

1. A newborn infant should have the first bath:
   a. Immediately
   b. Just prior to discharge
   c. After the vitamin K injection
   d. After temperature stabilization
2. Standard umbilical cord care for the mother *at home* is:
   a. Clean cord with alcohol three times a day.
   b. Clean cord with warm water and air dry.
   c. Apply petroleum jelly–covered gauze every 4 hours.
   d. Apply triple dye after the bath.
3. A 30-year old gravida 1, para 1 (G1, P1) mother who is attempting to nurse a 1-day-old infant is concerned that the infant is too sleepy to breastfeed. The most developmentally appropriate nursing intervention is to:
   a. Unwrap the infant.
   b. Place the infant skin-to-skin with the mother.
   c. Let the infant sleep; try nursing at a later time.
   d. Feed every 2 hours regardless of behavioral feeding cues.

A 39-week-gestation, 3270-g (7-pound, 2-ounce) infant was born to a 17-year-old Latina, gravida 1, para 1 (G1, P1). Labor and birth events were unremarkable. The infant's body was pink with blue extremities, HR 120, cough with suctioning, flexed muscle tone, and strong cry at 1 minute of life.

4. What is the initial Apgar score?
   a. 10
   b. 9
   c. 7
   d. 6
5. The most developmentally appropriate intervention to ensure that this infant is in a neutral thermal environment in the delivery room is to:
   a. Place in an incubator.
   b. Place in a radiant warmer.

   c. Place in an open crib, double wrapped with a hat.
   d. Dry thoughly and place prone skin-to-skin on mother's bare chest and cover wth a warm blanket.
6. What is the most frequent mechanism of heat loss in the newborn infant?
   a. Convection
   b. Conduction
   c. Radiation
   d. Evaporation
7. Which statement is *not true* about breast milk?
   a. Breast milk contains 30 kcal/ounce.
   b. Breast milk is economical.
   c. Breast milk provides protection against diarrhea.
   d. Breast milk provides protection against otitis media.
8. When should resuscitation be started in the delivery room?
   a. After the 1-minute Apgar score is obtained
   b. Immediately, if respirations are absent or ineffective
   c. Immediately, if HR is less than 80 bpm
   d. After 90 seconds of attempted tactile stimulation
9. In what sequence (1 to 5) should the activities occur for initial resuscitation of an infant?
   ___ 1. Position infant's head.
   ___ 2. Suction mouth.
   ___ 3. Dry infant.
   ___ 4. Place infant under preheated radiant warmer.
   ___ 5. Suction nose.

ANSWERS TO STUDY QUESTIONS

1. d
2. b
3. b

4. b
5. d
6. d

7. a
8. b
9. 4, 3, 1, 2, 5

REFERENCES

American Academy of Pediatrics (2007). Prevention of neonatal ophthalmia. In L. K. Pickering, C. J. Baker, D. W. Kimberlin, & S. S. Long (Eds.), *Redbook: Report of the committee on infectious diseases* (27th ed.). Elk Grove Village, IL: American Academy of Pediatrics.

American Academy of Pediatrics (2005). Policy statement. Breastfeeding and the use of human milk. *Pediatrics 115*(2), 496–506.

American Academy of Pediatrics Committee on Fetus and Newborn (2006). Policy statement: Controversies concerning vitamin K and the newborn. *Pediatrics, 112*(1), 191–192.

American Heart Association and American Academy of Pediatrics (2006). 2005 American Heart Association guidelines for cardiopulmonary resuscitation and emergency cardiovascular care of pediatric and neonatal patients: Neonatal resuscitation guidelines. *Pediatrics, 117*(5), e1029–e1038.

Association of Women's Health, Obstetric and Neonatal Nurses (2001). *Neonatal skin care. Evidence based clinical practice guideline*. Washington DC: Author.

Beal, J. (2005). Evidence for best practices in the neonatal period. *MCN The American Journal of Maternal-Child Nursing, 30*(6), 397–403.

Blackburn, S. (2006). Placental, fetal and transitional circulation revisited. *Journal of Perinatal and Neonatal Nursing, 20*(4), 290–294.

Bloomfield, D., Dinolfo, E., & Kokotos, F. (2009). Care of the newborn after delivery. In T. McInerny, H. Adam, D. Campbell, D. Kamat, & K. Kelleher (Eds.), *American Academy of Pediatrics textbook of pediatric care* (pp. 800–808). Elk Grove Village, IL: American Academy of Pediatrics.

Brazelton, T. (1999). Behavioral competence. In G. B. Avery, M. A. Fletcher, & M. G. MacDonald (Eds.), *Neonatalogy: Pathophysiology and management of the newborn* (pp. 321–332). Philadelphia: Lippincott Williams & Wilkins.

Canadian Paediatric Society. (2004). Position statement: Screening guidelines for newborns at risk for low blood glucose. *Paediatric Child Health 9*(10), 723–729.

Colyar, M. (2003). *Well-child assessment for primary care providers*. Philadelphia: F.A. Davis.

Dubowitz, L., Dubowitz, V., & Goldberg, C. (1970). Clinical assessment of gestational age in the newborn infant. *Journal of Pediatrics, 77*, 1–10.

Eiger, M. (2009). Feeding infants and children. In T. McInerny, H. Adam, D. Campbell, D. Kamat, & K. Kelleher (Eds.), *American Academy of Pediatrics textbook of pediatric care* (pp. 212–219). Elk Grove Village, IL: American Academy of Pediatrics.

Engle, W. A., & Boyle D.W. (2005). Delivery room management and transitional care. In L. Osborn, T. DeWitt, T. First, & J. Zenel (Eds.), *Pediatrics* (pp. 1250–1260). Philadelphia: Saunders.

Fuloria, M., & Kreiter, S. (2002). The newborn examination: Part I. Emergencies and common abnormalities involving the skin, head, neck, chest, respiratory and cardiovascular systems. *American Family Physician, 65*(1), 61–68.

Galligan, M. (2006). Proposed guidelines for skin to skin treatment of neonatal hypothermia. *Maternal-Child Nursing, 31*(5), 298–304.

Gaylord, N., & Yetman, R. (2009). Perinatal conditions. In C. Burns, A. Dunn, M. Brady, N. Star, & C. Blosser (Eds.), *Pediatric primary care* (4th ed, pp. 1035–1079). St. Louis: Saunders.

Hackman, P. S. (2001). Recognizing and understanding the cold stressed term infant. *Neonatal Network, 20*(8), 35–41.

Heird, W. (2007). The feeding of infants and children. In R. Kliegman, R. Behrman, H. Jensen, & B. Stanton (Eds.), *Nelson textbook of pediatrics* (18th ed, pp. 214–225). Philadelphia: Saunders.

Hernandez, J., & Thilo, E. (2005). Routine care of the full term newborn. In L. Osborn, T. DeWitt, L. First, & J. Zenel (Eds.), *Pediatrics* (pp. 1277–1289). Philadelphia: Saunders.

Hunt, C., & Hauck, F. (2007). Sudden infant death syndrome. In R. Kliegman, R. Behrman, H. Jensen, & B. Stanton (Eds.), *Nelson textbook of pediatrics* (18th ed., pp. 1736–1742). Philadelphia: Saunders.

Krebs, N., & Primak, L. (2006). Pediatric nutrition and nutritional disorders. In R. Kliegman, K. Marcdante, H. Jenson, & R. Behrman (Eds.), *Nelson essentials of pediatrics* (5th ed, pp. 131–155). Philadelphia: Saunders.

Lin, R. L., Tinkle, L. L., & Janniger, C. K. (2005). Skin care of the healthy newborn. *Cutis, 75*, 25–30.

London, M., Wieland-Ladewig, P., Ball, J., & Bindler, R. (2007). The physiologic responses to newborn birth. In *Maternal and child nursing care* (pp. 645–669). Upper Saddle River, NJ: Pearson Education, Inc.

McGrath, J. (2006). Family centered developmental care begins before birth: Little things can make a big difference. *Journal of Perinatal & Neonatal Nursing, 20*(3), 195–196.

Moore, E.R., Anderson, G.C., & Bergman, N. (2007). Early skin to skin contact for mothers and their healthy newborn infants. *Cochrane Database of Systematic Reviews*. Issue 3 Art No.: CD003519. DOI: 1002/14651858: CD 003519. Pub 2.

Pinheiro, J. (2009). Assessment and stabilization at delivery. In T. McInerny, H. Adam, D. Campbell, D. Kamat, & K. Kelleher (Eds.), *American Academy of Pediatrics textbook of pediatric care* (pp. 653–665). Elk Grove Village, IL: American Academy of Pediatrics.

Schanler, R. (2009). Breastfeeding the newborn. In T. McInerny, H. Adam, D. Campbell, D. Kamat, & K. Kelleher (Eds.), *American Academy of Pediatrics textbook of pediatric care* (pp. 809–823). Elk Grove Village, IL: American Academy of Pediatrics.

Schwartz, R., & Guthrie, K. (2008). Infant pacifiers: An overview. *Clinical Pediatrics, 47*(4), 327–331.

Stoll, B. (2007). The newborn infant. In R. Kliegman, K. Marcdante, H. Jenson, & R. Behrman (Eds.), *Nelson essentials of pediatrics* (5th ed., pp. 675–682). Philadelphia: Saunders.

VandenBerg, K. (2007). State systems development in high risk newborns in the neonatal intensive care unit: Identification and management of sleep, alertness and crying. *Journal of Perinatal & Neonatal Nursing, 21*(2), 130–139.

Walker, M. (2007). Breast-feeding: Good starts, good outcomes. *Journal of Perinatal & Neonatal Nursing, 21*(3), 191–197.

Zupan, J., Garner, P., & Omari AAA. (2004). Topical umbilical cord care at birth. *Cochrane Database of Systematic Reviews.* Issue 3. Art. No. CD001057. DOI: 10.1002/14651858: CD001057. Pub 2.

17 The Infant at Risk

Jacqueline M. McGrath and Whitney Hardy

OBJECTIVES

1. Identify the risk factors and maternal and fetal history for complications related to gestational age and birthweight issues in the neonate such as prematurity, postmaturity, and small for gestational age (SGA) and large for gestational age (LGA) infants.
2. Describe physical characteristics of preterm, late preterm, postterm, SGA, and LGA infants.
3. Recognize potential problems related to preterm, late preterm, postterm, SGA, and LGA infants.
4. Describe the immediate assessment parameters and management of the premature infant.
5. Identify risk factors and the maternal and fetal history that are predictive of respiratory distress syndrome (RDS).
6. Describe the specific pathophysiology, assessment parameters, and mangement of RDS.
7. Identify risk factors and the maternal and fetal history that are predictive of transient tachypnea of the newborn (TTN).
8. Describe the specific pathophysiology, assessment parameters, and mangement of TTN.
9. Identify risk factors and the maternal and fetal history that are predictive of meconium aspiration syndrome (MAS).
10. Describe the specific pathophysiology, assessment parameters, and mangement of MAS.
11. Identify risk factors and the maternal and fetal history that are predictive of persistent pulmonary hypertension of the newborn (PPHN).
12. Describe the specific pathophysiology, assessment parameters, and mangement of PPHN.
13. Describe the maternal and neonatal factors that contribute to jaundice in the neonate, and distinguish among the various causal factors and related outcomes of jaundice in the neonate.
14. Describe the physiologic process of the production, conjugation, and elimination of bilirubin in the neonate; the differences between conjugated and unconjugated bilirubin; and assessment parameters and mangement of hyperbilirubinemia.
15. Describe the maternal and neonatal factors that contribute to congenital anomalies in the neonate, and distinguish the differences among the various causal factors and related outcomes.
16. Describe the specific pathophysiology, assessment parameters, and mangement of common congenital anomalies in the neonatal period.

INTRODUCTION

Most newborns will transition to extrauterine life without a problem. However, even when transition is uneventful, the first 48 hours of life is when vigilant observation and anticipatory caregiving are essential. Most infants with serious illness present at birth or within the first 48 hours during the transition to extrauterine life. The challenge for the caregiver is to be able to discriminate the subtle signs of disease from the dynamically changing characteristics of normal transition and adaptation to the environment. Without excellent nursing care and good family education, early discharge might lead to some of these infants not being identified and thus being susceptible to poorer outcomes. Some of the most common disease processes that can appear in the newborn period include gestational age and birthweight-related issues, hypothermia, hypoglycemia, RDS, TTN, MAS, PPHN, sepsis, congenital anomalies, hyperbilirubinemia, and drug exposure of the infant. Newborn sepsis is discussed in Chapter 20, and the drug-exposed infant is covered in Chapter 25. For ease of discussion, gestational age and birthweight-related issues are addressed first followed by prematurity, respiratory and cardiac conditions, hyperbilirubinemia, and the most common congenital anomalies. However, it is important to note that these processes can occur concurrently, and in reality often infants diagnosed with any one of the previously noted newborn disease processes are more susceptible to the others.

SMALL FOR GESTATIONAL AGE INFANTS

INTRODUCTION

A. **An infant is defined as SGA when the weight is below the 10th percentile** (Anderson & Hay, 2005; Townsend, 2005).

B. **The SGA infant may also be known as having intrauterine growth restriction (IUGR).**

C. **Not all IUGR infants are SGA; IUGR from placental insufficiency usually reduces birthweight more than length and to a greater degree than head circumference; the greater the severity of IUGR, the greater is the deviation of weight, length, and (less so) head circumference as compared with population norms** (Anderson & Hay, 2005; Rosenberg, 2008).

D. **The SGA infant can be preterm, term, or postterm.**

E. **Conditions (alone or in combination) associated with SGA babies are as follows** (Hendrix & Berghella, 2008):

   1. Maternal conditions
      a. Chronic hypertension (associated with a four- to eightfold increase in the incidence of abruptio placentae)
      b. Anemia
      c. Cardiorespiratory disease
      d. Drug exposure (diethylstilbestrol, antineoplastics, narcotics, and illicit drugs)
      e. Smoking (frequently associated with abruptio placentae, placenta previa, prematurity, and respiratory distress) and alcohol consumption
      f. Young adolescent (10 to 14 years of age) or advanced maternal age (older than 35 years)
      g. Asthma

   2. Fetal conditions
      a. Chromosomal abnormalities
      b. Heart disease and hemolytic disease
      c. Intrauterine infection: toxoplasmosis, rubella, cytomegalovirus, and herpes simplex (TORCH)
      d. Malformations
      e. Multiple gestation

   3. Factors affecting the intrauterine environment
      a. Preeclampsia or eclampsia
      b. Decreased uteroplacental blood flow
      c. Diabetes mellitus
      d. Morphologic abnormalities
      e. Chorioamnionitis

   4. Placental conditions
      a. Abruptio placentae
      b. Placenta previa

   5. Environmental conditions
      a. High altitude
      b. Therapeutic x-ray exposure

F. **Conditions altering fetal growth produce insults that affect all organ systems and are known to produce two patterns of growth that depend on the timing of the insult to the developing embryo or fetus** (Rosenberg, 2008).

   1. Conditions affecting early gestation (generally less than 28 weeks) occur at a time when rapid cell proliferation (hyperplasia) occurs.
      a. An insult at this stage results in organs with cells of normal size but fewer numbers of cells than if the insult had not occurred.
      b. Infants are symmetrically grown (weight, length, and head circumference plot similarly on a growth curve) and all organ systems are small.
      c. Generally these infants have the poorest long-term prognosis and commonly have chromosomal abnormalities; postnatal nutrition is unable to correct for growth deficits; symmetrically grown SGA babies may never catch up in size when compared with unaffected children.

   2. Later in gestation (greater than 28 weeks), growth occurs as a combination of rapid cell proliferation (hyperplasia) but also as a result of increases in cell size (hypertrophy).
      a. An insult at this stage typically results in intrauterine malnutrition; organ systems have normal numbers of cells that are smaller.

    b. The brain and heart are larger in proportion to body size as a whole, whereas the liver, spleen, adrenals, thymus, and placenta are small.

    c. This type of infant is asymmetrically grown in that head size and length are spared, but overall weight and organ sizes are diminished.

    d. Generally, the asymmetrically IUGR infant has a better prognosis than one who is symmetrically IUGR; in utero malnutrition, however, is associated with increased risk of intrauterine death (Rosenberg, 2008; Townsend, 2005).

    e. Optimal postnatal nutrition generally restores normal growth potential because the number of body cells is normal.

G. The SGA infant may present with problems from the moment of birth (Rosenberg, 2008; Townsend, 2005).

    1. Fewer reserves are available to help the fetus tolerate the rigors of labor and delivery, leading to the development of fetal asphyxia or meconium passage in utero and the need for resuscitation at delivery.

        a. Uteroplacental circulation is often impaired. A small placenta may have diminished capability for gas exchange, nutrient delivery, and removal of waste products from the fetal circulation.

        b. Cardiac glycogen stores may already be reduced, leading to the development of fetal bradycardia.

        c. Uterine contractions may add an additional hypoxic stress on the chronically hypoxic fetus with a marginally functioning placenta.

    2. The combination of intrapartum and neonatal asphyxia places the infant at increased risk for a continuum of central nervous system insults that are the sequelae of perinatal asphyxia.

    3. Decreased glycogen stores increase the potential for early development of hypoglycemia and temperature instability in the transition period (see later discussion of preterm infants).

    4. Polycythemia frequently occurs as a result of chronic subacute hypoxia and dehydration.

H. Congenital anomalies are more frequently associated with intrauterine insult early in gestation during organogenesis; mortality rates for term SGA infants are five times that of term, appropriately grown infants resulting from the occurrence of major congenital anomalies (Mandruzzato et al, 2008).

I. The SGA infant is more frequently exposed to intrauterine infections such as rubella, cytomegalovirus (CMV), and toxoplasmosis; risk for impaired fetal gas exchange related to inadequate umbilical cord perfusion, hypoxia, and hypercarbia (Rosenberg, 2008).

J. Immune function in the SGA infant may be depressed as in older children with postnatal onset of malnutrition (Anderson & Hay, 2005; Mandruzzato et al, 2008).

K. The prognosis for SGA infants must consider adverse perinatal consequences in addition to being SGA; when perinatal problems are minimal or avoided because of early optimal obstetric intervention, the SGA neonate may still demonstrate developmental handicaps, especially in head growth restriction (Rosenberg, 2008).

L. Socioeconomic status and environment are the major determinant of developmental outcome at 2 years of age and older; SGA infants born to families of higher socioeconomic status demonstrate fewer developmental differences on follow-up, whereas those born to poorer families have significant developmental handicaps (Mandruzzato et al, 2008).

CLINICAL PRACTICE

A. Assessment

    1. History (Rosenberg, 2008; Townsend, 2005)

        a. Antenatal findings

          (1) Maternal weight gain

          (2) Age and socioeconomic status

          (3) Maternal illnesses or conditions

             (a) Renal

             (b) Cardiac; hypertension

             (c) Phenylketonuria (PKU)

          (4) Substance use or abuse such as alcohol, illicit drugs, or tobacco

        (5) Pregnancy conditions
           (a) Oligohydramnios
           (b) Multiple gestation
        (6) Elevated TORCH titers or other signs of infection
    b. Intrapartum findings
        (1) Length of gestation
        (2) Color, consistency, and amount of amniotic fluid
        (3) Fetal heart rate patterns suggestive of distress
  2. Physical findings (Rosenberg, 2008; Townsend, 2005)
    a. Soft-tissue wasting and dysmaturity
        (1) Decreased amount of breast tissue
        (2) Diminished subcutaneous fat tissue
        (3) Loose, dry, and cracked skin, with decreased turgor
        (4) Diminished muscle mass especially noticeable in the buttocks and extremities
        (5) Scaphoid abdomen resulting from shrinkage of the abdominal contents
    b. Smaller-than-average weight, length, and head circumference
        (1) The symmetric IUGR infant is smaller in all growth parameters (weight, length, and head circumference).
        (2) The asymmetric IUGR infant is smaller-than-average weight and average head circumference and length.
           (a) Large head-to-body ratio
           (b) Poor head control
  3. Presenting behavioral findings seen at or soon after delivery depend on the occurrence of asphyxia (postasphyxial encephalopathy) (Rosenberg, 2008; Townsend, 2005).
    a. Mild degree (duration less than 24 hours) exhibited by hyperalertness and sympathetic overactivity
    b. Moderate degree exhibited by lethargy, stupor, hypotonia, suppressed primitive reflexes, and seizures
    c. Severe degree manifested by coma, flaccid tone, suppressed brainstem function, seizures, and increased intracranial pressure
  4. Placental examination (Hendrix & Berghella, 2008)
    a. Abnormal cord insertion
    b. Placental hemangiomas, multiple infarcts, or chronic abruptio placentae
    c. Placenta previa
  5. Diagnostic procedures (Townsend, 2005)
    a. Weight, length, and head circumference
    b. Gestational age assessment and plotting of growth parameters on curve
    c. Serial bedside glucose assessment
    d. Assessment for infection (see Chapter 20 for a complete discussion of sepsis)
        (1) Complete blood count (CBC) with differential and platelets (also assess for polycythemia)
        (2) Viral studies
           (a) TORCH titer
           (b) Urine for CMV titer and culture
           (c) Nasopharyngeal culture for rubella
        (3) Possible lumbar puncture
        (4) Possible total and direct bilirubin levels
        (5) Coagulation studies if indicated by thrombocytopenia or petechia
B. Interventions/Outcomes (Rosenberg, 2008; Townsend, 2005)
  1. Interventions are described for the most common problems: birth asphyxia; respiratory distress; temperature instability; blood glucose instability; nutritional support; polycythemia; infection related to possible exposure to intrauterine infection (see Chapter 20 for complete discussion of newborn sepsis).
    a. Anticipate the need for and provide neonatal resuscitation according to Neonatal Resuscitation Program (NRP) guidelines as indicated by condition at the time of delivery.
    b. Monitor and record trends in transition vital signs, blood pressure, and clinical parameters; anticipate clinical manifestations such as tachypnea, respiratory distress, acidosis, cardiovascular instability, cyanosis, and hypoxemia.

    c. Provide oxygen as indicated based on pulse oximeter saturation monitoring, blood gas values, and close observation.

    d. Provide stabilization care in a neutral thermal environment (NTE), and allow the infant to stabilize and self-correct mild acidosis, clear lung fluid, stabilize blood glucose, and stabilize blood pressure.

    e. Monitor infant's body temperature: axillary should be in the range of 36.4° to 37° C (97.6° to 98.6° F).

    f. Examine the environment for potential sources of heat loss to prevent cold stress; for example, prewarm equipment, and avoid exposure to drafts.

    g. Monitor incubator or warmer bed temperature and heater output; the nurse should be concerned if heater output is constant.

    h. Monitor blood glucose levels if temperature instability occurs (to determine if hypoglycemia is causing temperature instability); anticipate blood glucose instability and hypothermia if the infant is fasting or as the infant transitions to bolus feedings; administer intravenous glucose (see discussion of hypoglycemia under care of preterm infant).

    i. Initiate early and frequent oral feedings (every 2 to 3 hours) if not contraindicated by respiratory status; provide a high-calorie formula (>20 calories/ounce [30 mL]) as ordered to provide additional nutrients.

    j. Obtain serum hemoglobin (normal 15 to 21.5 g/dL) and hematocrit (normal 45% to 65%) levels.

    k. Observe for signs and symptoms of polycythemia.
       (1) Ruddy appearance
       (2) Cyanosis; may be more pronounced with activity or crying
       (3) Tachypnea
       (4) Persistent hypoglycemia
       (5) Apnea or bradycardia
       (6) Jaundice

    l. Consider partial exchange transfusion for polycythemia when an infant is symptomatic to relieve capillary congestion and hyperviscosity.

  2. Outcomes

    a. Infant's 5-minute Apgar score is 7 to 10.

    b. Vital signs, blood pressure, blood glucose, and clinical parameters are stable.

    c. Oxygen saturation is maintained within normal limits.

    d. Normal body temperature is maintained.

    e. Neutral thermal environment is maintained.

    f. Infant shows no signs of cold stress, for example, increased oxygen consumption, hypoglycemia, and/or respiratory distress.

    g. Blood glucose levels are maintained at greater than 40 mg/dL.

    h. Oral feedings are tolerated well.

    i. Intravenous (IV) dextrose infusion, if indicated, maintains blood sugar within normal limits.

    j. Infant's initial weight loss stabilizes within 3 to 5 days of life, and weight increases thereafter at an average of at least 15 to 30 g (0.5 to 1 ounce) per day.

    k. Serum hematocrit is less than 65%.

    l. Signs and symptoms of hypoglycemia and polycythemia are absent.

    m. Neonate's intake is sufficient to achieve a urine output greater than 1.5 mL/kg/hr.

HEALTH EDUCATION

A. Inform parents of possible causes of IUGR.

B. Assist parents with guilt if chronic illness is a factor or if mother used substances known to compromise fetal growth.

C. Make parents aware of the discharge parameters for their newborn.

D. Instruct parents or family members on managing infant at home.
  1. Preparation of higher-caloric formula or frequent breastfeeding
  2. Performance of gavage feeding
  3. Use of developmental therapist to screen for developmental milestones and help optimize development

LARGE FOR GESTATIONAL AGE INFANTS

INTRODUCTION

A. The LGA infant is one whose weight is above the 90th percentile for gestational age (Townsend, 2005).
B. LGA babies may be preterm, term, or postterm.
C. Birthweight more than 4000 grams (8 pounds, 14.5 ounces) often reflects a genetic predisposition, except for the infant of a diabetic mother (IDM).
   1. Large parents tend to have large babies.
   2. Some Native Americans are more likely to have LGA infants.
D. Large size of the fetus may predispose the mother to an operative delivery.
E. If an LGA infant is born vaginally, the incidence of operative vaginal delivery (forceps or vacuum-assisted delivery) is higher than in the non-LGA infant; birth trauma is higher when compared with non-LGA babies and may include:
   1. Fracture of the clavicle or humerus
   2. Brachial plexus injuries
   3. Facial palsy
   4. Depressed skull fracture
   5. Cephalohematoma
F. The LGA fetus may show evidence of nonreassuring fetal heart rate patterns during a prolonged and difficult second stage of labor; neonatal respiratory depression may occur at the time of the delivery.
   1. Shoulder or body dystocia may occur.
   2. Particulate meconium-stained amniotic fluid may occur with risk of aspiration.
G. LGA infants are at risk for hypoglycemia related to early depletion of glycogen stores (see Chapter 22 for a complete discussion regarding the IDM).

CLINICAL PRACTICE

A. Assessment
   1. History
      a. Maternal
         (1) Previous delivery of an LGA neonate
         (2) Large weight gain during pregnancy
         (3) Diabetes (classes A through C) during the pregnancy
         (4) Prolonged or difficult labor and birth, particularly a long second stage
         (5) Ultrasonography that confirms fetal macrosomia
      b. Infant
         (1) Birthweight above the 90th percentile for gestational age
         (2) Type of delivery
            (a) Cesarean birth
            (b) Vaginal delivery with possible shoulder or body dystocia
            (c) Vacuum extraction or forceps-assisted delivery
         (3) Apgar scores at 1 and 5 minutes suggestive of neonatal respiratory depression
         (4) Particulate meconium-stained amniotic fluid
   2. Physical findings (Townsend, 2005)
      a. Weight greater than 90th percentile for gestational age
      b. Presence of caput succedaneum on the head
         (1) Localized soft tissue swelling over the presenting scalp area
         (2) Is present at birth and does not increase in size
         (3) Typically disappears within 12 to 48 hours
      c. Presence of a cephalohematoma
         (1) Increased incidence with vacuum extraction
         (2) Soft, fluctuant swelling in which the margins are limited to a cranial bone; does not cross suture lines
         (3) Increases in size for 2 to 3 days after birth

      (4) Disappears 6 to 8 weeks after birth

      (5) May be associated with complications

         (a) Jaundice, hyperbilirubinemia, or both

         (b) May be accompanied by a skull fracture with resultant subdural or subarachnoid hemorrhage

         (c) May be accompanied by intracranial hemorrhage

  d. Evidence of facial nerve damage, resulting from intrapartum pressure on facial nerves related to abnormal fetal position or forceps trauma

      (1) The eye on the affected side does not completely close as it normally does while the infant is crying.

      (2) The forehead does not wrinkle.

      (3) The side of the face is smooth.

      (4) The corner of the mouth droops.

  e. Evidence of brachial plexus injury as a result of overextension and torsion of the neck at the time of delivery resulting in overstretching, hemorrhage or tearing, or complete avulsion of the cervical nerve roots from the spinal cord

      (1) Erb's palsy (the most common type) as a result of upper cervical nerve root damage (C-5 and C-6)

         (a) Muscles of the upper arm are paralyzed.

         (b) The affected arm hangs limp, adducted, and internally rotated at the shoulder; movements that cannot be accomplished are:

           [i] Abduction and external rotation at the shoulder

           [ii] Flexion at the elbow and supination

         (c) Affected arm is pronated at the elbow and wrist is flexed, with strong palmar grasp present.

         (d) Deep tendon reflexes are absent.

         (e) Moro response is unilateral.

         (f) Occasionally associated with unilateral diaphragmatic paralysis, as evidenced by:

           [i] Asymmetry of chest expansion

           [ii] Tachypnea

           [iii] Cyanosis and/or dyspnea

      (2) Klumpke's palsy (rare) as a result of lower cervical root damage (C-8 to T-1 nerve roots)

         (a) The condition is limited to the wrist and hand.

         (b) The grasp reflex is abolished, the hand is held limply flexed, and voluntary movements of the wrist cannot be made.

         (c) Often associated with this are the manifestations of paralysis of the cervical sympathetic nerve (Horner's syndrome) on the same side.

           [i] Miosis of the pupil

           [ii] Slight lid droop

           [iii] Variations in local temperature, color, and sweating may appear later.

      (3) Complete brachial palsy (rare) as a result of injury to all roots from C-5 to T-1, producing entire paralysis of the arm and complete loss of sensation

  f. Evidence of clavicular or humeral fracture, either complete or incomplete

      (1) Decreased movement of affected side or arm may be seen when startle reflex is elicited.

      (2) Infant may cry in pain when affected area is manipulated; crepitus may be elicited.

      (3) Visible angulation or hematoma over the fracture site

      (4) Hypermobility of the bone

      (5) X-ray study confirms the diagnosis.

  g. Evidence of hypoglycemia (see later discussion under Preterm Infant)

  h. Signs of respiratory distress (see later discussion of respiratory distress)

      (1) Effort, character, and rate of respirations (increased, labored, greater than 60 breaths per minute)

      (2) Retractions: supraclavicular, intercostal, and substernal

      (3) Nasal flaring

      (4) Grunting

3. Diagnostic procedures
   a. Serum glucose
   b. X-ray study to assess for skeletal birth injuries
   c. X-ray study to assess for cause of respiratory distress
   d. Ultrasound scan or computed tomography (CT) for possible head injuries if cephalohematoma or depressed skull fracture is noted

B. **Interventions/Outcomes**
   1. Interventions are described for the most common problems: birth asphyxia; meconium aspiration (see later discussion); respiratory distress (see later discussion); birth trauma; temperature instability; blood glucose instability; nutritional support; hyperbilirubinemia; infection (see Chapter 20 for complete discussion of newborn sepsis).
      a. See discussion of hypoglycemia under care of preterm infant.
      b. See discussion of nutritional support under care of SGA infant
      c. See discussion of meconium aspiration.
      d. See discussion of respiratory distress.
      e. See discussion of temperature instability under care of preterm infant.
      f. On initial and repeat physical examination, note the following:
         (1) Size and position of caput or cephalohematoma
         (2) Evidence of skeletal bone fracture
         (3) Evidence of facial palsy or brachial plexus injury
      g. Observe for jaundice secondary to bruising or trauma (see discussion of hyperbilirubinemia).
      h. Provide treatment for any incidence of palsy.
         (1) Begin physical therapy and splinting early to prevent formation of contractures.
         (2) Provide gentle range-of-motion exercises to the affected extremity periodically.
         (3) Teach parents how to handle the infant without causing additional injury, provide range-of-motion exercises, and put on and take off splints.
      i. Provide treatment for fractured clavicle.
         (1) Obtain x-ray film for confirmation.
         (2) Immobilize affected arm and shoulder.
         (3) Support back and arm when lifting the infant.
         (4) Teach parents to expect a small bump over the fracture site to appear as healing occurs.
   2. Outcomes
      a. Infant's 5-minute Apgar score is 7 to 10.
      b. Vital signs, blood pressure, blood glucose, and clinical parameters are stable.
      c. Oxygen saturation is maintained within normal limits.
      d. Normal body temperature is maintained.
      e. Neutral thermal environment is maintained.
      f. Infant shows no signs of cold stress; for example, increased oxygen consumption, hypoglycemia, and/or respiratory distress.
      g. Blood glucose levels are maintained at greater than 40 mg/dL.
      h. Oral feedings tolerated well
      i. IV dextrose infusion, if indicated, maintains blood sugar within normal limits.
      j. Infant's initial weight loss stabilizes within 3 to 5 days of life, and weight increases thereafter at an average of at least 15 to 30 g (0.5 to 1 ounce) per day.
      k. Effects of trauma are minimized.
      l. Discomfort related to fracture is minimized or improved.
      m. Bilirubin levels remain within normal range or return to normal if phototherapy is instituted.

HEALTH EDUCATION

A. **Remind parents of the infant's immaturity and fragility despite her or his large size.**
B. **If the delivery was traumatic for the mother, she may need extra recuperation time before assuming total care of the infant.**
C. **Assist the parents to lift, position, and care for their large infant, especially for breastfeeding.**
D. **Instruct parents or family members regarding birth trauma, expected resolution, handling or treatment, and follow-up.**

E. Provide information about possible causes of macrosomia.

F. Provide feeding guidelines to prevent potential overfeeding or underfeeding.

POSTTERM INFANTS

INTRODUCTION

A. **A postterm pregnancy is one that extends beyond 41 completed weeks' gestation** (Avery & Richardson, 1998).

B. **Postterm neonates may be LGA, average for gestational age (AGA), SGA, or dysmature, depending on placental function.**
   1. If the placenta continues to function well, the fetus will continue to grow for the extra time in utero, which results in an LGA neonate with typical problems of LGA neonates (as previously stated).
   2. If placental function decreases, the fetus may not receive adequate nutrition and wasting of subcutaneous fat, muscle, or both occurs (Doherty & Norwitz, 2008).
      a. As the placenta loses its ability to nourish the fetus (placental insufficiency), the fetus uses stored nutrients for nutrition and wasting occurs; the body is lean, with thin extremities and little subcutaneous fat.
      b. This condition occurs in three forms
         (1) Chronic placental insufficiency
            (a) No meconium staining occurs.
            (b) Infant appears malnourished with skin changes.
            (c) Infant has an apprehensive look, reflecting hypoxia.
         (2) Acute placental insufficiency
            (a) Infant has a malnourished and apprehensive appearance.
            (b) Green meconium staining of the skin, umbilical cord, and placental membranes occur.
         (3) Subacute placental insufficiency
            (a) Skin and nails are stained golden yellow (resulting from breakdown of green meconium to hydrolyzed meconium, which is golden or yellow).
            (b) Umbilical cord, placenta, and placental membranes may be greenish brown.

C. **Because of the incidence of placental degeneration, postterm neonates are susceptible to perinatal asphyxia and meconium passage** (Doherty & Norwitz, 2008).
   1. Prenatal asphyxia often results in meconium passage in utero with or without fetal gasping.
   2. Aspiration of particulate meconium is highly likely to occur at the time of delivery with the first breath.
   3. The maternal care providers and neonatal resuscitation team plan together to provide management of the meconium (see later discussion of MAS). NRP guidelines are used to guide resuscitation care as needed.
   4. Intrauterine hypoxia may trigger increased red blood cell (RBC) production, leading to polycythemia, which results in the following:
      a. Sluggish perfusion of organ systems
      b. Hyperbilirubinemia resulting from breakdown of excessive numbers of RBCs

D. **Postterm neonates are susceptible to hypoglycemia because of the rapid depletion of glycogen stores.**

E. **Postterm neonates experience skin and integument changes** (Townsend, 2005).
   1. The skin is parchment-like and scaly.
   2. Loss of perfusion to the skin during prenatal asphyxia causes the top three layers of skin to die and slough, causing a macerated appearance.
   3. Loss of subcutaneous fat predisposes the neonate to increased extrarenal fluid loss and increased risk for hypothermia.
   4. Hair is abundant; nails are abnormally long; Wharton's jelly is decreased, and the umbilical cord is thin.

F. **Amniotic fluid volume is decreased, leading to potential fetal distress while in labor** (Doherty & Norwitz, 2008).
   1. Asphyxial renal changes cause fetal urine production to decrease; a low amniotic fluid index (AFI) may be present (AFI <5 suggests severe oligohydramnios).

2. In utero umbilical cord compression is more likely to occur if the amount of amniotic fluid to cushion the cord is reduced and the cord is thin, and is exhibited as decelerations, bradycardia, or both.

3. Prenatal passage of meconium in the circumstance of reduced amniotic fluid volume means that the meconium is thicker and the risk of aspiration is increased.

CLINICAL PRACTICE

A. **Assessment**
   1. History (Townsend, 2005)
      a. Estimated day of conception (EDC)
      b. Gestational age assessment based on prenatal ultrasonography, if available
      c. Color, consistency, and amount of amniotic fluid
      d. Placental grading, if available (see Chapters 3 and 8 for further discussion regarding placental functioning and grading)
         (1) Grades are based on deposits of calcium in the placenta that may interfere with adequate transfer of nutrients and oxygen to the fetus.
         (2) Grades II and III are mature.
      e. Irregular fetal heart rate patterns in labor
         (1) Variable decelerations, which are often the result of decreased amniotic fluid volume
         (2) Late decelerations and decreased or absent variability, which are indicative of nonreassuring fetal heart rate patterns
         (3) Bradycardia
      f. Apgar scores
      g. Cord blood gases
   2. Physical findings (Townsend, 2005)
      a. Skin is leathery, wrinkled, cracked, and peeling and frequently stained with meconium.
      b. Vernix is absent except in protected areas (scant amounts in neck and groin creases only).
      c. Fingernails are long and frequently meconium stained.
      d. Lanugo is absent.
      e. Creases cover the entire soles of the feet.
      f. Breast buds are large (greater than 1 cm in diameter) and the areolae are full and raised.
      g. Ear cartilage is thick and firm; ears stand away from the head.
      h. Has a wide-eyed and alert appearance, with more time spent in alert states.
      i. Postterm SGA neonates frequently appear hungry, with frantic rooting and fist sucking.
      j. Postterm LGA infants may be lethargic and have poor sucking ability.
      k. Signs and symptoms of respiratory distress may be present.
      l. Signs of birth trauma may be present in large infants.
   3. Diagnostic procedures
      a. Gestational age assessment plotted by growth parameters on growth curve
      b. Bedside blood glucose test monitoring
      c. Chest x-ray film to evaluate possible aspiration
      d. If respiratory distress is present, monitor oxygenation.
         (1) Oxygen saturation monitoring
         (2) Arterial blood gas assay

B. **Interventions/Outcomes**
   1. Interventions are described for the most common problems: glucose instability; nutritional support; meconium aspiration; respiratory distress; temperature instability; poor skin integrity
      a. See discussion of hypoglycemia under Care of Preterm Infant.
      b. See discussion of nutritional support under Care of SGA Infant.
      c. See discussion of meconium aspiration.
      d. See discussion of respiratory distress.
      e. See discussion of temperature instability under Care of Preterm Infant.
      f. Skin integrity may be decreased related to the absence of protective vernix and prolonged exposure to amniotic fluid (see discussion of skin integrity under Care of the Preterm Infant).

HEALTH EDUCATION

A. Inform parents of the consequences or sequelae of resuscitation as it applies to their newborn.
B. Refer to neurodevelopmental follow-up as indicated.
C. Provide parents or family members with information about any trauma sustained at birth.
D. Explain that postterm infants may need to feed more frequently (i.e., every 2 to 3 hours).

PRETERM INFANTS

INTRODUCTION

A. A preterm infant is one who is born before the end of 37 completed weeks' gestation (Moos, 2004).
B. Preterm infants, particularly those born before 34 weeks' gestation, represent a prototype of high-risk infants because of immaturity of all organ systems, numerous physiologic handicaps, and significant morbidity and mortality (Townsend, 2005). Late preterm infants are also at risk and need to be followed more closely because findings suggest that short- and long-term development is affected (Engle, Tomashek, & Wallman, 2007; Kelly, 2006).
C. **Risk factors** (Moos, 2004)
  1. Premature birth is frequently associated with maternal social deprivation and socioeconomic risk factors that promote catecholamine release, leading to decreased uterine blood flow and uterine irritability.
     a. Poverty, work away from home, teen pregnancy, and single motherhood have been identified as high-risk factors for preterm delivery (Balchin & Steer, 2007).
     b. Race (especially African American) continues to be a major risk factor for prematurity.
     c. Smoking and the use of illicit drugs, such as cocaine and crystal methamphetamine, have direct effects on placental and uterine blood flow and are commonly associated with uterine contractions, maternal hypertension, and placental abruption.
  2. Many women who deliver prematurely after spontaneous premature labor have an intraamniotic infection; bacterial vaginosis is a major risk factor for premature delivery, and early diagnosis and treatment of such infections have been shown to reduce the incidence of premature delivery.
  3. As the number of fetuses per pregnancy increases, the mean gestational age at delivery decreases; the mechanism of prematurity probably relates to the increase in intrauterine volume as well as the increased rate of volume change with multiple gestation.
  4. Bicornuate uterus and septate uterus are associated with increased incidence of prematurity.
  5. Prenatal maternal complications increase the risk for preterm birth.
     a. Maternal cardiorespiratory disease, hypoxia, hemorrhage, shock, hypotension, and hypertension
     b. Severe maternal anemia
     c. Maternal diabetes may result in preterm delivery because of fetal and maternal indications (Barnes-Powell, 2007).
     d. Abnormal placental conditions affect oxygen transfer from mother to fetus and result in asphyxial insult to the developing fetal lung.
D. **Clinical problems of the premature neonate are directly associated with the degree of organ maturity at birth; prematurity is not a disease but rather a lack of organ maturity.**
  1. Without full development, organ systems are not usually capable of functioning at a level needed to maintain extrauterine homeostasis.
  2. The more immature or lower the gestational age, the greater the risk of complications and system failure.
E. **The respiratory system is one of the last to mature; therefore, the preterm infant is at risk for numerous respiratory problems (see later discussion of respiratory distress for complete discussion of issues).**
F. **The cardiovascular system undergoes transition at birth from the fetal to the neonatal circulatory pattern; preterm delivery can adversely affect this transition** (Lott, 2007).

1. Transition is a response, in part, to the increased level of oxygen in the circulation once air breathing has begun; if oxygen levels remain low, the fetal pattern of circulation may persist, causing blood flow to bypass the lungs (Agarwal, Deorari, & Paul, 2008).
   a. Preterm infants have a high incidence of patent ductus arteriosus (PDA) (Dagle et al, 2009) (see more detailed discussion of PDA later).
   b. The foramen ovale may remain open if pulmonary vascular resistance is high.
2. The heart is relatively protected from hypoxia in utero; injury, if present, is generally reflected after delivery as cardiomegaly, with signs of cardiovascular insufficiency.
3. Preterm infants may have impaired regulation of blood pressure in the face of apnea, bradycardia, mechanical ventilation, and other types of neonatal intensive care unit (NICU) care (Blackburn, 2007).
   a. Fluctuations in cerebral blood flow are common. These fluctuations predispose the fragile blood vessels in the brain to rupture, causing intracranial hemorrhage.
   b. Fluctuations can cause loss of brain blood flow, resulting in ischemia. These fluctuations also predispose the preterm infant to develop retinopathy of prematurity.

G. **The immune system is both immature and inexperienced, making the preterm infant susceptible to infections** (Blackburn, 2007).
   1. Immunologic ability depends in part on immunoglobulins (Ig), such as IgG, IgM, and IgA.
   2. Preterm infants often have a deficiency of IgG because of delivery before transplacental transfer (occurs at approximately 34 weeks' gestation).
   3. IgA (the primary Ig in colostrum) is not available to the preterm infant if he or she does not receive breast milk or colostrum.
   4. On occasion, preterm delivery comes about as a result of maternal infection with pathogenic bacteria; the preterm infant is especially prone to developing group B beta-hemolytic *Streptococcus* infection.
   5. The risk for infection in the preterm infant is also increased because of disruption of skin integrity and instrumentation in the course of NICU care.

H. **The immature liver may be highly inefficient in conjugating bilirubin, leading to hyperbilirubinemia; drug metabolism in the liver may be markedly altered, increasing the risk of drug intolerance** (Blackburn, 2007; see more detailed discussion of hyperbilirubinemia later).

I. **The preterm infant has great difficulty maintaining body temperature** (McGrath, 2007b).
   1. The preterm infant is at great risk for excessive heat loss resulting from the following:
      a. Decreased or inadequate subcutaneous fat
      b. Large head-to-body ratio
      c. Lack of muscle tone and flexion
      d. Increased transepidermal evaporative losses
   2. Brown fat is not available or is inadequate to generate heat because sufficient stores are not available for use until after approximately 30 weeks' gestation.
   3. Cold stress quickly depletes what brown fat and glycogen stores are present, resulting in the following:
      a. Increased metabolic needs
      b. Increased oxygen consumption
      c. Consequences that include metabolic acidosis, hypoxemia, and hypoglycemia
   4. Poor nutrient intake is commonly associated with temperature instability.

J. **The preterm renal system is immature, resulting in the following** (Blackburn, 2007):
   1. Decreased ability to concentrate urine
   2. Lack of selectiveness in filtration
   3. Decreased glomerular filtration rate (GFR)
      a. Decreased drug clearance
      b. Increased likelihood of fluid retention
      c. Increased likelihood to develop fluid and electrolyte disturbances

K. **Periventricular intraventricular hemorrhage (PIVH) and ischemic changes are of particular significance in the preterm infant weighing less than 1500 g (3 lb 5 oz); more severe cases of PIVH tend to have poorer long-term neurodevelopmental outcomes** (Volpe, 2008).

L. **Necrotizing enterocolitis (NEC) is of particular significance in preterm infants with birthweights less than 1500 g (3 pounds, 5 ounces) with time of onset inversely related to gestational age and birthweight; signs and symptoms often begin with feeding intolerance and proceed to the classic signs and symptoms (similar to sepsis) and abdominal x-ray changes** (Bradshaw, 2009).

M. Hypocalcemia occurs in 30% to 90% of preterm infants.
N. Hypoglycemia is common among premature infants (Barnes-Powell, 2007; Stanley, 2006).
1. Functionally, hypoglycemia is defined as a serum glucose concentration of approximately 40 mg or less.
2. Perinatal conditions commonly associated with hypoglycemia are common among preterm, late preterm, and SGA infants.
   a. Diabetic mother
   b. Prematurity or SGA status
   c. Perinatal stress or hypoxia
   d. Cold stress
   e. Congenital heart disease or congestive heart failure
   f. Maternal drug therapy (beta-sympathomimetics, propranolol)
3. Signs and symptoms, if present, are nonspecific and appear at various serum glucose concentrations in different infants; they are often confused with infection and respiratory distress.
   a. Abnormal cry
   b. Lethargy
   c. Apnea
   d. Hypothermia
   e. Hypotonia
   f. Jitters
   g. Tremors
   h. Tachypnea
   i. Seizures
   j. Cardiac arrest

CLINICAL PRACTICE

A. Assessment
1. Maternal historical risk factors (Balchin & Steer, 2007)
   a. Premature labor treated with bedrest and tocolytics
   b. Multiple gestation
   c. Infections (see Chapter 20 for more detailed discussion of newborn sepsis)
   d. Antepartum bleeding
   e. Pregnancy-induced hypertension (PIH)
   f. Premature rupture of membranes (PROM)
   g. Cervical insufficiency or incompetence
   h. Psychosocial stress or high-risk maternal behaviors
   i. No prenatal care
   j. Poor nutrition
   k. Use of illicit drugs
   l. Domestic abuse
   m. Motor vehicle accident
2. Physical findings (Kelly, 2006)
   a. Neurologic: hypotonic resting posture (predominance of extensor muscle tone and underdevelopment of flexor muscle tone)
   b. Head
      (1) Larger in proportion to the body compared with the term infant
      (2) Skull bones soft and spongy, especially along suture lines
      (3) Fontanelles wide and soft with overriding sutures
      (4) Ears lacking development of cartilage
      (5) Scalp hair matted and woolly in appearance
   c. Skin
      (1) Skin is thin and edematous at early gestations, but thickness and opacity increase with advancing gestational age.
      (2) Transparent in early gestations so that the underlying capillary bed shows through, giving the infant a ruddy look; veins are readily visible.

   (3) Lanugo is fine and barely visible at early gestations, is thickest and most abundant between 28 and 30 weeks, and slowly disappears, beginning in the lower back as gestation advances.

   (4) Skin is susceptible to breakdown because of decreased cohesion between the dermis and epidermis.

   d. Breasts and nipples

   (1) Are barely visible at early gestations.

   (2) Areola becomes raised at about 34 weeks and increases in size as the breast bud enlarges.

   (3) A small bud is palpable at about 36 weeks' gestation and slowly increases in size with advancing gestational age.

   e. Sole creases develop first in the anterior third of the sole and slowly advance downward with advancing gestational age.

   f. Genitalia

   (1) The preterm male has a small scrotum with few rugae and testes that are high in the inguinal canal; presence of rugae increases, and testes descend into the scrotum with advancing gestational age.

   (2) The preterm female has a prominent clitoris and labia minora; the labia majora enlarge with advancing gestational age.

   g. Thermal instability (putting the infant at risk for heat loss) results from the following (McGrath, 2007b):

   (1) Larger surface-to-weight ratio

   (2) Immature muscle tone and decreased muscular activity

   (3) Diminished stores of white fat and brown fat

   (4) Poor nutrient intake

      (a) Infant has a scrawny appearance.

      (b) Lack of insulating properties of white fat allows for more rapid transfer of heat from the infant's core to the environment.

      (c) Reduced amounts of brown fat (deposited between 30 and 36 weeks' gestation) mean that chemical thermogenesis in the preterm infant (the usual, nonshivering method of heat production in newborns) is unreliable.

   h. An immature respiratory control center is exhibited by periods of apnea, periodic breathing, or both.

   (1) Apnea is an absence of respiration lasting more than 20 seconds accompanied by a fall in heart rate (usually to 80 beats per minute [bpm] or less) and with resultant cyanosis, hypotonia, and metabolic acidosis.

   (2) Periodic breathing is exhibited as breathing pauses, sometimes lasting more than 20 seconds, but without bradycardia, cyanosis, hypotonia, or acidosis.

   i. RDS, or hyaline membrane disease, may be present, is inversely related to gestational age, and is compounded when asphyxia is present (see Care of Infant with Respiratory Distress).

   j. Hypoglycemia may be present because of a lack of glycogen stores necessary to meet the infant's metabolic demands (see earlier discussion of hypoglycemia), exhibited by (Stanley 2006):

   (1) Lethargy

   (2) Tachycardia

   (3) Increased respiratory effort

   (4) Jitteriness

   k. Presence of a patent ductus arteriosus (PDA), which may be intermittent, as evidenced by:

   (1) Systolic cardiac murmur in area of upper left sternal border

   (2) Desaturation on pulse oximetry with or without color change

   (3) Increase in peripheral pulses

   (4) Increase in respiratory rate

   l. Signs and symptoms of infection may be present (see Chapter 20 for further discussion of newborn sepsis).

3. Diagnostic procedures

   a. Heart and respiratory rates

   b. Axillary, skin, and rectal temperatures

    c. Oxygen saturation levels by pulse oximetry and arterial blood gas assays
        (1) Oxygen saturation should be 90% to 92% in most cases.
        (2) Normal PaO_2 should be in the 50s to 60s.
    d. Blood
        (1) Glucose
        (2) CBC with differential
        (3) Electrolytes including calcium, blood urea nitrogen (BUN) and serum creatinine
        (4) Bilirubin concentrations
        (5) Cultures
    e. Urine output (normal 1 to 3 mL/kg/hr); specific gravity (normal 1.002 to 1.010)
    f. Chest radiographs
    g. Head and abdominal circumference
    h. Daily weights
B. Interventions/Outcomes
  1. Interventions for common problems of prematurity include those for temperature instability; blood glucose instability; respiratory distress (see later discussion); nutritional support; PDA (see later discussion); hyperbilirubinemia (see later discussion); renal insufficiency; environmental stress; infection related to possible exposure to intrauterine infection (see Chapter 20 for complete discussion of newborn sepsis).
    a. Monitor temperature.
        (1) Place neonate on servo-control mode under radiant warmer or in isolette with thermistor (located over the right upper quadrant of the abdomen) to achieve NTE.
        (2) Monitor heater output (be aware that continuous high heater output on servo-control mode in the face of normal skin surface temperatures is an alert to potential physiologic alterations in the neonate) (McGrath, 2007b)
        (3) Measure axillary, skin, and core temperatures as necessary (axillary temperatures are preferable and are as accurate as a core temperature if taken correctly) (McGrath, 2007b)
    b. Evaluate the environment for potential sources of heat loss or gain through conduction, convection, radiation, and evaporation.
        (1) Do not bathe the neonate without first evaluating the consequences of cold stress on the neonate's clinical condition.
        (2) Prewarm linens and equipment that will come into contact with the neonate.
        (3) Keep neonate's head covered with a cap.
        (4) Remain vigilant to the presence of radiant heat loss to cold walls or windows and convection heat loss in the path of air conditioning vents.
    c. Anticipate and prevent blood glucose instability (Stanley, 2006).
        (1) Bedside blood glucose levels (e.g., Accuchek, One Touch, Chemstrip) should be routinely measured at specific intervals (every 1 to 4 hours) in premature infants and others who have risk factors for hypoglycemia through the first several days of life.
        (2) Serum levels should be checked when the bedside value is less than 40 mg/dL in symptomatic infants.
            (a) If greater than 32 weeks' gestation with no respiratory distress offer formula or $D_{10}W$ (to raise and sustain the blood glucose level) every 2 to 3 hours.
            (b) Gavage feed an infant who refuses to suck, has tachypnea (respiratory rate greater than 60), or has poor coordination of suck, swallow, and breathing.
            (c) Administer parenteral $D_{10}W$ if blood glucose does not respond to oral feeding.
        (3) Continuous IV glucose infusion at maintenance rates (70 to 80 mL/kg/day), started early in symptomatic premature infants who are not yet hypoglycemic, will preclude the need for bolus glucose infusions that often result in flip-flopping serum glucose concentrations.
        (4) Bolus IV glucose ($D_{10}W$ at 2 mL/kg over several minutes) followed by a continuous infusion at maintenance rates often restores the serum glucose level within several minutes without producing unwanted flip-flop of the serum glucose level.
    d. Provide nutritional support as appropriate for body requirements and gestational immaturity
        (1) Monitor neonate's nutritional parameters (Kelly, 2006)
        (2) Intake (IV and oral) and output (urine, stool, or other) on an hourly basis
        (3) Body weight on a daily basis

(4) Head circumference and length on a weekly basis; document weight, length, and head circumference on a weekly basis on standard growth chart to assess for trends.

(5) Offer oral feedings, as tolerated and as ordered.

    (a) Oral feed if suck, swallow, and breathing coordination is present, neonate is in an awakened state, and stamina is good

    (b) Via breastfeeding as tolerated

    (c) Via intermittent bolus gavage (via intermittent insertion or indwelling tube)

    (d) Via continuous gavage (via indwelling tube)

(6) Monitor fluid and electrolyte levels regularly as needed.

    (a) Weight

    (b) Bedside monitoring of serum glucose level

    (c) Serum electrolyte values

    (d) Physical examination to determine hydration status

(7) Offer opportunities for nonnutritive sucking on a premature-size pacifier and social interaction as tolerated during feedings.

(8) Monitor for tolerance of feedings, noting characteristics, amount, and frequency of alterations.

    (a) Vomiting or regurgitation

    (b) Abdominal distention

    (c) Gastric residual (aspirated before next feeding): observe for color (bloody, bile-stained, or other); partially digested or not; and/or *mucusy* or not

    (d) Stools: observe for water loss; bloody; and/or explosive

    (e) Apnea or bradycardia related to reflux

    (f) Signs and symptoms of hypoglycemia

        [i] Jitters and tremors

        [ii] Lethargy and hypotonia

        [iii] Abnormal cry and tachypnea

        [iv] Bedside glucose screening test result less than 40 mg/dL

(9) Provide total parenteral nutrition (TPN) and lipids, when enteral feedings are contraindicated, administered via peripheral vein IV (maximum dextrose concentration is 12.5%) or via central catheter (central line or percutaneous central line).

e. Support skin integrity because of skin immaturity.

(1) Turn and reposition neonate every 3 to 4 hours and check skin integrity if tolerated.

(2) Keep skin clean, dry, and free from abrasions.

(3) Never use oil-based lotions or creams, alcohol, or benzoin on the very low-birthweight (VLBW) neonate or on dry skin of any neonate.

(4) Wipe off povidone-iodine (Betadine) with sterile water and cotton balls after procedures when it is used.

(5) Use hydrogel products to affix thermistor probes or leads; do not use tape on VLBW neonates.

(6) Remove hydrogel products and tape with sterile water and soak them off; if adhesive remover must be used, wash it off with sterile water immediately after.

(7) Use baby soap, sterile water, and cotton balls for diaper care.

(8) Consider using commercial skin barrier products whenever repeated taping to the skin is required and over areas of skin breakdown.

(9) Use positioning aids (e.g., bolster, nest, rolled blanket) to position neonate for comfort and to relieve pressure over bony prominences.

(10) Avoid friction or tearing of skin surfaces.

f. Evaluate environment for sources of excessive insensible water loss (IWL), and implement measures as needed to decrease IWL.

(1) Use heat shield or plastic wrap blanket under radiant warmer.

(2) Move to double-walled isolette as soon as possible after stabilization under radiant warmer.

(3) Provide warmed, humidified oxygen as needed.

(4) Ensure increased fluid intake under phototherapy as ordered.

g. Monitor urine output (check for mL/kg/hr) by weighing each diaper.

(1) Dipstick for protein and blood and check for specific gravity (concentration),

      (2) Monitor for signs and symptoms of overhydration or fluid overload.
         (a) Peripheral edema; taut and shiny skin
         (b) Bounding pulses
         (c) Increased blood pressure
      (3) Monitor for signs and symptoms of dehydration.
         (a) Poor skin turgor
         (b) Dry mucous membranes
         (c) Sunken fontanelles
      (4) Estimate IWL when clinical conditions or therapies are present that increase IWL.
         (a) Radiant warmer
         (b) Phototherapy
         (c) Respiratory distress
         (d) Skin breakdown
         (e) Ambient temperature above thermoneutrality
         (f) Fever
         (g) Increased activity
      (5) Monitor enteral and parenteral nutrition/fluid intake as ordered.
  h. Provide for minimal stimulation with appropriate sedation, if needed, to conserve energy stores.
      (1) Activity intolerance secondary to prematurity compromises effective ventilation, oxygenation, and caloric use.
      (2) Caretaking activities should be clustered to provide adequate periods of rest, but care should be taken to provide breaks between procedures when the infant demonstrates signs of stress.
      (3) Minimal handling should be observed by all personnel; unnecessary touching should be avoided to provide maximum opportunity for the parents for bonding (see Health Education).
      (4) Infant should be handled gently, with slow, purposeful movements rather than abrupt, jerky movements.
      (5) Sedation may be ordered for infants whose spontaneous activity level puts the infant at risk for respiratory distress.
      (6) Prone positioning has been shown to optimize respiratory status and decrease stress in the preterm infant.
2. Outcomes
  a. Neonate's axillary temperature is maintained within normal limits (36.4° to 37.1°C [97.6° to 98.8°F]).
  b. Optimal equipment to maintain thermal neutrality for infant is provided.
  c. No signs of cold stress are observed.
  d. The infant demonstrates intake of sufficient calories, as indicated by:
      (1) Weight gain of 15 to 30 g/day (0.5 to 1 ounce/day)
      (2) Head circumference growth averages 0.5 to 1 cm (0.2 to 0.4 inch) per week.
      (3) Spontaneous activity level that does not compromise weight gain
  e. The infant does not exhibit signs and symptoms of feeding intolerance or hypoglycemia.
  f. The infant is maintained on enteral feedings, as tolerated; if unable to tolerate enteral feedings, appropriate IV nutrition will be established and maintained.
  g. The infant demonstrates signs and symptoms of adequate hydration (absence of underhydration or overhydration).
      (1) Urine output between 1 and 2 mL/kg/hr
      (2) Electrolyte values within normal limits (WNL)
      (3) Weight loss in the first few days of life, followed by a weight gain of 15 to 30 g/day (0.5 to 1 ounce/day)
      (4) Absence of excessive generalized edema
      (5) Urine specific gravity ranges from 1.002 to 1.010.
      (6) Protein and blood are absent in the urine.
  h. The neonate is able to self-console by nonnutritive sucking on a pacifier and to show increased tolerance for social interaction.
  i. The neonate maintains good skin integrity as evidenced by lack of abrasions, skin breakdown, or local irritation or infection.

LATE PRETERM INFANT

INTRODUCTION

A. **The late preterm infant is born between 34 and 36 6/7 weeks' gestation** (Jorgensen, 2008a; 2008b).

B. **Late preterm infants make up 70% of the preterm infant population and the number may be increasing due to obstetric practices, such as inductions, elective cesarean sections, and increased number of multiple gestation infants** (Ramachandrappa & Jain, 2008; Yoder, Gordon, & Barth, 2008).

C. **Late preterm infants are often the size of some full-term infants and are often treated as such.**

D. **Late preterm infants are not physiologically or behaviorally mature and experience issues similar to preterm infants** (Engle et al, 2007).
   1. Temperature instability
   2. Difficulty with bottle and/or breastfeeding.
   3. Hyperbilirubinemia (see later discussion).
   4. Hypoglycemia (Laptook & Jackson, 2006).
   5. Respiratory distress (see later discussion).
   6. Sepsis

CLINICAL PRACTICE

See discussion of preterm infants for management strategies, interventions and outcomes with these infants. Often not ill enough to justify care in the NICU, the late preterm neonate is often cared for in the normal newborn nursery; thorough assessment of risk and health status, interventions, and parent education for these babies should be individualized (Campbell, 2006; Pappas & Walker, 2010). Certain criteria should be in place before these infants are discharged home.

A. **Discharge criteria** (Pappas & Walker, 2010)
   1. Normoglycemic
   2. Temperature stability
   3. Stable or decreasing bilirubin
   4. Feeding to sustain growth
   5. Feeding plan in place and parent(s) educated on plan
   6. Scheduled home care and follow-up appointments (i.e., lactation support, weight checks, home treatment for hyperbilirubinemia).

HEALTH EDUCATION

Preterm Infants

A. **Provide individualized instruction regarding the infant's respiratory diagnosis, handling and treatment considerations, and monitoring and treatment that will be continued in the home.**

B. **Teach parents to prepare high-calorie formulas or supplementation to breastfeeding to ensure adequate weight gain and growth, and instruct them if the infant is to be fed around the clock on a fixed schedule.**

C. **Teach parents to prepare and administer discharge medications.**

D. **Inform parents about the extent, outcome, and prognosis after PIVH or ischemic changes because they may need referral for persistent neurodevelopmental delays.**

Late Preterm Infants

A. **Instruct parents when and how often to see primary health care provider.**

B. **Instruct parents in temperature assessment and maintenance at home; avoid over and under dressing**

C. **Feeding plan (minimum number or volume of feeding/day)**

D. **Assessment for jaundice and dehydration**

E. **Education on respiratory syncytial virus (RSV) prophylaxis and prevention**

F. **Long-term outcomes/risks:**
1. Increased risk for Sudden Infant Death Syndrome (SIDS) (as much as 50%) (Darnall, Ariagno, & Kinney, 2006)
2. Increased risk for at least one hospital readmission within the first 6 to 12 months of life, especially if never admitted to the NICU (Cuevas, Silver, Brooten, Youngblut, & Bobo, 2005; Jain & Cheng, 2006)
3. Potential for growth and developmental delay (Chyi, Lee, Hintz, Gould, & Sutcliffe, 2008)

RESPIRATORY DISTRESS

INTRODUCTION

A. **Causes of Respiratory Distress.** The cause of respiratory distress in the newborn may have its beginnings in the failure of one or more major body systems. Conditions that result in the structural and functional failure of a major body system result in mild to profound respiratory distress in the newborn, regardless of size and gestational age. The following is a discussion of the five most common body systems involved in the causes of respiratory distress in general and specifically RDS (Sinha, Gupta, & Donn, 2008).
1. Cardiac diseases
   a. Congenital heart disease (CHD)
   b. Congestive heart failure (CHF)
   c. Patent ductus arteriosus (PDA)
2. Hematologic disorders
   a. Anemia
   b. Hemorrhage
   c. Polycythemia
3. Metabolic disorders
   a. Acidosis
   b. Hypoglycemia
   c. Hyperglycemia
   d. Hypocalcemia
   e. Hypothermia
   f. Hyperthermia
   g. Hypermagnesemia
   h. Congenital hyperthyroidism
4. Central nervous system disorders
   a. Hemorrhage
      (1) Intracranial, subdural hemorrhage (SDH), subarachnoid hemorrhage (SAH)
      (2) Intraventricular and periventricular hemorrhage (IVH and PVH)
   b. Infection
   c. Neonatal depression related to maternal drugs given during labor
      (1) Magnesium sulfate
      (2) Analgesics
   d. Neonatal substance-withdrawal syndrome
   e. Asphyxia
5. Respiratory disorders
   a. Most common conditions
      (1) RDS
      (2) TTN
      (3) Aspiration syndromes
         (a) MAS
         (b) Blood aspiration
         (c) Amniotic fluid aspiration
         (d) PPHN
   b. Pneumonia
   c. Spontaneous pneumothorax occurs in 1% to 2% of live births; only symptomatic in 1 in 1500 live births (Sinha et al, 2008). Symptoms may include tachypnea, minimal retractions,

grunting, nasal flaring, and cyanosis; diminished air entry on affected side, shifting of cardiac impulse, and muffled heart tones may also be noted.

CLINICAL PRACTICE

Although knowledge and understanding of these conditions are helpful in diagnosing and treating respiratory distress, this section focuses specifically on several respiratory conditions, including RDS, TTN, MAS, and PPHN.

Respiratory Distress Syndrome

A. **Introduction: RDS is the major cause of respiratory distress in the newborn, and prematurity is the single most important risk factor** (Sinha et al, 2008).
   1. RDS, sometimes referred to as hyaline membrane disease (HMD), accounts for 20% to 30% of all neonatal deaths and approximately 50% to 70% of all premature deaths; RDS occurs in 60% of babies born at less than 28 weeks' gestation, 50% of those born at 28 to 34 weeks, and in less than 5% of those born after approximately 34 weeks.
      a. Its incidence is inversely proportional to gestational age and occurs most frequently in infants of less than 1200 g (2 pounds, 10.5 ounces) birthweight and 30 weeks' gestation.
      b. Surfactant deficiency is the principal factor leading to the development of RDS.
   2. Prenatal maternal complications increase the risk for preterm birth and increase the risk of respiratory distress in the preterm infant by negatively affecting the fetal pulmonary circulation.
   3. The ability to stabilize the chest wall is directly related to increasing gestational age (GA); therefore, the preterm infant is at risk for chest wall deformation and atelectasis, which can result in hypoxemia, hypercarbia, and apnea.
   4. Immaturity of the respiratory system and its control centers places the preterm infant at risk for apnea of prematurity, a paradoxical response to low oxygen, high carbon dioxide, or both in which the preterm infant fails to breathe more quickly but instead stops breathing.
   5. Other causes of respiratory problems in the preterm infant (Sinha et al, 2008)
      a. TTN, in which delayed clearance of fetal lung fluid occurs manifested by rapid breathing, retractions, grunting, and cyanosis
      b. PPHN, in which hypoxemia and acidemia caused by failure to completely change from the fetal to the neonatal circulatory pattern occurs
      c. Bronchopulmonary dysplasia (BPD), in which oxygen therapy and intermittent mandatory ventilation combine to bring about chronic lung disease
   6. Pathophysiology: surfactant deficiency
      a. Surfactant is a complex mixture of phospholipids and proteins that binds to the alveolar surface of the lungs and forms a coating over the inner surface of the alveoli and decreases the surface tension, preventing collapse at the end of expiration (Halliday, 2008; Turell, 2008).
      b. Alveolar development occurs between 24 and 28 weeks' gestation, which results in the following (Hermansen & Lorah, 2007):
         (1) Increases in pulmonary vascularization
         (2) Development of ability for gas exchange
         (3) Development and proliferation of type II respiratory cells responsible for surfactant production and synthesis
      c. Surfactant deficiency results in the following (Halliday, 2008; Turell, 2008)
         (1) Increased surface tension, leading to alveolar collapse
         (2) Diffuse atelectasis
         (3) Loss of functional residual capacity
         (4) Decreased lung compliance
         (5) Right-to-left intrapulmonary shunting through the ductus arteriosus with increased pulmonary vascular resistance (PVR)
   7. Complications of RDS include the following:
      a. PDA incidence increases with decreasing gestational age (see later in this chapter for a complete discussion of PDA).
      b. Air leak syndromes (e.g., pneumothorax, pneumomediastinum, pneumopericardium) occur in 5% to 30% of infants with RDS (Sinha et al, 2008)

    c. IVH occurs in approximately 15% to 20% of infants weighing less than 1500 g (3 1bs, 5 oz) (Volpe, 2008).

    d. BPD occurs in approximately 23% of infants with RDS (Lefkowitz & Rosenberg, 2008).

    e. Retinopathy of prematurity (ROP) occurring in infants with RDS is increasing and is currently estimated to be between 20% and 25%; most of these cases regress, with the incidence of severe disease estimated to be between 5% and 10% (Pollan, 2009); prevention of premature birth is the best preventive of ROP; after a preterm birth, oxygen should be used only in amounts sufficient to avoid hypoxia.

B. Assessment

  1. History (risk factors) (Heinzmann et al, 2009; Sinha et al, 2008)

    a. At less than 28 weeks' gestation, 60% of neonates demonstrate clinical signs of RDS.

    b. At 28 to 32 weeks' gestation, 50% of neonates demonstrate clinical signs of RDS.

    c. At 37 weeks' gestation and older, 3% to 5% of neonates demonstrate clinical signs of RDS.

    d. At birth 10% to 15% of infants who weigh less than 2500 g (5 pounds, 8 ounces) demonstrate RDS; the highest incidence occurs among the group with the lowest birthweight (Hermansen & Lorah, 2007; Sinha et al, 2008)

    e. RDS is increased:

      (1) In males versus females (1.5 times' higher incidence)

      (2) Among whites versus nonwhites

      (3) In IDMs; insulin is antagonistic to surfactant production

      (4) In the presence of asphyxia, regardless of gestational age

      (5) When birth is by cesarean section, especially in the absence of labor, related to the lack of a thoracic squeeze

      (6) In the second-born of twins, which may be related to the second-born's longer stay in the birth canal, with the second twin receiving an excess of amniotic fluid with the birth of the first twin

    f. RDS is decreased with:

      (1) Prolonged or premature rupture of membranes (PROM)

      (2) IUGR

      (3) PIH

      (4) Maternal heroin addiction

      (5) Prenatal corticosteroids

  2. Physical findings: Symptoms of RDS frequently occur within 4 to 24 hours after delivery; symptoms are usually apparent in the delivery room; typically, the clinical course of RDS worsens during the first 48 hours after birth, and respiratory function generally begins to improve within 72 hours after birth.

    a. Intercostal, subclavicular, and substernal retractions occur because of the compliant chest wall of the preterm infant, in addition to relatively noncompliant lungs ("seesaw" respirations).

    b. Expiratory grunting, heard as a result of partial vocal cord closure, increases transpulmonary pressures in an attempt to improve lung volume capacity.

    c. Nasal flaring is often present as the infant attempts to decrease nasal airway resistance.

    d. Tachypnea with a respiratory rate of greater than 60 breaths per minute is common.

    e. Decreased breath sounds or unequal breath sounds are usually heard.

    f. Poor air entry is heard on auscultation.

    g. Fine rales may be heard bilaterally or unilaterally.

    h. Generalized cyanosis may be seen because of impaired ventilation and intrapulmonary and intracardiac shunting.

      (1) Peripheral cyanosis alone is common in newborns and is usually not significant.

      (2) The degree of cyanosis depends on the following:

        (a) Hemoglobin concentration

        (b) Status of the peripheral circulation

        (c) Color of the infant and the available light to visualize the cyanosis

    i. Tachycardia with a heart rate of 150 to 180 bpm may occur.

    j. Hypothermia may occur despite an NTE.

    k. Hypoglycemia with a glucose level of less than 20 mg/dL in the preterm infant may be noted.

    l. Hypotension is a frequent indication of severe RDS.

    m. Hypotonia results in a limp and flaccid infant.

    n. Apnea occurs frequently in the severely compromised infant.

3. Diagnostic procedures
    a. Apgar scores may not reflect the severity of RDS.
    b. Maturity assessment
        (1) Lecithin/sphingomyelin (L/S) ratio of greater than 2:1 indicates mature lungs in the absence of a diabetic pregnancy (Hermansen & Lorah, 2007).
        (2) The presence of phosphatidylglycerol (PG) confirms maturity and is especially important to ascertain lung maturity in the presence of maternal conditions such as diabetes.
            (a) Is present at 37 weeks' gestation and levels rise to term
            (b) If greater than 1%, indicates mature lungs
        (3) Shake test or foam stability index (FSI) may be performed on amniotic fluid at the maternal bedside to quickly determine the presence of surfactant.
    c. Chest x-ray initially may appear better than the clinical course would suggest; the classic chest x-ray film findings include the following:
        (1) Reticulogranular (ground-glass) pattern
        (2) Air bronchograms that demonstrate diffuse alveolar collapse surrounding open bronchi
        (3) Decreased lung volumes
        (4) Possible cardiomegaly
    d. Arterial blood gas (ABG) assays show hypoxemia and hypercapnia.
C. **Interventions**
    1. Provide appropriate supportive measures for the neonate, to offer optimal respiratory support.
        a. Resuscitation in the delivery room should follow NRP guidelines. Oxygen should be provided only as needed and blended based on assessment of infant (Rabi, Rabi, & Yee, 2007).
        b. Ensure ready availability of bag and mask setup and bulb and wall suction in the event that the infant requires intermittent mandatory ventilation or suction to clear the airway.
        c. Assess the neonate's respiratory effort with regard to rate, character, effort, and signs of respiratory distress.
        d. Maintain position of the neonate so that the upper airway is not obstructed.
        e. Intubate with the appropriate size of endotracheal tube (ETT); choice of tube size is determined by the neonate's weight, as follows (Bachman, Marks, & Rimensberger, 2008):
            (1) Less than 1001 g: 2.5 mm
            (2) 1001 to 2000 g: 3 mm
            (3) 2001 to 3000 g: 3.5 mm
            (4) More than 3001 g: 4 mm
        f. Transfer infant to the NICU if mechanical ventilation is required.
        g. Administer continuous positive airway pressure (CPAP) to infants, as needed, who do not require mechanical ventilation. May be administered via ETT or nasal prongs (Bancalari & Claure, 2008). CPAP may resolve some of the atelectasis, decrease intrapulmonary shunting, and improve ventilation to alveoli already open.
        h. Place infant in appropriate concentration of oxygen via oxygen hood or nasal cannula as determined by an ABG assay if mechanical ventilation or CPAP is not needed.
            (1) Oxygen should always be warmed and humidified to prevent infant heat loss and drying of mucous membranes.
            (2) Oxygen concentrations should be monitored continuously and documented per facility protocol (Shiao & Ou, 2007).
    2. Monitor continuously to determine trends.
        a. Cardiorespiratory monitor with 15-second apnea delay
        b. Oxygen saturation
    3. Assist with obtaining and review diagnostic tests to determine likely causes of respiratory distress (including any or all of the following: hypoglycemia, pneumonia, and RDS).
    4. Provide airway patency by the removal of secretions using accepted guidelines per facility protocol (Marechal, Barthod, Lottin, Gautier, & Jeulin, 2007).
        a. Use a catheter of appropriate size (a 5- or 6-mm catheter is recommended, if possible) to pass infant's airway.
        b. Determine depth of suctioning by size of infant or length of ETT tube; carefully pass the suctioning catheter, which will prevent damage to the mucosa; never deep suction, but

rather, suction to 0.5 cm below the length of the ETT (Marechal et al, 2007; Youngmee & Yonghoon, 2003). Never deep suction the infant, which may cause damage to the tracheal tissues.

   c. Set the vacuum gauge at 50 to 80 cm of water pressure.
   d. Suction only as needed; assess need to suction by the following:
      (1) Breath sounds
      (2) Type and amount of secretions
      (3) Tolerance and clinical status
   e. Have two people perform the procedure as necessary.
   f. Preoxygenate no more than 10% above baseline oxygen requirements and hyperinflate before suctioning.
      (1) Begin 1 minute before suctioning.
      (2) Continue during and after procedure until the infant reaches presuctioning heart rate and oxygen saturation baseline.
   g. Avoid repeated passes of the catheter if possible.
5. To minimize the risk of suctioning, continuously monitor the infant's tolerance of the suctioning procedure by observing for the signs and symptoms of:
   a. Hypoxia resulting in decreased oxygen saturation
   b. Bradycardia, dysrhythmias, or both
   c. Mucosal ulceration and hemorrhage secondary to the trauma of repeated suctioning
6. Provide continuous monitoring of infant's condition.
   a. All infants should be connected to continuous cardiorespiratory monitors to detect abnormalities in heart rate and rhythm, as well as apnea and bradycardia.
   b. Blood pressure should be monitored in all infants with RDS; normal blood pressure varies with size and gestational age.
   c. An ABG assay should be performed as needed.
   d. Ongoing infant respiratory status should be assessed every 1 to 4 hours as needed.
      (1) Auscultation of breath sounds
      (2) Quality of air entry
      (3) Respiratory effort and spontaneous respiratory rate
   e. Serial chest x-ray films should be obtained as appropriate to assess disease progression.
7. Administer exogenous surfactant per physician or facility protocol as needed to support lung function until the infant's own supply is produced (Halliday, 2008; Turell, 2008).
   a. Administration in the delivery room (early) has been shown to be more beneficial than late administration (Halliday, 2008; Turell, 2008)
   b. Administration protocol should be drug specific; not all surfactants are the same; dose, timing, and delivery systems may vary, as well as cost.
8. Prevent or treat hypotension.
   a. Systemic hypotension results in pulmonary and systemic vasoconstriction and will prevent adequate tissue perfusion and gas exchange.
   b. Administer fluids to prevent or treat hypovolemia. If more pressure support is needed the neonatal team should be notified and the infant should be prepared for transfer.
9. Prevent or treat hypothermia (McGrath, 2007b).
   a. Hypothermia causes cold stress in the neonate, which results in vasoconstriction and subsequent lowering of PaO_2.
   b. Maintain an NTE: defined as the condition under which the amount of heat produced is equal to the least amount of heat lost to the environment, with the least metabolic stress.
10. Prevent or treat metabolic acidosis.
   a. Metabolic acidosis causes constriction of pulmonary vessels and decreased lung perfusion.
   b. Administer IV fluids, as indicated.
   c. Prevent excessive water loss.
   d. Request support from neonatal team if infant does not respond to above interventions.
11. Prevent or treat hypoglycemia (see Care of Preterm Infant).
12. Prevent or treat anemia (see Care of Preterm Infant).
13. Provide for minimal stimulation with appropriate sedation, if needed, to conserve energy stores (see Care of Preterm Infant).

D. **Outcomes**
1. The neonate is appropriately and adequately resuscitated in the delivery room with minimal asphyxia, hypothermia, shock, and acidosis.
2. The infant receives the appropriate ventilatory support.
    a. The appropriate size of ETT is used, based on weight.
    b. Mechanical ventilation, CPAP, or oxygen is administered as needed.
3. The infant's vital signs are WNL.
    a. Heart rate between 120 and 180 bpm
    b. Respiratory rate between 40 and 60 breaths per minute
    c. Blood pressure WNL for size and gestational age
4. The neonate demonstrates minimal respiratory distress.
    a. Bilateral breath sounds
    b. Good air entry
    c. Consistent respiratory effort with spontaneous respirations
    d. Minimal retractions
    e. Absence of grunting and nasal flaring
    f. Absence of central or generalized cyanosis
5. The neonate demonstrates adequate pulmonary and tissue perfusion.
    a. Well oxygenated, with normal PaO_2
    b. Absence of metabolic acidosis
    c. Normal systemic blood pressure
    d. Absence of hypothermia
    e. Absence of hypoglycemia
    f. Normal hematocrit and hemoglobin levels
6. The infant receives minimal tactile stimulation.
    a. Caretaking activities will be grouped together.
    b. The infant will not be medically touched except to provide necessary care, and parental touch will be encouraged.
    c. Parents demonstrate knowledge of their infant's activity tolerance by minimizing stress during bonding activities.
    d. The infant is handled gently and carefully.
    e. Sedation is given to infants who demonstrate excess activity resulting in failure to adequately ventilate or oxygenate and whose caloric expenditure is in excess of caloric intake.

Transient Tachypnea of the Newborn (TTN)

A. **Introduction: TTN is sometimes referred to as wet lung syndrome, retained lung fluid (RLF), and RDS type II** (Guglani, Lakshminrusimha, & Ryan, 2008).
1. Pathophysiology: excess fluid in the lungs, failure to clear normal fetal lung fluid, or both (Takaya et al, 2008).
    a. Fluid accumulates in the peribronchial lymphatics and bronchovascular spaces.
    b. Excess fluid may be related to the following:
        (1) Aspiration
            (a) Amniotic fluid
            (b) Secretions; tracheal fluid
        (2) Factors that promote the formation of interstitial lung fluid
            (a) Decreased plasma colloid osmotic pressure (hypoalbuminemia)
            (b) Increased interstitial colloid osmotic pressure (transudation of plasma proteins)
            (c) Increased capillary hydrostatic pressure
    c. Fetal lung fluid is normally cleared via the following:
        (1) Expulsion during delivery
        (2) Absorption after delivery related to pulmonary circulation and lymphatic drainage
    d. Failure to clear fetal lung fluid is usually caused by the lack of a "thoracic squeeze" to expel the fluid during delivery.
2. There is no known residual pulmonary dysfunction; however, spontaneous pneumothorax may occur.

B. **Assessment**
   1. History (risk factors) (Takaya et al, 2008)
      a. TTN infants tend to be term or near term (36 weeks' and longer gestation) with mature lungs, as indicated by L/S ratio.
      b. TTN is increased (Guglani et al, 2008):
         (1) In large infants with a birthweight of more than 4000 g (8 pounds, 14 ounces)
         (2) In infants born by cesarean section
         (3) In breech births
         (4) In the second-born of twins
         (5) When labor and delivery are rapid and preclude the opportunity for an effective thoracic squeeze (especially in the small infant)
         (6) With a maternal history of heavy sedation
         (7) In infants with polycythemia, delayed cord clamping, or both; hyperviscosity of blood leads to sluggish circulation in the pulmonary vessels.
         (8) In infants suffering from hypothermia at or shortly after birth
            (a) Hypothermia causes pulmonary vasoconstriction.
            (b) Vasoconstriction causes the infant to experience hypoxemia and increased oxygen consumption, which produces respiratory distress.
   2. Physical findings: symptoms of TTN are usually present within the first hours of life (most often within 30 minutes); typically, the clinical course of TTN occurs during the first 12 to 72 hours of life and the disease is self-limiting.
      a. Transient tachypnea with a respiratory rate of 60 to 140 breaths per minute (rarely lasts longer than 48 to 96 hours)
      b. Grunting, nasal flaring and/or mild intercostal retractions
      c. Possible mild cyanosis
      d. Breath sounds that may be slightly decreased because of reduced air entry
      e. Absence of rales
      f. Chest that may appear hyperexpanded or barrel shaped
   3. Diagnostic procedures: TTN is a diagnosis of exclusion.
      a. A diagnosis of TTN can be ascertained only after resolution of symptoms within the first 4 days.
      b. Chest x-ray film reveals the following:
         (1) Increased lung fluid, with fluid in the interlobar tissues
         (2) Prominent vascular marking (so-called hairy heart)
         (3) Flat diaphragm, with increased lung volume
         (4) Mild pleural effusions may be demonstrated.
         (5) Occasional presence of mild cardiomegaly
         (6) Occasionally, the initial chest x-ray film (within the first 3 hours of life) appears similar to RDS.
      c. ABG assay
         (1) Mild hypoxemia
         (2) $PaCO_2$: normal to mildly elevated (less than 50 mm Hg)
         (3) pH: usually normal
C. **Interventions/Outcomes**
   1. Interventions
      a. Assisted ventilation is seldom required (Guglani et al, 2008; Takaya et al, 2008).
      b. Provide appropriate oxygen therapy to maintain ABG values WNL.
         (1) TTN infants rarely require more than 70% fraction of inspired oxygen (FIO_2) (usually 35% to 40%).
         (2) Providing CPAP for the first few hours with severe pulmonary involvement may be useful.
   2. Outcomes
      a. The infant receives the appropriate concentration of oxygen.
      b. The infant's ABG values are WNL.
      c. The infant demonstrates minimal respiratory distress.
         (1) Respiratory rate between 40 and 60 breaths per minute
         (2) Minimal retractions
         (3) Bilateral breath sounds with good air entry

(4) Absence of grunting and nasal flaring

(5) Absence of generalized cyanosis

Meconium Aspiration Syndrome

A. Introduction

1. Meconium aspiration is the most common of the aspiration syndromes (Walsh & Fanaroff, 2007; Wiedemann, Suagstad, Barnes-Powell, & Duran, 2008).

2. Pathophysiology: Two overlapping phenomena occur with MAS.
   a. Pneumonitis and pneumonia, with or without air leak
      (1) Bile salts and pancreatic enzymes and other particles in the meconium cause a chemical pneumonitis.
      (2) Meconium occludes the distal airways and acts as a ball-valve mechanism that allows air in but obstructs airflow out during expiration; this leads to air trapping and air leak (pneumothorax).
   b. Three general mechanisms in the fetus result in passage of meconium.
      (1) Direct hypoxic bowel stimulation
         (a) Passage of meconium into the amniotic fluid may be the result of some intrauterine insult that causes fetal distress.
         (b) Hypoxia and acidosis may result in relaxation of the anal sphincter and passage of meconium.
      (2) Spontaneous gastrointestinal (GI) motility: Spontaneous normal physiologic defecation may occur in the term or postterm infant.
      (3) Vagal stimulation with or without specific cause (often the result of cord compression)
   c. After the passage of meconium into the amniotic fluid, the fetus may swallow or aspirate the meconium into the mouth, pharynx, and trachea.
      (1) With hypoxia, the fetus demonstrates normal or irregular respiratory movements.
      (2) Intrauterine aspiration can occur in infants with overwhelming distress.
      (3) The greatest risk for aspiration is at delivery; if meconium-stained fluid is present in the mouth and pharynx when the infant draws the first breath (Wiedemann et al, 2008)
   d. In addition to the mechanical damage done by the meconium itself, asphyxia is by far the most damaging aspect of MAS (MAS infants without asphyxia do better clinically) (Walsh & Fanaroff, 2007).
      (1) Meconium aspiration may be the primary presenting event, but prolonged fetal asphyxia may have occurred before the meconium aspiration.
      (2) Asphyxia may lead to the following conditions:
         (a) Edema of the airways
         (b) Necrosis of the airways
         (c) Vascular collapse of the alveoli
         (d) Pulmonary hemorrhage

3. Incidence of MAS
   a. Approximately 12% of all births include the presence of meconium-stained amniotic fluid (Wiedemann et al, 2008).
   b. Meconium may be aspirated from the trachea in approximately 35% of these infants or approximately 4% of all live births.
   c. Infants who are depressed at birth or make poor attempts to take the first breath should be intubated in the delivery room and suctioning of the trachea should occur to remove meconium below the vocal cords; infants who do attempt to breathe and clear their own airway should be allowed to do so without intervention. Approximately one third of infants with meconium below the vocal cords become ill and require intensive care (Wiedemann et al, 2008).

4. Prevention
   a. Antenatal diagnosis and treatment of fetal asphyxia is critical to the prevention of MAS (Walsh & Fanaroff, 2007).
   b. Intrapartum amnioinfusion, particularly when oligohydramnios is an issue, should be considered for prevention (Walsh & Fanaroff, 2007).
      (1) Decreases rate of cesarean section
      (2) Decreases morbidities related to MAS

(3) Decreases cord compression

(4) Dilutes meconium and may decrease its toxicity

5. Complications of MAS include:

   a. Air leak syndrome such as pneumothorax, pneumomediastinum, or both occurs in 20% to 30% of MAS infants (Wiedemann et al, 2008).

   b. Pneumonia

   c. Infection

   d. PPHN

   e. Pulmonary instititial emphysema (PIE)

   f. Less commonly, severe asphyxia, thrombocytopenia, pulmonary hemorrhage

B. **Assessment**

1. History

   a. MAS infants tend to be primarily term, postterm, or SGA; the condition rarely occurs before 38 weeks' gestation (Wiedemann et al, 2008).

   b. Perinatal factors associated with or predisposing to MAS include (Bhat & Rao, 2008):

      (1) Prolonged labor

      (2) Fetal bradycardia and distress

      (3) Breech presentation

      (4) Presence of meconium-stained amniotic fluid

      (5) Delivery by cesarean section

      (6) Low Apgar scores (less than 6)

      (7) IUGR

      (8) Decreased fetal movements

2. Physical findings (El Shahed, Dargaville, Ohisson, & Soll, 2007)

   a. Severity of MAS correlates with:

      (1) Consistency of meconium

         (a) Early in the labor, heavy "pea soup" consistency

         (b) Late in the labor, passage of large particles

      (2) Amount of meconium

         (a) More than 2 mL in pharynx

         (b) More than 2 mL in trachea

   b. Meconium staining of skin, umbilical cord, and nails

   c. Hyperexpansion of the chest (barrel shaped)

   d. Signs and symptons of respiratory distress occur in up to 50% of MAS infants.

   e. Clinical signs of CHF

3. Diagnostic procedures

   a. ABG assays show hypoxemia with respiratory or metabolic acidosis or both.

   b. Chest x-ray film

      (1) Lungs are hyperinflated (9 to 11 ribs expanded).

      (2) Nonuniform, coarse, and patchy infiltrates radiate from one hilum into the peripheral lung fields.

      (3) Infiltrates associated with focal areas of irregular aeration may be present; some appear atelectatic or consolidated, and others appear emphysematous (air trapping).

      (4) Pleural effusions may be seen in MAS infants.

C. **Interventions/Outcomes**

1. Interventions

   a. Impaired ventilation and oxygenation in response to inadequate respiratory effort secondary to MAS

      (1) Perform amnioinfusion before delivery.

      (2) Provide appropriate delivery room care to prevent aspiration of any meconium found in the mouth and pharynx.

      (3) Once delivered, if the infant is depressed (i.e., anticipated 1-minute Apgar of less than 7), the vocal cords should be visualized with a laryngoscope, and the trachea should be suctioned; this selective approach has decreased the need for intubation by 40% without an increase in incidence of MAS (Bhat & Rao, 2008).

   b. Provide appropriate supportive measures for the neonate to offer optimal respiratory support.

      (1) Provide ventilatory support and transport to a tertiary nursery, if needed.

      (2) Provide for high oxygenation (PaO_2 of 75 to 90 mm Hg) to prevent vasoconstriction.

(3) Provide pharmacologic assistance, as needed, to achieve desired ventilation and oxygenation of the infant (Basu, Kumar, & Bhatia, 2007).

    (a) Surfactant inactivation can be overcome by instillation of exogenous surfactants; may require three or more doses (El Shahed et al, 2007).

    (b) Sedation to prevent hyperactivity that can compromise oxygenation

    (c) Vasodilators to increase pulmonary blood flow to allow for improved oxygenation

  c. Provide continuous monitoring of infant's condition.

    (1) Cardiorespiratory monitoring

    (2) Transcutaneous and oximetry monitoring

    (3) ABG assay

    (4) Ongoing respiratory status assessments

    (5) Serial chest films

  d. Prevent and treat conditions that may occur secondary to inadequate ventilation and oxygenation.

    (1) Systemic hypotension may be treated with the following:

      (a) Additional fluids

      (b) Vasopressors

    (2) Persistent metabolic acidosis may be treated with the following:

      (a) Additional fluids

      (b) Buffer agents as needed, to maintain a pH between 7.45 and 7.50

    (3) Anemia: transfuse with blood products, as indicated.

    (4) Infection (Basu et al, 2007)

      (a) Meconium is an excellent growth medium for bacteria.

      (b) Administration of prophylactic antibiotics may be indicated.

2. Outcomes

  a. The infant receives adequate delivery room care to prevent MAS.

    (1) Suctioned on the perineum before delivery of the thorax

    (2) Intubation and tracheal suctioning after birth only if the infant is depressed

  b. The infant is appropriately ventilated.

    (1) Mechanical ventilation, as needed

    (2) CPAP

  c. The infant is adequately oxygenated, as evidenced by:

    (1) PaO_2 of 75 to 90 mm Hg

    (2) The infant does not progress to or demonstrate signs of the severe consequences of MAS (persistent pulmonary hypertension, pneumonia, or air leaks).

  d. The infant receives pharmacologic support, as needed, to achieve adequate ventilation and oxygenation.

  e. The infant is continuously monitored.

  f. The infant does not demonstrate conditions secondary to inadequate oxygenation.

    (1) Hypotension

    (2) Metabolic acidosis

    (3) Anemia

    (4) Infection

Persistent Pulmonary Hypertension of the Newborn (PPHN)

A. Introduction: PPHN is described as hypoxemia with "persistent physiologic characteristics of fetal circulation in the absence of recognizable cardiac, pulmonary, hematologic, or central nervous system disease" (Latini, DelVecchio, DeFelice, Verrotti, & Bossone, 2008, p. 1507).

  1. Pathophysiology: failure to make the transition from high PVR and low pulmonary blood flow normally found in utero, to low PVR and high pulmonary blood flow normally found after transition to extrauterine life

    a. Usually the foramen ovale and ductus arterious remain open, with high blood flow shunting through these ducts that is sometimes bidirectional.

    b. Results in profound hypoxemia; mechanisms that maintain the fetal state are relatively unknown but may be related to alterations in nitric oxide, arachidonic acid metabolism, and systemic acidosis (Hernandez-Diaz, Van Mater, Werier, Lounik, & Mitchell, 2007).

    c. Theories suggest that indomethacin and aspirin, which are cyclooxygenase blockers, may contribute because exposure of the fetus to these drugs may prevent the decrease in PVR that occurs after initiation of ventilation.

    d. Research suggests that increased levels of immunoreactive endothelin-1, as well as insufficient production of endogenous endothelium-derived relaxin factor, may contribute to continued vasoconstriction (Silvani & Camporesi, 2007).

B. Assessment

  1. History (risk factors) (Hernandez-Diaz et al, 2007)

    a. MAS

    b. Birth asphyxia, postdates

    c. RDS

    d. Pneumonia

    e. Metabolic acidosis

    f. Infection (group B *Streptococcus*)

    g. Acute hypoxia with delayed resuscitation, hypoglycemia, or hypothermia

  2. Physical findings (Latini et al, 2008)

    a. Cyanosis over entire body or differential cyanosis may be seen.

    b. Respiratory distress with tachypnea

    c. Normal or decreased blood pressure (BP) or asymmetric BP with right arm being greater than left lower extremity

    d. Tricuspid insufficiency murmur may be present (harsh).

  3. Diagnostic procedures

    a. Hypoxia test: preductal and postductal PaO_2 with preductal and postductal oximetry

    b. Glucose status

    c. ABG assay: pH status; respiratory or metabolic or mixed acidosis usually present

    d. Chest x-ray film reveals variable heart size depending on cause of PPHN and whether heart defects are present; lung findings are also dependent on primary lung disease.

    e. Echocardiography may reveal:

      (1) Echo-increase in pulmonary artery (PA) pressure, shunting right to left or bidirectional at foramen ovale; may be shunting right to left at ductus or bidirectional at ductus.

      (2) Tricuspid insufficiency

      (3) Right ventricular hypertrophy may be present.

C. Interventions/Outcomes

  1. Interventions

    a. Prevention is best, with early and effective resuscitation and correction of acidosis and hypoxia.

    b. Assisted ventilation with hyperoxia may be used as needed to increase passive oxygen diffusion across alveolar membrane and promote vasodilation. Call the neonatal team and transfer to NICU as needed to best support the infant (Latini et al, 2008).

    c. Decrease environmental stimulation because these infants are often quite sensitive to handling and stress from the environment.

      (1) Decrease activity.

      (2) Decrease noise and light.

      (3) Cluster caregiving.

      (4) Use sedation as needed.

      (5) Manage and treat before painful procedures.

  2. Outcomes

    a. The infant receives the appropriate concentration of oxygen for PVR to decrease and pulmonary vascular blood flow to increase.

    b. The infant's ABG values are WNL.

    c. The infant demonstrates minimal respiratory distress.

      (1) Respiratory rate between 40 and 60 breaths per minute

      (2) Bilateral breath sounds with good air entry

      (3) Absence of generalized cyanosis

HYPERBILIRUBINEMIA

INTRODUCTION

Causes of Hyperbilirubinemia

Physiologic jaundice is a condition that is common in the term newborn infant during the second or third day of life (second to ninth day in preterm neonates) and is not considered to be pathologic unless bilirubin levels exceed the normal physiologic limitations of a healthy neonate; pathologic hyperbilirubinemia, which can be defined only by serum concentrations of unconjugated bilirubin, has diverse causes that are frequently, but not always, interlinked; jaundice is a manifestation of bilirubin accumulation in extravascular tissues.

A. **Incidence of physiologic jaundice during the first week of life**
   1. Almost all neonates have elevated serum bilirubin levels greater than 2 mg/dL (the normal level in adults is 1.3 mg/dL or less) (Maisel, 2006)
   2. Elevated serum bilirubin levels greater than 5 mg/dL occur in 60% of neonates (Maisel, 2006)
   3. Hyperbilirubinemia, as it occurs in physiologic jaundice, may confer some biologic advantage to the neonate.
      a. Beneficial effects of bilirubin molecules might be noted at a cellular level (Maisel, 2006).
      b. Bilirubin has a potent antioxidant effect.
      c. Neonates have deficient levels of most antioxidant substances.
   4. Breastfeeding jaundice appears in the first days of life and is called such because it appears to be related to early ineffective breastfeeding practices that lead to (Maisel, 2006):
      a. Decreased volume of fluid intake
      b. Decreased caloric intake of fluid
      c. Dehydration
      d. Delayed passage of meconium
   5. Breast milk jaundice occurs after 3 to 5 days of life, with a steady increase in serum bilirubin that usually peaks at approximately 2 weeks (5 to10 mg/dL) and then decreases slowly; this type of jaundice appears to be related to the composition of the breast milk that results in enhanced enterohepatic circulation, although this is speculative (Maisel, 2006).

B. **Bilirubin production and conjugation**
   1. Bilirubin has two forms:
      a. Unconjugated or indirect
         (1) Fat soluble
         (2) Toxic to tissues
      b. Conjugated or direct
         (1) Water soluble
         (2) Nontoxic to tissues
   2. The majority of bilirubin comes from the destruction of hemoglobin.
   3. Process of bilirubin conjugation
      a. Within the circulatory system, unconjugated bilirubin tightly bound to albumin is transported to the liver, where the conjugation process takes place.
      b. Bilirubin is then released from the albumin binding site and undergoes the following:
         (1) Transfer across the hepatocyte membrane
         (2) Cytoplasmic protein binding
            (a) Within the liver, bilirubin is bound to ligandin and other hepatic proteins.
            (b) This binding helps prevent a backup of bilirubin into the general circulation.
         (3) Transport (while bound to protein)
            (a) Smooth endoplasmic reticulum is the site of conjugation process.
            (b) Process of conjugation transforms the poorly soluble, unconjugated bilirubin into a water-soluble form that can be excreted by the neonate; this process requires oxygen and glucose.
         (4) Excretion (after conjugation) into the bile, into the intestine, and finally into stool
            (a) Some bilirubin is excreted through the kidneys as urobilinogen.
            (b) In the intestine, the enzyme glucuronidase may break the ester linkage of the bilirubin, causing it to become unconjugated.
            (c) The newly unconjugated bilirubin may be reabsorbed into the neonate's circulation, necessitating a repetition of the entire conjugation process.

4. Neonatal hyperbilirubinemia can occur from the following:
    a. An increased load of circulating bilirubin resulting from:
        (1) Polycythemia
        (2) Isoimmune hemolytic disease
        (3) Structural and enzyme defects of RBCs
        (4) Drug toxicity (chemical hemolysis)
        (5) Extravascular hemolysis
    b. Impaired hepatic function (e.g., defective uptake, conjugation, or excretion)
        (1) Deficient glucuronyl transferase activity
        (2) Biliary obstruction or biliary atresia
        (3) Infection
        (4) Metabolic problems: galactosemia, breast milk jaundice and hypothyroidism
    c. Perinatal complications, such as asphyxia, hypothermia, and hypoglycemia
    d. Decreased albumin binding sites, because of preterm birth and/or competition with drugs having an affinity for the binding sites
    e. Delayed meconium passage
5. Rate of bilirubin level increase
    a. Must exceed 4 to 6 mg/dL before it is visible as jaundice.
    b. In physiologic jaundice:
        (1) Bilirubin level increase first appears after 24 hours of age in term neonates and after 48 hours of age in preterm neonates.
            (a) Reaches peak at day 3 or 4 and returns to a normal level by the end of day 7 in term neonates
            (b) Reaches peak at day 5 or 6 and returns to a normal level by the end of day 9 or 10 in preterm neonates
            (c) Pattern for breastfed infants is slightly different; peak level often occurs on day 4 and the decline may be slower.
        (2) Indirect bilirubin value does not usually exceed 12 mg/dL.
        (3) Direct bilirubin does not usually exceed 1 to 1.5 mg/dL.
        (4) Daily increases of bilirubin do not usually exceed 5 mg/dL.
    c. In pathologic jaundice, elevated bilirubin levels:
        (1) Appear within the first 24 hours of life
        (2) Persist beyond the age for return to a normal level in term and preterm neonates
        (3) No specific serum level can be used for diagnosis.
    d. Kernicterus is a preventable neurologic syndrome with lifelong sequelae; it is caused by severe and inadequately treated hyperbilirubinemia during the neonatal period (Bhutani & Johnson, 2009).
        (1) Bilirubin encephalopathy is the most serious complication of hyperbilirubinemia.
        (2) Yellow staining of brain tissue occurs and creates morphologic changes in brain cells, which results in irreversible damage.
        (3) Approximately one half of affected neonates do not survive.
        (4) Condition is generally thought to occur at bilirubin levels in excess of 20 mg/dL in full-term neonates.
        (5) Early signs include:
            (a) Extreme jaundice
            (b) Alterations in level of consciousness (lethargy)
            (c) Tone (hypotonia, then later, hypertonia)
            (d) Abnormal movement (opisthotonos)
            (e) Poor feeding
            (f) High-pitched crying
        (6) The long-term sequelae include:
            (a) Cerebral palsy
            (b) Sensorineural hearing loss
            (c) Gaze paresis
            (d) Dental dysplasia
            (e) Kernicterus
            (f) Mental retardation

C. **Phototherapy**
   1. Treatment is widely used to manage and control rising bilirubin levels (Stokowski, 2006).
     a. Unclothed neonate, with eye shields, is placed in an infant incubator within 45 to 50 cm (18 to 20 inches) of the bank of lights and turned every 2 hours.
     b. Treatment can also be performed with a fiberoptic blanket attached to an illuminator and wrapped around the neonate's torso and extremities.
       (1) Allows use of an open crib
       (2) Eye shields are not needed.
       (3) Neonate can be held.
       (4) Can be used for home phototherapy (Stokowski, 2006)
   2. Mechanism of phototherapy action
     a. Treatment is thought to reduce serum bilirubin levels by facilitating biliary excretion of unconjugated bilirubin.
     b. Treatment causes the formation of photoisomers, which are more water soluble and therefore more easily excreted in stool and urine.
       (1) Unconjugated bilirubin is rapidly converted to photobilirubin and lumirubin.
       (2) Photobilirubin and lumirubin are rapidly taken up by the liver and transported into the bile.
       (3) Process occurs independent of hepatic conjugation of bilirubin.
     c. White, daylight, cool blue, and special blue are among the various types of phototherapy lights available.
       (1) Lights with high-energy output, ranging between 420 and 450 nm in the blue spectrum, are the most effective.
       (2) Optimal energy output light levels should be monitored to ensure that levels are maintained to achieve maximum efficiency.
     d. Home monitoring and treatment
       (1) Bilirubin levels can be determined in the hospital as well as during a home visit by using transcutaneous bilirubinometry (TcB).
         (a) Procedure uses a noninvasive, portable instrument.
         (b) Predicts serum bilirubin levels in the neonate by using reflective measurements on the skin to determine the amount of yellow in the skin.
         (c) Measurement can correlate well with serum bilirubin levels; however, error rates can be high because of a variety of neonatal factors (Maisel, 2006).
           [i] Gestational age of neonate
           [ii] Birthweight
           [iii] Skin pigmentation because of different ethnic origin
           [iv] Phototherapy treatment (Stokowski, 2006)
         (d) TcB should be used only as a screening tool to determine when a laboratory measurement of serum bilirubin is needed (Maisel, 2006).
       (2) In some circumstances, home phototherapy can be provided and thus avoid separation of neonate from parents.

D. **Treatment controversies surrounding physiologic jaundice exist.**
   1. The trend has been to decrease interventions and to observe and manage neonates as outpatients.
   2. Research has shown that healthy full-term neonates in the absence of significant hemolysis or other underlying medical conditions with serum bilirubin levels of approximately 18 mg/dL do not have any detrimental effects with an expectant observation treatment approach (Bhutani & Johnson, 2009; Maisel, 2006).
   3. The American Academy of Pediatrics (AAP) Practice Guidelines for Management of Hyperbilirubinemia in the Healthy Term Newborn provides guidelines for identifying at-risk infants and intervention and treatment strategies; in April 2001, The Joint Commission (TJC) issued a Sentinel Event Alert regarding the increased incidence of kernicterus. Proposed risk reduction strategies include:
     a. Predischarge bilirubin measurement, with standing orders allowing nurses to order total serum bilirubin (TSB) levels or TcB levels for newborns (Bhutani & Johnson, 2009; Maisel, 2006).
     b. Use of a percentile-based nomogram to predict the risk of hyperbilirubinemia and implement strategies for follow-up, which may be helpful in provision of care (Bhutani & Johnson, 2009) (Figure 17-1)

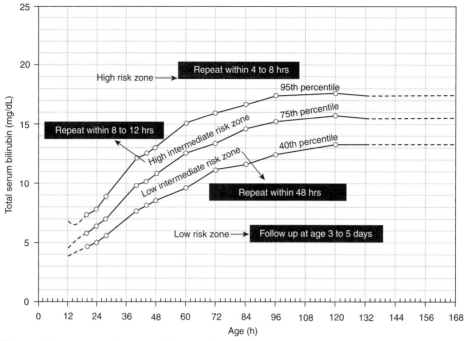

FIGURE 17-1 ■ An approach to time follow-up for repeat jaundice and bilirubin evaluation based on pre-discharge bilirubin testing. (From Bhutani, V.K., & Johnson, L. [2009]. A proposal to prevent severe neonatal hyperbilirubinemia and kernicterus. *Journal of Perinatology, 29,* S61-S67.)

    c. Follow-up for all newborns within 48 hours after discharge by a physician or trained health care provider who is experienced in the care of newborns to provide follow-up physical assessment and ongoing lactation support to ensure adequacy of intake for breastfed infants (Bhutani & Johnson, 2009; Maisel, 2006).

    d. Providing parents with adequate educational materials at discharge regarding jaundice, feeding adequacy, and symptoms to watch for (Stokowski, 2006)

CLINICAL PRACTICE

A. Assessment
  1. History
    a. Maternal
      (1) Mother's blood type can have an effect on a neonate's bilirubin levels by causing intravascular hemolysis via an antigen-antibody reaction.
        (a) Rh disease
        (b) ABO incompatibility
        (c) Positive Coombs' test result
      (2) Insulin-dependent diabetic mother
        (a) Neonate has an increased RBC mass at birth.
        (b) Breakdown of a high number of aged RBCs results in excessive amounts of bilirubin in the neonate.
      (3) Maternal and paternal ethnicity
        (a) Asian and Native American neonates have a higher incidence of hyperbilirubinemia.
        (b) Mean serum levels of unconjugated bilirubin in Asian and Native American neonates are higher than the mean levels for neonates of other ethnic origins (Maisel, 2006).
          [i] Mean serum levels of unconjugated bilirubin for the former are 10 to 14 mg/dL.
          [ii] This mean is approximately double that of neonates of other ethnic origins.
        (c) African American and white neonates tend to have lower mean levels of bilirubin.

        (4) Maternal drugs used during the last 3 months of pregnancy

           (a) The following drugs interfere with the binding of bilirubin to albumin in neonates:

               [i] Sulfonamides

               [ii] Salicylates

               [iii] Ibuprofen

           (b) Synthetic oxytocin (Pitocin) is associated with a higher incidence of neonatal jaundice.

        (5) 70% possibility of recurrence in subsequent siblings of an infant diagnosed with breast milk jaundice (Maisel, 2006)

           (a) Breast milk jaundice occurs in 0.5% to 2% of breastfed term infants (Maisel, 2006).

           (b) Affected breast milk contains substances that inhibit the activity of glucuronyl transferase in the neonatal liver.

           (c) Bilirubin levels continue to rise on the fourth and fifth days, when physiologic jaundice should be subsiding.

               [i] Rise to peak concentrations of between 10 and 27 mg/dL between 10 and 15 days of age

               [ii] Gradually decrease from peak levels to normal levels between 3 and 12 weeks of age (Maisel, 2006)

  b. Labor and delivery history

        (1) Use of the following drugs:

           (a) Synthetic oxytocin (Pitocin)

           (b) Diazepam

           (c) Bupivacaine (in epidural anesthesia)

        (2) Delayed umbilical cord clamping

           (a) Allows an excessive amount of blood to be transfused from the placenta to the neonate

           (b) Increase in quantity of RBCs results in the following:

               [i] Sequestration of greater numbers of aged RBCs

               [ii] Excessive amounts of bilirubin from breakdown of aged RBCs (Maisel, 2006)

        (3) Operative delivery: Ecchymosis and extravascular hemolysis may be increased by use of forceps or vacuum extractor.

  c. Perinatal complications

        (1) Cephalohematoma

        (2) Cerebral hemorrhage

        (3) Pulmonary hemorrhage

        (4) Any occult bleeding

        (5) Maternal-fetal transfusion

        (6) Hypoxia

           (a) Causes increase in free fatty acids.

           (b) Free fatty acids compete with bilirubin for albumin-binding sites.

        (7) Infection and sepsis (bacterial, viral, or protozoal)

           (a) Hemolysis

           (b) Hemolytic anemia

        (8) Low Apgar scores at 1 minute and at 5 minutes may indicate a complication.

  d. Postnatal complications

        (1) Caloric deprivation, causing weight loss, results from:

           (a) Infrequent feedings

           (b) Poor suck-and-swallow reflex

           (c) Decrease in gastric motility and enzymatic activity

        (2) Glucose-6-phosphate dehydrogenase (G6PD) deficiency

           (a) Is an enzymatic deficiency

           (b) Disrupts erythrocyte metabolism and causes hemolysis

           (c) Occurs primarily among African Americans, Filipinos, Sephardic Jews, Sardinians, Greeks, and Arabs (Maisel, 2006).

           (d) Manifests as jaundice on the second or third day of life and persists into the second or third week of life.

2. Physical findings

  a. Visible jaundice progresses in a cephalocaudal direction and can be seen first in facial skin, sclera, and gums, and later in the torso and lower extremities.

    b. Bilirubin levels
       (1) Elevated umbilical cord blood bilirubin level
       (2) Pattern of jaundice onset, length, and duration
    c. SGA condition that is associated with infection
    d. Small head circumference (microcephaly) that is associated with infection
    e. Cephalohematoma, ecchymosis, and abrasions are indicative of a traumatic delivery process.
    f. Pallor that is suggestive of hemolytic anemia
    g. Poor feeding or difficulty with breastfeeding
    h. Lethargy; difficult to awaken for feedings
    i. Petechiae that are suggestive of the following:
       (1) Congenital infection
       (2) Overwhelming sepsis
       (3) Severe hemolytic disease
    j. Plethora that is associated with polycythemia
    k. Vomiting that is suggestive of the following:
       (1) Sepsis
       (2) Pyloric stenosis
    l. Hepatosplenomegaly that is suggestive of the following:
       (1) Chronic intrauterine infection
       (2) Hemolytic anemia
   m. Congenital anomalies: Increased incidence of jaundice is found in infants with trisomies.
3. Diagnostic procedures
    a. Maternal blood group and indirect Coombs' test to rule out possibility of ABO or Rh incompatibility
    b. Serologic assays to rule out congenital syphilis
    c. Hemoglobin to rule out the following:
       (1) Anemia
       (2) Polycythemia: hemoglobin concentration higher than 22 g/dL
    d. CBC with differential
       (1) Elevated reticulocyte count suggests hemolytic disease.
       (2) RBC morphology
          (a) Spherocytes suggest ABO incompatibility.
          (b) RBC fragmentation suggests disseminated intravascular coagulopathy (DIC).
       (3) WBC count
          (a) Less than 5000/mm^3 suggests infection.
          (b) Increase in bands to more than 2000/mm^3 suggests infection.
       (4) Platelets: Thrombocytopenia suggests infection.
       (5) Sedimentation rate values in excess of 5 mm^3 during first 48 hours is suggestive of infection or ABO incompatibility.
       (6) Elevated direct bilirubin (conjugated) level suggests infection or severe Rh incompatibility.
B. Interventions/Outcomes
  1. Interventions
    a. Increase fluid intake to offset the following:
       (1) Increase in metabolic rate caused by phototherapy (Stokowski, 2006)
       (2) Significant increase in water loss through the skin
       (3) Increase in water content of frequent stools
       (4) Water loss caused by hyperthermia
    b. Offer neonate frequent feedings.
       (1) Feed as often as tolerated (approximately every 2 hours).
       (2) Increase calories to offset rapid intestinal transit time (frequent stooling) and decreased intestinal absorption of milk.
    c. Maintain thermal homeostasis while infant is under phototherapy lights by using a servo-control mechanism such as an isolette or radiant warmer.
       (1) Hypothermia stimulates the release of free fatty acids, which compete for albumin binding sites.
       (2) Hyperthermia increases the neonate's metabolic rate.

d. Monitor for impaired neonatal skin integrity related to diarrhea, urinary excretions of bilirubin, and exposure to phototherapy lights (Stokowski, 2006).
   (1) Diapering of the neonate may be accomplished by using a paper face mask with the metal strip removed.
      (a) Allows maximal skin exposure for phototherapy lights
      (b) Provides protection for genitals and bedding
      (c) Shields a minimum of jaundiced skin
   (2) It is typical for stools to be loose, greenish, frequent, and expelled with force.
   (3) It is important to protect neonate's skin from excoriation by thoroughly removing urine and feces with each diaper change.
   (4) It is important to change diapers frequently.
   (5) It is important to keep neonate's skin clean and dry by frequently checking bedding for dampness or stool soiling.
e. Protect the neonatal cornea from phototherapy light exposure through continuous wearing of protective eye shields.
   (1) Protect neonate's eyes from phototherapy lights by applying eye shields to prevent eye damage.
   (2) Secure placement of the eye shields tightly enough to prevent slippage and accidental eye exposure but not so tightly that constraint and excessive pressure are placed on the neonate's eyes.
   (3) Remove eye shields when neonate is not under phototherapy lights.
      (a) For feedings
      (b) For procedures not performed under phototherapy lights
   (4) Make sure the neonate's eyes are closed when applying the eye shields.
   (5) Change eye shields frequently and watch for any signs of conjunctivitis, such as:
      (a) Purulent discharge
      (b) Edema
f. Assess for impaired parenting related to parent-infant separation secondary to phototherapy treatments (Stokowski, 2006).
   (1) Encourage parents to participate in the caretaking responsibilities of their neonate.
   (2) Encourage parents to hold their neonate for short periods.
   (3) Encourage parents to provide gentle stroking and touching of their neonate while he or she is under phototherapy lights.
2. Outcomes
   a. Fluid intake is increased.
   b. Neonate remains well hydrated while under phototherapy lights.
   c. Neonate maintains a normal temperature while under the phototherapy lights.
   d. Neonate is covered and kept warm when not under phototherapy lights (i.e., for feedings and other procedures).
   e. Neonate's skin remains clean and dry while under phototherapy lights.
   f. No signs of redness or excoriation are present on the neonate's skin.
   g. Neonate wears protective eye shields at all times while under phototherapy lights.
   h. No signs of excessive eye shield pressure are present on neonate's skin around the eyes.
   i. No signs of conjunctivitis are present in neonate.
   j. Parents actively participate in caretaking activities with their neonate.
   k. Parents provide soothing tactile stimulation to their neonate while he or she is under phototherapy lights.

HEALTH EDUCATION

A. **The technologic advances made in newborn care during the past 30 years have markedly decreased morbidity and mortality in this group of high-risk infants.**
   1. Technologic advances have brought a heightened sensitivity to the psychological and emotional effect felt by the family of a sick neonate.
   2. This awareness has introduced the need for a family-centered approach to newborn care (McGrath, 2007a).
   3. In addition to the physiologic care of the sick neonate, health care workers need to address the psychologic needs of family members during this experience.

4. Parental attachment to the infant with respiratory distress, hyperbilirubinemia, or both, is especially difficult.
   a. The infant may be premature.
   b. Normal interaction may be severely curtailed.
   c. An infant who is sick enough to be in a special care or intensive care unit on a ventilator, or receiving oxygen support or phototherapy may not give cues adequate to arouse parental attachment.
5. Provide information in nontechnical terms to parents about serum bilirubin levels while the neonate is being monitored, and encourage their questions and concerns about their neonate's condition.

B. **The birth of a newborn who is sick represents a unique crisis for the family and perinatal health care team** (McGrath, 2007a).
   1. The family must simultaneously adjust to the immediate situation and begin the normal developmental process of parenthood.
   2. Situational factors have an important bearing on the family's ability to cope with this present crisis and can affect the overall outcome.
      a. The behavior and attitude of the hospital staff
      b. The sensitivity used in the transfer process either to another facility or the NICU
      c. The flexibility in unit visitation and extended family involvement
      d. The instruction received by the family related to their infant's unique characteristics and behavior
      e. The staff's sensitivity to the family's responses and adaptation to crisis
      f. The use of emotionally supportive intervention programs in the nursery
      g. The development of appropriate discharge planning to provide adequate follow-up for the family

C. **Discharge planning for the infant with respiratory distress or hyperbilirubinemia may include the following:**
   1. Family education
      a. Use of equipment needed in the care of the infant (e.g., oxygen, suctioning devices, phototherapy)
      b. Praise for parents' caretaking abilities of infant while in the hospital; parents are not visitors
      c. When and how to perform chest physiotherapy
      d. Dosage, route of administration, side effects, and planned duration of use of all medications
      e. Nutritional information to maintain adequate calorie and fluid balance
         (1) Type of formula (if used instead of breast milk)
         (2) How and when to feed the infant
         (3) Possible alternative feeding methods
         (4) If and when to provide oxygen during the feedings
      f. Support for mother's or father's attempts to feed the neonate and encourage frequent feedings to provide neonate with adequate hydration and increased calories
      g. The use of home monitoring, if needed
      h. Infant cardiopulmonary resuscitation (CPR)
      i. Recognition of signs and symptoms of illness in the newborn
      j. Normal newborn care
   2. Acquisition and maintenance of specialized equipment that may be needed to care for the infant at home, including:
      a. Oxygen and oxygen equipment
      b. Suction machine and supplies
      c. Home monitoring equipment
      d. Phototherapy
   3. All information and education given to the family should be in written form, if possible; in addition, whenever possible, return demonstrations by the family reinforce learning.
   4. Parents should be instructed about signs, symptoms, and treatment of hyperbilirubinemia that may occur at home as a result of early discharge program (Bhutani & Johnson, 2009; Maisel, 2006; Stokowski, 2006).
      a. Monitoring neonate's behaviors that may be indicative of increasing bilirubin levels
      b. Blanching neonate's skin to determine degree of jaundice

    c. Placing the neonate's bassinet or cradle near a window during the daytime to take advantage of natural sunlight

    d. Monitoring feeding and level of consciousness

    e. Maintaining sufficient hydration level in neonate

    f. Advising when to take the neonate to the health care provider for further evaluation of bilirubin levels

D. Long-term follow-up of the infant with respiratory distress or hyperbilirubinemia is essential.

    1. Parents must have telephone numbers of the medical facility and personnel to call 24 hours a day in case of problems or equipment failure.

    2. Before hospital discharge, parents need to have information regarding follow-up appointments and referrals for long-term care.

COMMON CONGENITAL ABNORMALITIES

NEURAL TUBE DEFECTS

A. Hydrocephalus

    1. Introduction

        a. Congenital hydrocephalus is an enlargement of the cerebral ventricles or subarachnoid spaces.

        b. Incidence of congenital hydrocephalus is 0.4 to 3.16 per 1000 newborns (Landingham, Nguyen, Roberts, Parent, & Zhang, 2008).

    2. Clinical practice

        a. Assessment

            (1) History

                (a) Fetal ultrasound testing shows an enlarged head.

                (b) Cephalopelvic disproportion (CPD)

            (2) Physical findings

                (a) Head circumference greater than the 90th percentile equates to a 95% likelihood of ventricular dilation (Landingham et al, 2008).

                (b) Enlarged or full fontanelles

                (c) Wide or split suture lines

                (d) Excessive rate of head growth

                (e) Vomiting might occur.

        b. Diagnostic procedures

            (1) Sequential ultrasound testing to evaluate ventricular size and rate of dilation

            (2) Magnetic resonance imaging (MRI) and CT for evaluation of cerebral parenchyma

        c. Interventions/Outcomes

            (1) Interventions

                (a) Clean and dry skin creases after feeding or vomiting.

                (b) Place infant on a waterbed or an egg-crate mattress.

                (c) Reposition neonate's head frequently.

                (d) Monitor any reddened areas, and position infant away from any potential problem areas.

            (2) Outcomes

                (a) Neonate's skin remains intact and shows no signs of beginning breakdown.

B. Spina bifida

    1. Introduction

        a. Spina bifida is a general term used to describe defects in closure of the neural tube associated with malformations of the spinal cord and vertebrae. Spina bifida is the most common congenital malformation of the CNS (Landingham et al, 2008).

        b. Spina bifida cystica includes three main types of defects

            (1) Meningocele

                (a) Presence of a sac containing meninges and cerebrospinal fluid (CSF); however, the spinal cord and nerve roots are normal in their structure and positioned within the spinal canal.

                (b) Typically infants will not show neurologic deficits.

            (2) Myelomeningocele (MN)

                (a) Most common form of spina bifida cystica; occurrence rate is 1 to 1.5 per 1000 live births (Vogel & Sturm, 2008)

(b) Presence of a sac containing meninges, CSF, spinal cord and/or nerve roots

(c) Typically infants will show neurologic deficit below level of lesion.

(d) Associated with Arnold-Chiari syndrome, which is the leading cause of death in patients with MN and hydrocephaly (Landingham et al, 2008).

(3) Myeloschisis: most severe; no cystic covering; the spinal cord is open and exposed.

2. Clinical practice

    a. Assessment

       (1) History

          (a) Elevated maternal serum alpha-fetoprotein levels

          (b) Ultrasound visualization of the defect

          (c) Familial history of spina bifida

          (d) Hydrocephalic fetus

       (2) Physical findings

          (a) Presence of a spinal lesion

          (b) Enlarged head circumference: hydrocephalus

          (c) Lack of spontaneous movement of the lower extremities

          (d) Hip clicks secondary to congenital hip dislocation

          (e) Clubfoot and scoliosis

          (f) Flaccid or spastic muscles in the lower extremities

          (g) Urine and stool leakage

    b. Interventions/Outcomes (for immediate care in the delivery room and prior to transport to more acute care)

       (1) Interventions

          (a) Place neonate only in prone or side-lying position.

          (b) Place neonate into sterile bowel bag, secure top at level of axilla; or cover defect with warm, normal saline–moistened sterile gauze, and place plastic wrap over dressing.

          (c) Keep meconium or urine away from lesion.

          (d) Administer antibiotics per orders.

       (2) Outcomes

          (a) Membranous sac stays intact.

          (b) Aseptic environment is maintained around and over the lesion.

          (c) Neonate does not show any signs of infection.

GASTROINTESTINAL CONGENITAL ANOMALIES

A. Cleft lip and cleft palate

    1. Introduction

        a. Cleft lip with or without cleft palate is the most common craniofacial anomaly affecting approximately 1 of every 600 live births (Johnson & Little, 2008).

        b. Cleft palate alone occurs in 1 of every 1000 newborns and occurs more frequently in females (Ciminello, Morin, Nguyen, & Wolfe, 2009).

        c. Cleft lip may be unilateral or bilateral. Cleft palate may involve just the soft palate or both the soft and the hard palates.

        d. Facial clefting is associated with an increased incidence of other abnormalities (Jaruratanairikul, Chichareon, Pattanapreechawong, & Sangsupavanich, 2007).

    2. Clinical practice

        a. Assessment

          (1) History

            (a) Maternal use of phenytoin, alcohol, retinoic acid, cigarette smoking

            (b) Family history of cleft lip and/or palate in siblings

            (c) More than 300 recognized syndromes include cleft lip and palate as a characteristic (Jaruratanairikul et al, 2007).

          (2) Physical findings

            (a) Unilateral or bilateral visible defect

            (b) Flattening or depression of midfacial contour in cleft lip

            (c) Fissure connecting oral and nasal cavities in cleft palate

            (d) Difficulty in sucking

  (e) Expulsion of formula or breast milk through the nares
  (f) Dehydration
  (g) Poor weight gain or weight loss
  b. Interventions/Outcomes (for care in the newborn nursery; some infants may require more acute care)
   (1) Interventions (Ciminello et al, 2009)
      (a) Feed with a special nipple and bottle set.
      (b) Burp frequently.
      (c) Feed in upright position with head and chest tilted slightly back to aid swallowing and discourage aspiration.
      (d) Limit feedings to 30 to 45 minutes to avoid poor weight gain due to fatigue.
      (e) Feed high-calorie-per-ounce formula to increase caloric intake.
      (f) Have mother attempt breastfeeding if only cleft lip is present.
      (g) Support parental coping and assist parents with grief over loss of idealized baby.
      (h) Encourage parents to verbalize feelings about the defect and the feeding frustrations.
      (i) Provide role modeling while interacting with the neonate so that parents can internalize positive interaction (Johnson & Little, 2008).
      (j) Refer parents to community agencies and support groups.
   (2) Outcomes
      (a) Neonate is gaining weight appropriate to age.
      (b) Neonate is not vomiting feedings.
      (c) Neonate is not excessively fatigued after feeding.
      (d) Parents are able to freely verbalize their feelings and frustrations about their infant.
      (e) Parents are involved in the neonate's care in the hospital and frequently seek information about the infant's progress.
      (f) Parents exhibit bonding behaviors with their infant.
B. Abdominal wall defects
  1. Introduction
   a. Omphalocele
    (1) Defect of the umbilical ring that allows evisceration of abdominal contents into an external peritoneal sac (Ledbetter, 2006)
    (2) Incidence is 1.5 to 3 per 10,000 live births (Ledbetter, 2006)
   b. Gastroschisis
    (1) Defect of the umbilical ring that allows evisceration of bowel through a defect in the abdominal wall with no membrane covering (Ledbetter, 2006)
    (2) The incidence is 0.4 to 3 per 10,000 live births (Ledbetter, 2006)
  2. Clinical practice
   a. Assessment
    (1) History
      (a) Polyhydramnios
      (b) Visualization on fetal ultrasonography
      (c) Elevated maternal serum alpha-fetoprotein
      (d) Preterm labor in the case of gastroschisis
    (2) Physical findings
      (a) Visible defect over the abdominal area
        [i] Omphalocele is covered with a sac consisting of peritoneum and amniotic membrane.
        [ii] Gastroschisis defect exposes viscera because of lack of any covering.
        [iii] Gastroschisis occurs almost exclusively to the right of the umbilicus.
      (b) About 50% of newborns born with omphalocele have cardiac, gastrointestinal, genitourinary, musculoskeletal, and CNS anomalies (Ledbetter, 2006).
   b. Interventions/Outcomes (for immediate care in the delivery room or prior to transfer to more acute care)
    (1) Interventions
      (a) Place neonate feet first into sterile bowel bag, and secure top at level of axilla.
      (b) Monitor temperature closely.
      (c) Place in isolette, and maintain NTE.

(d) Administer IV fluids and albumin per institutional protocol.

(e) Maintain nothing per mouth (NPO) status.

(f) Maintain integrity of sterile bowel bag or moist sterile dressing.

(g) Monitor glucose levels and electrolytes.

(h) Insert nasogastric tube to decompress bowel.

(2) Outcomes

(a) Omphalocele sac remains intact.

(b) Herniated viscera remains normal in color and moist.

[i] Hydration is maintained.

[ii] No further advancement of bowel herniation through defect

(c) Neonate's temperature remains WNL.

C. Congenital diaphragmatic hernia

1. Introduction

a. Congenital diaphragmatic hernia (CDH) is a malformation that consists of herniation of abdominal contents into the thorax cavity via a defect in the diaphragm. The exact etiology of CDH is not fully understood. CDH might be caused by maldevelopment of one or more components of the diaphragm occurring during the embryonic stage of development (Haricharan, Barnhart, Cheng, & Delzell, 2009).

b. Incidence of CDH is approximately 2.5 to 3.8 per 10,000 live births with a mortality rate of 45% in live-born infants (Kays, 2006). CDH and neonatal lung lesions often occur together. Abdominal contents in the thorax cause a mediastinal shift that can result in impairment of cardiovascular function.

(1) Interference with venous return to the heart

(2) Reduction in cardiac output

(3) Metabolic acidosis

2. Clinical practice

a. Assessment

(1) History

(a) Term or postterm

(b) Polyhydramnios common

(2) Physical findings (Haricharan et al, 2009)

(a) Large or barrel chest

(b) Scaphoid abdomen (Kays, 2006)

(c) Respiratory distress (ranges from mild to life threatening)

[i] Difficulty in initiating respiration

[ii] Gasping respirations

[iii] Retractions and nasal flaring

[iv] Cyanosis

[v] Decreased or absent breath sounds on the side of the hernia

(d) Displacement of the cardiac impulse to one side of the chest

(e) Bowel sounds heard in the chest

(f) Asymmetric chest expansion

(3) Diagnostic procedures

(a) Chest radiograph film: Diaphragmatic margin is absent on the defective side with presence of loops of intestine in the chest cavity, which might be gas filled, giving a multicystic appearance; mediastinal shift to the side opposite of defect (Haricharan et al, 2009)

(b) Arterial blood gas assay: hypoxemia, respiratory acidosis, and metabolic acidosis

b. Interventions/Outcomes (for immediate care and prior to transport to more acute care)

(1) Interventions

(a) Delivery room resuscitation

[i] Neonate should be immediately intubated; bag-and-mask ventilation must be avoided because air can be forced into the intestine, which will further compromise lung space in the chest.

[ii] Mechanical ventilation pressures should be kept at a minimal level to avoid pneumothorax.

[iii] Administer 100% oxygen to increase the PaO_2 and decrease persistent pulmonary hypertension.

[iv] Hyperoxygenate to minimize hypoxemia.
[v]   Ventilate with small tidal volumes at a rapid respiratory rate to provide oxygenation and decrease risk of pneumothorax.
[vi] Administer IV vasopressors as ordered.
[vii] Sedate as needed to minimize oxygen needs.
  c. Gastric decompression should be immediately initiated by inserting a large-bore nasogastric tube and advancing it as far as possible.
    (1) Positioning
      (a) Elevate head of bed to minimize abdominal organ pressure on diaphragm.
      (b) Turn the neonate onto the affected side to allow unaffected lung to expand.
3. Outcomes
  a. Neonate's respiratory effort receives optimal support until emergency surgical intervention occurs (Haricharan et al, 2009).
  b. Neonate remains hyperoxygenated as evidenced by blood gases.
  c. Blood pressure remains within the ordered parameters.
  d. Adequate sedation is maintained.

CONGENITAL CARDIAC LESIONS

INTRODUCTION

The incidence of congenital cardiovascular malformations is approximately 5 to 8 per 1000 live-born infants. Genetic disorders that might cause heart defects are categorized into three major groups (Lott, 2007).
A. Chromosomal disorders, including Di George syndrome, trisomy 21 (Down syndrome), and Turner syndrome
B. Single-gene disorders, which might be either autosomal dominant or autosomal recessive
C. Polygenic disorders resulting from multiple genetic or environmental influences
D. Cardiac defects or lesions are categorized as:
  1. Acyanotic: Oxygenated blood is shunted to the body, but the infant remains "pink."
  2. Cyanotic: Unoxygenated blood is shunted to the body causing the infant to be "blue."

CLINICAL PRACTICE

A. Acyanotic defects
  1. Patent Ductus Arteriosus (PDA)
    a. Introduction
      (1) An anatomic and functionally open shunt exists between the pulmonary artery and the aorta.
      (2) PDA occurs in 5% to 10% of all cases of congenital heart disease in full-term neonates (Lott, 2007).
      (3) PDA occurs in 37% of infants weighing 501 to 1500 g (1 lb, 2½ oz to 3 lbs, 5 oz) (Dagle et al, 2009).
      (4) PDA becomes functionally closed within the first 12 hours of life in the full-term infant. The closure is complete by 2 to 3 weeks of life (Agarwal et al, 2008).
    b. Assessment
      (1) Physical findings
        (a) A harsh systolic murmur, which becomes continuous, is heard at the left upper sternal border and posteriorly.
        (b) An active precordium is common.
        (c) Bounding peripheral pulses
        (d) Pulse pressure is widened with a low diastolic pressure.
      (2) Diagnostic procedures
        (a) Chest radiograph film: Findings depend on shunt size; in moderate or large shunts, heart enlargement might be present.
    c. Interventions/Outcomes (Sadowski, 2010)
      (1) Management depends on whether the shunt is hemodynamically significant. In premature infants, the PDA may prolong ventilator use beyond the dictates of the initial lung disease.

(2) Conservative measures are generally used initially, which may minimize exposure to pharmacologic agents. However, delaying treatment may decrease response to nonsteroidal antiinflammatory drugs.

    (a) Fluid restriction

    (b) Diuretics: If used with fluid restriction, may lead to electrolyte imbalance, dehydration, and caloric deprivation.

    (c) Positive end–expiratory pressure (PEEP) is useful in reducing left-to-right shunt via PDA.

(3) Medical management uses a nonsteroidal antiinflammatory agent that inhibits COX-1 and/or COX-2; treatment choices are indomethacin and ibuprofen lysine; usually used with preterm infants.

(4) Surgical management

    (a) Standard approach is surgical ligation via a thoracotomy.

    (b) New techniques include placement of a stainless-steel spring coil or Da occlusion device via cardiac catheterization or minimally invasive video-assisted thoracoscopic surgery that allows for PDA closure using two titanium clips placed with a trocar (Dutta & Albanese, 2006).

2. Atrial septal defects

  a. Introduction

    (1) An atrial septal defect (ASD) is an opening in the septum between the atria that occurs as a result of improper septal formation in early fetal cardiac development. An incompetent or malformed foramen ovale is the most common defect.

    (2) Atrial septal defects account for 5% to 10% of all congenital heart disease. Incidence in Down syndrome is 20% (Lott, 2007).

    (3) Permits shunting of blood between the two atria

  b. Assessment

    (1) Physical findings—dependent on severity of defect

      (a) Low-pitched diastolic murmur best heard at the left lower sternal border.

      (b) Widely split S_2

    (2) Diagnostic procedures

      (a) Chest radiograph film: cardiomegaly and increased vascular markings due to increased blood flow to the lungs as a result of shunting of blood from the left side of the heart to the right side

      (b) Electrocardiogram: usually sinus rhythm with ostium primum and secundum, but can show prolonged P-R interval with right atrial hypertrophy and P-wave changes

  c. Interventions (Sadowski, 2010)

    (1) If defect is small, clinical follow-up is indicated because the defect may close spontaneously.

    (2) If the defect is large, or with intractable CHF, surgical repair is done with the patient on cardiopulmonary bypass.

3. Ventricular septal defect

  a. Introduction

    (1) A ventricular septal defect (VSD) is an opening in the septum between the right and left ventricles that results from imperfect ventricular formation during early fetal development.

    (2) VSD is the most commonly occurring form of CHD, with an incidence of 20% to 25% among neonates with cardiac defects. VSD frequently occurs in association with other congenital heart diseases.

  b. Assessment

    (1) Physical findings

      (a) Neonates with a small VSD usually show no signs other than a holosystolic murmur in the area of the left lower sternal border. The infant might have normal growth and development patterns.

      (b) An infant with a large VSD will also have a holosystolic murmur that is frequently accompanied by a thrill.

    (2) Diagnostic procedures

      (a) Chest radiograph film: might be normal with small VSD. If larger, will show cardiomegaly and increased vascular markings due to increased blood flow to the lungs as a result of the shunting from the left side of the heart to the right side.

(b) Electrocardiogram: left ventricular hypertrophy; right ventricular hypertrophy if pulmonary hypertension is present. Echocardiogram: direct visualization of left to right shunting.

   c. Interventions (Sadowski, 2010)

     (1) 50% to 75% of small lesions close spontaneously; 20% of large defects become smaller or close.

     (2) With mild CHF, treatment consists of digoxin and diuretics.

     (3) Surgery is indicated if patient has failure to thrive or intractable CHF.

4. Coarctation of the aorta

   a. Introduction

     (1) Coarctation of the aorta is a narrowing of the upper thoracic aorta that produces an obstruction to the flow of blood through the aorta.

     (2) Simple coarctation presents with no other intracardiac lesions and can present with or without a PDA. Complex coarctation presents with other intracardiac lesions.

     (3) Coarctation of the aorta accounts for 8% of all cases of congenital heart disease. About 30% of infants with Turner syndrome present with coarctation of the aorta (Lott, 2007).

     (4) The coarctation can be juxtaductal, which is opposite to the location of the ductus arteriosus; preductal, which is proximal to the ductus arteriosus; or postductal, which is distal to the ductus arteriosus.

   b. Assessment

     (1) Physical findings depend on location of the coarctation.

       (a) Diminished or absent femoral pulses

       (b) Blood pressure more than 20 mm Hg; higher in upper extremities than in lower extremities (Wolfe, Boucek, Schaffer, & Wiggins, 1997)

       (c) Blowing systolic murmur at the left upper sternal border and axilla

       (d) Respiratory distress

       (e) Pallor

       (f) Poor weight gain during the first 2 to 6 weeks of life

     (2) Diagnostic procedures

       (a) Chest radiograph film: might show cardiomegaly with pulmonary venous congestion (Beekman, 2001)

       (b) Electrocardiogram: might be normal. However, in symptomatic neonates, the electrocardiogram might show evidence of left ventricular hypertrophy.

   c. Interventions (Sadowski, 2010)

     (1) Aggressive medical management of CHF

     (2) Prostaglandin E_1 (PGE_1) to dilate ductus arteriosus (preductal lesion)

     (3) Palliative balloon angioplasty in critically ill neonate, followed by surgery

     (4) Isolated postductal coarctation: control of CHF first, then delayed surgical correction

     (5) Surgical correction

B. Cyanotic defects

  1. Tetralogy of Fallot

   a. Introduction. Tetralogy of Fallot (TOF) is the most common type of cyanotic heart lesion, accounting for 10% of all cases of congenital heart disease (Lott, 2007), characterized by a combination of four defects.

     (1) Ventricular septal defect

     (2) An overriding aorta

     (3) Right ventricular outflow obstruction

     (4) Hypertrophy of the right ventricle

   b. Assessment

     (1) Physical findings

       (a) Respiratory distress, mainly tachypnea

       (b) Cyanosis: Degree is directly related to the extent of right ventricular outflow obstruction.

         [i] If there is severe right ventricular outflow tract obstruction and the ductus is patent, the neonate might have minimal cyanosis.

[ii] Spontaneous closure of the ductus arteriosus results in a severe decrease in pulmonary blood flow and significant cyanosis.

[iii] Crying or feeding increases cyanosis and respiratory distress due to increased shunting of unoxygenated blood from the right side of the heart to the left as a result of pulmonary artery obstruction.

(c) Harsh systolic murmur located at the left upper and lower sternal borders (Siwik, Patel, & Zahka, 2001)

(d) Signs of congestive heart failure if the VSD is large

(e) As the ductus arteriosus closes, the infant might exhibit hypoxemia if there is significant pulmonary stenosis.

(2) Diagnostic procedures

(a) Chest radiograph film: might be normal or decreased pulmonary vascular markings. Heart might have a boot-shaped appearance secondary to upturning of the apex related to right ventricular hypertrophy.

(b) Electrocardiogram: right atrial hypertrophy

(c) Echocardiogram: right ventricular wall thickening and visualization of the overriding aorta and the VSD

c. Interventions

(1) Current trend is complete repair of the TOF, which includes repair of pulmonary stenosis and closure of the VSD (Siwik et al, 2001).

(2) Palliative surgical interventions such as a Blalock-Taussig shunt and a central shunt can be used to control cyanosis. These shunts temporarily increase blood flow to the pulmonary artery from the aorta.

2. Transposition of the Great Arteries

a. Introduction

(1) Transposition of the great arteries (TGA) accounts for 5% of congenital heart disease (Lott, 2007).

(2) The aorta originates from the right ventricle and the pulmonary artery originates from the left ventricle.

(3) Survival is dependent on early diagnosis and aggressive treatment. An abnormal communication between the two separate circulations must be present or created if the infant is to survive. If the patent foramen ovale is closing, it should be reopened in the cardiac catheterization lab with a procedure called a balloon atrial septostomy. A PDA also maintains blood flow between the two independent circulations.

b. Assessment

(1) If untreated, the infant will become critically ill, including hypoxemia and heart failure, which may result in death.

(2) As the communication between the independent circulations closes, the infant becomes prominently cyanotic.

(3) Other symptoms might include progressive cyanosis that worsens with crying and feeding. Tachycardia, tachypnea, and a pansystolic murmur are present (Lott, 2007).

(4) Diagnostic procedures

(a) Chest radiograph may initially be normal in the neonate, but eventually shows an oval cardiac silhouette, mild cardiomegaly, and increased pulmonary vascular markings (Lott, 2007).

(b) Electrocardiogram might show ventricular hypertrophy.

(c) Echocardiogram is diagnostic and might show a small aorta and small left ventricle.

c. Interventions

(1) No supplemental oxygen to prevent closure of the PDA

(2) Correction of acidosis, inotropic therapy, and PGE_1 via continuous intravenous infusion

(3) Immediate transport to an appropriate facility with cardiac expertise. Surgically, a physiologic correction of the vessels, called an arterial switch, needs to be performed.

3. Hypoplastic left heart syndrome or single ventricle

a. Introduction

(1) Hypoplastic left heart syndrome includes various defects that are either valvular or vascular obstructive lesions on the left side of the heart that impede left-sided filling or emptying. As a result of the obstruction during intrauterine growth, a very small quantity of blood fills the left ventricle, causing hypoplasia of the left ventricle (Lott, 2007).

(2) Mitral atresia or aortic atresia rapidly causes congestive heart failure, and death can occur within a couple of days when ductus arteriosus typically closes.

(3) Infants with communicating atrial and VSDs might live longer, but require immediate surgical intervention.

(4) Hypoplastic left heart syndrome accounts for 7% to 9% of all congenital heart defects (Lott, 2007).

(5) These neonates are dependent on the PDA, and as it closes the neonate's condition deteriorates rapidly, leading to death.

  b. Assessment

(1) Birthweight can be normal.

(2) Neonate is commonly asymptomatic at birth but can become symptomatic within 1 to 2 days of life.

(3) Respiratory distress includes tachypnea and dyspnea.

(4) Diminished pulses, pallor, cyanosis, and mottling leading to vascular collapse and acidosis are seen as the PDA begins to close.

(5) Most neonates have a soft, systolic, ejection murmur (Lott, 2007).

(6) Diagnostic procedures

    (a) Chest radiograph film: radiograph may be normal. Vascular markings are variable. Aortic arch to the right is common (Lott, 2007).

    (b) Electrocardiogram: sinus tachycardia and right ventricular hypertrophy

  c. Interventions

(1) This lesion was once thought to be a lethal abnormality and inoperable, but now long-term, staged, palliative surgery is effective (Lott, 2007). Other options include cardiac transplantation.

(2) The neonate requires immediate transfer to an appropriate pediatric facility with cardiac expertise.

(3) Medical support might include inotropic therapy, PGE_1 IV infusion to maintain a PDA, and hypoventilation (reduced oxygen concentration).

(4) Maintenance of a delicate acid-base balance in the blood is essential for these fragile neonates.

HEALTH EDUCATION

A. General parental and family adaptation to an ill newborn (McGrath, 2007a)

1. Orient parents or family members to the nursery environment, including nursing, medical, and ancillary staff who will come into contact with their newborn; visiting and operational policies and procedures that will affect them; and telephone numbers to call to access care providers.

2. Help parents or family members recognize that grief is an appropriate response to the loss of the fantasized newborn.

  a. Discuss stages of grief.

  b. Teach that reactions to loss have individual and cultural differences.

  c. Be alert for inappropriate denial, which signals a dangerous lack of progress through the stages of grief.

3. Encourage parents or family members to express feelings and to deal openly with feelings of anger, fear, sadness, guilt, blame, frustration, and loss of self-esteem.

4. Encourage parents or family members not to become trapped in feelings of guilt, blame, or low self-esteem.

5. Remind parents or family members to support each other in their unique reactions to the situation.

6. Help parents or family members obtain accurate information about the infant's treatment, care, prognosis, and outcomes.

7. Help mobilize support among the extended family, friends, and religious community.
   a. Provide information about local and national support groups.
   b. Refer the family to clergy and other social services as needed.
8. Promote attachment between parents or family members and infant.
9. Demonstrate safe methods of interaction and direct care that parents or family may provide.
10. Support and encourage the mother's attempts to express breast milk, if she desires.
11. Help parents or family members interpret infant responses and recognize cues of satisfaction, overstimulation, and distress.
12. Teach parents to bathe, clothe, position, feed, and monitor the newborn according to individual needs, and support and encourage parents as they learn new skills.
13. Teach the parents or family members infant CPR.
14. Perform discharge planning and teaching from the time of admission.
    a. Offer parents a rooming-in option as available in anticipation of discharge.
    b. Assist parents or family members to plan for care to be provided in the home.
15. Follow up with telephone calls and home visits after discharge.

CASE STUDIES AND STUDY QUESTIONS

A 2300-g (5-pound, 1.5-ounce) infant girl is born to a 25-year-old gravida 1 woman, now para 1 (G1, P1) by spontaneous vaginal delivery. The infant's length is 44 cm (17.5 inches), and her head circumference is 30.5 cm (12 inches). No abnormalities are noted on physical examination. Maternal history and a gestational age assessment reveal the neonate to be at approximately 38 weeks' gestation and that she is SGA.

1. What might you expect to find in the mother's history?
   a. Weight gain of 15.9 kg (35 pounds)
   b. A history of smoking one pack of cigarettes per day
   c. Documented class A diabetes
2. What implications do the infant's measurements have?
   a. The insult occurred early in gestation, during the hyperplasia phase.
   b. The insult occurred late in gestation, during the hypertrophy phase.
   c. The insult occurred during labor and delivery.
3. To what should the nurse be alert when caring for this infant?
   a. Possible skull fracture
   b. Positive drug screen
   c. Hypothermia

A 4100-g (9-pound, 1.5-ounce) boy is born after a difficult forceps delivery. The prenatal history reveals an uncomplicated pregnancy of 40 weeks' gestation. The infant's length is 53.3 cm (21 inches), and his head circumference is 37 cm (14.6 inches). Gestational age assessment reveals the infant to be LGA.

4. On physical examination, what might you expect to find with this infant?
   a. Clubfoot
   b. Brachial plexus injury
   c. Diminished Babinski reflex
5. In actuality, the nurse finds the infant has a fractured clavicle, which is confirmed by x-ray. What may have led the nurse to this conclusion?
   a. Asymmetric startle reflex
   b. Extreme jitteriness
   c. History of forceps delivery
6. For what should the nurse be alert when caring for this infant?
   a. Hypothermia
   b. Respiratory distress
   c. Hypoglycemia

An 18-year-old G1, P1 woman is delivered of a 2000-g (4-pound, 6.5-ounce) boy by cesarean section. The infant is assessed to be AGA of 34 weeks. No abnormalities are noted on physical examination.

7. This infant is at risk for what condition?
   a. Hyperglycemia
   b. Premature closure of the ductus arteriosus
   c. Respiratory distress syndrome
8. What might the nurse expect to find in the mother's history?
   a. Premature labor treated with tocolytics
   b. Gestational diabetes
   c. Exposure to rubella in the first trimester
9. What might be detected in this infant during the first few days of life?
   a. Congenital syphilis
   b. Cephalohematoma
   c. Hyperbilirubinemia

A 32-year-old gravida 3, now para 3 (G3, P3) woman delivered a 3250-g (7-pound, 3-ounce) girl through meconium-stained fluid at 42 weeks' gestation. The infant's initial presentation is that she is limp, cyanotic, has minimal respirations, and has a heart rate less than 100 bpm. She was intubated and suctioned by the neonatal team. Although she was suctioned through the endotracheal tube, no meconium was seen below the cords. With oxygen and stimulation, her Apgar scores at 1 and 5 minutes were 7 and 9, respectively.

10. What is the most serious consequence that might result from this delivery?
    a. Patent ductus arteriosus
    b. Meconium aspiration
    c. Hyaline membrane disease
11. What would the nurse expect to see on examination of this infant?
    a. Abundant lanugo
    b. Absence of sole creases
    c. Leathery, cracked, and wrinkled skin
12. What should the nurse do to protect this infant's skin from further trauma?
    a. Avoid the use of tape except when absolutely necessary.
    b. Use powders and oils frequently.
    c. Wear gloves when handling the infant.
13. Why is hyperbilirubinemia of special concern in preterm infants?
    a. Immature liver function
    b. Poor vascular system
    c. Immature endocrine function
14. What physiologic factor contributes to greater risk for alterations in skin integrity in preterm infants?
    a. Immature immunologic system
    b. Malfunctioning of regulatory organs, such as the kidneys and respiratory tract
    c. Decreased cohesion between the dermis and epidermis
15. Gavage feedings are frequently needed to meet the nutritional needs of preterm infants because:
    a. Lactose enzyme activity is not adequate.
    b. Suck, swallow, and breathing reflexes are uncoordinated.
    c. Hyperbilirubinemia is likely.
16. A 42-week postterm neonate was born with greenish discoloration of the nails and skin and greenish secretions in the nasal passages. Why might the infant be transferred to a level 3 nursery?
    a. To determine the reason for the postmaturity

b. To observe more closely for skin color changes
    c. To manage severe respiratory problems that develop
17. Factors that contribute to impaired fetal growth include:
    a. Class A and C maternal diabetes
    b. Grade III placenta
    c. Multiple births
18. What problem may the LGA infant experience?
    a. PDA
    b. Facial nerve damage
    c. Poor suck, swallow, and breathing coordination
19. Which characteristic best describes an SGA infant with a late in gestation insult?
    a. Long fingernails that extend over the ends of the fingers
    b. Prone to meconium aspiration syndrome
    c. Wasted and thin at birth with loose and scaling skin

Ms. J., a gravida 2, para 1 (G2, P1) woman, delivered an infant boy vaginally at 35 weeks' gestation. The infant weighed 2500 g (5 pounds, 8 ounces); the fetal heart rate appeared fine during labor, although an L/S ratio was reported at 1.8:1. Ms. J. has gestational diabetes.

20. Surfactant production for an infant with RDS is inhibited because of:
    a. Prematurity
    b. Infection
    c. Hypoglycemia
21. The best indicator of an infant's need for oxygen is:
    a. Respiratory rate
    b. Skin color
    c. Arterial PaO_2
22. What is characteristic of neonates with RDS?
    a. Have a deficiency of pulmonary surfactant
    b. Are postmature
    c. Have sternal excursions
23. Which statement is NOT true about RDS?
    a. It is characterized by atelectasis.
    b. It may be induced by hypothermia in a preterm infant.
    c. With adequate supportive care, it is self-resolving in approximately 72 hours.
24. In RDS, blood may not be well oxygenated because of all of the following *except*:
    a. A patent ductus arteriosus
    b. Decreased pulmonary resistance
    c. Atelectasis of the alveoli

25. Which prenatal factor is most likely to predispose the neonate to develop respiratory distress?
    a. Maternal diabetes
    b. Gestation of 34 weeks
    c. Fetal scalp pH of 7.20
26. True or False: Acidosis and hypothermia may lead to decreased pulmonary blood flow, which perpetuates decreased production of surfactant and may cause RDS.
27. A condition that usually occurs in term infants and cesarean section deliveries, is manifested by tachypnea, and is caused by retained lung fluid is called:
    a. Pneumonia
    b. TTN
    c. Meconium aspiration
28. When suctioning a limp neonate born through meconium-stained amniotic fluid, what is suctioned first?
    a. Both nares
    b. Stomach
    c. Trachea
29. An infant with PPHN and a PDA is at risk for developing:
    a. Pulmonary hemorrhage
    b. Hepatomegaly
    c. Pleural effusions
30. You are preparing to care for several infants recently born. Which infant is at greatest risk for TTN?
    a. Spontaneous vaginal delivery; 40 weeks' gestation
    b. Cesarean section delivery; 41 weeks' gestation
    c. Vaginal delivery with maternal anesthesia; 38 weeks' gestation

Baby M. was delivered after a 16-hour induced labor. Maternal membranes were artificially ruptured, fluid was clear, and a Pitocin infusion was initiated. The mother was afebrile throughout the labor. The second stage of labor was 2 hours, 45 minutes. Review of the mother's prenatal and labor history yielded the following information:

> Blood type is A+.
> Venereal disease research laboratory (VDRL) is nonreactive.
> Alpha-fetoprotein is normal.
> Average BP is 116-124/76-82.
> Total weight gain was 12.25 kg (27 pounds).
> Medications are prenatal vitamins, iron, and aspirin for stress headaches.
> Gestational age is 40 6/7 weeks.
> Nonstress test is reactive.

Baby M. had the umbilical cord wrapped twice around her neck and required stimulation to initiate breathing and administration of oxygen by face mask. Apgar scores were 7 at 1 minute and 8 at 5 minutes.

31. From this information, which factor places Baby M. at increased risk for hyperbilirubinemia?
    a. Ruptured membranes for 16 hours
    b. Postmaturity
    c. Labor induced with Pitocin
32. All of the following factors indicate that Baby M. is at greater risk for hyperbilirubinemia *except:*
    a. Gestational age of 40 6/7 weeks
    b. Mother taking aspirin for her headaches
    c. Respirations having to be stimulated and oxygen administered

On her second day of life, Baby M. required phototherapy treatment. Her mother was being discharged from the hospital and came to the nursery to breastfeed her infant before leaving. Baby M.'s mother was crying and did not want to go home without her infant. Baby M.'s father was trying to comfort his wife.

33. While Baby M. is under the phototherapy lights, it is important to:
    a. Keep the infant under the lights at all times so that there will be maximal effectiveness in the shortest period.
    b. Discontinue Baby M.'s breastfeeding because the fluid content of breast milk is deficient for a neonate undergoing phototherapy.
    c. Prevent hypothermia, hyperthermia, or both in Baby M.
34. Baby M.'s mother is crying, expresses fear about her infant's health, and does not want to leave. Which intervention would be the *least* effective?
    a. Encourage the mother to come in to feed her infant as often as possible.
    b. Emphasize the temporary nature of hyperbilirubinemia, and explain the monitoring of Baby M.'s bilirubin levels.
    c. Remind the mother that newborns require demanding care, which is very fatiguing to a new mother, and that she should take this added opportunity to rest and recover.

Baby L. was born to a 21-year-old gravida 1, para 1 (G1, P1) Vietnamese mother. He was born vaginally after a difficult delivery due to shoulder dystocia. At admission, his weight was 4400 g

(9 pounds, 11.5 ounces). Physical and neurologic examination placed him at 40 weeks of gestation. His physical examination revealed an unequal Moro reflex with decreased movement of the left arm and crepitus at the left neck area. Bluish marking was also noted across the lower back.

35. What is the correct gestational classification for Baby L.?
    a. LGA with risk for hypoglycemia
    b. AGA with risk for hypothermia
    c. SGA with risk for hypoglycemia
36. The historical and physical findings for Baby L. might suggest:
    a. Torticollis
    b. Fractured clavicle
    c. Erb's palsy
37. What is the most likely cause of the bluish marking across the lower back?
    a. Purpura
    b. Birth trauma
    c. Mongolian spot

Baby R. is a 6-hour-old female born to a 28-year-old mother with a history of pregnancy-induced hypertension. Baby R. was born 5 weeks premature and has a birthweight of 1450 g (3 pounds, 3 ounces). On admission to the newborn nursery, the infant's respiratory rate was 74, and she was noted to have mild intercostal and substernal retractions with adequate air entry on auscultation. Auscultation of her heart revealed a harsh murmur that was best heard in the area of the left upper sternal border.

38. Baby R.'s history and presentation are most indicative of:
    a. Coarctation of the aorta
    b. Atrial septal defect
    c. Patent ductus arteriosus
39. All of the following statements regarding gastroschisis are true *except*:
    a. There is an increased incidence of preterm birth associated with gastroschisis.
    b. There is no skin covering the eviscerated organs.
    c. Intestinal atresias are frequently associated with gastroschisis.
40. A term infant develops severe respiratory distress immediately after birth. On physical examination, the chest is hyperexpanded, and the point of maximal impulse (PMI) is shifted to the right. What is the most likely cause for this infant's respiratory distress?
    a. Diaphragmatic hernia
    b. Right pneumothorax
    c. Transposition of the great arteries

ANSWERS TO STUDY QUESTIONS

1. b	11. c	21. c	31. c
2. a	12. a	22. a	32. a
3. c	13. a	23. c	33. c
4. b	14. c	24. b	34. c
5. a	15. b	25. b	35. a
6. c	16. c	26. True	36. c
7. c	17. c	27. b	37. c
8. a	18. b	28. c	38. b
9. c	19. c	29. a	39. c
10. b	20. a	30. b	40. a

REFERENCES

Agarwal, R., Deorari, A. K., & Paul, V. K. (2008). Patent ductus arteriosus in preterm neonates. *Indian Journal of Pediatrics, 75*(3), 277–280.

Anderson, M. S., & Hay, W. W. (2005). Intrauterine growth restriction and the small-for-gestational-age infant. In M. G. MacDonald, M. D. Mullet, & M. M. K. Seshia (Eds.), *Avery's neonatology: Pathophysiology and management of the newborn* (pp. 515–516). Philadelphia: Lippincott.

Avery, M., & Richardson, D. (1998). History and epidemiology. In H. Tauesch, & R. Ballard (Eds.), *Avery's diseases of the newborn* (pp. 413–428). Philadelphia: Saunders.

Bachman, T. E., Marks, N. E., & Rimensberger, P. C. (2008). Factors effecting adoption of new neonatal and pediatric respiratory technologies. *Intensive Care Medicine, 34*(1), 174–178.

Balchin, I., & Steer, P. J. (2007). Race, ethnicity and immaturity. *Early Human Development, 83*(12), 749–754.

Bancalari, E., & Claure, N. (2008). Non-invasive ventilation in the preterm infant. *Early Human Development*, *84*(12), 815–819.

Barnes-Powell, L. L. (2007). Infants of diabetic mothers: Effects of hyperglycemia on the fetus and neonate. *Neonatal Network*, *26*(5), 283–290.

Basu, S., Kumar, A., & Bhatia, B. D. (2007). Role of antibiotics in meconium aspiration syndrome. *Annals of Tropical Paediatrics*, *27*(2), 107–113.

Beekman, R. (2001). Coarctation of the aorta. In H. Allen, H. Gutgessel, E. Clark, & D. Driscoll (Eds.), *Heart disease in infants, children and adolescents* (6th ed., pp. 988–1010). Philadelphia: Lippincott, Williams & Wilkins.

Bhat, R. Y., & Rao, A. (2008). Meconium-stained amniotic fluid and meconium aspirate syndrome: A prospective study. *Annals of Tropical Paediatrics*, *28*(3), 199–203.

Blackburn, S. T. (2007). *Maternal, fetal, and neonatal physiology: A clinical perspective* (3rd ed.). St. Louis: Saunders.

Bhutani, V. K., & Johnson, L. (2009). A proposal to prevent severe neonatal hyperbilirubinemia and kernicterus. *Journal of Perinatology*, *29*, S61–S67.

Bradshaw, W. T. (2009). Necrotizing enterocolitis: Etiology, presentation, management, and outcomes. *Journal of Perinatal and Neonatal Nursing*, *23*(1), 87–94.

Campbell, M. (2006). Development of a clinical pathway for near-term and convalescing premature infants in a level II nursery. *Advances in Neonatal Care*, *6*(3), 150–164.

Chyi, L., Lee, H., Hintz, S., Gould, J., & Sutcliffe, T. (2008). School outcomes of late preterm infants: Special needs and challenges of infants born at 32 to 36 weeks. *Journal of Pediatrics*, *153*(1), 5–6.

Ciminello, F. S., Morin, R. J., Nguyen, T. J., & Wolfe, S. A. (2009). Cleft lip and palate: Review. *Comprehensive Therapy*, *35*(1), 37–43.

Cuevas, K., Silver, D., Brooten, D., Youngblut, J., & Bobo, C. (2005). The cost of prematurity: Hospital charges at birth and frequency of rehospitalizations and acute care visits over the first year of life. *American Journal of Nursing*, *105*(7), 56–65.

Dagle, J. M., Lepp, N. T., Cooper, M. E., Schaa, K. L., Kelsey, K. J. P., Orr, K. L., et al. (2009). Determination of genetic predisposition to patent ductus arteriosus in preterm infants. *Pediatrics*, *123*, 1116–1123.

Darnell, R., Ariagno, R., & Kinney, H. (2006). The late preterm infant and the control of breathing, sleep, and brainstem development: A review. *Clinics in Perinatology*, *33*(4), 883–914.

Doherty, L., & Norwitz, E. R. (2008). Prolonged pregnancy: When should we intervene? *Current Opinion in Obstetrics and Gynecology*, *20*, 519–527.

Dutta, S., & Albanese, C. (2006). Minimal access surgery in the neonate. *NeoReviews*, *7*(8), e400–e409.

El Shahed, A. I., Dargaville, P., Ohisson, A., & Soll, R. F. (2007). Surfactant for meconium aspiration syndrome in full term/near term infants. *Cochrane Database of Systematic Reviews*, July 18(3), CD002054.

Engle, W. A., Tomashek, K. M., Wallman, C. The Committee on the Fetus and Newborn. (2007). "Late preterm" infants: A population at risk. *Pediatrics*, *120*, 1390–1401.

Guglani, L., Lakshminrusimha, S., & Ryan, R. M. (2008). Transient tachypnea of the newborn. *Pediatric Reviews*, *29*, e59–e65, DOI: 10.1542/pir.29-11-e59.

Halliday, H. L. (2008). Surfactant, past, present and future. *Journal of Perinatology*, *28*, S47–S58.

Haricharan, R. N., Barnhart, D. C., Cheng, H., & Delzell, E. (2009). Identifying neonates at a very high risk for mortality among children with congenital diaphragmatic hernia managed with extracorporeal membrane oxygenation. *Journal of Pediatric Surgery*, *44*, 87–93.

Heinzmann, A., Brugger, M., Engels, C., Promperier, H., Superti-Furge, A., Strauch, K., & Krueger, M. (2009). Risk factors of neonatal respiratory distress following vaginal delivery and cesarean section in the German population. *Acta Paediatrics*, *98*(1), 25–30.

Hendrix, N., & Berghella, V. (2008). Non-placental causes of intrauterine growth restriction. *Seminars in Perinatology*, *32*(3), 161–165.

Hermansen, C. L., & Lorah, K. N. (2007). Respiratory distress in the newborn. *American Family Physician*, *76*(7), 987–994.

Hernandez-Diaz, S., Van Mater, L. J., Werier, M. M., Lounik, C., & Mitchell, A. A. (2007). Risk factors for persistent pulmonary hypertension in newborns. *Pediatrics*, *120*(2), e272–e282.

Jain, L., & Cheng, J. (2006). Emergency department visits and rehospitalizations in late preterm infants. *Clinics in Perinatology*, *33*(4), 935–945.

Jaruratanairikul, S., Chichareon, V., Pattanapreechawong, N., & Sangsupavanich, P. (2007). Cleft lip and/or palate: 10 years experience at a pediatric cleft center in southern Thailand. *Cleft Palate-Craniofacial Journal*, *45*(6), 597–602.

Johnson, C. Y., & Little, J. (2008). Folate intake, markers of folate status and oral clefts: Is the evidence converging? *International Journal of Epidemiology*, *37*, 1041–1058.

Jorgenson, A. M. (2008a). Late preterm birth: A rising trend—Part one of a two part series. *AWHONN: Nursing for Women's Health*, *12*(4), 310–315.

Jorgenson, A. M. (2008b). Late preterm birth: Clinical complications and risk—Part two of a two part series. *AWHONN: Nursing for Women's Health*, *12*(4), 318–331.

Kays, D. W. (2006). Congenital diaphragmatic hernia and neonatal lung lesions. *Surgical Clinics of North America*, *86*(2), 329–352.

Kelly, M. M. (2006). Basics of prematurity. *Journal of Pediatric Health Care*, 20(4), 238–244.

Landingham, M. V., Nguyen, T. V., Roberts, A., Parent, A. D., & Zhang, J. (2008). Risk factors of congenital hydrocephalus: A 10 year retrospective study. *Journal of Neurology, Neurosurgery, and Psychiatry*, 80, 213–217.

Laptook, A., & Jackson, G. L. (2006). Cold stress and hypoglycemia in the late preterm ("near term") infant: Impact on nursery admission. *Seminars in Perinatology*, 30(1), 24–27.

Latini, G., DelVecchio, A., DeFelice, C., Verrotti, A., & Bossone, E. (2008). Persistent pulmonary hypertension of the newborn: Therapeutical approach. *Mini Reviews of Medical Chemistry*, 8(14), 1507–1513.

Ledbetter, D. J. (2006). Gastroschisis and omphalocele. *Surgical Clinics of North America*, 86(2), 249–260.

Lefkowitz, W., & Rosenberg., S. H. (2008). Bronchopulmonary dysplasia: Pathway from disease to long-term outcomes. *Journal of Perinatology*, 28(12), 837–840.

Lott, J. W. (2007). Cardiovascular system. In C. Kenner, & J. W. Lott (Eds.), *Comprehensive neonatal care: An interdisciplinary approach* (4th ed., pp. 39–55). St. Louis: Saunders.

Maisel, M. J. (2006). Neonatal jaundice. *Pediatrics in Review*, 27(12), 443–454.

Mandruzzato, G., Antsaklis, A., Botet, F., Chervenak, F. A., Figueras, F., Grunebaum, A., Puerto, B., Skupski, D., & Stanojevic, M. (2008). Intrauterine growth restriction (IUGR). *Journal of Perinatal Medicine*, 36(4), 277–281.

Marechal, L., Barthod, C., Lottin, J., Gautier, G., & Jeulin, J. C. (2007). Measurement system for gesture characterization during chest physiotherapy act on newborn babies suffering from bronchiolitis. *Conference proceedings of the IEEE English Medical & Biologic Society*, 5771–5774.

McGrath, J. M. (2007a). Family centered care. In C. Kenner, & J. Wright Lott (Eds.), *Comprehensive neonatal care: An interdisciplinary approach* (4th ed.). Philadelphia: Saunders.

McGrath, J. M. (2007b). Neonatal thermoregulation. In J. Verger, & R. Lebet (Eds.), *AACN procedure manual for pediatric acute and critical care* (pp. 1390–1398). St. Louis: Mosby.

Moos, M. K. (2004). Understanding prematurity: Sorting facts from fiction. *AWHONN Lifelines*, 8(1), 32–37.

Pappas, B., & Walker, B. (2010). Care of the late preterm infant. In M. Verklan, & M. Walden (Eds.), *AWHONN'S Core curriculum for neonatal intensive care nursing* (4th ed., pp. 447–452). St. Louis: Saunders.

Pollan, C. (2009). Retinopathy of prematurity: An eye toward better outcomes. *Neonatal Network*, 28(2), 93–101.

Rabi, Y., Rabi, D., & Yee, W. (2007). Room air resuscitation of the depressed newborn: A systematic review and meta-analysis. *Resuscitation*, 72(3), 353–363.

Ramachandrappa, A., & Jain, L. (2008). Elective cesarean section: Its impact on neonatal respiratory outcome. *Clinics in Perinatology*, 35(2), 373–393.

Rosenberg, A. (2008). The IUGR newborn. *Seminars in Perinatology*, 32(3), 219–224.

Sadowski, S. (2010). Cardiovascular disorders. In M. Verklan, & M. Walden (Eds.), *AWHONN'S Core curriculum for neonatal intensive care nursing* (4th ed., pp. 534–588). St. Louis: Saunders.

Shiao, S. Y., & Ou, C. N. (2007). Validation of oxygen saturation monitoring in neonates. *American Journal of Critical Care*, 16(2), 168–178.

Silvani, P., & Camporesi, A. (2007). Drug-induced pulmonary hypertension in newborns: A review. *Current Vascular Pharmacology*, 5(2), 129–133.

Sinha, S. K., Gupta, S., & Donn, S. M. (2008). Immediate respiratory management of the preterm infant. *Seminars in Fetal and Neonatal Medicine*, 13(1), 24–29.

Siwik, E., Patel, C., & Zahka, K. (2001). Tetrology of Fallot. In H. Allen, H. Gutgessel, E. Clark, & D. Driscoll (Eds.), *Heart disease in infants, children and adolescents* (6th ed, pp. 880–902). Philadelphia: Lippincott, Williams & Wilkins.

Stanley, C. A. (2006). Hypoglycemia in the neonate. *Pediatric Endocrinology Reviews*(4 Suppl 1), 76–81, Dec.

Stokowski, L. A. (2006). Fundamentals of phototherapy for neonatal jaundice. *Advances in Neonatal Care*, 6(6), 303–312.

Takaya, A., Igarashi, M., Nakajima, M., Mikake, H., Shima, Y., & Suzuki, S. (2008). Risk factors for transient tachypnea of the newborn in infants delivered vaginally at 37 weeks or later. *Journal of Nippon Medicine & Scholarship*, 75(5), 269–273.

Townsend, S. F. (2005). The large-for-gestational-age and the small-for-gestational-age infant. In P. J. Thureen, J. Deacon, & J. A. Hernandez (Eds.), *Assessment and care of the well newborn* (2nd ed., pp. 273–278). Philadelphia: Saunders.

Turell, D. C. (2008). Advances with surfactant. *Emergency Medical Clinics of North America*, 26(4), 921–928.

Vogel, L. C., & Sturm, P. (2008). Management of patients with developmental and hereditary spinal cord disorders. *Topics in Spinal Cord Injury Rehabilitation*, 14(2), 53–62.

Volpe, J. J. (2008). *Neurology of the newborn* (5th ed.). Philadelphia: Saunders.

Walsh, M. C., & Fanaroff, J. M. (2007). Meconium stained fluid: Approach to the mother and the baby. *Clinics in Perinatology*, 34(4), 653–665, viii.

Wiedemann, J. R., Suagstad, A. M., Barnes-Powell, L., & Duran, K. (2008). Meconium aspirate syndrome. *Neonatal Network*, 27(2), 81–87.

Wolfe, R., Boucek, M., Schaffer, M., & Wiggins, J. (1997). Cardiovascular diseases. In W. Hay, J. Groothuis, A. Hayward, & M. Levin (Eds.), *Current pediatric diagnosis and treatment* (13th ed., pp. 474–536). Stamford, CT: Appleton & Lange.

Yoder, B. A., Gordon, M. C., & Barth, W. H., Jr. (2008). Late preterm birth: Does the changing obstetrical paradigm alter the epidemiology of respiratory complications? *Obstetrics & Gynecology, 111*(4), 814–822.

Youngmee, A., & Yonghoon, J. (2003). The effects of the shallow and the deep endotracheal suctioning on oxygen saturation and heart rate in high-risk infants. *International Journal of Nursing Studies, 40*(2), 97–104.

COMPLICATIONS OF CHILDBEARING

18 Intimate Partner Violence

Kathryn Records

OBJECTIVES

1. Discuss the prevalence of violence against women in the United States.
2. Describe the cycle of violence, and differentiate between the various phases.
3. List behaviors of the abuser in each of the phases of the violence cycle.
4. Identify the types of physical injuries that battered women sustain, and discuss how pregnancy alters the body parts targeted by the abuser.
5. Discuss the psychological injuries that battered women sustain.
6. Identify how cultural differences and socioeconomic status influence the prevalence of intimate partner violence (IPV) in the United States.
7. Describe common characteristics of men who are abusers and of women who are victims of abuse.
8. Recognize key elements to be included in the assessment of all women and additional data to be collected from a woman at high risk for abuse.
9. List physical, psychological, and nonverbal findings in a woman that are consistent with abuse in her relationship.
10. Describe and discuss primary, secondary, and tertiary intervention strategies used to provide care to abused women.
11. Design a plan of care that maximizes the abused woman's ability to protect herself and her children and to make informed decisions on which she can act.
12. Identify resources and referrals that are available for victims of IPV.

INTRODUCTION

A. **Health care providers need to understand the types of violence that women experience in order to provide informed care.**
   1. IPV, family violence, battering, and partner or spousal abuse all describe the physical, sexual, or psychological harm caused by a current or former partner or spouse (Centers for Disease Control and Prevention [CDC], 2008). IPV includes some or all of the following (Saltzman, Fanslow, McMahon, & Shelley, 2002):
      a. Physical violence
      b. Sexual violence
      c. Threats of physical or sexual violence
      d. Psychological or emotional violence, including economic coercion (Fawole, 2008)
B. **Health care providers interact with women experiencing IPV on a daily basis, often without being aware of it.**
   1. The true incidence of IPV perpetrated against women in the United States is unknown because a large amount of it remains undetected and unreported.
      a. The mandatory reporting mechanism for IPV involving an adult woman only exists in five states, whereas nearly all states require reporting of IPV if it occurs concurrently with a crime (Phelan, 2007).
      b. IPV is, however, considered a felony in all states.
      c. Domestic violence accounts for more injuries to women than car accidents, muggings, and rapes combined (CDC, 2008).
      d. One third of women seen in emergency rooms report current physical abuse or battering (Kramer, Lorenzon, & Mueller, 2004).

    e. Up to 31% of women using primary care clinics report one or more types of abuse within the past year (Kramer et al, 2004).

    f. IPV has been recognized as a health problem of major proportions in the United States and Canada.

       (1) In the United States, estimates are that 1.9 million women are assaulted annually by an intimate partner (Tjadin & Thoennes, 2000).

       (2) In Canada, 21% of women have experienced IPV within the past year (Romans, Forte, Cohen, Du Mont, & Hyman, 2007).

       (3) Each year, more than 500,000 women injured as a result of IPV require medical treatment (Tjaden & Thoennes, 2000).

       (4) Women in same-sex relationships also experience IPV (Hassouneh & Glass, 2008).

C. Cycle of violence

  1. Pioneer research about abuse of women was conducted by Lenore Walker in 1979 (Walker, 1982).

    a. Her research gave detailed accounts of women's abuse and how the abuse progressed in a relationship.

    b. She discovered a cyclic pattern of progression of abuse in female-male relationships that is now identified as the cycle of violence (Figure 18-1).

  2. Abusive behavior, especially battering, exhibits a three-phase cyclic pattern. Although this illustration focuses on male abuser and female victim, females can also be abusers.

    a. Phase 1 is characterized as a period of increasing tension in the abuser, marked by the following behaviors:

       (1) Increased anger directed toward the woman

       (2) Increased blame attributed to the woman

       (3) Escalated arguments with the woman

       (4) Woman may feel like she has to keep her partner or spouse calm.

    b. Phase 2 is the acute battering incident in which the batterer demonstrates an uncontrollable discharge of the built-up tension.

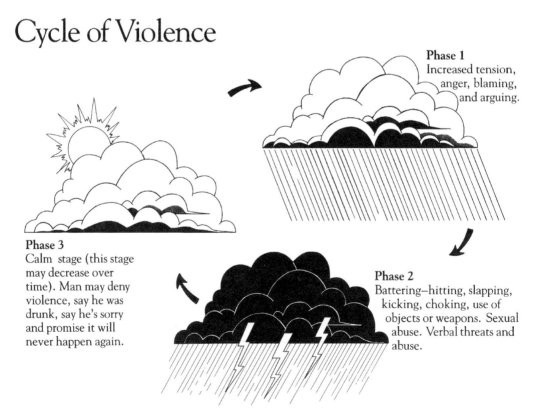

Cycle of Violence

Phase 1
Increased tension, anger, blaming, and arguing.

Phase 3
Calm stage (this stage may decrease over time). Man may deny violence, say he was drunk, say he's sorry and promise it will never happen again.

Phase 2
Battering–hitting, slapping, kicking, choking, use of objects or weapons. Sexual abuse. Verbal threats and abuse.

FIGURE 18-1 ■ March of Dimes brochure on preventing battering during pregnancy. (Developed under a March of Dimes Birth Defects Foundation grant at Texas Woman's University, Houston.)

(1) This phase can last from a few minutes to hours, sometimes even several days.
(2) Physical battering behaviors are as follows:
    (a) Slapping
    (b) Pinching
    (c) Kicking
    (d) Punching
    (e) Choking
    (f) Stomping
    (g) Pushing
    (h) Biting
    (i) Throwing the woman across a room or up against a wall
    (j) Bone fracturing
    (k) Mutilating with objects such as knives, broken glass, razor blades, and tools
    (l) Burning with objects such as an iron, scalding liquids, cigarettes, or caustic substances
    (m) Shooting with a gun
    (n) Sexually abusing or mutilating
(3) Psychological battering behaviors are as follows:
    (a) Threats
    (b) Intimidation
    (c) Name calling
    (d) Destroying things of value to the woman
    (e) Destroying her personal belongings
    (f) Throwing her things out the door or window
    (g) Humiliation
    (h) Derogatory remarks
    (i) Verbal "put downs"
    (j) Remarks intended to decrease her self-esteem
    (k) Remarks to make her doubt her worth, her abilities, and her decision making
    (l) Taking away "privileges" normally afforded to adults and conditionally granting permission to temporarily get them back
    (m) Isolating her from family, friends, and adult contacts
    (n) Treating her as a child
(4) The batterer frequently justifies his battering behaviors by stating that the purpose is to teach the woman a lesson.
(5) Most injuries are to the woman's face, arms, and buttocks; during pregnancy, injuries may be frequently seen around the abdomen.

c. Phase 3 is the calm stage; also called the honeymoon stage.
(1) The batterer is usually remorseful and profusely apologetic.
(2) He may shower her with gifts.
(3) He solemnly promises that the abuse will never happen again.
(4) He may deny or minimize the violence that occurred in phase 2.
(5) He promises the woman that everything will be different from this time on.
(6) He may profess his intense love for her.

d. The behaviors exhibited in phase 3 of the cycle of violence offer the woman hope and are a powerful and positive reinforcement for staying in the relationship.
(1) This restores the woman's hope that he will change.
(2) She has a tendency to deny the inevitable recurrence of the abuse.

D. Types of injuries
  1. Physical injuries to an abused woman may include the following:
    a. Bruises and abrasions
    b. Hematomas, particularly periorbital
    c. Bites
    d. Broken teeth
    e. Lacerations, particularly around the mouth, lips, eyes, and other parts of the face
    f. Perforation of the tympanic membrane
    g. Scalp lacerations, hematomas, tufts of hair missing
    h. Fractured ribs or limbs

        i. Fractured nose

        j. Concussion

        k. Stab wounds

        l. Gunshot wounds

        m. Death

  2. Other physical problems occur in response to repeated abuse. Abused women report an increased prevalence of:

        a. Gastrointestinal disorders

        b. Sleep disorders

        c. Chronic pain disorders

        d. Headaches; migraines

        e. Sexually transmitted infections (STIs) (Kramer et al, 2004)

        f. Vaginal bleeding

  3. Psychological injuries to a battered woman may include the following:

        a. Anxiety and increased fear

        b. Insomnia

        c. Lethargy

        d. Feelings of helplessness and hopelessness

        e. Severe mood swings

        f. Panic attacks or night terrors

        g. Depression

        h. Posttraumatic stress syndrome

        i. Self-abuse

           (1) Alcoholism

           (2) Drug abuse

           (3) Eating disorders

         j. Diminished self-esteem

        k. Suicide attempts

E. Cultural and socioeconomic differences

  1. Violence against women cuts across all socioeconomic and ethnic lines (Rodriguez, 1994).

  2. Poverty and oppression are significant factors in the prevalence of violent behavior; the following factors have been associated with a higher incidence of IPV:

        a. Low income with subsequent stress

        b. Limited resources of all kinds

        c. Unemployment

        d. Low-prestige jobs

  3. The meaning of violence in various cultures is difficult to determine because cultures vary in their perceptions and definitions of abuse (Hanrahan, Campbell, & Ulrich, 1993; Mattson & Rodriguez, 1999).

  4. Minority women, in general, are less likely to use shelters and more likely to use the health care system combined with support from family and friends (Noel & Yam, 1992). The culture is viewed as an oppressed group, and access to health care can be very limited (Rynerson, 2007; Suarez & Ramirez, 1999).

  5. Cultural influences on awareness of abuse

        a. African American

           (1) No convincing evidence has been found that greater violence against women exists among this group (Hattery, 2008); however, women are more likely to report violence when it does occur.

           (2) Men who live in an impoverished neighborhood are three times as likely to commit IPV as compared with their counterparts who do not live in impoverished areas (Cunradi, Caetano, Clark, & Schafer, 2000).

           (3) IPV may be triggered by threats to the men's masculinity, such as unemployment, difficulty keeping a job, and racial domination (Smith, 2008).

           (4) The risk of abuse may be high when the woman has more education than the man if he views this as a threat to his masculinity (Smith, 2008).

           (5) Women fear that disclosing abuse will bring disgrace or increased discrimination to the entire community (Campbell et al, 2006).

        b. Hispanic

(1) Families are more egalitarian in their decision making than in past years, especially when women work outside the home or have higher education levels (Klevens et al, 2007).
(2) Generally, sex roles are clearly defined.
(3) Mexican-American women perceive fewer types of behavior as being abusive (Torrés, 1991).
(4) Women typically share their experiences of abuse with their families and friends; although responses are variable, families most often prefer to remain uninvolved beyond providing tangible aid or confronting the abuser (Klevens et al, 2007).
(5) Through religious and cultural images, Hispanic women often believe abuse is their "lot in life to suffer"; they are defined by their family roles, and their primary obligation is to preserve the family at all costs (Flores-Ortiz, 1993; Mattson & Rodriguez, 1999).
(6) Acculturation is an important influence on IPV for men and women, although the relationship differs. Men with low acculturation levels experience high stress and increased involvement in IPV, whereas women who are highly acculturated have an increased risk for IPV (Caetano, Ramisetty-Mikler, Caetano Vaeth, & Harris, 2007).
(7) The culture is viewed as an oppressed group, and access to health care can be very limited (Rynerson, 2007; Suarez & Ramirez, 1999).

   c. Native American
(1) Rates of IPV among Native American women are more than double the rates among African American, white, and Asian women (Rennison, 2001).
(2) Native American women may experience more forms of potentially lethal violence than women from all other ethnic and racial groups (Tjaden & Thoennes, 2000).
(3) Few studies seek to understand IPV across more than one tribe or region, failing to take into account the tremendous heterogeneity across more than 500 U.S. tribes, many of whom have their own culture, traditions, lifestyles, and language (Bohn, 2003).
(4) Native Americans' 400-year history of oppression, violence, poverty, limited resources, isolation, and disenfranchisement may contribute to the violence within Native American families (Bohn, 2003).

F. Characteristics of abusers
1. The progression of aggression continuum (O'Leary, 1993)
   a. Verbal aggression, such as yelling and name calling
   b. Followed by lesser forms of physical aggression, such as pushing and slapping
   c. Followed by true violent behavior, such as punching and beating
   d. In extreme situations, continuum ends with murder.
2. Intergenerational transmission of violence
   a. Abuser and woman generally learn about IPV in their family of origin.
(1) Witnessing violence in childhood triples one's risk of becoming a batterer in adulthood (Ehrensaft & Cohen, 2003).
(2) Most abusers report childhood memories of harsh physical punishment as a means of discipline (Rynerson, 2007).
   b. Childhood sexual abuse increases the risk of physical and sexual abuse in adulthood, thereby perpetuating the cycle of intergenerational abuse (Noll, Horowitz, Bonanno, Trickett, & Putnam, 2003).
   c. An acceptable awareness is—as a child in a violent family—that people who love each other can be violent.
   d. Children who witness parental violence are especially susceptible to psychological and social consequences with lifelong effect, including:
(1) Posttraumatic stress disorders
(2) Depressive disorders
(3) Attention-deficit hyperactive disorder
(4) Irritability, aggression, and quickness to anger
(5) Boys are more likely to act out; girls are more likely to internalize (Ruiz & Mattson, 2003).
   e. Some research suggests that exposure of the neonate and very young children to violence alters central nervous system development, predisposing the child to more impulsive, reactive, and violent behavior (Ruiz & Mattson, 2003).
3. Family structure can shape the attitude toward IPV.
   a. Gender inequality with ascribed gender roles

(1) A woman's place is in the home.
(2) A woman is dependent on a man as provider and protector.
   b. Power and violence serve to maintain a patriarchal view that gives authority to men.
4. Possible causes of aggression in an abuser (O'Leary, 1993)
   a. Verbal aggression
      (1) Need to control (Figure 18-2)
      (2) Misuse of power
      (3) Jealousy
      (4) Relationship discord
   b. Physical aggression
      (1) Violence as an acceptable means of remaining in complete control of the relationship
      (2) Modeling of violent behavior seen or experienced as a child
      (3) Alcohol abuse, drug abuse, or both
   c. Severe physical aggression
      (1) Severe personality disorder
      (2) Emotional lability
      (3) Poor self-esteem with a fragile sense of self
      (4) Aggressive personality
   d. Fear of abandonment is a common trait among abusers.

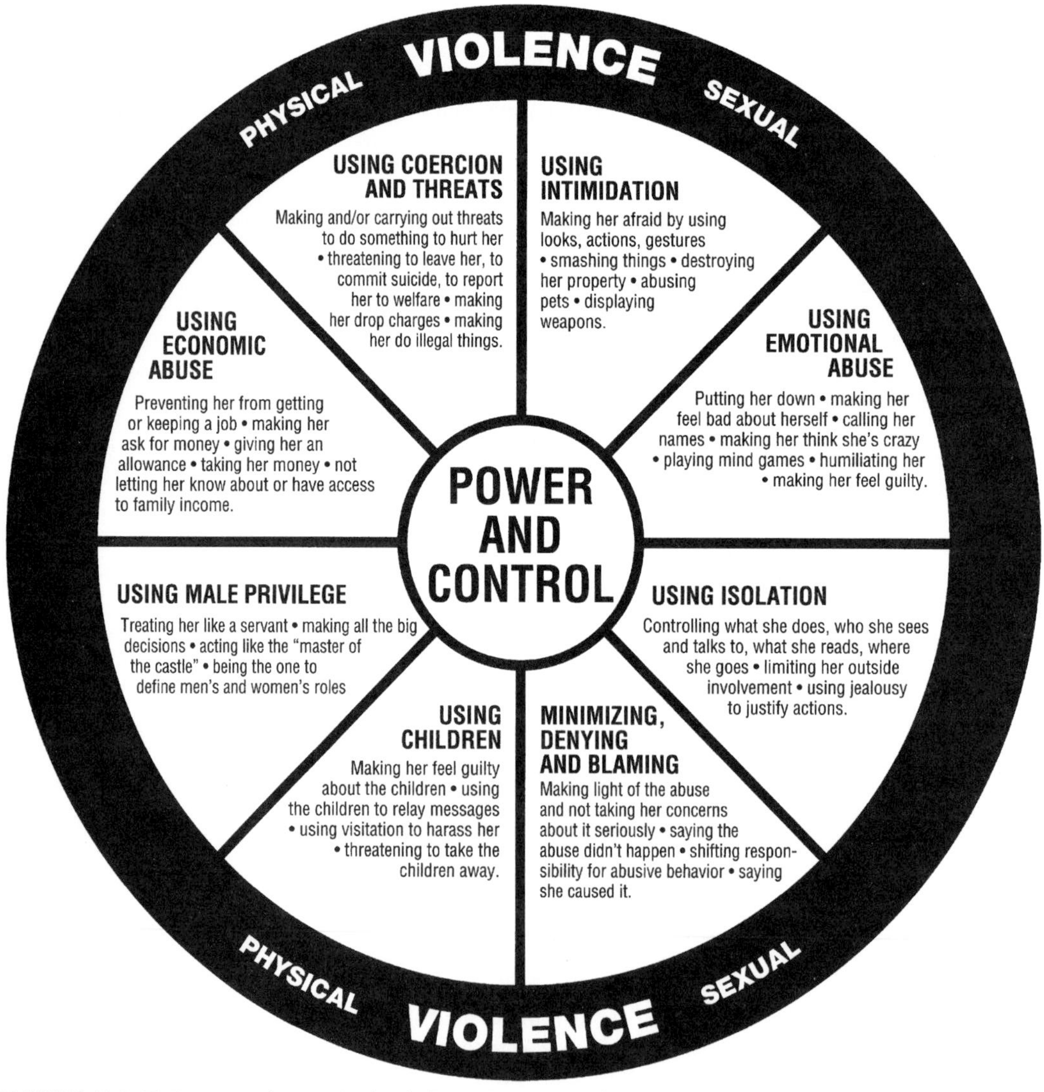

FIGURE 18-2 ■ Power and control wheel. (From Domestic Abuse Intervention Project, 206 West Fourth St., Duluth, MN 55806.)

G. Characteristics of women in abusive relationships
  1. An abused woman frequently accepts blame and responsibility for the violence.
  2. She believes she is not a "good enough" wife or partner in the relationship.
  3. She believes she needs to try harder to please her abuser.
  4. She exhibits a blend of loyalty, fear, terror, and learned helplessness.
  5. Most abused women have very low self-esteem and fear societal rejection if the abuse is revealed.
  6. Abused women seem to demonstrate a high level of traditional feminine traits, which are as follows:
      a. Nurturing
      b. Compassion
      c. Sympathy
      d. Yielding
  7. Abused women who are more likely to seek help are divided into three groups (Rynerson, 2007):
      a. Women who are beaten frequently and severely
      b. Women who have not experienced or witnessed family violence in their family of origin
      c. Women who can see an alternative to life in their abusive relationships

H. Estimates of IPV during pregnancy vary widely and have significant effects
  1. A nationally represented cohort of pregnant women revealed that over one third experienced IPV during pregnancy or after birth (Charles & Perreira, 2007); as many as 324,000 women each year experience IPV during a pregnancy (Gazmararian et al, 2000).
  2. Violence may induce preterm birth (Rodrigues, Rocha, & Barros, 2008), although results are not conclusive across studies (Fried, Cabral, Amaro, & Aschengrau, 2008); physical abuse may be the specific type of abuse that leads to preterm birth and injury or death to the fetus.
  3. IPV is a leading cause of pregnancy-related death (Chang, Berg, Saltzman, & Herndon, 2005).

I. IPV during pregnancy
  1. Pregnancy is often the trigger for the beginning or escalation of violence in a relationship.
      a. Stresses of pregnancy may strain a troubled relationship beyond normal coping abilities.
      b. The abuser may harbor jealousy of the fetus.
         (1) Resents intrusion into the relationship
         (2) Resents the woman's attention to the fetus
      c. Physical violence may be an attempt to end the pregnancy.
      d. A pregnant woman who is battered is unlikely to have strong social support on which she can rely (Christian, 1995).
  2. The body parts targeted for abuse tend to change during pregnancy.
      a. Pregnant women are likely to have more multiple injury sites than nonpregnant women.
      b. Physical abuse is directed to the breasts, genitalia, and especially to the abdomen.
      c. An increase in sexual assault is common.
      d. Risk of injury to the fetus is very high.
  3. When battering occurs during pregnancy, a high risk exists of the following sequelae:
      a. Continued battering after the birth
      b. Child abuse
  4. When violence occurs during pregnancy, the woman may experience conflicting psychological and social processes (Lutz, Curry, Robrecht, Libbus, & Bullock, 2006).
      a. As women try to complete the developmental task of ensuring safe passage for themselves and their babies, they are confronted by the realities of their abuse.
      b. These conflicting experiences may encourage a woman to work harder to have a good relationship with her spouse or partner.
      c. Women may report feeling as if they are living in two separate worlds—an external one with the pregnancy that everyone can see and a private internal world of abuse.

CLINICAL PRACTICE

A. Assessment
  1. Pregnancy presents a unique opportunity for health care providers to recognize abuse and to appropriately intervene. The first task is for providers to examine their own feelings and beliefs about abuse, which may be difficult.

    a. Physical abuse has long been minimized by the public.

    b. The media portray violence in music, magazines, videos, and films.

    c. Many people believe that IPV is a private affair and should be worked out by the couple.

    d. Many people believe that abuse is justified in certain circumstances, or that women can easily leave an abusive relationship if they want to.

    e. Care providers with a history of abuse or living in abusive relationships may feel that if they can do it, so can other victims.

    f. The care provider *must* believe that IPV is a serious health problem with negative sequelae for women and their infants if he or she is to effectively screen for abuse.

B. **History of abuse can be obtained from the prenatal history or from the woman.**

    1. Approach the topic of assessment by telling the woman that all women are screened for abuse.

    2. If she hesitates when asked to answer yes or no, offer her the choice of sometimes.

    3. Do not pressure her to respond to the abuse questions; she will choose when, where, and with whom to share her history.

    4. Look for the following indicators:

        a. Previous assault; a man who abuses a woman before pregnancy is likely to continue the abuse during pregnancy.

        b. Injuries inflicted by weapons; look for scars from blunt traumas, as well as weapon wounds.

        c. Injuries consistent with assault that are inadequately explained

        d. History of depression or suicide attempts by the woman or her male partner

            (1) Depression is common among survivors of childhood or adult violence

            (2) Depression may be attributed to pregnancy or postpartum stressors during childbearing, rather than to the underlying abusive relationship.

            (3) Both abuser and abused have a higher incidence of suicide attempts.

        e. Legal or illegal substance use by the woman or her partner

            (1) Many violent episodes involve the use of alcohol or drugs by the abuser.

            (2) Abused women may use alcohol and drugs to cope with the abuse.

            (3) Tranquilizer or sedative use may be prescribed for the victim.

        f. Eating disorders

        g. Complications of previous pregnancies, which include:

            (1) Spontaneous abortions

            (2) First- or second-trimester bleeding

            (3) Poor weight gain

            (4) Preterm labor or birth

            (5) Low birthweight

            (6) Abruptio placentae

        h. Late or inadequate prenatal care; abused women are twice as likely as nonabused women to delay entry into prenatal care.

        i. Sexually transmitted infections, group B *Streptococcus*, pelvic inflammatory disease, or both

        j. Change in appointment pattern

            (1) Appointments that are missed

            (2) Multiple medical visits for injuries or anxiety symptoms; look for repeated visits for vague or somatic complaints, including headaches, insomnia, back, chest or pelvic pain, choking sensation, or false preterm labor (McFarlane & Parker, 1995)

        k. Reports of pet abuse

            (1) Abuse or threats of abuse toward women's pets, children's pets, or both may occur as a method of "keeping them in line."

            (2) Some women will not seek help because they worry about leaving pets behind.

C. **Physical findings and observations that may indicate abuse** (McFarlane & Parker, 1995):

    1. Early signs of abuse take many forms and may be considered warning signs.

        a. Partner is overly possessive and jealous.

        b. Partner is threatened by the woman's success or by her pregnancy.

        c. Partner is cruel and violent in other relationships.

        d. Partner may enjoy teasing or scaring the woman.

        e. Partner may be impatient or rough with the woman.

2. Look for the following indicators:
   a. Injuries consistent with assault that are inadequately explained (see earlier discussion for assault-like injuries)
   b. Painful vaginal examination; women with a history of child or sexual abuse may experience difficulty, including pain and tenseness.
   c. Anxious behaviors
      (1) Crying
      (2) Sighing
      (3) Minimizing statements
      (4) Searching and engaging eye contact (fear)
      (5) No eye contact (not applicable in certain cultures)
      (6) Inappropriate laughing, giggling, or both
   d. Comments about emotional abuse
   e. Comments about a "friend" who is abused
   f. Woman's behavior in presence of her partner
      (1) The woman may appear afraid of her partner.
      (2) She may defer to her partner.
      (3) She checks out her responses with her partner.
   g. Partner's behavior in presence of the woman
      (1) He may hover and be very unwilling to leave her unattended.
      (2) He may speak for her.
      (3) He may make derogatory comments about her appearance and behavior.
      (4) He is anxious and wants to minimize the woman's time with the care provider.
D. **Interventions:** The overall goal is that the mother and fetus do not suffer injury; thus the interventions are directed at acknowledging the abuse (assessment screening), ensuring the woman's and the fetus's safety (information concerning protection), and empowering the woman to make changes (increase her coping skills). Assessing for abuse carries the responsibility for intervention after a positive response; at a minimum, all agencies should have referral sources available, as well as information on available legal options. In working with abused women, the nurse must be aware of state reporting procedures and be available to assist the woman in filing a report if she so requests.
   1. Primary prevention includes assessing all women for potential or actual abuse.
      a. This intervention should occur at the first contact with the health care delivery system (i.e., prenatal care, labor and delivery suite, emergency room).
      b. Assessment for abuse at each visit is important.
         (1) Because of guilt, shame, embarrassment, and fear, some abused women deny the abuse during the initial assessment, but later the woman may feel comfortable in sharing the information.
         (2) Some abuse may not occur until the second or third trimester.
      c. A suitable atmosphere of quiet, privacy, and trust should be created for this questioning, away from the partner, whose presence might endanger the woman.
         (1) Assure her that her disclosure is confidential.
         (2) All states do not have mandatory reporting laws; if in a state that does not, inform her that the legal authorities will not be notified unless she wishes it.
      d. Ask specific, nonjudgmental, open-ended questions that encourage the woman to disclose abuse and yet do not label her as an "abused woman."
         (1) The questions should reflect the full spectrum of abuse.
         (2) Questions should be concrete and direct.
      e. An abuse assessment screen has been developed by the Nursing Research Consortium on Violence and Abuse (McFarlane & Parker, 1995) and addresses the following three questions:
         (1) Within the last year, have you been hit, slapped, kicked, or otherwise physically hurt by someone? If yes, by whom?
         (2) Since you've been pregnant, have you been hit, slapped, kicked, or otherwise physically hurt by someone? If yes, by whom?
         (3) Within the last year, have you been forced by anyone to have sexual activities? If yes, by whom?

    f. Prefacing the assessment by comments can convey the message that the nurse cares about a woman who is abused and is prepared to help her; examples of comments are as follows:

        (1) "Many women experience abuse."

        (2) "You are not alone."

        (3) "Sometimes abuse happens for the first time during pregnancy."

    g. An essential intervention for all abused women is assessing for their safety, including the safety of the woman, her infant and other children, and family members.

        (1) Asking directly about whether she feels safe is crucial; abused women can judge their own safety.

        (2) The Danger Assessment tool can be used to help the woman determine the danger she and others may be in (King et al, 1993) (Figure 18-3).

        (3) If a woman's safety is in question, this concern should be shared with her.

            (a) Desired assistance should be provided.

            (b) An important point to keep in mind is that a woman is in most danger of homicide when the relationship is changing or ending, even if it is not ending for violence-related reasons (Nicolaidis et al, 2003).

        (4) Women should also be assessed for thoughts of suicide.

2. After the woman has told her story of abuse, it is important to validate her experience and empower her to discuss her options and decisions.

    a. Her decision may or may not be to leave the abuser; only she knows when it is feasible or safe.

    b. Secondary intervention should be aimed at assisting the woman in choosing what is best for her from many options.

    c. A crucial intervention is helping abused women mobilize social support.

Danger Assessment

Several risk factors have been associated with homicides (murder) of both batterers and battered women in research that has been conducted after the killings have taken place. We cannot predict what will happen in your case, but we would like you to be aware of the danger of homicide in situations of severe battering and for you to see how many of the risk factors apply to your situation. (The "he" in the question refers to your husband, partner, ex-husband, ex-partner, or whoever is currently physically hurting you.)

Please check YES or NO for each question below

YES   **NO**

____ ____ 1. Has the physical violence increased in frequency over the past year?

____ ____ 2. Has the physical violence increased in severity over the past year and/or has a weapon or threat with a weapon been used?

____ ____ 3. Does he ever try to choke you?

____ ____ 4. Is there a gun in the house?

____ ____ 5. Has he ever forced you into sex when you did not wish to do so?

____ ____ 6. Does he use drugs? By drugs I mean "uppers" or amphetamines, speed, angel dust, cocaine, "crack," street drugs, heroin, or mixtures.

____ ____ 7. Does he threaten to kill you and/or do you believe he is capable of killing you?

____ ____ 8. Is he drunk every day or almost every day? (In terms of quantity of alcohol.)

____ ____ 9. Does he control most of all your daily activities? For instance, does he tell you whom you can be friends with, how much money you can take with you shopping, or when you can take the car?

         (If he tries, but you do not let him, check here ____.)

____ ____ 10. Have you ever been beaten by him while you were pregnant?

         (If never pregnant by him, check here ____.)

____ ____ 11. Is he violently and constantly jealous of you?

         (For instance, does he say, "If I can't have you, no one can.")

____ ____ 12. Have you ever threatened or tried to commit suicide?

____ ____ 13. Has he ever threatened or tried to commit suicide?

____ ____ 14. Is he violent outside of the home?

TOTAL YES ANSWERS

      THANK YOU. PLEASE TALK TO YOUR NURSE, ADVOCATE, OR
      COUNSELOR ABOUT WHAT THE DANGER ASSESSMENT
      MEANS IN TERMS OF YOUR SITUATION.

FIGURE 18-3 ■ March of Dimes Danger Assessment questionnaire. (From Campbell, J. [1986]. Nursing assessment for risk of homicide with battered women. *Advances in Nursing Science*, 8[4], 36-51.)

(1) Identify other friends or relatives that might have been in a similar situation or who may be willing to help.

(2) Referrals can be made to local shelters, battered women's organizations, and legal advocacy resources (see Resources for Professionals).

d. Another intervention is to provide adequate documentation of the abuse in the medical records.

(1) The record should show that the woman revealed that she was abused by her partner and sought help.

(2) The record should include the relationship of the abuser to the woman and detail the specifics of the emotional, sexual, or physical abuse.

(3) Injuries should be explicitly described, with photographs if appropriate; a body map can be used to sketch the location of old and new injuries.

3. Tertiary intervention means assisting the abused woman in making long-term plans for her life.

a. Constant support and intervention, coupled with advocacy by shelter staff or formerly battered women, are most effective in mobilizing a woman's resources.

b. When a woman is ready to leave the relationship, she needs affirmation of her choice and encouragement in her independence; she should have the following available:

(1) Telephone numbers for a shelter and the police

(2) Plan for quick escape

(3) Packed bag with keys, money, and important papers (see Health Education for a safety plan)

c. Women experiencing repeated abuse may feel emotionally unstable and depressed and harbor feelings of low self-esteem.

(1) Nurses can advocate for individual or group counseling to help women address these reactions.

(2) Nurses can help women strengthen their emotional health while learning new coping strategies.

d. It is important to ensure continued health care for the woman and her infant, as well as her other children.

HEALTH EDUCATION

A. **The top priority of health education is to emphasize safety for the abused woman, her fetus, and her other children whether she decides to leave or to stay in the relationship; she should have the following items immediately ready for use at any time:**

1. Free calls to the National Domestic Violence Hot Line: 800-799-SAFE; TTY: 800-787-3224.

a. Help is available 24 hours a day, 365 days a year, in 170 languages.

b. Internet access to the National Domestic Violence Hotline at www.ndvh.org

2. Safety plan

a. Hide money.

b. Hide extra set of house and car keys. Both money and keys should be placed in a location that is easily retrievable by the woman, but not likely to be found by the man (e.g., with nearby neighbor or family, or a place in or out of the house not frequented by partner).

c. Establish code with family and friends (e.g., words to use if woman calls so she does not have to explain situation or say she is being abused).

d. Ask neighbor to call police if violence begins.

e. Remove weapons.

f. Have the following documents available:

(1) Social security numbers (his, hers, children's)

(2) Rent and utility receipts

(3) Birth certificates (hers and children's)

(4) Driver's license

(5) Bank account numbers

(6) Insurance policies and numbers

(7) Marriage license

g. Have prescription drugs and refill numbers for her and children.

      h. Have valuable jewelry and keepsakes.

      i. Have important telephone numbers.

      j. Hide bag with extra clothing.

B. Women need to be educated that abuse of any kind is a violation of their basic human rights.

    1. They need to know how to access protective services.

    2. They also need to know how to access affordable legal services.

C. Educate the woman about the cycle of violence and how to recognize signs of escalating danger.

D. Provide referrals for support services to empower the abused woman.

E. Encourage the woman to consider the following:

    1. Self-defense courses

    2. Assertiveness courses

    3. Self-help groups

    4. Educational or skills development courses

F. Resources professionals need to provide health education.

    1. Health care providers need ongoing and regularly scheduled continuing education.

      a. Health Resource Center on Domestic Violence

        (1) Technical assistance to individuals or organizations setting up IPV training programs or developing IPV protocols

        (2) Provides assistance on how to respond to IPV in a safe and effective manner

        (3) Available via phone: 800-313-1310

      b. National Directory of Shelters: national listing of shelters, safe homes, and community programs: (303) 839-1852

      c. Continuing education and staff updating: AWHONN has a prepared program for educating health professionals about intimate partner violence; AWHONN: 800-673-8499; www.awhonn.org.

    2. Care providers need clear, specific, and regularly updated materials.

      a. Designate who will review the materials available for patients and how often this review should occur.

      b. Providers may appreciate having a specific resource material available with local phone numbers.

        (1) Safety checklist (Furniss, McCaffrey, Parnell, & Rovi, 2007)

        (2) Protocols (Furniss et al, 2007)

      c. Materials for patients should be designed with attention to protecting their safety (e.g., palm or shoe size).

        (1) Review recommendations from AWHONN.

        (2) Review recommendations from the Centers for Disease Control and Prevention.

        (3) Review March of Dimes materials.

        (4) Designate who will review the materials and how often.

    3. Communication training

      a. Staff may need training in effective interviewing styles for IPV victims.

      b. Role playing may be useful if using a variety of abuse victim scenarios.

      c. "You are not alone" and "You do not deserve to be treated in this way" are powerful messages and effective communication.

      d. Never use a family member as an interpreter. Practice working with an interpreter.

    4. Office or unit design issues

      a. Make sure the setting is one in which the woman has complete privacy for abuse screening.

      b. Establish policies that enable the woman to be interviewed separately from family or friends.

        (1) Send overly attentive partners to complete insurance information while "feminine hygiene takes place" (Furniss et al, 2007).

      c. Place posters and discrete palm cards in restrooms that only women use (Furniss et al, 2007).

      d. Allow flexibility in workload assessments to accommodate the additional time that may be required for abuse assessments.

      e. Support colleagues

        (1) Hearing abuse stories can be unsettling.

        (2) Continued contact with abused women who do not leave their abuser can be frustrating.

        (3) Provide a safe outlet for colleagues who may need to vent their feelings.

CASE STUDY AND STUDY QUESTIONS

Ms. S. is 20 years of age, unmarried, and 6 months pregnant. She lives with her boyfriend, Mr. K., who is also 20 years of age and is the father of her unborn infant. Mr. K. works at a local restaurant, where he washes dishes. Ms. S. does not work, and their income is very limited. She has come to the clinic for her first prenatal visit. Mr. K. is with her and says he wants to stay with her throughout the visit.

1. Ms. S. is late in seeking prenatal care. Why is this one of the indicators of potential abuse?
   a. She may not value her unborn child.
   b. She may not have realized that she should seek early prenatal care.
   c. She may have been trying to conceal signs of abuse before this visit.
   d. She did not want her family to know she was pregnant.
2. Mr. K. has some potential indicators of an abuser, which include all of the following *except:*
   a. His young age
   b. His low-paying job
   c. His constant presence during her clinic visit
   d. He is not her husband.

Mr. K. leaves the room briefly to go to the bathroom. When asked about her relationship with Mr. K., Ms. S. says that it is good most of the time. She says he has a bad temper and sometimes gets very mad at her. She says it is usually over some dumb thing she has done or said, so she deserves it. She said she thinks she just needs to try harder not to do and say those things anymore.

3. Her response is typical of abused women because they frequently:
   a. Cannot admit to others that abuse is taking place
   b. Take the blame for invoking the abuse
   c. Are trying harder to be a better partner or wife to the abuser
   d. All of the above
4. Ms. S.'s pregnancy is high risk because of late prenatal care. If physically abused, what added risk occurs?

   a. Fetus might have a genetic disorder.
   b. Gestational diabetes
   c. Polyhydramnios
   d. Fetus might be physically injured.

Ms. S. returned to the clinic 2 weeks later for a scheduled ultrasound examination. Mr. K. was unable to be with her. He insisted that she reschedule her appointment, but she did not. She was anxious to find out the sex of the infant. Exposure of her abdomen revealed several bruises, all in various states of healing. She tried to explain the presence of the bruises as merely the result of her clumsiness. With further questioning, she broke down in tears and admitted that Mr. K. slapped her, pulled her by her hair, kicked her, and hit her in the stomach. He was extremely mad that she did not reschedule the appointment. She said that she had sure learned her lesson and would never do that again. She also said he is all over it now and has been wonderfully sweet to her. He promised to never do that again.

5. Mr. K.'s actions are examples of all of the phases of:
   a. The circle of abuse
   b. The cycle of violence
   c. The abuser-abuse-victim syndrome
   d. The abuse, cover-up, make-up theory
6. The abuser typically tries to minimize the acute abuse episode. This was evident when Ms. S. said that:
   a. He is all over it now.
   b. He has been wonderfully sweet to her.
   c. She sure learned her lesson.
   d. He promised never to do that again.
7. The abdominal trauma she endured is:
   a. Not dangerous to the fetus because labor did not start and no vaginal bleeding occurred
   b. A typical target for the physical abuse of a pregnant woman
   c. Usually harmless because of the amniotic sac and fluid
   d. Less painful for a woman who is pregnant because of the extra cushioning for her vital organs

ANSWERS TO STUDY QUESTIONS

1. c
2. a
3. d
4. d

5. b
6. c
7. b

REFERENCES

Bohn, D. K. (2003). Lifetime physical and sexual abuse, substance abuse, depression, and suicide attempts among Native American women. *Issues in Mental Health Nursing, 24*, 333–352.

Campbell, J., Campbell, D. W., Gary, F., Nedd, D., Price-Lea, P., Sharps, P. W., et al. (2006). African American women's responses to intimate partner violence: An examination of cultural context. *Journal of Aggression, Maltreatment, & Trauma, 16*(3), 277–295.

Caetano, R., Ramisetty-Mikler, S., Caetano Vaeth, P. A., & Harris, T. R. (2007). Acculturation, stress, drinking, and intimate partner violence among Hispanic couples. *U.S. Journal of Interpersonal Violence, 22*(11), 1431–1447.

Centers for Disease Control and Prevention (2008). *Intimate partner violence: Definitions. National Center for Injury Prevention and Control, Division of Violence Prevention*. Bethesda, MD: Author.

Chang, J., Berg, C. J., Saltzman, L. E., & Herndon, J. (2005). Homicide: A leading cause of injury deaths among pregnant and postpartum women in the United States, 1991-1999. *American Journal of Public Health, 95*, 471–477.

Charles, P., & Perreira, K. (2007). Correlates of intimate partner violence during pregnancy and 1 year postpartum. *Journal of Family Violence, 22*(7), 609–619.

Christian, A. (1995). Home care of the battered pregnant woman: One battered woman's pregnancy. *Journal of Obstetric, Gynecologic, and Neonatal Nursing, 24*(9), 836–842.

Cunradi, C. B., Caetano, R., Clark, C., & Schafer, J. (2000). Neighborhood poverty as a predictor of intimate partner violence among White, Black, and Hispanic couples in the United States: A multilevel analysis. *Annals of Epidemiology, 10*(5), 297–308.

Ehrensaft, M., & Cohen, P. (2003). Intergenerational transmission of partner violence: A 20-year prospective study. *Journal of Consulting & Clinical Psychology, 7*, 741–753.

Fawole, O. I. (2008). Economic violence to women and girls: Is it receiving the necessary attention? *Trauma, Violence, & Abuse, 9*(3), 167–177.

Flores-Ortiz, Y. (1993). *La mujer y la violencia*: A culturally based model for the understanding and treatment of domestic violence in Chicana/Latina communities. In Mujeres Activas en Letras y Cambio Social (Ed.), *Chicana critical issues* (pp. 169–182). Berkeley, CA: Chicana/Latina Research Center.

Fried, L. E., Cabral, J., Amaro, J., & Aschengrau, A. (2008). Lifetime and during pregnancy experiences of violence and the risk of low birth weight and preterm birth. *Journal of Midwifery & Women's Health, 53*(6), 522–528.

Furniss, K., McCaffrey, M., Parnell, V., & Rovi, S. (2007). Nurses and barriers to screening for intimate partner violence. *MCN The American Journal of Maternal-Child Nursing, 32*(4), 238–243.

Gazmararian, J., Petersen, R., Spitz, A., Goodwin, M., Saltzman, L., & Marks, J. (2000). Violence and reproductive health: Current knowledge and future research directions. *Maternal & Child Health Journal, 4*(2), 79–84.

Hanrahan, P., Campbell, J., & Ulrich, Y. (1993). Theories of violence. In J. Campbell, & J. Humphreys (Eds.), *Nursing care of survivors of family violence* (pp. 5–42). St. Louis: Mosby.

Hassouneh, D., & Glass, N. (2008). The influence of gender role stereotyping on women's experiences of female same-sex intimate partner violence. *Violence Against Women, 14*(3), 310–325.

Hattery, A. J. (2008). *Intimate partner violence*. New York: Routledge.

King, M., Torres, S., Campbell, D., Ryan, J., Sheridan, D., Ulrich, Y., et al. (1993). Violence and abuse of women: A perinatal health care issue. *AWHONN Clinical Issues in Perinatal and Women's Health Nursing, 4*(2), 163–173.

Klevens, J., Shelley, G., Clavel-Arcas, C., Barney, D. D., Tobar, C., Duran, E. S., Barajas-Mazahen, R., Esparza, J. (2007). Latinos' perspectives and experiences with intimate partner violence. *Violence Against Women, 13*(2), 141–158.

Kramer, A., Lorenzon, D., & Mueller, G. (2004). Prevalence of intimate partner violence and health implications for women using emergency departments and primary care clinics. *Women's Health Issues, 14*, 19–29.

Lauderdale, J. (2003). Transcultural perspectives in childbearing. In M. Andrews, & J. Boyle (Eds.), *Transcultural concepts in nursing care* (4th ed., pp. 95–131). Philadelphia: Lippincott Williams & Wilkins.

Lutz, K. F., Curry, M. A., Robrecht, L. C., Libbus, M. K., & Bullock, L. (2006). Double binding, abusive intimate partner relationships, and pregnancy. *Canadian Journal of Nursing Research, 38*(4), 118–134.

Mattson, S., & Rodriguez, E. (1999). Battering in pregnant Latinas. *Issues in Mental Health Nursing, 20*(4), 405–422.

McFarlane, J., & Parker, B. (1994). Preventing abuse during pregnancy: An assessment and intervention protocol. *American Journal of Maternal-Child Nursing, 19*(6), 321–324.

McFarlane, J., & Parker, B. (1995). *Abuse during pregnancy: A protocol for prevention and intervention. March of Dimes Nursing Monograph*. White Plains, NY: March of Dimes.

Nicolaidis, C., Curry, M. A., Ulrich, Y., Sharps, P., McFarlane, J., et al. (2003). Could we have known? A qualitative analysis of data from women who survived an attempted homicide by an intimate partner. *Journal of General Internal Medicine, 18,* 788–794.

Noel, N., & Yam, M. (1992). Domestic violence: The pregnant battered woman. *Nursing Clinics of North America, 4*(27), 871–884.

Noll, J. G., Horowitz, L. A., Bonanno, G. A., Trickett, P. K., & Putnam, F. W. (2003). Revictimization and self-harm in females who experienced child sexual abuse: Results from a prospective study. *Journal of Interpersonal Violence, 18*(12), 1452–1471.

O'Leary, K. (1993). Through a psychological lens: Personality traits, personality disorders, and levels of violence. In R. Gelles, & D. Loseke (Eds.), *Current controversies on family violence* (pp. 142–180). Newbury Park, CA: Sage.

Phelan, M. B. (2007). Screening for intimate partner violence in medical settings. *Trauma, Violence, and Abuse, 8*(2), 199–213.

Rennison, C. (2001). *Violent victimization and race, 1993–1998. (NCJ No. 176354).* Washington, DC: U.S. Department of Justice, Office of Justice Programs, National Institute of Justice.

Rodrigues, T., Rocha, L., & Barros, H. (2008). Physical abuse during pregnancy and preterm delivery. *American Journal of Obstetrics and Gynecology, 198*(2), 171.e1–171.e6.

Rodriguez, M. (1994). Domestic violence. *Western Journal of Medicine, 161*(1), 60–61.

Romans, S., Forte, T., Cohen, M. M., Du Mont, J., & Hyman, I. (2007). Who is most at risk for intimate partner violence? A Canadian population-based study. *Journal of Interpersonal Violence, 22*(12), 1495–1514.

Ruiz, E., & Mattson, S. (2003). Observation, self-efficacy and anger: Latino children and domestic violence. In *Communicating nursing research conference proceedings: Responding to societal imperatives through discovery & innovation* (Vol. 3, p. 291). Portland, OR: Western Institute of Nursing.

Rynerson, B. (2007). Violence against women. In D. L. Lowdermilk, & S. E. Perry (Eds.), *Maternity & women's health care* (9th ed., pp. 125–144). St. Louis: Mosby.

Saltzman, L. E., Fanslow, J. L., McMahon, P. M., & Shelley, G. A. (2002). *Intimate partner violence surveillance: Uniform definitions and recommended data elements, version 1.0.* Atlanta: Centers for Disease Control and Prevention, National Center for Injury Prevention and Control. Accessed February 25, 2009. Available from: www.cdc.gov/ncipc/pubres/ipv_surveillance/intimate.htm.

Smith, E. (2008). African American men and intimate partner violence. *Journal of African American Studies, 12*(2), 156–179.

Suarez, L., & Ramirez, A. (1999). Hispanic/Latino health and disease. In R. Huff, & M. Kline (Eds.), *Promoting health in multicultural populations* (pp. 115–136). Thousand Oaks, CA: Sage.

Tjaden, P., & Thoennes, N. (2000). *Extent, nature, and consequences of intimate partner violence.* Washington, DC: U.S. Department of Justice.

Torrés, S. (1991). A comparison of wife abuse between two cultures: Perceptions, attitudes, nature, and extent. *Issues in Mental Health Nursing, 12*(1), 113–131.

Walker, L. (1982). *The battered woman.* New York: Harper & Row.

19 Hypertensive Disorders in Pregnancy

Dustine Dix

OBJECTIVES

1. Describe the characteristics of gestational hypertension, preeclampsia, eclampsia, and chronic hypertension.
2. List the risk factors for the development of preeclampsia.
3. Review the pathophysiology and physiologic alterations associated with preeclampsia and HELLP syndrome.
4. Identify assessment and physical examination techniques used in clinical practice.
5. Describe the care management of the woman with mild and severe preeclampsia.
6. Evaluate the use of anticonvulsant and antihypertensive medications.
7. Identify the priorities for management of eclamptic seizures.
8. Describe the care management of a woman with chronic hypertension.
9. Review postpartum care and women's health issues.

INTRODUCTION

A. **Hypertensive disorders are the most common complication that occur during pregnancy** (Sibai, 2007).
   1. Hypertension complicates 5% to 10% of all pregnancies.
   2. Hypertensive disorders occur in 37.8 per 1000 births (Martin et al, 2005).
      a. Highest rates: Native American (46.5 per 1000) and African American (41.5 per 1000) women
      b. Intermediate rate: Hispanic women (25.9 per 1000)
      c. Lowest rate: Asian or Pacific Islander women (19.6 per 1000)
   3. Hypertensive disorders are a major cause of maternal and fetal or neonatal morbidity and mortality (Sibai, 2007).
      a. Account for 10% to 15% of maternal deaths worldwide (Askie, Duley, Henderson-Smart, & Stewart, 2007)
   4. Potential maternal complications include placental abruption, intracranial hemorrhage, hepatic and renal dysfunction, disseminated intravascular coagulation (DIC), adult respiratory distress syndrome (ARDS), hypervolemia, and inhalation of gastric content (Grujić & Milasinović, 2006).
   5. Potential neonatal complications include intrauterine growth restriction, prematurity, and necrotizing enterocolitis.
B. **Classification of hypertensive disorders of pregnancy**
   1. Hypertensive disorders in pregnancy are classified into five groups (Gilbert, 2007; Peters, 2008; Sibai, 2007).
   2. Gestational hypertension
      a. Development of hypertension without proteinuria
      b. Hypertension develops after 20 weeks' gestation and resolves by 12 weeks' postpartum
      c. Hypertension is defined as:
         (1) Systolic blood pressure of 140 mm Hg or greater
         (2) Diastolic blood pressure of 90 mm Hg or greater
   3. Preeclampsia
      a. Most common hypertensive disorder of pregnancy
      b. Development of hypertension and proteinuria after 20 weeks of gestation
      c. Vasospastic, multisystem disease process
      d. Classified as mild or severe, depending on the severity of organ dysfunction

   4. Eclampsia
       a. Seizure activity or coma in a woman with preeclampsia
   5. Chronic hypertension
       a. Hypertension prior to pregnancy or that develops before 20 weeks' of gestation
   6. Preeclampsia superimposed on chronic hypertension
       a. Occurs in 21% of women with chronic hypertension
       b. Increased maternal or fetal morbidity rates
C. Risk factors for developing preeclampsia (Gilbert, 2007; Peters, 2008; Sibai, 2007)
   1. Occurs most often with first pregnancies
   2. Age extremes (younger than 19 or older than 40 years)
   3. First pregnancy with a new partner
   4. Preexisting medical conditions
       a. Chronic hypertension, renal disease, diabetes, or collagen disease
   5. Antiphospholipid antibody syndrome
   6. Exposure to abundance of trophoblast tissue
       a. Multi-fetal pregnancies
       b. Hydatidiform mole
   7. History of severe preeclampsia
       a. Recurrence rate in subsequent pregnancy ranges from 22% to 35%
   8. Family history of preeclampsia
   9. Obesity
       a. Increases the risk threefold
       b. Women with a body mass index (BMI) greater than 35 have a fourfold increased risk.
   10. Periodontal disease
D. The etiology of preeclampsia is unknown (Sibai, 2007).
   1. Theories of etiology
       a. Abnormal trophoblast invasion
       b. Coagulation abnormalities
       c. Vascular endothelial damage
       d. Cardiovascular maladaptation
       e. Dietary deficiencies or excesses
       f. Immunologic factors
       g. Genetic predisposition
E. Normal physiologic adaptations to pregnancy (Dix, 2007; Gilbert, 2007; Peters, 2008; see also Chapter 5 for further discussion)
   1. Cardiovascular/hemodynamic
       a. Systemic vasodilation
       b. Increased blood plasma volume (30% to 50%), which is greater than red cell mass expansion
       c. Hemodilution leads to physiologic anemia of pregnancy
       d. Increased cardiac output, stroke volume, heart rate, and oxygen consumption
       e. Decreased systemic vascular resistance; diastolic blood pressure (BP) drops 7 to 10 mm Hg by midgestation
       f. Decreased plasma colloid osmotic pressure; increased venous capillary hydrostatic pressure
       g. Fluid shifts to extracellular space in dependent limbs, resulting in edema.
       h. Increased clotting factors, and decreased serum albumin levels
   2. Renal
       a. Increased renal plasma flow and glomerular filtration rate
       b. Decreased serum creatinine, increased creatinine clearance
   3. Endocrine
       a. Increased estrogen production results in increased renin, angiotensin II, and aldosterone levels.
       b. Progesterone blocks effect of aldosterone.
       c. Increased vasodilator prostaglandins and nitric oxide levels
       d. Resistance to angiotensin II (vasopressor that causes an increase in BP)
F. Pathophysiology of preeclampsia has two stages (Gilbert, 2007; Peters, 2008).
   1. Disruptions in placental perfusion
       a. The trophoblast cells of the placenta alter the spiral arteries to accommodate increased blood flow.

    b. The vessels seen in preeclampsia are abnormally thick walled and have higher resistance.

    c. Lesions develop within the vessels, along with an increase in placental infarcts.

    d. These abnormalities result in decreased placental perfusion.

  2. Maternal syndrome

    a. Hypersensitivity to vasoactive hormones

    b. Vasoconstriction occurs, which decreases the plasma volume and cardiac output.

    c. Results in hypertension and increased peripheral resistance

    d. Leads to hemoconcentration, increased hematocrit, and development of microthrombi

    e. The blood vessel walls are damaged, which leads to endothelial cell dysfunction.

    f. Vasospasm and poor perfusion impede blood flow to all organ systems.

    g. These abnormalities result in multiorgan system dysfunction (Figure 19-1)

G. Physiologic alterations with preeclampsia (Gilbert, 2007; Peters, 2008)

  1. Uteroplacental perfusion

    a. Restricted intrauterine growth, and small-for-gestational age infants

    b. Premature birth

    c. Placental abruption

  2. Cardiovascular/hemodynamic

    a. Decreased serum albumin and plasma colloid osmotic pressure

    b. Endothelial cell damage leads to increased capillary permeability.

    c. Fluid shifts result in edema, possible rapid weight gain and risk of pulmonary edema.

    d. Endothelial cell damage leads to the activation of the clotting cascade and risk of DIC.

    e. Decreased platelet production can result in thrombocytopenia.

  3. Renal

    a. Reduced kidney perfusion decreases the glomerular filtration rate.

    b. This damages the glomerular membrane, increasing permeability to proteins (albumin).

    c. Blood urea nitrogen (BUN), serum creatinine, and serum uric acid levels increase.

    d. Reduced uric acid and creatinine clearance can lead to acute tubular necrosis and oliguria.

  4. Central nervous system (CNS)

    a. Fibrin deposits, hemorrhages, and cerebral edema lead to increased CNS irritability.

    b. Manifests as headache, hyperreflexia with clonus and seizure activity

  5. Ophthalmic

    a. Retinal arteriolar vasospasms leads to scotomata (blurred spots), photophobia, or double vision.

  6. Hepatic

    a. Fibrin deposits and hepatic ischemia result in elevated liver enzymes.

    b. Manifests as epigastric or right upper quadrant pain, nausea and vomiting.

H. HELLP syndrome (Gilbert, 2007; Peters, 2008; Sibai, 2007)

  1. A severe complication that occurs in 5% of women with preeclampsia

  2. HELLP is an acronym

    a. *H*—Hemolysis of red blood cells

    b. *EL*—Elevated Liver enzymes (aspartate transaminase [AST], alanine transaminase [ALT])

    c. *LP*—Low Platelet count ($<100,000/mm^3$)

  3. Pathophysiology of HELLP syndrome

    a. Endothelial cell damage leads to fibrin deposits and adherence of platelets in blood vessels.

    b. Red blood cells are damaged passing through narrowed blood vessels and hemolyzed

    c. Leads to decreased red blood cell and platelet count

    d. Hyperbilirubinemia and hemolytic anemia may develop.

    e. Fibrin deposits in the liver result in impaired function and elevated liver enzymes.

    f. Hemorrhagic necrosis can result in a subcapsular hematoma (rare occurrence, but life threatening).

  4. Signs of HELLP syndrome usually develop in the third trimester, or within 48 hours after birth.

    a. Most often present with influenza-like symptoms and malaise

    b. Epigastric or right upper quadrant pain, possibly jaundice

    c. Nausea or vomiting

    d. Headache

    e. Bruising or hematuria

  5. Perinatal mortality rates range from 7.4% to 20.4%.

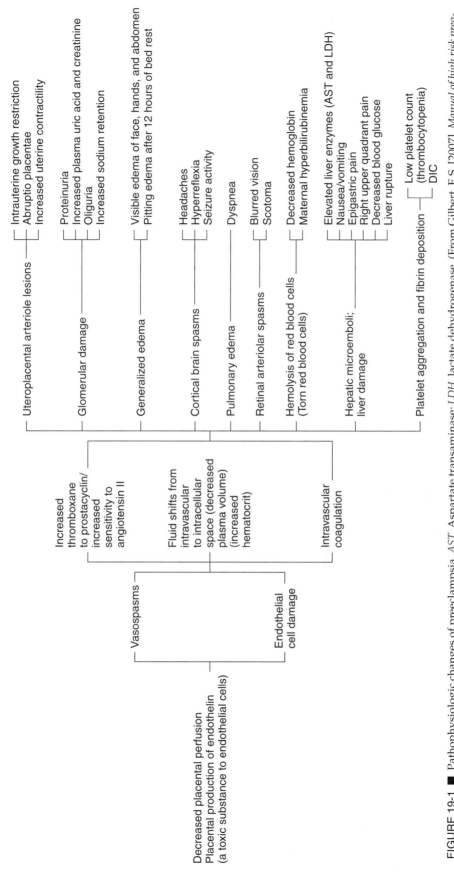

FIGURE 19-1 ■ Pathophysiologic changes of preeclampsia. *AST,* Aspartate transaminase; *LDH,* lactate dehydrogenase. (From Gilbert, E.S. [2007]. *Manual of high risk pregnancy & delivery* [4th ed.]. St. Louis: Mosby.)

CLINICAL PRACTICE

A. Predicting or preventing preeclampsia
1. No reliable test has been developed as a routine screening tool for preeclampsia (Dix, 2007; Peters, 2008).
   a. Several studies found that women were more likely to develop preeclampsia with low levels of placental growth factor (PIGF) in their urine, and high levels of two proteins in their blood (soluble endoglin and fms-like tyrosine kinase) (Cockey, 2005; Hellwig, 2007).
   b. Preeclampsia was correlated with very low levels of 25-hydroxyvitamin D in an epidemiologic study (Ravin, 2008).
2. Use of antioxidants, calcium, magnesium, zinc; restricted protein or sodium intake and fish oil supplementation have not been found to be helpful in preventing or reducing the severity of preeclampsia (Sibai, 2007).
   a. Low-dose aspirin therapy (60 to 75 mg a day) demonstrated a small to moderate benefit in the reduction of preeclampsia and was found to have no harmful effects (Gilbert, 2007).
3. The best method of prevention is early detection.
B. Assessment (Dix, 2007; Duckitt & Harrington, 2005; Peters, 2008; Sibai, 2007)
1. History
   a. Age, parity, and estimated date of confinement (EDC)
   b. Medical and obstetric history
   c. Family history
2. Risk factors
   a. First pregnancy or new partner with this pregnancy
   b. Multiple gestation
   c. Age extremes (younger than 19 or older than 40 years)
   d. Obesity
   e. Preexisting renal disease, diabetes, collagen disease, or chronic hypertension
   f. Personal or family history of preeclampsia
3. Social history
   a. Marital status
   b. Cultural beliefs
   c. Drug, tobacco, and alcohol use
      (1) Tobacco use may decrease risk of preeclampsia, but it increases risk of low birthweight, placental abruption, and overall maternal health
      (2) Advised to avoid alcohol and tobacco, and limit caffeine intake.
   d. Activity level: exercise—amount and frequency
      (1) Advised to engage in 30 minutes of moderate exercise on most days.
4. Nutritional status
   a. Dietary intake
      (1) Nutritious well-balanced diet with foods high in roughage
      (2) 60 to 70 g protein and 1200 mg calcium
      (3) No sodium restriction, limit excessively salty foods
      (4) Advised to drink six to eight 8-ounce glasses of water per day
5. Review of systems
   a. Baseline blood pressure, weight, and presence of edema
C. Physical examination (Dix, 2007; Gilbert, 2007; Peters, 2008; Sibai, 2007)
1. Blood pressure
   a. Use correct cuff size; cuff should cover 80% of the upper arm or be 1.5 times the length of the upper arm.
      (1) A small cuff results in elevated readings.
      (2) A large cuff results in falsely low readings.
   b. BP measurement is altered by position.
      (1) BP is lowest (by 10 to 20 mm Hg) in a lateral recumbent position.
      (2) BP is highest when supine or standing, and intermediate when sitting.
      (3) Sitting position is recommended for prenatal assessments.
   c. The arm should be supported on a desk at the level of the heart.
   d. BP may vary by >10 mm Hg with each arm; record the higher reading.

    e. Diastolic pressure should be recorded at:

      (1) Korotkoff phase V (disappearance of sound)

      (2) Not Korotkoff phase IV (muffling sound)

    f. If the BP is elevated, allow the woman to rest for 5 to 10 minutes, then retake it.

    g. Measurements with an automated device should be checked with a manual device.

2. Edema

    a. Dependent edema (lowest or most dependent parts of the body) is common during pregnancy.

    b. Assessment of degree of edema

      (1) Minimal edema of lower extremities—1+

      (2) Marked edema of lower extremities—2+

      (3) Edema of lower extremities, face and hands—3+

      (4) Generalized edema including abdomen and sacrum—4+

    c. Pitting edema leaves a small indentation or pit after finger pressure is applied to the area

      (1) 2-mm indentation: 1+

      (2) 4-mm indentation: 2+

      (3) 6-mm indentation: 3+

      (4) 8-mm indentation: 4+

3. Weight gain

    a. Average weight gain during pregnancy is 25 to 35 pounds

    b. Excessive weight gain is 2 pounds per day or 5 pounds per week

4. Deep tendon reflexes (DTRs; usually patellar reflex)

    a. Classification of DTRs

      (1) No response: 0

      (2) Sluggish or diminished: 1+

      (3) Active or normal: 2+

      (4) Brisk: 3+

      (5) Brisk with beats of clonus: 4+

    b. Assessment of clonus

      (1) Briskly dorsiflex the foot while slightly flexing the knee.

      (2) Apply continuous pressure to the sole of the foot.

      (3) Involuntary oscillations are seen between flexion and extension.

      (4) Recorded as number of beats (e.g., three beats clonus)

5. Renal status

    a. Dipstick a clean-catch urine specimen for the presence of protein.

      (1) Mild preeclampsia: 2+ or 3+

      (2) Severe preeclampsia: 3+ or 4+

    b. A 24-hour urine collection can measure the quantity of protein.

      (1) Mild preeclampsia: proteinuria of 3 to 4 g

      (2) Severe: proteinuria of ≥5 g

    c. Alkaline, concentrated, or dilute urine can yield a false reading.

      (1) Normal specific gravity is 1.030, with a pH <8.

    d. Urine contaminated with bacteria, blood, and amniotic fluid can yield a false-positive for proteinuria.

    e. Measure intake and output.

      (1) Oliguria is less than 30 mL/hr or 120 mL for 4 hours

6. Pulmonary status

    a. Count respiratory rate, and auscultate lungs for wheezing and crackles.

    b. Observe skin color, mucous membranes, and oxygenation with a pulse oximeter.

    c. At risk for pulmonary edema (especially when oliguria develops)

    d. Signs of pulmonary edema:

      (1) Dyspnea

      (2) Tightness of the chest

      (3) Shallow respirations

      (4) Productive or nonproductive cough

7. Cardiovascular status

    a. Check capillary refill time (<3 seconds is normal).

    b. Assess temperature of extremities and peripheral pulses.

8. Maternal subjective signs of severe preeclampsia
   a. Severe headaches or pressure in the head (usually frontal)
   b. Scotomata (blurred spots), photophobia, or double vision
   c. Nausea and vomiting (especially if new)
   d. Epigastric pain (heartburn) or right upper quadrant pain
   e. Edema of the face or abdomen or pitting edema
9. Fetal status
   a. Measure fundal height in centimeters from symphysis pubis to top of fundus.
      (1) Between 20 and 32 weeks, the fundal height should approximate the gestational age.
   b. Assess fetal heart rate with Doppler or electronic fetal monitor.
      (1) Normal baseline rate of 110 to 160 bpm
      (2) Note presence of accelerations and absence of decelerations.
   c. Fetal movement counting
   d. Nonstress testing (NST)
   e. Biophysical profile (BPP)
   f. Serial ultrasound evaluation
      (1) Amniotic fluid index (AFI)
      (2) Fetal growth
   g. Amniocentesis to assess pulmonary maturity (L/S ratio of 2:1)
10. Uteroplacental perfusion
    a. Doppler flow studies
    b. Assess for signs of placental abruption.
       (1) Uterine tenderness
       (2) Hypersystole
       (3) Sustained abdominal pain
       (4) Dark red vaginal bleeding
       (5) Increasing fundal height
11. Laboratory tests (Table 19-1)
    a. Complete blood count (CBC) with platelet count
    b. Clotting studies (bleeding time, prothrombin time (PT), partial thromboplastin time (PTT), and fibrinogen)
    c. Liver enzymes (lactate dehydrogenase [LDH], AST, ALT)
    d. Chemistry panel (BUN, creatinine, creatinine clearance, uric acid)

INTERVENTIONS

A. **Mild preeclampsia**
   1. Goals of management (Barton & Sibai, 2008; Dix, 2007; Gilbert, 2007; Sibai, 2007)
      a. Identify women at risk for preeclampsia.
      b. Reassess at each prenatal visit:
         (1) BP, weight gain, presence and location of edema
         (2) Urine dipstick for protein
         (3) Fetal status (heart rate, fundal height, fetal kick counts)
      c. Allow time for the fetus to mature.
   2. The woman suspected of preeclampsia may be hospitalized for 1 to 2 days.
      a. Thorough evaluation of maternal and fetal status to determine severity
         (1) Physical assessment
         (2) Signs of severe preeclampsia (headaches, blurred vision, epigastric pain)
         (3) Laboratory tests and 24-hour urine for protein.
         (4) Fetal assessment (NST, ultrasound, biophysical profile)
         (5) Signs of placental abruption
   3. Mild preeclampsia: plan of care
      a. Multidisciplinary plan developed with the woman and her family.
      b. Greater than 36 weeks' gestation:
         (1) Cervical ripening as indicated and induction of labor
      c. Less than 36 weeks' gestation:
         (1) Expectant management with close maternal and fetal surveillance

■ TABLE 19-1
■ ■ **Laboratory Tests Affected by Preeclampsia and HELLP Syndrome**

	Pregnancy	**Preeclampsia**
Hemoglobin	10-12 g/dL	Decreased in HELLP
Hematocrit	32%-40%	Increased Decreased in HELLP
Platelets	150,000-400,000/mm^3	Decreased
Fibrinogen	300-600 mg/dL	Decreased
Fibrin split products	Absent or minimal	Increased
PT	10-14 sec	Unchanged
PTT	20-31 sec	Unchanged
Bleeding time	1-3 min (Duke)	Unchanged
	2-4 min (Ivy)	Decreased
	2-8 min (Template)	Increased
Hemolysis Peripheral smear	N/A	HELLP Schistocytes or burr cells present
Factors VII, VIII, IX, X	Increased	Increased
Factors XI, XIII	Decreased	Decreased
Renal		
Creatinine	0.4-1 mg/dL	Increased
BUN	5-10 g/dL	Increased
Uric acid	<6 mg/dL	Increased in HELLP
Creatinine clearance	130-180 mL/min	Decreased in HELLP
Uric acid clearance	10% of creatinine clearance	
Hepatic		
Alkaline phosphatase	60-480 IU/mL	Increased in HELLP
Albumin	2.8-3.7 g/dL	Decreased
Bilirubin	Slight elevation from 0.2-0.9 mg/dL	Increased in HELLP
AST (SGOT)	5-40 IU	Increased in HELLP
ALT (SGPT)	3-21 IU	Increased in HELLP
LDH	90-200 IU	Increased in HELLP

ALT, Alanine transaminase; *AST,* aspartate transaminase; *BUN,* blood, urea, and nitrogen; *HELLP,* hemolysis, elevated liver enzymes, and low platelets; *IU,* international units; *LDH,* lactate dehydrogenase; *N/A,* not applicable; *PT,* prothrombin time; *PTT,* partial thromboplastin time; *SGOT,* serum glutamic-oxaloacetic transaminase; *SGPT,* serum glutamic-pyruvate transaminase.

4. Home health care
    a. Criteria
        (1) In stable condition, without signs of severe preeclampsia.
        (2) Reassuring fetal status
    b. Daily maternal self-assessment
        (1) Weight, BP, and first-voided urine to dipstick for protein
        (2) Fetal movement counting
        (3) Signs of severe preeclampsia
        (4) Signs of labor and placental abruption
    c. A home health nurse calls daily and visits twice a week.
    d. Weekly prenatal visits and laboratory tests as ordered
5. Activity restriction
    a. Modified bedrest in the lateral position for the duration of the pregnancy
        (1) Resting on the left side enhances venous return.

    (2) Leads to increased renal and uterine blood flow, diuresis, and decreased BP
  b. Maternal risks associated with bedrest
    (1) Muscle atrophy and weight loss
    (2) Cardiovascular deconditioning and thrombophlebitis
    (3) Prolonged postpartum recovery
 6. A high-risk pregnancy can be very stressful for a woman and her family.
  a. Concerns
    (1) Need for long-term bedrest, activity restrictions, and boredom
    (2) Separation from family when hospitalized
    (3) Inability to work and loss of financial support
    (4) Ability to manage household, family activities, and childcare
  b. Provide emotional support and encouragement
  c. Refer to web (www. sidelines.org) and community-based support groups.

B. Severe preeclampsia
 1. Goals of management (Gilbert, 2007; Sibai, 2007; Sibai & Barton, 2007)
  a. Ensure maternal safety.
  b. Assess degree of maternal and fetal risk.
    (1) Hospitalization: preferably in a tertiary care center
    (2) Through evaluation of maternal and fetal status (see Mild Preeclampsia)
  c. Formulate plan for delivery based on risk.
  d. Prevent eclampsia and other serious complications.
 2. Severe preeclampsia: plan of care
  a. Greater than 34 weeks' gestation:
    (1) Induction of labor or cesarean section if indicated
  b. Less than 34 weeks' gestation:
    (1) Pharmacologic therapy to prevent seizures and control BP
    (2) Continuous maternal and fetal surveillance for indicators of worsening condition
    (3) Evaluation of diagnostic tests demonstrating organ dysfunction
 3. Indicators for immediate delivery
  a. Signs of fetal distress or deterioration
  b. Uncontrolled blood pressure
  c. Thrombocytopenia, or elevated liver enzymes with epigastric pain and tenderness
  d. HELLP syndrome
  e. Placental abruption
  f. Oliguria and/or pulmonary edema
  g. Eclampsia

C. Pharmacologic therapy (Table 19-2)
 1. Anticonvulsive therapy (Gilbert, 2007; Sibai, 2007)
  a. Magnesium sulfate is the drug of choice in the prevention and treatment of seizures.
    (1) Administered intravenously as a secondary infusion (piggyback) by infusion pump
    (2) 40 g of magnesium sulfate/1000 mL intravenous (IV) fluid = 1 g/25 mL.
    (3) Intramuscular (IM) route is not recommended. IM dose: 5 g, every 4 hours using Z-track technique
    (4) Antidote: calcium gluconate 5 to 10 mEq IV push over 1 to 2 minutes (only as ordered)
  b. Phenytoin can be used if magnesium sulfate is contraindicated.
 2. Antihypertensive therapy
  a. Initiated when systolic blood pressure >160 mm Hg and diastolic pressure >110 mm Hg
  b. Risks associated with blood pressure >160/110 mm Hg
    (1) Renal, hepatic, cardiocerebrovascular (left ventricular failure, cerebral hemorrhage)
  c. Most commonly used drugs are hydralazine and labetalol, then nifedipine (procardia).
 3. Corticosteroid therapy
  a. Betamethasone enhances fetal lung maturity between 24 and 34 weeks' gestation.
    (1) Dose: 12.5 mg IM, repeat in 24 hours
    (2) Benefits are seen after 24 hours of administration and last for 7 days.

D. Intensive hemodynamic monitoring (Gilbert, 2007)
 1. Hemodynamic monitoring is not a routine standard of practice.
 2. Only indicated in the presence of pulmonary edema, or oliguria unresponsive to fluid challenge or severe hypertension unresponsive to medications

■ TABLE 19-2

■■ **Drugs Used for Hypertensive Disorders in Pregnancy**

Medication/Action	Dosage/Route	Potential Side Effects	Nursing Interventions
MAGNESIUM SULFATE: SEIZURE PROPHYLAXIS			

Decreases acetylcholine released by nerve impulse; thereby depresses CNS and provides anticonvulsant effect
Acts peripherally as a vasodilator with transient decrease in BP
Use with caution when renal function is impaired
Contraindicated with myocardial damage, heart block, or myasthenia gravis
	IV loading dose 4-6 g over 15-30 minutes, followed by maintenance infusion of 2 g/hr	Headache
		Flushing
		Diaphoresis
		Lethargy
		Nausea
		Blurred vision
			Monitor for signs and symptoms of magnesium toxicity:
			  Respirations <16
			  Oxygen saturation <95%
			  Slurred speech
			  Chest pain
			Monitor for fetal decreased variability

	Serum Magnesium Levels	**(mEq/L)**	
	Normal	1.5-2	
	Therapeutic	4-7	
	ECG changes	5-10	
	Loss of reflexes	8-12	
	Respiratory distress	15	
	Cardiac arrest	25	
HYDRALAZINE HYDROCHLORIDE (APRESOLINE): ANTIHYPERTENSIVE AGENT			
Reduces BP by relaxing smooth muscle Resultant vasodilation reduces peripheral vascular resistance; increases cerebral and renal blood flow Decreases uteroplacental blood flow May be contraindicated with cardiac disease because of side effects of tachycardia, increased cardiac output, and oxygen consumption	For acute dosing: 5-10 mg IV push over 1-2 min; can repeat every 20 min for a maximum of 30 mg	Tachycardia Dizziness Headache Palpitations	Check BP every minute for 5 min, then every 5 min for 30 min Goal is to maintain diastolic BP between 90 and 100 mm Hg Hypotension might decrease uteroplacental perfusion Monitor fetal heart rate continuously Assess intake and output Use with caution if tachycardia is present

(Continued)

■ TABLE 19-2
▨▨ **Drugs Used for Hypertensive Disorders in Pregnancy—cont'd**

Medication/Action	Dosage/Route	Potential Side Effects	Nursing Interventions
LABETALOL HYDROCHLORIDE (NORMODYNE): ANTIHYPERTENSIVE Alpha- and beta-blocker, decreased peripheral resistance without significant change in cardiac output or causing tachycardia Contraindicated with asthma and congestive heart failure	IV bolus doses: initial dose 20 mg; if needed can give 40 mg 10 min later, then 80 mg 10 min after that to a maximum of 300 mg	Orthostatic hypotension Dizziness Nausea/vomiting Headaches Sweating Bronchospasm Dyspnea	Check BP every minute for 5 min, then every 5 min for 30 min Less excessive hypotension, tachycardia, and rebound hypertension than hydralazine Monitor for fetal bradycardia and neonatal respiratory depression
NIFEDIPINE (PROCARDIA): ANTIHYPERTENSIVE Calcium channel blocker dilates arterioles and decreases systemic vascular resistance by relaxing arterial smooth muscle May potentiate CNS effects of magnesium sulfate	10 mg orally and repeat in 30 min if needed	Headache Flushing	See hydralazine Use caution if the woman is also receiving magnesium sulfate

3. A pulmonary artery (Swan-Ganz) catheter may be placed to evaluate central vein and pulmonary artery pressures.

E. **Care of women with preeclampsia receiving magnesium sulfate** (Dix, 2007; Gilbert 2007; Simpson & Creehan, 2008)
   1. General guidelines: frequency of vital signs and assessments as ordered and per institutional policy
   2. Baseline assessment prior to staring infusion
      a. Vital signs, oxygen saturation with a pulse oximeter, level of consciousness (LOC)
      b. Deep tendon reflexes, clonus, edema, proteinuria
      c. Signs of severe preeclampsia
      d. Assessment of fetal and uterine status
   3. Insert a Foley catheter with urine meter for accurate measurement of output.
      a. Magnesium sulfate is excreted by the kidneys.
      b. Toxicity can develop quickly with impaired renal function.
   4. Discuss the rationale and side effects with the woman and her family.
      a. Initially she may feel flushed, hot, and sedated.
      b. Provide emotional support to help allay anxiety.
   5. Frequency of nursing assessments after infusion started
      a. Every 15 minutes: BP during loading dose (the nurse should stay at the bedside during the bolus dose), every 30 minutes on maintenance dose
      b. Every 30 minutes: oxygen saturation
      c. Every hour: respiratory rate, pulse, LOC, DTRs, intake and output (I&O)
      d. Every 4 hours: temperature if membranes are intact, every 2 hours if ruptured
      e. Every 8 hours: signs of worsening condition, degree of edema
      f. Continuous electronic fetal monitoring
   6. Maintain fluid balance to reduce the risk of pulmonary edema.
      a. Infuse IV fluids only as ordered
      b. Total IV and oral fluids should not exceed 125 mL/hr.
   7. Evaluate laboratory studies and magnesium levels.
   8. Monitor for signs of magnesium toxicity.
   9. Neonatal response to magnesium sulfate
      a. Magnesium crosses the placenta.
      b. The newborn infant may have depressed respirations and hyporeflexia.
      c. Pediatric team should attend the birth in event of resuscitation.
   10. Initiate seizure precautions.
      a. Bedrest in side-lying position
      b. Maintain a quiet, darkened environment.
      c. Place emergency supplies at bedside.
      d. Test oxygen and suction equipment.
      e. Keep side rails up.

F. **Eclampsia** (Dix, 2007; Gilbert, 2007)
   1. 70% of seizures occur during pregnancy and labor.
   2. Usual warning signs of impending eclampsia
      a. Severe persistent headaches
      b. Epigastric pain
      c. Hyperreflexia with clonus
      d. Restlessness
   3. Seizures can also develop without any warning signs.
   4. Convulsive activity
      a. Begins with facial twitching
      b. Generalized muscle rigidity
      c. Tonic-clonic convulsions
      d. Respirations cease, resulting in hypoxia.
      e. Hypotension and coma ensue.
      f. Disorientation and amnesia follow.
      g. May become incontinent of urine and stool
   5. Nursing care during a convulsion
      a. Remain with the woman and call for help.
      b. Note time of onset and duration of seizure.

      c. Lower the head of the bed and turn her head to the side.

      d. Do not try to insert a tongue blade.

  6. Nursing care after a convulsion

      a. First stabilize the woman.

        (1) Assess for airway, breathing, and pulse.

        (2) Suction secretions in mouth to clear airway.

        (3) Insert an oral airway.

        (4) Place in the side-lying position.

        (5) Administer oxygen at 10 L/min.

        (6) Administer magnesium sulfate IV as ordered.

        (7) Pad side rails.

      b. Assess fetal and labor status.

        (1) The membranes may rupture and birth may be imminent.

        (2) Assess for signs of placental abruption.

  7. After stabilization of mother and fetus, prepare for delivery.

G. Chronic hypertension (Cunningham et al, 2005; Gilbert, 2007; Sibai, 2007)

  1. Chronic hypertension affects 4% to 5% of pregnant women.

      a. 90% have primary (essential) hypertension.

      b. 10% have secondary hypertension related to a medical condition.

  2. Preconception counseling

      a. Evaluate cause, severity, and any target organ damage (kidneys, heart, and eyes).

      b. Lifestyle modifications

        (1) Smoking and alcohol cessation

        (2) Aerobic exercise until pregnant

        (3) Weight loss

        (4) Dietary modifications: maximum of 2.4 g of sodium per day

  3. Classified as mild or severe

      a. Prehypertension: systolic 120-139 or diastolic 80-90

      b. Stage 1: hypertension—systolic 140-150 or diastolic 90-99

      c. Stage 2: hypertension—systolic greater than 150 or diastolic greater than 100

  4. Complications associated with chronic hypertension in pregnancy

      a. Placental abruption

      b. Superimposed preeclampsia (21%)

      c. Fetal growth restriction and small-for-gestational-age infants

      d. Increased perinatal mortality (three- to fourfold)

      e. Renal failure

      f. DIC

  5. Chronic hypertension in pregnancy plan of care

      a. Classified as either high or low risk for pregnancy complications

      b. Frequent assessments of maternal and fetal well-being

      c. Antihypertensive medication

        (1) Methyldopa (Aldomet) is the drug of choice.

        (2) Alternative drugs: beta-blockers (labetalol) or calcium channel blockers (nifedipine)

  6. Timing of the birth is dependent on the maternal and fetal status.

  7. Increased risks during postpartum period

      a. Pulmonary edema

      b. Heart failure

      c. Encephalopathy

H. Postpartum and women's health care (Barton & Sibai, 2008; Dix, 2007; Gilbert, 2007)

  1. 30% of cases of eclampsia and HELLP syndrome occur after delivery.

  2. Magnesium sulfate is continued postpartum as ordered and per institutional policy.

      a. Signs of resolution include diuresis and decreased edema.

      b. Increased risk of uterine atony and heavy vaginal bleeding secondary to relaxation of smooth muscle side effect; frequently assess uterine tone and lochia flow.

  3. Facilitate family bonding of infant born prematurely.

      a. Provide the family with photographs of infant.

      b. Keep the family informed of the infant's status.

   c. Encourage the father to visit the neonatal intensive care unit (NICU).
   d. When the mother's condition has stabilized, accompany her to the NICU.
4. Discharge teaching (Simpson & James, 2005)
   a. Provide emotional support and encouragement.
   b. Assess coping mechanisms and initiate appropriate referrals.
   c. Birth of a premature infant can be very stressful for the woman and her family.
   d. Parents often feel emotionally drained by the fluctuations in the infant's status.
   e. Emotional stress can decrease the ability to process information.
   f. Incorporate family members during discharge teaching.
   g. Supplement teaching with written information.
5. Increased risk of adverse outcomes in subsequent pregnancy (Barton & Sibai, 2008; Duckitt & Harrington, 2005)
   a. Preterm delivery
   b. Fetal growth restriction
   c. Placental abruption
   d. Fetal death
6. Sevenfold increase of developing hypertensive disorders in subsequent pregnancy
   a. Increased maternal surveillance and frequency of prenatal visits.
   b. Closely monitor for signs of severe hypertension and preeclampsia.
   c. Serial ultrasound evaluation for fetal growth and amniotic fluid volume
   d. Home blood pressure monitoring
7. Increased risk for cardiovascular disease later in life (Gilbert, 2007; von Dadelszen, Menzies, & Magee, 2005)
   a. Women with early-onset and/or severe preeclampsia are at highest risk.
   b. Annual lipid profiles and urine tests for albumin
   c. Education regarding lifestyle modifications to reduce risk
8. Need for improved prenatal screening, preventive, and treatment strategies (Wagner, Barac, & Garovic, 2007)
   a. Reduce the incidence and severity of hypertensive disorders in pregnancy.
   b. Improve the health of women long term.

HEALTH EDUCATION

Teaching for Self-Care (Dix, 2007; Gilbert, 2007)

A. **Mild preeclampsia: instructions for home care**
   1. Daily assessments
      a. After you wake up in the morning, urinate in the specimen pan and dipstick test your urine for protein.
      b. Weigh yourself using the same scale.
      c. Take your blood pressure (using the same arm) every 4 to 6 hours during the day.
         (1) Sit down and support your arm on a table.
         (2) If your blood pressure is elevated, rest for 5 to 10 minutes and take it again.
      d. Twice a day assess fetal activity level.
         (1) After eating a meal, lie on your side for 2 hours
         (2) Count the number of kicks and movements that you feel, until 10 movements are counted.
      e. Fill out a daily log of your assessments and take it with you to your next prenatal visit.
      f. Call your health care provider immediately for any of the following:
         (1) Increase in blood pressure
         (2) Proteinuria 2+
         (3) Weight gain greater than 2 pounds/day or 5 pounds/week
         (4) Fewer than four fetal movements in 1 hour
         (5) Severe headache
         (6) Blurred vision or seeing spots
         (7) Pain in the abdomen or on the right side
         (8) Signs of labor or leakage of amniotic fluid
         (9) Vaginal bleeding

     g. You can expect your home health nurse to call you daily.
  2. One or two times a week
     a. It is very important to keep your scheduled prenatal appointments.
     b. You can expect your home health nurse to visit you.
B. Nutrition and health habits
  1. Eat a healthy, nutritious, well-balanced diet with plenty of protein and dairy products.
  2. Eat foods high in fiber or roughage (bran, raw fruits, and vegetables).
  3. Avoid salty foods (luncheon meats, pretzels, potato chips, pickles).
  4. Drink six to eight glasses of water per day.
  5. Limit caffeine intake (coffee, tea, soda, or cocoa).
  6. Avoid alcohol and tobacco.
C. Coping with bedrest
  1. Limit your activity and try to sleep for 12 hours at night.
  2. Rest in the side-lying position.
     a. Allows more blood to flow to your uterus
     b. Helps decrease your blood pressure and swelling
  3. Drink 8 glasses of water a day.
  4. If you become constipated, your doctor may order a stool softener.
  5. To help reduce boredom, place a box or table within reach to store magazines, books, puzzles, and crafts.
  6. Twice a day perform exercises to improve your muscle tone and circulation.
     a. Circle your hands and feet.
     b. Gently tense and relax your arm and leg muscles.
  7. Involve your family and friends to help you with care of the household and children.
  8. To help cope with stress
     a. Listen to soothing music.
     b. Relax your body, one muscle at a time.
     c. Imagine some pleasant scene, word, or image.

CASE STUDIES AND STUDY QUESTIONS

Ms. M. is a 22-year-old, gravida 1, para 0 (G1, P0) woman at 30 weeks' gestation. During a routine prenatal visit her BP is 146/94 mm Hg, which at her last prenatal visit had been 130/88. Her urine dipstick reveals 2+ protein. She has dependent edema, and denies headache, blurred vision, or epigastric pain. Ms. M. is admitted to the hospital for 2 days for a thorough assessment of maternal-fetal status. All of her labs are within normal limits (WNL), except for proteinuria. Her plan of care includes expectant management at home to allow time for the fetus to mature.

1. Her signs and symptoms are associated with which type of hypertensive disorder?
   a. Severe preeclampsia
   b. Mild preeclampsia
   c. HELLP syndrome
   d. Gestational hypertension
2. Which is *not* a risk factor for developing preeclampsia?
   a. Age extremes
   b. First pregnancy
   c. Stressful job
   d. Periodontal disease

3. Which physiologic alteration occurs during preeclampsia?
   a. Increased serum albumin and plasma colloid osmotic pressure
   b. Decreased peripheral vascular resistance
   c. Reduced plasma volume and increased hematocrit
   d. Increased platelet production
4. Which recommendation for activity levels at home is correct?
   a. Sleep 8 hours each night.
   b. No activity restrictions
   c. Complete bedrest
   d. Modified bedrest in the side-lying position
5. Which recommendation for maternal self-assessments at home is correct?
   a. Check weight and BP daily.
   b. Call the office when contractions are 2 minutes apart.
   c. Call the office for proteinuria of 1+.
   d. Assess fetal activity level before eating a meal.

Two weeks later Ms. M. is admitted to Labor and Delivery. Her BP is 154/96 and her weight gain in the last 2 weeks has been 10 pounds

(5 pounds/week). Ms. M. complains about a severe headache and blurred vision. She has 2+ edema, and 3+ protein in her urine.

6. Her signs and symptoms are associated with which type of hypertensive disorder?
   a. Mild preeclampsia
   b. Severe preeclampsia
   c. Chronic hypertension
   d. Gestational hypertension

Precautions are taken to prevent seizures and she is given a 4-g loading dose of magnesium sulfate followed by a 2-g/hr maintenance dose. Orders are written for an indwelling catheter with a urine meter, BP checks every 15 minutes during loading dose, then every 30 minutes with oxygen saturation, hourly respiratory rate, pulse, LOC, DTRs, I&O, and continuous fetal monitoring. Laboratory work includes a complete blood count (CBC), liver enzymes, and renal function studies.

7. A subjective sign of severe preeclampsia is:
   a. Dependent edema
   b. Fatigue
   c. Headache
   d. Cough
8. A common side effect of magnesium sulfate is:
   a. Decreased fetal heart rate (FHR) baseline rate
   b. Decreased uteroplacental blood flow
   c. Smooth muscle relaxation
   d. Sympathetic nervous system stimulation
9. A sign of magnesium toxicity is:
   a. Slurred speech
   b. Respirations are 20 per minute.
   c. Reflexes are 2+.
   d. Feeling flushed or hot
10. What is *not* recommended when a woman is placed on seizure precautions?
    a. Bedrest in side-lying position
    b. Maintain a quiet, darkened environment.
    c. Encourage all family members to visit.
    d. Keep side rails up.
11. What is *not* an indicator for immediate delivery?
    a. Signs of fetal distress or deterioration
    b. Thrombocytopenia, or elevated liver enzymes with epigastric pain and tenderness
    c. HELLP syndrome
    d. Urine output of 40 mL/hr

Ms. T., a 29-year-old, G2, P1 woman with chronic hypertension and superimposed preeclampsia, at 34 weeks' gestation, is admitted to Labor and Delivery. Her baseline BP had been 130/90 mm Hg; 1 week ago, her BP was 160/105 and today it is 170/110 mm Hg. She gained 5 pounds in 1 week, has 3+ pitting edema, and 2+ protein in her urine. Her usual hypertension medications are methyldopa (Aldomet) and hydralazine. Her laboratory studies are WNL except for proteinuria. During the admission process Ms. T. has a grand mal seizure.

12. What is *not* an appropriate nursing activity during a seizure?
    a. Remain with the woman and call for help.
    b. Note time of onset and duration of seizure.
    c. Lower the head of the bed and turn her head to the side.
    d. Insert a tongue blade.
13. What is the priority nursing intervention *immediately* after a convulsion?
    a. Assess for airway, breathing, and pulse.
    b. Administer oxygen at 10 L/min.
    c. Cover her with a blanket.
    d. Pad the side rails.
14. A potential complication from a seizure is:
    a. Pulmonary edema
    b. Renal damage
    c. Pulmonary embolism
    d. Placental abruption

Ms. D. is a 32-year-old G1, P0 woman at 33 weeks' gestation. She had an elevated BP of 140/90 mm Hg for 2 weeks, with proteinuria and generalized edema, and has stayed at home on bedrest. She was hospitalized with severe epigastric pain. Laboratory values demonstrated an abnormal peripheral smear, elevated liver enzymes (AST >70 IU/L and LDH >600 IU/L), and a platelet count <100,000/mm^3.

15. The acronym of HELLP syndrome stands for:
    a. Hemolysis, eclampsia, and low platelets
    b. Hemolysis, elevated liver enzymes, and low platelets
    c. Hyperbilirubinemia, elevated liver enzymes, and low platelets
    d. Hyperbilirubinemia, eclampsia, and low platelets
16. When do the signs of HELLP syndrome usually develop?
    a. During the first trimester
    b. During the second trimester
    c. During the third trimester
    d. 72 hours after birth
17. Which are *not* signs of HELLP syndrome?
    a. Influenza-like symptoms and malaise
    b. Epigastric or right upper quadrant pain
    c. Bruising
    d. Visual disturbances

ANSWERS TO STUDY QUESTIONS

1. b	7. c	13. a
2. c	8. c	14. d
3. c	9. a	15. b
4. d	10. c	16. c
5. a	11. d	17. d
6. b	12. d	

REFERENCES

Askie, L. M., Duley, L., Henderson-Smart, D. J., & Stewart, L. A. (2007). Anti-platelet agents for prevention of preeclampsia: A meta-analysis of individual patient data. *Lancet, 369,* 1791–1798.

Barton, J. R., & Sibai, B. M. (2008). Prediction and prevention of recurrent preeclampsia. *Obstetrics and Gynecology, 112*(2 Pt 1), 359–372.

Cockey, C. (2005). Predicting preeclampsia. *AWHONN Lifelines, 9*(1), 25–26.

Cunningham, F., Leveno, K., Bloom, S., Hauth, J., Gilstrap, L., & Wenstrom, K. (2005). *Williams obstetrics* (22nd ed.). New York: McGraw-Hill.

Dix, D. N. (2007). Hypertensive disorders in pregnancy. In D. Lowdermilk, & S. Perry (Eds.), *Maternity & women's health care* (9th ed., pp. 784–803). St. Louis: Mosby.

Duckitt, R., & Harrington, D. (2005). Risk factors for preeclampsia at antenatal booking: Systematic review of controlled studies. *British Medical Journal, 33*(7491), 565.

Gilbert, E. S. (2007). *Manual of high risk pregnancy & delivery* (4th ed.). St. Louis: Mosby.

Grujić , I., & Milasinović , L. (2006). Hypertension, preeclampsia and eclampsia-monitoring and outcome of pregnancy. *Medicinski Pregle, 59*(11–12), 556–559.

Hellwig, J. P. (2007). Predicting preeclampsia. *AWHONN Lifelines, 10*(6), 456.

Martin, J., Hamilton, B., Sutton, P., Ventura, S., Menacker, F., & Munson, M. (2005). Births: Final data for 2003. *National Vital Statistics Reports, 54*(2), 1–116.

Peters, R. M. (2008). High blood pressure in pregnancy. *Nursing for Women's Health, 12*(5), 412–421.

Ravin, C. R. (2008). Vitamin D and health. What does the latest research show? *Nursing for Women's Health, 12*(1), 70–74.

Sibai, B. M. (2007). Hypertension. In S. Gabbe, J. Niebyl, & J. Simpson (Eds.), *Obstetrics: Normal and problem pregnancies* (5th ed., pp. 863–912). Philadelphia: Churchill Livingstone.

Sibai, B. M., & Barton, J. R. (2007). Expectant management of severe preeclampsia remote from term: Patient selection, treatment, and delivery indications. *American Journal of Obstetrics and Gynecology, 196*(6), 514.e1–514.e9.

Simpson, K., & Creehan, P. (2008). *AWHONN Perinatal Nursing* (3rd ed.). Philadelphia: Lippincott Williams & Williams.

Simpson, K., & James, D. (2005). *Postpartum care.* White Plains, NY: March of Dimes.

von Dadelszen, P., Menzies, J., & Magee, L. A. (2005). The complications of hypertension in pregnancy. *Minerva Medica, 96*(4), 287–302.

Wagner, S. J., Barac, S., & Garovic, V. D. (2007). Hypertensive pregnancy disorders: Current concepts. *Journal of Clinical Hypertension, 9*(7), 560–566.

20 Maternal Infections

Barbara A. Moran

OBJECTIVES

1. Identify causative pathogens and describe primary signs and symptoms of perinatal infections.
2. Identify risk groups for acquired immunodeficiency syndrome (AIDS) and other sexually transmitted infections (STIs).
3. Correlate history and physical findings with early indicators of maternal infection.
4. Recognize clinical signs and symptoms of perinatal infections.
5. Discuss potential fetal complications associated with maternal infections.
6. Formulate nursing interventions from information obtained in the history.
7. Define health-education strategies to prevent maternal infections.

INTRODUCTION

Maternal and perinatal infections are common complications of pregnancy. Some infections affect only the mother, such as urinary tract infections (UTIs) and trichomonas infections. Others such as rubella, cytomegalovirus (CMV), and parvovirus infections have little effect on the mother but cause significant fetal injury; and others such as gonorrhea culture (GC), syphilis, toxoplasmosis, rubella, group B streptococcus, pyelonephritis, chorioamnionitis, and human immunodeficiency virus (HIV) may cause serious problems for mother and infant (Duff, 2007). Fetal infections may be acquired transplacentally; organisms may also ascend into the birth canal or be acquired during the passage through the vagina at the time of birth.

Preconception counseling is imperative in preventing many infections such as rubella, rubeola and varicella. These vaccines should not be administered during pregnancy. The (CDC) recommends all pregnant women receive the influenza vaccine at any time during pregnancy because pregnant women often become more ill with influenza (www.cdc.gov/vaccines/vpd.html).

TORCH (Table 20-1)

INTRODUCTION

A. TORCH is an acronym for a group of five infectious diseases.
  1. Toxoplasmosis
  2. Other (hepatitis B)
  3. Rubella
  4. CMV
  5. Herpes simplex virus (HSV)
B. Each disease is teratogenic.
  1. Each crosses the placenta.
  2. Each may adversely affect the developing fetus.
  3. The effect of each varies, depending on developmental stage at time of exposure.

CLINICAL PRACTICE

A. Assessment
  1. History
    a. Influenza-like illness

Text continued on p. 454

■ TABLE 20-1
■ TABLE 20-1
■ **TORCH Diseases**

Infection	Agent	Mode of Transmission	Detection	Maternal Effects	Neonatal Effects	Incidence and Prevention
Toxoplasmosis	Single-celled protozoal parasite *Toxo-plasma gondii*	Transplacental Eating raw meat, touching hands or mouth after handling under-cooked meat containing *T. gondii* secreted in feces of infected cats *Cysts* are destroyed with heat	Serologic antibody testing IgM-specific antibody IgGA serocon-version from negative to positive Most accurate confirmation of active infec-tion is a rise in IgG titer in two appropriately spaced tests	Most infections in humans are asymptomatic However, may include fatigue, muscle pains, pneumonitis, myocarditis and lymphadenopathy	Severity varies with gesta-tional age Congenital infection can occur if a woman develops acute toxoplasmosis during pregnancy (most likely in the third trimester) Sequelae include low birth-weight, hepatosplenomegaly, icterus, anemia, neurologic disease, and chorioretinitis	Approximately 40%-50% of U.S. adults have antibodies Incidence of congenital toxoplasmosis infection in U.S. is 1 in 1000-8000 More than 60 million people in the U.S. carry the parasite Frequency of seroconversion during pregnancy is <5%, and approximately 3 in 1000 infants show evidence of congenital infection Cook meat to a safe temperature Peel or thoroughly wash fruits and vegetables ACOG does not recommend routine screening except for pregnant women with HIV infection
Hepatitis B	HBV incubation is 4 weeks to 6 months following exposure	Direct contact with the blood or body fluids of an infected person Sexual Perinatal Percutaneous Transplacental Blood, stool, amni-otic fluid,	HBsAg identified 7-14 days after exposure HBsAg present with HBsAg indicates nonin-fectious stage	Course of the disease is not altered during pregnancy Symptoms are seen in only 30%-50% of patients; these include low-grade fever, nausea, anorexia, jaundice,	Transmission to the neonate appears to occur as a result of exposure to infected blood and genital secretions during delivery Infants infected at birth have a 90% risk of becoming chronically infected with HBV (carrier) and 25% risk of developing significant	HBV causes 40%-45% of all U.S. cases of hepatitis. Incidence in pregnancy is 1-2 per 1000 Estimated that 1 to 1.25 million people in the U.S. are chronically infected with HBV Approximately 8000 acute HBV infections were

Disease	Mode of Transmission	Diagnosis	Signs and Symptoms	Effects on Fetus/Newborn	Comments
(Hepatitis B, continued)	and saliva transmission Shared razors, toothbrushes, towels, and other personal items		hepatomegaly, malaise, premature labor, and premature birth No specific treatment, but may include bedrest and a high-protein, low-fat diet	liver disease, yet if they receive prophylaxis at birth, 95% can be prevented Increased risk of transmission to infant if mother is HBcAg-positive (indicating acute infection) Stillbirth Clinical illness is relatively infrequent Most (90%-95%) of those infected are symptomatic and become chronic hepatitis B carriers	reported to CDC Acute infection occurs in 1-2 per 1000 pregnancies Minimize exposure of physical contact Heptavax-B vaccine ***Vaccine not contraindicated during pregnancy*** Screen all pregnant women

Rubella (German measles)
Rubella virus incubation is 12-19 days
	Nasopharyngeal secretions
	Transplacental
		Rubella-specific IgM antibodies
		Rubella antibody titer of 1:8 or more indicates immune status
			Erythematous maculopapular rash on face, neck, arms, and legs lasting 3 days
			Lymph node enlargement
			Slight fever, malaise, headache, and arthralgia
			History of exposure 3 weeks earlier
				Overall risk of congenital rubella syndrome is approximately 20% for primary maternal infection in the first trimester
				Approximately 50% of infants exposed to the virus within 4 weeks of conception will manifest signs of congenital infection
				When infection occurs in second 4-week period after conception, approximately 25% of fetuses will be infected; when infection develops in third month, approximately 10% of fetuses will be infected
				Spectrum anomalies:
				  Deafness (60%-75%)
				  Eye defects (10%-30%)
				  CNS anomalies (10%-25%)
				  Cardiac malformation (10%-20%)
					Last epidemic in 1965; since introduction of vaccine in late 1960s rubella is rare
					Absence of rubella antibody indicates susceptibility
					Estimated that 6%-25% of women are susceptible
					Occurs more commonly in springtime
					Vaccinate immediately postpartum and use contraception for a minimum of 3 months after vaccination
					Vaccine is contraindicated during pregnancy

(Continued)

■ TABLE 20-1
■ TORCH Diseases—cont'd

Infection	Agent	Mode of Transmission	Detection	Maternal Effects	Neonatal Effects	Incidence and Prevention
Cytomegalovirus (CMV)	DNA virus of the herpes-virus group	Transmitted horizontally by droplet infection and contact with saliva and urine, vertically from mother to fetus-infant, and as a sexually transmitted infection Intimate contact with infected secretions (breast milk, cervical mucus, semen, saliva, tears, and urine)	Serology of CMV specific IgM antibody	Most infections are asymptomatic, but approximately 15% of adults have a mononucleosis-like syndrome characterized by fever, pharyngitis, lymphadenopathy, and polyarthritis	Infection is most likely to occur with primary maternal infection Timing of infection during pregnancy is major determinant of outcome (first and second trimester being more severely affected) Low birthweight, IUGR, microcephaly CNS abnormalities, mental and motor retardation, intracranial calcification, sensorineural deafness, blindness with chorioretinitis, mental retardation, hepatosplenomegaly, and jaundice	As with other viruses, maternal immunity to CMV does not prevent recurrence Found in 0.5%-2% of all neonates Incidence of primary CMV infections in pregnant women in the U.S. varies from 1%-3% Rigorous personal hygiene throughout pregnancy
Herpes simplex virus (HSV)	Herpesvirus type 1 (more common with oral lesions) and type 2 (more common in genital lesions) Incubation is 2-10 days	Ascending infection Intimate mucocutaneous exposure Transmission is more likely to occur from men to women Passage through an infected birth canal	Tissue culture (swab specimen from vesicles) and immunofluorescent staining of the cell can differentiate HSV-1 from HSV-2 Swelling, redness, and painful lesions	Painful genital vesicle lesions Vesicles on cervix, vagina or external genital area Primary infection is commonly associated with fever, malaise, and myalgia; numbness, tingling, burning, itching, and pain	Rare transplacental transmission has resulted in miscarriage Estimated mortality of 50% if neonatal exposure is with active primary infection Neurologic morbidity such as chorioretinitis, microcephaly, mental retardation, seizure, and apnea	Estimated 1 million Americans are newly infected with genital HSV annually Seroprevalence of HSV is approximately 25% Approximately 1%-2% of pregnancies 1 in 3000-20,000 live births for the development of neonatal herpes Prophylactic treatment with oral acyclovir, valacyclovir,

or famciclovir may be appropriate in women with frequent recurrent infections in pregnancy

If symptoms or lesions are present, cesarean delivery should be performed

Avoid genital contact when male partner has penile lesions

Use condoms

with lesions; lymphadenopathy; and urinary retention

ACOG, American College of Obstetricians and Gynecologists; *CDC*, Centers for Disease Control and Prevention; *CNS*, central nervous system; *DNA*, deoxyribonucleic acid; *IUGR*, intrauterine growth restriction; *HBsAg*, hepatitis B surface antigen; *HBV*, hepatitis B virus; *HIV*, human immunodeficiency virus; *Ig*, immunoglobulin.

Centers for Disease Control and Prevention. (2009). Cytomegalovirus. Available online at: www.cdc.gov/cmv/pregnancy.html.

Centers for Disease Control and Prevention. (2009). *FAQ's for health professionals.* Available online at: www.cdc.gov/hepatitis/HBV/HBVfaq.htm#oview.html.

Davies & Gibbs. 2008, p. 340.

www.cdc.gov/cmv/pregnancy.html.

www.cdc.gov/hepatitis/HBV/HBVfaq.htm#oview.html.

www.marchofdimes.com/professionals/14332_1201.asp.

www.marchofdimes.com/professionals/14332_1225.asp.

www.marchofdimes.com/professionals/14332_1226.asp.

www.marchofdimes.com/professionals/14332_1228.asp.

      b. Fever of unknown origin

      c. Exposure to sick children

      d. Rash

      e. Painful genital lesions

      f. Close contact with possibly infected cats (outside-dwelling cats)

      g. Chronic fatigue

      h. Blood or secretion exposure

      i. Raw meat ingestion

  2. Physical findings

      a. Lymphadenopathy: suboccipital, postauricular, cervical

      b. Rash: pink or red maculopapules

      c. Ulcerated, painful lesions on the cervix, vagina, and genital area

      d. Low-grade temperature

      e. Headache

      f. Malaise

      g. Anorexia

      h. Jaundice

      i. Hepatomegaly

      j. Arthralgias or arthritis

      k. Nausea and vomiting

      l. Clay-colored stool

  3. Psychosocial findings

      a. Anxiety

      b. Fear

      c. Apprehension

  4. Diagnostic tests and findings

      a. Complete blood count (CBC)

      b. TORCH screen

      c. Immunoglobulin G (IgG)–specific antibody (i.e., rubella-specific IgG to document prior infection)

      d. IgM-specific antibody (i.e., rubella-specific IgM to confirm recent infection; it becomes detectable approximately 1 week after onset of illness and persists for approximately 1 month).

      e. Culture lesions

      f. Hepatitis B surface antigen (HBsAg) is present in blood 30 to 50 days after exposure and 7 to 21 days before the onset of jaundice.

      g. Hepatitis B early antigen (HBeAg): the presence of early antigen denotes a high degree of infectivity.

      h. Enzyme-linked immunosorbent assay (ELISA)

      i. Liver function

         (1) Elevated bilirubin levels

         (2) Elevated transaminase enzyme levels

      j. Serial sonography (to detect intrauterine growth restriction [IUGR])

B. Interventions

  1. Encourage preconceptional counseling and advice on appropriate immunizations.

  2. During prenatal visits, instruct the patient on good handwashing and cleaning of all kitchen surfaces, especially after handling raw meat; avoid eating insufficiently cooked meat; avoid contact with cat feces in litter boxes during pregnancy, and avoid gardening in soil contaminated with cat feces

ACQUIRED IMMUNODEFICIENCY SYNDROME (Table 20-2)

INTRODUCTION

A. Major public health issue

  1. AIDS is caused by HIV, a virus passed from one person to another through blood and sexual contact. It was first recognized in 1981. The percentage of AIDS cases among female adults and adolescents (age >13 years) increased from 7% in 1985 to 27% in 2007

Text continued on p. 459

■ TABLE 20-2

■ ■ **Sexually Transmitted Infections**

Infection	Agent	Detection	Maternal Effects	Neonatal Effects	Treatment	Incidence
Acquired immunodeficiency syndrome (AIDS)	HIV retrovirus	Enzyme-linked immunosorbant assay (ELISA); highly sensitive and inexpensive If ELISA is positive, repeat; then a Western blot or immunofluorescent antibody assay	Acute phase of infection usually occurs 4-6 weeks following HIV exposure Studies have shown no effect of pregnancy on the progression of HIV disease Complications include preterm delivery, preterm PROM, IUGR, increased perinatal mortality and postpartum endometritis Fever, malaise, fatigue, anorexia, nausea, vomiting, diarrhea, weight loss, and generalized lymphadenopathy Opportunistic infections include *Pneumocystis jiroveci* pneumonia, *Mycobacterium avium* complex, pulmonary tuberculosis, toxoplasmosis, candidiasis, and CMV infection	Multiple factors associated with perinatal HIV transmission: low CD4 count, chorioamnionitis, preterm delivery, and illicit drug use Avoid instruments during birth, leave fetal membranes intact, avoid fetal scalp electrode, avoid episiotomy and assisted vaginal delivery 25%-30% chance of transmission from infected mother, unless mother is treated If HIV positive as newborn, repeat antibody testing at 6 months	All patients should be encouraged to screen on first prenatal visit Current treatment guidelines recommend administration of at least three antiretroviral drugs. Zidovudine (ZDV), & AZT should be administered IV during labor and given orally to the baby for at least 6 weeks after delivery. Antiretroviral prophylaxis has reduced perinatal transmission to <2% ***Check for latest guidelines from CDC***	First recognized in 1981 and appears to have originated in Africa Increasing incidence in women An estimated 16.4 million women worldwide are living with HIV For women, heterosexual contact accounted for 80% of new diagnosis
Human papillomavirus (condyloma acuminatum)	Human papillomavirus (HPV) Some strains cause warts, others highly associated with cervical cancer	Cervical cytologic testing Colposcopy used as adjunct in equivocal situation Single or multiple, irregular, painless	May enlarge during pregnancy If enlarged, may interfere with delivery; therefore, may need a cesarean section	Approximately 2%-5% of all births are at risk for neonatal HPV exposure Potential transmission of laryngeal papillomata	Small lesions: trichloroacetic acid (TCA) 80%-90%; cryotherapy; CO_2 laser therapy; electrocautery; podophyllin; or 5-fluorouracil (5-FU)	Most common sexually transmitted infection in the U.S. causing 5.5 million new cases each year Incidence in college-age women is nearly 50%

(Continued)

■ TABLE 20-2
■■ **Sexually Transmitted Infections—cont'd**

Infection	Agent	Detection	Maternal Effects	Neonatal Effects	Treatment	Incidence
	More than 200 HPV genotypes have been identified	papules in the genital or perianal area Transmitted sexually and/or vertically		Vaginal delivery is estimated to carry a 0.04% risk of laryngeal infection to the neonate	**(contraindicated in pregnancy)** Large lesions: surgical excisions In pregnancy, small lesions do not require treatment, but larger lesions may be treated with TCA or surgically removed by cryotherapy, laser, electrocautery or excision	Estimated 20 million Americans are currently infected with HPV Prevalence of increasing incidence noted in STD clinics and private offices Risk factors: number of sexual partners, age of first intercourse (<16 considered greater risk), number of sexual partners male partner has had, age of first male partner (older, greater risk) Peak occurrence between ages 15 and 35 Associated with other STIs
Chylamydia	Bacteria: *Chlamydia trachomatis*	Endocervical and rectal-vaginal culture	Approximately 75% of women are asymptomatic Mucopurulent cervicitis, bartholinitis, salpingitis, friable cervix, and postpartum endometritis Up to 40% of women with untreated chlamydia will develop PID; 20% will become	Up to 50% of infants exposed during delivery develop conjunctivitis 10% of exposed infants develop pneumonia	Azithromycin 1 g in a single dose or doxycycline 100 mg orally twice a day for 7 days Simultaneous treatment of partner Test of cure 2 weeks after therapy	An estimated 3-4 million cases occur annually in the U.S. An estimated 30% of pregnant women are infected Increase in adolescent and young adult population, multiple

Infection	Etiology/Incubation	Diagnosis	Clinical Manifestations	Fetal/Neonatal Effects	Treatment	Comments
			infertile; 18% will experience chronic pelvic pain and 9% will experience tubal pregnancy Occasional effects include PROM, preterm labor, IUGR, and chorioamnionitis		Erythromycin ophthalmic ointment for newborns	sex partners, and non barrier contraceptive methods May be associated with other STIs
Gonorrhea	Bacteria: *Neisseria gonorrhoeae*, gram-negative diplococcus Incubation: 10 days	Endocervical and rectal-vaginal culture	Asymptomatic to mildly symptomatic localized infection of urethra, endocervix, rectum, or any combination Acute PID May cause severe disseminated infection: arthritis, dermatitis, pericarditis, endocarditis, and meningitis Dysuria, urinary frequency, PPROM, chorioamnionitis, and endometritis	Purulent conjunctivitis Sepsis or meningitis	Ceftriaxone (125 mg IM) single dose or ciprofloxacin 500 mg orally in a single dose or ofloxacin 400 mg orally in a single dose Treat sex partners Treat infant with either silver nitrate or tetracycline ophthalmic preparation ***Check with CDC for latest guidelines***	One of the most common STIs—second only to chlamydia infection More than 1 million cases are reported in U.S. each year Primarily seen in women with multiple sex partners and history of other STIs
Syphilis	Bacteria: spirochete—*Treponema pallidum* Incubation: 10-90 days (average 21 days)	VDRL RPR Positive screening needs to be confirmed with FTA-ABS Will have positive tests within 4 weeks of initial infection Secondary syphilis—increased liver enzymes	Primary chancre–painless ulcerative lesion Secondary syphilis–fever and malaise, red macules on palms or soles of feet Generalized lymphadenopathy Early latent positive serology <1 year duration Late latent >1 year Cardiovascular syphilis and neurosyphilis Malodorous, frothy, discolored vaginal discharge 75% have symptoms, including pruritus, vaginal bleeding, dysuria, and dyspareunia	Transplacental transmission Effects vary on gestation Stillbirth IUGR Prematurity (caused by preterm labor) Frequency of vertical transmission varies with stage of maternal disease	Benzathine penicillin G 2.4 million units IM as a single dose Penicillin allergy: doxycycline 100 mg PO twice daily for 2 weeks. ***Check with CDC for latest guidelines***	Responsible for approximately 25% of cases of vaginitis Estimated 3 million cases per year More common in women with multiple sex partners Also nonvenerably acquired

(Continued)

■ TABLE 20-2
■■ **Sexually Transmitted Infections—cont'd**

Infection	Agent	Detection	Maternal Effects	Neonatal Effects	Treatment	Incidence
Trichomonas	Protozoan: *Trichomonas vaginalis*	"Wet prep" saline examination Pap smear Urinalysis	Malodorous, frothy, discolored vaginal discharge 75% have symptoms, including pruritus, vaginal bleeding, dysuria, and dyspareunia	Infant contact though infected vagina Usually asymptomatic or short lived	Metronidazole (Flagyl) for mother and partner (avoid during first trimester) Single dose of 2 g; 250 mg tid x 7 days; or 500 mg bid x 7 days Local therapy	Responsible for approximately 25% of cases of vaginitis Estimated 3 million cases per year More common in women with multiple sex partners Also nonvenereally acquired
Bacterial vaginosis	Polymicrobial massive overgrowth of anaerobic bacteria *Gardnerella vaginalis*, *Mobiluncus* species.	Thin, gray, homogeneous, malodorous vaginal discharge "wet prep" for clue cells–vaginal epithelial cell covered with bacteria pH >4.5; fishy odor	Associated with preterm labor, PROM, chorioamnionitis, endometritis and UTIs	No specific risks other than secondary to prematurity	Metronidazole (Flagyl) 250 mg tid x 7 days for mother and sex partner (avoid during first trimester) Clindamycin 300 mg tid x 7 days	Responsible for approximately 45% of cases of vaginitis

CDC, Centers for Disease Control and Prevention; *CMV,* cytomegalovirus; *FTA-ABS,* fluorescent treponemal antibody absorption; *HIV,* human immunodeficiency virus; *IM,* intramuscular; *IUGR,* intrauterine growth restriction; *PID,* pelvic inflammatory disease; *PPROM,* Preterm premature rupture of membranes; *PROM,* premature rupture of membranes; *RPR,* rapid plasma reagin; *STD,* sexually transmitted disease; *STI,* sexually transmitted infection; *UTI,* urinary tract infection; *VDRL,* Venereal Disease Research Laboratory

Davies & Gibbs, 2008. p. 340
Department of Health and Human Services, 2007, HIV/AIDS surveillance report
Department of Health and Human Services, 2007, Sexually transmitted disease surveillance
Duff, 2007
Eschenbach, 2008
Minkoff, 2008
Ramin & Landers, 2007
www.cdc.gov/hiv.html
www.cdc.gov/hiv/resources/factsheets/us/html
www.cdc.gov/hiv/topics/surveillance/incidence.html
www.cdc.gov/hiv/topics/surveillance/resources/qa/surv_rep.html
www.cdc.gov/std/stats07/trends.html
www.cdc.gov/STD/STDfact-STDs&pregnancy.html
www.marchofdimes.com/professionals/14332_1223.asp.
www.marchofdimes.com/professionals/14332_1226.asp.
www.nichd.nih.gov/health/topics/aids_hiv.cfm.

(Figure 20-1). The incidence of AIDS among female adults and adolescents rose steadily through 1993, when the AIDS surveillance case definition was expanded, and leveled off at approximately 13,000 AIDS cases each year from 1993 through 1996. In 1996, the incidence among women and adolescent girls began to decline, primarily because of the success of antiretroviral therapies. Cases have remained level since 2000 (www.cdc.gov/hiv/topics/surveillance/resources/slides/women/index.htm).

B. **HIV**
  1. Agent: retrovirus (ribonucleic acid [RNA] virus)
     a. A virus containing RNA that has the ability to produce deoxyribonucleic acid (DNA) in its cellular host
     b. HIV destroys blood cells CD4 T cells (helper cells) that are crucial to the normal function of the human immune system; loss of these cells in people with HIV is an extremely powerful predictor of the development of AIDS.
  2. Transmission
     a. By exposure to blood and blood products or byproducts
        (1) Transfusions: This mode of transmission has dramatically decreased since screening of donated blood for HIV started in 1985.
        (2) Needle sharing among addicts
        (3) Accidental inoculation in health care workers
     b. Perinatal exposure
        (1) Transplacental
        (2) Intrapartal
        (3) Breast milk
     c. Sexual contact factors that increase the rate of transmission include (Bernstein, 2007)
        (1) Lack of condoms
        (2) Sexual contact with an uncircumcised man
        (3) High number of sexual contacts
        (4) Presence of genital sores
        (5) Advanced disease
        (6) Presence of other sexually transmitted infections, particularly those that cause genital ulcers (herpes, syphilis, chancroid)

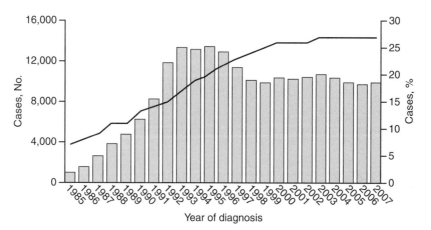

Year of diagnosis

Note: Data have been adjusted for reporting delays.

*Percentage of all cases that were diagnosed among females.

FIGURE 20-1 ■ Estimated numbers and percentages of AIDS cases among female adults and adolescents 1985-2007—United States and dependent areas (www.cdc.gov/hiv/topics/surveillance/resources/slides/women/index.htm).

   d. Factors associated with increased perinatal HIV transmission (Bernstein, 2007)
      (1) Mother with AIDS
      (2) Preterm delivery
      (3) Decreased maternal CD4 count
      (4) High maternal viral load
      (5) Chorioamnionitis
      (6) Blood exposure due to episiotomy, vaginal laceration, forceps delivery
   e. Highest concentrations of HIV have been isolated from blood, semen, and cerebrospinal fluid.
   f. HIV also is found in vaginal secretions, saliva, tears, breast milk, amniotic fluid, and urine; contact with saliva or tears has not been shown to result in infection.
   g. HIV is *not* transmitted through casual contact (e.g., water, food, environmental services).

C. Counseling and early diagnosis are recommended for the following:
  1. Persons who consider themselves at risk for infection
  2. Women of childbearing age who are at risk for infection
  3. Persons attending STI clinics and drug abuse clinics
  4. Women seeking family planning services
  5. Tuberculosis patients and selected patients who received transfusions of blood and blood components between 1978 and 1985
  6. The CDC operates a free telephone service that is available 24 hours a day, 7 days a week (800-342-2437); services for Spanish-speaking audiences and the deaf are also available.

D. Statistics
  1. In 2006 it was estimated that there were 56,300 new HIV infections (CDC, 2008).
  2. Rates of reported AIDS cases (per 100,000) among female adults and adolescents are shown in Figure 20-2. The highest rates were found in the District of Columbia, U.S. Virgin Islands, Maryland, New York, and Florida. Rates were lowest in states in the Midwest.

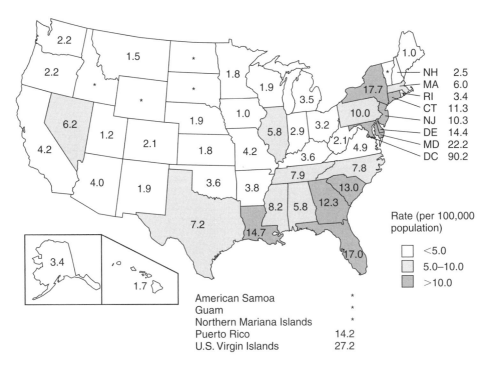

*Rates were not calculated for areas reporting fewer than 5 AIDS cases in females in 2007.

FIGURE 20-2 ■ AIDS rates for female adults and adolescents reported in 2007—United States and dependent areas (www.cdc.gov/hiv/topics/surveillance/resources/slides/women/index.htm).

3. Today women account for more than one quarter of all new HIV/AIDS diagnoses. Women of color are especially affected by HIV infection and AIDS. For female adults and adolescents, in 2007, the AIDS diagnosis rate (AIDS cases per 100,000) for African-American females (39.8) was 22 times as high as the rate for white females (1.8). The estimated number of AIDS cases diagnosed among females in 2007 was similar for Hispanic/Latino and white females; however, the rate for Hispanic/Latino females (8.9) was nearly 5 times as high as the rate for white females (Figure 20-3).

4. Among female adults and adolescents diagnosed with HIV/AIDS in 2007, 83% of the 10,977 HIV/AIDS cases were attributed to high-risk heterosexual contact, 16% to injection drug use, and 1% to other risk factors (Figure 20-4).

Race/Ethnicity	Cases	Rate (Cases per 100,000 population)
American Indian/Alaska Native	46	5.0
Asian*	93	1.6
Black/African American	6,243	39.8
Hispanic/Latino†	1,452	8.9
Native Hawaiian/Other Pacific Islander	12	7.1
White	1,600	1.8
Total‡	9,579	7.5

Note: Data have been adjusted for reporting delays.

*Includes Asian and Pacific Islander legacy cases.
†Hispanics/Latinos can be of any race.
‡Includes 132 female adults and adolescents of unknown race or multiple races.

FIGURE 20-3 ■ Estimated numbers of AIDS cases and rates for female adults and adolescents, by race/ethnicity 2007—50 states and the District of Columbia (www.cdc.gov/hiv/topics/surveillance/resources/slides/women/index.htm).

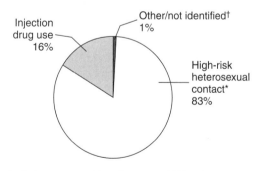

Note: Data include persons with a diagnosis of HIV infection regardless of their AIDS status at diagnosis. Data from 34 states with confidential name-based HIV infection reporting since at least 2003. Data have been adjusted for reporting delays and missing risk-factor information.

*Heterosexual contact with a person known to have, or to be at high risk for, HIV infection.
†Includes blood transfusion, perinatal exposure, and risk factor not reported or not identified.

FIGURE 20-4 ■ Percentages of HIV/AIDS cases among female adults and adolescents, by transmission category 2007—34 states (www.cdc.gov/hiv/topics/surveillance/resources/slides/women/index.htm).

CLINICAL PRACTICE

A. Assessment
1. History
   a. Fatigue
   b. Malaise
   c. Fever
   d. Night sweats
   e. Diarrhea
   f. Weight loss
   g. Anorexia
   h. Cognitive changes
   i. Neurologic disorders
   j. History of blood transfusion before 1985
   k. Oral or gingival lesions
   l. Nasal congestion
   m. Cough and shortness of breath
   n. Recurrent or persistent vaginal infections
   o. Lymphadenopathy
   p. Menstrual cycle disturbance (substance abuse and weight loss may cause oligomenorrhea and amenorrhea)
   q. Tuberculosis (TB); including association with persons with TB
   r. Intravenous (IV) drug abuse
   s. Prostitution
   t. Sexual behavior: number of sexual partners, sexual orientation, contraceptive use, and specific sexual practices
   u. Partner who is an IV drug user or is bisexual
2. Physical findings
   a. Elevated temperature (38.5° C [101.3° F])
   b. Lymphadenopathy
   c. Oral or gingival lesions
   d. Vaginitis caused by *Candida, Trichomonas,* and bacterial vaginosis that may not respond to therapy
   e. Presence of opportunistic infection
      (1) *Pneumocystis jiroveci* pneumonia
      (2) Kaposi's sarcoma; reddish-blue or purple lesions on hard palate; rare in women with AIDS
      (3) Candidiasis (thrush)
         (a) White patches on mucous membrane
         (b) Candida esophagitis; more common in women
      (4) Disseminated mycobacterial infections
      (5) Ulcerative herpes simplex
      (6) Salmonella
      (7) Hepatitis
      (8) CMV
      (9) Toxoplasmosis
      (10) Human papillomavirus (HPV) condyloma
      (11) Syphilis
      (12) TB
      (13) *Staphylococcus aureus;* most common cause of bacterial skin disease
      (14) Diarrhea lasting greater than 1 month
      (15) Herpes zoster (shingles), involving at least two distinct episodes
      (16) Listeriosis
      (17) Pelvic inflammatory disease, particularly if complicated by tubo-ovarian abscess
3. Psychosocial findings
   a. Anxiety
   b. Fear
   c. Lack of social support and social isolation

       d. Stress

       e. Depression

       f. Emotional instability

       g. Denial

       h. Financial problems

       i. Possible lack of food, clothing, and basic childcare or health care

       j. Transportation problems

   4. Diagnostic procedures

       a. The initial serologic screening test is ELISA, which is highly sensitive and inexpensive. If the ELISA is positive, repeat. After two positive ELISA assays, a Western blot or immunofluorescent antibody assay is performed for confirmation.

       b. Other tests

          (1) CBC with differential and platelet count (to monitor anemia, leukocytopenia, and thrombocytopenia)

          (2) Type, Rh factor, and antibody screen

          (3) Rubella titer

          (4) HBsAg

          (5) Purified protein derivative (PPD) or radiograph (incidence of active TB is markedly elevated among HIV-infected patients)

          (6) Immunoglobulin levels are elevated.

          (7) Papanicolaou (Pap) smear: increased incidence of invasive cervical cancer

          (8) Gonorrhea, chlamydia cultures, and TORCH screen

          (9) Ultrasonography every trimester for IUGR, congenital abnormalities, and placental problems

         (10) Venereal Disease Research Laboratory (VDRL) testing

         (11) Urinalysis: may reveal proteinuria resulting from AIDS nephropathy

         (12) Blood chemistries

            (a) Elevated blood urea nitrogen (BUN) and creatinine levels may indicate presence of AIDS-related renal disease.

            (b) Abnormal liver enzymes may indicate liver infiltration by opportunistic infection.

            (c) Elevated total protein may indicate hypergammaglobulinemia.

            (d) Decreased albumin may indicate poor nutrition.

         (13) Antigen capture assay

         (14) Viral culture

B. Interventions

   1. The U.S. Public Health Service recommends that HIV-infected pregnant women be offered a combination of drug treatments to include zidovudine (ZDV). This can be initiated as early as the 14th week of pregnancy (Bernstein, 2007).

   2. Treatment is updated frequently; therefore, check for the latest guidelines from the CDC at www.cdc.gov/hiv/html.

       a. The use of ZDV can substantially reduce the risk of mother-to-child transmission of HIV in some patients to <2% from approximately 30% (Bernstein, 2007).

       b. Medical care of the HIV-infected pregnant woman requires coordination and communication between the HIV specialist caring for the woman and her obstetrician.

   3. Provide information about HIV antibody testing and benefits of early diagnosis.

       a. A pregnant woman should be tested for HIV infection in early pregnancy after she is notified that she will be tested as part of the routine panel of prenatal tests, unless she decides to opt out of the screening (CDC, 2008). All pregnant women should be tested.

       b. Inform the patient that antibodies generally appear within 3 months after infection with HIV but may take up to 6 months in some women.

   4. Provide information about the infection and how it is transmitted in an open and nonjudgmental manner; make safer sex a routine part of health teaching for all patients.

   5. Discuss high-risk behaviors for HIV transmission.

   6. Provide information on implications of HIV infection versus the disease of AIDS.

   7. Counsel patient about the risk to sexual partners and lack of risk to casual contacts at home and work; explain precautions regarding blood and body fluids.

   8. Give written information on the foregoing at a level that the patient can understand; refer to support groups and appropriate websites.

9.   Assure patient of confidentiality; ask her to consider if and to whom she wishes to disclose diagnosis (if she wants family or partner to know), and document this information.
10. Explain all procedures and treatments.
     a.   Counsel about risk of HIV transmission to infant.
     b.   Provide information on ZDV to reduce risk of perinatal infection.
     c.   Discuss CDC guidelines for treatment during pregnancy; refer to the latest CDC guidelines on their website at www.cdc.gov/hiv.
     d.   Emphasize adherence of taking medications as directed.
11. Discuss nutrition needs to include supplemental vitamins, ferrous sulfate, folic acid (if low folate levels), increase need for protein. Refer the patient to a nutritionist.

SEXUALLY TRANSMITTED INFECTIONS

INTRODUCTION

STIs remain a major public health problem in the United States. The CDC estimates that approximately 19 million new infections occur each year. The majority of these new infections are among young people 15 to 24 years of age. The two most frequently reported STIs in the United States are chlamydia and gonorrhea. CDC's 2007 STD surveillance report indicates persistent racial disparities in infection rates, with African Americans bearing the burden. Disparities may be in part because racial and ethnic minorities are more likely to seek care in public health settings that report STIs. However, this cannot explain the significant differences (www.cdc.gov/std/stats07/trends.html).

A. **STIs include the following** (see Table 20-2):
    1.   Gonorrhea
    2.   Syphilis
    3.   HPV
    4.   Chlamydia
    5.   Trichomonas
    6.   Candida
B. **Definition**
    1.   STIs are any diseases spread by sexual contact between partners.
    2.   Transmission occurs through contact with the genitalia, mouth, or rectal area of an infected person.
C. **High-risk population** (Ramin & Landers, 2007)
    1.   Sexually active adolescents have the highest rate of STIs. Gender differences make more efficient transmission from men to women.
    2.   Women with multiple sex partners
    3.   Indigent women with no prenatal care
D. **Statistics**
    1.   In the United States it is estimated that >1.1 million new infections of chlamydia, >300,000 new cases of gonorrhea, >11,000 new cases of syphilis, 5 million new cases of HPV, and 3 million new infections of trichomonas occur each year (www.cdc.gov/std/stats07/trends.htm). Reasons include:
         a.   Sexually active adolescents have the highest rates of STIs of any age group.
         b.   Number of sexual partners has increased.
         c.   Most common method of birth control is oral contraceptives, which do not protect against STIs.
         d.   Many avoid treatment and, if treated, do not inform partner.
    2.   Most cases occur among persons younger than 25 years of age.

CLINICAL PRACTICE

A. **Assessment**
    1.   History: Sexual history needs to be taken in a nonjudgmental manner.
         a.   Previous STI infection of self or partner
         b.   Multiple sexual partners
         c.   Sex with new partner in the preceding 2 months
         d.   Sexual partners with penile discharge, condyloma, or ulcer
         e.   Dysuria

      f. Fever

      g. Dyspareunia

      h. Vaginal discharge, itching, or odor

      i. Exposure to infected sexual partner

      j. Recent use of antibiotics or other medications

      k. Allergy history (allergic reactions to soap or medications often mimic STI lesions).

  2. Physical findings

      a. Purulent urethral or cervical discharge

      b. Friable cervix

      c. Genital lesion that may or may not be painful

      d. Tender uterus, adnexal structures, or both

      e. Pain on motion of cervix

      f. Inguinal adenopathy

      g. Low-grade temperature

      h. Disseminated lymphadenopathy

      i. Rash on palms and soles of feet in secondary syphilis

      j. Genital warts

      k. Poor personal hygiene

  3. Psychosocial findings

      a. Anxiety

      b. Fear

      c. Confusion

      d. Difficulty in communicating

      e. Guilt

  4. Diagnostic tests and findings

      a. Positive cervical, oral, or rectal culture for gonorrhea

      b. Positive cervical culture for chlamydia or streptococcus

      c. Gram stain showing gram-negative diplococci

      d. VDRL or rapid plasma reagin (RPR) test for general screening

      e. Fluorescent treponemal antibody absorption (FTA-ABS) test for specific testing

      f. Tissue cultures

      g. Potassium hydroxide (KOH) smear and wet prep (to identify trichomonas, monilia, and "clue cells")

      h. Culture of herpes lesions

      i. Microscopic darkfield examination for motile spirochetes

B. Interventions

  1. Provide factual information about cause, mode of transmission, and rationale for treatment of the related STI.

  2. Explain importance of taking prescribed medication and completion of entire course, even if symptoms subside.

  3. Instruct patient in warning signs of complications (e.g., fever, increased pain, bleeding).

  4. Advise the patient to abstain from intercourse until she and partner are free of infection.

  5. Advise the patient of importance of having her sexual partners evaluated and treated.

URINARY TRACT INFECTION AND PYELONEPHRITIS

INTRODUCTION

A. Includes:

  1. Asymptomatic bacteriuria during pregnancy and cystitis—most common bacterial infection encountered during pregnancy

  2. Acute pyelonephritis

B. Anatomic and physiologic changes

  1. A change in urine composition occurs that supports bacterial growth.

  2. Dilation of the upper part of ureter occurs—renal calyces and pelvis, as well as the ureters.

  3. Enlarging uterus compresses ureters.

  4. Smooth muscle relaxation effect of progesterone leads to stasis of urine and delayed emptying.

C. **Predisposing history**
  1. History of UTIs before pregnancy
  2. History of childhood UTIs
  3. Advanced maternal age
  4. Low socioeconomic status
  5. Underlying chronic diseases
  6. Hypertension: studies demonstrate mixed association
  7. Risk factors include sickle cell trait, preeclampsia, diabetes, and poor hygiene.
D. **Statistics** (Duff, 2007)
  1. Asymptomatic bacteriuria is found in 5% to 10% of pregnant women.
  2. Incidence of pyelonephritis in pregnancy is 1% to 2%; however, it will develop in 25% to 30% of cases of bacteriuria, if untreated.
  3. Approximately 75% to 80% of cases of pyelonephritis occur on the right side.
  4. Acute pyelonephritis may cause premature labor and delivery and causes postpartum endometritis.
  5. Approximately 20% to 30% of pregnant women with acute pyelonephritis develop a recurrent urinary tract infection later in pregnancy.

CLINICAL PRACTICE

A. **Assessment**
  1. History
     a. Previous asymptomatic bacteriuria or UTIs, voiding habits, and urine continence
     b. Recent catheterization
     c. Frequent intercourse
     d. Presence of predisposing diseases such as hypertension, diabetes, sickle cell trait, or kidney disease
     e. Abdominal or pelvic surgery or trauma to the pelvis
  2. Physical findings
     a. Dysuria
     b. Frequency
     c. Hematuria
     d. Fever or chills
     e. Urgency
     f. Suprapubic pain
     g. Nocturia
     h. Malaise
     i. Malodorous urine
     j. Flank pain or tenderness
     k. Low abdominal pain and tenderness: may be mistaken for labor, chorioamnionitis, appendicitis, placental abruption, or infarcted myoma.
     l. Nausea, vomiting, or diarrhea
     m. Tender urethra and trigone (bladder neck)
     n. Spiking or elevated temperature, 37.2° to 38.9° C (99° to 102° F) (with pyelonephritis, may be greater than 38.9° C [102° F])
     o. Decreased bowel sounds (with pyelonephritis)
  3. Psychosocial findings: anxiety
  4. Diagnostic findings
     a. Urine: midstream, clean-catch specimen
        (1) Pyuria (more than 5 white blood cells (WBCs) per high-power field)
        (2) Hematuria
        (3) Bacteria: more than 100,000 colonies/mL of a single organism from a midstream clean catch
           (a) *Escherichia coli* can account for majority (80% to 90%) of UTIs (Duff, 2007).
           (b) A mixed culture suggests a specimen contamination.
           (c) Other organisms found may include the following:
              [i] *Chlamydia*
              [ii] *Proteus*

                [iii] *Klebsiella*
                [iv] *Enterobacter*
                [v] Group B streptococci
                [vi] Staphylococci

    b. CBC with differential
        (1) Elevated WBC count (12,000 to 20,000 WBCs) and 80% polymorphonuclear leukocytes (PMNs)
        (2) Anemia (from chronic bacteriuria)
        (3) Serum creatinine
    c. Fever and anatomical location of the pain and tenderness are the findings most commonly used to tentatively distinguish cystitis from pyelonephritis.

B. Interventions
  1. All pregnant women should have urine cultures at the first prenatal appointment.
  2. Provide information related to the following:
    a. Signs and symptoms of a UTI (pain with urination, urgency, frequency) and importance of reporting them to health care provider; importance of adequate hydration: 8 to 10 glasses of water each day; correct method of wiping perineal area; prompt voiding; possible effects of UTI on pregnancy (e.g., preterm labor)
    b. Importance of completing treatment with antibiotics must be explained so patient will take all of her medications; single-dose therapy is not as effective in pregnant women as in nonpregnant women. Three-day courses of treatment appear to be comparable to a 7- to 10-day course (Duff, 2007). Refer to the CDC Guidelines for Treatment at www.cdc.gov/std /treatment/2006/rr5511.pdf for the latest treatment regimen.
    c. Obtain follow-up urine cultures; continuous surveillance for recurrent bacteriuria by repeated urine cultures is essential.
    d. Instruct the patient on signs and symptoms of early labor, and tell her to report them promptly.

OTHER INFECTIOUS DISEASES

INTRODUCTION

A. Other communicable diseases include the following (Table 20-3):
  1. Measles
  2. Mumps
  3. Chickenpox
  4. Influenza
  5. Mononucleosis
  6. Upper respiratory infection (URI)
  7. Parvovirus

B. Effects
  1. Pregnant women are exposed to the same communicable diseases as the general population.
  2. Mother and fetus must be considered.
  3. Effect of infection varies depending on disease and stage of pregnancy during which infection occurs.

CLINICAL PRACTICE

A. Assessment
  1. History
    a. Previous exposure
    b. Lack of immunization
  2. Physical findings
    a. Stuffy nose or nasal discharge
    b. Watery eyes
    c. Fever, chills, or low-grade fever

■ TABLE 20-3
■ ■ **Other Infectious Diseases**

Infection	Agent	Detection	Maternal Effects	Neonatal Effects	Incidence
Varicella (chickenpox) zoster (shingles)	Virus: VZV member of herpesvirus family Incubation: 10-21 days May be latent in dorsal root ganglia and reactivated years later to cause herpes zoster or shingles	Portal of entry is respiratory tract Transmitted via aerosolized respiratory droplets Transplacental vesicular secretions are highly contagious Contagious from 1-2 days before the onset of the characteristic rash through the crusting over of all the lesions (4-5 days after onset of the rash)	No evidence that pregnancy specifically influences the spectrum of initial signs and symptoms Varicella is a febrile systemic illness associated with generalized pruritic rash Offer calamine lotion and antipyretics Death per case ratio is 50:100,000 in adults compared with 2:100,000 in children Risk of premature labor caused by high temperature Risk of varicella pneumonia appears to increase during pregnancy Postexposure prophylaxis is available through the use of VZIG, which is shown to reduce the maternal risks of varicella infection–associated complications if administered within 72-96 hours after exposure	Congenital varicella syndrome (usually exposed before 20 weeks) may cause congenital malformations by transplacental infection–cutaneous scars, limb hypoplasia, muscle atrophy, malformed digits, psychomotor retardation, microcephaly, chorioretinitis Vertical transmission rate estimated between 2%-10% Fetal exposure later in pregnancy is associated with congenital varicella lesions If mother contracts infection 5-7 days or less before delivery, administer VZIG to reduce the occurrence and severity of varicella	All women should be assessed for immunity High rate of seropositive women (93%-95%) Generally occurs during the late winter or early spring Incidence estimated at 0.7 per 1000 pregnancies If seronegative, an attenuated live-virus (Varivax) before conception ***Vaccine not recommended for pregnant women*** Preconception vaccinations–delay pregnancy for 3 months Avoid exposure Passive immunization with VZIG–give within 96 hours of exposure–safe during pregnancy
Mumps	Paramyxovirus Incubation: 14-18 days, but may vary from 7 to 23 days	Respiratory secretions	Fever, myalgia, and swelling and tenderness of salivary glands One third may not have symptoms Spontaneous abortion rate is increased twofold	Infection during first trimester associated with spontaneous miscarriage Teratogenicity is unknown, but probably rare or nonexistent Debate about possible association between intrauterine mumps and endocardial fibroelastosis	Up to 80%-90% of adults are seropositive Incidence during pregnancy is between 0.8 and 10 cases per 10,000 pregnancies ***Mumps vaccine is contraindicated during pregnancy***

Influenza	Virus: influenza virus Incubation: 24-72 hours	Respiratory secretions Spread from person to person when an infected person coughs or sneezes	Usually brief but incapacitating disease Pregnancy can increase the risk for complications of influenza Effects include fever, headache, extreme tiredness, dry cough, sore throat, runny or stuffy nose, and muscle aches Deaths occur from secondary bacterial pneumonia	No firm evidence exists that influenzavirus causes congenital malformations	Approximately 10%-20% of U.S. residents get influenza Peak influenza season in the U.S. occurs from late December through March ***Vaccination against influenza is recommended by the CDC and ACOG for all pregnant women*** ***Antiviral drugs to treat early influenza in adults not recommended for pregnant women***
Measles (rubeola)	RNA virus Incubation is 10-14 days	Highly contagious Droplet and airborne routes Can survive up to 2 hours in the air Communicable from 4 days before to 4 days after rash appears	Fever, malaise, cough, runny nose, red watery eyes Symptoms begin 2-7 days after exposure Rash occurs 2-4 days later beginning on face Rash lasts 4-7 days	Does not appear to be teratogenic There is a 20%-60% risk of spontaneous abortion and preterm delivery following measles during pregnancy. If miscarriage does not occur, does not appear to be associated with an increased risk of fetal malformations Increased mortality in preterm and term infants with neonatal measles Evaluate fetus (with sonogram) for microcephaly, growth restriction and oligohydramnios If mother has had infection 7-10 days before birth, infant should receive IM immunoglobulin	Marked decline with improved vaccinations Second vaccination for older children and college students Vaccination contraindicated during pregnancy Susceptible women are vaccinated routinely postpartum

(Continued)

■ TABLE 20-3
■ Other Infectious Diseases—cont'd

Infection	Agent	Detection	Maternal Effects	Neonatal Effects	Incidence
Tuberculosis (TB)	Bacteria: *Mycobacterium tuberculosis*	Respiratory secretions	Cough, pain in chest, coughing up blood, weakness, weight loss, chills, fever, night sweats 5%-10% risk of contracting active disease if infected Some drugs contraindicated during pregnancy such as streptomycin	Untreated TB represents a greater hazard to a fetus than does treatment Neonatal TB carries a high morbidity and mortality rate At birth, evaluate for congenital TB	Approximately one third of world's population infected with TB 8 million new cases diagnosed annually and 3 million deaths annually worldwide TB skin testing is safe throughout pregnancy ***Check latest CDC guidelines for treatment***
Group B Streptococcus	*Streptococcus agalactiae*-gram-positive organism	Colonizes the female genital tract and rectum Vertical transmission occurs during labor Horizontal transmission occurs after birth	UTI, pyelonephritis, chorioamnionitis, preterm labor, vaginal discharge, postpartum endometritis, postcesarean wound infection and endocarditis Women who tested positive for GBS in a previous pregnancy should not be assumed to be colonized and should be retested in present pregnancy	Common cause of sepsis, meningitis and pneumonia Transmission rate from mother to baby at birth is 50%-75% Risk factors include prematurity, maternal intrapartum fever (ROM >12-18 hr), previously infected infant with GBS, GBS in this pregnancy	***CDC recommends routine cultures of vagina and rectum between 35 and 37 weeks' gestation*** and if positive, give antibiotics such as ampicillin or penicillin Approximately 30%-50% of pregnant women are carriers of GBS Prevalence of neonatal GBS is 0.5 per 1000 live births
Parvovirus B19 (fifth disease)	DNA virus	Respiratory droplets Possible through infectious particles on surfaces Transplacental Serologic testing can detect IgG and IgM antibodies	Bright red macular rash and erythroderma that affects the face giving a "slapped face" appearance; elevated temperature; arthralgia affecting hands, wrists, and knees; and malaise Associated with miscarriage	Fetal death is rare when maternal infection occurs after 20 weeks of gestation but the fetal mortality rate is approximately 11% when maternal B19 infection occurs during the first 20 weeks of pregnancy Diagnosis with ultrasound will show evidence of fetal hydrops	Highly contagious Confirmation of infection is by parvovirus-specific IgM Typically occurs in elementary schools and daycare populations in the late winter and early spring Risk of women with primary infection during first 20 weeks of pregnancy is 15%-17%

Disease	Organism	Transmission/Source	Clinical Features	Fetal/Neonatal Effects	Comments
Listeriosis	*Listeria monocytogenes* gram-positive aerobic motile bacillus	Isolated from soil, water, and sewage. Food-borne transmission is important	May not be symptomatic. Fever, muscle aches, nausea, or diarrhea. Headache, stiff neck, confusion	Neonate is particularly susceptible to infection and mortality approaches 50%. Early onset: diffuse sepsis with multiorgan involvement. Associated with high still-birth rate and high neonatal mortality rate. Late onset: meningitis neurologic sequelae	Approximately 65% of pregnant women have evidence of prior infection and are immune. CDC estimates nearly 2500 U.S. individuals annually are ill with listeriosis and more than 500 will die. From 1%-5% of adults carry *Listeria* in their feces. Penicillin G and ampicillin are effective
Lyme disease	*Borrelia burgdorferi*	Tick-borne infection	Multisystem illness characterized by a distinct lesion and rash, fatigue, muscle and joint pain, swollen lymph nodes, arthritis, rare cardiac irregularities	Experience with pregnancy is limited. No adverse effects on fetus when mother received appropriate antibiotic treatment	Tetracycline is an effective agent for eradicating *B. burgdorferi* but is ***contraindicated in pregnancy***

ACOG, American College of Obstetricians and Gynecologists; *CDC*, Centers for Disease Control and Prevention; *DNA*, deoxyribonucleic acid; *GBS*, group B streptococcus; *IgM*, immunoglobulin M; *IM*, intramuscular; *ROM*, rupture of membranes; *UTI*, urinary tract infection; *VZV*, varicella-zoster virus; *VZIG*, varicella-zoster immune globulin.

www.cdc.gov/GroupBStrep/guidelines/recommendations.html.
www.cdc.gov/NCIDOD?dvrd/revb/respiratory/B19&preg.html.
www.cdc.gov/nczved/dfbmd/disease_listing/listeriosis_gi.html.
www.cdc.gov/tb/pubs/tbfactsheets/pregnancy.htm.
www.cdc.gov/vaccines/vdp.html.
www.fsis.usda.gov/Fact_Sheets/Protect_Your_Baby/index.asp.
www.health.ri.gov/disease/communicable/lyme/symptoms.php.
www.marchofdimes.com/professionals/14332_1185.asp.
www.marchofdimes.com/professionals/14332_1205asp.
www.marchofdimes.com/professionals/14332_25586.asp.
www.perinatology.com/exposures/Infection/Mumps.htm.

  d. Enlarged lymph nodes
  e. Fatigue, malaise
  f. Myalgia (muscle aches)
  g. Skin rash (macules, papules, or vesicles)
  h. Sore throat and cough
  i. Adenopathy
  j. Parotitis (swollen salivary glands)
  3. Psychosocial findings
   a. Anxiety
   b. Fear
   c. Apprehension
  4. Diagnostic findings
   a. CBC (increased WBC count)
   b. Throat culture
   c. Mononucleosis spot test and heterophile test
   d. Disease-specific serology antibody tests of IgG and IgM
   e. Virus isolation
   f. Serologic testing: ELISA or fluorescent antibody membrane antigen (FAMA)
B. **Interventions**
  1. Provide information about the signs and symptoms of the communicable disease, its mode of transmission and prevention, and the importance of reporting exposure to health care provider.
  2. Provide written material containing information at appropriate level for the patient.
  3. Reinforce need for the patient to take all of medication.
  4. Provide information about the safety of vaccines during pregnancy.

CHORIOAMNIONITIS

INTRODUCTION

A. **Definition**
  1. Inflammation of the chorion and amnion occurs either before or during labor. Also called amnionitis or intraamniotic infection.
  2. Mononuclear leukocytes and PMNs infiltrate the membranes.
  3. Organisms are usually present in vagina (most commonly streptococcus).
  4. Chorioamnionitis occurs in approximately 1% to 5% of term pregnancies; in patients with preterm birth may approach 25% (Duff, 2007).
B. **Chorioamnionitis is associated with the following** (Duff, 2007):
  1. Premature rupture of membranes
  2. Prolonged rupture of membranes
  3. Young age, low socioeconomic status, nulliparity
  4. Preexisiting infections of the lower genital tract
  5. Multiple vaginal exams
  6. About 5% to 10% of infants born to mothers with chorioamnionitis have pneumonia or bacteremia.
C. **Management**
  1. Identification of the infecting organism
  2. Parenteral antibiotic therapy
  3. Delivery of the infant
  4. Vaginal delivery preferred, but cesarean section may be performed in presence of severe infection

CLINICAL PRACTICE

A. **Assessment**
  1. History
   a. Premature rupture of membranes before the onset of labor
   b. Prolonged rupture of membranes during or before the onset of labor

    c. Prenatal infection
    d. Poor prenatal care

2. Physical findings
    a. Maternal fever (39° C [102.2° F] in mild infection and 40° C [104° F] in severe infection)
    b. Maternal and fetal tachycardia (usually >180 beats/minute) in absence of other localized signs of infection
    c. Fetal monitoring tracing consistent with hypoxia
    d. Chills
    e. Uterine pain and tenderness
    f. Foul-smelling vaginal discharge
    g. Hypotension
    h. Tachycardia

3. Psychosocial findings
    a. Fear
    b. Anxiety

4. Diagnostic findings
    a. Amniotic fluid (bacteria and neutrophils seen)
    b. Culture of amniotic fluid and cervix: possible pathogens include the following:
      (1) Group A and B streptococci
      (2) *Neisseria gonorrhoeae*
      (3) *Chlamydia*
      (4) *Staphylococcus aureus*
      (5) *Haemophilus influenzae*
      (6) *Escherichia coli*
      (7) Anaerobic gram-positive cocci
    c. CBC: increased WBC count (>15,000/mm^3 with preponderance of leukocytes)
    d. Urinalysis to rule out UTI

B. **Interventions**
1. Reinforce information provided by the physician on the possible course of labor, including possibility of cesarean section.
2. Provide accurate information about chorioamnionitis and potential risks.

HEALTH EDUCATION

A. **Encourage preconceptional counseling on potential infections and give information on appropriate immunizations.**
B. **Test pregnant women for potential infections as part of the prenatal panel of lab tests.**
C. **Educate patient about the importance of reporting symptoms to health care providers.**
D. **Instruct the patient of the importance of completing the course of any antibiotic or other medication prescribed for self/partners.**
E. **If medication is provided, instruct patient on any potential side effects.**

CASE STUDIES AND STUDY QUESTIONS

TORCH

Mrs. S., a health care worker in a daycare setting, is a 27-year-old multigravida whose last menstrual period was 11 weeks ago. Her 3-year-old daughter experienced a fever and rash 5 days earlier. Two days later the pediatrician established a diagnosis of rubella. On examination, Mrs. S. is found to be healthy, and her uterus is 10 to 11 weeks in size. She does not remember having had rubella. Her friend told her to be tested for TORCH. She wants to know what it is.

1. What does TORCH stand for?
2. What laboratory test might determine her susceptibility?
    a. CBC
    b. Rubella titer
    c. Nasopharyngeal swab
3. For what other TORCH disease might she be at risk?
    a. AIDS
    b. CMV
    c. Toxoplasmosis
    d. Rubeola

4. What will reduce her chances of exposure?
   a. Cooking chicken until it is well done
   b. Using a mask to protect her from airborne diseases
   c. Rigorous personal hygiene while at work and home
   d. Taking acyclovir
   e. Undergoing serial cervical cultures
      (1) a, c, d
      (2) b, d
      (3) a, b, c
      (4) None of the above

Acquired Immunodeficiency Syndrome

Ms. D. is a 21-year-old primigravida (G1) who had her last menstrual period 12 weeks ago. She is in for her initial prenatal visit. Her uterus is approximately 12 weeks in size and her blood pressure is 110/72 mm Hg. During your discussion with Ms. D., she expresses some concern over the possibility of being exposed to AIDS. She states she has had only one sexual partner and they have been in a monogamous relationship for 2 years. When questioned, her concern stems from the fact that a colleague at work recently tested positive for HIV.

5. As part of your assessment, what other information do you need to know?
   a. Does she live with other people?
   b. Has she eaten at her colleague's home?
   c. Sexual history of her partner
6. In your discussion with Ms. D. about AIDS, you may tell her (answer the following true or false):
   a. AIDS is spread only through sexual contact.
   b. The occurrence of AIDS in women has not been increasing.
   c. She may take ZDV prophylactically.
   d. Symptoms of AIDS include fatigue, night sweats, and lymphadenopathy.
7. If it is established that Ms. D.'s partner had previous partners, what would you recommend for general screening?
   a. ELISA
   b. Western blot
   c. T cell count
8. If this test result were positive, what test would confirm HIV infection?
   a. ELISA
   b. Western blot
   c. T-cell count
9. HIV has been found in all of the following *except:*
   a. Saliva
   b. Tears
   c. Sweat
   d. Semen

Sexually Transmitted Infections

Ms. G. is a 17-year-old single primigravida (G1) who is seen for her first prenatal visit at 20 weeks' gestation. Her history is unremarkable with the exception of treatment for gonorrhea 1 year previously. Examination of the skin, head, ears, nose, and throat yields normal results. Ms. G. is afebrile, her pulse is 88 beats/minute, and her blood pressure is 118/72 mm Hg. The size of her uterus corresponds with gestational age by dates. There is a small amount of yellow discharge at the cervix. The vulva appears red and inflamed.

10. What is the causative agent of gonorrhea?
    a. Gram-negative diplococcus
    b. Gram-positive diplococcus
    c. Protozoa
    d. Spirochete
11. Determine whether the following statements are true or false.
    a. Because Ms. G. does not appear to have symptoms, you need not worry about gonorrhea or chlamydia.
    b. Untreated gonorrhea may cause premature rupture of membranes (PROM).
    c. Gonorrhea has been on the decline for the last 5 years because of better hygiene.
    d. An allergic reaction to soap or medications can mimic STI symptoms.

Urinary Tract Infection and Pyelonephritis

Ms. A. is a 23-year-old gravida 2, para 1 (G2, P1) woman whose last menstrual period was 24 weeks ago. She has had one prenatal visit. She now complains of increasing urinary frequency for 5 days and of burning on urination for 2 days. For the last 24 hours, she has had a constant aching pain in her back and right side, along with chills and fever. Her temperature is 38.9° C (102° F), her pulse is 110 beats per minute, and her blood pressure is 110/70 mm Hg. There is marked costovertebral angle tenderness on the right. Her uterus measures 23 cm, the fetal heart rate is 146 beats/minute, and her cervix is long and closed. Based on urine laboratory values, she is diagnosed as having acute pyelonephritis.

12. Select three physiologic changes that occur during pregnancy that predispose women to UTI.
    a. Changes in urine composition
    b. Dilation of the upper third of ureters
    c. Decreased frequency of urination
    d. Compression of ureters by enlarging uterus
    e. Increased intake of liquids

(1) a, b, c
(2) b, c, e
(3) a, b, d
(4) b, c, d

13. A history of _____ places a pregnant woman at an increased risk for UTI.
    a. childhood UTIs
    b. chronic disease and hypertension
    c. prior UTIs
    d. a, c
    e. a, b, c

Mrs. V. is a 24-year-old schoolteacher approximately 14 weeks' pregnant with her first baby. She is concerned about many of the diseases she may be exposed to and asks many questions.

14. How is chickenpox transmitted?
    a. Aerosolized droplets
    b. Blood and mucus
    c. Skin-to-skin contact

15. Mumps is caused by what agent?
    a. Paramyxovirus
    b. Protozoa
    c. RNA virus

16. What is the incubation period for measles?
    a. 5 to 9 days
    b. 10 to 14 days
    c. 15 to 20 days

Ms. R. is a 16-year-old single primigravida (G1) who is admitted at 36 weeks' gestation with a temperature of 39.4° C (103° F), uterine tenderness, chills, and a blood pressure of 102/72 mm Hg. Fetal heart rate is 180 beats/minute. Fetal monitoring tracing shows minimal variability but no decelerations. Catheterized urinalysis is unremarkable. CBC shows hemoglobin values of 10.5 g/dL, hematocrit of 36%, and WBC count 22,000/mm^3 with 85% PMNs, 10% bands, and 5% lymphocytes.

17. All of the following are possible pathogens associated with chorioamnionitis *except*:
    a. *Escherichia coli*
    b. Group A and B streptococci
    c. *Toxoplasma gondii*

18. All of the following are diagnostic for chorioamnionitis *except*:
    a. Culture of cervix
    b. Amniotic fluid smear
    c. Vaginal smear

19. Chorioamnionitis is associated with premature rupture of membranes and what other factor?
    a. Cerclage use
    b. Prolonged rupture of membranes
    c. Inadequate hydration

20. Determine whether the following statements are true or false.
    a. Mononuclear leukocytes and PMNs infiltrate the chorion.
    b. Teenage unwed pregnancy and poor nutrition are factors that predispose to chorioamnionitis.
    c. A cesarean section is the preferred method of delivery in a patient with chorioamnionitis.

ANSWERS TO STUDY QUESTIONS

1. Toxoplasmosis, other (hepatitis B), rubella, cytomegalovirus, herpes simplex
2. b
3. b
4. 3
5. c

6. a. False
   b. False
   c. False
   d. True
7. a
8. b
9. c
10. a

11. a. False
    b. True
    c. False
    d. True
12. 3
13. e
14. a
15. a

16. b
17. c
18. c
19. b
20. a. True
    b. True
    c. False

REFERENCES

Bernstein, H. (2007). Maternal and perinatal infection—Viral. In S. Gabbe, J. Niebyl, & J. Simpson (Eds.), *Obstetrics: Normal and problem pregnancies* (5th ed.). St. Louis: Churchill Livingstone.

Centers for Disease Control and Prevention. (2007). *Sexually transmitted disease surveillance 2007.* Available online at: www.cdc.gov/std/stats07/chlamydia.htm.

Centers for Disease Control and Prevention. (2007). *Sexually transmitted disease surveillance 2007.* Available online at: www.cdc.gov/std/stats07/gonorrhea.htm.

Centers for Disease Control and Prevention. (2007). *Sexually transmitted disease surveillance 2007.* Available online at: www.cdc.gov/std/stats07/syphilis.htm.

Centers for Disease Control and Prevention. (2007). *Sexually transmitted disease surveillance 2007.* Available online at: www.cdc.gov/std/stats07/other.htm.

Centers for Disease Control and Prevention. (2007). *Sexually transmitted disease surveillance 2007.* Available online at: www.cdc.gov/std/stats07/womenandinf.htm.

Centers for Disease Control and Prevention. (2007). *Trends in reportable sexually transmitted diseases in the United States, 2007.* Available online at: www.cdc.gov/std/stats07/trends.htm.

Centers for Disease Control and Prevention. (2008). *Estimates of new HIV infections in the United States.* Available at: www.cdc.gov/hiv/topics/surveillance/resources/factsheets/incidence/htm. Accessed December 14, 2009.

Centers for Disease Control and Prevention. (2008). *MMWR analysis provides new details on HIV incidence in U.S. populations.* Available online at: wwws.cdc.gov/hiv.html.

Centers for Disease Control and Prevention. (2009). *Group B strep prevention.* Available online at: www.cdc.gov/GroupBStrep/guidelines/recommendations.htm.

Centers for Disease Control and Prevention. (2009). *HIV incidence.* Available online at: www.cdc.gov/hiv/topics/surveillance/incidence.htm.

Centers for Disease Control and Prevention. (2009). *Parvovirus B19 infection and pregnancy.* Available online at: www.cdc.gov/NCIDOD?dvrd/revb/respiratory/B19&preg.htm.

Centers for Disease Control and Prevention. (2009). *Questions and answers: The 15% increase in HIV diagnosis from 2004-2007 in 34 states and general surveillance report questions.* Available online at: www.cdc.gov/hiv/topics/surveillance/resources/qa/surv_rep.html.

Centers for Disease Control and Prevention. (2009). *STDs and pregnancy.* Available online at: www.cdc.gov/STD/STDfact-STDs&pregnancy.htm.

Centers for Disease Control and Prevention. (2009). *Varicella vaccine—Q&A about pregnancy.* Available online at: www.cdc.gov/vaccines/vpd.html.

Centers for Disease Control and Prevention. (2009). *HIV/AIDS among women.* Available online at: www.cdc.gov/hiv/resources/factsheets/us/html.

Centers for Disease Control and Prevention. (2009). *FAQ's for health professionals.* Available online at: www.cdc.gov/hepatitis/HBV/HBVfaq.htm#oview.

Centers for Disease Control and Prevention. (2009). *Cytomegalovirus.* Available online at: www.cdc.gov/cmv/pregnancy.htm.

Davies, J., & Gibbs, R. (2008). Obstetric and perinatal infections. In R. Gibbs, B. Karlan, A. Haney, & I. Nygaard (Eds.), *Danforth's obstetrics and gynecology* (10th ed). Philadelphia: WoltersKluwer/Lippincott Williams & Wilkins.

Duff, P. (2007). Maternal and perinatal infection—Bacterial. In S. Gabbe, J. Niebyl, & J. Simpson (Eds.), *Obstetrics: Normal and problem pregnancies* (5th ed.). Philadelphia: Churchill Livingstone.

eMedicine. (2009). *Pregnancy: Urinary tract infections.* Available online at: www.emedicine.medscape,com/article/797066-overview.html.

Eschenbach, D. (2008). Pelvic and sexually transmitted infections. In R. Gibbs, B. Karlan, A. Haney, & I. Nygaard (Eds.), *Danforth's obstetrics and gynecology* (10th ed.). Philadelphia: Wolters Kluwer/Lippincott Williams & Wilkins.

March of Dimes. (2009). *Chickenpox in pregnancy.* Available online at: www.marchofdimes.com/professionals/14332_1185.asp.

March of Dimes. (2009). *Cytomegalovirus infection in pregnancy.* Available online at: www.marchofdimes.com/professionals/14332_1226.asp.

March of Dimes. (2009). *Cytomegalovirus infection in pregnancy.* Available online at: www.marchofdimes.com/professionals/14332_1195.asp.

March of Dimes. (2009). *Fifth disease in pregnancy.* Available online at: www.marchofdimes.com/professionals/14332_25586.asp.

March of Dimes. (2009). *Genital herpes and pregnancy.* Available online at: www.marchofdimes.com/professionals/14332_1201.asp.

March of Dimes. (2009). *Group B strep infection.* Available online at: www.marchofdimes.com/professionals/14332_1205.asp.

March of Dimes. (2009). *Rubella (German measles).* Available online at: www.marchofdimes.com/professionals/14332_1225.asp.

March of Dimes. (2009). *Toxoplasmosis.* Available online at: www.marchofdimes.com/professionals/14332_1228.asp.

March of Dimes. (2009). *HIV and AIDS in pregnancy.* Available online at: www.marchofdimes.com/professionals/14332_1223.asp.

Merck. (2009). *Urinary tract infection in pregnancy.* Available online at: www.merck.com/mmpe/sec18/ch261/ch261p.html.

Minkoff, H. (2008). Human immunodeficiency virus. In R. Gibbs, B. Karlan, A. Haney, & I. Nygaard (Eds.), *Danforth's obstetrics and gynecology* (10th ed.). Philadelphia: Wolters Kluwer/Lippincott Williams & Wilkins.

National Institute of Child Health and Human Development. (2009). *AIDS/HIV.* Available online at: www.nichd.nih.gov/health/topics/aids_hiv.cfm.

U.S. Department of Health and Human Services. (2007). *HIV/AIDS surveillance report.* Atlanta: Centers for Disease Control and Prevention.

U.S. Department of Health and Human Services. (2007). *Sexually transmitted disease surveillance 2007.* Atlanta: Centers for Disease Control and Prevention.

Ramin, K., & Landers, D. (2007). Maternal and perinatal infection: The sexually transmitted diseases chlamydia, gonorrhea, and syphilis. In S. Gabbe, J. Niebyl, & J. Simpson (Eds.), *Obstetrics: Normal and problem pregnancies* (5th ed.). Philadelphia: Churchill Livingstone.

Additional Resources

American Social Health Association (ASHA): www.ashastd.org.

Centers for Disease Control and Prevention: www.cdc.gov.

Centers for Disease Control and Prevention National AIDS Clearinghouse: www.cdc.gov/hiv.

March of Dimes: www.marchofdimes.com.

National Herpes Hotline: www.herpesonline.org/articles/herpes_hotline.html.

Office on Women's Health: www.4woman.gov/owh.

World Health Organization: www.who.int/en.

Also, state or local health departments have a variety of resources and patient information materials.

21 Hemorrhagic Disorders

S. Kim Genovese

OBJECTIVES

1. Define the hemorrhagic complications of placenta previa, abruptio placentae, disseminated intravascular coagulation (DIC), and gestational trophoblastic disease.
2. Identify the classical signs and symptoms of placenta previa, abruptio placentae, DIC, and trophoblastic disease.
3. List the appropriate nursing interventions for care of the perinatal patient with a hemorrhagic disorder.
4. Correlate patient response with desired response to treatment to anticipate subsequent care.
5. Assemble the appropriate health care provider team and coordinate the health care team as long as is necessary.

INTRODUCTION

A. **Hemorrhagic disorders are obstetric emergencies. They are the leading cause of perinatal patient admissions to intensive care units. Maternal morbidity and mortality are significantly affected** (Fuller & Bucklin, 2007; Martin, Hamilton, Ventura, Menacker, & Park, 2002; Ventura, Martin, Curtin, Menacker, & Hamilton, 2001). **Between 17% and 25% of all pregnancy-related deaths can be directly attributed to hemorrhage** (Chang, Elam-Evans, & Berg, 2003).
   1. Bleeding complicates one in five pregnancies
   2. Incidence and type of bleeding varies by trimester.
      a. Most maternal deaths from obstetric hemorrhage after first trimester of pregnancy occur secondary to placental abruption.
      b. Risk of mortality is related to maternal age and race, with highest rates among U.S. African American women.
B. **The maternal mortality rate for 2006 was 13.3 deaths per 100,000 live births. African American women have a substantially higher risk of maternal death than white women with a maternal mortality rate of 32.7, roughly 3.4 times the rate for white deaths per 100,000 live births. The maternal mortality rate for Hispanic women was 10.2 deaths per 100,000 live births** (National Vital Statistics Report, 2009).
   1. The ranked order causes of death after a live birth are uterine atony, complications from DIC, and abruptio placentae.
   2. The ranked order causes of death after stillbirth are abruptio placentae and uterine rupture.
   3. 68% of maternal deaths secondary to hemorrhage occur within 48 hours after the pregnancy ends.
C. **Obstetric hemorrhage is defined as a 10% decrease in hematocrit, total blood loss of more than 1000 mL, or need for transfusion therapy** (Benedetti, 2002). **Class 2 hemorrhage is characterized by a 1200- to 1500-mL blood loss and early compensatory changes of tachypnea and tachycardia** (Francois & Foley, 2007).

PLACENTA PREVIA

A. **Placenta previa is an implantation of the placenta in the lower uterine segment, near or over the internal cervical os. The underlying cause of placenta previa is unknown.**
   1. Reported incidence affects approximately 0.5% to 1% (1 in 200) of births; among grand multiparous women it is increased 2% (Clark, 2004; Hull & Resnik, 2009).

2. Recurrence risk following one pregnancy complicated by a previa ranges from 4% to 8% (Konje & Taylor, 1999).
3. There is a direct relationship between the number of previous cesarean births and risk of placenta previa, probably due to uterine scarring (Benedetti, 2002; Clark, 2004; Gilbert, 2007; Hull & Resnik, 2009; Konje & Taylor, 1999).
B. **Classifications for placenta previa**
   1. Classifications for placenta previa are based on the degree to which the internal cervical os is covered by the placenta. The four types of placenta previa identified are:
      a. Low-lying placenta: reserved for those situations in which the exact relationship of placenta to the cervical os has not been determined
      b. Marginal previa: edge of the placenta is within 2 to 3 cm of the internal cervical os but does not cover it
      c. Partial (incomplete) previa: partial or an incomplete placental coverage of the cervical os
      d. Complete placenta previa: placenta covers part or all of the internal cervical os in the third trimester
   2. Advanced ultrasound technology has allowed more accurate assessments of placental location in relation to the cervical os. The more contemporary ultrasound classification used is that the os is covered or marginal.
C. **The degree of occlusion of the internal cervical os may depend on the degree of cervical dilation, so what may appear to be low-lying or marginal on ultrasound examination prior to the onset of labor can become more serious as labor progresses.**

CLINICAL PRACTICE

Assessment

A. **The classical sign of placenta previa is painless vaginal bleeding in the second or third trimester of pregnancy.**
   1. History
      a. Presents with confirmed placenta previa or vaginal bleeding
         (1) Previously diagnosed by ultrasonogram
            (a) About 12% to 25% of women might be diagnosed with placenta previa or low-lying placenta before 30 weeks' gestation.
            (b) Low-lying and placenta previa before 30 weeks usually resolves (up to 75%) or migrates.
            (c) If the placental edge is 15 mm or more over the internal os at 12 to 16 weeks' gestation, the incidence of third-trimester previa becomes 5.1% (Taipale, Hiilesmaa, & Ylostalo, 1997).
         (2) Documentation on antepartal record
         (3) History of one or more previous pelvic bleeding episodes
            (b) Peak incidence for initial bleeding episode is early third trimester.
               [i] 33% become symptomatic before 30 weeks' gestation.
               [ii] 33% become symptomatic after 36 weeks.
         (4) Increased risk for incidence (Hull & Resnik, 2009):
            (a) Previous placenta previa; 83 times the increased risk
            (b) Advanced maternal age greater than 40; 93 times the increased risk (Ananth, Demissie, Smulian, & Vintzileos, 2003)
            (c) Previous cesarean birth: 1.5 to 15 times the increased risk (Clark, 2004; Silver, Landon, & Rouse, 2006).
            (d) Short interval between pregnancies and multiparity (Cunningham et al, 2005)
            (e) Previous abortions with curettage; risk increased 1.3 times
            (f) Smoking, amount dependent, with a 1.4- to 3-fold increased risk
            (g) Race; Asian women have a 1.9 times greater risk
            (h) Large placenta related to multiple gestation, diabetes, or erythroblastosis fetalis
   2. **Physical assessment**
      a. Vaginal bleeding, which is typically bright red and painless

    (1) Vaginal bleeding, with or without uterine contractions, due to placental separation from cervical os or lower uterine segment and the inability of the uterus to contract at the vessel sites; the initial bleed is rarely profuse and usually stops spontaneously; bleeding recurs later.

    (2) Presence of clots usually indicates normal coagulation process.

    (3) Absence of clots might indicate evolving coagulopathy, either hypofibrinogenemia or thrombocytopenia.

    (4) Painful bleeding can occur when the placenta abrupts away from the uterine tissue, even with a placenta previa.

    (5) Vaginal examination with speculum is postponed until ultrasound confirmation of diagnosis.

    (6) Monitor amount, color, and frequency of vaginal bleeding.

b. Abdominal assessment

    (1) Abdominal palpation should indicate a soft, relaxed nontender uterus with normal tone.

    (2) Abdominal tone can be tense with the laboring patient.

    (3) Transabdominal ultrasound confirms diagnosis in 93% to 97% of cases. Difficulty with interpretation in the obese patient, with a posteriorly implanted placenta and with an engaged cephalic presentation.

c. Hemodynamic changes; risk associated with blood loss

    (1) Vital signs may initially remain normal; due to pregnancy blood volume changes can accommodate up to 40% blood loss before showing signs of a hypovolemic state and shock (Francois & Foley, 2007).

    (2) Maternal blood loss can occur rapidly; approximately 700 to 1000 mL/min (10% to 15% of maternal cardiac output) of blood flow is directed to the uterine vasculature and placenta during pregnancy (Sosa, 2001).

    (3) Maternal blood loss results in decreased oxygen-carrying capacity, which directly affects oxygen delivery to maternal organ systems and indirectly affects oxygen delivery to the fetus.

        (a) Placental blood flow is directly proportional to uterine perfusion pressures; uterine perfusion pressures are proportional to maternal systemic blood pressure.

        (b) Maternal hemorrhage, if not identified and corrected, leads to a hypovolemic state, decreasing maternal cardiac output and systemic perfusion pressures (Benedetti, 2002).

        (c) Decreased maternal systemic blood pressure leads to decreased uterine perfusion pressures and fetal compromise.

        (d) Decreased oxygenation and hypoperfusion can set up cascade of events predisposing to multiorgan dysfunction syndrome (MODS) (Benedetti, 2002).

    (4) Fetal oxygenation decreases proportionally to changes in maternal cardiac output generation and systemic perfusion pressures (Blackburn, 2007; Feinstein & Atterbury, 2003).

        (a) Fetal risks from maternal hemorrhage include blood loss, anemia, hypoxemia, hypoxia, anoxia, and preterm birth.

        (b) Fetal blood loss is always significant because of the small fetal blood volume (80 to 100 mL/kg).

        (c) Disruption of uteroplacental blood flow can result in a progressive deterioration of fetal status; the degree of fetal compromise is directly related to the total volume of blood loss and duration of the bleeding episode (Sosa, 2001).

d. Shock as a result of significant blood loss

    (1) Rising pulse rate: initially is full and easily palpable; as bleeding continues, pulse becomes weak and thready

    (2) Increase in respiratory rate; desaturation of hemoglobin as measured by lowered pulse oximetry is a later finding and might overestimate value if vasoconstriction is present in the extremity in which measurement is taken

    (3) Skin changes to pallor, cold and clammy with mottling as a result of systemic vasoconstriction to shunt perfusion to essential organs

    (4) Falling blood pressure; hypotension is a late finding

    (5) Decreasing urinary output secondary to acute left ventricular dysfunction and renal hypoperfusion

        (a) A key indicator in early significant blood loss

      (6) Decreasing level of consciousness with increasing anxiety, apprehension, and restlessness

      (7) Changes in laboratory findings consistent with acute blood loss

  e. Fetal heart rate (FHR) response to maternal bleeding or shock

      (1) Loss of variability and accelerations

      (2) Abnormal FHR and loss of variability

          (a) Initial compensatory tachycardia

          (b) Subsequent bradycardia; fetal cardiac output is rate dependent, and therefore when baseline rate decreases by 50%, fetal cardiac output decreases by 50%.

          (c) Sinusoidal pattern, indicating fetal anemia, hypoxia, and acidemia

          (d) Persistent late decelerations indicating impaired uteroplacental perfusion

      (3) If maternal status remains unstable, and bleeding is allowed to continue, intrauterine demise is possible.

  f. Complications associated with placenta previa

      (1) Coagulopathy is rare (Wing, Paul, & Millar, 1996).

      (2) Abnormal implantation of placenta invading uterine wall

          (a) Placenta accreta is an abnormality of invasion of the trophoblast beyond normal boundary of the Nitabuch's fibrinoid layer. Placenta accreta occurs in 5% to 10% of pregnancies with a previa (Lockwood & Funai, 1999).

             [i] Prevalence of accreta is increasing and is closely correlated with number of cesarean births a woman has undergone (Benedetti, 2002; Gilbert, 2007).

             [ii] One prior cesarean: risk of accreta is 10% to 25%; risk is greater than 50% with two or more cesarean births

             [iii] Presence of accreta significantly increases risk of severe hemorrhage and peripartal hysterectomy (Flamm, 2001).

          (b) Placenta increta: Invasion of trophoblast extends into the myometrium.

          (c) Placenta percreta: Invasion of trophoblast extends beyond the serosa.

      (3) Postpartum hemorrhage due to placental implantation in the less muscular, lower uterine segment, which contracts poorly and lacerates easily during delivery and manual removal of placenta.

      (4) Uterine rupture

      (5) Abnormal placental development and abnormal cord insertion are rare but significant causes of fetal bleeding (see Chapter 11 for complete discussion of placental variations).

          (a) Vasa previa: Fetal vessels cross the placental membranes in the lower uterine segment and cover the cervical os.

          (b) Velamentous cord insertion: Fetal vessels run across chorion and amnion without protective Wharton's jelly before entering the placental surface.

          (c) Succenturiate placenta: one or more small accessory lobes of placental vascular tissue in membranes that are attached to main placenta by fetal vessels

          (d) Classic presentation of vasa previa, velamentous cord insertion, or succenturiate placenta is vaginal bleeding with rupture of membranes, followed quickly by abrupt change in fetal heart rate and fetal death.

          (e) Increased fetal mortality rate

          (f) Greater risk of compression, rupture, or both, when velamentous vessels are close to cervix

  g. Fetal malpresentation in third trimester (Neilson, 2001)

      (1) Nonpolar fetal lie is common; includes transverse lie, breech, and unengaged vertex.

      (2) With placenta implanted in lower uterine segment, fetal presenting part remains at high station late in pregnancy.

3. Psychosocial findings

  a. Maternal stress factors

      (1) Anxiety

      (2) Fear of pregnancy loss

      (3) Fear for self

      (4) Confusion and panic

      (5) Difficulty in making decisions

  b. Loss of pregnancy and loss of own life and health questioned

  c. Feelings of helplessness

4. Diagnostic procedures
   a. Ultrasonography accuracy 93% to 98% by combination of abdominal, transperineal, and transvaginal techniques
      (1) Need more than one view to locate placenta, including lateral uterine walls, for diagnosis of placenta previa.
      (2) Differentiate placenta previa from abruptio placentae or other causes of bleeding.
      (3) Determine if placenta previa and abruptio placentae coexist.
      (4) Approximately 7% to 10% of women are asymptomatic when placenta previa is found on routine ultrasonogram.
      (5) Magnetic resonance imaging (MRI) is occasionally used to diagnose placenta previa; especially diagnostic for posterior uterine wall placenta
      (6) Doppler color flow aids diagnosis of placental vessel abnormalities associated with placenta previa, such as velamentous insertion of cord.
   b. Avoid speculum and digital vaginal examinations to diagnose placenta previa.
      (1) Speculum examination might be performed after placenta previa has been ruled out by ultrasonography.
      (2) Digital examination risks perforation or abruption of placenta previa.
      (3) If speculum examination is absolutely necessary, should be performed with *double set-up* procedure in room equipped for an emergency cesarean section if profound bleeding occurs.
   c. If there is significant blood loss, clotting problems develop; therefore, evaluate baseline clotting values.
   d. Clotting studies (e.g., prothrombin time [PT], partial thromboplastin time [PTT], platelets, D-dimer, complete blood count [CBC], fibrinogen, fibrin split products [FSPs], or fibrin degradation products or clotting screen such as CBC, platelets, and D-dimer.
   e. Test for presence of fetal RBCs in maternal blood sampling or vaginal blood using rapid tests (4 to 7 minutes): Ogita (most sensitive at 20% fetal blood), APT (sensitive at 60%), Loendersloot (sensitive at 60%), or more lengthy tests (1 hour): Kleihauer-Betke stain or hemoglobin electrophoresis.
B. **Interventions/Outcomes**
   1. Painless vaginal bleeding
      a. Immediate interventions
         (1) Avoid vaginal examinations.
         (2) Monitor maternal pulse and blood pressure.
            (a) Assess trends in vital signs: hemodynamic status is stable or further fluid resuscitation is needed.
            (b) Use electrocardiogram (ECG) monitor or maternal rate mode on electronic fetal monitor (EFM), as needed.
            (c) Monitor central venous pressure (CVP) or pulmonary pressures with Swan-Ganz catheter if bleeding progresses.
         (3) Establish intravenous (IV) line with large-bore intracatheter (16 gauge preferable, or 18 gauge).
            (a) Rapidly administer nondextrose crystalloids, such as Ringer's lactate or normal saline to stabilize and increase blood volume.
         (4) Monitor urinary output.
            (a) Measure specific gravity.
         (5) Blood draw analysis
            (a) Type and crossmatch for initial two units of packed cells.
            (b) Clotting studies as ordered
            (c) CBC and chemistry profile as ordered
            (d) Observe for clotting of blood.
         (6) Administer oxygen at 8 L per mask (10 to 12 L if rebreather bag used).
         (7) Measure or estimate blood loss. Weighing pads is a method of accurate assessment of blood loss, but not frequently practiced.
            (a) Metric scale: 1 g = 1 ml
            (b) Nonmetric scale: 1 ounce = 29/30 ml
         (8) Engage health care team in management
      b. Anticipated expectant care management (Gilbert, 2007)

(1) Initial hospitalization for evaluation of maternal and fetal status.

(2) Activity restriction might be ordered, requiring bedrest with bathroom privileges; as maternal and fetal status allows, the patient may be allowed limited periods of ambulation.

(3) Continuous monitoring for active vaginal bleeding.

(4) Venous access site maintained during hospitalization

(5) Monitor laboratory values of hemoglobin/hematocrit levels and coagulation profile; maternal status determines need to hold blood in blood bank for possible type and cross-match.

(6) Continuous EFM initially and during bleeding episodes.

(7) Biophysical profile (BPP) or nonstress test (NST) with amniotic fluid index (AFI), followed by a weekly modified BPP.

(8) Antenatal corticosteroids to enhance fetal pulmonary maturity between 24 and 34 weeks' gestation

(9) Monitor for signs and symptoms of preterm labor and intrauterine infection; uterine irritability or preterm labor can be treated with tocolytics, such as magnesium sulfate, if patient is otherwise stable (Baron & Hill, 2002).

(10) Preparation for emergency cesarean section delivery if necessary. Transfer to a tertiary perinatal center if necessary to manage care effectively.

c. Outcomes of improved tissue perfusion: decreased and/or stopped blood loss

(1) Stabilized and improved vital signs

(2) Improved or stable color and warmth of skin and hemodynamic parameters

(3) Clotting studies stable

(4) Respiratory rate normal and breathing unlabored

(5) Few or no uterine contractions

2. Maternal blood loss leading to ineffective fetal perfusion and oxygenation

a. Ongoing interventions

(1) Continuously monitor FHR, preferably with EFM, to evaluate variability.

(2) Observe for abnormal FHR patterns (see Chapter 12 for further discussion of FHR patterns).

(a) Loss of variability; accelerations

(b) Sinusoidal pattern

(c) Tachycardia

(d) Persistent late decelerations

(e) Terminal bradycardia

(3) Place patient in lateral position or wedge to left.

(4) Treat patient for alteration in tissue perfusion as indicated.

(a) Oxygen therapy

(b) Fluids and blood products

(c) Position change

(d) Tocolysis

(5) Anticipate cesarean delivery and maintain close observation for postpartum hemorrhage.

(6) Provide home care instructions and preparation.

b. Outcomes for optimal fetal perfusion

(1) Normal or improved FHR patterns

(2) Normal or improved FHR variability

(3) Home care instructions and preparation provided

3. Maternal anxiety

a. Immediate interventions

(1) Speak calmly to patient and support persons.

(2) Explain condition as diagnosed using pictures, images, and resources of health care team.

(3) Explain interventions and reason they are being performed.

(a) Observation during time frame to allow for fetal growth and organ maturity

(b) Administration of tocolysis to treat and prevent premature uterine contractions

(c) Immediate responses for profuse bleeding and fetal compromise

(d) Reassurances and instructions for home care with patient and support system

    b. Antepartal home care maintenance
      (1) Anticipate discharge from health care facility:
        (a) 72 hours after last bleeding episode
        (b) If no indicators of preterm labor
        (c) If evidence of fetal well-being
        (d) If mechanism in place to return to hospital immediately if active bleeding resumes
      (2) Focus on accurate assessments and appropriate referral.
      (3) Criteria for home care management vary with primary perinatal provider and home care agency (Baron & Hill, 2002; Gilbert, 2007; Simpson & Creehan, 2001).
      (3) Ongoing assessments include assessment of vaginal bleeding; evaluation of fetal well-being and uterine activity; warning signs of preterm labor, including possible home uterine monitoring; daily or at least twice weekly home visits for comprehensive maternal-fetal evaluation; timing of appropriate laboratory assessment; fetal kick counts (after 24 weeks gestation), vaginal bleeding, uterine activity, maternal activity level, and adherence to prescribed nursing care plan (Simpson & Creehan, 2001).
    c. Outcomes related to maternal anxiety
      (1) Patient reports less anxiety.
      (2) Observe relaxed body posture and expressions that are less tense.
      (3) Patient can describe home care plans, recognition of signs and symptoms requiring immediate attention or transport, and preparations for immediate hospitalization.

C. Health education
  1. Education for diagnosis of second-trimester placenta previa
    a. Assess patient's readiness for discharge to residential location.
      (1) Has access to immediate transportation if bleeding recurs
      (2) Residing at location within reasonable distance of hospital
        (a) Distance established by physician
    b. Assess patient's understanding of diagnosis of placenta previa.
      (1) Use pictures to explain diagnosis.
      (2) Answer questions as they arise.
      (3) Involve family members and support team as patient requests.
    c. Review symptoms that will necessitate a return to hospital.
      (1) Bleeding
        (a) Document amounts in metric or nonmetric units (e.g., 2 cups); pad count.
        (b) Describe appearance of clots (e.g., dark red, falls apart).
        (c) Describe feeling of dizziness, difficulty breathing, and pallor.
      (2) Uterine and abdominal pain
        (a) Uterine contractions
        (b) Rupture of membranes
    d. Review factors that contribute to reducing risk of intrauterine growth restriction.
      (1) Good nutrition
      (2) Avoidance of smoking
      (3) Rest and avoid fatigue.
      (4) Avoid supine hypotension.
        (a) Tilt to side, even with semi-Fowler position.
        (b) Side-lying positions
        (c) Upright positions if ordered
    e. Avoid insertion of anything into vagina and coitus until physician approved.
    f. Explain importance of follow-up.
      (1) Repeat ultrasounds
        (a) Placental status and position
        (b) Fetal growth
  2. Education for diagnosis of late third-trimester placenta previa
    a. Explain reasons for hospitalization.
      (1) Cervical changes occur as delivery approaches.
      (2) Bleeding increases with cervical changes.
        (a) Need for transfusion availability
        (b) Need for close observation and/or blood testing
      (3) Observation of labor status

(a) Tocolytics, as indicated

(b) Cesarean section availability

(4) Need for fetal observation and testing

(a) FHR monitoring

(b) Fetal lung maturity

(c) Ultrasound testing

(5) Monitor status of fetus at delivery.

(a) Neonatal resuscitation available and anticipated

(b) Immediate neonatal care available if preterm

(6) Provide preparatory educational videotapes and reading materials regarding the following:

(a) Labor and delivery

(b) Infant care: breast vs. bottle-feeding

(c) Nutrition

(d) Postpartum self-care

ABRUPTIO PLACENTAE

A. **Abruptio placentae is the premature separation of a normally implanted placenta from the decidual lining of the uterus after 20 weeks' gestation.**

1. Separation can be partial or complete.

2. The resultant loss of blood can be revealed (external) or concealed (internal) depending on the dissection of membrane edges away from the uterine wall.

B. **Incidence is reported as ranging from 0.3% to 1.6%** (Ananth, Oyelese, Yeo, Pradham, & Vintzileos, 2005; Baumann, Blackwell, Schild, Berry, & Friedrich, 2000).

1. Average rate of abruption is 1 case per 120 births (0.83%) (Clark, 2004; Hull & Resnik, 2009; Sosa, 2001).

2. In pregnancies complicated by abruption, approximately 1 out of 420 births are severe enough to threaten fetal viability (Clark, 2004; Hull & Resnik, 2009).

CLINICAL PRACTICE

Assessment

A. **The classical sign of abruptio placentae is the pregnant woman presenting with painful vaginal bleeding.**

1. History

a. Presents with history of signs and symptoms of vaginal bleeding; external bleeding, or enlarging uterus (without external bleeding). Vaginal bleeding is present in up to 70% to 80% of women presenting with abruption (Benedetti, 2002).

b. Complains of painful, tense abdomen that may be accompanied by uterine contractions. Increased uterine tone and tenderness might be absent unless the abruption is a grade 2 or grade 3 (Benedetti, 2002).

(1) Occurs in 1 in 150 deliveries; extent of abruption varies and might be expressed in a grading system.

(2) Recurrence rate ranges from 5% to 17%, which yields a relative risk of 30 times higher than in the general population (Clark, 2004; Konje & Taylor, 1999).

(3) Perinatal mortality rate is 20%.

(4) Overall, 12% of stillbirths are due to abruptio placentae.

(5) Racial incidence: African American 1 in 595, white 1 in 876, Latino 1 in 1473

c. Increased risk for incidence

(1) Maternal hypertension, whether chronic, gestational, or preeclampsia/eclampsia: five times more likely to have abruption

(2) Cigarette smoking: most preventable risk factor. Ananth et al. (2005) report an overall 90% increase in the risk of abruption with maternal smoking.

(a) Decidual necrosis found

(b) Dose-related effects on birthweight

(c) Worse if more than 40 years of age (compared with teen years) (Cnattingius, 1997)

(3) Multiparity, especially women younger than 30 years of age

(4) Abortions, spontaneous and elective

(5) Illicit drug use

    (a) Cocaine

    (b) Methamphetamine

(6) Short fetal umbilical cord

(7) Abdominal trauma: Symptomatic response might be delayed.

    (a) Blunt abdominal trauma places a woman at increased risk for abruption.

        [i] 5% incidence with minor trauma

        [ii] Up to 50% incidence with major injuries

        [iii] Because of the increased risk of placental abruption following maternal trauma, continuous fetal heart rate monitoring is recommended until the woman is stabilized. The American College of Obstetricians and Gynecologists (ACOG, 2000) recommends a minimum of 2 to 6 hours of fetal monitoring after maternal abdominal trauma.

    (b) Fetal-maternal bleed is of concern if blood type is Rh D^u negative.

    (c) Trauma includes amniocentesis, uterine catheter, accidents, and assaults.

(8) Rupture of membranes

    (a) Premature and prolonged risk increases 5 to 10 times; fetal distress is increased if rupture preceded by bleeding.

    (b) Sudden uterine decompression as with second twin or in polyhydramnios

    (c) Chorioamnionitis (Kramer et al, 1997).

(9) Uterine leiomyoma located behind placenta (Cunningham et al, 2005).

2. **Physical assessment**

  a. Bleeding with or without abdominal tenderness

    (1) Grading for placental abruption (Konje & Taylor, 1999)

      (a) Grade 0 = asymptomatic; small retroplacental clot noted after birth; normal maternal-fetal assessment findings; normal laboratory findings

      (b) Grade I = minimal vaginal bleeding; minimal uterine tenderness and mild tetany; no coagulopathy; maternal-fetal hemodynamic status stable

      (c) Grade II = external vaginal bleeding might or might not be present; tetanic contractions; maternal hemodynamic stability with tachycardia; nonreassuring fetal heart rate pattern; hypofibrinogenemia (15 to 250 mg/dL)

      (d) Grade III = heavy vaginal bleeding; bleeding may be concealed; tetanic, painful uterus; persistent abdominal pain; maternal-fetal hemodynamic instability; hypofibrinogenemia (<150 mg/dL); coagulopathy present

    (2) Prediction of an abruptio placentae is difficult; grade I is subtle and difficult to diagnose.

    (3) Antepartum testing results tend to be normal until placenta significantly abrupts.

    (4) Ultrasonography used to rule out placenta previa; however, it is not diagnostic during acute phase of abruption.

  b. Continuous dull back pain and abdominal pain may be present.

  c. Intermittent abdominal cramping may be present.

  d. Uterine contractions: frequent and mild; tonus might be elevated; must be differentiated from preterm labor.

  e. Symptoms of significant bleeding from abruptio placentae

    (1) Rising pulse rate with falling blood pressure; hypotension with tachycardia is a late finding.

      (a) Blood pressure drops to normal range with hypertensive patients.

      (b) True blood pressure returns after intravascular volume replaced.

      (c) Noninvasive automatic blood pressure/pulse monitoring less accurate in hypotensive state; verify values.

    (2) Pale, clammy skin

    (3) Increasing uterine distention and tone

      (a) Abdominal girth and fundal height might increase.

      (b) More common with concealed bleeding

        (4) Concealed (internal) bleeding in 10% of patients
           (a) Bleeding is behind placenta with margins adherent or membranes attached to uterine wall.
           (b) Blood might break through membranes into amniotic cavity.
           (c) When fetal head is in the lower uterine segment, external bleeding might be obstructed.
           (d) Can be self-limiting and not expand during pregnancy
        (5) Nausea and vomiting
        (6) Shock
        (7) Renal output decreases until hypovolemia treated
     f. FHR changes
        (1) Increased baseline rate initially
        (2) Decreased baseline variability
        (3) Late deceleration pattern
        (4) Decreased baseline rate
        (5) Absence of heart rate; fetal death occurs when 50% or more of blood volume from placenta is lost.
3. Psychosocial findings
     a. Maternal stress factors
        (1) Anxiety
        (2) Fear of loss or injury of pregnancy
        (3) Fear for self
        (4) Confusion
        (5) Pain
     b. Maternal behavioral factors
        (1) Patient has difficulty in communicating facts and concerns.
        (2) Patient expresses pain verbally, by body posture, or both.
        (3) Patient expresses fear of events and situation.
4. Diagnostic procedures
     a. Observe for coagulation abnormalities with clotting studies (PT, PTT, platelet count, D-dimer, fibrinogen, FSP).
     b. Obtain results of alkaline denaturation tests that mark presence of fetal blood: Ogita, APT, or Loendersloot (Odunsi, Bullough, Henzel, & Polanska, 1996); D-dimer level is twice as high and useful in diagnosing abruptio placentae; thrombomodulin and CA125 markers are under study and might prove helpful (Cunningham et al, 2005).
     c. Consider ultrasonography for placental condition, if possible, and to differentiate from placenta previa.
        (1) Ultrasonography for diagnosis of abruptio placentae can be unreliable; 25% of cases are confirmed; false-positive results can occur if lacunae or normal lakes of placental blood are viewed.
        (2) Several minutes after delivery, placenta begins to reveal clotted blood over an area of depression.
     d. Palpation of abdomen might reveal:
        (1) Tenderness
        (2) Rigidity
        (3) Elevated tonus
        (4) Frequent uterine contractions
5. Complications
     a. Couvelaire uterus
        (1) Bleeds into and sometimes through the myometrium beneath serosa into the tube, broad ligament, and ovaries and across the serosa into the peritoneum
        (2) Abrupts in center of placenta; blood is trapped
        (3) Immediate blood loss is concealed.
        (4) Unclotted blood flows into the amniotic sac; amniotic fluid becomes a port-wine color.
        (5) Actual versus observed blood loss estimates are disparate, and therefore actual loss is underestimated.
     b. Fetal growth restriction
     c. Fetal anoxia and demise

    d. Fetal exsanguination

    e. Prematurity

    f. Maternal shock

    g. Maternal or neonatal coagulopathy (or both)

        (1) Hypofibrinogenemia (less than 150 mg/dL)

        (2) Elevated FSP (greater than 100 mg/mL)

        (3) Positive D-dimer levels

        (4) Thrombocytopenia

    h. Maternal renal failure; usually reversible; proteinuria resolves

    i. Hypoxic damage to liver, adrenal glands, and anterior pituitary (Sheehan syndrome)

    j. Postpartum hemorrhage

B. Interventions/Outcomes related to abruptio placentae

    1. Blood loss resulting in poor maternal tissue perfusion

        a. Immediate interventions

          (1) Monitor maternal pulse and blood pressure.

            (a) Monitor progressive changes to avoid shock.

          (2) Establish one or more IV lines with 18-gauge or larger intracatheter.

          (3) Rapidly administer parenteral crystalloids or colloids as ordered (e.g., Ringer's lactate or plasmanate).

          (4) Measure and estimate blood loss.

            (a) Weigh blood loss on metric scale (1 g = 1 ml) or on nonmetric scale (1 ounce = 29 ml).

            (b) Measure and mark height of fundus on the abdomen, especially if bleeding is concealed.

          (5) Avoid vaginal examinations until placenta previa has been ruled out; specific order is advised.

          (6) Administer oxygen via face mask at 8 to 10 L/min.

          (7) Position supine with wedge under hip and Trendelenburg if condition intensifies

          (8) Assist with CVP or insertion of Swan-Ganz catheter as needed; recommended ranges vary.

            (a) CVP 5 to 12 mm Hg

            (b) Pulmonary arterial pressure (PAP) 10 to 20 mm Hg

            (c) Pulmonary wedge pressure (PWP) less than 6 to 8 mm Hg

          (9) Insert Foley catheter: 30 to 60 ml/hr output is desired.

         (10) Prepare for immediate cesarean delivery based on the following:

            (a) Gestational age, viability of fetus, and status of fetus

            (b) Maternal condition (e.g., anemia, hypoxia)

         (11) Prepare for amniotomy if vaginal delivery anticipated

            (a) Might hasten delivery of a fetus of adequate size

            (b) Might decrease bleeding

         (12) Observe labor progress.

            (a) Uterine contractions often stronger

            (b) Oxytocin used if contractions are inadequate or absent

         (13) Type and crossmatch for 2 to 4 units of packed red blood cells (PRBCs); administer blood products as necessary and ordered.

            (a) More than 10 units is considered to be a massive transfusion.

            (b) After administration of 4 to 6 units, reevaluate clotting studies and potassium level for replacement of clotting factors.

        b. Outcomes: improved tissue perfusion shown by the following:

          (1) Improved vital signs

          (2) Improved or stable clotting studies; improved or no anemia

          (3) Improved or stable color and warmth of skin

          (4) Decreased blood loss; no hypovolemia

          (5) Normal respiratory rate and unlabored breathing; no hypoxia

          (6) Improved comfort level

    2. Anxiety related to fear for self and fetus

        a. Ongoing interventions

          (1) Speak calmly to patient and support persons.

          (2) Reassure with information about events and efforts of team

(3) Explain status of problem and plan.
   (a) Imminent delivery
   (b) Observation
(4) Answer questions directly.
   b. Outcomes
      (1) Patient expresses fewer concerns and fears.
      (2) Patient's body posture and facial expression are less tense.
C. Health education
   1. Abruptio placentae diagnosis education
      a. Assess patient's knowledge about abruptio placentae.
      b. Explain problem of placental separation before delivery using diagrams.
         (1) Risk to fetus
         (2) Risk to mother
      c. Describe symptoms to be reported immediately to health care providers.
         (1) Increased blood loss
         (2) Increased pain and contractions
         (3) Difficulty in breathing and dizziness
         (4) Rupture of membranes
      d. Define plan of care.
         (1) Fluid replacement
         (2) Blood product replacement, as needed
         (3) Need to monitor FHR and maternal status or changes
         (4) Reason for ultrasound scan
         (5) Preoperative preparation for possible cesarean section
         (6) Close observation of both mother and infant after delivery

DISSEMINATED INTRAVASCULAR COAGULATION

A. DIC (defibrination syndrome, defibrination coagulopathy, consumption coagulopathy) is a pathologic form of clotting that is diffuse and consumes large amounts of clotting factors, causing widespread external or internal bleeding or both (Benedetti, 2002; Fuller & Bucklin, 2007; Gonik, 1999; Horn, Davies, & Kean, 2000; Kilpatrick & Laros, 1999; Maresh, James, & Neales, 2000).
   1. Overactivation of clotting cascade and the fibrinolytic system
   2. Depletion of soluble clotting factors and platelets; lysis, or breakdown, of fibrinogen, which creates low fibrinogen levels and elevated FSP (or FDPs, fibrin degradation products).
B. Not a primary disease process, but it is a secondary process activated by a number of serious illnesses
C. Pathophysiology is dependent on inciting event and represents a failure of normal hemostatic function.
   1. Activation of intravascular coagulation and fibrinolytic pathway results in simultaneous fibrin clot formation and clot lysis.
   2. Microthrombi occlude small vessels, which results in tissue ischemia.
D. Possible clinical consequences of DIC
   1. Hemorrhage secondary to platelet consumption and depletion of clotting factors with potentiation by the anticoagulant effects of FDP or FSP
   2. Tissue hypoxia and ischemic necrosis secondary to obstruction of the microvasculature by fibrin plugs
   3. Microangiopathic hemolysis due to destruction of erythrocytes within the microvasculature

CLINICAL PRACTICE

A. Assessment
   1. History
      a. Patient presents with previous obstetric complications such as the following (Fuller & Bucklin, 2007):

      (1) Abruptio placentae

      (2) Intrauterine fetal death

      (3) Preeclampsia/eclampsia and HELLP (hemolysis, elevated liver [enzymes], low platelets) syndrome

      (4) Sepsis/systemic inflammatory response syndrome (SIRS)

      (5) Anaphylactoid syndrome of pregnancy (formerly called amniotic fluid embolism [AFE])

      (6) Gestational trophoblastic disease

      (7) Placenta accreta

      (8) Couvelaire uterus with concealed (internal) abruptio placentae

      (9) Hypovolemic shock after obstetric hemorrhage

         (a) Large blood loss with treatment of crystalloid and 5 to 10 units of PRBCs

         (b) Platelets and clotting factors depleted

     (10) Cardiopulmonary arrest

  b. Patient presents with medical complication during pregnancy, such as the following:

      (1) Thrombocytopenia

      (2) Vascular disorders

      (3) Acid-base imbalance

      (4) Malignancy

      (5) Hemolytic transfusion reaction; intravascular hemolysis

2. Physical findings: Diagnosis is based on clinical findings and laboratory markers (Cunningham et al, 2005; Kilpatrick & Laros, 2004; Labelle & Kitchens, 2005).

  a. Bleeding

      (1) Might occur from gums, nose, puncture sites, bladder, uterus, incision sites, episiotomy; might continuously ooze

      (2) Typically without clot formation

      (3) Abdomen may distend after cesarean section.

      (4) Increases the risks of thrombosis or hemorrhage, especially if low-grade DIC is present

      (5) Petechiae or purpura present

  b. Signs and symptoms of shock

      (1) Pale, clammy skin

      (2) Rising thready pulse rate and falling blood pressure

      (3) Altered level of response and consciousness

      (4) Organ hypoperfusion and tissue ischemia (e.g., respiratory distress, renal failure)

  c. Abnormal clotting study results (some, but not all, might be abnormal); platelets and activated partial thromboplastin time (aPTT) are cost-effective screenings, especially for preeclampsia.

      (1) Fibrinogen level less than 100 mg/dL; normal is 300 to 600 mg/dL during pregnancy

      (2) Platelet count less than 50,000; normal is 150,000 to 400,000 mm^3; symptomatic when less than 100,000 mm^3.

      (3) FSP present, elevated, or both; normal is 10 fg/mL.

      (4) D-dimer is positive in 34% of cases and is a specific diagnostic test.

      (5) Plasma antithrombin III (AT III) consumption

      (6) Elevated fibrinopeptide A

      (7) Abnormal PT and PTT (values might vary with method)

         (a) Thrombin time (TT) is 15 seconds.

         (b) PT is 11 seconds and at least 60%.

         (c) Whole blood clotting time (WBCT) is 4 to 12 minutes.

         (d) Activated coagulation time (ACT) by hand is 75 to 90 seconds.

         (e) PTT is 26 to 39 seconds.

      (8) Blood vessel and RBC damage

         (a) Arteriolar vasospasms damage the endothelial layer of small blood vessels, forming lesions that allow platelet aggregation and formation of a fibrin network.

         (b) When RBCs are forced through the fibrin network under high pressure, the cell membrane is morphologically damaged, causing schistocytes or abnormally shaped RBCs and hemolysis.

      (9) Leukocytosis

     (10) Positive result on protamine sulfate test, a coagulation test based on FSP

     (11) Abnormal clot retraction

       d. FHR patterns indicative of fetal distress
         (1) Loss of variability
         (2) Tachycardia or bradycardia
         (3) Late decelerations
         (4) Occasional sinusoidal pattern
  3. Psychosocial findings
       a. Maternal anxiety
         (1) Related to self
         (2) Related to infant
       b. Maternal sense of impending doom
       c. Maternal altered consciousness and response
  4. Diagnostic procedures
       a. Complete clotting studies
       b. Liver studies
       c. Arterial blood gas studies
       d. Type and crossmatching for blood products
       e. Measurement of fundal height as appropriate (see Physical Findings)
       f. Palpation for uterine tone and contractions

B. Interventions/Outcomes
  1. Ineffective maternal tissue perfusion from DIC
       a. Immediate interventions
         (1) Draw blood for clotting studies and send to laboratory.
            (a) Serial levels might be helpful in diagnosis.
            (b) Studies might be repeated as needed.
         (2) Cultures if sepsis is suspected
         (3) Establish IV line with large-bore intracatheter (16- or 18-gauge).
         (4) Administer fluid volume and blood products as ordered to replace and maintain circulating blood volume and clotting factors.
            (a) Anticipate aggressive fluid replacement therapy.
            (b) Crystalloids, colloids, albumin, plasmanate, cryoprecipitate, platelets, fresh frozen plasma, prothrombin, and packed erythrocytes might be used.
         (5) Monitor vital signs, including quality of respiratory rate and baseline characteristics.
         (6) Administer oxygen via face mask at 8 L/min; support cardiorespiratory system as needed.
         (7) Position patient for comfort and stabilization.
         (8) Administer medications as ordered.
            (a) Heparin use is rare and controversial; it is given to normalize PTT and prevent thrombosis.
               [i] Heparin effectiveness improves when AT III is more than 70%.
               [ii] Usual heparin dose is 2500 to 5000 units every 4 to 12 hours.
            (b) Other medications: AT III concentrates and antiplatelet drugs
       b. Outcomes: improved tissue perfusion shown by the following:
         (1) Decreased blood loss
         (2) Improved results in clotting studies
         (3) Improved vital signs
         (4) Normal or improved respirations
         (5) Improved color and warmth of skin
  2. Interventions to monitor ineffective fetal perfusion (if undelivered) related to maternal blood loss
       a. Interventions
         (1) Continuously monitor fetal heart for rate, variability, and sinusoidal pattern.
         (2) Avoid supine position when positioning patient for comfort.
         (3) Treat mother for alteration in tissue perfusion.
       b. Outcomes
         (1) Normal or improved FHR and variability

C. Health education
  1. Education about DIC
       a. Assess patient's knowledge of DIC and causative factors.

    b. Explain that blood is not clotting properly.
    c. Explain necessity for observation and tests.
        (1) Fetal monitoring
        (2) Coagulation factors
        (3) Signs of increased bleeding
        (4) Signs of other complications
    d. Prepare patient for events related to changing status.
        (1) Explain present plan of care.
        (2) Explain anticipated plan if condition intensifies.
    e. Explain immediate actions that will progress.
        (1) Fluid replacement
        (2) Laboratory testing and blood product replacement
        (3) Foley catheter insertion
        (4) Use of CVP or Swan-Ganz catheter to evaluate response to interventions and status
    f. Prepare patient for possibility of imminent events, such as:
        (1) Cesarean section
        (2) Postdelivery surgery
        (3) Critical care equipment and personnel

GESTATIONAL TROPHOBLASTIC DISEASE

A. **Gestational trophoblastic disease (GTD) describes a spectrum of trophoblastic diseases that have common clinical findings, such as abnormal proliferative tissues and abnormally high human chorionic gonadotropin (hCG) levels.**
B. **Hydatidiform mole (molar pregnancy) is characterized by chronic or acute bleeding and a uterus that is large for gestational age. It is characterized as complete or partial mole. Hydatidiform mole occurs 1 in 1200 pregnancies in the United States, with a higher incidence reported in Asian countries** (Berman, DiSaia, & Tewari, 2004).
C. **Gestational trophoblastic neoplasia (GTN) is persistent trophoblastic tissue that is assumed to be malignant** (Berman et al, 2004; Gilbert, 2007). **It is staged as low risk, intermediate risk, and high risk** (ACOG, 2004). **This is a curable gynecologic malignancy when there is early diagnosis** (Berman et al, 2004).
D. **Classifications have varied over the years, but the symptoms are unchanged for the hydatidiform mole and GTN.**

CLINICAL PRACTICE

A. Assessment
  1. History
    a. Excessively enlarged uterus in relation to the last menstrual period (LMP)
    b. Gestational hypertension prior to 24 weeks' gestation
    c. Differentiate type of hydatidiform mole (molar pregnancy).
        (1) Complete (classic)
          (a) Absence of maternal genetic tissue: no nucleus in fertilized egg
          (b) No fetus, placenta, amniotic membranes, or fluid
          (c) 20% neoplasia rate
          (d) Other microscopic differences from incomplete type occur.
        (2) Incomplete (partial)
          (a) Embryonic or fetal parts and an amniotic sac
          (b) Triploid karyotype: 69 chromosomes often present with extra paternal haploid set
          (c) 5% neoplasia rate
        (3) Increased risk for incidence
          (a) Women older than 40, or early teens
          (b) Previous history of ovulation stimulation with clomiphene (Clomid)
          (c) Genetic predisposition of gene translocation error
          (d) Risk of recurrence is 1% to 2%.

        (4) Invasive mole (chorioadenoma destruens)
          (a) Severity is intermediate between mole and choriocarcinoma: usually a locally invasive lesion
          (b) Occurs when trophoblastic tissue continues to grow
          (c) Trophoblastic tissue locally invades:
            [i] Uterine myometrium
            [ii] Pelvic blood vessels
            [iii] Vagina (occasionally)
          (d) Occurrence rate is 15% after hydatidiform mole.
    d. Choriocarcinoma
        (1) Highly malignant, with widespread metastasis to:
          (a) Lungs
          (b) Brain
          (c) Liver
          (d) Kidneys
          (e) Intestines
          (f) Spleen
          (g) Vagina
        (2) Not always preceded by molar pregnancy
          (a) About 25% of diagnosed choriocarcinoma is preceded by spontaneous abortion.
          (b) About 20% of cases of diagnosed choriocarcinoma occur after normal pregnancy when abnormal tissue proliferates.
        (3) About 5% of molar pregnancies turn into choriocarcinoma—normal value of serum interleukin-2 (SIL-2R) assay excludes choriocarcinoma.
        (4) High levels of human chorionic gonadotropin (hCG) persist after delivery, and serum granulocyte-macrophage colony-stimulating factor (GM-CSF) elevates when malignant.
  2. Physical findings
    a. Chronic or acute bleeding occurs by 12 weeks' gestation.
        (1) Overt or concealed bleeding
        (2) Brown (prune-juice colored) or bright red blood
    b. Rapidly enlarging uterus in relation to LMP.
        (1) Palpation is difficult because of soft tissue.
        (2) Ovaries might be enlarged and tender.
    c. Fetal heart rate is absent.
        (1) A single heartbeat is detected when the molar pregnancy affects one in a twin pregnancy.
    d. Increased risk of antepartal complications
        (1) Excessive nausea and vomiting
        (2) Abdominal cramping
        (3) Anemia
        (4) Preeclampsia at 9 to 12 weeks' gestation
  3. Diagnostic tests
    a. Elevated serial beta-hCG levels
    b. Ultrasonography confirmation
        (1) Shows molar pregnancy as numerous disorganized echoes or as abnormal gestational sacs
        (2) Diffuse "snowstorm" echo pattern
  4. Invasive neoplasia
    a. Neoplasia: chorioadenoma destruens or choriocarcinoma
        (1) Prognosis can be good or poor, depending on the extent of disease.
        (2) Condition often develops early as a blood-borne trophoblast.
        (3) Lungs are invaded in 75% of metastases.
          (a) Cough and bloody sputum are present.
          (b) Evidence of original lesion might disappear.
        (4) Also invades vagina (50%), vulva, kidney, liver, brain, ovaries, and bowel
        (5) Good prognosis
          (a) Detected and therapy started within 4 months of onset

(b) hCG levels less than 40,000 (mIU/ml) correct label (milli international unit/ml)

(c) No prior chemotherapy

(d) Cure rate of 90% to 100% when the foregoing are present

(6) Poor prognosis

(a) Detected at more than 4 months' duration

(b) hCG levels of greater than 40,000 (mIU/ml) or rising indicate extensive disease

(c) Prior chemotherapy failure

(d) Metastasis to brain and liver (irradiation might be useful)

(e) Occurs after a term pregnancy

(f) Remission rate is 45% to 65% when the above-listed factors (a through e) are present

(g) Death is usually a result of hemorrhage.

5. Complications

a. Adult respiratory distress syndrome (2% to 11%)

(1) Pulmonary edema

(2) Pulmonary emboli

b. Preeclampsia at less than 24 weeks' gestation

c. Hyperthyroidism; thyrotoxicosis

d. Theca-lutein cysts

e. Sepsis (20% to 50%)

B. **Interventions/Outcomes**

1. Insufficient knowledge of trophoblastic disease and loss of pregnancy state

a. Immediate interventions

(1) Assess patient's knowledge of her specific trophoblastic disease.

(2) Clarify and verify knowledge base of the state of molar pregnancy.

(3) Encourage compliance with a close follow-up regimen (see Health Education for specifics of follow-up).

(4) Discuss contraceptive options and reason to prevent pregnancy for 1 year (see Chapter 15 for a complete discussion of contraception).

(5) Encourage patient to verbalize concerns about cancer threat.

b. Outcomes

(1) Patient complies with follow-up plan.

(2) Patient maintains contraception plan for 1 year.

C. **Health education**

1. Gestational trophoblastic disease

a. Provide information on condition, symptoms, and cause; explain the following:

(1) Abnormal formation of a pregnancy

(2) Cause unknown

(3) Presence of placental tissue and absence of fetal tissue

(4) Symptoms of nausea, vomiting, cramping, and bleeding

b. Describe events to expect during evacuation procedures.

(1) Vacuum curettage as the preferred procedure

(a) Medication for pain

(b) Cramping and bleeding

(c) Environment and equipment to be used

(2) Hysterectomy procedure is performed when:

(a) Excessive bleeding is present.

(b) Patient is more than 40 years of age.

c. 1-year follow-up plan consists of:

(1) hCG levels

(a) Weekly for 3 weeks

(b) Monthly for 6 months

(c) Every 2 months for 6 months

(d) No pregnancy for 1 year

(2) Chest radiograph

d. Acknowledge family concerns and provide information about resources for support.

CASE STUDIES AND STUDY QUESTIONS

Ms. A., a 29-year-old, gravida 6, para 1 (G6, P1) woman, has been admitted to a local level-I hospital at 26 weeks' gestation complaining of painless vaginal bleeding. Vital signs are stable, hematocrit is 30.5%, and an ultrasound scan reveals a complete placenta previa. She is given IV magnesium sulfate and oral terbutaline for mild uterine contractions and transferred to a level-III (tertiary) regional hospital. After 12 days hospitalization, no further bleeding is noted and Ms. A. is discharged to home on bed rest. She lives within 15 minutes of the hospital.

Upon readmission for bleeding at 29 weeks, about 200 mL of vaginal blood is noted. Ms. A. is started on a graduated-dose regimen of magnesium sulfate, 5 g the first hour, 4 g the second hour, 3 g the next hour, and then a maintenance dose. At this time, an ultrasound scan reveals a complete previa, grade II placenta, and transverse fetal lie.

On the tenth day of admission, uterine contractions and increased amounts of bleeding begin. Her hematocrit is 25.9%, hemoglobin value is 8.5 g/dL, vital signs are stable, and an NST is reactive. On day 14 she experiences spontaneous rupture of membranes (SROM) with clear amniotic fluid, increasing uterine contractions, persistent bloody drainage; ultrasonography shows an oblique lie. A cesarean section is performed, and the placenta previa is noted to have abrupted free of the internal os. The combined blood loss before and during surgery is estimated at 2000 mL.

In the recovery room, lochia rubra is light to moderate, the fundus is firm at the umbilicus, and oxygen saturation (SaO$_2$) is 98% to 99%. Ms. A. receives a continuous infusion of Ringer's lactate with 20 units of oxytocin, morphine sulfate for pain, an additional 2 units of PRBCs, and prophylactic ampicillin.

1. The initial hospital admission exam of Ms. A. should omit examination of:
   a. Fetal heart tones
   b. Vaginal bleeding
   c. Vaginal exam
   d. Blood pressure
2. As Ms. A.'s nurse, you should know that a transverse lie:
   a. Is an isolated condition
   b. Indicates an occiput presentation of either left occipitotransverse (LOT) or right occipitotransverse (ROT)
   c. Has an increased incidence with placenta previa
   d. Will be rotated by her physician to a normal presentation

3. Measuring her hematocrit periodically:
   a. Will prevent undue blood loss
   b. Reflects the normal hemodilution of her pregnancy
   c. Reflects the need for cryoprecipitate
   d. Serially reflects her blood loss from placenta previa
4. As Ms. A.'s high-risk antepartum nurse, which action would you initiate?
   a. Enrollment in hospital preterm infant care program
   b. Instruction before discharge to home about the danger signs of bleeding and cramping
   c. Chain-of-command process to deny discharge to home order
   d. Enrollment in hospital childbirth exercise program

Ms. P. is a 21-year-old Laotian Hmong, G4, P3 woman, with a history of one cesarean section followed by two vaginal births after cesarean (VBAC) who appears at the hospital complaining of vaginal bleeding. She is uncertain of her estimated date of confinement (EDC), and an ultrasound scan places her at 27 to 28 weeks' gestation with an anterior fundal placenta and breech presentation. Her vital signs are stable, hematocrit is 34.1%, hemoglobin value is 11.5 g/dL, and during the next 2 weeks, Ms. P. experiences small amounts of dark, bloody discharge with occasional scant, bright red mucus-like bleeding.

Ms. P. remains hospitalized and receives a tapering magnesium sulfate regimen; oral terbutaline, 2.5 mg every 3 hours; oral indomethacin, 25 mg every 6 hours; and steroids for stimulating fetal lung maturity.

On day 14 she has increased mucus and bloody discharge, low back pain, and cramps, and she seems tense. She refuses lunch. Now the uterine tone is palpable and cervical changes are noted; the FHR is 160 with decreased variability, and variable decelerations occur with uterine contractions.

A decision is made to perform a cesarean section. Ms. P. is now at 29 to 30 weeks' gestation. During the surgery, a 20% to 25% abruption is noted with a 200-g retroplacental clot; estimated blood loss at delivery is 800 mL. A 1360-g (3-pound) girl with Apgar scores of 5 and 6 is delivered, and no immediate respiratory distress is noted.

Although Ms. P. recovers well, her second-day hematocrit is 22%, and her hemoglobin value is 7.3 g/dL; 2 units of PRBCs are administered. On postpartum day 3 she is discharged in stable condition with a hematocrit of 30% and a hemo-globin value of 9.7 g/dL.

5. As her intrapartum nurse you:
   a. Recognize the potential of abruptio pla-centae and request an ultrasound scan.
   b. Reassure her that her infant is fine right now.
   c. Request a Kleihauer-Betke blood test.
   d. Recognize the symptoms of uterine rup-ture and request an emergency cesarean section.

6. At delivery a retroplacental clot was noted near the center of the placenta. If Ms. P. con-tinued to bleed from the clot site, she would have been likely to develop:
   a. Iatrogenic thrombocytopenia
   b. Revealed bleeding
   c. Couvelaire uterus
   d. Uterine rupture

7. If Ms. P. had not undergone a cesarean, and was in labor, the following scenario might have occurred. At 9 cm, she suddenly loses consciousness; she becomes cyanotic; she has shallow, irregular respirations and a rapid, thready pulse; and the FHR is decreased to 50 beats per minute. These are symptoms of:
   a. Precipitous delivery
   b. Abruptio placentae
   c. Impending cardiac arrest
   d. Supine hypotension

8. This situation:
   a. Is associated with consumptive coagulopathy
   b. Is associated with abruptio placentae
   c. Occurs frequently with abruptio placentae
   d. Describes an unrealistic event

Ms. G. is a 15-year old G1, P0, 167.6 cm, 73.5 kg (5 feet, 6 inches, 162 pounds) woman who is 14 weeks' gestation by figured EDC from LMP. Her fundal height is 20 cm with a positive B-hCG. She has had an initial prenatal examination with her primary care practitioner. No ultrasounds have been done. She smokes one pack of ciga-rettes a day. She presents to the emergency room with nausea, vomiting, anxiety, and dark brown bleeding resembling the color of prune juice. Her mother is at her bedside and concerned about her daughter's condition.

9. A stat transabdominal ultrasound is com-peted after Ms. G.'s bladder is filled per catheter. The ultrasound results indicate no fetal heart rate and a diffuse "snowstorm" pattern. This is indicative of the diagnosis of:
   a. Partial placenta previa
   b. Hydatidiform molar pregnancy
   c. 40% placental abruption
   d. Normal gestational assessment for 14 weeks' gestation

10. Ms. G.'s discharge instructions after this pregnancy will include:
    a. Frequent B-hCG levels for 1 year
    b. Resume ovulation stimulation with clomi-phene (Clomid).
    c. Prevent pregnancy for 5 years.
    d. Select an intrauterine device (IUD) as a contraceptive technique.

ANSWERS TO STUDY QUESTIONS

1. c
2. c
3. d
4. b
5. a

6. c
7. c
8. b
9. b
10. a

REFERENCES

American College of Obstetricians and Gynecologists (Ed.), (1998). *Postpartum hemorrhage (Educational Bulletin No. 243)*. Washington, DC: ACOG.

American College of Obstetricians and Gynecologists (Ed.), (1999). *Prevention of Rh D alloimmunization (Practice Bulletin No. 4)*. Washington, DC: ACOG.

American College of Obstetricians and Gynecologists (Ed.), (2000). *Obstetric aspects of trauma management (Practice Bulletin No. 251)*. Washington, DC: ACOG.

American College of Obstetricians & Gynecologists (Ed.), (2004). *Diagnosis and treatment of gestational trophoblastic disease (Practice Bulletin No. 53)*. Wash-ington, DC: ACOG.

Ananth, C., Demissie, K., Smulian, J., & Vintzileos, A. (2003). Placenta previa in singleton and twin births in the United States, 1989 through 1998: A comparison of risk factor profiles and associated conditions. *American Journal of Obstetrics & Gynecology, 188*(1), 275–282.

Ananth, C., Oyelese, Y., Yeo, L., Prahdan, A., & Vintzileos, A. (2005). Placental abruption in the United States, 1979 through 2001: Temporal trends and potential determinants. *American Journal of Obstetrics & Gynecology, 192*(1), 191–198.

Baron, F., & Hill, W. C. (2002). Managing placenta previa and abruptio placentae on an outpatient basis. In W. C. Hill (Ed.), *Ambulatory obstetrics* (pp. 65–72). Philadelphia: Lippincott Williams & Wilkins.

Baumann, P., Blackwell, S. C., Schild, C., Berry, S. M., & Friedrich, H. J. (2000). Mathematic modeling to predict abruptio placentae. *American Journal of Obstetrics & Gynecology, 183*(4), 815–822.

Benedetti, T. J. (2002). Obstetric hemorrhage. In S. G. Gabbe, J. R. Niebyl, & J. L. Simpson (Eds.), *Obstetrics: Normal and problem pregnancies* (4th ed, pp. 503–538). New York: Churchill Livingstone.

Berman, M., DiSai, P., & Tewari, K. (2004). Pelvic malignancy, gestational trophoblastic neoplasm, and nonpelvic malignancies. In R. Creasy, R. Resnik, & J. Iams (Eds.), *Maternal-fetal medicine: Principles and practice* (5th ed.). Philadelphia: Saunders.

Blackburn, S. T. (2007). *Maternal, fetal, & neonatal physiology: A clinical perspective* (3rd ed.). St. Louis: Saunders.

Carter, S. (1999). Overview of common obstetric bleeding disorders. *Nurse Practitioner, 24*(3), 50–51, 54, 57–58.

Centers for Disease Control and Prevention (2003). Pregnancy-related mortality surveillance—United States, 1991–1999. CDC Surveillance Summaries, February 21, 2003. *MMWR Morbidity and Mortality Weekly Report, 52*(SS02), 1–8.

Chang, J., Elam-Evans, L., & Berg, C. J. (2003). Pregnancy-related mortality surveillance—United States, 1991-1999. *MMWR Morbidity and Mortality Weekly Report, 52*(1), 2003.

Chichakli, L. O., Atrash, H. K., MacKay, A. P., Musani, A. S., & Berg, C. J. (1999). Pregnancy-related mortality in the United States due to hemorrhage: 1979–1992. *Obstetrics & Gynecology, 94*(5 Pt 1), 721–725.

Clark, S. L. (2004). Placenta previa and abruptio placenta. In R. Creasy, & R. Resnik (Eds.), *Maternal-fetal medicine: Principles and practice* (5th ed.). Philadelphia: Saunders.

Cnattingius, S. (1997). Maternal age modifies the effect of maternal smoking on intrauterine growth retardation but not on late fetal death and placental abruption. *American Journal of Epidemiology, 145*(4), 319–323.

Conklin, K. A., & Backus, A. M. (1999). In D. H. Chestnut (Ed.), *Obstetric anesthesia: Principles and practice* (2nd ed., pp. 17–42). St. Louis: Mosby.

Connolly, A. M., Katz, V. L., Bash, K. L., McMahon, M., & Hansen, W. (1997). Trauma and pregnancy. *American Journal of Perinatology, 14*(6), 331–336.

Copeland, L., & Landon, M. (2007). Malignant diseases and pregnancy. In S. Gabbe, J. Niebyl, & J. Simpson (Eds.), *Obstetrics: Normal and problem pregnancies* (5th ed.). New York: Churchill Livingstone.

Coppens, M., & James, D. K. (1999). Organization of prenatal care and identification of risk. In D. K. James, P. J. Steer, C. P. Weiner, & B. Gonik (Eds.), *High risk pregnancy: Management options* (2nd ed., pp. 11–22). Philadelphia: Saunders.

Cunningham, F., Leveno, K., Bloom, S., Hauth, J., Gilstrap, L., & Wenstrom, K. (2005). *Williams obstetrics* (22nd ed.). New York: McGraw-Hill.

Curet, M. J., Schermer, C. R., Demarest, G. B., Bieneik, E., & Curet, L. (2000). Predictors of outcome in trauma during pregnancy: Identification of patients who can be monitored for less than 6 hours. *Journal of Trauma, 49*(1), 18–25.

Daddario, J. B. (1999). Trauma in pregnancy. In L. K. Mandeville, & N. H. Troiano (Eds.), *High-risk and critical care intrapartum nursing* (2nd ed.). Philadelphia: Lippincott.

Davies, S. (1999). Amniotic fluid embolism and isolated disseminated intravascular coagulation. *Canadian Journal of Anesthesia, 46*(5 Pt 1), 456–459.

Davies, S. (2001). Amniotic fluid embolus: A review of the literature. *Canadian Journal of Anesthesia, 48*(1), 88–98.

Dildy, G. A., III (2002). Postpartum hemorrhage: New management options. *Clinical Obstetrics and Gynecology, 45*(2), 330–344.

Feinstein, N., & Atterbury, J. L. (2003). Intrinsic influences on the fetal heart rate. In N. Feinstein, K. L. Torgersen, & J. L. Atterbury (Eds.), *AWHONN fetal heart monitoring: Principles and practices* (3rd ed.). Dubuque, IA: Kendall-Hunt.

Flamm, B. L. (2001). Vaginal birth after cesarean: Reducing medical and legal risks. *Clinical Obstetrics and Gynecology, 44*(3), 622–629.

Francois, K., & Foley, M. (2007). Antepartum and Postpartum Hemorrhage. In S. Gabbe, J. Niebyl, & J. Simpson (Eds.), *Obstetrics: Normal and problem pregnancies* (5th ed.). New York: Churchill Livingstone.

Franklin, C. M., Darovic, G. O., & Dan, B. B. (2002). Monitoring the patient in shock. In G. O. Darovic (Ed.), *Hemodynamic monitoring: Invasive and noninvasive clinical application* (3rd ed.). Philadelphia: Saunders.

Fuller, A. J., & Bucklin, B. (2007). Blood component therapy in obstetrics. *Obstetrics and Gynecology Clinics of North America, 34*(2007), 443–458.

Gilbert, E. S. (2007). *Manual of high risk pregnancy & delivery* (4th ed.). St. Louis: Mosby.

Goddijn-Wessel, T. A., Wouters, M. G., Van de Molen, E. S., Spuijbroek, M. D., Steegers-Theunissen, R. P., Blom, H. J., et al. (1996). Hyperhomocysteinemia: A risk factor for placental abruption or infarction. *European Journal of Obstetrics, Gynecology, and Reproductive Biology, 66*(1), 23–29.

Gonik, B. (1999). Intensive care monitoring of the critically ill pregnant patient. In R. Creasy, & R. Resnick (Eds.), *Maternal-fetal medicine* (4th ed.). Philadelphia: Saunders.

Hankins, G. D. V., & O'Day, M. P. (1997). Disseminated intravascular coagulation. In S. L. Clark, D. B. Cotton, G. D. V. Hankins, & J. P. Phelan (Eds.), *Critical care obstetrics* (3rd ed., pp. 551–563). Boston: Blackwell Scientific.

Horn, E., Davies, J., & Kean, L. (2000). Other hematologic conditions. In D. K. James, P. J. Steer, C. P. Weiner, & B. Gonik (Eds.), *High risk pregnancy: Management options* (2nd ed.). Philadelphia: Saunders.

Hull, A. D., & Resnik, R. (2009). Placenta previa, placenta accreta, abruptio placentae and vasa previa. In R. Creasy, R. Resnik, & J. Iams (Eds.), *Creasy & Resnik's maternal-fetal medicine: Principles and practice* (6th ed., pp. 725–737). Philadelphia: Saunders.

Jackson, M., & Branch, D. W. (2003). Alloimmunization in pregnancy. In S. G. Gabbe, J. R. Niebyl, & J. L. Simpson (Eds.), *Pocket companion to accompany Obstetrics: Normal and problem pregnancies* (pp. 545–569). Philadelphia: Churchill Livingstone.

Kilpatrick, S., & Laros, R. (2004). Maternal hematologic disorders. In R. Creasy, R. Resnik, & J. Iams (Eds.), *Maternal-fetal medicine: Principles and practice* (5th ed.). Philadelphia: Saunders.

Konje, J. C., & Taylor, D. J. (1999). Bleeding in late pregnancy. In D. K. James, P. J. Steer, C. P. Weiner, & B. Gonik (Eds.), *High risk pregnancy: Management options* (2nd ed., pp. 111–128). Philadelphia: Saunders.

Koonin, L. M., MacKay, A. P., Berg, C. J., Atrash, H. K., & Smith, J. C. (1997). Pregnancy-related mortality surveillance—United States, 1987–1990. CDC surveillance summaries, August 8, 1997. *MMWR Morbidity and Mortality Weekly Report, 46*(SS04), 17–36.

Kramer, M. S., Usher, R. H., Pollak, R., Boyd, M., & Usher, S. (1997). Etiologic determinants of abruptio placentae. *Obstetrics & Gynecology, 89*(2), 221–226.

Labelle, C., & Kitchens, C. (2005). Disseminated intravascular coagulation: Treat the cause not the lab values. *Cleveland Clinic Journal of Medicine, 72*(5), 377–397.

Lanni, S. M., & Seeds, J. W. (2002). Malpresentations. In S. G. Gabbe, J. R. Niebyl, & J. L. Simpson (Eds.), *Obstetrics: Normal and problem pregnancies* (4th ed., pp. 493). New York: Churchill Livingstone.

Lockwood, C. J., & Funai, E. F. (1999). In J. T. Queenan (Ed.), *Management of high-risk pregnancy* (4th ed., pp. 466–474). Malden, MA: Blackwell Science.

Maresh, M., James, D., & Neales, K. (2000). Critical care of the obstetric patent. In D. K. James, P. J. Steer, C. P. Weiner, & B. Gonik (Eds.), *High risk pregnancy: Management options* (2nd ed.). Philadelphia: Saunders.

Martin, J. A., Hamilton, B. E., Ventura, S. J., Menacker, F., & Park, M. M. (2002). *Births: Final data for 2000.* Hyattsville, MD: National Center for Health Statistics National Vital Statistics Reports, *50*(5).

Murphy, S. L. (2000). *Deaths: Final data for 1998.* Hyattsville, MD: National Center for Health Statistics National Vital Statistics Reports, *48*(11).

National Vital Statistics Report (April 2009). Deaths: Final data for 2006. U.S. Department of Health and Human Services. *Centers for Disease Control and Prevention, 57*(14), DHHS Publication No. PHS 2009–1120.

Neilson, J. (2001). Interventions for suspected placenta previa (Cochrane Review). In *The Cochrane Library* Oxford: Update Software, Issue 2.

Odunsi, K., Bullough, C. H., Henzel, J., & Polanska, A. (1996). Evaluation of chemical tests for fetal bleeding from vasa previa. *International Journal of Gynaecology and Obstetrics, 55*(3), 207–212.

Pak, L. L., Reece, E. A., & Chan, L. (1998). Is adverse pregnancy outcome predictable after blunt abdominal trauma? *American Journal of Obstetrics and Gynecology, 179*(5), 1140–1144.

Penning, D. (2001). Trauma in pregnancy. *Canadian Journal of Anaesthesia, 48*, R7.

Samuels, P. (1997). Acute care of thrombocytopenia and disseminated intravascular coagulation complicating pregnancy. In M. Foley, & T. Strong (Eds.), *Obstetric intensive care.* Philadelphia: Saunders.

Secor, V. H. (1996). *Multiple organ dysfunction & failure: Pathophysiology and clinical implications* (2nd ed.). St. Louis: Mosby.

Seeds, J. W., & Walsh, M. (2002). Malpresentations. In S. G. Gabbe, J. R. Niebyl, & J. L. Simpson (Eds.), *Obstetrics: Normal and problem pregnancies* (4th ed.). New York: Churchill Livingstone.

Silver, L. E., Hobel, C. J., Lagasse, L., Luttrull, J., & Platt, L. (1997). Placenta previa percreta with bladder involvement: New considerations and review of the literature. *Ultrasound in Obstetrics and Gynecology, 9*(2), 131–138.

Silver, R. M., Landon, M. B., & Rouse, D. J. (2006). Maternal morbidity associated with multiple repeat cesarean deliveries. *Obstetrics & Gynecology, 107*(6), 1226–1232.

Simpson, K. R., & Creehan, P. A. (2001). Guidelines for home care management of high-risk pregnancy conditions. In K. R. Simpson, & P. A. Creehan (Eds.), *AWHONN perinatal nursing* (2nd ed., pp. 292–296). Philadelphia: Lippincott Williams & Wilkins.

Sosa, M. E. B. (2001). High risk pregnancy, bleeding disorders. In K. R. Simpson, & P. A. Creehan (Eds.), *AWHONN perinatal nursing* (2nd ed., pp. 190–206). Philadelphia: Lippincott Williams & Wilkins.

Taipale, P., Hiilesmaa, V., & Ylostalo, P. (1997). Diagnosis of placenta previa by transvaginal sonographic screening at 12–16 weeks in a nonselected population. *Obstetrics & Gynecology, 89*(3), 364–367.

VandeKerkhove, K., & Johnson, T. (1998). Bleeding in the second half of pregnancy. In M. Pearlman, & J. Tintinalli (Eds.), *Emergency care of the woman* (pp. 77–98). New York: McGraw-Hill Health Professions Division.

Ventura, S. J., Martin, J. A., Curtin, S. C., Menacker, F., & Hamilton, B. E. (2001). *Births: Final data for 1999.* Hyattsville, MD: National Center for Health Statistics National Vital Statistics Reports, 49(1).

Wing, D., Paul, R., & Millar, L. (1996). Management of the symptomatic placenta previa: A randomized, controlled trial of inpatient versus outpatient expectant management. *American Journal of Obstetrics & Gynecology, 175*(4 Pt 1), 806–811.

Yap, O. W., Kim, E. S., & Laros, R. K., Jr. (2001). Maternal and neonatal outcomes after uterine rupture in labor. *American Journal of Obstetrics & Gynecology, 184*(7), 1576–1581.

22 Endocrine and Metabolic Disorders

Lucy R. Van Otterloo

OBJECTIVES

1. Describe maternal and fetal complications associated with endocrine and metabolic disorders in pregnancy.
2. Recognize alterations in pregnancy associated with various endocrine and metabolic disorders.
3. Identify signs and symptoms associated with endocrine and metabolic disorders diagnosed prior to conception or during pregnancy that require specific nursing interventions and care for the childbearing woman and her fetus.
4. Evaluate significant clinical signs and symptoms characterized by various endocrine and metabolic disorders during the childbearing period.
5. Plan assessments and interventions essential in caring for the childbearing woman with an endocrine or metabolic disorder.
6. Implement specific educational content and strategies to empower the childbearing woman with an endocrine or metabolic disorder to knowledgeably participate in her plan of care throughout the childbearing experience.

DIABETES MELLITUS

A. **Definition**
   1. Chronic, systemic endocrine disorder of insulin production or of the body's response to insulin
   2. Caused by absent or inadequate insulin secretion or increased cellular resistance to insulin, resulting in its impaired utilization.
   3. Characterized by an abnormal metabolism of carbohydrates, proteins, fats, and electrolytes, resulting in hyperglycemia and other systemic metabolic disturbances
   4. Might be associated with severe neurologic, cardiovascular, ocular, renal, and microvascular complications
   5. Classified according to cause rather than treatment
   6. Complicates more than 200,000 pregnancies per year in the United States (American Diabetes Association [ADA], 2009a)
B. **Symptoms**
   1. Excessive thirst and hunger
   2. Frequent urination
   3. Fatigue
   4. Blurred vision
   5. Weight loss
   6. Recurrent infections
   7. Often asymptomatic in its early stages
C. **Classification**
   1. Type 1 diabetes mellitus (formerly insulin-dependent diabetes mellitus [IDDM])
      a. Cause is an absolute deficiency of insulin secretion by the pancreatic beta cells
      b. Might occur by an autoimmune process involved in beta-cell destruction, genetic defects, and disease of the pancreas, endocrinopathies, and use of certain drugs
      c. Usually appears before the age of 30 years
      d. Has an abrupt onset of symptoms requiring prompt medical treatment
      e. Approximately 5% of those diagnosed with diabetes have type 1 diabetes.

2. Type 2 diabetes mellitus (formerly non–insulin-dependent diabetes mellitus [NIDDM])
   a. Cause is a combination of resistance to insulin action and an inadequate compensatory insulin secretory response
   b. Type 2 diabetes is diagnosed primarily in adults older than 30 years of age, but is now seen more frequently in children. Is often associated with obesity and sedentary lifestyle.
   c. Disease is typically symptom-free for many years, with slow onset and gradual progression of symptoms.
   d. Type 2 diabetes increases with age, accounting for approximately 95% of all diagnosed cases of diabetes.
   e. Disease is managed with diet and exercise: The use of oral hypoglycemic medications and/or insulin might also be indicated when hyperglycemia persists. Almost all need insulin for optimum control during pregnancy.
3. Gestational diabetes mellitus (GDM)
   a. Defined as any degree of glucose intolerance with onset or first recognition during pregnancy (Metzger et al, 2007); further categorized into A1 (controlled with diet and exercise) and A2 (controlled with diet, exercise and requiring the addition of oral meds and/or insulin)
   b. Estimated to occur in approximately 4% of pregnancies; however, prevalence might range from 1% to 14%, depending on the population studied and diagnostic test used (ADA, 2009a). Accounts for approximately 90% of all diabetes in pregnancy.
   c. Women diagnosed with GDM are at increased risk for developing diabetes (DM2) later in life.
   d. Symptoms are generally mild and not life-threatening in the pregnant woman.
   e. Maternal hyperglycemia is associated with increased fetal morbidity secondary to fetal hyperinsulinemia, which potentiates fetal size (large for gestational age [LGA] or macrosomia greater than 4500 g); therefore, maintenance of normal glucose levels is required for optimal perinatal outcome (Table 22-1).
4. Impaired fasting glucose (IFG) and impaired glucose tolerance (IGT)
   a. Characterized by hyperglycemia at a level lower than what qualifies as a diagnosis of diabetes.
   b. Symptoms of diabetes are absent.
   c. Infants born to women with IGT are at increased risk for being LGA.
D. **Maternal metabolism and pathophysiology in pregnancy**
   1. Changes in carbohydrate, protein, and fat metabolism in normal pregnancy are profound, mediated in part by the developing fetus and production of placental hormones.
   2. First half of pregnancy is considered an anabolic phase (protein and fat storage).
      a. In pregnant women without diabetes, this is associated with increased estrogen and progesterone secretion, leading to pancreatic beta-cell hyperplasia and hyperinsulinemia.
      b. Increased insulin production leads to an increased tissue response to insulin and increased uptake and storage of glycogen and fat in the liver and other tissues.

■ TABLE 22-1
■ ■ **Blood Glucose Values in Pregnancy**

	Ideal*	Goal
Fasting blood glucose	60-89 mg/dL	<90 mg/dL
1 hour postprandial	100-129 mg/dL	<140 mg/dL
Mean blood glucose	87 mg/dL	<100 mg/dL
Hemoglobin A_{1c}	2%-5%	<7%

*These values are demonstrated in women with neither diabetes nor carbohydrate intolerance during pregnancy.
Sources: Metzger B.E., Lowe L.P., Dyer A.R., Trimble E.R., Chaovarindr U., Coustan D.R., Hadden D.R., McCance D.R., Hod M., McIntyre H.D., Oats J.J., Persson B., Rogers M.S., Sacks D.A., (2008). HAPO Study Cooperative Research Group: Hyperglycemia and adverse pregnancy outcomes. *New England Journal of Medicine*, 358(19), 1991-2002;
Combs, C.A., Gavin, L.A., Gunderson, E., Main, E.K., & Kitzmiller, J.L. (1992). Relationship of fetal macrosomia to maternal postprandial glucose control during pregnancy. *Diabetes Care*, 15, 1251-1257.

3. Second half of pregnancy is characterized by a catabolic phase (protein and fat breakdown) with increased insulin resistance due to the production of placental hormones (prolactin, human chorionic somatomammotropin [HCS]), cortisol, and growth hormones, which are diabetogenic and act as insulin antagonists; in women who cannot meet the increasing demands for insulin production, this leads to altered carbohydrate metabolism and progressive hyperglycemia; characteristics of this catabolic phase include:
   a. Increased production of HCS
   b. Elevated levels of estrogen, progesterone, blood triglycerides, free fatty acids, and serum cortisol
   c. Tendency for decreased glycogenesis and increased lipolysis, gluconeogenesis, and ketone production; maternal lipolysis provides maternal fuel needs while sparing glucose for fetal use, creating a starvation-like state in the mother (accelerated starvation of pregnancy)
4. The developing fetus continuously removes glucose and amino acids from the maternal circulation.
   a. Glucose and amino acids are readily transported across the placenta to the developing fetus; insulin is not easily transported.
   b. Maternal hyperglycemia leads to fetal beta-cell hyperplasia and fetal hyperinsulinemia.
      (1) Fetal hyperinsulinism functions as a growth hormone for the developing fetus.
      (2) Fetal hyperinsulinism contributes to increased fetal size and leads to a decrease in surfactant production, with potential development of respiratory distress syndrome in the neonate.
5. The constant transport of maternal glucose levels across the placenta leads to lowered blood glucose levels (hypoglycemia) and explains the lower fasting blood glucose levels observed during normal pregnancy. Note: Fasting blood glucose levels decline 10% to 20% in the first trimester when fetal demands for glucose are low.

E. **Primary goals in the treatment of diabetes and pregnancy**
   1. Achieve and maintain normal maternal glucose levels. Note: Normal blood glucose levels are lower during pregnancy than in the nonpregnant state.
   2. Promptly identify and manage complications associated with diabetes and pregnancy in the childbearing woman, fetus, and neonate.

CLINICAL PRACTICE

Pregestational Diabetes (Type 1 and Type 2 Diabetes)

A. **Assessment**
   1. Definition and prognosis
      a. Type 1 diabetes is primarily a chronic autoimmune disorder resulting from the destruction of the pancreatic beta-cells, which usually leads to absolute insulin deficiency.
      b. Type 2 diabetes arises because of insulin resistance, sometimes combined with relative insulin deficiency.
      c. Predisposition is genetically determined.
   2. Incidence
      a. Incidence of pregestational diabetes is approximately 1% of all pregnancies and affects 10,000 to 14,000 women annually (American College of Obstetricians and Gynecologists [ACOG], 2005).
      b. Pregestational diabetes accounts for 10% of all diabetic pregnancies.
   3. Prognosis
      a. Pregnant women with pregestational diabetes might be categorized prognostically according to the classic system of White, with some minor modifications (Table 22-2).
      b. The quality of metabolic regulation (diabetic control) throughout pregnancy and the presence or absence of serious complications of diabetes, especially nephropathy, hypertension, and heart disease, account for most of the risks associated with diabetes in pregnancy rather than the genetic characteristics of the maternal diabetes.
      c. Observe for complications associated with diabetes: ketoacidosis, preeclampsia, and pyelonephritis.

■ TABLE 22-2
■ ■ **Modified White's Classification of Diabetes in Pregnancy**

Class	Age of Onset	Duration	Vascular Disease	Treatment
A	Any	Any	None	Diet alone
A1	During pregnancy		None	Diet alone
A2	During pregnancy		None	Insulin
B	≥20	<10	None	Insulin
C	10-19	or 10-19	None	Insulin
D	≤10	or >20	Benign (hypertension, background retinopathy)	Insulin
F	Any	Any	Nephropathy	Insulin
R	Any	Any	Proliferative retinopathy	Insulin
H	Any	Any	Cardiac disease	Insulin
T	Any	Any	Renal transplant	Insulin

(1) Diabetic ketoacidosis (DKA) affects about 5% to 10% of diabetic pregnancies (ACOG, 2005); associated with:
   (a) Poor glycemic control
   (b) Hyperemesis gravidarum contributing to dehydration
   (c) Tocolytic therapy (beta-sympathomimetic agents)
   (d) Infections (most common)
   (e) Insulin pump failure
(2) Risk of preeclampsia increases with diabetes; complicates 15% to 20% of diabetic pregnancies versus 5% of nondiabetic pregnancies (ACOG, 2005)
(3) Maternal infections occur more frequently in diabetic pregnancies than in nondiabetic pregnancies.

4. History
   a. Preconceptual assessments for preexisting diabetics
      (1) Classification of diabetes in pregnancy
      (2) Blood glucose control, HbA_{1c} (glycosylated hemoglobin), and frequency of self-blood glucose monitoring (SBGM)
      (3) Presence of vascular complications and current vascular status; evaluation of renal, retinal, neural, and cardiac status is recommended if duration of diabetes is longer than 5 years.
      (4) Thyroid panel (type 1 diabetic women only)
      (5) Neuropathy, retinopathy, nephropathy and CVD treatment if indicated
      (6) Adequacy of current diet and plans for dietary adjustments in pregnancy
         (a) Recommended total calorie intake is 30 kcal/kg prepregnant weight of nonobese individuals given as three meals and three snacks (ACOG, 2005). For obese women with a body mass index (BMI) greater than 30, a calorie restriction to approximately 24 kcal/kg actual weight per day (ACOG, 2005)
         (b) Recommended dietary composition is 40% to 45% carbohydrate, 12% to 20% protein, and 35% to 40% unsaturated fat (Reece & Homko, 2008).
      (7) Medications should be evaluated. Current insulin regimen might need to be adjusted to attain euglycemia. Note: Women with type 2 diabetes on oral hypoglycemic agents might need to be controlled on insulin prior to conception (contributing to an increase in weight prior to pregnancy); oral agents (glyburide, metformin) in pregnancy may be considered if compliance with insulin regimen is questionable (Langer, Yogev, Xenakis, & Rosenn, 2005; Rowan, Hague, Gao, Battin, & Moore, 2008).

(8) Understanding of self-care responsibilities and comprehensive collaborative management of diabetes in pregnancy to promote optimal perinatal outcomes

(9) Current lifestyle and related health habits

    (a) Exercise

    (b) Current method of family planning

b. Prenatal assessments

(1) Adequacy of dietary intake; pattern and composition of intake

(2) SBGM

    (a) Frequency and method of testing

    (b) Pattern and recorded results of SBGM

    (c) Ability to adjust insulin requirements based on changing pattern of blood glucose levels

    (d) HbA_{1c}, usually each trimester

(3) Insulin administration and intensified insulin therapies

    (a) Multiple injections

        [i] Tight control in type 1 diabetes is recommended. The documented methods to achieve tight control include multiple (three or more) daily injections or treatment with an insulin pump (Diabetes Control and Complications Trial [DCCT], 1993).

        [ii] Multiple injections of regular or lispro (rapid-acting) insulin before meals. Intermediate-acting insulin administered with the evening meal or at bedtime. Lispro has a more rapid onset, an earlier peak, and a shorter duration than regular insulin (ACOG, 2005) and has been shown to be more effective in achieving desired glucose levels and reducing the risk of fetal macrosomia (Perkins, Dunn, & Jagasia, 2007).

    (b) Continuous subcutaneous insulin infusion using an insulin pump with administration of basal rate and bolus doses

    (c) Dosage adjustments according to changing insulin requirements during pregnancy to maintain euglycemia; typically, insulin requirements increase by two to three times beginning at approximately 18 weeks, peaking at 36 weeks' gestation.

    (d) Human forms of insulin recommended; less likely to result in insulin antigenicity

(4) Episodes of maternal hypoglycemia and hyperglycemia

    (a) Might experience increase in episodes of hypoglycemia; signs of hypoglycemia might be altered and not as readily perceived in pregnancy because the release of normal counter-regulatory hormones can be suppressed

    (b) Assessment of ketones in the urine is recommended:

        [i] In the morning (first morning specimen)

        [ii] When blood glucose levels are greater than 200 mg/dL

        [iii] During illness

(5) Urinalysis (UA) and urine culture (UC) are usually obtained each trimester, or if symptoms are present.

(6) Evaluation of fetal status

    (a) Ultrasound testing

        [i] Pregnancy dating (estimation of gestational age)

        [ii] Fetal growth and development; assess for:

            • Intrauterine growth restriction (IUGR)

            • Hydramnios

            • Fetal macrosomia

        [iii] Assessment for congenital anomalies: increased risk of neural tube defects and congenital heart disease

    (b) Maternal serum alpha-fetoprotein (MS-AFP)

    (c) Biophysical profile (BPP)

    (d) Nonstress testing (NST)

    (e) Maternal assessment of fetal activity and fetal movement counts

    (f) Amniocentesis for lecithin/sphingomyelin (L/S) ratio and phospholipid phosphatidylglycerol (PG) to assess fetal lung maturity and optimize timing of delivery; indicated if induction is planned before 39 weeks' gestation

      (g) Doppler studies using Doppler umbilical and uterine artery velocimetry to assess pregnancies at risk for placental vascular disease; might be particularly helpful in the early detection of fetal growth restriction in women with diabetes and vasculopathy.

5. Physical findings

  a. Maternal effects and complications

    (1) Altered insulin requirements

    (2) Metabolic disturbances related to hyperemesis, nausea and vomiting of pregnancy, and diabetogenic effects of pregnancy

      (a) Increased risk of hypoglycemia, especially in first trimester

      (b) Increased risk of ketoacidosis, especially in second trimester

    (3) Increased risk of maternal infection related to hyperglycemia

      (a) Urinary tract infection

      (b) Chorioamnionitis

      (c) Postpartum endometritis

    (4) Progression and possible acceleration of vascular disease secondary to alterations in diabetic control, including retinopathy, nephropathy, and neuropathy

    (5) Hydramnios; related to fetal anomalies and fetal hyperglycemia

    (6) Preeclampsia or gestational hypertension

    (7) Increased maternal mortality and morbidity, associated with the following:

      (a) Ischemic heart disease

      (b) Advanced vascular disease

      (c) Ketoacidosis

      (d) Hypoglycemia

      (e) Labor disturbances and dystocia; related to fetal increased size and shoulder dystocia

      (f) Complications of cesarean birth

      (g) Postpartum hemorrhage and subsequent anemia; related to:

        [i] Birth trauma

        [ii] Uterine atony secondary to prolonged labor

        [iii] Fetal macrosomia

        [iv] Hydramnios

        [v] Infection

  b. Fetal effects and complications

    (1) Increased incidence of congenital malformations and anomalies, including cardiac, skeletal, neurologic, genitourinary, and gastrointestinal; related to maternal hyperglycemia during organogenesis (first 6 to 8 weeks of pregnancy)

      (a) The incidence of anomalies can be correlated with $HgbA_{1c}$ levels in the mother.

      (b) It is suggested that levels be kept below 7% to reduce the incidence of anomalies (Slocum, 2007).

    (2) Growth disturbances

      (a) Large fetal size; related to fetal hyperinsulinemia (increased risk in mothers without vascular disease; White's classes A to C (see Table 22-2)

        [i] Unlike other LGA neonates, the organs of the infant of a diabetic mother (IDM) are affected by the macrosomia (organomegaly), and body fat is increased (ACOG, 2005).

        [ii] A cesarean section might be warranted if the fetus is estimated to weigh more than 4500 g, to avoid traumatic injury from a vaginal birth (ACOG, 2005).

      (b) IUGR; related to maternal vasculopathy and decreased placental perfusion (increased risk in mothers with vascular disease; White's classes D to T (see Table 22-2) (see Chapter 17 for further discussion of risks associated with size and age)

    (3) Fetal asphyxia; related to fetal hyperglycemia and fetal hyperinsulinemia

    (4) Birth trauma; related to fetal macrosomia and shoulder dystocia

    (5) Stillbirth, especially after 36 weeks' gestation in pregnancies complicated by:

      (a) Poor blood glucose control

      (b) Large fetal size

      (c) Maternal vascular disease

      (d) Ketoacidosis

   c. Neonatal effects and complications
      (1) Prematurity; related to preterm birth associated with maternal complications
      (2) Respiratory distress syndrome; related to delayed fetal lung maturity and preterm birth
         (a) Excess insulin produced by the pancreas of the fetus results in delayed surfactant production, probably by interfering with the lung's ability to use phospholipids by blocking receptor sites.
            [i] This delay in surfactant production is found primarily in classes A to C of diabetic amniotic fluid.
            [ii] Diabetic infants with vascular disease seldom develop respiratory distress syndrome (RDS); chronic stress of poor intrauterine perfusion leads to increased production of steroids, which accelerates lung maturation (Ricci, 2007).
         (b) To avoid iatrogenic RDS, it is suggested that the usual parameters of lung maturity be adjusted for IDMs.
            [i] An amniotic fluid L/S ratio of two or greater does not always ensure that lung maturity has been achieved (Ricci, 2007).
            [ii] The presence of PG is reassuring (see Chapter 17 for a complete discussion of respiratory distress).
      (3) Metabolic and hematologic disturbances; related to maternal hyperglycemia
         (a) Hypoglycemia
            [i] Glucose molecules readily cross the placenta, but insulin does not readily cross.
            [ii] The fetus responds by producing large quantities of insulin, leading to hyperinsulinemia.
            [iii] When the umbilical cord is cut after delivery, the supply of glucose rapidly diminishes, yet the level of insulin remains constant, leading to neonatal hypoglycemia.
            [iv] Glucose levels should be monitored frequently in the newborn (as per institutional protocol); levels should be greater than 40 mg/dL. If less, offer breast milk or formula; if necessary, intravenous (IV) glucose infusion.
         (b) Hypocalcemia
            [i] Defined as serum calcium less than 7 mg/dL
            [ii] Is usually manifested in first 2 to 3 days of life
            [iii] Might occur as result of birth injury or decreased magnesium level, which suppresses parathyroid hormone production, thus decreasing calcium levels (Ricci, 2007)
         (c) Hypomagnesemia
         (d) Polycythemia and hyperbilirubinemia
            [i] Polycythemia is due to the decreased ability of HbA_{1c} in the mother's blood to release oxygen; subsequent breakdown of increased red blood cells (RBCs) predisposes to hyperbilirubinemia.
            [ii] Might result from fetal hypoxia, increase in fetal erythropoietin, sequestered blood from birth injuries, and/or impairment of hepatic function by neonatal hypoglycemia that interferes with bilirubin conjugation (see Chapter 17 for a complete discussion of hyperbilirubinemia)
      (4) Cardiomyopathy and anomalies; related to maternal hyperglycemia (see the previous discussion and Chapter 17 for more information about congenital anomalies)
6. Psychosocial considerations
   a. Adaptation to presence of chronic illness
   b. Presence and adequacy of support systems: partner, family, significant others
   c. Adequacy of coping responses associated with diagnosis of high-risk pregnancy
   d. Presence of psychosocial problems such as depression, anxiety, and eating disorders
   e. Financial concerns related to need for more intensive monitoring of pregnancy
   f. Planned or unplanned pregnancy
   g. Family's response to pregnancy
   h. Feelings regarding high-risk status of pregnancy
   i. Availability of specialized health care team for management of pregnancy
7. Diagnostic procedures
   a. HbA_{1c} (blood test that reflects mean blood glucose levels during the previous 4 to 8 weeks)

    b. Renal evaluation

    c. Ophthalmologic evaluation

    d. Cardiovascular assessment

B. Interventions/Outcomes

  1. Altered metabolism of carbohydrates, proteins, fats, and electrolytes

    a. Interventions

      (1) Assess caloric intake and dietary pattern using 24-hour recall; review importance of regularity of meals when taking insulin.

      (2) Encourage monitoring blood glucose levels and recording results of testing at least four to seven times daily (before and after meals and at bedtime). Note: Abnormal glucose results are most frequently caused by:

        (a) Improper user technique

        (b) Anemia; might falsely elevate results

      (3) Assist with regulation of insulin dosage according to changing physiologic needs and blood glucose levels throughout pregnancy.

        (a) Might switch to human forms of insulin

        (b) Intensify insulin regimen with multiple injections three or four (or more) times daily.

        (c) Might initiate insulin pump therapy

      (4) Encourage urine testing for ketones to identify starvation ketosis or developing ketoacidosis:

        (a) On first morning specimen

        (b) For blood glucose levels greater than 200 mg/dL

        (c) During maternal illness

        (d) When glucose control is altered. Note: Persistent ketonuria might indicate the need for an additional snack or change in insulin regimen.

      (5) Review signs and symptoms for maternal hypoglycemia, which might be altered during pregnancy; and the prevention and management of hypoglycemic episodes (patients should be instructed to have a source of fast-acting carbohydrate with them at all times, such as six to eight LifeSavers, 120 mL [4 ounces] of fruit juice, or 2 tablespoons of raisins).

        (a) Mild

          [i] Tremors

          [ii] Tachycardia

          [iii] Diaphoresis

          [iv] Paresthesia

          [v] Excessive hunger

          [vi] Pallor

          [vii] Shakiness (associated with adrenergic system response)

        (b) Moderate

          [i] Headache

          [ii] Mood change

          [iii] Irritability

          [iv] Inability to concentrate

          [v] Drowsiness

          [vi] Confusion

          [vii] Impaired judgment

          [viii] Slurred speech

          [ix] Staggering gait

          [x] Double or blurred vision (associated with adrenergic plus neuroglycopenic symptoms)

        (c) Severe

          [i] Disorientation

          [ii] Unconsciousness

          [iii] Seizures

    b. Outcomes

      (1) Appropriate amounts of carbohydrate (CHO), proteins, and unsaturated fats are consumed to maintain blood sugar levels within individualized goals.

      (2) Blood glucose levels remain within individualized goals determined for optimal maternal and fetal outcome.

          (3) Insulin dosages are regulated according to changing physiologic needs and maternal blood glucose levels throughout pregnancy.

          (4) Urine is tested for ketones in the morning, when blood glucose levels are 200 mg/dL or higher, during maternal illness, and when blood glucose control is altered.

          (5) Signs and symptoms of maternal hypoglycemia and ketoacidosis are recognized promptly and managed appropriately during pregnancy.

2. Anxiety due to high-risk pregnancy status

   a. Interventions

      (1) Clinical assessments

         (a) Blood-pressure monitoring

         (b) Presence of visual disturbances

         (c) Signs and symptoms of preeclampsia and urinary tract infections (UTIs)

      (2) Prompt identification of alterations in clinical assessments and referral for appropriate medical and obstetric management

      (3) Review potential effects of diabetes on pregnancy to promote understanding of risks and ways to control or minimize them.

   b. Outcomes

      (1) Alterations in blood pressure, presence of visual disturbances, and signs and symptoms of preeclampsia and UTIs are promptly assessed.

      (2) Appropriate referrals for medical and obstetric management of clinical alterations in pregnancy are obtained to minimize potential maternal, fetal, and neonatal complications.

      (3) Effects of diabetes on pregnancy outcome and risk reduction strategies are reviewed.

3. Feelings of powerlessness related to fetal outcome

   a. Interventions

      (1) Discuss strategies for maintenance of optimal glycemic control during pregnancy.

      (2) Provide information about tests and procedures for fetal assessment and surveillance.

      (3) Encourage active participation in decision making and planning for medical and obstetric care throughout pregnancy.

      (4) Discuss feelings about pregnancy and self-monitoring practices for management of diabetes during pregnancy.

   b. Outcomes

      (1) Patient maintains optimal blood glucose control during pregnancy.

      (2) Patient receives information about tests and procedures for fetal assessment.

      (3) Patient actively participates in decision making and planning for medical and obstetric care throughout pregnancy.

      (4) Patient expresses her feelings about her pregnancy and self-monitoring practices for management of diabetes during pregnancy.

4. Plan of diabetes self-care and obstetric management of diabetes during pregnancy

   a. Interventions

      (1) Discuss the rationale for blood glucose control and importance of euglycemia before conception and during pregnancy.

      (2) Review self-care practices.

         (a) Blood glucose monitoring and frequency of testing

         (b) Insulin administration; adjustment of insulin dosages based on blood glucose levels

         (c) Regular daily mild exercise program

         (d) Dietary adjustments and management during pregnancy

      (3) Refer for dietary counseling to ensure optimal diet for glycemic control and fetal growth and development.

      (4) Discuss plan of care for obstetric management and fetal surveillance.

   b. Outcomes

      (1) Patient can verbalize rationale for blood glucose control and importance of euglycemia before conception and during pregnancy.

      (2) Patient demonstrates proper techniques and frequency for blood glucose monitoring and insulin administration, adjusts insulin dosages based on blood glucose determinations, and modifies dietary intake during pregnancy.

      (3) Patient receives dietary counseling to ensure optimal diet for glycemic control and fetal growth and development.

(4) Patient can verbalize a recommended plan of care for obstetric management and fetal surveillance.
5. Elevated serum glucose levels, changes in circulation
   a. Interventions
      (1) Monitor maternal glycemia.
      (2) Assess fetal well-being, including results of NST, AFP, BPP, Doppler studies, and ultrasound testing.
      (3) Encourage maternal assessment of fetal movement using daily fetal movement counts.
   b. Outcomes
      (1) Patient demonstrates dietary management, blood glucose monitoring, and insulin dosage adjustments to maintain euglycemia.
      (2) Fetal status and well-being are monitored via NST, BPP, Doppler studies, and ultrasound testing.
      (3) Patient participates in assessment of fetal well-being using daily movement counts and records, and reports changes in the pattern of fetal activity.
6. Demands of recommended diabetes and obstetric care during pregnancy
   a. Interventions
      (1) Assess maternal support systems and the presence and involvement of significant others in assisting the patient with self-care behaviors and practices.
      (2) Assess alterations in maternal work or employment status and potential economic effect of pregnancy, including financial concerns and expenses.
      (3) Encourage active participation of significant others in prenatal care and testing.
      (4) Discuss family's responses to pregnancy.
   b. Outcomes
      (1) Patient describes support systems and the presence and involvement of significant others in the performance of self-care behaviors and practices during pregnancy.
      (2) Patient expresses financial concerns related to alterations in maternal work or employment status during pregnancy.
      (3) Patient's significant others will actively participate in prenatal care and testing.
      (4) Patient discusses family's responses to pregnancy.

HEALTH EDUCATION

Pregestational Diabetes Mellitus

A. **Preconceptual**
   1. Discussion of potential maternal and fetal risks associated with diabetes and pregnancy, effects of diabetes on pregnancy, and pregnancy on diabetes
   2. Discussion of financial expenses and other demands related to the increased surveillance of maternal and fetal status during pregnancy
   3. Discussion of rationale for interdisciplinary team approach and role of each team member in the management of diabetes and pregnancy
   4. Discussion of rationale for optimal blood glucose control before conception to ensure optimal timing of conception and early diagnosis of pregnancy. Note: Research has demonstrated that near-normal blood glucose levels at the time of conception and in the early weeks of gestation might significantly reduce the increased incidence of congenital anomalies associated with infants of mothers with diabetes (Slocum, 2007).
   5. Review of self-care practices and self-monitoring expectations during pregnancy, including diet, intensification of insulin regimen, and multidisciplinary plan for medical and obstetric management
B. **Prenatal**
   1. Reinforcement of multidisciplinary plan for medical and obstetric management during pregnancy
   2. Ongoing assessment of blood glucose levels and adjustment of insulin requirements to ensure euglycemia
   3. Discuss minimization and prompt recognition of potential maternal and fetal complications associated with diabetes and pregnancy

4. Exercise is encouraged 30 to 60 minutes per day to increase insulin sensitivity. Monitor blood glucose before and after exercise. If glucose is less than 100 mg/dL, consume carbohydrate to prevent hypoglycemia (ADA, 2009b).

C. **Postpartum**
   1. A precipitous decrease in insulin requirements in the immediate postpartum period is related to delivery of placenta and cessation of contra-insulin hormones associated with pregnancy; usually persists for at least 72 hours after birth.
   2. Breastfeeding is encouraged in women with diabetes.
      a. Improves glucose metabolism and promotes high-density lipoprotein (HDL) cholesterol
      b. Might be associated with decreased insulin requirements (up to 27%)
      c. Necessitates increased calories and continued dietary modifications to ensure adequate nutrition during lactation and milk production
      d. Might experience increased incidence of mastitis, sore nipples secondary to candidiasis, and hypoglycemic episodes. Note: Maternal hypoglycemia is most likely to occur 1 hour after breastfeeding, and women with preexisting diabetes should be encouraged to eat a small snack just before breastfeeding.
      e. Hypoglycemia decreases milk production and might lead to problems with establishing milk supply and maintaining lactation.
   3. Discuss birth control and preconception care for next pregnancy.

GESTATIONAL DIABETES MELLITUS

A. **Definition**
   1. Carbohydrate intolerance of variable severity with onset or first recognition during pregnancy
   2. Patient might need diet, exercise, and/or insulin for optimum control.
   3. Diabetes mellitus might persist after pregnancy. Screening should occur 6 to 12 weeks's postpartum.
   4. Glucose intolerance might have antedated the pregnancy.
   5. Some studies suggest oral meds may be used in lieu of insulin (Langer et al, 2005; Rowan et al, 2008).

B. **Incidence**
   1. Occurs in approximately 7% of all pregnant women (ADA, 2009a)
   2. Affects 135,000 women per year (ADA, 2009a)
   3. Accounts for 90% of diabetic pregnancies
   4. African Americans, Hispanics, Asian Americans, Pacific Islanders, and Native Americans are at increased risk for GDM (Perkins et al, 2007).

CLINICAL PRACTICE

A. **Assessment**
   1. History (preconceptual risk factors associated with GDM)
      a. Previous delivery of an LGA or macrosomic (>4500 g) infant
      b. Previous infant with congenital anomaly
      c. Previous unexplained intrauterine fetal demise (IUFD) or neonatal death
      d. History of GDM in previous pregnancy
      e. History of hydramnios in prior pregnancy
      f. Poor reproductive history (i.e., history of preterm birth or recurrent spontaneous abortions)
      g. Family history of diabetes (i.e., parent or sibling with diabetes)
      h. Age 35 years or older
      i. BMI greater than 29 (maternal obesity) (ADA, 2009a)
      j. Hypertension
      k. Ethnic background: African American, Asian, Pacific Islander, Hispanic, and Native American
   2. Physical findings and associated risk factors in current pregnancy
      a. Maternal effects
         (1) Development of hydramnios, suspected large fetal size, or increased fundal height relative to dating of pregnancy

          (2) Persistent glycosuria on two successive prenatal visits

          (3) Proteinuria

          (4) Urinary frequency after first trimester

          (5) Recurrent monilial infections

          (6) Reported feelings or behaviors of excessive thirst or hunger

    b. Fetal and neonatal effects

          (1) Increased fetal size; associated with operative delivery, birth trauma, and shoulder dystocia

          (2) Neonatal hypoglycemia

          (3) Neonatal hypocalcemia

          (4) Neonatal polycythemia

          (5) Neonatal hyperbilirubinemia

          (6) Respiratory distress syndrome

          (7) Infants of mothers with fasting and postprandial hyperglycemia are at greatest risk for intrauterine death or neonatal mortality.

          (8) Overall perinatal mortality has been reported to be 6.4% when GDM is untreated; studies suggest that there is no increase in perinatal mortality when GDM is managed appropriately and maternal glucose levels are normal.

          (9) Increased risk of childhood obesity

3. Psychosocial considerations—adaptation to diagnosis and management of GDM (see previous section on Pregestational Diabetes, Psychosocial Considerations)

4. Diagnostic procedures

    a. Glucose screening

          (1) The American College of Obstetricians and Gynecologists (ACOG) recommends universal screening (ACOG, 2001); however, published data indicate that universal screening is not cost effective. Recommendation by ADA (2009a) is for selective screening for GDM of pregnant women with one or more of the following criteria:

             (a) Age more than 25 years

             (b) Obesity (BMI of 29 or higher)

             (c) Family history of type 2 diabetes (first-degree relative)

             (d) Ethnic group with a high prevalence of type 2 diabetes

             (e) History of abnormal glucose tolerance

             (f) History of poor obstetric outcome

             (g) Presence of glycosuria

             (f) Diagnosis of polycystic ovary syndrome (PCOS)

             (g) Delivery of an LGA infant

          (2) Testing protocol

             (a) Women meeting the criteria should undergo a glucose challenge test between the 24th and 28th week of gestation; an earlier screen should be performed on those women with identified risk factors.

             (b) Remain seated, no smoking, administer 50 g of oral glucose, given without regard to time of day or interval since the last meal.

             (c) Measure venous plasma glucose 1 hour later; level should be less than 140 mg/dL; any value equal to or greater than 140 mg/dL requires a full 3-hour diagnostic oral glucose tolerance test (OGTT). A glucose threshold of 140 identifies approximately 80% of GDM, and using a threshold value of 130 results in about 10% more abnormal screens. Either threshold is acceptable (ADA, 2009a).

    b. OGTT

          (1) Diagnosis of GDM is based on results of the 100-g OGTT during pregnancy. OGTT should be performed in the morning after an overnight fast of at least 8 hours. Criteria set by the American Diabetes Association (Carpenter & Coustan, 1982) for evaluation of results are:

Fasting	95 mg/dL
1 hour	180 mg/dL
2 hour	155 mg/dL
3 hour	140 mg/dL

      (2) Definitive diagnosis requires that two or more of the venous plasma (or serum) glucose concentrations be met or exceeded.

      (3) Studies suggest that a single abnormal test value should be regarded as a pathologic finding with increased risk for adverse outcomes, and therefore patients should be treated similarly to the patient with GDM (Crowther et al, 2005; McLaughlin, Blake, Cheng, & Caughey, 2006).

B. Interventions/Outcomes

  1. Altered metabolism

    a. Interventions

      (1) Review normal changes in carbohydrate metabolism during pregnancy and significance of impaired glucose tolerance to developing fetus.

      (2) Discuss rationale for normalizing blood glucose levels during pregnancy, and review the effects of elevated blood glucose levels on fetal growth and development and neonatal outcome.

      (3) Monitor fasting and postprandial blood glucose levels. Note: The recommended frequency of monitoring blood glucose levels varies in women with GDM.

      (4) Instruct patient in self-monitoring of blood glucose levels and recording results; review instructions and monitoring techniques. Note: The decision to initiate SBGM for women with GDM might vary according to maternal age, gestational age, degree of metabolic abnormality on the OGTT, whether the administration of insulin is required, and other risk factors.

      (5) If indicated, instruct patient in proper technique for administration of insulin and how to record insulin dose and time of injection.

    b. Outcomes

      (1) Patient states normal changes in carbohydrate metabolism during pregnancy and significance of impaired glucose tolerance to developing fetus.

      (2) Patient can verbalize rationale for normalization of blood glucose levels during pregnancy and describes the effects of elevated blood glucose levels on fetal growth and development and neonatal outcomes.

      (3) Alterations in fasting and postprandial blood glucose levels are recognized and managed with dietary modifications, exercise, and insulin administration.

      (4) Patient demonstrates proper technique in SBGM and records results accurately.

      (5) If indicated, patient demonstrates proper technique in administration of insulin and records insulin dose and time of injection.

  2. Anxiety due to high-risk pregnancy status

    a. Interventions

      (1) Provide information regarding effects of elevated blood glucose levels on developing fetus and rationale for normalizing maternal glucose levels.

      (2) Discuss dietary modifications, exercise, and SBGM to promote normalization of blood glucose levels.

      (3) Encourage active participation in self-monitoring practices and decision making about plan for managing GDM.

      (4) Discuss results of fetal assessment tests and procedures for evaluation of fetal status and well-being.

    b. Outcomes

      (1) Patient can state effects of elevated blood glucose levels on developing fetus and rationale for normalizing maternal glucose levels.

      (2) Patient modifies her dietary intake, adopts a regular exercise plan, and self-monitors blood glucose levels to promote normalization of blood glucose levels.

      (3) Patient actively participates in self-monitoring practices and decision making regarding the plan for managing GDM.

      (4) Patient is informed of results of fetal assessment tests and procedures for evaluation of fetal status and well-being.

  3. Emotional reactions related to diagnosis of high-risk pregnancy

    a. Interventions

      (1) Encourage maternal expression of feelings and concerns related to diagnosis of GDM.

      (2) Discuss alterations in anticipated plan for obstetric care, and provide support to minimize potential complications related to unexpected interventions necessitated in pregnancy.

       (3) Refer to behavioral medicine specialist for support with emotional aspects of diabetes management (stress, change) as well as psychosocial barriers to adherence and to care (eating disorders, depression, and anxiety) (California Diabetes and Pregnancy Program [CDAPP], 2008).

  b. Outcomes

       (1) Patient expresses her feelings and concerns about the diagnosis of GDM.

       (2) Patient describes alterations in anticipated plan for obstetric care and identifies sources of support to minimize potential complications related to unexpected interventions necessitated in pregnancy.

       (3) Patient is referred to appropriate specialist for added emotional support.

4. Macrosomia

  a. Interventions

       (1) Monitor blood glucose levels.

       (2) Monitor fetal status and development using NST, BPP, and ultrasound testing. Note: Twice-weekly NST, weekly BPP, or weekly NST alternated with BPP may be initiated as early as 32 weeks.

       (3) Encourage maternal assessment of fetal movement using daily fetal movement counts.

  b. Outcomes

       (1) Patient participates in monitoring of blood glucose levels.

       (2) Fetal status and development are monitored using NST, BPP, and ultrasound testing.

       (3) Patient participates in the assessment of fetal well-being using daily fetal movement counts and reports changes in the pattern of fetal activity.

5. Management plan and self-care activities

  a. Interventions

       (1) Review rationale for normal blood glucose levels in pregnancy.

       (2) Discuss plan for normalizing blood glucose levels, including dietary management, exercise, blood glucose monitoring, and possible insulin administration.

         (a) Recommended calorie intake is 30 kcal/kg ideal body weight.

           [i] Typically provides additional 300 to 400 calories per day

           [ii] Calorie restrictions might be recommended for the overweight woman with GDM to minimize the likelihood of fetal macrosomia and prevent or decrease exogenous insulin requirements.

           [iii] Weight loss and ketonuria should be avoided.

         (b) Exercise assists in glucose normalization in women with type 2 diabetes, women with GDM, and obese women with carbohydrate intolerance; benefits include improved insulin sensitivity and glucose utilization with potential prevention of need for insulin or reduction in insulin requirements.

         (c) Recommendations for the initiation and frequency of SBGM for women with GDM vary; generally, all women with GDM requiring insulin require SBGM.

         (d) Insulin is usually prescribed if fasting or postprandial blood glucose levels are persistently elevated despite dietary modifications.

           [i] Initiate insulin therapy with mild hyperglycemia when post-meal values are greater than 120 or fasting values are greater than 90 on two or more occasions during a 2-week period (Gilmartin, Ural, & Repke, 2008).

           [ii] Insulin might also be recommended for women with an elevated fasting blood glucose level on the 3-hour OGTT.

  b. Outcomes

       (1) Patient can verbalize rationale for normal blood glucose levels in pregnancy.

       (2) Patient demonstrates normalization of blood glucose levels through dietary management, exercise, blood-glucose monitoring, and possible administration of insulin, if prescribed.

6. Nutritional requirements: providing adequate dietary intake for maternal and fetal needs without causing excessive maternal weight gain

  a. Interventions

       (1) Refer patient for dietary counseling to ensure proper diet for normalization of blood glucose levels and optimal fetal growth and development.

       (2) Encourage patient to record dietary intake and blood glucose results.

    b. Outcomes

        (1) Patient receives dietary counseling to ensure proper diet for normalization of blood glucose levels and optimal fetal growth and development.

        (2) Patient records dietary intake and blood glucose levels.

  7. Demands of optimal diabetes and obstetric care during pregnancy

    a. Interventions

        (1) Encourage patient to express concerns related to plan for management of GDM and presence of family support to encourage adherence to dietary recommendations and maintain blood glucose control.

        (2) Provide anticipatory guidance about the frequency of prenatal appointments and testing for evaluation of maternal glycemic status and the need for additional fetal assessment tests and surveillance.

        (3) Assess effect of the diagnosis of GDM on the family.

    b. Outcomes

        (1) Patient expresses her concerns about the plan for diabetes management during pregnancy and describes presence of family support to encourage adherence to dietary recommendations and maintenance of blood glucose control.

        (2) Patient receives anticipatory guidance about the frequency of prenatal appointments and testing for evaluation of maternal glycemic status and the need for additional fetal assessment tests and surveillance.

        (3) Appropriate resources and support are available to the family to minimize the effect of the diagnosis of GDM and its management on the family.

HEALTH EDUCATION

Gestational Diabetes—Postpartum

A. Breastfeeding should be encouraged in women with GDM because breastfeeding improves glucose utilization and promotes HDL cholesterol.

B. Women diagnosed with GDM should be closely observed postpartum to detect diabetes early in its course.

  1. Reclassification of maternal glycemic status should be performed at 6 weeks' postpartum (ADA, 2009a). If glucose levels are normal, reassessment of glycemia should be undertaken every 3 years. Women with IFG or IGT should be tested annually for diabetes.

  2. Initially, explain that evaluation should occur at the first 6-week postpartum visit with a 2-hour OGTT with a 75-g glucose load.

  3. Explain that the incidence of abnormal glucose tolerance at 6 to 8 weeks's postpartum in women with previous GDM varies between 20% and 65%, depending on the population.

  4. Discuss the criteria for the diagnosis of diabetes mellitus in the nonpregnant state (Table 22-3).

▨ **TABLE 22-3**

▨ ▨ **Criteria for Diagnosis for Diabetes Mellitus**

Normal	IFG or IGT	Diabetes Mellitus
FPG <110 mg/dL	FPG 100-125	FPG ≥126 mg/dL
75-g, 2h OGTT	75-g, 2h OGTT	75-g, 2h OGTT
2h PG <140 mg/dL	2h PG 140-199	2h PG ≥200 mg/dL or Symptoms of DM and PG ≥200 mg/dL (no regard to last meal)

DM, Diabetes mellitus; *FPG,* fasting plasma glucose; *IFG,* impaired fasting glucose; *IGT,* impaired glucose tolerance; *OGTT,* oral glucose tolerance test; *PG,* phosphatidylglycerol.
From American Diabetes Association. (2009b). Position statement: Diagnosis and classification of diabetes mellitus. *Diabetes Care,* 32(1), 103-105.

C. Preventive health measures emphasizing the importance of weight management through diet and regular exercise should be promoted. Note: Women with GDM and their children are at increased risk for developing hypertension, obesity, and overt diabetes; weight reduction can reduce these risks.

D. The history of GDM confers a 60% to 70% chance of GDM in subsequent pregnancies.

E. Approximately 40% of women diagnosed with GDM develop overt diabetes within 20 years of index pregnancy; maintaining ideal body weight, eating a healthful diet, and regular exercise might decrease the likelihood of developing overt diabetes or delay its onset.

HYPERTHYROIDISM

A. Hyperthyroidism is caused by hyperfunctioning of thyroid gland, so that the thyroid gland produces excessive amounts of thyroid hormone. Overactivity of hypothalamus, pituitary, or thyroid gland can cause hyperthyroidism (ACOG, 2002).

B. Graves' disease (an autoimmune process) is the most common cause of hyperthyroidism during pregnancy. It is typified by "production of thyroid-stimulating immunoglobulin (TSI) and thyroid-stimulating hormone binding inhibitory immunoglobulin (TBII) and acts on thyroid-stimulating hormone (TSH) receptor to inhibit thyroid stimulation" (ACOG, 2002, p. 387).

C. Diagnosis and management of thyroid disease in pregnancy is complicated by the normal physiologic changes of pregnancy that mimic hyperthyroidism and a hypermetabolic state. Hyperdynamic symptoms are characteristic of normal pregnancy and of hyperthyroidism.

   1. Increased metabolic rate
   2. Increased protein-bound iodine values
   3. Increased iodine uptake; plasma iodine decreases during pregnancy
   4. Increased thyroid-binding globulin (TBG) due to reduced hepatic clearance and estrogen stimulation of TBG synthesis
   5. Increased size of thyroid gland
   6. Increased total thyroxine (TT_4) and total triiodothyronine (TT_3) (most significant thyroid hormones)

D. Various metabolic and hormonal changes that occur in pregnancy affect the thyroid gland.

   1. Presence of placental estrogen alters thyroid function studies, such as the total thyroxine (TT_4) and triiodothyronine resin uptake (T_3RU).
   2. Thyroid is stimulated by human chorionic gonadotropin (hCG) in the first trimester (Casey & Leveno, 2006).
   3. Other metabolic changes can be seen in thyroid function tests during pregnancy (Table 22-4).

E. Incidence of hyperthyroidism in pregnancy is approximately 0.2%. In Graves' disease, there is an increase in levels of free thyroxine (FT_4) or free thyroxine index (FTI) (see Table 22-4). Other causes of hyperthyroidism include increased TSH, gestational trophoblastic neoplasia, hyperfunctioning thyroid adenoma, goiter, subacute thyroiditis (ACOG, 2002), and hyperemesis gravidarum (Casey & Leveno, 2006).

F. Fetal synthesis of thyroid hormones

   1. Synthesis begins at 10 to 12 weeks and is controlled by pituitary TSH by 20 weeks' gestation.
   2. Fetal serum levels of TSH, TBG, FT_4, and FT_3 increase during pregnancy.

G. Treatment of hyperthyroidism is complicated by the presence of the fetus.

   1. Inadequate treatment is associated with risk for preterm deliveries, low birthweight, and fetal loss.
   2. The fetus might be jeopardized by surgery or antithyroid medications. If maternal drug treatment is not effective or if drug intolerance exists, partial thyroidectomy or total resection of the maternal thyroid gland might be indicated. If necessary, maternal surgery is usually recommended after the first trimester to decrease the risk of spontaneous abortion. Postoperative hypothyroidism is common, affecting at least 20% of women with hyperthyroidism.

■ TABLE 22-4

■ ■ **Changes in Thyroid Function Test Results in Normal Pregnancy and in Thyroid Disease**

Maternal Status	TSH	FT_4	FTI	TT_4	TT_3	T_3RU
Pregnancy	No change	No change	No change	Increase	Increase	Decrease
Hyperthyroidism	Decrease	Increase	Increase	Increase	Increase or no change	Increase
Hypothyroidism	Increase	Decrease	Decrease	Decrease	Decrease or no change	Decrease

FT_4, Free thyroxine; *FTI,* free thyroxine index; *T_3RU,* triiodothyronine resin uptake; *TSH,* thyroid-stimulating hormone; *TT_3,* total triiodothyronine; *TT_4,* total thyroxine. From American College of Obstetricians and Gynecologists. (2002). Thyroid disease in pregnancy. *Practice Bulletin,* 387-396.

3. Patients with Graves' disease can have TSI or TBII that can stimulate or inhibit fetal thyroid, possibly resulting in either neonatal hypothyroidism or hyperthyroidism. Also, fetal thyrotoxicosis should be considered in maternal Graves' disease (ACOG, 2002).
4. Hyperthyroidism in pregnancy is treated with thioamides. Drugs that inhibit synthesis of thyroid hormones such as propylthiouracil (PTU) or methimazole can be used to decrease thyroid synthesis (ACOG, 2002).
   a. The dosage of PTU is gradually tapered to the smallest effective dosage to prevent unnecessary maternal and fetal hypothyroidism.
   b. Maintain free T_4 or FTI in upper limits of normal range.
   c. PTU is usually well tolerated by the mothers, but infrequent side effects might occur.
      (1) Rash
      (2) Nausea
      (3) Pruritus
      (4) Hepatitis
      (5) Arthralgias
      (6) Vasculitis
      (7) Thrombocytopenia
      (8) Agranulocytosis
   d. Can breastfeed while taking PTU (ACOG, 2002)
H. **Associated with increased risk for congestive heart failure, preeclampsia and postpartum hemorrhage if poorly controlled**
I. **When diagnosed during pregnancy, hyperthyroidism might be transient or permanent; spontaneous remissions might occur during pregnancy.**
J. **Thyroid storm is an extreme hypermetabolic state that has a high risk of maternal heart failure occurring in 1% of patients with hyperthyroidism during pregnancy. It is considered a medical emergency.**
   1. Signs and symptoms include fever, extreme tachycardia, changes in mental status, nervousness, seizures, nausea, vomiting, diarrhea, and cardiac arrhythmia.
   2. If untreated, thyroid storm can result in shock, coma, or maternal heart failure.
   3. Pharmacologic treatment includes drugs that will suppress thyroid function.
      a. PTU
      b. Saturated solution of potassium iodide and sodium iodide
      c. Dexamethasone
      d. Propranolol (beta-blockers)
      e. Phenobarbital (for extreme restlessness)
   4. Supportive treatment includes:
      a. Oxygen
      b. Intravenous solutions
      c. Use of antipyretics
      d. Fetal monitoring
      e. Continuous maternal cardiac monitoring (ACOG, 2002)
K. **Thyroid nodules in pregnancy should be investigated to rule out malignancy due to an increased risk for malignancy during pregnancy.**

CLINICAL PRACTICE

A. **Assessment**
   1. History
      a. Clinical symptoms
         (1) Weakness
         (2) Muscle tremors
         (3) Palpitations
         (4) Heat intolerance and sensitivity
         (5) Increased appetite
         (6) Failure to gain weight or actual weight loss
         (7) Fatigue
         (8) Insomnia
         (9) Frequent stools
         (10) Nervousness and hyperactivity
         (11) Excessive perspiration
         (12) Exophthalmos
         (13) Enlargement of the thyroid gland (goiter)
      b. Infertility
         (1) Anovulation and amenorrhea might occur if hyperthyroidism is not treated.
         (2) When treated, hyperthyroidism is not usually associated with infertility.
   2. Physical findings
      a. Maternal effects
         (1) Resting pulse greater than 100 beats per minute (bpm)
         (2) Proximal muscle wasting
         (3) Separation of the distal nail from the nailbed
         (4) Eye signs
            (a) Stare with exophthalmos
            (b) Lid lag
            (c) Lid retraction
            (d) Chemosis
         (5) Goiter: diffusely enlarged, soft gland
         (6) Soft skin with fine hair
         (7) Increased skin warmth
         (8) Development of thyroid storm or thyrotoxic crisis
            (a) Medical emergency that presents clinically with:
               [i] High fever
               [ii] Tachycardia
               [iii] Severe dehydration
               [iv] Profuse sweating
               [v] Restlessness
               [vi] Nausea and vomiting associated with abdominal pain
               [vii] Possible pulmonary edema or congestive heart failure
               [viii] Hypotension
               [ix] Stupor
            (b) Most commonly occurs in pregnant women when hyperthyroidism has not been detected or is poorly controlled
            (c) Precipitating factors include:
               [i] Infection
               [ii] Labor
               [iii] Cesarean birth
            (d) Requires prompt treatment with IV fluids, oxygen, and pharmacologic treatment
         (9) Increased incidence of preeclampsia if poorly controlled
         (10) Side effects associated with antithyroid medications
      b. Fetal and neonatal effects
         (1) Increased incidence of preterm labor and delivery
         (2) Increased risk of small for gestational age (SGA) or low birthweight (LBW) infants
         (3) Small increase in perinatal mortality

      (4) Maternal use of antithyroid medication might impair fetal thyroid function and cause hypothyroidism, goiter, or mental deficiencies.

      (5) If hyperthyroidism is untreated, rates of spontaneous abortion, intrauterine death, and stillbirth increase.

      (6) Rare occurrence of fetal thyrotoxicosis in presence of maternal thyroid storm

      (7) If untreated, iodine-deficient hypothyroidism increases risk of congenital cretinism.

  3. Psychosocial considerations (same as Pregestational Diabetes, Psychosocial Considerations)

  4. Diagnostic procedures

    a. Laboratory findings: elevated FTI, elevated FT_4, elevated TT_4, and decreased T_3RU (see Table 22-4)

    b. Maintaining the fetus in a euthyroid state, especially in the last trimester, is recognized as essential for brain development; the FTI is a useful index of fetal thyroid status.

    c. Neonates born to mothers with hyperthyroidism undergo serum thyroxine determinations at birth and are observed closely during the first 2 weeks of life for signs and symptoms of hyperthyroidism.

B. Interventions/Outcomes

  1. Anxiety

    a. Interventions

      (1) Assess maternal anxiety level, including behavioral and physiologic changes.

      (2) Encourage maternal expression of feelings and concerns.

      (3) Inform the patient of all procedures and expectations, presenting accurate information and answering her questions.

      (4) Encourage active participation in decision making about the therapeutic regimen.

    b. Outcomes

      (1) Behavioral and physiologic changes associated with maternal anxiety do not compromise the patient's ability to participate in the therapeutic regimen prescribed during pregnancy.

      (2) Patient expresses feelings and concerns about pregnancy and its outcome.

      (3) Patient can describe accurate information about procedures and expectations during pregnancy.

      (4) Patient actively participates in decision-making process concerning implementation of the therapeutic regimen.

  2. Altered metabolism

    a. Interventions

      (1) Perform head-to-toe assessment.

      (2) Monitor for cardiovascular signs and symptoms.

        (a) Vital signs

        (b) Electrocardiogram (ECG)

        (c) Arterial blood gases

        (d) Arterial oxygen saturation

      (3) Assess for signs and symptoms of pulmonary edema.

        (a) Dyspnea

        (b) Rales

        (c) Persistent cough

        (d) Mechanical ventilation might be needed

      (4) Assess for hyperthermia: If maternal fever increases, treat immediately.

    b. Outcomes

      (1) Cardiovascular/respiratory systems are stable.

      (2) Maternal temperature remains normal.

      (3) Reassuring fetal heart rate pattern is noted.

  3. Therapeutic regimen to optimize maternal and fetal outcomes

    a. Interventions

      (1) Assess and facilitate understanding of effects of hyperthyroidism on pregnancy and fetal development, including possible fetal goiter and hypothyroidism.

      (2) Discuss plan for frequent monitoring of FTI and TT_4 to ensure that lowest possible amount of antithyroid medication is administered for control of patient's symptoms while minimizing fetal exposure to antithyroid medications.

(3) Perform clinical assessment to determine adequacy of maternal response to antithyroid medications.
   (a) Pulse below 100
   (b) Reflexes 2+ to 3+
   (c) Loss of tremor
   (d) Normal weight gain
   (e) Normal fetal growth
(4) Review complications of antithyroid therapy.
   (a) Purpuric skin rash
   (b) Pruritus
   (c) Fever
   (d) Nausea
   (e) Rarely, agranulocytosis (usually after 1 to 2 months of therapy)
(5) Instruct the patient to report fever, sore throat, or other symptoms of infection.
(6) Provide accurate information about all procedures, tests, and interventions planned during pregnancy and after birth of the infant.
(7) Inform the patient of the results of laboratory tests and provide information about fetal status and well-being.
(8) Review dietary requirements in pregnancy to reinforce adequate nutritional intake and facilitate fetal growth and development. Note: Increased metabolic state requires increased calories and protein intake.
(9) Instruct the patient about the signs and symptoms of preterm labor.
(10) Review the signs and symptoms of hyperthyroidism, the use of self-monitoring diaries, and self-assessment records.

b. Outcomes
(1) Patient can verbalize an understanding of effects of hyperthyroidism on pregnancy and fetal development, including possible fetal goiter and hypothyroidism.
(2) Patient can verbalize a plan for frequent monitoring of total free T_4 levels to ensure lowest possible amount of antithyroid medication is administered for control of her symptoms while minimizing fetal exposure to antithyroid medications.
(3) Patient demonstrates therapeutic response to antithyroid medications.
(4) Patient can state possible complications of antithyroid therapy, including skin rash, pruritus, fever, and nausea.
(5) Patient reports fever, sore throat, or other symptoms of infection.
(6) Patient receives accurate information about all procedures, tests, and interventions planned during pregnancy and after birth of infant.
(7) Patient is informed of fetal status and well-being throughout pregnancy and at birth.
(8) Patient reports adequate nutritional intake during pregnancy.
(9) Patient can verbalize signs and symptoms of preterm labor.
(10) Patient actively participates in monitoring and recording signs and symptoms of hyperthyroidism during pregnancy.

4. Medical management with antithyroid drugs
a. Interventions
(1) Monitor fetal growth and development through ultrasound testing and fundal height measurement.
(2) Fetal heart rate (FHR) monitored in utero as metabolic guide for the following:
   (a) Fetal hyperthyroidism (FHR greater than 160)
   (b) Fetal hypothyroidism (FHR less than 120)
(3) Assess maternal serum for FTI and TT_4 levels for possible adjustment of dosage for propylthiouracil (PTU) therapy.
   (a) The lowest possible amount is used to control symptoms; the patient is kept mildly hyperthyroid or within the high end of the normal range of pregnancy to minimize potential detrimental effects to the fetus.
   (b) Keeping the fetus in euthyroid state, especially near term, is recognized as essential for brain and neurologic development.
(4) Assess patient for signs and symptoms of preterm labor.
(5) Perform fetal movement counts to assess fetal well-being.
(6) Assess for fetal hydrops.
(7) Assess fetal heart rate for sinusoidal patterns or tachycardia.

b. Outcomes
(1) Fetal growth and development and FHR are within normal parameters.
(2) Maternal total free T_4 levels are maintained in the prescribed range to control symptoms (the patient might be mildly hyperthyroid).
(3) Signs and symptoms of preterm labor are promptly reported and managed to minimize incidence of preterm birth.
(4) Fetal activity and movement indicate fetal well-being.

HEALTH EDUCATION

Hyperthyroidism

A. Preconceptual
1. Assessment of adequacy of antithyroid medications with baseline laboratory values
2. Discussion of potential maternal and fetal complications associated with hyperthyroidism in pregnancy, including thyroid storm

B. Prenatal
1. Discuss the need for careful history-taking and physical assessment of the patient's symptoms at each prenatal visit.
2. Explain treatment with antithyroid drugs in pregnancy and close monitoring to determine minimal dosage required to control symptoms.
3. Discuss information regarding fetal status and potential maternal and fetal complications associated with hyperthyroidism in pregnancy.
4. Explain and discuss the presence of congenital goiter or signs of airway obstruction necessitating intubations at birth; evaluation of thyroid function of the newborn.
5. Provide nutritional counseling to meet additional calorie requirements.

C. Postpartum
1. Patients taking antithyroid medications such as PTU may breastfeed if the infant's thyroid status is closely monitored (every 2 to 4 weeks).
2. Infants exposed to small amounts of antithyroid medications do not usually become hypothyroid.

HYPOTHYROIDISM

A. Definition
1. This is a rare condition (1 to 3/1000) in pregnancy because women with hypothyroidism ovulate irregularly, frequently are infertile, and experience menstrual dysfunction or amenorrhea.
2. Hypothyroidism is caused by inadequate thyroid hormone production.
3. Increased likelihood of having another autoimmune disease; 5% to 8% of patients with hypothyroidism have type 1 diabetes.

B. Etiology
1. Primary hypothyroidism is due to the following:
   a. Hashimoto's thyroiditis; production of antithyroid antibodies including thyroid antimicrosomal and antithyroglobulin antibodies (ACOG, 2002)
   b. Therapy with antithyroid drugs
   c. Iodine deficiency associated with goiters (most common cause of hypothyroidism worldwide)
   d. Destruction of the thyroid gland (by radiation or previous surgery)
2. Secondary hypothyroidism is from pituitary-hypothalamic disease.

C. Prognosis for the mother and fetus is favorable with successful hormone replacement.
1. Levothyroxine (Synthroid) is most often prescribed in pregnancy.
2. Dosage is gradually increased until normal levels of TSH and thyroxine are reached.
3. Thyroid hormones cross placenta in small amounts early in gestation. The fetus is dependent on maternal thyroid hormones until 12 weeks' gestation, after which fetal production begins.

D. High fetal mortality and morbidity are characteristics of the hypothyroid state when replacement therapy is inadequate or not instituted during pregnancy.

E. Thyroidectomy for women who fail thioamide treatment can be performed during pregnancy.

F. Radioactive iodine (^{131}I) is contraindicated in pregnancy.

G. Avoid breastfeeding for at least 120 days after ^{131}I treatment.

CLINICAL PRACTICE

A. **Assessment**
   1. History
      a. Fatigue and malaise; lack of energy
      b. Cold intolerance
      c. Lethargy
      d. Headache
      e. Constipation
      f. Paresthesias
      g. Mental impairment
      h. Infertility, if thyroid function is significantly impaired
      i. Increased incidence of spontaneous abortion (risk doubled if maternal hypothyroidism is untreated), preeclampsia, anemia, abruptio placentae, postpartum hemorrhage, and stillbirth
   2. Physical findings
      a. Maternal effects
         (1) Dry, scaly skin
         (2) Thin, brittle nails
         (3) Alopecia or hair loss
         (4) Poor skin turgor
         (5) Delayed deep tendon reflexes (slow relaxation phase)
         (6) Carpal tunnel syndrome
         (7) Enlarged thyroid gland (goiter)
         (8) Can progress to increased weight gain, mental impairment, voice changes, and insomnia
         (9) Thyroid nodules should be further evaluated for possible thyroid cancer because malignancy during pregnancy occurs in 40% of these nodules (ACOG, 2002).
      b. Fetal and neonatal effects
         (1) If mother is treated, infants might be low birthweight, but usually without evidence of hypothyroidism.
         (2) If mother is untreated, fetal loss is 50%.
         (3) Increased risk of congenital goiter
         (4) Increased risk of true cretinism
         (5) Increased incidence of congenital anomalies (risk tripled if maternal hypothyroidism is untreated)
   3. Psychosocial considerations (same as Pregestational Diabetes, Psychosocial Considerations)
   4. Diagnostic procedures
      a. Diagnosis is confirmed by the presence of low total T_4, free T_4, and T_3RU.
      b. TSH is above normal (see Table 22-4).
      c. Monitor levels of TSH or FT_4/FTI during pregnancy for thyroid disease.
      d. Screen newborn for T_4 levels.

B. **Interventions/Outcomes**
   1. Anxiety
      a. Interventions: same as Hyperthyroidism
      b. Outcomes: same as Hyperthyroidism
   2. Altered metabolism
      a. Interventions
         (1) Assess for temperature stabilization and regulation.
         (2) Assess for activity level due to decreased metabolic rate.

  b. Outcomes
  (1) Temperature is stable.
  (2) Maternal response to levothyroxine will be therapeutic.
  (3) Fetal heart rate is reassuring.
3. Therapeutic regimen to optimize maternal and fetal outcomes
  a. Interventions
  (1) Assess and facilitate the patient's understanding of the effects of hypothyroidism on pregnancy and fetal development.
  (2) Provide accurate information about all procedures, tests, and interventions planned during pregnancy and after birth of the infant. Note: Thyroid hormones administered endogenously or exogenously do not cross the placenta in significant amounts.
  (3) Inform the patient of fetal status and well-being, including plans for monitoring the neonate's thyroid status to detect any abnormalities after birth.
  (4) Instruct the patient in self-monitoring fetal activity via daily fetal movement counts.
  b. Outcomes
  (1) Patient can verbalize an understanding of pregnancy and normal growth and development of the fetus.
  (2) Patient receives accurate information about all procedures, tests, and interventions planned during pregnancy and after birth of the infant.
  (3) Patient is informed of fetal and neonatal status and well-being throughout pregnancy and during and after birth.
  (4) Patient participates in assessment of fetal well-being by performing daily fetal movement counts.
4. Thyroid replacement therapy
  a. Interventions
  (1) Monitor fetal growth and development by ultrasound screening.
  (2) Assess maternal serum total T_4 and T_3RU levels for possible adjustment of dosage to keep within the normal range during pregnancy and to minimize detrimental effects to fetus.
  b. Outcomes
  (1) Fetal growth and development are within normal parameters.
  (2) Maternal serum free T_4 levels are maintained in the prescribed range to ensure a euthyroid state throughout pregnancy.

HEALTH EDUCATION

Hypothyroidism

A. **Preconceptual**
  1. Explanation and assessment of adequacy of thyroid replacement as indicated by the free T_4 index (plasma-free T_4 index) and achievement of clinical and biochemical euthyroidism
  2. Discussion and assessment of fertility and ovulation
  3. Discussion of potential maternal and neonatal complications associated with hypothyroidism in pregnancy; with adequate hormonal replacement, outcomes for the mother and fetus are improved
B. **Prenatal**
  1. Explain the need for a careful history-taking and physical assessment of the patient's symptoms at each prenatal visit.
  2. Explain that treatment should begin as soon as possible with thyroid replacement medication.
    a. During pregnancy, thyroid replacement must be adequate for maternal needs and for adequate fetal growth and development.
    b. The plasma-free T_4 index is used to monitor the adequacy of replacement therapy during pregnancy.
    c. Placental transfer of thyroid hormone replacement is negligible.
    d. Long-term T_4 replacement therapy during pregnancy usually continues at the same dosage prescribed before pregnancy.

3. Inform patient about fetal status and potential maternal and fetal complications associated with hypothyroidism in pregnancy.
4. Tests and procedures indicated during pregnancy and used for assessment of the neonate at birth should be explained and discussed with the patient.
   a. Monitoring the plasma T_4 index
   b. Adjusting dosage of thyroid medication
C. **Postpartum**
   1. Long-term T_4 replacement therapy after birth is usually resumed at the same dosage prescribed before pregnancy.
   2. Results of tests and procedures performed to assess the neonate should be discussed with the patient.

ADRENAL DISORDERS

Hyperadrenocorticism (Cushing's Syndrome)

A. **General overview**
   1. Many parameters of adrenal function are altered during pregnancy.
   2. Normal physiologic changes in pregnancy mimic adrenal disease.
      a. Abdominal striae
      b. Edema
      c. Increased pigmentation
      d. Decreased glucose tolerance
   3. Physiologic hypercortisolism occurs in normal pregnancy and is associated with the following:
      a. Progressive rise in circulating levels of adrenocorticotropic hormone (ACTH) (does not cross the placenta)
      b. Dexamethasone suppressibility
      c. Increased plasma cortisol levels by two to three times in pregnancy (can cross the placenta)
B. **Definition**
   1. Adrenal hyperfunction occurs most commonly as Cushing's syndrome, a rare disorder of steroid overproduction, primarily corticotropin, that occurs with pituitary or adrenal tumors or adenomas or with adrenal hyperplasia secondary to elevated ACTH secretion.
   2. Adrenal hyperfunction also occurs with exogenous steroid administration (women with this syndrome are generally infertile because of ovulatory failure; this condition is extremely rare in pregnancy).
   3. In most cases Cushing's syndrome is rare during pregnancy with fewer than 150 cases during pregnancy; usually adenoma is the underlying cause (Lindsay & Nieman, 2005).
C. **Etiology due to long-term overabundance of glucocorticoid**
   1. Abnormality of pituitary gland adenomas, producing excess amounts of ACTH, the hormone that stimulates adrenal glands to produce cortisol
   2. Adrenal hyperplasia
   3. Large doses of glucocorticoids given for asthma, rheumatoid arthritis, or other chronic diseases
D. **Diagnosis**
   1. Radiographs to locate any tumors
   2. 24-hour urinary tests to measure corticosteroid hormones
   3. Computed tomography (CT) scan
   4. Magnetic resonance imaging (MRI)
   5. Dexamethasone-suppression test
   6. Corticotropin-releasing hormone (CRH) stimulation test
E. **Effects on pregnancy: Data are limited regarding maternal prognosis in pregnancy because most women with this condition are infertile.**
   1. Maternal effects/complications
      a. Abnormal glucose tolerance test (25%) (Biller et al, 2008)
      b. Pulmonary edema
      c. Hypertension in most patients (68%) (Biller et al, 2008)
      d. Myopathy
      e. Increased risk for postoperative wound infection or dehiscence

2. Fetal and neonatal effects
   a. Increased incidence of spontaneous abortions
   b. Increased stillbirths and neonatal mortality (6%) (Biller et al, 2008)
   c. Intrauterine growth restriction (21%) (Biller et al, 2008)
   d. Premature births (43%) (Lindsay & Nieman, 2005)
   e. Suppression of fetal/neonatal adrenals
   f. Patients with poorly controlled hyperplasia have increased production of androgens; fetus is at risk for adrenogenital syndrome.

CLINICAL PRACTICE

A. **Assessment**
   1. History
      a. Emotional lability
      b. Psychiatric disorders
      c. Glucose intolerance
      d. Excessive weight gain, primarily in face, neck, trunk, and abdomen
      e. Menstrual irregularities
      f. Infertility
   2. Physical findings
      a. Centripetal obesity with muscle wasting and proximal myopathy
      b. Acne
      c. Striae
      d. Hirsutism
      e. Moon face, facial rounding
      f. "Buffalo hump" (increased fat over the dorsal vertebrae)
      g. Hypertension
      h. Muscle loss and weakness
      i. Glucose intolerance; increased blood glucose in diabetes
   3. Psychosocial considerations
      a. Emotional lability, depression, panic attacks, and paranoia
      b. Insomnia
      c. Psychiatric disorders
   4. Fetal/neonatal effects
      a. Increased prematurity by 43%
      b. Increased spontaneous abortions, stillbirths, and neonatal mortality
      c. Possible suppression of fetal adrenals
   5. Diagnostic procedures
      a. Plasma cortisol level is elevated.
      b. Dexamethasone suppression test result is abnormal.
      c. Ultrasonography might indicate adrenal tumors of the adrenal glands.
B. **Interventions/Outcomes**
   1. Anxiety
      a. Interventions: same as in Hyperthyroidism
      b. Outcomes: same as in Hyperthyroidism
   2. Therapeutic regimen to optimize maternal and fetal outcomes
      a. Interventions
         (1) Assess patient's understanding of effects of adrenal hyperfunction on pregnancy and fetal development.
         (2) Provide accurate information about all procedures, tests, and interventions planned during pregnancy and after birth of the infant.
         (3) Inform patient of fetal status and well-being.
         (4) Instruct patient regarding the signs and symptoms of preterm labor and self-monitoring of fetal activity with daily fetal movement counts.
      b. Outcomes
         (1) Patient can verbalize an understanding of the effects on pregnancy and normal growth and development of the fetus.

        (2) Patient receives accurate information about all procedures, tests, and interventions planned during pregnancy and after birth of the infant.

        (3) Patient is informed of fetal status and well-being throughout pregnancy and at birth.

        (4) Patient reports any signs or symptoms of preterm labor and any decrease or significant change in fetal movement patterns.

3. Suppression of adrenal function and maternal hypertension
   a. Interventions
      (1) Monitor fetal growth and development.
      (2) Monitor signs and symptoms of preterm labor.
      (3) Monitor and treat maternal hypertension (see Chapter 19).
   b. Outcomes
      (1) Fetal growth and development are within normal parameters.
      (2) Preterm labor will be recognized early, and management will be instituted promptly to minimize incidence of preterm birth.
      (3) Maternal hypertension will be recognized early and management will be instituted promptly.

HEALTH EDUCATION

Hyperadrenocorticism (Cushing's Syndrome)

A. **Preconceptual**
   1. Assessment and discussion of fertility and ovulation
   2. Discussion of potential maternal and neonatal complications associated with adrenal hyperfunction in pregnancy
B. **Prenatal**
   1. Explain the need for a careful history-taking and physical assessment of the patient's symptoms at each prenatal visit.
   2. Provide endocrine consultation to determine the cause of the syndrome.
   3. Inform regarding fetal status and potential maternal and fetal complications associated with adrenal hyperfunction in pregnancy, including increased risk of preterm labor and stillbirth

ADRENAL INSUFFICIENCY

A. **Definition**
   1. Classified as either primary or secondary adrenal insufficiency; further classified as congenital or acquired
   2. Primary adrenal insufficiency occurs when the adrenal gland itself is dysfunctional and is uncommon in pregnancy. Secondary adrenal insufficiency is seen with pituitary lesions. There is a lack of CRH from the hypothalamus or lack of ACTH secretion from the pituitary.
   3. Acquired occurs with autoimmune destruction of the adrenals usually caused by diseases such as tuberculosis, fungal disease, or, more rarely, metastatic cancer. Any severe sepsis might precipitate adrenal insufficiency. Congenital causes might include congenital adrenal hypoplasia or hyperplasia or defects in ACTH receptor.
   4. Diagnosis is usually established before pregnancy, and the woman is on maintenance steroid replacement when conception occurs.
   5. Long-term use of glucocorticoids (for asthma, inflammatory bowel, or rheumatic disease) might precipitate adrenal insufficiency due to chronic suppression of CRH-ACTH-adrenal axis (Lindsay & Nieman, 2005).
B. **Effects on pregnancy**
   1. Maternal effects
      a. Mild cases might go undetected during pregnancy, and the patient might go on to adrenal crisis with stress of labor or illness.
      b. Risk of adrenal crisis is increased in the postpartum period because of the inability to mount an adrenal response to the stress of delivery.
      c. Hyperkalemia, hyponatremia, and hypoglycemia

  2. Fetal and neonatal effects
     a. Increased incidence of SGA and LBW infants
     b. Depressed adrenal function related to maternal therapy with steroids
     c. IUGR

CLINICAL PRACTICE

A. Assessment
  1. History
    a. Weakness
    b. Fatigue
    c. Nausea and vomiting, diarrhea
    d. Anorexia
    e. Apathy
    f. Altered mental status
  2. Physical findings (Note: Some of these signs and symptoms might occur in normal pregnancy; suspect adrenal insufficiency if the symptoms are unusually severe or persistent.)
    a. Weight loss
    b. Hypotension
    c. Hyperpigmentation
    d. Fever
    e. Fatigue and depression
    f. Salt craving with chronic primary adrenal insufficiency
    g. Acute dehydration
    h. Hypoglycemia
  3. Psychosocial considerations (same as Pregestational Diabetes, Psychosocial Considerations)
  4. Diagnostic and therapeutic procedures
    a. For previous diagnosis, stabilize on glucocorticoids and increase for labor and delivery, surgery, or other severe stress
    b. Diagnosis is confirmed by serum cortisol concentration less than 18 mcg/dL with increased serum ACTH and plasma renin activity, or a concentration lower than the level obtained 60 minutes following cosyntropin administration. Because plasma cortisol increases during gestation, this value might be in the normal, nonpregnant range and still represent a deficiency. Cosyntropin administration is controversial but might be specified. The standard CRH-stimulation test is reliable in diagnosis and differential diagnosis of adrenal insufficiency. If serum cortisol is low with elevated ACTH, antiadrenal antibodies can confirm an autoimmune cause for the disorder (Lindsay & Nieman, 2005).
    c. Laboratory studies
      (1) Electrolytes
      (2) Fasting blood sugar
      (3) Serum ACTH
      (4) Plasma renin activity
      (5) Serum cortisol
      (6) Serum aldosterone
    d. Imagining studies
      (1) CT scan
      (2) Abdominal radiographs (usually contraindicated and avoided in pregnancy)
    e. Glucocorticoid replacement therapy recommended; use of mineralocorticoids might be suggested for replacement of aldosterone deficiency.
    f. Increase dose of steroids before delivery and 24-hour postpartum with patients on chronic therapy.
B. Interventions/Outcomes
  1. Anxiety
    a. Interventions: same as Hyperthyroidism
    b. Outcomes: same as Hyperthyroidism
  2. Therapeutic regimen to optimize maternal and fetal outcomes
    a. Interventions

      (1) Assess and facilitate understanding of effects of adrenal hypofunction on pregnancy and fetal development.

      (2) Provide explanations regarding possible needs for altering or increasing dosage of adrenocortical hormones during pregnancy.

        (a) Minor illnesses

        (b) Acute adrenal crisis

        (c) At time of delivery (either vaginal or cesarean birth)

        (d) In the postpartum period

      (3) Review signs and symptoms of acute adrenal crisis

        (a) Nausea and vomiting

        (b) Abdominal pain

        (c) Fever

        (d) Hypotension

        (e) Shock

      (4) Provide accurate information about all procedures, tests, and interventions planned during pregnancy and after birth of the infant.

      (5) Inform patient of fetal status and well-being.

      (6) Review dietary requirements for adequate nutritional intake and to promote normal fetal growth and development during pregnancy.

  b. Outcomes

      (1) Patient can verbalize an understanding of risks associated with adrenal hypofunction to self and fetus.

      (2) Patient can state a rationale and management plan for alterations in adrenocortical hormone therapy during pregnancy and childbirth.

      (3) Patient can verbalize the signs and symptoms of acute adrenal crisis.

      (4) Patient receives accurate information about all procedures, tests, and interventions planned during pregnancy and after birth of the infant.

      (5) Patient is informed of fetal status and well-being throughout pregnancy and at birth.

      (6) Patient verbalizes adequate nutritional intake during pregnancy.

3. Maternal steroid replacement therapy

  a. Interventions

      (1) Monitor fetal growth and development.

      (2) Assess adrenal function at birth.

  b. Outcomes

      (1) Fetal growth and development are within normal parameters.

      (2) Neonatal adrenal function is assessed at birth.

HEALTH EDUCATION

Hypoadrenocorticism (Addison's Disease)

A. Preconceptual

  1. Discuss assessment of adequacy of adrenocortical hormone replacement as indicated by serum cortisol levels.

  2. Assess and discuss fertility and ovulation.

  3. Discuss potential maternal and neonatal complications associated with adrenal hypofunction in pregnancy; with adequate steroid replacement, outcomes for the mother and neonate are improved.

B. Prenatal

  1. Explain that the need for a careful history-taking and physical assessment of the patient's symptoms at each prenatal visit are important in the diagnosis of adrenal hypofunction (Addison's disease).

  2. Explain that treatment with steroid replacement should begin as soon as possible.

  3. Information regarding potential maternal and neonatal complications associated with adrenal hypofunction in pregnancy should be discussed, as well as alterations in dosage of prescribed adrenocortical hormones to minimize potential complications of acute adrenal crisis and to provide adequate glucocorticoid coverage during birth and in the postpartum period.

MATERNAL PHENYLKETONURIA

A. **Definition**
1. Phenylketonuria (PKU) (also known as hyperphenylalaninemia) is a rare metabolic disorder resulting from a deficiency of the liver enzyme phenylalanine (Phe) hydroxylase (PAH).
2. PKU is a genetic disease with an autosomal recessive genetic trait (defect). There is an inborn error of metabolism, in which the body's ability to efficiently metabolize Phe is impaired because of an enzyme hepatic deficiency (Phe hydroxylase).
3. Phenylalanine is an essential amino acid found in all protein foods; deficiency of Phe hydroxylase prevents metabolization of Phe and causes Phe to rise in the bloodstream. The enzyme deficiency keeps this essential amino acid from being synthesized and converted to tyrosine (Gambol, 2007).
4. In classic PKU, the absence of Phe hydroxylase results in the accumulation of Phe and its metabolites in the blood and urine, inhibiting normal brain development. Excessive levels of Phe lead to severe and irreversible mental retardation.
5. When untreated, children normal at birth become severely mentally retarded, exhibit a variety of behavioral abnormalities, and are at increased risk for congenital heart disease (Gambol, 2007).
6. Clinical manifestations of PKU besides mental retardation might include facial dysmorphism, microcephaly, developmental and speech delays, irritability, vomiting, "musty odor," eczema, hyperactivity, schizoid-like behavioral patterns, and seizures (Maillot, Cook, Lilburn, & Lee, 2007).

B. **Incidence and screening**
1. Incidence of PKU is reported to be 1 in 15,000 live births in the United States (Gambol, 2007; National Institutes of Health [NIH] Consensus Development Panel, 2001).
2. Approximately 300 to 400 infants with PKU are born each year in the United States.
3. Approximately 3000 U.S. women of childbearing age have been successfully treated for PKU.
4. Guthrie test is the most common and inexpensive screening test. A few drops of newborn blood is placed on filter paper. The test is considered positive when Phe rises above 120 μmoL/L.

C. **Management of classic PKU**
1. "Diet for life" approach: Phe levels greater than 10 mg/dL should be treated before the neonate is 7 days old. Medical nutritional therapy for newborns with levels between 7 to 10 mg/dL. No consensus concerning optimal levels of blood Phe. Most common in the United States are 2 to 6 mg/dL for patients younger than 12 years of age and 2 to 10 mg/dL for those older than 12 years.
2. Mothers are encouraged to breastfeed their infants: initially infants are placed on a Phe-restricted diet limiting infant formula and breast milk. The infant is fed a special milk preparation such as Lofenalac or Albumaid XP until Phe levels are at acceptable ranges. Then precalculated amounts of breast milk or formula can be added to the diet while observing the Phe levels. Breast milk has lower levels of Phe than formulas, allowing for greater intake of breast milk and still remain in the therapeutic Phe range (Giovannini, Verduci, Salvatici, Fiori, & Riva, 2007).
3. Monitor monthly or more frequently if needed.
4. Diet has been highly successful in preventing mental retardation.

D. **Maternal PKU**
1. Because women identified as newborns with PKU have been successfully treated with dietary management and have reached childbearing age, the emergence of maternal PKU has been recognized as another form of PKU.
2. Associated fetal and neonatal effects are caused when elevated maternal serum Phe levels cross the placenta and overwhelm the fetus' ability to metabolize Phe. NOTE: This occurs even in the presence of a normal genetic makeup in the fetus; however, there is also a higher incidence of hyperphenylalaninemic infants born to mothers with PKU. The placenta aids in maintaining higher levels of amino acids (Gambol, 2007; NIH Consensus Development Panel, 2001).
3. Maternal PKU prevents the normal expression of liver Phe hydroxylase during fetal development, creating phenotypic hyperphenylalaninemia.
4. Management of maternal PKU
   a. Key to successful management of maternal PKU is the institution of the specific low-Phe diet before conception. Patients are advised to continue to maintain a restricted Phe diet.
      (1) Ideally, the program of dietary therapy is coordinated in collaboration with a PKU clinic.

(2) In the past it was believed to be safe to discontinue the Phe diet after age 6; however, because of the effects of increased Phe on intellectual and neurologic function and effects on fetuses, the Phe diet is recommended throughout life.

(3) The recommended low-Phe diet is highly restrictive, allowing only measured amounts of low-protein cereals, fruits, vegetables, fats, and grains and requiring the consumption of a special formula that is unpalatable to many women. Dairy products, meats, nuts, and aspartame must be avoided, and prescribed supplements must be taken. Vitamin B_{12} and folic acid are recommended prior to conception (Maillot et al, 2007; NIH Consensus Development Panel, 2001).

b. Poor adherence to dietary restrictions and medical recommendations to stop the Phe diet continue to contribute to adverse effects on children born to mothers with PKU. Further, serious consequences to a fetus exposed to elevated Phe can occur.

c. Acceptable suggested range in the United States is 2 to 6 mg/dL; British and German standards are even lower (NIH Consensus Development Panel, 2001).

d. Suggested frequency of monitoring by NIH Consensus Development Panel (2001):
  (1) Once a week during first year
  (2) Twice monthly ages 1 through 12
  (3) Monthly after age 12
  (4) Twice weekly during pregnancy

E. Effects on pregnancy
  1. Maternal effects
    a. None specific to pregnancy
    b. Requirements of low-Phe diet and careful dietary management during pregnancy
  2. Fetal and neonatal effects
    a. Women with classic PKU and other forms of PKU classified with Phe concentrations exceeding 20 mg/dL are at increased risk of having infants with:
      (1) Mental retardation or cognitive impairment
      (2) Intrauterine and postnatal growth restriction
      (3) Low birthweight
      (4) Microcephaly
      (5) Congenital heart defects
      (6) Other malformations
      (7) Spontaneous abortions
    b. Fetal Phe levels are about 50% higher than maternal levels.
    c. Incidence of hyperphenylalaninemia among infants born to mothers with PKU is increased as a result of impaired expression of liver Phe hydroxylase during fetal development.
    d. Depending on the zygosity of the father for PKU, the infant either inherits the disease or is a carrier.

CLINICAL PRACTICE

A. Assessment
  1. History
    a. Identification of childhood PKU, ideally prior to conception
    b. Dietary assessment and counseling: A low-Phe diet is mandatory before conception and metabolic control is necessary across the life span.
  2. Physical findings: None is specific to maternal PKU, although serum Phe levels might be elevated if diet is not restricted.
  3. Psychosocial considerations
    a. Feelings regarding high-risk status of pregnancy due to maternal condition that might affect fetal growth and development
    b. Concerns about low-Phe diet and adhering to it during pregnancy
    c. Access to clinic or health care provider specializing in care and support of women with maternal PKU
  4. Diagnostic procedures
    a. Serum Phe levels are carefully monitored three times a week during pregnancy.
    b. The goal of dietary management is to maintain levels between 2 and 6 mg/dL.

5. Encourage the option to breastfeed. Breastfeeding was once discouraged for women with PKU. Breast milk contains 40 mg/dL of phenylalanine compared with infant formula of 85 mg/dL. Can pump and bottle-feed premeasured amounts and give with prescribed special formula, or can weigh infant before and after breastfeeding and supplement with Phe-free metabolic formula.

B. **Interventions/Outcomes**
   1. Maternal Phe levels
      a. Interventions
         (1) Monitor fetal growth and development.
         (2) Assess maternal serum Phe levels.
            (a) The level recommended is 2 to 6 mg/dL.
            (b) Ideally this level is achieved at least 3 months before conception.
         (3) Refer patient for genetic counseling.
         (4) Encourage compliance with low-Phe diet.
         (5) Prenatal vitamins are not recommended.
         (6) Monitor plasma levels of tyrosine, and other amino acids, zinc, iron, and selenium levels once a month.
      b. Outcomes
         (1) Fetal growth and development are within normal parameters.
         (2) Maternal serum Phe levels are maintained in the prescribed range throughout pregnancy.
         (3) Patient receives information relevant to fetal outcome and genetic inheritance through genetic counseling.
         (4) Patient adheres to low-Phe diet.
   2. Anxiety
      a. Interventions: same as in Hyperthyroidism
      b. Outcomes: same as in Hyperthyroidism
   3. Therapeutic regimen to minimize potential effects of PKU on developing fetus
      a. Interventions
         (1) Assess understanding of low-Phe diet and food-exchange lists.
         (2) Refer for dietary counseling and adaptation of diet to ensure adequate dietary intake for pregnancy and normal growth and development of fetus.
         (3) Provide accurate information about all procedures, tests, and interventions planned during pregnancy and after birth of the infant.
         (4) Inform patient of fetal status and well-being.
         (5) Assess and inform about option to breastfeed.
      b. Outcomes
         (1) Patient can verbalize an understanding of low-Phe diet and food-exchange lists.
         (2) Patient receives information about adequate dietary intake for pregnancy and normal growth and development of the fetus.
         (3) Patient receives accurate information about all procedures, tests, and interventions planned during pregnancy and after birth of the infant.
         (4) Patient is informed of fetal status and well-being throughout pregnancy and at birth.
   4. Imbalanced nutrition
      a. Interventions
         (1) Assess understanding of low-Phe diet and food-exchange lists.
         (2) Refer patient for dietary counseling and adaptation of diet to ensure adequate dietary intake for pregnancy and normal growth and development of fetus.
            (a) Diet combines low-protein foods (primarily fruits and vegetables) with special formulas containing all amino acids except Phe.
            (b) Prenatal vitamins should not be prescribed because all except folic acid are provided in special dietary formulas used to treat PKU.
            (c) Folic acid supplements should be provided separately.
         (3) Monitor patient's ability to follow dietary requirements and reported intake.
         (4) Monitor maternal weight gain and fetal growth during pregnancy.
      b. Outcomes
         (1) Patient can verbalize an understanding of low-Phe diet and food-exchange lists.
         (2) Patient's dietary intake is adequate for pregnancy and normal growth and development of the fetus.

(3) Patient verbalizes her ability to follow dietary requirements and reports actual dietary intake as prescribed.

(4) Patient demonstrates adequate weight gain with appropriate fetal growth during pregnancy.

HEALTH EDUCATION

Maternal Phenylketonuria

A. Preconceptual

1. Counseling regarding the potential risks associated with maternal PKU, including the genetic assessment of risk to potential children of the inheritance of PKU and the effects of elevated Phe levels on fetal development

2. Discussion of information regarding the potential dangers to the developing fetus from untreated maternal PKU as well as the fetal protection offered by dietary treatment beginning before conception and maintained throughout pregnancy

3. Counseling regarding the need for family planning so that a low-Phe diet can be initiated prior to conception. Note: It is particularly important that this information is also presented to adolescents with childhood PKU so that unintentional pregnancy might be prevented and appropriate dietary requirements can be instituted prior to conception.

4. Discussion of the importance of early identification of pregnancy and information regarding the specific dietary treatment and therapeutic regimen prescribed before conception and during pregnancy

5. Ideally, preconceptual referral to a PKU clinic for genetic counseling, biochemical analysis, nutritional formulas, and support for comprehensive and multidisciplinary management of maternal PKU

B. Prenatal

1. Counseling regarding the importance of maintaining a prescribed low-Phe diet to optimize pregnancy and neonatal outcomes

2. Ongoing explanations and education regarding rationale for prescribed tests and procedures to assess fetal growth and well-being

C. Postpartum

1. Assessment and screening of neonate to evaluate PKU status

2. Institution of low-Phe diet for neonate with PKU (usually recommended to be initiated before 3 weeks of age)

3. May breastfeed along with low-Phe diet

4. Counseling regarding the need for family planning to prevent unintended pregnancy and to encourage return to low-Phe diet before conception; many centers specializing in the care of persons with PKU recommend indefinite continuation of the PKU diet for women with PKU throughout their childbearing years and lifetime.

CASE STUDY AND STUDY QUESTIONS

J.S., a 31-year-old Hispanic primigravida, presents to the maternity clinic for her routine prenatal care visit at 26 weeks' gestation. She complains of urinary frequency and excessive thirst. Her fundal height measures 28 cm. She began her pregnancy 25 pounds overweight, but has maintained appropriate weight gain thus far. The 50-g glucose tolerance test J.S. took last week revealed a plasma level of 160 mg/dL. A subsequent OGTT was positive for gestational diabetes. J.S. is now taking insulin injections twice a day. The nurse provided information on self–blood glucose monitoring and administering insulin injections correctly. J.S. states she is worried about how her diabetes will affect the pregnancy. She is concerned about what changes she will have to make in her daily routine and what the pregnancy outcome will be.

1. The nurse assesses J.S.'s anxiety about the possible effects of diabetes on pregnancy and tells her that the *most* important factor

in achieving a successful pregnancy with minimal complications is:

a. The length of time she has had diabetes

b. The absence of vascular complications

c. Maintenance of near-normal blood glucose levels throughout pregnancy

d. Frequency of self-monitoring of blood glucose levels

2. J.S. asks the nurse how her diabetes will affect her baby. The *best* explanation is:

a. "Your baby may be smaller than average at birth."

b. "Your baby will probably be larger than average at birth."

c. "As long as you control your blood sugar, your baby will not be affected at all."

d. "Your baby might have high blood sugar for several days."

3. J. S. is following a program of regular exercise, which includes walking and swimming. What instructions should be included in a teaching plan for her?

a. Exercise either just before meals or wait until 2 hours after a meal.

b. Carry hard candy (or simple sugar) when exercising.

c. If her blood sugar is 130 mg/dL, eat 20 g of carbohydrate.

d. If her blood sugar is more than 120 mg/dL, drink a glass of whole milk.

4. The nurse prepares J.S. for additional laboratory work, clinical assessments, and consults that will be obtained during her care. These additional tests and referrals may include all of the following *except:*

a. Biophysical profile

b. Dietary counseling

c. Fetal glucose utilization index

d. Glycosylated hemoglobin (HbA$_{1c}$)

5. J.S. is concerned about the episodes of hypoglycemia that have occurred at night during the previous week. The nurse explains that this commonly occurs early in pregnancy for what reason?

a. The fetus produces insulin that crosses the placenta and decreases maternal insulin requirements.

b. The placenta produces hormones that decrease maternal insulin requirements during pregnancy.

c. The fetus is constantly using maternal glucose for its growth and development.

d. The metabolic changes associated with pregnancy predispose women with diabetes to experience decreased needs for insulin during pregnancy.

6. Specific guidelines should be followed when planning a diet with a diabetic woman to

ensure a euglycemic state. An appropriate diet would reflect:

a. About 40 calories/kg or prepregnancy weight daily

b. A caloric distribution among three meals and at least two snacks

c. A minimum of 350 mg of carbohydrate daily

d. A protein intake of at least 30% of the total kcal in a day

7. Infants born to women with gestational diabetes are at increased risk for:

a. Fetal macrosomia

b. Neonatal hyperglycemia

c. Neonatal seizures

d. Congenital anomalies

8. Ms. W. presents to labor and delivery at 36 weeks' gestation with the possible diagnosis of thyroid storm. Which signs and symptoms are characteristic of thyroid storm?

a. Fatigue, sudden weight loss, heat intolerance, extreme weakness

b. Low blood pressure, bradycardia, lethargy, generalized interstitial edema

c. Blurred vision, hypertension, epigastric pain, severe headache

d. High fever, tachycardia, dehydration, profuse sweating, restlessness

9. Ms. O. was diagnosed with Addison's disease 3 years ago. Since then she has been managed with prednisone for maintenance steroid replacement. She is admitted to labor and delivery at 40 weeks' gestation and is in labor. In addition to monitoring Ms. O.'s progress in labor and fetal status, which clinical signs and symptoms should be closely monitored during labor, during delivery, and in the immediate postpartum period?

a. Nausea and vomiting, abdominal pain, fever, hypotension, shock

b. Hyperventilation, dehydration, odor of acetone on breath, impaired mental status

c. High fever, tachycardia, dehydration, congestive heart failure

d. Hypertension, central nervous system irritability, edema, proteinuria

10. Why is the institution of a low-Phe diet indicated before conception and during pregnancy in a woman with PKU?

a. To prevent the inheritance of this disease by the developing fetus

b. To minimize the incidence of mental retardation, microcephaly, congenital heart defects, and growth restriction in the developing fetus

c. To prevent the expression of liver Phe hydroxylase during fetal development

ANSWERS TO STUDY QUESTIONS

1. c	5. c	9. a
2. b	6. b	10. b
3. b	7. a	
4. c	8. d	

REFERENCES

American College of Obstetricians and Gynecologists (2001). ACOG Practice Bulletin. *Gestational diabetes, 30*, 525–538.

American College of Obstetricians and Gynecologists (2002). ACOG Practice Bulletin. *Thyroid disease in pregnancy*, 387–396.

American College of Obstetricians and Gynecologists (2005). ACOG Practice Bulletin. *Pregestational diabetes mellitus, 60*, 675–684.

American Diabetes Association (ADA). (2009a). Diagnosis and classification of diabetes mellitus. *Diabetes Care, 32*(1), 62–67.

American Diabetes Association (ADA). (2009b). Position statement: Standards of medical care in diabetes. *Diabetes Care, 32*(1), 15–16, 40-41.

Biller, B. M., Grossman, A. B., Stewart, P. M., Melmed, S., Bertagna, X., Bertherat, J., Buchfelder, M., Colao, A., Hermus, A. R., Hofland, L. J., Klibanski, A., Lacroix, A., Lindsay, J. R., Newell-Price, J., Nieman, L. K., Petersenn, S., Sonino, N., Stalla, G. K., Swearingen, B., Vance, M. L., Wass, J. A., & Boscaro, M. (2008). Treatment of adrenocorticotropin-dependent Cushing's syndrome: A consensus statement. *Journal of Clinical Endocrinology and Metabolism, 93*(7), 2454–2462.

California Diabetes and Pregnancy Program (CDAPP). (2008). *Sweet success guidelines for care*. Sacramento, CA: California Department of Public Health; Maternal Child Adolescent Health Division.

Carpenter, M. W., & Coustan, D. R. (1982). Criteria for screening tests for gestational diabetes. *American Journal of Obstetrics & Gynecology, 144*, 768–773.

Casey, B. M., & Leveno, K. J. (2006). Thyroid disease in pregnancy. *Obstetrics & Gynecology, 108*(5), 1283–1292.

Combs, C. A., Gavin, L. A., Gunderson, E., Main, E. K., & Kitzmiller, J. L. (1992). Relationship of fetal macrosomia to maternal postprandial glucose control during pregnancy. *Diabetes Care, 15*, 1251–1257.

Crowther, C. A., Hiller, J. E., Moss, J. R., McPhee, A. J., Jeffries, W. S., & Robinson, J. S. (2005). The Australian Carbohydrate Intolerance Study in Pregnant Women (ACHIOS) Trial Group: Effect of treatment of gestational diabetes on pregnancy outcome. *New England Journal of Medicine, 352*, 2477–2486.

Diabetes Control and Complications Trial (DCCT) Research Group. (1993). The effect of intensive treatment of diabetes on the development and progression of long-term complications in insulin-dependent diabetes mellitus. *New England Journal of Medicine, 329*(14), 977–986.

Gambol, P. J. (2007). Maternal phenylketonuria syndrome and case management implications. *Journal of Pediatric Nursing, 22*(2), 129–137.

Gilmartin, A. B., Ural, S. H., & Repke, J. T. (2008). Gestational diabetes mellitus. *Reviews in Obstetrics & Gynecology, 1*(3), 129–134.

Giovannini, M., Verduci, E., Salvatici, E., Fiori, L., & Riva, E. (2007). Phenylketonuria: Dietary and therapeutic challenges. *Journal of Inherited Metabolic Disease, 30*(2), 145–152.

Langer, O., Yogev, Y., Xenakis, E. M. J., & Rosenn, B. (2005). Insulin and glyburide therapy: Dosage, severity level of gestational diabetes, and pregnancy outcome. *American Journal of Obstetrics & Gynecology, 192*, 134–139.

Lapolla, A., Dalfra, M. G., & Fedele, D. (2005). Insulin therapy in pregnancy complicated by diabetes: Are insulin analogs a new tool? *Diabetes Metabolism Research and Reviews, 21*, 241–252.

Lindsay, J. R., & Nieman, L. K. (2005). The hypothalamic-pituitary-adrenal axis in pregnancy: Challenges in disease detection and treatment. *Endocrine Reviews, 26*(6), 775–799.

Maillot, F., Cook, P., Lilburn, M., & Lee, P. J. (2007). A practical approach to maternal phenylketonuria management. *Journal of Inherited Metabolic Diseases, 30*, 198–201.

McLaughlin, G., Blake, D. O., Cheng, Y. W., & Caughey, A. B. (2006). Women with one elevated 3-hour glucose tolerance test value: Are they at risk for adverse perinatal outcome? *American Journal of Obstetrics & Gynecology, 194*, 16–19.

Metzger, B. E., Buchanan, T. A., Coustan, D. R., de Leiva, A., Dunger, D. B., Hadden, D. R., Hod, M., Kitzmiller, J. L., Kjos, S. L., Oats, J. N., Pettitt, D. J., Sacks, D. A., & Zoupas, C. (2007). Summary and recommendations of the fifth international workshop conference on gestational diabetes mellitus. *Diabetes Care, 30*(Suppl 2), S251–S260.

Metzger, B. E., Lowe, L. P., Dyer, A. R., Trimble, E. R., Chaovarindr, U., Coustan, D. R., Hadden, D. R., McCance, D. R., Hod, M., McIntyre, H. D., Oats, J. J., Persson, B., Rogers, M. S., & Sacks, D. A. (2008). HAPO Study Cooperative Research Group; Hyperglycemia and adverse pregnancy outcomes. *New England Journal of Medicine, 358*(19), 1991–2002.

National Institutes of Health (NIH) Consensus Development Panel. (2001). Phenylketonuria screening and management. *Pediatrics, 108*(4), 972–982.

Perkins, J. M., Dunn, J. P., & Jagasia, S. (2007). Perspectives in gestational diabetes mellitus: A review of screening, diagnosis, and treatment. *Clinical Diabetes, 25*(2), 57–62.

Reece, E. A., & Homko, C. J. (2008). Diabetes mellitus and pregnancy. In R. S. Gibbs, B. Y. Karlan, A. F. Haney, & I. E. Nygaard (Eds.), *Danforth's obstetrics and gynecology* (10th ed). Philadelphia: Wolters Kluwer/Lippincott Williams & Wilkins.

Ricci, S. (2007). *Essentials of maternity, newborn, and women's health nursing.* Philadelphia: Lippincott Williams & Wilkins.

Rowan, J. A., Hague, W. M., Gao, W., Battin, M. R., & Moore, M. P. (2008). Metformin versus insulin for the treatment of gestational diabetes. *New England Journal of Medicine, 358,* 19.

Slocum, J. M. (2007). Preconception counseling and type 2 diabetes. *Diabetes Spectrum, 20,* 117–123.

23 Trauma in Pregnancy

Lucy R. Van Otterloo

OBJECTIVES

1. State the normal physiologic changes that potentially affect the evaluation of a pregnant trauma patient.
2. Identify the major mechanisms of injury that affect the pregnant trauma patient.
3. Describe the components of the primary and secondary survey for a pregnant trauma patient.
4. List interventions to prevent maternal and fetal mortality resulting from trauma.
5. Develop a plan of care for a pregnant patient experiencing blunt or penetrating trauma.
6. Demonstrate knowledge of the physiologic changes of pregnancy and the specific mechanisms of injury in the assessment, diagnosis, planning, intervention, and evaluation of a pregnant trauma patient and her fetus.
7. Interpret physiologic assessment and diagnostic findings to establish priorities for the care of the pregnant trauma patient and her fetus.
8. Identify health promotion needs, and promote behavioral changes that produce healthy outcomes of pregnancy.

INTRODUCTION

A. Incidence and epidemiology
   1. Trauma is the fourth leading cause of death worldwide and the leading cause of maternal death during pregnancy.
      a. In the United States, 6% to 7% of all pregnant women experience some sort of trauma, with the greatest frequency in the last trimester (Tweddale, 2006).
      b. Trauma is more likely to cause maternal death than any other medical complication of pregnancy (Mattox & Goetzl, 2005).
      c. The most common cause of maternal death by trauma is serious abdominal injury leading to hemorrhagic shock and head injury (Ikossi, Lazar, Morabito, Fildes, & Knudson, 2005).
      d. The most common cause of fetal death is maternal death and maternal shock; fetal demise results 80% of the time when the mother experiences hemorrhagic shock (McGowan Repasky, 2007).
   2. Injury to the pregnant patient can result from forces causing blunt or penetrating trauma.
      a. Blunt trauma is the most frequent cause of maternal and fetal injury (McGowan Repasky, 2007).
      b. The most common causes of blunt trauma are motor vehicle accidents (MVAs), falls, and assaults.
         (1) Blunt trauma might result from force applied to the abdomen from direct impact or as a result of secondary injury from abdominal organ displacement and hemorrhage from coup-contrecoup event (Tweddale, 2006).
         (2) Rapid compression, deceleration, or shearing forces can also result in abruptio placentae (McGowan Repasky, 2007).
         (3) Blunt abdominal trauma can lead to retroperitoneal bleeding as well as pelvic fractures, abruption, rupture, or premature onset of labor (Muench & Canterino, 2007).
      c. Penetrating trauma occurs most frequently from gunshot or stab wounds, with gunshot wounds being more common.
      d. Fetal injury is more common during the third trimester when the head is relatively fixed in the pelvis and less amniotic fluid is present to buffer energy transfer (Tweddale, 2006).
      e. The incidence of intentional injury from domestic violence rises during pregnancy (El Kady, Gilbert, Xing, & Smith, 2005).

        (1) Women who claim fall injuries but whose patterns of injuries do not correlate might have been abused.

        (2) Screening for abuse assessment should be done privately.

B. Important concepts for trauma in pregnancy

  1. The initial goal in trauma evaluation is maternal stabilization.

    a. Resuscitation during pregnancy proceeds as in any other trauma patient.

    b. The primary assessment includes the ABCs: Airway, Breathing, Circulation, and cervical spinal precautions, as well any emergent interventions needed to support the ABCs.

    c. The secondary assessment includes a full set of vital signs (including fetal heart rate [FHR]), brief overall examination (maternal and fetal), and important historical data; further injury-focused assessments are completed once all of the injuries are identified.

  2. Trauma in pregnancy involves two patients: woman and fetus.

    a. Minor injuries to the woman might cause significant or fatal injury to the fetus.

    b. Maternal outcome in trauma corresponds to the injury, whereas fetal outcome depends on the injury and the maternal physiologic response.

    c. Early recognition of pregnancy assists in identification of pregnancy-related changes that might alter assessment findings and mask signs of shock (Ikossi et al, 2005).

  3. Proper seatbelt use prevents ejection during motor vehicle collisions; ejection from vehicles frequently results in head trauma with high maternal and fetal death rates.

  4. Risk factors predictive of fetal death include young age, history of smoking or alcohol use, placental abruption, maternal ejection from MVA, maternal death, maternal hypotension, maternal hypoxia, younger gestational age, lack of restraints from MVA, and an injury severity score greater than 9 (Aboutanos et al, 2007; El Kady, 2007; Muench & Canterino, 2007).

  5. Frequently, trauma cases involve litigation; accurate, well-documented records protect patients as well as the health care system.

C. Important physiologic considerations for trauma in pregnancy (altered physiologic state of the pregnant patient alters the patient's response to trauma) (Muench & Canterino, 2007).

  1. Cardiovascular changes

    a. Blood volume increases 50%, and of this, plasma volume increases 30% to 40% and red blood cell volume only increases 20% to 30%, leading to a physiologic anemia in pregnancy (Gordon, 2007; Tsuei, 2006).

      (1) By the third trimester, maternal cardiac output peaks at 50% above nonpregnant values, which is indicated by an increase in baseline normal heart rates of 10 to 15 beats per minute (bpm).

      (2) Blood pressure change also occurs with a 5 to 15 mm Hg drop in the systolic and diastolic readings (Muench & Canterino, 2007).

      (3) The maturing fetus causes marked increases in uterine blood flow, which can comprise 20% of cardiac output at term (Tsuei, 2006); maternal perfusion pressure is needed to maintain uterine blood flow.

    b. Pregnant women in shock might not have cool, clammy skin typical of shock because of normal maternal vasodilation in the first and second trimesters (Tweddale, 2006).

      (1) The physiologic changes in pregnancy might delay the usual vital sign changes of hypovolemia; blood loss of up to 1500 mL can occur without a change in maternal vital signs.

      (2) A 15% to 30% reduction of uterine blood flow can occur without change in maternal blood pressure; fetal compromise can occur before there are any changes in maternal vital signs.

    c. Compression of the inferior vena cava, from the fetus, when the mother is in a supine position (after 20 weeks' gestation) can result in a systolic blood pressure drop of up to 30 mm Hg and a 28% cardiac output decrease (Tsuei, 2006); by displacing the uterus to the left when a supine position or spinal immobilization is required, the compression can be relieved (Figure 23-1).

    d. Because the fetal heart rate is often the first vital sign to change, all pregnant trauma patients need continuous fetal heart rate monitoring.

  2. Respiratory changes affect maternal and fetal outcome when trauma occurs.

    a. Hormonal and mechanical (enlarging uterus) changes combine to produce hyperventilation (Ladewig, London, & Davidson, 2010).

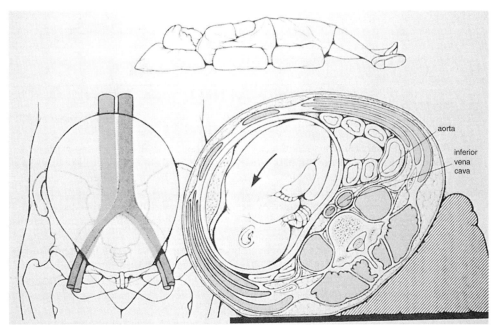

FIGURE 23-1 ■ Left lateral positioning displaces the uterus and decreases compression of major abdominal vessels. (From McQuillan, K.A., Flynn Makic, M.B., & Whalen, E. [2008]. *Trauma nursing: From resuscitation through rehabilitation* [4th ed.]. Philadelphia: Saunders.)

(1) The elevation of the diaphragm by the gravid uterus results in a 20% decrease in functional residual capacity (FRC); increased maternal oxygen consumption, and diminished oxygen reserves occur, increasing susceptibility to hypoxia (Ramsay, 2006).

(2) Minute ventilation and tidal volume are increased 40% and respiratory rate will increase, leading to a predisposition for rapid hypoxemia with apnea (Torgersen & Curran, 2006).

b. PaO_2 is normal or slightly increased, but the $PaCO_2$ decreases to 27 to 32 mm Hg; a compensated respiratory alkalosis occurs with the pH remaining in the normal range due to increased excretion of bicarbonate by the kidneys (Yeomans & Gilstrap III, 2005).

(1) Anxiety and pain can cause respiratory rate increases that result in hypocapnia and can lead to faintness and perioral numbness.

(2) Capillary engorgement of the mucosa causes swelling of the respiratory tract, severely compromising the airway, making intubation more difficult (Muench & Canterino, 2007).

c. Maternal hypoxia (diminished oxygen reserve) affects fetal oxygenation; therefore, fetal heart rate changes might indicate maternal hypoxia; arterial blood gas measurement is the best indicator of maternal status (Witcher, 2006).

3. Gastrointestinal changes occur during pregnancy.

a. The small bowel is pushed up by the uterus, and the large bowel moves posteriorly; penetrating trauma might injure multiple loops of bowel (Cunningham et al, 2005).

(1) Diminished bowel sounds might be normal or indicate intraperitoneal injury (Smith, 2009).

(2) Chronic distention of the parietal peritoneum by the uterus reduces the symptoms of intraperitoneal bleeding, such as rigidity and guarding (Chames & Pearlman, 2008).

b. Progesterone causes smooth muscle relaxation, and lower esophageal sphincter tone is decreased (Tsuei, 2006), increasing the need for a nasal gastric tube in the trauma pregnant patient.

c. The enlarged uterus is vulnerable to injury but can protect the maternal abdominal organs (spleen, liver, kidneys, bowel).

4. The genitourinary system changes in pregnancy increase the risk of injury.
   a. The bladder moves from the pelvic area to the abdominal area by 12 weeks' gestation, increasing the risk of traumatic injury (Constanty & Cruz, 2006). Figure 23-2 shows uterine size and location, reflecting gestational age.
   b. Renal blood flow increases in pregnancy, the serum creatinine and blood urea nitrogen values are lower, and hydronephrosis is common due to the smooth muscle–relaxing properties of progesterone.
5. The hematologic changes that occur in pregnancy put the pregnant trauma patient at risk for disseminated intravascular coagulopathy.
   a. Platelet levels might be normal or slightly lower than normal.
   b. Fibrinogen levels are doubled by the third trimester.
   c. There is an increase in clotting factors VII, VIII, IX, and X that can result in hypercoagulopathy and increased thromboembolic risk (Constanty & Cruz, 2006).
6. The pelvis becomes more flexible during pregnancy, and a widening occurs.
   a. An unsteady gait caused by the widening pelvis and increased abdomen might predispose the pregnant patient to falls (Schiff, 2008).
   b. A widened symphysis pubis by the third trimester decreases the risk for pelvic fractures (Smith, 2009).

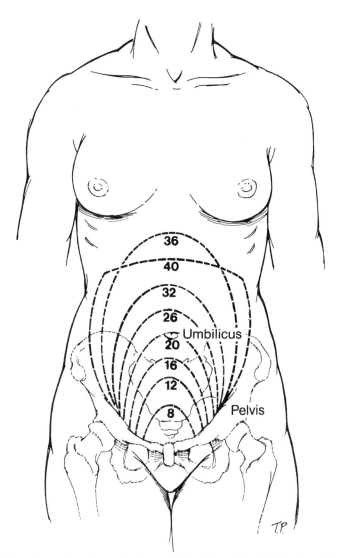

FIGURE 23-2 ■ Uterine size and location, reflecting gestational age. (From McQuillan, K.A., Flynn Makic, M.B., & Whalen, E. [2009]. *Trauma nursing: From resuscitation through rehabilitation* [4th ed.]. Philadelphia: Saunders.)

D. **Types of trauma injuries**
   1. Maternal injuries
      a. Head injuries
      b. Chest injuries
      c. Abdominal and pelvic injuries
      d. Spinal trauma
      e. Burns and inhalation injuries
      f. Fracture/sprain/dislocation
      g. Soft tissue injuries
   2. Fetal injuries
      a. Skull fractures
      b. Other direct fetal injury
      c. Fetal death
E. **Cause or mechanism of injury**
   1. Motor vehicle accidents (MVAs)
      a. MVAs account for most traumas and are the leading cause of more serious maternal injury (66% to 67%) (El Kady, 2007; Schiff & Holt, 2005).
      b. Lack of seatbelt use contributes to increased morbidity and mortality (Sirin, Weiss, Sauber-Schatz, & Dunning, 2007) by increasing the number of patients who have been ejected from the vehicle as well as the number receiving blunt head and abdominal trauma.
      c. Head and blunt abdominal injuries are the most common causes of maternal death.
      d. Maternal death is the most common cause of fetal death.
      e. MVAs are the most frequent cause of blunt injury, which can result in abruptio placentae, uterine rupture, and preterm labor.
      f. Pelvic fracture occurs most often with an MVA and can cause massive bleeding as well as fetal skull fracture.
   2. Falls
      a. Falls are the second most common cause of blunt trauma in pregnancy (26%) (Schiff, 2008).
      b. Head and spinal cord injuries, and fractures of the pelvis and lower extremities are common because a pregnant woman is likely to fall on her buttock or side (Schiff, 2008).
      c. Observation for abruptio placentae is important.
      d. Details of the fall, such as the height of the fall and landing surface material, can be important factors to consider when assessing for injuries.
   3. Assaults
      a. Assaults are rapidly edging out falls as the second leading cause of injury to pregnant women, especially in urban areas; assaults cause blunt and penetrating injuries.
      b. Assaults might cause death, direct maternal or fetal injury, preterm labor, and abruptio placentae.
      c. Domestic violence affects up to 20% of women (American Academy of Pediatrics [AAP] and American College of Obstetricians and Gynecologists [ACOG], 2007); domestic violence is rarely an isolated event and often escalates in pregnancy (see Chapter 18 for a complete discussion of intimate partner violence in pregnancy); any nonvehicular trauma in pregnancy warrants domestic violence screening (El Kady et al, 2005).
      d. Younger pregnant women (ages 15 to 24) are more likely to be hospitalized for assault than older pregnant women (El Kady et al, 2005).
   4. Burns and inhalation
      a. The incidence of burns is low, but burns are detrimental to fetal survival (Tweddale, 2006).
         (1) Burns are generally caused from flames or hot liquids.
         (2) Fetal survival is influenced by gestational age and maternal survival, as well as the total body surface area (TBSA) burned.
      b. Inhalation injuries and carbon monoxide intoxication should always be suspected in the burn victim.
         (1) Carbon monoxide poisoning impairs the release of oxygen from the mother to the fetus and from the fetal hemoglobin to fetal tissue (Kennedy, McMurtry Baird, & Troiano, 2008).
         (2) Concentration of carboxyhemoglobin is 10% to 15% higher in the fetus than in the mother, and the fetal half-life of carbon monoxide is twice as long as that of the maternal half-life (Kennedy et al, 2008).

(3) Automobile exhaust and faulty heating systems are also major causes of carbon monoxide poisoning (the leading cause of all poisoning deaths).

5. Gunshot and stab wounds

    a. Gunshot wounds are the more common of the two and usually require surgical exploration and repair.

    b. The uterine muscle absorbs energy from penetrating bullets, which decreases the velocity and lessens the likelihood of visceral injury (Tweddale, 2006).

    c. Penetrating wounds to the uterus can cause significant injury to the fetus (70%), but they generally result in a good maternal outcome (Mattox & Goetzl, 2005).

    d. With penetrating injury above the umbilicus after the second half of pregnancy, there is an increased likelihood of injury to the bowel.

F. **Complications**

    1. Premature labor

    2. Abruptio placentae

        a. Occurs in as many as 50% of patients with major injuries (Tsuei, 2006)

        b. Occurs in as many as 5% of patients with minor injuries (Tsuei, 2006)

    3. Uterine rupture

    4. Maternal cardiopulmonary arrest/fetal delivery

CLINICAL PRACTICE

A. **Assessment**

    1. History

        a. A brief history is obtained if possible, including chief complaint, mechanism of injury, previous assessment, and treatment.

        b. Mechanism of injury

            (1) Blunt injury

                (a) Motor vehicle accident

                    [i] Position in vehicle (driver, passenger, front, rear)

                    [ii] Restraints used (shoulder harness, lap belt, three-point restraint, helmet)

                    [iii] Speed of all vehicles involved in collision

                    [iv] Point of impact: head on, rear, or side collision (T-bone) and amount of intrusion into the passenger compartment

                    [v] Airbag deployment

                    [vi] Ejection from vehicle versus extrication required

                (b) Assault

                    [i] Blunt trauma versus penetrating instrument

                    [ii] Single or multiple assaults

                    [iii] Area of injury

                (c) Fall

                    [i] Height of fall

                    [ii] Landing surface

                    [iii] Body part impacted

                    [iv] Was fall broken or was it direct impact?

            (2) Penetrating injury

                (a) Stab wound

                    [i] Offending object, type

                    [ii] Length and width of object

                    [iii] Direction of assault

                    [iv] Depth of penetration

                (b) Ballistic or gunshot wound

                    [i] Type and caliber of weapon

                    [ii] Low or high velocity

                    [iii] Distance from weapon to victim-range

                    [iv] Trajectory

             (3) Burns

                (a) Causative agent (direct flame, hot liquid, chemical, electric, radiation)

(b) Extent of burn (total amount of body surface area burned)

(c) Depth of burn (partial or full thickness)

(d) Carbon monoxide exposure

(e) Inhalation damage/hoarseness of voice

2. Primary maternal assessment: rapid, brief assessment of the patient to identify any life-threatening problem requiring immediate intervention per Trauma Nursing Core Course guidelines (Emergency Nurses Association [2007]) (Figure 23-3)

   a. A—airway

      (1) Open and clear

         (a) Patient able to speak

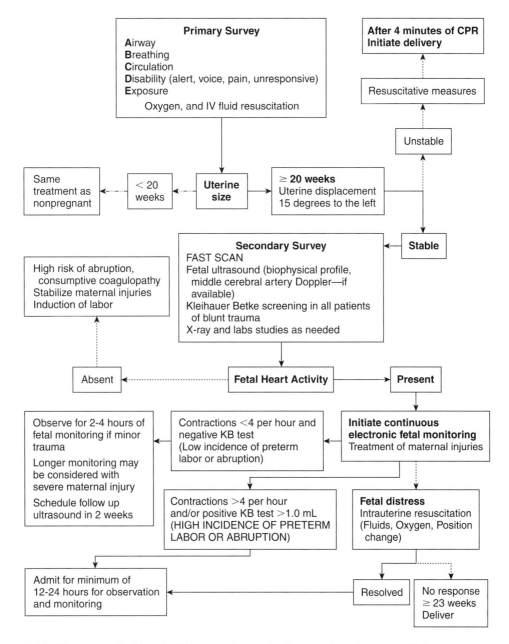

***Modifications to algorithm should be based on mechanism of maternal trauma and injury

FIGURE 23-3 ■ Maternal trauma algorithm. *CPR*, Cardiopulmonary resuscitation; *FAST SCAN*, focus assessment sonographic trauma scan; *IV*, intravenous; *KB*, Kleihauer-Betke. (From Muench, M.V., & Canterino, J.C. [2007]. Trauma in pregnancy. *Obstetrics and Gynecology Clinics of North America*, 34[3], 555-583.)

          (b) No stridor

          (c) No visible foreign matter in the upper airway

     (2) Obstructed

          (a) Patient unable to speak

          (b) Stridor, noisy, or absent respirations

          (c) Vomitus, teeth, blood, secretions, or debris in upper airway

          (d) Substernal and intercostal retractions

          (e) Decreased level of consciousness

          (f) Soft tissue damage to the face and neck

          (g) Cyanosis and dusky mucous membranes and nailbeds

     (3) Interventions if airway obstruction

          (a) Jaw-thrust maneuver to open airway

          (b) Gentle oral suction to remove vomitus, blood, secretions, and so on

          (c) Insertion of oral or nasal airway to maintain airway if needed

     (4) Cervical spine precautions

          (a) Maintain cervical spine precautions or initiate them if not previously done.

          (b) Cervical collar, head block, backboard, and straps in correct placement needed

  b. B—breathing

     (1) Effective

          (a) Spontaneous rise and fall of chest

          (b) Unlabored respirations

          (c) Equal chest expansion

          (d) No accessory muscle use

     (2) Ineffective

          (a) Apnea or agonal respirations less than 10 per minute

          (b) Shallow, ineffective respirations

          (c) Unequal or absent breath sounds

          (d) Asymmetry of chest wall expansion, severe retractions

          (e) Tracheal shift or distended neck veins

          (f) Obvious chest wounds, such as an open pneumothorax; impaled object in chest; multiple rib fractures

          (g) Decreased level of consciousness

          (h) Cyanosis and dusky mucous membranes and nailbeds

     (3) Interventions if breathing ineffective

          (a) 100% oxygen with nonrebreather mask

          (b) Bag-valve mask with 100% oxygen

          (c) Assist with needle thoracotomy or chest tube insertion if pneumothorax or tension pneumothorax is suspected.

          (d) Cover open wound with three-sided dressing.

          (e) Stabilize impaled object (but do not remove).

          (f) Assist with intubation if needed.

  c. C—circulation

     (1) Effective

          (a) Palpable radial pulse between 60 and 100 bpm

          (b) Normal capillary refill time (less than 2 seconds)

          (c) Pink, warm, and dry skin

          (d) Patient alert and oriented

     (2) Ineffective

          (a) Unable to palpate peripheral pulses

          (b) Obvious external hemorrhage

          (c) Delayed capillary refill (more than 2 seconds)

          (d) Decreased level of consciousness

          (e) Pale, cool, moist skin

     (3) Interventions if circulation is ineffective

          (a) Stop any obvious external sources of bleeding.

          (b) Start two large-bore (14- to 16-gauge) intravenous (IV) lines and run warmed fluid (lactated Ringer's or normal saline) in rapidly.

        (c) Transfuse blood products as ordered, O-negative, until type-specific blood is available.

        (d) Administer volume expanders such as Hespan as ordered.

        (e) Assist with emergency thoracotomy if needed.

        (f) Cardiopulmonary resuscitation if needed for circulatory support

  d. D—deficit (brief neurologic examination)

    (1) AVPU assessment method

        (a) A: alert

        (b) V: responds to verbal stimuli

        (c) P: responds to painful stimuli

        (d) U: unresponsive

    (2) Can follow commands; moves all extremities; note any numbness or tingling noted by patient

    (3) Brief pupil examination looking for pupil size, symmetry, and reaction to light

3. Secondary maternal assessment: Brief, complete head-to-toe survey is performed to determine all injuries, obvious as well as hidden.

  a. E—expose and environmental controls

    (1) Remove all clothing for examination.

        (a) Clothes should be cut off in the interest of time.

        (b) If the patient is unstable, particularly with a suspected spinal injury, cut clothing off.

    (2) Keep patient warm with blankets, warmed IV fluids, and warming lights.

  b. F—five interventions, full set of vital signs, facilitate family presence

    (1) Obtain vital signs: blood pressure (BP)—auscultated BPs (both arms if chest injuries are suspected); heart rate (HR), respiratory rate, and temperature; include FHR.

    (2) Obtain pulse oximetry.

    (3) Apply cardiac monitor.

    (4) Draw blood for type and crossmatch and other lab tests.

    (5) Consider indwelling urinary catheter.

    (6) Consider oral or nasal gastric tube.

    (7) Facilitate family presence (i.e., notification of family or significant other).

  c. G—give comfort measures.

    (1) Pain medications as ordered

    (2) Verbal assurances/psychosocial support

    (3) Touch/repositioning

  d. H—history and head-to-toe examination focused on identifying all injuries per Emergency Nurses Association's Trauma Nursing Core Course (2007) guidelines

    (1) Any pertinent maternal history

        (a) Medications and allergies

        (b) Maternal history: gravida, parity, abortion, living children

        (c) Additional data regarding the details and mechanism of injury

    (2) Any pertinent fetal history

        (a) Fetal movement since incident

        (b) Any problems with pregnancy

    (3) Head-to-toe brief examination to identify all injuries using inspection, palpation, percussion, and auscultation skills

        (a) General appearance of patient: abnormal posturing, other unusual body positioning or alignment, and unusual odors

        (b) Head and face

           [i] Surface wounds, ecchymosis, edema, deformity, and tenderness

           [ii] Pupils: size, equality, and reactivity

           [iii] Raccoon eyes (periorbital ecchymosis caused by dissection of blood from a basilar skull fracture)

           [iv] Drainage (clear or bloody) from nose or ears

           [v] Battle's sign (ecchymosis over mastoid process behind the ear)

           [vi] Nasal deformity or tenderness

           [vii] Neck, surface wounds and edema, tracheal deviation, and distended neck veins

      (c) Neck
- [i] Surface wounds and edema
- [ii] Trachea position
- [iii] Distended neck veins
- [iv] Subcutaneous emphysema
- [v] Tenderness and crepitus (especially posteriorly)

      (d) Chest
- [i] Subcutaneous emphysema
- [ii] Surface wounds and ecchymosis
- [iii] Impaled objects
- [iv] Bilateral and symmetric chest rise
- [v] Accessory muscle use
- [vi] Breath sounds and heart sounds
- [vii] Pain on palpation, crepitus, and deformity

      (e) Abdomen and flanks
- [i] Note the shape of the abdomen (deformity or irregular size might indicate uterine rupture).
- [ii] Bowel signs auscultated (before palpation of abdomen to prevent false-positive findings)
- [iii] Surface wounds, ecchymosis, seatbelt marks; any injuries from airbag deployment
- [iv] Impaled objects
- [v] Distention, rigidity, and tenderness; uterine contractions
- [vi] Uterine tenderness or increased uterine tone on palpation; fetal movement; fetal heart rate

      (f) Pelvis and genitalia
- [i] Surface wounds, ecchymosis, and edema of perineum or genitalia
- [ii] Instability or tenderness on gentle squeeze of anterior iliac crests and/or symphysis pubis
- [iii] Bleeding from the urinary meatus, vagina, or rectum; vaginal protrusions (amniotic sac/fetal parts)
- [iv] Pain and/or urge to void; urge to bear down (Valsalva maneuver)

      (g) Extremities
- [i] Surface wounds, edema, and/or ecchymosis
- [ii] Deformities: open or closed fractures
- [iii] Bony crepitus on palpation
- [iv] Skin color, temperature, and presence of distal pulses
- [v] Spontaneous motor function of all extremities
- [vi] Gross sensory function of all extremities

      (h) Posterior surface
- [i] Observe cervical spine precautions, and log-roll patient to assess for presence of injuries on posterior body.
- [ii] Surface wounds of back, flanks, buttocks, or thighs
- [iii] Pain or deformity on palpation of entire spinal column

4. Fetal assessment (should occur simultaneously with maternal secondary assessment)
   a. Fetal heart rate is the best indicator of fetal and maternal condition source.
      (1) Assess fetal heart rate (Doppler or ultrasound); 120 to 160 bpm is normal.
      (2) Continuous electronic fetal monitoring is ideal for essential ongoing fetal assessment.
   b. Fundal height (to assess gestational age)
   c. Fetal movement
5. Focused obstetric assessment
   a. Spontaneous rupture of membranes
   b. Vaginal bleeding
      (1) Assess vaginal fluid for amniotic fluid by testing the pH (7.0 to 7.5).
      (2) Place fluid on slide and observe for fern effect when dried.
   c. Labor status
      (1) Contractions
      (2) Cervical dilation, effacement, station, and presenting part

      d. Abruptio placentae
          (1) Assess for presence of abdominal pain, uterine tenderness, and bleeding
          (2) Lack of these symptoms does not preclude the possibility of abruption (Tsuei, 2006)
      e. Uterine rupture
      f. Nonreassuring fetal heart tones
   6. Focused obstetric history
      a. Present pregnancy
          (1) Gestational age (last menstrual period [LMP]) and expected date of confinement (EDC)
          (2) Complications of current pregnancy
      b. Past obstetric history
      c. Events preceding injury (suspected intimate partner abuse)
   7. Glasgow Coma Scale score (Table 23-1)
   8. Psychosocial findings
      a. Anxiety or fear about life of fetus
      b. Anxiety or fear about own well-being and ability to care for infant
      c. Guilt about being injured and causing potential harm to fetus
      d. Injuries inconsistent with reported history, anxiety regarding abusive significant other
B. Diagnostic procedures
   1. Laboratory
      a. Complete blood count (CBC), differential, and platelet count
      b. Blood type and crossmatch
      c. Sodium, potassium, and chloride determinations
      d. Glucose, blood urea nitrogen (BUN), and creatinine determinations
      e. Clotting factors: prothrombin time (PT), partial thromboplastin time (PTT), fibrinogen, and fibrin split products

■ TABLE 23-1
■ ■ **Glasgow Coma Scale**

Finding	Score
EYE OPENING	
Spontaneous	4
To voice	3
To pain	2
None	1
BEST VERBAL RESPONSE	
Oriented	5
Confused	4
Inappropriate words	3
Incomprehensible sounds	2
None	1
BEST MOTOR RESPONSE	
Obeys commands	6
Purposeful movement (pain)	5
Withdrawal (pain)	4
Flexion (pain)	3
Extension (pain)	2
None	1

Total score from each section equals the Glasgow Coma Scale score. Maximum score is 15; lowest score is 3.

    f. D-dimer: blood test to rule out active blood clot formation; positive or elevated means further testing is needed

    g. Amylase and liver function tests

    h. Urinalysis

    i. Arterial blood gases, serum bicarbonate (altered levels correlate with fetal outcome) (Tweddale, 2006)

    j. Blood alcohol and/or toxicology studies

    k. Urine or serum beta–human chorionic gonadotropin (hCG)

    l. Tests for presence of fetal erythrocytes in maternal blood sampling or in vaginal blood (indicates fetal-maternal hemorrhage)

        (1) Kleihauer-Betke (KB) stain or hemoglobin electrophoresis takes 1 hour (not needed in minor trauma [Cahill et al, 2008], but should be completed in major trauma).

        (2) More rapid tests (4 to 7 minutes) might be more useful in the emergency room.

            (a) Ogita (most sensitive at 20% fetal blood)

            (b) Apt test (sensitive at 60%)

            (c) Loendersloot (sensitive at 60%)

2. Radiology

    a. Perform studies as indicated; radiation risk to fetus should not interfere with lifesaving interventions for mother.

    b. Avoid duplicate films.

    c. Uterus should be shielded with lead apron whenever possible.

    d. IV pyelogram (IVP) dye does not cross placenta.

3. Computed tomography (CT) scan

    a. Using sequential slices of tissue with small gaps between cuts decreases radiation exposure.

    b. Shield for nonabdominal scans.

    c. Assess for bleeding and solid organ injury, occult fracture diagnosis.

4. Magnetic resonance imaging (MRI) (might be used because of its advantages over CT)

    a. MRI uses no ionizing radiation.

    b. Vascular structures can be evaluated without the need to inject iodinated contrast medium.

    c. Imaging of deep pelvic structures does not depend on a urine-filled bladder.

    d. Ability to identify flowing blood and distinguish blood from other fluid collections (AAP/ACOG, 2007)

    e. Takes longer than CT scan; patient must be relatively stable

5. Ultrasonography

    a. Triage tool for the pregnant patient with blunt abdominal trauma (Tweddale, 2006)

    b. A safe, noninvasive bedside study for maternal and fetal assessment (Tweddale, 2006)

    c. Detects uterine rupture (Tweddale, 2006) as well as free fluid in the blunt abdominal trauma patient (Tsuei, 2006)

    d. Can identify fetal activity, determine fetal heart rate, and diagnose fetal death.

    e. Determines:

        (1) Gestational age (accuracy varies with trimester)

        (2) Fetal position

        (3) Amount of amniotic fluid

        (4) Multiple gestations

        (5) Fetal weight estimation

        (6) Placental location and possible placental abruption (not 100% accurate)

6. Electronic fetal monitor and uterine monitoring (for more than 20 to 24 weeks' gestational age)

    a. Note baseline heart rate and variability (variability is a sign of fetal well-being) (Burke Sosa, 2007).

    b. Monitor uterine contractions (observe for trauma-induced preterm labor).

    c. Monitoring fetal heart rate detects trends such as bradycardia (ominous sign) and prolonged tachycardia, which might indicate fetal distress.

    d. Assists in diagnosing abruptio placentae.

    e. Nonreassuring signs might be an indication of occult maternal distress (Witcher, 2006).

  f. Is recommended for all pregnant patients with viable pregnancies after trauma, regardless of physiologic status and location or severity of injury (Burke Sosa, 2007; Tweddale, 2006)

  g. Fetal monitoring for a minimum of 4 hours if no FHR abnormality or maternal complications or up to 24 hours until fetal well-being is established (Burke Sosa, 2007; Tweddale, 2006)

 7. Diagnostic peritoneal lavage (DPL) surgical technique to diagnose intraperitoneal bleeding

  a. Indications include:

   (1) Altered level of consciousness

   (2) Unexplained shock

   (3) Major chest injuries

   (4) Signs and symptoms of intraabdominal bleeding

  b. Will not assess retroperitoneal or intrauterine injuries

  c. Insert an indwelling urinary catheter and oronasal gastric tube before the procedure.

  d. Procedure

   (1) Peritoneal catheter is inserted with direct visualization using the open technique to avoid the gravid uterus (Tsuei, 2006) with the insertion site above the umbilicus.

   (2) Aspiration of gross blood is considered positive.

    (a) If aspiration is negative, 1 L of warmed lactated Ringer's solution or normal saline solution is infused over 10 to 15 minutes into the peritoneal cavity.

    (b) The solution bag is lowered to gravity drainage, and the return fluid is analyzed for the presence of blood cells, amylase, bile, food fiber, or feces.

   (3) Surgical intervention is needed for positive results.

C. Interventions/Outcomes

 1. Chest injury

  a. Interventions

   (1) Position patient in supine position and immobilize the cervical spine if not done.

    (a) Manual stabilization (Figure 23-4)

    (b) Rigid cervical collar

    (c) Apply rolled blankets to side of neck; place patient on backboard and secure with straps and tape.

   (2) Open airway with jaw thrust or chin lift, keeping head in neutral, midline position.

   (3) Remove loose objects, and suction gently if needed to clear airway.

   (4) Maintain open airway with appropriate adjunct (oropharyngeal or nasopharyngeal airway); consider endotracheal intubation.

   (5) Consider insertion of nasogastric tube for gastric decompression and airway protection.

  b. Outcomes

   (1) Airway is open and clear; patient is able to speak.

   (2) Patient exhibits no stridor.

   (3) No foreign matter is visible in the upper airway.

   (4) Cervical spine precautions are maintained.

 2. Breathing difficulties

  a. Interventions

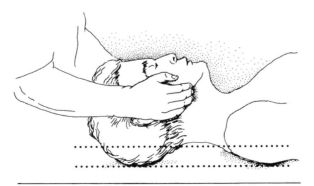

FIGURE 23-4 ■ Manual stabilization of the cervical spine.

(1) If patient is not breathing:
  (a) Provide positive-pressure ventilation with bag-valve-mask device and 100% oxygen.
  (b) Assist with endotracheal intubation.
(2) If breathing is present but ineffective:
  (a) Administer oxygen by nonrebreather mask at 12 to 15 L/min to keep reservoir bag inflated.
  (b) Assist ventilations with bag-valve-mask device with 100% oxygen as necessary.
  (c) Identify and intervene for specific life-threatening injuries.
    [i] Tension pneumothorax
      • Severe respiratory distress
      • Restlessness; agitation
      • Tracheal shift
      • Distended neck veins
      • Absent breath sounds
      • Immediate needle thoracotomy on affected side
    [ii] Open pneumothorax
      • Sucking or gurgling chest wound
      • Severe respiratory distress
      • Cyanosis
      • Apply three-sided sterile occlusive dressing; monitor for development of tension pneumothorax.
    [iii] Flail chest
      • Severe respiratory distress
      • Cyanosis
      • Paradoxical chest wall movement
      • Assist with intubation and mechanical ventilation.
      • Prevent IV fluid overload.
    [iv] Massive hemothorax
      • Severe respiratory distress
      • Signs of hypovolemic shock (previous conditions ruled out)
      • Assist with insertion of large-bore chest tube on affected side at fifth or sixth intercostal space.
(3) Monitor arterial blood gas and pulse oximetry readings.
  b. Outcomes
  (1) Rise and fall of chest is spontaneous.
  (2) Respirations are not labored.
  (3) Chest wall expansion is equal and symmetric.
  (4) Trachea is midline.
  (5) No accessory muscles are used.
  (6) Skin is pink, warm, and dry.
  (7) Patient is alert and oriented.
  (8) Pulse oximetry readings are at 100% on oxygen and blood gas results within normal pregnancy range.
3. Decreased cardiac output related to severe blood loss
  a. Interventions
  (1) If pulse is absent:
    (a) Begin cardiopulmonary resuscitation.
    (b) Initiate advanced life support measures.
    (c) Prepare for emergency open thoracotomy to control intrathoracic hemorrhage.
    (d) Administer blood as ordered; prepare for autotransfusion.
    (e) Prepare for surgery after open thoracotomy.
  (2) If pulse is present but ineffective:
    (a) Control obvious external bleeding by direct pressure, elevation of extremities, application of pressure on arterial pressure points, and tourniquet only as a last resort.
    (b) Establish two 14- to 16-gauge IV lines with Y-type blood administration tubing, and administer warmed normal saline or lactated Ringer's solution.

[i] Assist with possible placement of central line.

[ii] Rapid transfusion device or pressurized IV bags

[iii] Fluids titrated to hemodynamic status

[iv] Burn injury fluid resuscitation

- 4 mL of crystalloid solution multiplied by the percentage of total body surface area burned multiplied by the patient's weight in kg to be given over first 24 hours
- Half of the total volume given in first 8 hours after burn injury

(c) Draw blood for hemoglobin/hematocrit, type and crossmatching, and other studies.

(d) Administer uncrossmatched, O-negative blood as ordered.

(e) Administer typed and crossmatched blood as soon as possible.

(f) Initiate continuous cardiac monitoring (reminder: heart rate increases 15 to 20 bpm during pregnancy).

(g) Place patient in left lateral position to prevent supine hypotension syndrome; might need to manually displace uterus or place supports under patient's right hip to tilt patient 30 degrees to the left side (see Figure 23-1 for left lateral positioning).

(h) Replacement of clotting factors must be considered when packed cells are given.

(i) Anticipate autotransfusion if hemothorax is present.

(j) Consider using pneumatic antishock garment (legs only). See Figure 23-5 for application.

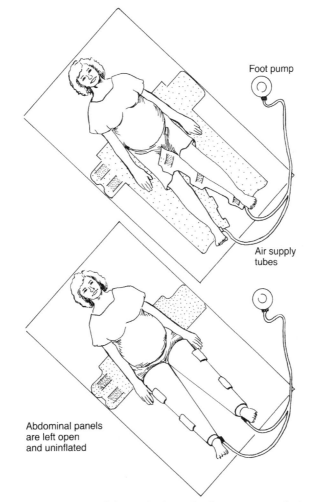

FIGURE 23-5 ■ Application of the medical antishock trousers suit during pregnancy.

        (k) Insert indwelling urinary catheter to monitor hourly output; urinary output is a sensitive indicator of tissue perfusion status and of the adequacy of fluid replacement.

  b. Outcomes

      (1) Patient has improved level of consciousness.

      (2) Skin is pink, warm, and dry.

      (3) Urinary output is more than 30 mL/hr.

      (4) Distal pulses are present and strong.

      (5) Capillary refill time is less than 2 seconds.

      (6) Heart rate and blood pressure are within normal pregnancy range.

4. Actual or potential loss of fetus

  a. Interventions

      (1) Establish trusting relationship by being nonjudgmental; stay with patient and explain all procedures and interventions.

      (2) Provide updates on maternal and fetal status and encouragement when appropriate.

      (3) Actively listen to patient's questions and responses.

      (4) Involve significant others.

      (5) Involve pastoral care service if patient or family requests; social worker, mental health nurse, or other support available in the hospital.

      (6) Answer questions regarding fetus honestly and realistically.

  b. Outcomes

      (1) Exhibits appropriate grieving behavior.

      (2) Verbalizes feelings and fears.

      (3) Patient is able to participate in decision making.

      (4) Physiologic symptoms of fear, such as increased heart rate, blood pressure, diaphoresis, hyperventilation, and complaints of heart palpitations are absent or significantly decreased.

5. Fetal tissue perfusion problems

  a. Interventions

      (1) Aggressive maternal resuscitation (leading cause of fetal death is maternal death)

      (2) Emergency (crash) cesarean section for a fetus of viable gestational age

        (a) Indications

          [i] Nonreassuring fetal heart rate tracing

            • Late and ominous decelerations of fetal heart rate; severe bradycardia or tachycardia

            • Blood on amniocentesis

            • Positive fetal erythrocytes in maternal blood

          [ii] Development of disseminated intravascular coagulation (DIC)

          [iii] Fetal malpresentation during premature labor

          [iv] Improving surgical access to save the mother

          [v] Placental abruption

          [vi] Uterine rupture

          [vii] Uncontrolled hemorrhage

          [viii] Maternal arrest (postmortem cesarean section)

        (b) Factors affecting fetal survival of postmortem cesarean section

          [i] Time interval between maternal arrest and fetal delivery is the most important factor (Katz, Balderston, & DeFreest, 2005); perform procedure within 4 minutes of maternal arrest or initiation of resuscitative measure.

          [ii] Fetal condition

          [iii] Maternal cause of death (e.g., severe hemorrhage)

          [iv] Fetal gestational age

         (c) Newborn resuscitation required (see Chapter 17 on newborn resuscitation)

      (3) Admit all pregnant patients with viable fetuses and with major injuries to the hospital for continuous fetal monitoring after resuscitation and stabilization for 24 to 48 hours; in particular, all abdominal injuries must be observed for 48 hours to rule out abruptio placentae.

  b. Outcome: Fetal perfusion is improved.

HEALTH EDUCATION

A. Prevention
1. Wearing a three-point seatbelt properly during pregnancy might prevent ejection or serious injury from collision with steering wheel or dashboard (Figure 23-6).
   a. Seatbelt should be worn with the shoulder strap positioned between breasts and above dome of uterus.
      (1) Lap belt is worn under the uterus and across the anterior spines of the pelvis.
      (2) Padding the seatbelt for comfort is discouraged because the belt can shift upward on impact, causing injury to the thinner portion of the fundus (Smith, 2009).
   b. Three-point restraints help prevent rapid deceleration, forward-flexion injuries that can cause shearing forces on the uterus.
   c. Lap belts used alone might cause injury to enlarged gravid uterus.
      (1) A pregnant patient should be advised that use of only a lap belt is preferable to using no restraint.
      (2) It is preferable that the pregnant patient rides in the back seat, however.
   d. If the pregnant woman is driving a car with an airbag, she should direct a tilting steering wheel away from the abdomen, move the front seat backward as far as possible, consider having the airbag disconnected, or sit in the back seat as a passenger.
2. Refer to public education programs regarding danger to mother and fetus when seatbelt is not worn; omission of seatbelt for all persons increases chance of ejection, which increases chance of death by 20 times; refer to programs for automotive infant restraint devices as needed.
3. Support enforcement of current laws that require seatbelt use.
4. Educate providers on risk factors, assessment for intimate partner violence injuries and illnesses, and identify referral resources for women identified in need of intervention and/or resources (see Chapter 18).

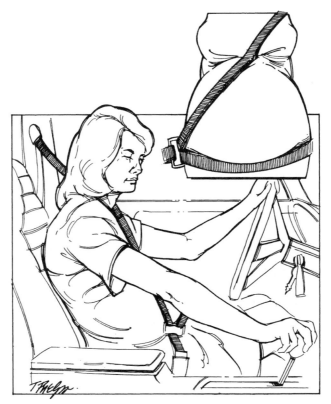

FIGURE 23-6 ■ Proper use of a seatbelt during pregnancy. (From McQuillan, K.A., Flynn Makic, M.B., & Whalen, E. [2008]. *Trauma nursing: From resuscitation through rehabilitation* [4th ed.]. Philadelphia: Saunders.)

B. Education

1. Prenatal care should include information about normal anatomic changes that predispose pregnant women to accidents.
2. Encourage frequent rest breaks while driving and/or riding in a car.
3. Safety measures in the home and workplace, such as avoiding climbing on chairs and ladders, should be instituted.
4. Counseling regarding possibility of spousal or partner abuse during pregnancy in confidential, supportive settings should be offered.
5. Provide information at an appropriate reading level and in a cultural context, with illustrations to clarify information and instructions.

CASE STUDIES AND STUDY QUESTIONS

1. Of all the mechanisms of injury associated with blunt trauma, the leading cause of maternal trauma is:
   a. Forceful bruising
   b. Spousal battering
   c. Motor vehicle accidents
   d. Falls
2. The primary survey in trauma focuses on:
   a. In-depth management and definitive care interventions
   b. Life-threatening priorities
   c. A thorough head-to-toe assessment
   d. Chief complaint, past medical history, and allergies
3. The reason for the increased incidence of falls in pregnant women as the pregnancy progresses is:
   a. Change in the center of gravity
   b. Orthostatic hypotension
   c. Neurovascular changes
   d. Anemia
4. What amount of blood loss may occur prior to observing any signs or symptoms of shock, due to the extra intravascular reserve accumulating during pregnancy?
   a. 800 mL
   b. 1000 mL
   c. 1500 mL
   d. 2000 mL
5. The best overall indicator for fetal well-being is:
   a. Fetal heart rate
   b. Type of injury
   c. Maternal tachycardia
   d. Lack of uterine contractions
6. What important physiologic change must be considered when determining a patient's response to trauma?
   a. Blood volume decreases during pregnancy.
   b. The bowel is pushed down by the uterus.
   c. The bladder is protected by the pelvis.
   d. Increased maternal oxygen consumption.
7. Preventive measures to reduce the risk of trauma during pregnancy include:
   a. Avoid climbing stairs.
   b. Wear lap belt only to decrease risk of uterine strain.
   c. Avoid climbing on chairs and ladders.
   d. Encourage patient not to drive during the third trimester.

D.H., a 26-year old primigravida at 36 weeks' gestation, was brought to the hospital by ambulance after a motor vehicle accident. She was driving her minivan when she was rear-ended by a pickup truck. D.H. was wearing a three-point seatbelt in the proper position and the airbag was deployed. Damage to her car was moderate. When she arrived at the emergency room, she was alert with no respiratory distress noted, but her skin was pale and clammy. Her blood pressure was 90/50, heart rate 98 bpm, respirations 30/min. Her chief complaint was abdominal pain "all over" and verbalized concern for her baby. She had what appeared to be a seatbelt contusion across the lower abdomen. Intravenous access was obtained with two large-bore catheters, and fluid resuscitation with 3 L of lactated Ringer's solution was administered. Oxygen was applied at 15 L/min by mask.

After it had been determined that D.H.'s airway, breathing, and circulation were intact, she was transferred to Labor and Delivery for further assessment and observation. Her family was notified of her admission. The secondary maternal assessment was performed. The assessment revealed abdominal tenderness, but no lacerations or active bleeding was noted.

Laboratory studies including CBC, type and crossmatch, and clotting factors were performed and ultrasound was negative for uterine rupture. Continuous electronic fetal monitoring revealed regular uterine contractions every 4 to 5 minutes, and a fetal heart rate of 135 bpm with minimal variability. Cervix remained closed, membranes intact. A Foley catheter was inserted, and urine was negative for blood.

After 3 hours of monitoring, the fetal heart rate dropped to 90 bpm. D.H. complained of increased abdominal pain and fundus was firm on palpation. An emergency cesarean section was performed immediately whereby a partial placental abruption was identified. D.H. recovered well and was discharged home on day 3 with her newborn girl in stable condition.

8. Which test is performed to detect hemorrhage of fetal cells within the maternal circulation?
   a. RhoGAM test
   b. Kleihauer-Betke test
   c. Vandersloot test
   d. Serum hCG
9. The most appropriate position for D.H. to be placed in to optimize maternal/fetal outcome is:
   a. Left lateral position to displace uterus
   b. Semi-Fowler's position to facilitate breathing
   c. Head down, left lateral position to prevent vomiting and possible aspiration
   d. Trendelenburg position to improve blood flow to the brain
10. Additional information regarding the mechanism of injury in the described accident might include all of the following *except:*
    a. The need for extrication
    b. The speed at which the vehicles were traveling
    c. The intersection at which the accident occurred
    d. Passenger space intrusion

L.K. was brought to the emergency room by her roommate after being stabbed in the upper abdomen by her boyfriend. She was 22 years old and 33 weeks' pregnant with her second child. She was seen at the county health clinic intermittently throughout her pregnancy. The stabbing occurred approximately 30 minutes prior to admission.

The emergency department staff noted that she had a very weak pulse with shallow, ineffective respirations and was unresponsive. Several small lacerations were noted on her hands and upper arms. She had an obvious knife wound to the upper abdomen with profuse bleeding. A pressure dressing was placed over the open wound. Respiratory support by bag-valve-mask with 100% oxygen was provided and two large-bore IV lines with lactated Ringer's was

initiated. Blood products were ordered and infusion of 2 units of packed red blood cells and 2 units of platelets started. The OB team was called to assist. Fetal heart tones were noted at 90 bpm. L.K.'s blood pressure was 90/40, pulse thready, and respirations 10 per min. L.K. was intubated and transferred to the OR for an emergency cesarean section.

A baby boy was delivered with Apgars of 1, 3, and 5 at 1, 5, and 10 minutes, respectively. Newborn resuscitation was required and baby was transferred to the neonatal intensive care unit (NICU) in critical condition because of respiratory failure and probable cerebral anoxia. The obstetric team continued to provide volume resuscitation and respiratory support to L.K. With the uterus emptied, L.K.'s circulating volume improved. Vital signs were stabilized and L.K. was transferred to the ICU for continued monitoring postdelivery. Collaborative care between the OB and ICU staff was provided to the patient.

11. What further assessment should be completed on a pregnant woman with a penetrating wound to the upper abdomen?
    a. Examination of the posterior uterine wall
    b. Fetal oxygenation studies
    c. Exploration of the small intestine
    d. Presence of vaginal bleeding
12. Factors affecting fetal survival of a postmortem cesarean section include:
    a. Time interval between maternal death and fetal delivery
    b. Fetal gestational age
    c. Cause of maternal death
    d. All of the above
13. Priorities in the initial care of L.K. include:
    a. Applying the pneumatic antishock garment and inflating the legs and abdominal compartments
    b. Establishing a patent airway and ventilating the patient by endotracheal intubation and administration of 100% oxygen
    c. Amniocentesis to determine fetal lung maturity
    d. Administration of crystalloid solution at 125 mL/hr
14. In addition to maternal death, indications for a crash cesarean section include all of the following *except:*
    a. All pelvic fractures
    b. After fetal heart tones have been confirmed
    c. Uterine rupture
    d. Late and ominous decelerations of fetal heart rate

ANSWERS TO STUDY QUESTIONS

1. c	6. d	11. c
2. b	7. c	12. d
3. a	8. b	13. b
4. c	9. a	14. a
5. a	10. c	

REFERENCES

Aboutanos, S. Z., Aboutanos, M. B., Dompkowski, D., Duane, T. M., Malhotra, A. K., & Ivatury, R. R. (2007). Predictors of fetal outcome in pregnant trauma patients: A five-year institutional review. *The American Surgeon, 73*(8), 824–827.

American Academy of Pediatrics (AAP) & American College of Obstetricians and Gynecologists (ACOG). (2007). *Guidelines for perinatal care* (6th ed.). Elk Grove Village, IL: Author.

Burke Sosa, M. -E. (2007). The pregnant trauma patient in the intensive care unit: Collaborative care to ensure safety and prevent injury. *Journal of Perinatal Neonatal Nursing, 22*(1), 33–38.

Cahill, A. G., Bastek, J. A., Stamilio, D. M., Odibo, A. O., Stevens, E., & Macones, G. A. (2008). Minor trauma in pregnancy—Is the evaluation warranted? *American Journal of Obstetrics & Gynecology, 198*, 208.e1–208.e5.

Chames, M. C., & Pearlman, M. D. (2008). Trauma during pregnancy: Outcomes and clinical management. *Clinical Obstetrics and Gynecology, 51*(2), 398–408.

Constanty, P. M., & Cruz, D. A. (2006). Trauma and the obstetrics patient: Collaboration in care. *Critical Care Nursing Clinics of North America, 18*, 273–278.

Cunningham, F., Leveno, K., Bloom, S., Hauth, J., Gilstrap, L., & Wenstrom, K. (2005). In *Williams obstetrics* (22nd ed.). New York: McGraw-Hill.

Cusick, S. S., & Tibbles, C. D. (2007). Trauma in pregnancy. *Emergency Medicine Clinics of North America, 25*, 861–872.

El Kady, D. E. (2007). Perinatal outcomes of traumatic injuries during pregnancy. *Clinical Obstetrics and Gynecology, 50*(3), 582–591.

El Kady, D. E., Gilbert, W. M., Xing, G., & Smith, L. H. (2005). Maternal and neonatal outcomes of assaults during pregnancy. *Obstetrics & Gynecology, 105*, 357–363.

Emergency Nurses Association. (2007). Initial assessment. In *Trauma nursing core course* (6th ed.). Des Plaines, IL: Emergency Nurses Association.

Gordon, M. C. (2007). Maternal physiology. In S. G. Gabbe, J. R. Niebyl, & J. L. Simpson (Eds.), *Obstetrics: Normal and problem pregnancies* (5th ed.). New York: Churchill Livingstone.

Ikossi, D. G., Lazar, A. A., Morabito, D., Fildes, J., & Knudson, M. M. (2005). Profile of mothers at risk: An analysis of injury and pregnancy loss in 1,195 trauma patients. *Journal of the American College of Surgeons, 200*(1), 49–56.

Katz, V., Balderston, K., & DeFreest, M. (2005). Perimortem cesarean delivery: Were our assumptions correct? *American Journal of Obstetrics & Gynecology, 192*, 1916–1921.

Kennedy, B. B., McMurtry Baird, S., & Troiano, N. H. (2008). Burn injuries and pregnancy. *Journal of Perinatal & Neonatal Nursing, 22*(1), 21–30.

Ladewig, P. A., London, M. L., & Davidson, M. R. (2010). *Contemporary maternal-newborn nursing care* (7th ed.). New York: Pearson.

Mattox, K. L., & Goetzl, L. (2005). Trauma in pregnancy. *Critical Care Medicine, 33*(10 Suppl), S385–S389.

McGowan Repasky, T. (2007). Obstetric trauma. In K. S. Hoyt, & J. Selfridge-Thomas (Eds.), *Emergency nursing core curriculum* (6th ed.). St. Louis: Saunders.

Muench, M. V., & Canterino, J. C. (2007). Trauma in pregnancy. *Obstetrics and Gynecology Clinics of North America, 34*(3), 555–583.

Ramsay, M. M. (2006). Normal values. In D. K. James, P. J. Steer, C. P. Weiner, & B. Gonik (Eds.), *High risk pregnancy: Management options* (3rd ed., pp. 1665–1734). Philadelphia: Saunders.

Schiff, M. A. (2008). Pregnancy outcomes following hospitalisation for a fall in Washington State from 1987 to 2004. *British Journal of Obstetrics and Gynecology, 115*, 1648–1654.

Schiff, M. A., & Holt, V. L. (2005). Pregnancy outcomes following hospitalization for motor vehicle crashes in Washington State from 1989 to 2001. *American Journal of Epidemiology, 161*, 503–510.

Sirin, H., Weiss, H. B., Sauber-Schatz, E. K., & Dunning, K. (2007). Seat belt use, counseling and motor-vehicle injury during pregnancy: Results from a multi-state population-based survey. *Maternal Child Health Journal, 11*(5), 505–510.

Smith, L. (2009). The pregnant trauma patient. In K. A. McQuillan, M. B. Flynn Makic, & E. Whalen (Eds.), *Trauma nursing: From resuscitation through rehabilitation* (4th ed.). St. Louis: Saunders.

Torgersen, K. L., & Curran, C. A. (2006). A systematic approach to the physiologic adaptations of pregnancy. *Critical Care Nursing Quarterly*, 29(1), 2–19.

Tsuei, B. J. (2006). Assessment of the pregnant trauma patient. *Injury: International Journal of the Care of the Injured*, 37, 367–373.

Tweddale, C. (2006). Trauma during pregnancy. *Critical Care Nursing Quarterly*, 29(1), 55–57.

Witcher, P. M. (2006). Promoting fetal stabilization during maternal hemodynamic instability or respiratory insufficiency. *Critical Care Nursing Quarterly*, 29(1), 70–76.

Yeomans, E. R., & Gilstrap, L. C., III. (2005). Physiologic changes in pregnancy and their impact on critical care. *Critical Care Medicine*, 33(10 Suppl), S256–S258.

24 Surgery in Pregnancy

Linda Callahan

OBJECTIVES

1. Describe the incidence of nonobstetric surgery performed during pregnancy in the United States.
2. Analyze alterations in the pregnant patient's physiology and the risks associated with anesthesia.
3. Discuss optimal timing for nonobstetric surgery when performed during pregnancy.
4. Describe potential complications of nonobstetric surgery for the pregnant patient.
5. Describe the potential effects of nonobstetric surgery and anesthesia on the fetus.
6. Assess the patient's response to surgery and the potential for preterm labor.
7. Outline important parameters of general maternal preoperative assessment.
8. Discuss basic and specific considerations in anesthetic choices for the pregnant patient requiring nonobstetric surgery.
9. Describe assessment of symptoms of the pregnant patient with acute cholecystitis.
10. Describe assessment of symptoms of appendicitis in the pregnant patient.
11. Describe assessment of symptoms of the pregnant patient with ovarian cyst/tumor requiring surgical intervention.
12. Discuss the use of laparoscopy as a surgical technique in pregnant patients in need of cholecystectomy or appendectomy.
13. Describe the patient at risk for cervical incompetence.
14. Define the function and types of surgical approaches to cervical cerclage.
15. Discuss procedure-specific assessment of the pregnant patient in need of cervical cerclage.
16. Discuss indications for endoscopic gastrointestinal procedures that might be present in the pregnant patient.
17. Discuss the risks that might be present for pregnant patients undergoing esophagogastroduodenoscopy (EGD) or endoscopic retrograde cholangiopancreatography (ERCP).
18. Outline methods for risk reduction in pregnant patients undergoing endoscopic gastrointestinal procedures.
19. Describe the potential maternal complications associated with intrauterine fetal surgery.
20. Discuss specific life-threatening fetal anomalies that might be amenable to treatment by intrauterine fetal surgery.
21. Describe the utility of intrauterine fetal surgery in correction of nonfatal fetal anomalies such as myelomeningocele or obstructive uropathy.
22. Select appropriate nursing actions based on acquired knowledge of the alterations in the pregnant patient's physiology, and integrate that knowledge into preoperative, intraoperative, and postoperative care.
23. Define psychosocial stressors affecting the pregnant patient undergoing surgery.
24. Describe the care of the pregnant surgical patient and her family based on analysis of the patient's needs in this emotionally and physically stressful situation.
25. Formulate nursing interventions to prevent postoperative surgical complications in the pregnant surgical patient.

INTRODUCTION

A. **Incidence of nonobstetric surgery performed during pregnancy ranges from 0.75% to 2%. Of this incidence approximately 42% occur in the first trimester, 35% in the second trimester, and 23% in the third trimester** (Birnbach & Browne, 2005; Mhuireachtaigh & O'Gorman, 2006).
   1. Incidence is probably underestimated in first trimester because pregnancy might be unrecognized at time of surgery.

B. Types of procedures
1. Laparoscopy for appendicitis is the most common first-trimester procedure. Incidence is estimated at 1 per 1500 to 2000 pregnancies (Mhuireachtaigh & O'Gorman, 2006).
2. Other situations that might lead to surgery during pregnancy include:
    a. Nongynecologic: acute cholecystitis (1 to 8 per 10,000 pregnancies [Mhuireachtaigh & O'Gorman, 2006]), intestinal obstruction, trauma with visceral injury, vascular accidents (ruptured aneurysms), peptic ulcer, rectal cancer, breast tumors, or other malignancies; rarely, maternal cardiac or neurosurgical conditions
    b. Gynecologic: cervical incompetence, ovarian cyst, torsion of fallopian tube, tubo-ovarian abscess, uterine myoma with degeneration or torsion
    c. Intrauterine fetal surgery as an intervention for certain prenatal congenital defects

CLINICAL PRACTICE

Anesthetic Considerations

A. Concepts essential to planning and management
1. Anesthetic management priorities
    a. Possibility of increased maternal morbidity
        (1) Risk of preterm delivery after surgery during pregnancy is approximately 8.8%.
        (2) Risk of spontaneous abortion after surgery is approximately 8% in the first trimester and 6.9% in the second trimester.
    b. Possibility of increased fetal risk from:
        (1) Effects of maternal disease or treatment modalities
        (2) Possible teratogenicity of anesthetic agents
        (3) Intraoperative decrease in uteroplacental flow: fetal hypoxia; uterine flow is not autoregulated and represents approximately 10% of maternal cardiac output by full term
        (4) Increased risk of preterm delivery
2. Pregnancy-induced changes in maternal physiology of importance during anesthesia and surgery
    a. Pregnancy-induced changes result from:
        (1) Increases in human chorionic gonadotropin, progesterone, and estrogen; responsible for most first-trimester changes
        (2) Mechanical effects of the gravid uterus
        (3) Increased metabolic demand
        (4) Hemodynamic changes due to presence of low-pressure placental circulation (Hill & Pickinpaugh, 2008)
    b. Cardiovascular changes
        (1) Increased pulse rate and stroke volume result in cardiac output increases of 30% to 50% during pregnancy.
        (2) By 8 weeks' gestation, 57% of the overall increase in cardiac output and 78% of the total increase in stroke volume have occurred (Hill & Pickinpaugh, 2008).
        (3) 90% of overall decrease in peripheral resistance has occurred by 24th week due to increased synthesis of vasodilators such as prostacyclin (Mhuireachtaigh & O'Gorman, 2006).
        (4) During the second trimester, the weight of the uterus compresses the inferior vena cava when mother is supine (25% to 30% decrease in venous return and cardiac output), which can produce supine hypotensive syndrome, especially in the face of anesthetics that abolish compensatory mechanisms (Kilpatrick & Monga, 2007).
        (5) A gravid uterus can also compress the aorta in a supine patient (leading to decreased uteroplacental blood flow and fetal compromise).
        (6) Combined hypotensive effect of general or regional anesthesia and aortocaval compression, leading to fetal asphyxia
        (7) Chronic vena caval obstruction in the third trimester predisposes to venous stasis, phlebitis, and lower-extremity edema (Hill & Pickinpaugh, 2008)
        (8) Distention of epidural venous plexus due to vena caval compression contributes to the spread of smaller amounts of local anesthetics administered epidurally during pregnancy.

 c. Respiratory changes

  (1) Under the influence of progesterone, alveolar ventilation is increased by 25% by 20 weeks' gestation due to a 15% increase in respiratory rate and an increase in tidal volume of 40%; increased 45% to 70% by term, leading to chronic respiratory alkalosis ($Paco_2$ is 28 to 32 mm Hg; slightly alkaline pH). Chronic respiratory alkalosis shifts maternal oxygen-hemoglobin dissociation curve to the right, promoting increased oxygen delivery to the fetus. The increase in arterial pH is limited by an increase in renal bicarbonate excretion (Kilpatrick & Monga, 2007; Mhuireachtaigh & O'Gorman, 2006).

  (2) Functional residual capacity (FRC) decreases 20%, leading to decreased oxygen reserve.

  (3) Decreased FRC, increased oxygen consumption, and decreased buffering capacity cause rapid hypoxemia and acidosis if stressed by hypoventilation or apnea.

  (4) Capillary engorgement of nasal and pharyngeal mucosa predisposes to bleeding, trauma, and obstruction.

 d. Hematologic changes

  (1) Blood volume expansion begins in first trimester, increases to 30% to 50% by term; increased plasma volume causes dilutional anemia. Moderate blood loss is well tolerated, but reserve is decreased when significant hemorrhage occurs.

  (2) Pregnancy-induced leukocytosis makes white blood cell (WBC) count an unreliable indicator of infection; might be as high as 15,000/µL during pregnancy with increases up to 20,000/µL during labor.

  (3) Hypercoagulable state of pregnancy (increased fibrinogen, factors II, VII, VIII, X, and XII) leads to high postoperative risk of thromboembolic events.

 e. Gastrointestinal changes

  (1) Lower esophageal sphincter incompetence and distortion of gastric and pyloric anatomy increases risk of esophageal reflux with possible aspiration and resultant pneumonia (Kilpatrick & Monga, 2007).

  (2) All pregnant patients, after 16 weeks' gestation, are considered to be at increased risk for aspiration (Mhuireachtaigh & O'Gorman, 2006).

3. Potential effects of surgery and anesthesia on the fetus

 a. Greatest risk to fetus is intrauterine asphyxia.

  (1) Transient decrease in maternal Pao_2 is well tolerated because of increased affinity of fetal hemoglobin for oxygen.

  (2) Maternal hypercarbia leads to fetal acidosis, which might cause fetal myocardial depression and hypotension (Hill & Pickinpaugh, 2008).

  (3) Maternal hypocarbia from stress-induced or positive-pressure hyperventilation might produce decreased fetal oxygenation due to resultant umbilical artery constriction and shift of the maternal oxygen-hemoglobin dissociation curve to the left (acidosis); administration of 100% oxygen to mother will result in oxygen tension in fetus of approximately 65 mm Hg, which is the maximum possible (Hill & Pickinpaugh, 2008).

  (4) Uteroplacental perfusion might be reduced as a result of maternal hypotension, which might occur in response to deep general anesthesia, sympathetic blockade from high spinal or epidural blockade, aortocaval compression, hemorrhage, or hypovolemia (Kilpatrick & Monga, 2007).

  (5) The administration of alpha-adrenergic vasopressor agents, preoperative anxiety, and/or very light levels of general anesthesia might produce increased maternal circulating catecholamines, which can lead to decreased uterine blood flow.

 b. Risk of teratogenicity

  (1) Drug-related factors

   (a) Greatest risk of structural abnormalities occurs with drug exposure from approximately day 31 to day 71 after the first day of the last menstrual period (LMP) (Mhuireachtaigh & O'Gorman, 2006).

   (b) Currently administered inhaled or local anesthetics, narcotics, and skeletal muscle relaxants in clinical concentration are not deemed to be teratogenic or carcinogenic (Mhuireachtaigh & O'Gorman, 2006).

   (c) Long-standing relative contraindication and concern over first-trimester use of benzodiazepine agents has been removed. Research failed to demonstrate link with increased incidence of cleft lip/palate (Mhuireachtaigh & O'Gorman, 2006).

(2) Non–drug-related factors
  (a) No congenital defects have been noted after brief periods of hypoxia, hypercarbia, or hypoglycemia.
  (b) Effect of maternal stress and anxiety is questionable because of the lack of supportive research.
  (c) Central nervous system congenital anomalies are associated with maternal fever (>39° C) (102.2° F) during the first half of pregnancy.
  (d) Ionizing radiation: No congenital defects from exposure below 10 rads (average chest radiograph exposure = 8 mrads).
  (e) The increased incidence of abortion, early delivery, and perinatal mortality associated with anesthesia and surgery might be attributed to the surgical site and/or underlying conditions; no clear relationship between outcome and type of anesthesia has been demonstrated.

B. **General maternal preoperative assessment**
  1. History and physical examination
    a. Gestational age
      (1) By date of LMP or ultrasound test
      (2) Palpation of uterine size; fundal height
    b. Urgency of need for surgery
    c. Presence of underlying chronic or acute illness
    d. Known drug allergies
    e. Current medications (prescription, over-the-counter, herbal, and recreational)
    f. Surgical history: previous procedures and responses to anesthesia
    g. Previous obstetric history
    h. Pain evaluation: location, intensity, characteristics, duration, and patient tolerance
    i. Vital signs
      (1) Temperature
      (2) Pulse
      (3) Respiration
      (4) Blood pressure
    j. Evaluation of fetal heart rate (FHR) by Doppler or continuous fetal monitoring
    k. Evaluation of uterine activity
      (1) Palpation and patient reported
      (2) Continuous fetal monitoring
    l. Respiratory status: dyspnea, evidence of distress, history of recent fever, or congestion, asthma, inhalant allergies, or smoking
    m. Cardiovascular status: presence of pregnancy-induced hypertension (PIH), history of rheumatic fever, or mitral valve dysfunction
    n. Hepatic status: history of hepatitis and alcohol consumption
    o. Renal status: history of bladder or kidney infection
  2. Psychosocial response
    a. Stress factors producing anxiety
      (1) Fear of loss or harm to fetus
      (2) Fear of harm to self
      (3) Lack of understanding of planned procedure, anesthesia options, and possible outcomes
    b. Behavioral factors
      (1) Desire to meet cultural expectation
      (2) Variable response to pain
      (3) Difficulty with open expression of fears and anxieties
  3. Laboratory and diagnostic procedures
    a. Ultrasonography
    b. Fetal monitoring
    c. Preoperative laboratory evaluation: complete blood count (CBC), urinalysis (UA), and type and crossmatch of blood products as indicated
    d. Electrocardiogram (ECG); chest radiograph (shielded) if indicated because of preexisting cardiovascular or pulmonary disease (e.g., floppy mitral valve, questionable aspiration pneumonitis, history of rheumatic fever)

C. Surgical choices: Open laparotomy versus laparoscopic approach

1. Overall safety of laparoscopy during the first half of pregnancy has been confirmed (Lu & Curet, 2007).
2. Laparoscopy is safe up to 26 to 28 weeks, when there is less risk of spontaneous abortion or premature labor due to manipulation. There is increased risk of uterine puncture during the third trimester due to large size of the uterus (Kilpatrick & Monga, 2007; Lu & Curet, 2007; Moreno-Sanz, Pascual-Pedreno, Picazo-Yeste, & Seoane-Gonzalez, 2007).
3. Risk may be lessened during laparoscopy if:
   a. Intraperitoneal pressure is maintained at 10 to 15 mm Hg or lower to protect uterine perfusion (Kilpatrick & Monga, 2007).
   b. Carbon dioxide should be used for production of pneumoperitoneum.
   c. Patient should be placed in reverse Trendelenburg in the left-side-down position, if possible.
   d. Intraoperative fetal monitoring is performed, if possible, because carbon dioxide used for insufflation can be absorbed, leading to fetal respiratory acidosis and hypercapnia (Kilpatrick & Monga, 2007; Moreno-Sanz et al, 2007).
4. Advantages of laparoscopy include better visualization, smaller incision, less pain, less operative time, decreased recovery time, earlier ambulation, and decreased risk of thromboembolic disease.
5. Open laparotomy is required when sufficient access is not possible with laparoscopy or when profound uterine relaxation is required to facilitate the planned procedure.

D. Anesthetic choices

1. Preoperative medication
   a. Low-dose benzodiazepine and/or narcotic to allay maternal anxiety
   b. Histamine receptor type 2 (H_2) antagonist and 30 mL of clear antacid as a precaution against acid aspiration after 16 weeks' gestation (Mhuireachtaigh & O'Gorman, 2006)
2. Choice of anesthetic technique
   a. Basic considerations
      (1) No studies correlate improved maternal or fetal outcome with any specific anesthetic technique.
      (2) Local and regional techniques are useful for cervical cerclage or urologic or lower-extremity procedures.
      (3) General anesthesia is required for most abdominal procedures.
   b. Specific considerations
      (1) After 18 to 20 weeks, left displacement of uterus is necessary when patient is positioned on the operating table to avoid supine hypotensive syndrome and aortocaval compression.
      (2) Basic perioperative monitoring: blood pressure, ECG, and pulse oximetry; general anesthesia requires the addition of capnography, temperature monitor, and nerve stimulator to assess skeletal muscle relaxation.
      (3) General anesthetic choices
         (a) High concentration oxygen plus a potent opioid (fentanyl or sufentanil) and/or a moderate concentration of a volatile agent (e.g., isoflurane, desflurane, sevoflurane), and a skeletal muscle relaxant
         (b) Nitrous oxide (N_2O) might be safely chosen, especially after the sixth week of gestation.
      (4) Regional anesthesia
         (a) Epidural and spinal anesthesia
            [i] Fetal hypoxia occurs if maternal systolic blood pressure drops below 100 mm Hg; in healthy pregnant women, 1 to 2 L of crystalloid fluid may be infused to prevent maternal hypotension.
            [ii] Patients with PIH experience decreased placental flow at higher systolic pressures than do normal pregnant women.
         (b) Increased vascularity and sensitivity to local anesthetics present during pregnancy; observe for signs of toxicity after injection (e.g., tingling, tinnitus, shivering, unexplained confusion or drowsiness). The therapeutic dose and the toxic plasma levels of local anesthetics are decreased approximately 30% during pregnancy (Mhuireachtaigh & O'Gorman, 2006).

3. Other intraoperative considerations
   a. FHR monitoring
      (1) If feasible, with external tocodynamometer intraoperatively and in immediate postoperative period to detect any need for administration of tocolytic agents.
      (2) Unexplained change in FHR: evaluate maternal position, blood pressure, oxygenation, acid-base balance, whether surgeon or retractor placement is impairing uterine perfusion.
      (3) Maternal hypothermia can cause a decrease in baseline fetal heart rate, as well as beat-to-beat variability, but it does not cause spontaneous decelerations.
      (4) Management plan must be in place regarding what to do in the face of persistent fetal distress (i.e., feasibility of cesarean section).
   b. Prevention of aortocaval compression
   c. Prevention of preterm labor
      (1) Procedures with minimal uterine manipulation occurring after the first trimester of pregnancy carry the lowest risk for preterm labor.
      (2) Prophylactic use of tocolytic agents is not without complications but has been suggested for patients at greatest risk (e.g., for cervical cerclage); if unsuccessful, beta$_2$-agonist tocolytic agents might complicate anesthesia because of production of tachycardia. Arg16 homozygosity of the beta$_2$-adrenergic receptor appears to confer better response to beta$_2$-agonist therapy for tocolysis (Landau, 2008).
   d. Compression hose should be placed on the patient to decrease the risk of deep vein thrombosis; low-molecular-weight heparin administration may be considered to protect against embolism (Moreno-Sanz et al, 2007).
E. **Interventions/Outcomes**
   1. Maternal and fetal physiologic dynamics related to surgery and anesthesia
      a. Interventions: preoperative
         (1) Monitor and record vital signs.
         (2) Provide intravenous (IV) hydration.
            (a) Maintenance by 16- or 18-gauge intracatheter infusion of nondextrose crystalloid solution (Ringer's lactate or normal saline)
            (b) 1 to 2 L might be ordered for volume expansion before administration of epidural or spinal anesthetic or if patient is fluid depleted due to illness.
         (3) Use left lateral positioning in the second and third trimesters to prevent aortocaval compression, which might result in decreased uteroplacental blood flow; if left lateral position is not possible, place a wedge (pillow or rolled blanket) under right hip to displace uterus to the left.
         (4) Use FHR monitoring: Doppler or external fetal monitor after 18 weeks gestation if positioning allows (Mhuireachtaigh & O'Gorman, 2006).
         (5) Assess preoperative laboratory test results for abnormalities that might alter or complicate perioperative care.
         (6) Communicate findings to other members of the healthcare team.
      b. Interventions: postoperative (in addition to those just mentioned)
         (1) Monitor vital signs frequently within the first 1 to 2 postoperative hours.
            (a) Overall, general anesthetics produce varying degrees of vasodilation and impair compensatory mechanisms, thereby increasing the potential for postoperative hypotension.
            (b) A major side effect of regional anesthesia (spinal or epidural) is hypotension due to sympathetic paralysis and resultant peripheral vasodilation; increased fluid and lateral positioning might stabilize this transient event.
         (2) Administer humidified oxygen via face mask (8 to 10 L/min).
            (a) Presence of some general anesthetic agents might depress respiration.
            (b) Pregnancy-induced increased mucosal vascularity of nose and throat predisposes patient to hoarseness and laryngeal edema following endotracheal intubation during general anesthesia.
         (3) Monitor and record intake and output (I&O).
         (4) Assess for thrombosis/phlebitis (Homan's sign) and apply antiembolic stockings.
         (5) FHR and uterine activity should be monitored to assess any alteration in fetal tissue perfusion.

(6) Adequate analgesics to manage pain should be administered systemically or by spinal/epidural injection, as appropriate.
  (a) Patient receiving analgesics might be unaware of onset of uterine contractions.
  (b) Apply comfort measures (e.g., positioning, use of pillows for support).
  (c) After cervical cerclage, position patient in slight Trendelenburg position to decrease cervical pressure.
  (d) Provide and instruct patient in incentive spirometry and coughing/deep breathing exercises.
(7) Avoid vasoconstrictors (might decrease uteroplacental blood flow).

  c. Outcomes
   (1) Patient's vital signs remain stable.
   (2) Patient maintains adequate oxygenation and circulation throughout the perioperative period.
   (3) Patient maintains adequate I&O.
   (4) Patient avoids thromboembolic phenomenon.
   (5) Patient experiences adequate pain control.
   (6) FHR remains within normal range.
   (7) Signs of impending preterm labor are recognized and treated properly.

2. Anxiety
  a. Interventions
   (1) During the preoperative and postoperative periods:
    (a) Assess patient's response and ability to cope with current situation.
    (b) Assess presence of social support systems and plan integration into patient care.
    (c) Provide opportunity for verbalization of fears, anxieties, and concerns.
    (d) Facilitate ability of surgeon, anesthesia provider, patient, and family to discuss surgical and anesthetic options.
    (e) Teach stress reduction techniques, and reinforce patient's ability to implement techniques.
    (f) Integrate mental health care team into patient care, if needed.
  b. Outcomes
   (1) Patient demonstrates positive coping strategies.
   (2) Social support system is involved with patient care.
   (3) Patient demonstrates stress reduction techniques.
   (4) Patient demonstrates knowledge of anesthetic choices, risks and benefits, and recommendations.

SPECIFIC SURGICAL PROCEDURES

Cholecystectomy

A. Introduction
  1. Incidence of acute cholecystitis during pregnancy is 1 to 8 per 10,000 gestations; is the cause of more than 90% of cholecystectomies performed during pregnancy (Mhuireachtaigh & O'Gorman, 2006).
    a. Increased bile lithogenicity and decreased motility occurs secondary to increased estrogen levels. By end of second trimester, progesterone levels produce smooth muscle relaxation and decreased tone (Dietrich, Hill, & Hueman, 2008).
    b. 3% develop gallstones during pregnancy, with 28% experiencing pain but only a limited number are sufficiently serious enough to require surgery (Kilpatrick & Monga, 2007; Mhuireachtaigh & O'Gorman, 2006).
  2. Previous pregnancies predispose to cholecystitis.
  3. Optimal timing of surgery is during second trimester (after highest risk of spontaneous abortion and organogenesis has passed and before enlarging uterus impairs surgical exposure (Birnbach & Browne, 2005).
  4. Maternal mortality (15%) and fetal loss (60%) have been associated with secondary pancreatitis; gallstone pancreatitis can be managed with an endoscopic retrograde cholangiogram. Most cases occur in the third trimester and are self-limiting (Dietrich et al, 2008; Kilpatrick & Monga, 2007).

5. Surgery should not be delayed if urgently indicated, such as in gallstone pancreatitis or unresolved cholecystitis. Gallstone pancreatitis is associated with a 70% incidence of recurrent symptoms and a 10% to 20% chance of fetal loss. Uncomplicated open cholecystectomy is associated with rare mortality, 5% fetal death, and 7% preterm labor (Birnbach & Browne, 2005; McAneny, 2008).

6. A laparoscopic surgical approach may be selected for cholecystectomy, adnexal disease, or appendectomy in the first trimester of pregnancy (Birnbach & Browne, 2005). This approach for cholecystectomy has been successful and safe in all trimesters (Dietrich et al, 2008) and is reported to significantly reduce the time of hospitalization, decrease the need for narcotic analgesics, and produce quicker return to regular diet compared with open laparotomy in pregnant women. Open laparotomy is the chosen approach later in pregnancy (Lu, Curet, El-Said, & Kirkwood, 2004).

7. Specific considerations of laparoscopic approach include:
   a. Additional risk of gastric reflux and aspiration due to upward pressure of pneumoperitoneum during surgery
   b. During immediate postoperative period, patient may experience shoulder or back pain from irritation by CO_2 used to produce pneumoperitoneum.

B. **Procedure-specific patient assessment (in addition to general maternal preoperative assessment)**
   1. History
      a. Assessment of pain: stabbing, colicky, or steady midepigastric pain that radiates to the right upper quadrant, right flank, or right shoulder
      b. Excessive flatulence, heartburn, or fatty-food intolerance
      c. Increased discomfort after meals
      d. Nausea or vomiting
      e. Medical and surgical history
      f. Obstetric history
      g. Gestational age by LMP or ultrasonography
   2. Physical examination
      a. Abdominal examination
         (1) Palpation: right upper quadrant rebound tenderness, positive Murphy's sign (pain in right midclavicular line on deep inspiration), rigidity, and uterine contractions (Kilpatrick & Monga, 2007)
         (2) Auscultation
            (a) Presence of bowel sounds
            (b) Peristaltic rushes (borborygmi) might indicate an intestinal obstruction.
      b. Vaginal examination
         (1) Presence or absence of vaginal bleeding: The patient should not experience bleeding with a diagnosis of cholecystitis.
         (2) Cervical examination to differentiate abdominal pain from preterm labor contractions
      c. Inspiratory effort often accentuates pain.
      d. Evaluate for volume deficit due to decreased oral intake, vomiting, or nasogastric suction.
   3. Laboratory/diagnostic procedures
      a. Laboratory tests
         (1) CBC with differential
            (a) WBC of 15,000 to 20,000 mm^3 might be normal in pregnancy.
            (b) Hemoglobin level should be stable (greater than 10 g/dL).
         (2) UA and urine culture to differentiate cholecystitis from pyelonephritis or cystitis
         (3) Electrolytes, liver function tests, and bilirubin
            (a) Hyperamylasemia is usually indicative of gallstone pancreatitis.
            (b) Serum alkaline phosphatase value may be increased to twice that of nonpregnant values (even higher values might occur in cholecystitis).
            (c) Severely elevated bilirubin, elevated lipase and amylase levels may indicate associated pancreatitis (Dietrich et al, 2008).
            (d) Jaundice and abnormal hepatic transaminase levels suggest choledocholithiasis (Dietrich et al, 2008).
      b. Ultrasonography: fetal viability; if cholelithiasis is present, dilated common bile duct and biliary tree will be present. Ultrasonography has 95% sensitivity detecting gallstones (Birnbach & Browne, 2005; Kilpatrick & Monga, 2007).
      c. Fetal monitoring to rule out preterm labor (see Chapter 12 for further discussion)

OVARIAN TUMORS: OVARIAN CYSTECTOMY OR OOPHORECTOMY

A. **Introduction**
   1. Hazards related to ovarian tumors—1% to 8% of adnexal masses diagnosed during pregnancy are malignant (Mhuireachtaigh & O'Gorman, 2006).
      a. Possibility of malignancy
      b. Torsion is more common in pregnancy (1% to 22%) (Bertolotto, Serafina, Toma, Zapetti, & Migaleddu, 2008; Leiserowitz, 2006).
      c. Rupture with hemorrhage
      d. Infection
   2. Corpus luteum cysts
      a. Corpus luteum cysts are most common during the first trimester.
      b. After first trimester, there is a decreased risk of spontaneous abortion from removal (Takeda, Sakai, Mitsui, & Nakamura, 2007).
   3. Benign ovarian tumors
      a. Dermoids
      b. Serous cystadenomas
      c. Mucinous cystadenoma
      d. Endometriomas ("chocolate cysts")
   4. Malignant ovarian tumors
      a. Dysgerminomas
      b. Granulosa cell tumors
   5. Ultrasound test is the most useful tool for diagnosis and evaluation.
   6. Surgical intervention indicated if tumor is:
      a. Solid
      b. Bilateral
      c. Hormonally active
      d. Symptomatic
      e. Increasing in size
B. **Procedure-specific patient assessment (in addition to general maternal preoperative assessment)**
   1. History
      a. Pain: Onset, location, and quality; may wax and wane (Kilpatrick & Monga, 2007); nausea and vomiting may also be present (Bertolotto et al, 2008).
      b. Presence of vaginal bleeding
      c. Gestational age by date of LMP or ultrasound test
      d. Presence of adnexal mass by palpation or ultrasound test
      e. Medical and surgical history, especially previous gynecologic history and surgery
      f. Obstetric history: previous pregnancies or complications
      g. Ability to urinate: as tumor enlarges, might cause urinary obstruction.
   2. Physical examination
      a. Presence of adnexal mass confirmed by pelvic examination, ultrasound test, or both
      b. Palpation of uterine contractions
      c. Presence of vaginal bleeding
      d. Cervical status: presence of dilation
      e. Fundal height: approximate for gestational age or increasing as tumor enlarges
      f. Abdominal examination: presence of ascites; distended bladder
   3. Diagnostic procedures
      a. Ultrasound test: fetal and adnexal mass evaluation (solid or cystic and estimation of size)
      b. Fetal monitoring to assess FHR and rule out preterm labor preoperatively and postoperatively

APPENDECTOMY

A. **Introduction**
   1. Incidence
      a. The most common cause of nonobstetric acute abdomen during pregnancy—incidence 0.05% to 0.1% (Moreno-Sanz et al, 2007)

    b. Surgery to remove the appendix occurs in approximately 1 in 1500 to 2000 pregnancies (Dietrich et al, 2008; Kilpatrick & Monga, 2007).

    c. Appendectomy accounts for 25% of nonobstetric surgeries in pregnancy. Appendicitis occurs with equal frequency in each trimester, but the incidence of perforation is as high as 43% in pregnant women in comparison to nonpregnant women (Cappell, 2007; Lu & Curet, 2007).

2. Symptoms

    a. Enlarged uterus makes interpretation of physical signs difficult.

    b. Right flank pain rather than right lower quadrant pain is often present. The appendix is thought to rise up into the abdomen during pregnancy, reaching the iliac crest by week 24, but this has been challenged in a prospective study comparing appendix location in pregnant women undergoing appendectomy and at cesarean section (Hodjati & Karerooni, 2003; Kilpatrick & Monga, 2007). Further research is needed to clarify this issue (Figure 24-1).

    c. Rebound tenderness has been noted to be less in late pregnancy; abdominal guarding is a less reliable symptom late in pregnancy due to the laxity of the abdominal wall muscles (Deitrich et al, 2008; Kilpatrick & Monga, 2007).

    d. Symptoms might be confused with:

        (1) Preterm labor

        (2) Pyelonephritis

    e. No cervical change should be present.

3. Peritonitis increases the incidence of preterm labor.

    a. Symptoms of perforation with peritonitis might be masked during pregnancy because of increased steroid levels, which decrease the normal inflammatory response.

    b. If perforation is present, preterm contractions are seen in up to 83% of cases, although preterm labor and delivery occur only 5% to 14% of the time. Fetal loss associated with appendectomy is 2.6% and increases to 10.9% in the presence of peritonitis (Dietrich et al, 2008).

    c. If perforation and peritonitis are absent, a laparoscopic approach might be chosen before 20 weeks' gestation; an open laparotomy will be chosen later in gestation or in complicated cases (Dietrich et al, 2008) (for laparoscopic considerations, see discussion of cholecystectomy).

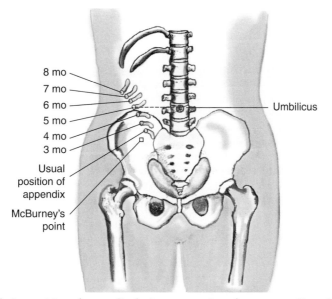

FIGURE 24-1 ■ Relative position of appendix during progression of pregnancy. (From Lowdermilk, D.L., & Perry, S.E. [2007]. *Maternity & women's health care* [9th ed.]. St. Louis: Mosby.)

B. Procedure-specific patient assessment (in addition to general maternal preoperative assessment)
1. History
   a. Gestational age by date of LMP or ultrasonography
   b. Symptoms
      (1) Nausea and vomiting
      (2) Fever
      (3) Periumbilical pain
      (4) Right flank pain
      (5) Anorexia
      (6) Constipation
      (7) Diarrhea
   c. Assessment of pain: location, duration, quality, and aggravating or alleviating factors
2. Physical examination
   a. Abdominal examination
      (1) Rebound tenderness: less prevalent in late pregnancy
      (2) Uterine contractions
   b. Check for evidence of vaginal bleeding
   c. Cervical examination for labor status
3. Diagnostic procedures
   a. Laboratory tests
      (1) CBC with differential
         (a) Hemoglobin level should be greater than 10.
         (b) WBC might not be helpful because values of 15,000 to 20,000 mm^3 occur in pregnancy and labor; however, a shift to the left (differential count of greater than 80% polymorphonuclear leukocytes) is a significant finding (Dietrich et al, 2008).
      (2) UA and urine culture
         (a) Help to differentiate urinary tract infection from the clinical picture.
         (b) In the second half of pregnancy, pyuria has been found in 20% of patients with appendicitis; sterile pyuria might result from the proximity of the appendix to the ureter or renal pelvis.
   b. Ultrasonography: to assess fetal well-being as well as to confirm the diagnosis. Magnetic resonance imaging (MRI) may be used to confirm diagnosis if ultrasound findings are equivocal (Dietrich et al, 2008).

CERVICAL CERCLAGE

A. Introduction
1. Cervical incompetence (Ludmir & Owen, 2007)
   a. Painless dilation of cervix during second trimester
   b. Associated with repeated second-trimester abortion in absence of contractions
   c. Short cervical length as assessed by vaginal sonography
2. Surgical technique that closes or supports cervix at level of internal os is done to support pregnancy to viability.
   a. McDonald's suture: Mersilene suture placed at cervicovaginal junction and removed for labor
   b. Shirodkar procedure: Mersilene tape encircles the cervix, is passed under the mucosa; might be removed for labor or to perform cesarean section
   c. Laparoscopic placement and removal of a transabdominal cerclage is a therapeutic option for patients with history of failed cerclage (Ludmir & Owen, 2007).
3. Optimal timing
   a. After first trimester, most practitioners choose between 14 and 18 weeks' gestation.
   b. After 20 weeks of gestation, preliminary research indicates a significant negative linear relationship between term at time of cerclage and prolongation of pregnancy.
   c. Suture usually removed electively at 37 weeks
4. Tocolytic therapy as an adjunctive therapy might be considered to treat preterm labor or uterine irritability.

B. **Procedure-specific patient assessment (in addition to general maternal preoperative assessment)**
   1. History
      a. Gestational age by date of LMP or ultrasound test
      b. Obstetric history of second-trimester cervical dilation or fetal losses
      c. Previous gynecologic surgery and cervical laceration
      d. History of premature rupture of membranes (PROM) in previous pregnancies
      e. History of vaginal bleeding
      f. Diethylstilbestrol (DES) exposure
   2. Physical examination
      a. Pelvic examination
         (1) Cervical dilation (less than or equal to 3 to 4 cm to be candidate for cerclage)
         (2) Evidence of infection (treatment of infection before cerclage)
         (3) Status of membranes (must be intact for cerclage)
      b. FHR: presence (confirming a viable fetus)
   3. Diagnostic procedures
      a. Ultrasonography: gestation, cervical length, and internal os dilation
      b. Palpation of uterus to assess uterine activity and/or use of external fetal monitor to determine presence of distress

ENDOSCOPIC GASTROINTESTINAL PROCEDURES

A. **Introduction**
   1. Incidence
      a. Approximately 12,000 pregnant women each year in the United States have strong indications for EGD; indications for sigmoidoscopy or colonoscopy exist in an additional 6000 pregnancies (Cappell, 2007).
      b. Approximately 1000 pregnant women each year demonstrate the need for therapeutic ERCP (Cappell, 2007).
   2. Risks of endoscopy during pregnancy include:
      a. Premature labor
      b. Potential teratogenesis from medications administered during the procedure
      c. Placental abruption or fetal trauma during placement of the endoscope in certain procedures
      d. Systemic hypotension/hypertension
      e. Transient maternal or fetal hypoxia
   3. Cholelithiasis occurs in approximately 8% of pregnancies.
      a. Cholecystectomy might be delayed until the postpartum period for uncomplicated cholelithiasis that responds to conservative medical treatment.
      b. Choledocholithiasis usually requires urgent therapy due to the potential for cholangitis or gallstone pancreatitis that might be life threatening. In this situation, therapeutic ERCP can be performed to avoid complex biliary surgery until after delivery. Lead shielding of the mother's abdomen, except the operative site, is essential to minimize radiation exposure (Cappell, 2007).
   4. Gastrointestinal bleeding is the primary indication for EGD during pregnancy.
      a. Increased incidence in susceptible patients might be due to increased variceal bleeding from portal hypertension secondary to gestational increases in plasma volume.
      b. Other indications for EGD include undiagnosed abdominal pain and prolonged vomiting (Cappell, 2007).
   5. Sigmoidoscopy does not induce labor or produce congenital abnormalities in medically stable pregnant women with indications, such as lower gastrointestinal bleeding, rectal mass, or rectal obstruction.
   6. Few safety data are available on colonoscopy during pregnancy, but partial colonoscopy may be considered for confirmation of suspected colonic cancer, for severe colonic bleeding, or prior to urgent colonic surgery (Cappell, 2007).
   7. Colon cancer is relatively rare during pregnancy with an incidence of 1 per 13,000 to 50,000 pregnancies (Cappell, 2007).
   8. Two thirds of colon cancer found during pregnancy are in the rectal area. This differs from nonpregnant women of the same age (Cappell, 2007).

B. **Procedure-specific patient assessment (in addition to general maternal preoperative assessment)**
   1. Risks to the mother/fetus
      a. EGD or ERCP can produce maternal respiratory compromise and resultant hypoxia from:
         (1) Medications administered
         (2) Vagally mediated bronchospasm due to stretching of the viscera
         (3) Laryngeal impingement during esophageal intubation with resultant pulmonary aspiration (Cappell, 2007)
      b. Sigmoidoscopy and colonoscopy can produce hypoxia due to:
         (1) IV sedation medications administered
         (2) Circulatory changes due to vagal responses to colonic distention
   2. Methods of risk management (Cappell, 2007)
      a. Defer endoscopy until after the first trimester if possible.
      b. Defer endoscopy until postpartum if possible.
      c. Administer smallest effective dose of all required medications during procedure.
      d. Involve patient in decisions about use of potentially fetotoxic drugs; always use drugs with greatest fetal safety, if possible.
      e. Consider use of qualified anesthesia provider (physician anesthesiologist or certified registered nurse anesthetist) to provide sedation during procedure.
      f. If bipolar cautery is used for hemostasis, biopsy, polypectomy, or papillotomy, be sure grounding pad is positioned so uterus is not directly between the cautery and the grounding pad to minimize fetal exposure.
   3. Laboratory/diagnostic procedures
      a. Endorectal ultrasound is useful to stage rectal carcinomas.
      b. MRI is preferred to abdominal CT to evaluate metastatic or regional disease.

INTRAUTERINE FETAL SURGERY

A. **Introduction**
   1. Birth defects account for more than 21% of all infant deaths; first intrauterine fetal surgery to repair a congenital defect took place in 1981.
   2. Decision requires balancing risk to mother and fetus against potential benefit to only the fetus.
   3. Maternal safety increased by use of fetoscopic approach over open hysterotomy
   4. Potential maternal complications associated with fetal surgery include:
      a. Preterm labor; increased need for intensive care unit (ICU) and/or prolonged hospitalization (Golombeck et al, 2006)
      b. Earlier gestational age at delivery
      c. Increased lifelong risk of uterine rupture following hysterotomy
      d. Increased risk of transfusion
   5. Research supports the use of fetal surgical procedures only in highly specialized tertiary centers due to the severity and very high risk of the procedures.
      a. Risks are considered to be so great to mother and fetus that prenatal correction of cleft lip or palate is deemed unjustified at present (Aronsarena, 2007).
      b. Failure of open fetal repair of congenital diaphragmatic hernia to increase survival and lack of success with several fetal tracheal occlusion techniques in producing fetal lung growth has led to opinion that fetal surgery to correct congenital diaphragmatic hernia cannot be recommended at this time (Kays, 2006).
B. **Specific anomalies amenable to fetal surgery**
   1. Twin-twin transfusion syndrome
      a. Results from unbalanced twin-to-twin transfusion between monochorionic twins, which leads to:
         (1) A recipient twin with polyhydramnios and hydrops, and
         (2) A donor twin who develops oligohydramnios, growth restriction, and increased mortality
      b. A similar pathology is twin reversal arterial perfusion syndrome in which:
         (1) One twin is acardiac/anencephalic and nonviable with a vascular anastomosis.
         (2) A normal twin develops heart failure due to the stress of providing cardiac output for both fetuses.
      c. Fetal mortality may be up to 90% if left untreated (Crombleholme et al, 2007).

   d. Fetoscopic laser ablation of abnormal placental vessels produces a 53% to 56% survival rate as compared to amnioreduction alone to treat this abnormality (Crombleholme et al, 2007).
   e. Selective fetoscopic laser photocoagulation of only vessels communicating between the two twins is associated with 30-day survival rates of 62% to 70% (Crombleholme et al, 2007).
2. Spina bifida/hydrocephalus
   a. Neural tube defects are among the most common congenital abnormalities.
      (1) Anencephaly and encephalocele account for 50% of all neural tube defects.
      (2) The remainder occurs along the spine with myelomeningocele being most prevalent (4.4 to 4.6 cases per 10,000 live births).
   b. Myelomeningocele occurs at end of the fourth week of gestation if the neural tube fails to close spontaneously. Early diagnosis is aided by measuring maternal alpha-fetoprotein levels with follow-up use of sonography in the second trimester (Chen, 2008).
   c. The "two-hit hypothesis" for the pathology: primary defect in closure of the neural tube plus secondary injury to exposed neural tissue from chronic mechanical trauma and amniotic fluid–induced chemical injury
   d. Hydroureteronephrosis and vesicoureteral reflux are present in 10% to 30% of fetuses with myelomeningocele (Salaam, 2006).
   e. Myelomeningocele: More than 400 have been repaired by fetal surgery; preliminary results indicate positive reversal of Chiari II malformation herniation, a decrease in shunt-dependent hydrocephalus; possible improvement in leg function. Randomized multicenter trial is soon to be completed (Sutton, 2008).
3. Obstructive uropathy
   a. First done with open fetal surgery at University of California, San Francisco, in 1981; now performed via percutaneous insertion of vesicoamniotic shunts
   b. Indication for surgery is presence of bilateral hydronephrosis with oligohydramnios.
   c. Posterior urethral valves are thin membranes of obstructive tissue. Research currently indicates visceroamniotic shunt placement to treat posterior urethral valves makes no difference to long-term outcomes of the fetus; therefore, primary valve ablation remains keystone of treatment (Salaam, 2006).
   d. Overall efficacy in preserving lung and kidney function is under study.
C. **Approaches and concerns in fetal surgery**
   1. Surgical approaches
      a. Minimal access fetal surgery is performed endoscopically with one small uterine trocar for placement under general or regional anesthesia.
      b. Hysterotomy is a procedure in which the uterus is opened to allow direct operation on the fetus.
         (1) Always requires general anesthesia to produce maximal uterine relaxation
         (2) Might open the uterus using electrocautery following assessment of placental location and fetal lie by ultrasonography
      c. Intraoperative management
         (1) Maternal safety
         (2) Avoidance of teratogenic anesthetic and ancillary drugs
         (3) Avoidance of fetal and maternal asphyxia
         (4) Adequate fetal anesthesia and monitoring
         (5) Adequate uterine relaxation
         (6) Prevention of premature labor
D. **Procedure-specific patient assessment (in addition to general maternal preoperative assessment): following determination of the surgical approach, the assessment, and the approach remain the same as endoscopic considerations and perioperative nursing interventions.**

HEALTH EDUCATION

Patient Education and Preparation for Perioperative Experience

A. **Involve patient in planned care.**
   1. Surgical options
   2. Anesthetic options

   3. Methods of pain control
   4. Postoperative care
B. **Teach signs and symptoms of preterm labor** (see Chapter 27 for further information).
C. **Discharge instructions should include:**
   1. Follow-up care as ordered by physician
   2. Report signs and symptoms of:
      a. Infection
      b. Fever
      c. Vaginal bleeding
      d. Excessive pain
   3. Report signs and symptoms of preterm labor.
   4. Discussion of importance of patient's awareness of and cooperation with the following:
      a. Antiembolic or support stockings
      b. Progressive ambulation and activity (or restrictions)
      c. Diet and fluid intake
      d. Adequate rest
      e. Avoidance of heavy lifting (including lifting children)
      f. Avoidance of constipation
   5. Review medications: dose, route, frequency, and potential side effects.
D. **Emphasize importance of social support and increased assistance at home during immediate postoperative period.**

SUMMARY

A. **The greatest risk to the fetus during nonobstetric surgery is intrauterine asphyxia.**
B. **No anesthetic technique or agent has been shown to make a significant difference in maternal or fetal outcome after nonobstetric surgery in the pregnant patient.**
C. **Management of the pregnant surgical patient should focus on prevention of hypoxemia, acidosis, hypotension, and hyperventilation.**

CASE STUDIES AND STUDY QUESTIONS

A 25-year-old gravida 1, para 0 (G1, P0) patient at 18 weeks of gestation arrives in the emergency room with a 2-day history of right flank pain, nausea and vomiting, and anorexia. She denies urinary frequency, urgency, or burning and states that her last bowel movement was 24 hours prior to admission. On examination, pain is elicited with deep palpation at the right flank and right lower abdominal quadrant. The uterus is soft and nontender. The pelvic examination reveals a long cervix without dilation, and the adnexa are not palpable.

Vital signs: oral temperature, 38.3° C (101° F); pulse 92/min; respiratory rate 16 breaths/min; blood pressure, 124/72; FHR, 140/min.

Admission laboratory values: hemoglobin, 12.4 g/dL; WBC, 24,000 mm^3; UA, clear. Patient is sent for an ultrasound test that reveals a viable singleton pregnancy at 18 weeks' gestation, with no evidence of separation of the placenta. A laparoscopic appendectomy is performed, and the postoperative course is without complication. A healthy infant is delivered without complication at term.

1. During surgery the *greatest* risk to the viability of the infant would be:
   a. Administration of beta-adrenergic vasopressors
   b. Severe maternal hypotension
   c. Exposure to general anesthetic agents
   d. Maternal hypothermia
2. During perioperative management of this patient:
   a. Therapy with tocolytic agents is essential.
   b. Dehydration is not a consideration because of her expanded blood volume.
   c. Left lateral uterine displacement should be applied to protect fetal blood flow.
   d. Steroids should be administered to prevent laryngeal edema.
3. In the immediate postoperative period the patient complains of right shoulder and chest pain; this is most likely due to:
   a. Irritation from retained abdominal CO_2
   b. Referred pain from onset of uterine contractions
   c. Right upper lobe aspiration
   d. Pneumothorax

4. In the immediate postoperative period, the patient complains of a scratchy throat and mild hoarseness. This is due to:
   a. Intraoperative damage to the vocal cords
   b. Normal, hormone-induced edema
   c. Mild, transient irritation from endotracheal tube placement during surgery
   d. Right upper-lobe pulmonary aspiration

5. Immediately after surgery, the patient receives narcotics for pain control. During this period of time, it is important to:
   a. Give as little as possible to avoid damage to the fetus.
   b. Get the patient to take oral medications as quickly as possible.
   c. Begin tocolytic therapy.
   d. Monitor carefully for unrecognized uterine contractions.

6. Immediately after the laparoscopic appendectomy, the patient's lungs sound slightly congested and it is reported that she vomited upon emergence from anesthesia and there is a possibility of aspiration of a small amount of gastric contents into her lungs. This event is probably due to:
   a. Carelessness by the anesthesia provider
   b. Increased pressure on the stomach and diaphragm during laparoscopy
   c. Failure of the patient to relate preoperative fluid intake accurately
   d. Fear and anxiety of the patient

7. Had this patient's appendix perforated, symptoms of the resultant peritonitis might have been blunted by:
   a. Pregnancy-induced rotation of the appendix with referred pain
   b. Lack of inflammatory response due to pregnancy-induced increases in steroid levels
   c. Prophylactic administration of tocolytic agents
   d. An increased tendency to wall off abscesses that exist during pregnancy

A 30-year-old G4, P1 patient at 18 weeks' gestation has arrived for evaluation at the antenatal clinic. She relates an obstetric history of a preterm birth at 32 weeks' gestation and two midtrimester losses at 18 and 22 weeks, respectively. Pelvic examination reveals a cervix that is 25% effaced and 1 cm dilated. The membranes are intact.

Vital signs: oral temperature, 37° C (98.6° F); pulse rate 90/min; respiratory rate 20/min; blood pressure, 120/68; FHR, 132/min.

Diagnostic ultrasound testing reveals a singleton, 18-week viable uterine pregnancy. The patient is scheduled for surgical placement of cervical cerclage in 2 days.

8. The criteria that make this patient an excellent candidate for immediate cerclage are:
   a. She is young and healthy.
   b. She has a positive history of cervical incompetence, and her membranes are intact.
   c. Once the membrane ruptures, it is more difficult to complete the procedure.
   d. She is not a good candidate because no labor contractions have begun.

9. The optimal time for cervical cerclage to be attempted is:
   a. 4 to 8 weeks
   b. 10 to 14 weeks
   c. 14 to 18 weeks
   d. 18 to 22 weeks

10. Throughout the entire perioperative period, tocolytic agents will be administered to this patient:
    a. Continuously
    b. If the membranes rupture
    c. Only if uterine irritability is demonstrated
    d. Adjunctively with narcotics to prevent pain

11. To eliminate pressure on the cervix in the immediate postoperative period, the patient:
    a. Should be placed in Trendelenburg position in bed
    b. Should be positioned on her side in reverse Trendelenburg position
    c. Should be catheterized for 48 hours
    d. Should be kept sedated for 24 hours

12. In preparation for discharge, it is most important that this patient be counseled to:
    a. Resume sexual activity immediately.
    b. Remain bedridden as much as possible.
    c. Take no medication of any kind.
    d. Avoid heavy lifting for any reason.

13. Cervical cerclage in this patient will be accomplished under spinal anesthesia. During the anesthesia and surgery, if the maternal blood pressure drops below 100 mm Hg, the most important factor to consider is:
    a. Administration of alpha-adrenergic vasopressors will be necessary.
    b. The increased risk of fetal hypoxia
    c. Too much local anesthetic has been injected by the anesthesia provider.
    d. The patient received inadequate preoperative fluid preparation.

14. During spinal or epidural anesthesia, maternal hypotension is due to:
    a. Transient anesthesia-induced paralysis of sympathetic outflow
    b. Transient anesthesia-induced paralysis of parasympathetic outflow
    c. Concurrent intraoperative administration of tocolytic agents
    d. Pregnancy-induced changes in peripheral resistance

ANSWERS TO STUDY QUESTIONS

1. b	5. d	9. c	13. b
2. c	6. b	10. c	14. a
3. a	7. b	11. a	
4. c	8. b	12. d	

REFERENCES

Aronsarena, O. A. (2007). Cleft lip and palate. *Otolaryngologic Clinics of North America*, *40*(1), 27–60.

Bertolotto, M., Serafina, G., Toma, P., Zapetti, R., & Migaleddu, V. (2008). Adnexal torsion. *Ultrasound Clinics 3*, 109–119.

Birnbach, D. J., & Browne, I. M. (2005). Anesthesia for obstetrics. In R. D. Miller (Ed.), *Miller's anesthesia* (6th ed., pp. 2307–2339). Philadelphia: Churchill Livingstone.

Cappell, M.S. (2007). Hepatic and gastrointestinal diseases. In S.G. Gabbe, J.L. Simpson, J.R. Niebyl, (eds), H. Galan, L. Goetzl, Eric R.M. Jauniaux, M. Landon (Associate Eds), *Obstetrics: Normal and problem pregnancies* (5th ed., pp.1107–1109). Philadelphia: Churchill Livingstone.

Chen, C. P. (2008). Prenatal diagnosis, fetal surgery, recurrence risks and differential diagnosis of neural tube defects. *Taiwan Journal of Obstetrics and Gynecology*, *47*(3), 283–290.

Crombleholme, T. M., Shera, D., Lee, H., Johnson, M., D'Alton, M., Porter, F., et al. (2007). A prospective, randomized, multicenter trial of amnioreduction vs. selective fetoscopic laser photocoagulation for the treatment of severe twin-twin transfusion syndrome. *American Journal of Obstetrics & Gynecology*, *197*, 396.e7–396.e9.

Dietrich, C. S., Hill, C. C., & Hueman, M. (2008). Surgical diseases presenting in pregnancy. *Surgical Clinics of North America*, *88*, 403–419.

Golombeck, K., Ball, R. H., Lee, H., Farrell, J. A., Farmer, D. L., Jacobs, V. R., Rosen, M. A., Filly, R. A., & Harrison, M. R. (2006). Maternal morbidity after maternal-fetal surgery. *American Journal of Obstetrics & Gynecology*, *194*(3), 834–839.

Hill, C. C., & Pickinpaugh, J. (2008). Physiologic changes in pregnancy. *Surgical Clinics of North America*, *88*, 391–401.

Hodjati, H., & Karerooni, T. (2003). Location of the appendix in the gravid patient: A re-evaluation of the established concept. *International Journal of Gynaecology and Obstetrics*, *81*(3), 245–247.

Kays, D. W. (2006). Congenital diaphragmatic hernia and neonatal lung lesions. *Surgical Clinics of North America*, *82*(2), 329–352.

Kilpatrick, C. C., & Monga, M. (2007). Approach to the acute abdomen in pregnancy. *Obstetrics and Gynecology Clinics of North America*, *34*, 389–402.

Landau, R. (2008). Pharmacogenetics and obstetric anesthesia. *Anesthesiology Clinics*, *26*, 183–195.

Leiserowitz, G. S. (2006). Managing ovarian masses during pregnancy. *Obstetric Gynecologic Surgery*, *61*(7), 463–470.

Lu, E. J., & Curet, M. J. (2007). Surgical Procedures in Pregnancy. In S. G. Gabbe, J. R. Niebyl, & J. L. Simpson (Eds.), *Obstetrics: Normal and problem pregnancies* (5th ed., pp. 619–622). Philadelphia: Churchill Livingstone.

Lu, E. J., Curet, M. J., El-Said, Y. Y., & Kirkwood, K. S. (2004). Medical versus surgical management of biliary tract disease in pregnancy. *American Journal of Surgery*, *188*, 755.

Ludmir, J., & Owen, J. (2007). Cervical incompetence. In S. G. Gabbe, J. R. Niebyl, & J. L. Simpson (Eds.), *Obstetrics: Normal and problem pregnancies* (5th ed., pp. 650–664). Philadelphia: Churchill Livingstone.

McAneny, A. (2008). Open cholecystectomy. *Surgical Clinics of North America*, *88*, 1273–1294.

Mhuireachtaigh, R. N., & O'Gorman, D. A. (2006). Anesthesia in pregnant patients for nonobstetric surgery. *Journal of Clinical Anesthesia*, *18*, 60–66.

Moreno-Sanz, C., Pascual-Pedreno, A., Picazo-Yeste, J. S., & Seoane-Gonzalez, J. B. (2007). Laparoscopic appendectomy during pregnancy: Between personal experiences and scientific evidence. *Journal of the American College of Surgeons*, *205*(1), 37–42.

Salaam, M. A. (2006). Posterior urethral valve: Outcomes of antenatal intervention. *International Journal of Urology*, *13*(10), 1317–1322.

Sutton, L. N. (2008). Fetal surgery for neural tube defects. *Best Practices and Research Clinical Obstetrics and Gynaecology*, *22*(1), 175–188.

Takeda, A., Sakai, K., Mitsui, T., & Nakamura, H. (2007). Management of ruptured corpus luteum cyst of pregnancy occurring in a 15-year-old girl by laparoscopic surgery with intraoperative autologous blood transfusion. *Journal of Pediatric and Adolescent Gynecology*, *20*, 97–100.

25 Substance Abuse in Pregnancy

Barbara A. Moran

OBJECTIVES

1. Discuss the scope of substance abuse in pregnancy.
2. Recognize signs of substance abuse.
3. Describe the effects of drug use during pregnancy on the developing fetus.
4. Elicit appropriate history and pertinent information from the patient.
5. Describe the special needs of the drug-dependent pregnant woman.
6. Recognize the teaching needs and appropriate referrals for the pregnant substance abuser.

SUBSTANCE ABUSE

INTRODUCTION

A. **Major public health issue**
   1. Drug use in pregnancy and its associated problems has become a major public health issue.
   2. Polydrug use, such as alcohol and tobacco with marijuana or cocaine, has become more common.
B. **Statistics**
   1. The overall rate of current illicit drug use among persons ages 12 or older in 2007 (8%) was similar to the rate in 2006 (8.3%) and has remained stable since 2002 (8.3%) (U.S. Department of Health & Human Services [USDHHS], 2008).
   2. Nearly 4% of pregnant women use illicit drugs such as marijuana, cocaine, and heroin (March of Dimes, 2006).
C. Outcomes of substance abuse are related to the following:
   1. Molecular weight influences whether the drug crosses the placenta.
   2. The first 8 weeks of pregnancy are the most critical in terms of embryonic development. During the third trimester, drug use has the greatest potential for impairing fetal growth.
   3. Route of ingestion
      a. Drugs taken orally might reduce the drug's ability to cross the placenta.
      b. Drugs taken intravenously and intranasally more readily cross the placenta.
      c. Intravenous (IV) drug use increases maternal and fetal exposure to human immunodeficiency virus (HIV).
   4. Adequacy of prenatal care
   5. Presence of obstetric or maternal complications
   6. Multiple drug use
   7. Lifestyle of mother, including poverty, homelessness or inadequate housing, lack of education, domestic violence, and social and emotional problems
   8. Nutritional status
   9. Many medical conditions, including anemia, bacteremia/septicemia, cardiac disease, cellulitis, depression, diabetes, edema, hepatitis B and C, tuberculosis (TB), hypertension, phlebitis, sexually transmitted infections (STIs), urinary tract infections, and vitamin deficiency compromise many drug-involved pregnancies.
   10. Obstetric complications include abruptio placentae, placenta previa, intrauterine death, spontaneous abortion, premature labor and delivery, premature rupture of membranes (PROM), intrauterine growth restriction (IUGR), and polyhydramnios.

D. **Effects on fetus**
   1. Generalized growth restriction and its associated complications
   2. Increase in the frequency of sudden infant death syndrome (SIDS)
   3. Signs of withdrawal, which can occur from birth to 6 days of life, include:
      a. High-pitched or shrill cry
      b. Gastrointestinal disturbances
      c. Tremulousness
      d. Excoriation of knees and elbows from increased restlessness and sleeplessness
      e. Perianal excoriation (chemical dermatitis due to acidic stool)
      f. Respiratory disturbances
         (1) Tachypnea
         (2) Nasal congestion
         (3) Frequent yawning
         (4) Sneezing
      g. Seizure activity
   4. Many of the signs of drug withdrawal in the neonate are similar to other neonatal problems, such as sepsis, hypoglycemia, and central nervous system (CNS) disorders; therefore, testing to rule out these conditions should be considered in addition to drug screening.

E. **Cocaine**
   1. Cocaine abuse and addiction is a complex problem involving biological changes in the brain as well as social, family, and environmental factors (National Institute of Drug Abuse and Addiction [NIDAA], 2008a).
   2. The estimated number and percentage of persons ages 12 and older who used cocaine in the past month in 2007 (2.1 million users or 0.8% of the population) were similar to those in 2006 (2.4 million or 1%) and 2002 (2 million or 0.9%) (USDHHS, 2008).
   3. Cocaine is found in the leaves of the *Erythroxylum coca* plant of Peru, Ecuador, and Bolivia; it can be snorted, sniffed, injected, or smoked; other names include coke, snow, flake, and blow.
   4. Cocaine blocks the reuptake of catecholamines at nerve terminals, which increases circulating concentrations of catecholamines in the blood, resulting in vasoconstriction, tachycardia, hypertension, and uterine contractions.
   5. Cocaine use is second only to marijuana in pregnant women who used an illicit drug during pregnancy.
   6. Crosses the placenta by diffusion
   7. Cardiovascular and neurologic complications, such as hypertension, tachycardia, myocardial ischemia, sudden death, dysrhythmias, subarachnoid hemorrhage, thrombocytopenia, and seizures have been described among parturients who abuse cocaine.
   8. Used during early months of pregnancy, may increase risk of miscarriage
   9. Acute cocaine use during the third trimester might result in preterm labor, abruptio placentae, a greater incidence of PROM, and an increased risk of meconium staining, precipitous delivery, premature and low birthweight infants.

F. **Heroin**
   1. Derived from seeds of the poppy plant *Papaver somniferum;* it produces an off-white or pale brown powder that can be sniffed, smoked, or injected parenterally; it is approximately 25 times stronger than morphine and crosses the placenta readily, appearing in fetal tissue within 1 hour of maternal consumption; may be called sugar, dope, horse, junk, white horse, or smack (National Institute of Drug Abuse [NIDA], 2009a)
   2. The number of heroin users decreased from 338,000 in 2006 to 153,000 in 2007, and the corresponding prevalence rate decreased from 0.14% to 0.06% (USDHHS, 2008).
   3. Heroin abuse during pregnancy and associated environmental factors have been associated with adverse consequences including low birthweight (NIDAA, 2008b).
   4. Primary effects are analgesia, sedation, feeling of well-being, and euphoria.
   5. Heroin is not generally thought to be a teratogen capable of producing congenital malformation.
      a. Easily crosses the placenta via simple diffusion
      b. Hazards of heroin to the fetus are thought to be the direct effects of the drug on the fetus and the maternal lifestyle associated with heroin use.
         (1) The woman typically does not seek early prenatal care—this is related to fear of detection of heroin use and to an absence or irregularity of menses caused by heroin that makes amenorrhea a norm in her life.

        (2) There is an increased maternal and fetal exposure to serious infection such as:

           (a) STIs

           (b) Hepatitis

           (c) HIV

  6. Neonatal effects of prenatal heroin exposure include the following:

    a. Neonatal abstinence syndrome

      (1) Causes severe neonatal withdrawal symptoms

      (2) Has an average onset of symptoms between 6 and 12 hours after birth, with an average peak of symptoms between 48 and 72 hours

    b. Withdrawal symptoms might persist in a subacute form for 4 to 6 months after birth.

    c. Increased incidence of meconium aspiration at birth

    d. Increased incidence of neonatal sepsis

    e. Symmetric IUGR

      (1) Low birthweight

      (2) Decreased length

      (3) Small head circumference

    f. Neurodevelopmental behavioral problems

      (1) Tremulous and irritable

      (2) Poor organizational responses to environmental stimuli

      (3) Poor motor control

      (4) Difficult to console

      (5) Poor suck and swallow coordination, which leads to poor feeding tolerance

G. Marijuana

  1. Marijuana was the most commonly used illicit drug (14.4 million past month users). In 2007, marijuana was used by 72.8% of illicit drug users and was the only drug used by 53.3% of them (DHHS, 2008).

  2. Among persons ages 12 and older, the overall rate of past month marijuana use in 2007 (5.8%) was similar to the rate in 2006 and the rates in earlier years going back to 2002 (USDHHS, 2008).

  3. Often called pot, grass, reefer, weed, herb, Mary Jane, MJ, skunk, blunt, dope, or joint (NIDAA, 2008a)

  4. Causes tachycardia and decreased blood pressure, resulting in orthostatic hypotension

  5. Research has shown that babies born to women who used marijuana during pregnancy display altered responses to visual stimuli, increased tremulousness, and a high-pitched cry, which may indicate problems with neurologic development (NIDAA, 2008c).

H. Methadone hydrochloride

  1. Developed as a substitute for morphine and heroin; frequently used to treat pregnant heroin-dependent women to prevent repeated episodes of heroin withdrawal in the fetus (National Institute of Drug Abuse International Program, 2009)

  2. Blocks the craving of withdrawal

  3. Is longer-acting and therefore is thought to stabilize the environment for the fetus, sustaining the addict and avoiding withdrawal, thus:

    a. Decreasing maternal complications

    b. Decreasing prematurity and low birthweight

  4. Methadone maintenance requires enrollment in a drug-treatment program, therefore increasing the likelihood of prenatal care.

  5. Mother may breastfeed infant if not infected with HIV, hepatitis, or TB; long-term effects on the neonate have not been determined.

CLINICAL PRACTICE

A. Assessment

  1. History

    a. Menstrual history: irregular menses in 60% to 90% of addicted women

    b. Obstetric/gynecologic history

      (1) Little or no prenatal care

      (2) Number of pregnancies and method of delivery, miscarriages, abortions, and living children

        (3) Gynecologic infections

        (4) STIs

        (5) Method of contraception

  c. Medical history

        (1) Preexisting medical conditions and treatments; the most common comorbid diagnoses for women are affective disorders, such as chronic or acute depression and anxiety disorders

        (2) Hospitalizations

        (3) Surgeries

        (4) History of physical or sexual abuse or family violence

        (5) Weight less than the 50th percentile and little or no weight gain during pregnancy

  d. Drug abuse history

        (1) Drugs currently used

        (2) Length of use

        (3) Age at onset

        (4) Duration

        (5) Frequency and route of administration

        (6) Date of last use

        (7) Any previous treatment

        (8) Family history of substance abuse

  e. Erratic appetite

  f. Poor nutrition

  g. Deterioration in personal hygiene

  h. Allergies

  i. Hepatitis

  j. Acquired immunodeficiency syndrome (AIDS) and other sexually transmitted infections

  k. History of child abuse, neglect, and/or sexual abuse

2. Physical findings

  a. Bloodshot eyes, conjunctivitis, and yellow sclera

  b. Slurred speech

  c. Dilated or constricted pupils

  d. Restlessness or fatigue

  e. Shortness of breath

  f. Poor dental hygiene, abscesses, and gum disease

  g. Rhinitis, nasal or sinus irritation, septal erosion, and loss of sense of smell

  h. Hepatomegaly, jaundice, or distended neck veins secondary to liver failure

  i. Scars from injuries or surgery

  j. Subcutaneous abscesses or cellulitis and rashes

  k. Needle marks and ecchymotic spots or scars

  l. Unsteady walk and impaired coordination

  m. Slowed reflexes

  n. Elevated blood pressure

  o. Tachycardia

  p. Altered moods and perceptions/inappropriate behavior

  q. Nausea

  r. Dizziness

  s. Odor of substance on clothing

  t. Burns on fingertips or singed eyebrows or eyelashes

  u. Phlebitis

  v. Placental abruption

3. Psychosocial findings

  a. Low self-esteem

  b. Depression

  c. Chronic anxiety

  d. Inability to maintain close relationships

  e. Family disorganization

  f. Manipulative behaviors

  g. Hostility or anger

  h. Homelessness

      i. Unplanned pregnancy

      j. Denial

      k. Late prenatal care, missed appointments, or late for appointments

      l. Difficulty following through on referrals

      m. Intimate partner violence (IPV)

  4. Diagnostic studies

      a. Complete blood count (CBC), differential, and urinalysis (UA)

      b. Toxicologic urine screening (detects cocaine ingestion within past 24 hours)

      c. Venereal Disease Research Laboratory (VDRL) test

      d. Cervical culture for gonorrhea and chlamydia

      e. Papanicolaou test (Pap smear)

      f. Hepatitis profile

      g. HIV testing

      h. Sonography (to detect IUGR)

      i. TB skin test

      j. Rubella titer

      k. Sickle cell screening (when appropriate)

      l. Blood type and antibody screen

      m. Alpha-fetoprotein (if between 16 and 20 weeks' gestation)

      n. Hepatitis panel (Hep B core antibody, Hep B surface antibody, Hep B surface antigen, Hep A antibody profile, Hep C antibody)

      o. Baseline liver and renal function tests

      p. Group B streptococcus culture

      q. Toxoplasmosis, cytomegalovirus, and herpes cultures

B. Interventions

  1. Identify substance abuse in patient.

      a. Unexplained late first obstetric visit or no prenatal care

      b. Multiple missed visits

      c. History of unexplained miscarriages, fetal growth restriction, stillbirths, abruptio placentae, and precipitous birth

      d. Children with developmental problems

      e. History of drug- or alcohol-related medical problems

      f. History of physical or sexual abuse

      g. Questions phrased positively to elicit honest responses (e.g., "To care for you and your baby, I need to know" or "I noticed track marks and I'm concerned for you and your baby and need to know")

  2. Give accurate and specific information on complications associated with drug use and the increase in morbidity and mortality in a nonjudgmental way.

      a. Explain that quitting or decreasing drugs at any time in pregnancy improves obstetric outcome.

      b. Explain dangers of operating vehicles or machinery while under the influence of drugs.

      c. Provide nutritional counseling, emphasizing protein intake; provide supplemental vitamins, iron and folate.

      d. Encourage listening to fetal heart rate by the mother and significant other at each visit.

      e. Show sonogram to the patient so she can visualize the fetus.

      f. Provide information on fetal growth and development.

      g. Reinforce patient's understanding with printed material at a level she can understand and use a variety of teaching methods to reinforce education.

      h. Discourage breastfeeding if the mother is using a substance that might pass through the breast milk.

  3. Infant

      a. Use an interdisciplinary team approach in a nonjudgmental and sensitive manner.

      b. Promote attachment by recommending attendance at childbirth preparation and parenting classes.

      c. Monitor and document daily nutritional intake for volume and calories; daily weight; hydration, daily output, urine, stool, and insensible water loss; oxygenation by pulse oximetry and capillary refill time.

      d. Determine suck, swallow, and breathing coordination; provide pacifier to meet increased sucking need.

    e. Assist family in supporting patient in a nonjudgmental and supportive fashion; help patient identify stresses in her family life.

    f. Give parents or guardians counseling regarding available resources and necessary follow-up care for the infant.

    g. Facilitate referral to child protective services, welfare, adoption, community health, or charity agencies as needed. (See Box 25-1.)

TOBACCO

INTRODUCTION

A. Smoking is a major public health problem and is the leading preventable cause of death in the United States. It kills approximately 438,000 people per year (Centers for Disease Control and Prevention [CDC], 2009c).

    1. Nicotine is highly addictive. The tar increases risk of lung cancer, emphysema, and bronchial disorders. The carbon monoxide increases cardiovascular disease (NIDA, 2009b).

    2. Nearly 73 million Americans used a tobacco product at least once in 2006 (NIDA, 2009b) and nearly 4 million American adolescents have used tobacco within the past month (NIDAA, 2006).

    3. More than 1 in 6 American women ages 18 years or older (17%) smoke cigarettes (American Cancer Society [ACS], 2008).

    4. Approximately 13% of women reported smoking during the last 3 months of pregnancy (CDC, 2009d).

    5. The rate of current use of any tobacco product among persons ages 12 and older decreased from 29.6% in 2006 to 28.6% in 2007, but the rates of current use of cigarettes, smokeless

---

■ BOX 25-1
■ **OBSTETRIC COMPLICATIONS ASSOCIATED WITH THE ADDICTED PATIENT**

COMPLICATIONS OF MOTHER

Abruptio placentae
Anemia
Cesarean delivery
Chorioamnionitis
Gestational diabetes
Maternal hypertension
Placental insufficiency
Postpartum hemorrhage
Precipitous delivery
Preeclampsia/eclampsia
Premature rupture of membranes
Preterm labor/delivery
Septic thrombophlebitis
Sexually transmitted infections
Spontaneous miscarriage
Stillbirths
Urinary tract infection
Uterine rupture

COMPLICATIONS OF NEWBORN

Apnea
Bradycardia
Detrimental maternal-infant bonding
Difficult to console
Exaggerated startle response
Generalized growth restriction
High-pitched cry
Hyperactivity
Hypoactivity
Hypoglycemia
Increased frequency of sudden infant death syndrome
Intracranial hemorrhage
Intrauterine growth restriction
Gastrointestinal disturbances
Low birthweight
Meconium aspiration
Neurobehavioral abnormalities (altered sleep patterns, irritability, jitteriness, tremors, depressed sucking)
Pneumonia
Poor feeding
Possible seizures
Respiratory distress syndrome
Small head circumference
Tachycardia
Tachypnea

tobacco, cigars, and pipe tobacco did not change significantly over that period. Between 2002 and 2007, past month use of any tobacco product decreased from 30.4% to 28.6%, and past month cigarette use declined from 26% to 24.2%. Rates of past month use of cigars, smokeless tobacco, and pipe tobacco were similar in 2002 and 2007 (USDHHS, 2008).

6. Among women ages 15 to 44, combined data for 2006 and 2007 indicated that the rate of past month cigarette use was lower among those who were pregnant (16.4%) than it was among those who were not pregnant (28.4%). However, among those ages 15 to 17, the rate of cigarette smoking for pregnant women was higher than for nonpregnant women (24.3% vs. 16%). A similar pattern in cigarette smoking was observed in the combined 2004-2005 data, although the difference among those ages 15 to 17 was not statistically significant in the data for those years (USDHHS, 2008).

B. **Maternal tobacco smoking during pregnancy adversely affects** (March of Dimes, 2008b):
   1. Prenatal and postnatal growth—pregnant women who smoke cigarettes are nearly twice as likely to have a low-birthweight baby as women who do not smoke. Smoking slows fetal growth and increases the risk of premature delivery.
      a. Increased risk of fetal mortality and morbidity
      b. Cognitive developmental delay
      c. Spontaneous abortion
      d. SIDS
      e. Long-term neurobehavioral effects
      f. Poor nutritional status of the mother associated with the anorexigenic effect of nicotine, carbon monoxide exposure
      g. Blood flow restriction to the placenta due to the vasoconstrictive effects of catecholamines released from the adrenals and nerve cells after nicotine activation
   2. According to the American Cancer Society, if all pregnant women in the United States stopped smoking, there would be an estimated 5% reduction in newborn deaths (ACS, 2008).

CLINICAL PRACTICE

A. **Assessment**
   1. History
      a. Prior tobacco use
      b. Current use
      c. Quantity of cigarettes smoked daily
      d. Family members who smoke
   2. Physical findings
      a. Cough
      b. Congestion
      c. Tobacco air (smell) surrounding patient
   3. Psychosocial findings
      a. Anxiety
      b. Guilt
      c. Denial
      d. Hostility or anger
      e. Depression
   4. Diagnostic procedure: ultrasonography (to detect IUGR)
B. **Interventions**
   1. Provide the patient with factual information about smoking and the health hazard to herself (ACS, 2008).
      a. Hemorrhage (from abruptio placentae and placenta previa)
      b. Sepsis (from ruptured membranes)
      c. Bronchitis, lung cancer, and other lung diseases
      d. Cancers of cervix, mouth, larynx, pharynx, esophagus, kidney, bladder, pancreas, stomach
      e. Hypertension and cardiovascular disease
      f. Spontaneous abortion
      g. Depletion of vitamin C level, which is needed to produce collagen and enhances absorption of iron

2. Provide the patient with factual information about the health hazard of smoking to the unborn child.
   a. Reduction in uteroplacental flow that might impair oxygen exchange across the placenta
   b. Abortion, stillbirth, and prematurity
   c. IUGR
   d. Low birthweight infant
   e. SIDS: occurs twice as frequently in children of smokers
   f. Low Apgar scores
   g. Neurobehavioral effects
   h. Increased frequency of apnea
   i. Possible withdrawal-like symptoms similar to those seen in babies of mothers who use illicit drugs (jittery and difficult to soothe)
3. Emphasize that the earlier a pregnant woman gives up smoking, the lower her risk of having a low-birthweight infant.
4. Provide specific suggestions for decreasing cigarette use.
   a. Assess when the patient is smoking (i.e., with meals, at social occasions, when bored).
   b. Support decreasing patient's intake by one cigarette per day.
   c. Substitute a healthy behavior for a cigarette (i.e., a walk, a nutritious snack).
   d. Assist the patient in identifying stressors that trigger smoking.
   e. Help the patient identify alternative ways of coping (i.e., relaxation or substitution of fruits or vegetables in place of cigarettes).
5. Refer the patient to appropriate programs for stress reduction and smoking cessation.
6. Refer for comprehensive approach to effective parenting.

ALCOHOL

INTRODUCTION

A. **Major public health problem**
   1. Alcohol remains the leading known preventable cause of mental retardation (http://pubs. niaaa.nih.gov/publications/fas/fas.htm).
   2. Most commonly used drug; drug of choice for most teenagers
   3. A cluster of birth defects resulting from prenatal alcohol exposure was recognized in 1973 and called fetal alcohol syndrome (FAS). Alcohol exposure in utero has been linked to a variety of other neurodevelopment problems, and alcohol-related neurodevelopment disorder (ARND) and alcohol-related birth defects (ARBDs) have been proposed to identify infants affected (National Institute of Alcohol Abuse and Alcoholism [NIAAA], 2000).
   4. Alcohol in a pregnant woman's bloodstream circulates to the fetus by crossing the placenta and interferes with the ability of the fetus to receive sufficient oxygen and nourishment for normal cell development in the brain and other body organs.
   5. Infants exposed to alcohol prenatally might have the following characteristics: small size for gestational age, facial abnormalities such as small eye openings, poor coordination, hyperactive behavior, learning disabilities, developmental disabilities, mental retardation or low IQ, problems with daily living, poor reasoning and judgment skills, and sleep and sucking disturbances in infancy.
B. **Statistics**
   1. Among pregnant women ages 15 to 44, an estimated 11.6% reported current alcohol use, 3.7% reported binge drinking, and 0.7% reported heavy drinking. These rates were significantly lower than those for nonpregnant women in the same age group (53.2%, 24.1%, and 5.5%, respectively). Binge drinking during the first trimester of pregnancy was reported by 6.6% of pregnant women ages 15 to 44. All of these estimates by pregnancy status are based on data averaged over 2006 and 2007 (USDHHS, 2008).
   2. Each year in the United States, up to 40,000 babies are born with fetal alcohol spectrum disorders (March of Dimes, 2008a).
   3. Current data do not support the concept of a "safe level" of alcohol consumption by pregnant women below which no damage to a fetus will occur. The U.S. Surgeon General, the March of Dimes, and the American Academy of Pediatrics recommend that all pregnant women and women who are planning to become pregnant not drink alcohol.

C. **Fetal alcohol syndrome**
  1. Prenatal exposure to alcohol can cause a range of effects that can occur in an infant of a woman who drank alcohol during pregnancy. This umbrella term is known as fetal alcohol spectrum disorders (FASDs) (USDHHS, 2007b). Rates of fetal alcohol syndrome (FAS) range from 0.2 to 1.5 per 1000 live births (CDC, 2009a). FAS is defined by four criteria: maternal drinking during pregnancy; a cluster of birth defects such as facial abnormalities; growth restriction; and brain damage, which often is manifested by intellectual difficulties or behavior problems. Alcohol-related neurodevelopmental disorder (ARND) refers to fetal alcohol exposure with signs of brain damage, but an absence of other indications of FAS. FASD is used to describe the problems associated with exposure to alcohol during pregnancy (NIAAA, 2000).
D. **Alcohol related neurodevelopmental disorder: Children with ARND have CNS abnormalities and behavior and cognitive abnormalities. They do not have the facial features and growth restriction that can be caused by Fetal Alcohol Effects (FAE); ARND can occur either alone or in combination with FAS or FAE** (March of Dimes, 2008a).
E. **Alcohol-related birth defects (ARBDs): Alcohol might cause one or more birth defects of the eyes, ears, heart, kidneys, and bones. ARBDs can occur either alone or in combination with FAS or FAE** (March of Dimes, 2008a).
  1. Factors contributing to different teratogenic effects might include:
     a. Genetic makeup
     b. Type, amount, and duration of alcohol consumption
     c. Access to prenatal care, education, and support services
     d. Maternal age, parity, and health

CLINICAL PRACTICE

A. **Assessment**
  1. History
     a. How to ask
        (1) Find an approach that is comfortable for you.
        (2) Be nonjudgmental.
        (3) Make it a routine part of prenatal care.
        (4) Know how to respond.
     b. Approaches to screening may include the following instruments (Morse, Gehshan, & Hutchins, 1997):
        (1) 4 P's
           (a) Have you ever used drugs or alcohol during this **P**regnancy?
           (b) Have you had a problem with drugs or alcohol in the **P**ast?
           (c) Does your **P**artner have a problem with drugs or alcohol?
           (d) Do you consider one of your **P**arents to be an addict or alcoholic?
        (2) T-ACE questions to identify women at high risk
           (a) How many drinks does it take to make you feel high? (**T**olerance)
           (b) Have people **A**nnoyed you by criticizing your drinking?
           (c) Have you felt you ought to **C**ut down on your drinking?
           (d) Have you ever had to drink first thing in the morning to steady your nerves or to get rid of a hangover? (**E**ye-opener)
  2. The U.S. Department of Health and Human Services, National Institutes of Health, National Institute of Alcohol Abuse and Alcoholism can provide an excellent guideline on assessing your patient at: http://pubs.niaaa.nih.gov/publications/practitioner/cliniciansguide2005/guide.pdf.
  3. High risk (USDHHS, 2007a)
     a. Women with substance abuse or mental health problems
     b. Women who have already had a child with FAS, FAE, ARND or ARBDs.
     c. Recent drug users
     d. Smokers
     e. Women who have multiple sex partners
     f. Recent victims of abuse and violence
  4. Physical findings
     a. Poor nutritional and hygiene status

      b. Hepatomegaly

      c. Tremors

      d. Edema

      e. Agitated behavior

      f. Memory difficulty

   5. Psychosocial findings

      a. Low self-esteem

      b. Anxiety and fear

      c. Depression

      d. Family disorganization

      e. Hostility or anger

      f. Denial

      g. Possible unplanned pregnancy

   6. Diagnostic studies

      a. Blood alcohol level (to establish presence of alcohol in system); a blood alcohol level of 0.08 is legally defined as intoxication in most of the United States.

      b. CBC

      c. Serum electrolytes

      d. Serial sonograms to detect IUGR

      e. VDRL and other STI testing

      f. Hepatitis profile

      g. HIV testing

B. Interventions

   1. Provide factual information about health hazards of alcohol to women and developing fetus. The National Institute on Alcohol Abuse and Alcoholism has excellent patient education materials (http://pubs.niaaa.nih.gov/publications/fas/fas.htm).

      a. Fetal risk factors

         (1) CNS involvement (including mental retardation)

         (2) Facial dysmorphia

         (3) Growth restriction (before and after birth)

         (4) Spontaneous abortion

         (5) Stillbirth

      b. Maternal risk factors

         (1) Cirrhosis

         (2) Increased obstetric complications

         (3) Infertility

         (4) Malnutrition

         (5) Withdrawal

         (6) Major factor in the spread of HIV and other sexually transmitted infections (STIs)

         (7) Unwanted pregnancy

   2. Inform the patient that decreasing and stopping alcohol intake at any point during pregnancy will improve the outcome.

      a. Comprehensive inpatient or outpatient treatment for alcohol and other drugs

      b. Case management

      c. Counseling and other mental health treatment

   3. Give written information at a level the woman will understand.

   4. May need medical and prenatal care, child care, transportation, follow-up by pediatric services (see Box 25-2).

HEALTH EDUCATION

A. Prevention

   1. Dispel myths that drugs, alcohol, and smoking are harmless; educate patient on the potential dangers of their use to mother and baby.

   2. Inform patient of contraindication of drug use while breastfeeding (include alcohol, amphetamines, cocaine, heroin, marijuana, and nicotine).

▓ BOX 25-2
▓ **POSSIBLE EFFECTS OF ALCOHOL USE DURING PREGNANCY**

Attention deficits	Microcephaly
Cardiac defects	Mild to moderate mental retardation
Cleft lip or palate	Poor coordination
Delayed motor and language development	Poor suck
Flat midface (hypoplasia of midface)	Prenatal and postnatal growth restriction
Fusion of cervical vertebrae	Restricted bone growth
Hyperactivity	Short palpebral fissures (small eye openings)
Increased infections	Sleep disturbances
Increased irritability	Small in size, height, and/or weight
Indistinct philtrum (groove above the upper lip)	Strabismus, ptosis, myopia
Kidney defects	Thin upper lip
Learning disabilities	

▓ BOX 25-3
▓ **RESOURCES**

- Centers for Disease Control and Prevention (CDC) Office on Smoking and Health; 1-800-232-4636 (1-800-CDC-INFO): www.cdc.gov/tobacco/quit_smoking/index.htm
- National Council on Alcoholism and Drug Dependence (NCADD): 1-800-NCA-CALL (622-2255)
- National Organization on Fetal Alcohol Syndrome: www.nofas.org
- National Clearinghouse for Alcohol and Dug Information: www.ncadia.samhsa.gov
- National Institute of Alcohol Abuse and Alcoholism (NIAAA): www.niaaa.nih.gov
- National Institute of Drug Abuse (NIDA): www.nida.nih.gov
- National Cancer Institute (NCI): www.cancer.gov
- March of Dimes (MOD): www.marchofdimes.com
- National Organization on Fetal Alcohol Syndrome (NOFAS): www.nofas.org

   3. Because no amount of alcohol has been proven safe during pregnancy, a woman should stop drinking immediately if she even suspects she could be pregnant, and she should not drink alcohol if she is trying to conceive.
B. **Referral to community**
   1. Refer pregnant women to specialized programs that address the medical, obstetric, psychologic, neonatal, and pediatric needs of women and their babies.
   2. Resources (see Box 25-3)

CASE STUDIES AND STUDY QUESTIONS

Substance Abuse

Mrs. G. is a 29-year-old gravida 2, para 0 (G2, P0) woman who is 18 weeks pregnant. She is married and very excited about the pregnancy. On her third prenatal visit you notice that she has nasal congestion and slightly slurred speech. There is no odor of alcohol. You suspect she might be using cocaine.

1. A toxicologic urine screen can detect cocaine ingestion within the past:
   a. 10 hours
   b. 24 hours
   c. 1 week
   d. 2 hours
2. A possible result of cocaine use is:
   a. IUGR
   b. Polyhydramnios

c. Polydipsia

d. Postterm pregnancy

3. It is probable that Mrs. G. is using cocaine intranasally. What is the significance of this?

a. It might reduce its ability to cross the placenta.

b. It more readily crosses the placenta.

c. It does not reach the placenta because it is exhaled immediately.

4. Answer the following as true or false.

a. Stillbirths are associated with the addicted patient.

b. Both PROM and abruptio placentae are associated with drug abuse during pregnancy.

c. Cocaine will not cause ill effects to the fetus if used only in the second trimester.

d. Maternal-infant bonding might be enhanced by some drug use because of the relaxation effect.

e. SIDS is not associated with addiction.

Smoking

Ms. U. is an 18-year-old primigravida whose last menstrual period was 21 weeks ago. Her history is unremarkable except for the fact that she smokes a pack of cigarettes a day. She believes smoking helps her control her weight and helps her relax. She has been told that smoking will not harm the baby. On examination, Ms. U. has gained 908 g (2 pounds) since the beginning of her pregnancy. Her blood pressure is 118/72, the fetal heart rate is 140 bpm. She has not noticed fetal movement.

5. What three detrimental compounds are found in cigarettes?

a. Carbon monoxide

b. Nicotine

c. Cyanide

d. Tar

e. Tannic acid

6. All of the following are major effects of smoking on pregnancy *except:*

a. Maternal vasoconstriction and reduced oxygen availability

b. Reduced oxygen-carrying capacity of erythrocytes

c. Fetal bradycardia

7. What are maternal risks attributed to smoking?

a. Abruptio placentae

b. Vitamin C depletion

c. Excessive weight gain

d. Bronchitis

8. Answer the following as true or false.

a. Impaired uteroplacental blood flow decreases oxygen exchange across the placenta.

b. Babies born to mothers who smoke will not have weight problems.

c. SIDS occurs less frequently in babies of mothers who smoke.

d. It is not important if a mother quits smoking in the second trimester because the damage is already done.

Alcohol

Mrs. J., 29 years old, delivered a 3203 g (7-pound, 1-ounce) boy 24 hours earlier. She says that she had been concerned during her pregnancy because she drank heavily in her first trimester before knowing she was pregnant. She begins to ask questions.

9. Answer the following as true or false.

a. Growth restriction might result from alcohol ingestion.

b. Spontaneous abortions occur more frequently in mothers who drink heavily.

c. Drinking after the first trimester is acceptable.

10. Features of fetal alcohol syndrome include all of the following *except:*

a. CNS damage

b. Flattened philtrum

c. Cardiac defects

d. Short fingers

11. When counseling a woman who is pregnant, what should you tell her?

a. Alcohol in the third trimester will not affect the fetus.

b. One glass of wine is considered safe.

c. There is no safe limit of alcohol during pregnancy.

ANSWERS TO STUDY QUESTIONS

1. b

2. a

3. b

4. a. True b. True c. False d. False e. False

5. a, b, c

6. c

7. a, b, d

8. a. True b. False c. False d. False

9. a. True b. True c. False

10. d

11. c

REFERENCES

American Cancer Society (2008). *Women and smoking.* Available at: www.cancer.org/docroot/PED/content/PED_10_2x_Women_and_Smoking.asp. Accessed May 14, 2009.

Centers for Disease Control and Prevention (CDC). (2007). *Preventing smoking during pregnancy.* Available at: www.cdc.gov/NCCdphp/publications/factsheets/Prevention/smoking.htm. Accessed February 28, 2009.

Centers for Disease Control and Prevention (CDC). (2009a). *Alcohol use among pregnant and nonpregnant women of childbearing age—United States, 1991-2005.* Available at: www.cdc.gov/mmwr/preveiw/mmwrhtml/mm5819a4.htm?s_cid=mm5819a4_e. Accessed July 7, 2009.

Centers for Disease Control and Prevention (CDC). (2009b). *Fetal alcohol spectrum disorders.* Available at: www.cdc.gov/ncbddd/fas/fasask.htm. Accessed February 23, 2009.

Centers for Disease Control and Prevention (CDC). (2009c). *Smoking and tobacco fact sheet: Women and smoking.* Available at: www.cdc.gov/tobacco/Data_statistics/fact_sheets/health_effects/tobacco_related_mortality.htm. Accessed May 22, 2009.

Centers for Disease Control and Prevention (CDC). (2009d). *Tobacco and pregnancy.* Available at: www.cdc.gov/reproductivehealth/tobaccoUsePregnancy/index.htm. Accessed May 22, 2009.

March of Dimes. (2006). *Illicit drug use during pregnancy.* Available at: www.marchofdimes.com/professionals/14332_1169.asp. Accessed February 20, 2009.

March of Dimes. (2008a). *Drinking alcohol during pregnancy.* Available at: www.marchofdimes.com/professionals/14332_1170.asp. Accessed February 20, 2009.

March of Dimes. (2008b). *Low birthweight.* Available at: www.marchofdimes.com/professionals/14332_1153.asp. Accessed May 15, 2009.

March of Dimes. (2008c). *Smoking during pregnancy.* Available at: www.marchofdimes.com/professionals/14332_1171.asp. Accessed February 29, 2009.

Morse, B., Gehshan, S., & Hutchins, E. (1997). *Screening for substance abuse during pregnancy: Improving care, improving health.* Arlington, VA: National Center for Education in Maternal and Child Health.

National Institute of Alcohol Abuse and Alcoholism (NIAAA). (2000). *Alcohol alert. No. 50.* Available at: http://pubs.niaaa.nih.gov/publications/aa50.htm. Accessed February 24, 2009.

National Institute of Alcohol Abuse and Alcoholism (NIAAA). (2006). *Drinking and your pregnancy.* Available at: http://pubs.niaaa.nih.gov/publications/fas/fas.htm. Accessed May 22, 2009.

National Institute of Drug Abuse (NIDA). (2009a). *Commonly abused drugs.* National Institute on Drug Abuse and Addiction. Atlanta: U.S. Department of Health and Human Services Available at: www.drugabuse.gov/drugpages/drugsofabuse.html. Accessed May 14, 2009.

National Institute of Drug Abuse (NIDA). (2009b). *Tobacco/nicotine.* Available at: www.drugabuse.gov/drugpages/nicotine.html. Accessed May 22, 2009.

National Institute of Drug Abuse and Addiction (NIDAA). (2006). *Research report series—Tobacco addiction.* Available at: www.drugabuse.gov/researchreports/nicotine/nicotine4html. Accessed May 14, 2009.

National Institute of Drug Abuse and Addiction (NIDAA). (2008a). *Research report series—Cocaine abuse and addiction.* Available at: www.Drugabuse.gov/ResearchReports/Cocaine/cocaine4.html. Accessed May 14, 2009.

National Institute of Drug Abuse and Addiction (NIDAA). (2008b). *Research report series—Heroin abuse and addiction.* Available at: www.drugabuse.gov/ResearchReports/Heroin/heroin4.html. Accessed May 14, 2009.

National Institute of Drug Abuse and Addiction (NIDAA). (2008c). *Research report series—Marijuana abuse.* Available at: www.drugabuse.gov/ResearchReports/marijuana/Marijuana4html. Accessed May 14, 2009.

National Institute of Drug Abuse International Program (2009). *Methadone research web guide.* Available at: internationaldrugabuse.gov/collaboration/guide_methadone. Accessed May 14, 2009.

National Institutes of Health. (2007). *Fact sheet: Fetal alcohol spectrum disorder.* Available at: www.nih.gov/about/researchresultsforthepublic/FetalAlcohol.pdf. Accessed May 22, 2009.

U.S. Department of Health and Human Services (USDHHS). (2005). *Helping patients who drink too much: A clinician's guide.* Available at: http://pubs.niaaa.nih.gov/publications/practitioner/cliniciansguide2005/guide.pdf. Accessed May 22, 2009.

U.S. Department of Health and Human Services (USDHHS). (2007a). *Preventing FASD: Healthy women, healthy babies.* Rockville, MD: USDHHS Publication No. (SMA) 07-4253. Available at: www.fasdcenter.samhsa.gov/documents/WYNK_Preventing_FASD.pdf. Accessed February 20, 2009.

U.S. Department of Health and Human Services (USDHHS). (2007b). *The physical effects of fetal alcohol spectrum disorders*. Rockville, MD: USDHHS Publication No. (SMA) 07-4253 Available at: www.fasdcenter.samhsa.gov/documents/wynk_physical_effects.pdf. Accessed February 20, 2009.

U.S. Department of Health and Human Services (USDHHS). (2008). *Results from the 2007 National Survey on Drug Use and Health:* National Findings Substance Abuse and Mental Health Services Administration (SAMHSA) Office of Applied Studies (OAS). Available at: www.oas.samhsa.gov/NSDUH/2k7NSDUH/2k7results.cfm. Accessed May 22, 2009.

26 Other Medical Complications

Margaret Yancy

OBJECTIVES

1. Describe the data to be documented in obtaining a history from pregnant patients with cardiac, respiratory, renal, hematologic, gastrointestinal, and hepatic complications.
2. Describe the fetal implications for pregnant patients with medical complications.
3. Describe the signs and symptoms and laboratory data that indicate cardiac, respiratory, renal, hematologic, gastrointestinal, and hepatic complications of pregnancy.
4. Formulate a plan of care consisting of interventions and health education based on nursing history and assessments for the pregnant patient with cardiovascular, respiratory, renal, hematologic, gastrointestinal, and hepatic complications.
5. Design a plan to teach principles necessary for maintenance of health for pregnant patients with cardiac, respiratory, renal, hematologic, gastrointestinal, and hepatic complications.
6. Define specific preconception health education strategies to maximize maternal and fetal outcomes for patients with cardiovascular, respiratory, renal, hematologic, and gastrointestinal complications.

INTRODUCTION

A. Women who enter pregnancy with a preexisting disease or a chronic condition are at risk for complications; the disease can complicate the course of pregnancy, or, alternatively, the pregnancy might worsen the disease process.
B. Women with medical complications of pregnancy often experience anxiety regarding the effect of the complication on the outcome of the pregnancy.

CLINICAL PRACTICE

A. Assessment
   1. History
      a. Duration and course of disease
      b. Treatment and medications
      c. Medical complications affecting previous pregnancies
   2. Physical findings
      a. Refer to specific disease or condition.
   3. Diagnostic procedures and laboratory tests
      a. Refer to specific disease or condition.
B. Interventions
   1. Discuss patient's fears and concerns about her pregnancy and its outcome.
      a. Provide reassurance and comfort.
      b. Encourage patient to ask questions about tests, medications, treatments, and physician orders.
      c. Explain all procedures and their purpose.
      d. Acknowledge patient's feelings and respond appropriately to her needs.
   2. Maintain clean, orderly, quiet, and stress-free environment.
   3. Discuss effects of prolonged hospitalization on the family process.
   4. Assess financial burden on family.

5. Assess family members' level of anxiety and knowledge of disease process; assess them as a support system for patient.
   a. Assist family members in reorganizing roles at home and setting priorities to maintain family integrity and to reduce stress.
   b. Aid family members in changing and maintaining realistic expectations of the patient.
   c. If patient is hospitalized, encourage her friends and family to visit frequently; instruct them about visiting hours.
6. Allow patient and family members to ventilate fears about pregnancy outcome.
7. Prepare patient and her family members for signs of depression, anxiety, and dependency.
8. Assess the patient's and family's spiritual needs and help them to meet those needs.
9. Arrange for a tour of special care nursery or for infant special care staff to visit with patient/family as appropriate; orient patient to have realistic expectations for newborn.
10. Encourage patient's interest in diversional activities (e.g., crafts, books, music).
11. Encourage patient and her family to participate in support groups and education programs.
12. Use additional resources as appropriate.
    a. Advanced practice nurses (clinical nurse specialist, nurse practitioner)
    b. Clinical psychologist
    c. Social worker
    d. Lay support and self-help groups
    e. Home health care
    f. Financial assistance programs
13. Determine patient's knowledge of her illness, its treatment, and preventive measures.
14. Assess patient and family members' readiness and ability to learn.
    a. Begin patient and family education regarding the disease and its effects on the mother and fetus.
15. Assess patient's adherence to prescribed treatment regimen and its effect on her lifestyle.
16. Discuss with patient and family signs and symptoms to report.
17. Explain the purpose of treatments, interventions, and tests.
18. Teach patient behavioral interventions and explain physiologic rationale as appropriate to her condition.
    a. Bedrest in lateral position
    b. Observance of prescribed medication regimen
    c. Maintenance of a quiet and stress-free environment as is possible
19. Explain to patient the rationale and procedure for fetal assessment tests such as:
    a. Nonstress test (NST)
    b. Biophysical profile (BPP)
    c. Amniocentesis

CARDIAC COMPLICATIONS

INTRODUCTION

A. **Cardiac disease of varying severity occurs in approximately 1% of all pregnancies and is the leading nonobstetric cause of maternal mortality** (Cunningham et al, 2001).
B. **Assessment and management of women with known cardiac disease should begin before conception to optimize the woman's health and determine the best time for pregnancy** (Arafab & McMurtry Baird, 2006; Dobbenga-Rhodes & Privé, 2006)
C. **The woman's cardiac problem, functional capacity, exercise tolerance, medication needs, history of arrhythmias, degree of cyanosis, and New York Heart Association (NYHA) classification should be taken into consideration when assessing risk stratification** (Arafab & McMurtry Baird, 2006; Blanchard & Shabetai, 2009; Dobbenga-Rhodes & Privé, 2006).
D. **Pregnancy causes significant alterations in maternal cardiovascular physiology; these hemodynamic changes have a profound effect on pregnant patients with cardiac disease; each of these changes increases cardiac work and might exceed the functional capacity of a diseased heart, resulting in pulmonary hypertension, pulmonary edema, congestive heart failure, or maternal death** (Arafab & McMurtry Baird, 2006; Gei & Hankins, 2001; **these changes include:**
   1. Increased heart rate
   2. Increased stroke volume

    3. Increased cardiac output
    4. Expanding blood volume
    5. Decreased systemic and peripheral vascular resistance
    6. Decreased pulmonary vascular resistance
    7. Decreased colloid oncotic pressure

E. **The risk of maternal mortality associated with specific cardiac lesions is outlined in** Box 26-1; **the potential for a successful pregnancy is also determined by the functional limitation with which the patient enters pregnancy; those patients entering pregnancy at NYHA functional class I or II usually do well during pregnancy** (Cunningham et al, 2001; Sui & Colman, 2001) (Table 26-1); **the risk of perinatal and maternal morbidity and mortality associated with cardiac disease during pregnancy depends on:**
    1. The specific cardiac lesion
    2. The functional abnormality produced by the lesion
    3. Development of pregnancy-related complications, such as infection, hemorrhage, or preeclampsia

F. **Cardiac disease during pregnancy may be categorized as congenital, acquired (rheumatic), or ischemic** (Blanchard & Shabetai, 2009; Gei & Hankins, 2001; Wenstrom & Malee, 1999).
    1. Congenital cardiac disease
       a. Is increasing due to advances in diagnosis and treatment, allowing more women with congenital heart defects to survive to reproductive age and achieve a successful pregnancy
       b. Includes atrial septal defect, ventricular septal defect, pulmonic stenosis, congenital aortic stenosis, coarctation of the aorta, tetralogy of Fallot, and Eisenmenger syndrome

---

BOX 26-1
MORTALITY RISK ASSOCIATED WITH PREGNANCY

GROUP I: MORTALITY < 1%

Atrial septal defect, uncomplicated

Ventricular septal defect, uncomplicated

Patent ductus arteriosus, uncomplicated

Pulmonic/tricuspid disease

Corrected tetralogy of Fallot

Porcine valve

Mitral stenosis, NYHA classes I and II

GROUP II: MORTALITY 5% TO 15%

Mitral stenosis with atrial fibrillation

Artificial valve

Mitral stenosis, NYHA classes III and IV

Aortic stenosis

Coarctation of aorta, uncomplicated

Uncorrected tetralogy of Fallot

Previous myocardial infarction

Marfan's syndrome with normal aorta

GROUP III: MORTALITY 25% TO 50%

Pulmonary hypertension

Coarctation of aorta, complicated

Marfan's syndrome with aortic involvement

NYHA, New York Heart Association.

From Clark, S., Cotton, D., Hankin, G., & Phelan J. (1994). *Handbook of critical care obstetrics.* Boston: Blackwell Scientific Publications.

■ TABLE 26-1
■ ■ **New York Heart Association Functional Classification of Cardiac Disease**

Class	Description
I	Patients with cardiac disease and no limitation of physical activity. Patients in this class neither have symptoms of cardiac insufficiency nor experience pain.
II	Patients with cardiac disease and slight limitation of physical activity. They are comfortable at rest, but if ordinary physical activity is undertaken, discomfort results in the form of excessive fatigue, palpitation, dyspnea, or anginal pain.
III	Patients with cardiac disease and marked limitation of physical activity. They are comfortable at rest, but less-than-ordinary activity causes discomfort in the form of excessive fatigue, palpitation, dyspnea, or anginal pain.
IV	Patients with cardiac disease and inability to perform any physical activity without discomfort. Symptoms of cardiac insufficiency or of the anginal syndrome might occur even at rest, and if any physical activity is undertaken, discomfort is increased.

2. Acquired cardiac disease
   a. Is mainly rheumatic in origin
   b. Incidence of rheumatic heart disease is decreasing, resulting in a decline in rheumatic valvular disease.
   c. Includes valvular lesions such as mitral stenosis and aortic stenosis
3. Ischemic cardiac disease (rare in pregnancy)
   a. Coronary artery disease
   b. Myocardial ischemic syndromes
   c. Myocardial infarction

G. **Fetus is at increased risk.**
   1. The fetus is at risk for hypoxia because of maternal hypoxemia.
   2. The incidence of prematurity, intrauterine growth restriction (IUGR), spontaneous abortion, and stillbirth is increased because of maternal hypoxemia.
   3. If the woman has congenital heart disease, there is an increased incidence of fetal congenital cardiac anomalies.

CLINICAL PRACTICE

A. **Assessment**
   1. History
      a. Category of heart disease: congenital, acquired, or ischemic
      b. Duration and course of disease
      c. NYHA Functional Classification of Cardiac Disease: degree of limitation of physical activity
      d. Previous surgeries
      e. Response to previous pregnancies
      f. Prescribed medications
   2. Physical findings
      a. Vital signs: blood pressure and apical/radial pulse
      b. Signs and symptoms of heart disease; Table 26-2 lists the signs and symptoms common to normal pregnancy compared with those of actual heart disease
      c. Signs and symptoms of cardiac decompensation (Gilbert, 2007)
         (1) Dyspnea severe enough to limit usual activity
         (2) Progressive orthopnea
         (3) Paroxysmal nocturnal dyspnea
         (4) Syncope during or immediately following exertion
         (5) Chest pain associated with activity
         (6) Sustained arrhythmia
         (7) Cyanosis

■ TABLE 26-2
■ ■ **Signs and Symptoms Common to Normal Pregnancy Compared with Signs and Symptoms of Actual Cardiac Disease**

Normal Pregnancy	Actual Cardiac Disease
Chest discomfort	Chest discomfort with myocardial ischemia
Dyspnea	Severe dyspnea that limits activity; paroxysmal nocturnal dyspnea
Orthopnea	Progressive orthopnea
Palpitations	Cardiac arrhythmia
Easy fatigability	Fatigue with chest pain and syncope
Dizzy spells	Dizzy spells plus other actual signs and symptoms
Syncope	Syncope with exertion
Systolic murmurs	Loud, harsh, systolic murmurs: grade III intensity, diastolic murmurs
Dependent edema	Dependent plus nondependent edema
Rales in lower lung fields	Rales that do not clear with deep inspiration; hemoptysis
Visible neck veins	Persistent neck vein distention
Cardiomegaly	Cardiomegaly plus hepatomegaly and ascites

  d. Signs and symptoms of congestive heart failure (CHF)
   (1) Right-sided congestive heart failure
    (a) Neck vein distention
    (b) Hepatomegaly
    (c) Dependent and nondependent edema
    (d) Weight gain
   (2) Left-sided CHF
    (a) Dyspnea
    (b) Orthopnea
    (c) Rales
    (d) Cough
    (e) Extreme fatigue
    (f) Chest pain
    (g) Syncope
    (h) Pallor
    (i) Cyanosis
    (j) Cardiac arrhythmias
  e. Laboratory and diagnostic studies
   (1) Arterial blood gas values or pulse oximetry, as indicated
   (2) Coagulation studies
   (3) Serum electrolytes
   (4) White blood cell count
   (5) Hemoglobin and hematocrit
   (6) Cardiac enzymes as indicated
   (7) Electrocardiogram
   (8) Cardiac ultrasonography
   (9) Echocardiogram
   (10) Chest radiograph
  f. Fetal assessment tests
B. Interventions
 1. Assess for risk of decreased cardiac output related to structural defects, CHF, or pulmonary edema.
  a. Monitor for signs and symptoms of decreased cardiac output (Carpenito, 1997).
   (1) Decreased and/or irregular pulse rate
   (2) Increased respiratory rate

      (3) Decreased blood pressure
      (4) Abnormal heart sounds
      (5) Decreased urine output (less than 30 mL/hr)
      (6) Changes in mentation
      (7) Abnormal lung sounds (crackles)
      (8) Cool, moist, cyanotic, mottled skin
      (9) Delayed capillary refill time
     (10) Neck vein distention
     (11) Weak peripheral pulses
     (12) Electrocardiogram (ECG) changes
     (13) Dysrhythmias
     (14) Decreased oxygen saturation

2. Teach patient to avoid stress and anxiety.
3. Instruct the patient in following a low-sodium diet to prevent fluid retention.
4. Monitor weight gain; encourage patient to avoid excessive weight gain, which causes increased cardiac workload.
5. Counsel patient to avoid physical exertion and encourage frequent rest periods in left lateral recumbent position.
   a. Assess activity tolerance.
   b. Assist patient in modifying schedule and spacing activities to allow for more rest.
   c. Maintain patient's activity level short of fatigue.
6. Encourage patient to obtain 8 to 10 hours of sleep per night and to take frequent rest periods during the day.
7. Assist patient with activities of daily living (ADL) and ambulation as necessary, or refer to appropriate social services for help with household responsibilities, as needed.
8. Administer cardiovascular medications as ordered; evaluate the patient's response to medication (Table 26-3 lists cardiovascular drugs used during pregnancy).
9. Provide nutritional counseling, encourage high-iron foods, and administer iron and vitamin supplements as ordered to prevent anemia.
   a. Iron and folic acid supplements are frequently needed, and hemoglobin and hematocrit levels should be carefully monitored.
10. Monitor for infection related to increased risk due to bacterial invasion, pulmonary congestion, or invasive procedures.
    a. Teach the patient to recognize the signs and symptoms of infection.
    b. Caution the patient to avoid exposure to infection.
    c. Antibiotic prophylaxis is frequently used to prevent bacterial endocarditis.
    d. Use strict aseptic technique during invasive procedures.
    e. Monitor for leukocytosis.
11. Assess for signs and symptoms of thromboembolism (Carpenito, 1997).
    a. Diminished or absent peripheral pulses
    b. Unusual warmth and redness or coolness and cyanosis
    c. Increasing leg pain
    d. Sudden severe chest pain, increased dyspnea, and tachypnea
    e. Positive Homans' sign
    f. Antiembolic stockings as ordered
12. Anticoagulant therapy (usually heparin) and monitoring of blood coagulation laboratory results to detect any preliminary indications or risk of abnormal bleeding
    a. Hematuria
    b. Bleeding gums
    c. Ecchymoses
    d. Petechiae (Carpenito, 1997)
13. Encourage patient to labor in lateral position; avoid lithotomy position during second stage of labor.
14. Provide effective pain control during labor and delivery to decrease cardiac workload.
15. Encourage gentle pushing to avoid erratic venous return associated with Valsalva effect.
16. Assess hemodynamic function and cardiac output during the intrapartum period and after delivery by implementing hemodynamic monitoring as ordered (e.g., cardiac monitor, arterial line, central venous pressure catheter, pulmonary artery catheter).

■ TABLE 26-3
■ ■ **Cardiovascular Drugs Used during Pregnancy**

Drug Group	Use During Pregnancy	Adverse Effects
Diuretic	Use as in nonpregnant women Should not be used prophylactically or to treat pedal edema unless there is associated pulmonary vascular congestion.	Might exacerbate preeclampsia by reducing uterine blood flow.
Inotropic agent	Pregnancy does not alter the indications for digitalis therapy. An increased dose might be required to achieve acceptable serum levels. Digitalis crosses the placenta and is excreted in breast milk, but fetal or infant toxicity is unusual.	Labor potentially earlier and shorter in women on digitalis.
	Beta-stimulating or dopaminergic agents should be reserved for life-threatening situations.	Might decrease uterine blood flow.
Vasodilators	Afterload-reducing agents: adverse fetal effect not reported with hydralazine. Avoid angiotensin-converting enzyme (ACE) inhibitors. Preload-reducing agents: nitrates indicated as in nonpregnant state. Nitroprusside justified in life-threatening situations. Little experience with pregnancy.	Hypotension may jeopardize uterine blood flow. Fetal renal development abnormalities with ACE inhibitors. Concern about, but no documentation of, cyanide toxicity with nitroprusside.
Antiarrhythmic agents	Indications for use as in nonpregnant state. Greatest experience with quinidine, but procainamide and disopyramide not clearly inferior. Lidocaine crosses the placenta, but no teratogenic effects have been reported.	Potential fetal dysrhythmias. Phenytoin can cause fetal abnormalities and should be avoided.
Beta-blocking agents	May be used to treat hypertension, angina, and supraventricular tachyarrhythmias when there are no reasonable alternatives. Close fetal and newborn monitoring required. Selective beta-blockers may result in fewer adverse fetal effects.	Can depress intrauterine growth. Newborn bradycardia, hypotension, hypoglycemia, and respiratory depression occur.
Calcium channel blockers	Verapamil and nifedipine can be used as blockers in nonpregnant state. Little information on diltiazem and almost none on newly introduced agents.	Might cause uterine relaxation.
Anticoagulants	Warfarin contraindicated at time of conception and during pregnancy because of teratogenic effect and because of placental and fetal bleeding.	Teratogenic effect 10%-20% in first trimester
	When anticoagulation required heparin via subcutaneous administration at home is preferred. It does not cross the placenta.	Maternal and placental bleeding.
	Acetylsalicylic acid can be used, but there is some increased risk of bleeding. No reported experience with dipyridamole or sulfinpyrazone.	Potential premature closure of ductus arteriosus by prostaglandin inhibition.

From Burrow, G., & Ferris, T. (1995). *Medical complications during pregnancy* (4th ed., p. 134). Philadelphia: Saunders.

17. Monitor intake and output carefully, and regulate intravenous (IV) fluids with an infusion pump to prevent fluid overload and possible pulmonary edema.
18. Minimize postpartum blood loss to prevent hypovolemia.

HEALTH EDUCATION

A. **Preconceptual counseling**
   1. Discuss the risk of pregnancy to the mother and the risks to the fetus.
   2. Discuss potentially teratogenic cardiovascular drugs.
      a. Warfarin
      b. Propranolol
      c. Thiazide diuretics
      d. Angiotensin-converting enzyme (ACE) inhibitors
   3. Discuss the advances that have improved the outcome for women with cardiac disease in:
      a. Medical and surgical therapy
      b. Fetal surveillance
      c. Neonatal care
B. **Discuss the importance of early, regular, and frequent medical supervision and encourage patient to be in the care of an obstetrician and a cardiologist.**
C. **Discuss the importance of a multidisciplinary team including cardiology, obstetrics, nursing, dietary, social service, and pediatrics/neonatology.**
   1. Include the woman and her family in care conferences.
D. **Teach patient about rationale for modifying her diet and activities and for taking prescribed medications.**
E. **Teach patient to limit exposure to infection.**
F. **Discuss the importance of obtaining antibiotic prophylaxis before dental and surgical procedures.**
G. **Teach patient to get adequate rest with frequent rest periods and to restrict activity to that which is just short of fatigue.**
H. **Assist patient to modify diet as prescribed.**
I. **Teach patient to avoid excessive weight gain.**
J. **Teach patient to maintain normal hemoglobin levels by eating increased amounts of high-iron and folic-acid–containing foods and taking supplements if needed.**
K. **Teach patient to report signs and symptoms of cardiac decompensation.**
L. **Discuss other topics as appropriate** (Arafab & McMurtry Baird, 2006).
   1. Timing of birth, method of delivery, and anesthesia options
   2. Endocarditis prophylaxis if needed
   3. Use of anticoagulant therapy if needed

RENAL COMPLICATIONS

INTRODUCTION

A. **Anatomic and physiologic changes that occur in the kidney during pregnancy include:**
   1. Marked dilation of the collecting system
   2. Stasis of urine in the upper part of the collecting system
   3. Delayed emptying
   4. Increase in renal plasma flow
   5. Increase in glomerular filtration rate (GFR)
   6. Changes in tubular reabsorption of glucose and amino acids so glycosuria and aminoaciduria are normal in pregnancy
   7. Decrease in blood urea nitrogen (BUN) and serum creatinine
   8. Decreased serum osmolality
   9. Increased uric acid filtration and secretion, leading to decreased levels of uric acid (Thorsen, 2002)

B. Renal disease during pregnancy falls into two categories: new onset of renal disease during pregnancy and chronic renal disease.
   1. New onset of renal disease during pregnancy
      a. Acute pyelonephritis
         (1) Approximately 4% to 10% of all pregnant women have asymptomatic bacteriuria, and if untreated, 25% to 40% will experience pyelonephritis; acute pyelonephritis affects 1% to 3% of pregnancies (Cunningham et al, 2001; Wenstrom & Malee, 1999; Williams & Davidson, 2009).
         (2) *Escherichia coli* is responsible for more than 80% of infections.
      b. Acute nephrolithiasis (renal stones) occurs in 1 of every 1000 deliveries.
      c. Acute renal failure
         (1) Incidence of 1 in 10,000 pregnancies
         (2) Multiple causes are categorized as:
            (a) Women with preexisting renal disease
            (b) Consequences of pregnancy-associated event
            (c) Consequences of a nonpregnant event (i.e., trauma) (Thorsen, 2002)
         (3) Most common cause is severe preeclampsia or following hemorrhagic shock.
      d. Nephrotic syndrome
         (1) Proteinuria greater than 3 g/day
         (2) Serum albumin less than 3 g/dL
         (3) Edema
         (4) Hyperlipidemia
   2. Chronic renal disease
      a. Chronic renal disease in pregnancy is uncommon, with the incidence of moderate to severe chronic renal disease estimated to be less then 1 in 1000 pregnancies (Ramin, Vidaeff, Yeomans, & Gilstrap, 2006).
      b. There are multiple causes of chronic renal disease each with its own pathophysiologic mechanisms.
      c. The degree of renal function impairment appears to be the most important determinant for pregnancy outcome. In patients with mildly impaired renal function, pregnancy does not usually accelerate renal damage (Cunningham et al, 2001; Ramin et al, 2006).
      d. Fetal outcomes are related to maternal renal function impairment and underlying disease (Vidaeff, Yeomans, & Ramin, 2008).
      e. Preexisting hypertension along with the degree of renal insufficiency are predictive of pregnancy outcome; hypertension is an indicator of poor pregnancy outcome (Ramin et al, 2006).
      f. Patients with renal transplants can sustain a pregnancy; pregnancy should not be considered for 2 years following implantation of a cadaver kidney, or 1 year after a live donor kidney, with the understanding that continuation of immunosuppressive therapy is essential (Thorsen, 2002).
C. Adverse consequences of pregnancy in renal disease
   1. Maternal consequences
      a. Hypertension
         (1) New onset
         (2) Increased severity
         (3) Superimposed preeclampsia
      b. Proteinuria
         (1) Worsens
         (2) Nephrotic syndrome can develop
      c. Decreased renal function
         (1) New onset
         (2) Accelerated rate of decline
   2. Fetal consequences
      a. Fetal loss
         (1) Spontaneous abortion
         (2) Stillbirth
         (3) Neonatal death
      b. Preterm birth
      c. IUGR

CLINICAL PRACTICE

A. Assessment
1. History
   a. Incidence of urinary tract infections (UTIs)
      (1) Pregnant women are at greater risk for UTI because of the physiologic changes of pregnancy.
         (a) Decreased bladder tone can cause stasis of urine.
         (b) Delayed or incomplete emptying of bladder
   b. Incidence and duration of acute and/or chronic renal disease
   c. History of medical conditions associated with acute renal failure
2. Physical findings
   a. Signs and symptoms of UTI
      (1) Dysuria
      (2) Frequency
      (3) Urgency of urination
      (4) Lower abdominal pain
   b. Signs and symptoms of pyelonephritis
      (1) Fever
      (2) Chills
      (3) Flank pain: sometimes reported as lower back pain
      (4) Costovertebral angle (CVA) tenderness
      (5) Urgency
      (6) Frequency
      (7) Nausea
      (8) Vomiting
      (9) Malaise
      (10) Dehydration
   c. Signs and symptoms of fluid overload and systemic vascular resistance
      (1) Vital signs
      (2) Peripheral edema
      (3) Distended neck veins
      (4) Breath sounds
   d. Neurologic signs and symptoms of rapid onset acute renal failure
      (1) Fatigue
      (2) Lethargy
      (3) Somnolence
      (4) Irritability
      (5) Disorientation
      (6) Tonic-clonic seizures
   e. Laboratory and diagnostic tests for renal disease
      (1) Urinalysis
         (a) Proteinuria: indicates glomerular damage
         (b) Hematuria: red cell casts indicate glomerular inflammation and injury
         (c) Pyuria: indicates inflammation/infection
      (2) Urine culture and sensitivity
      (3) Serum creatinine
      (4) Creatinine clearance
      (5) 24-hour urine protein
      (6) BUN
      (7) Uric acid
      (8) Electrolytes
      (9) Intravenous pyelography (IVP)
      (10) Renal ultrasonography
      (11) Arterial blood gases as indicated
      (12) ECG as indicated
      (13) Pulse oximetry as indicated

   f. Fetal assessment
      (1) Because of the strong association of renal disease with IUGR, fetal surveillance is important.
      (2) Fetal heart rate monitoring, biophysical profile (BPP), ultrasonography, and fetal lung maturity if severity of maternal disease warrants early delivery

B. **Interventions**
   1. Monitor for risk for infection related to anatomic and physiologic changes of the renal system in pregnancy.
      a. Monitor for signs and symptoms of infection (UTI or pyelonephritis).
      b. Administer antibiotics as ordered.
      c. Maintain adequate hydration; encourage oral intake, and if necessary, administer IV fluids as ordered.
      d. Assess for maternal bacteremia via blood culture.
      e. Assess for maternal septic shock by monitoring vital signs for tachycardia and hypotension.
      f. Monitor for contractions and other signs and symptoms of preterm labor.
      g. Obtain follow-up urine culture.
   2. Monitor fluid volume related to inability of the kidney to regulate fluid balance.
   3. In chronic renal disease monitor for signs and symptoms of improvement or deterioration in renal status by observing the following parameters:
      a. Urinalysis reports
      b. Kidney function tests: serum creatinine, BUN, uric acid, and creatinine clearance
      c. Complete blood count (CBC)
      d. Electrolytes
      e. Intake and output
      f. Proteinuria
      g. Blood pressure values
      h. Dependent edema and sacral edema
      i. Daily weight
      j. Skin turgor, color, and temperature
      k. Color, odor, and appearance of urine
   4. Position in left lateral position when on bedrest.
   5. Administer prescribed medications (e.g., antihypertensives).
   6. Maintain prescribed sodium restrictions.
   7. Adjust the patient's daily fluid intake as ordered, and distribute fluid intake fairly evenly throughout the day.
   8. Observe for signs and symptoms of superimposed preeclampsia.
   9. Observe for signs and symptoms of renal insufficiency (Carpenito, 1997).
      a. Increased BUN
      b. Increased serum creatinine; decreased creatinine clearance
      c. Nausea and vomiting
      d. Systemic edema
      e. Urticaria
      f. Anemia
      g. Elevated blood pressure
      h. Fatigue and lethargy
      i. Headache
      j. Electrolyte imbalance (sodium, potassium, calcium, phosphorus, magnesium)
      k. Mental confusion or apathy
      l. Urine output less than 30 mL/hr
      m. Metabolic acidosis
   10. Monitor for signs and symptoms of metabolic acidosis.
      a. Rapid, shallow respirations
      b. Headaches
      c. Nausea and vomiting
      d. Low plasma pH
      e. Behavioral changes, drowsiness, and lethargy
   11. Consult with dietitian for an appropriate diet.
   12. Monitor for impaired comfort related to bladder spasm or renal colic; risk for renal calculi

13. Monitor for signs and symptoms of calculi.
    a. Sediment in urine
    b. Flank or loin pain
    c. Hematuria
    d. Abdominal pain, distention, nausea, and diarrhea (Carpenito, 1997)
14. Strain urine for calculi as indicated.
15. Instruct the patient to increase fluid intake, if not contraindicated.
16. Assess pain-precipitating factors, and document deviation from baseline.
    a. Quality
    b. Region radiation
    c. Severity
    d. Duration
    e. Relieving factors
17. Have patient evaluate pain intensity on a 1 to 10 scale (10 being most severe).
    a. Observe, report, and record verbal and nonverbal expressions of pain, fear, and anxiety.
18. Provide and encourage rest periods and a restful environment.
19. Medicate patient with analgesics, antispasmodics, and antibiotics as ordered.
    a. Assess effectiveness of pain medications.
20. Provide comfort measures.
21. Teach patient and her family about factors that contribute to pain experience.
22. Assess patient's urgency and frequency of urination and nocturia.
23. Palpate patient's bladder for distention.
24. Provide preoperative and postoperative care if surgery is required for ureteral obstruction.

HEALTH EDUCATION

A. **Preconceptual counseling**
   1. Discuss increased risk of fetal loss and preeclampsia with patients already demonstrating proteinuria and hypertension.
   2. Discuss increased incidence of anovulation, menstrual irregularities, loss of libido, and decreased fertility among patients with underlying chronic renal disease.
   3. Discuss effects of pregnancy on progression of chronic renal disease.
   4. Discuss need for early and frequent fetal surveillance.
B. **Teach patient self-monitoring of weight gain, edema, and blood pressure.**
C. **Teach patient to avoid exposure to infection.**
D. **Educate patient regarding prophylactic antibiotic therapy.**
E. **Discuss increased risk of anemia and fluid imbalance, and the importance of adequate nutrition and compliance with prescribed diet and fluid intake.**
F. **Teach patient to recognize and report signs of fluid and electrolyte imbalance and superimposed preeclampsia.**
G. **Discuss the importance of early, regular, and frequent medical supervision, and encourage patient to be in the care of an obstetrician and nephrologist.**
H. **Discuss the importance of a multidisciplinary team including nephrology, obstetrics, nursing, dietary, social service, and pediatrics/neonatology.**
   1. Include the woman and her family in care conferences
I. **Teach proper front-to-back perineal hygiene.**
J. **Teach all women to recognize and report the symptoms of UTI.**
K **Teach patient signs and symptoms of premature labor and increased uterine irritability and when to report.**

RESPIRATORY COMPLICATIONS

INTRODUCTION

Pulmonary diseases have become more prevalent in the general population and therefore in pregnant women. Normal physiologic changes of pregnancy can cause a woman with a history of compromised respirations to decompensate. The outcome of a pregnant woman with respiratory complications depends on the adequacy of ventilation and oxygenation as well as early detection of decompensation. Hypoxia is the major fetal threat.

A. Asthma

1. Asthma is the most common form of lung disease that can affect pregnancy and its affects approximately 4% to 8% of pregnancies (Murdock, 2002; National Asthma Education and Prevention Program [NAEPP], 2007; Rey & Boulet, 2007).

2. Asthma is a reversible syndrome characterized by varying degrees of airway obstruction, bronchial hyperresponsiveness, and bronchial edema (Dombrowski & Schatz, 2008; Wendel, 2001).

3. Well-controlled asthma during pregnancy allows women to continue a normal pregnancy with little or no increased risk to their health or that of their fetuses (Murdock, 2002; Whitty & Dombrowski, 2009).

4. Pregnancy has variable effects on the course of asthma with a third each becoming worse, improving, or remaining unchanged; the course of asthma in a previous pregnancy predicts the course in a subsequent pregnancy in approximately 60% of women; typically the more severe the disease, the more likely it is to worsen (Cunningham et al, 2001; Murdock, 2002; Wenstrom & Malee, 1999).

5. The goal of asthma therapy during pregnancy is to prevent maternal hypoxic episodes and maintain adequate oxygenation of the fetus.

6. Arterial blood gases should be interpreted according to normal values for pregnancy.
   a. pH: 7.40 to 7.45
   b. Po_2: 100 to 108
   c. Pco_2: 28 to 31 (Murdock, 2002)

7. Asthma should be as aggressively treated during pregnancy as at any other time because the benefits of asthma control far outweigh the risks of medication usage. The National Asthma Education and Prevention Program (NAEPP, 2007) found that it is safer to treat pregnant women with asthma medications than to allow these women to have symptoms and exacerbations.

8. Virtually all of the commonly used asthma medications are considered safe during pregnancy; however, data are scarce on the safety of leukotriene modifiers in pregnancy (NAEPP, 2007; Rey & Boulet, 2007).

9. Asthma in pregnancy is associated with an increase in:
   a. Perinatal mortality
   b. Preterm birth
   c. Low birthweight
   d. IUGR
   e. Neonatal hypoxia (National Asthma Education Program, 1993)

10. Treatment of asthma is based on four management components (NAEPP, 2007):
    a. Assessment and monitoring of asthma signs and symptoms, including pulmonary function studies
    b. Avoidance of triggers and other factors contributing to asthma severity
    c. Pharmacologic therapy using the stepwise approach
    d. Education to promote self-management

11. Goals of therapy and special considerations in pregnant women with asthma include (NAEPP, 2007):
    a. Optimal control of asthma symptoms, including nocturnal symptoms
    b. Maintain normal or near normal pulmonary function.
    c. Manage exacerbations aggressively.
    d. Avoid delay in diagnosis and treatment.
    e. Assess medication needs and response to therapy frequently and avoid adverse effects from asthma medications.
    f. Assess for rhinitis, gastric reflux, and other comorbidities.
    g. Encourage smoking cessation.

12. Discuss the importance of a multidisciplinary team including pulmonology, obstetrics, nursing, dietary, social service, and pediatrics/neonatology.
    a. Include the woman and her family in care conferences

13. Refer to the National Asthma Education and Prevention Program (2007) for a comprehensive discussion of management of patients with asthma during pregnancy.

B. Tuberculosis

1. Tuberculosis (TB) is caused by infection with the acid-fast bacillus *Mycobacterium tuberculosis;* the bacillus is carried on droplet nuclei and spread by airborne transmission. TB remains a major health problem and has undergone a resurgence related to an influx of women from

Asia, Africa, Mexico, and Central America; homelessness; drug abuse; poverty; and human immunodeficiency virus (HIV) (Cunningham et al, 2001).

2. Pregnancy is not altered by the patient's tuberculosis, and pregnancy itself is not a risk factor for tuberculosis. With the advent of effective chemotherapy treatment for active TB, pregnant women have the same good prognosis as their nonpregnant counterparts.

3. Pregnancy, however, does complicate treatment of multidrug-resistant tuberculosis because several of the antimycobacterial drugs are contraindicated during pregnancy and untreated, infectious multidrug-resistant tuberculosis may be vertically and laterally transmitted (Whitty & Dombrowski, 2009).

4. Screening is recommended for pregnant women who fall into a high-risk group (Cunningham et al, 2001).
   a. Foreign-born persons from high-prevalence countries
   b. Medically underserved low-income populations; high-risk racial/ethnic minorities
   c. Persons with HIV infection
   d. Alcoholics and IV drug users
   e. Those with close contact to infectious cases
   f. Persons with medical conditions that increase the risk of TB

5. The method of screening is the tuberculin skin test using purified protein derivative (PPD); the antituberculosis drugs recommended for use in pregnancy are isoniazid (INH), ethambutol, and rifampin (Cunningham et al, 2001; Lake, 2001).
   a. If the induration is more than 5 mm, and if any of the following risk factors are present, the test is positive.
      (1) HIV infection
      (2) Recent contact with person who has infectious TB
      (3) Abnormal chest radiograph typical of old TB infection
      (4) Recipients of organ transplants on immunosuppressant therapy
      (5) Other immunosuppressed individuals receiving the equivalent of more than 15 mg/day of prednisone for more than 1 month
   b. If the induration is more than 10 mm and any of the following risk factors are present, the test is positive.
      (1) Immigrants who have arrived within the last 5 years from countries with high prevalence
      (2) Injection drug use
      (3) High-risk medical conditions
      (4) Residents or employees of hospitals, shelters, correctional facilities
      (5) Children younger than 4 years
      (6) Adolescents, infants, or children exposed to adults in high-risk categories
   c. If the person has no risk factors, the induration must be more than 15 mm for the test to be positive.

6. The cornerstone of treatment for tuberculosis is maintaining and completing treatment (Lake, 2001).

7. Congenital tuberculosis remains relatively rare; neonatal tuberculosis might reflect acquisition of infection in utero (i.e., congenital) or during the first few weeks of life from a contagious mother or other person. Neonatal tuberculosis has a high morbidity and mortality rate (Simpkins, Hench, & Bhatia, 1996). Newborns born to mothers with TB should be evaluated and treated per the guidelines of the American Thoracic Society and the Centers for Disease Control and Prevention (1994).

8. Breastfeeding can begin and can continue during treatment. The mother with active tuberculosis must be separated from her baby until she is bacteriologically negative and the baby has undergone appropriate prophylaxis (Lake, 2001).

CLINICAL PRACTICE

A. Assessment
   1. History
      a. Specific form of respiratory disease
      b. Duration and course of disease

      c. For women with asthma: history of status asthmaticus, hospitalization, and endotracheal intubation

      d. Duration and severity of shortness of breath and dyspnea

      e. Degree of exercise and activity limitations

      f. Type of cough

      g. Amount of hemoptysis

      h. Amount, color, and consistency of sputum

      i. Duration and severity of wheezing and chest tightness

      j. Duration and severity of fever, chills, and night sweats

      k. Medication use (prescribed and over-the-counter)

      l. Smoking history (amount, length of time)

      m. Exposure to respiratory infections

  2. Physical findings

      a. Rate, rhythm, and depth of respirations

      b. Auscultation of the lungs

      c. Skin color

      d. Blood pressure and pulse

      e. Level of consciousness

      f. Intake and output (I&O)

  3. Diagnostic procedures

      a. Arterial blood gases; pulse oximetry

      b. Chest radiograph (with abdominal shield)

      c. CBC

      d. Pulmonary function tests

         (1) Forced expiratory volume in 1 second (FEV_1) by spirometry

         (2) Peak expiratory flow rate (PEFR) by peak flowmeter

      e. Sputum smear and culture

  4. Fetal assessment for signs and symptoms of fetal hypoxia

B. Interventions

  1. Administer supplemental oxygen as indicated.

  2. Position in semi- or high-Fowler's position with lateral tilt and supported arms for adequate breathing and decreased dyspnea.

  3. Auscultate lung fields for baseline, and monitor frequently.

  4. Observe respiration for rate, rhythm, and regularity.

  5. Administer prescribed medications and respiratory treatments.

      a. Bronchodilators

      b. Antibiotics

      c. Antiinflammatory agents

      d. Antituberculosis drugs (refer to Table 26-4 for drugs and dosages for antituberculosis drugs)

  6. Monitor and trend:

      a. Arterial blood gas analysis

      b. Pulse oximetry

      c. PEFR

  7. Assess for productive and nonproductive cough.

  8. Teach the patient effective coughing technique.

  9. Assist in coughing and deep breathing, administer incentive spirometer, and note effectiveness of treatment.

 10. Maintain adequate hydration to help liquefy secretions.

 11. Assess fluid volume status by:

      a. Orthostatic vital signs

      b. Capillary refill time

      c. Thirst

      d. Skin turgor and mucous membranes

 12. Assess activity tolerance.

 13. Assist patient in modifying her schedule and spacing her activities to allow time for more rest.

 14. Maintain patient's activity level just short of fatigue.

 15. Provide long periods for sleep at night and frequent rest periods during the day.

 16. Assist patient with ADLs and ambulation as required.

■ TABLE 26-4
■ ■ **Commonly Used Antituberculosis Drugs**

Drug	Daily Dose (Adults) (mg/kg/day)	Major Toxicity
Isoniazid	5 (maximum 300 mg)	Hepatitis Peripheral neuropathy
Rifampin	10 (maximum 600 mg)	Hepatitis Flulike syndrome Thrombocytopenia Orange discoloration of secretions Alteration of other drug levels (e.g., OCP)
Ethambutol	15-25	Optic neuritis*
Pyrazinamide[†]	15-30 (maximum 2 g)	Hepatitis Arthralgias Hyperuricemia
Streptomycin[†]	15 (maximum 1 g)	Ototoxicity[‡] Nephrotoxicity[‡]

*Conduct baseline and monthly monitoring of visual acuity and color vision.
[†]Do not use in pregnancy.
[‡]Perform baseline audiometry and renal function studies.
From Simpkins, S., Hench, C., & Bhatia, G. (1996). Management of the obstetric patient with tuberculosis. *Journal of Obstetric, Gynecologic, & Neonatal Nursing, 25*(4), 309.

17. Provide steroid supplementation for 24 to 48 hours prior to delivery, as indicated, in asthmatic women who have undergone recent steroid therapy.
18. Prevent increased oxygen consumption related to painful contractions by medicating the woman adequately during labor.
19. Prevent patient from hyperventilating during labor by providing coaching and support.
20. Implement respiratory isolation while patient is considered infectious; patients with TB are not considered infectious if they meet all the following criteria:
    a. Adequate therapy received for 2 to 3 weeks
    b. Favorable clinical response to therapy
    c. Three consecutive negative sputum smear results from sputum collected on different days (Carpenito, 1997)
21. Instruct the patient to cough and expectorate into disposable tissues to prevent disease transmission.
22. Provide support and counseling for the new mother who is isolated at delivery and separated from her neonate.
23. Consult social services as needed to arrange temporary care of the infant outside the home until the infant and the mother have received adequate treatment.

HEALTH EDUCATION

Asthma (Box 26-2)

A. **Explain disease and therapy goals.**
B. **Teach patient to avoid exposure to allergens and infection.**
C. **Teach patient how to use a peak flowmeter to manage symptoms.**
D. **Clarify when primary provider should be contacted** (Carpenito, 1997).
    1. When medications have to be increased to control symptoms
    2. Persistent cough; difficulty breathing, with or without wheezing
    3. Peak flows less than 80% of normal

▒ BOX 26-2
▒ **PATIENT SELF-CARE STRATEGIES FOR ASTHMA**

Know own patterns of asthma symptoms (e.g., dyspnea, wheezing, tightness in the chest, recurrent cough persisting more than 1 week).

Evaluate severity of symptoms on a scale of 1 to 10.

Monitor daily peak expiratory flow rate (PEFR).

Monitor daily symptoms in relation to PEFR, weather patterns, activity level, and medications.

Practice relaxation and breathing techniques.

Identify and avoid precipitating factors including bronchial irritants (e.g., active and passive smoking, personal use of scented cosmetics, aerosols).

Adjust activity patterns according to climatic conditions.

Take medications as prescribed.

Use metered-dose inhaler medications properly and with a spacer if appropriate.

Learn what triggers asthma by keeping a symptom diary.

Identify and prioritize strategies that work best.

Develop a crisis-management plan.

Maintain a daily exercise program.

Place reasonable limits on activity to avoid hypoxemia.

Receive annual influenza vaccine in the fall if after the third trimester.

Control weight gain during and following pregnancy.

From Geiger-Bronsky, M. (1992). Asthma and pregnancy: Opportunities for enhancing outcomes. *Journal of Perinatal & Neonatal Nursing*, 6(2), 43.

E. **Discuss signs and symptoms to report.**
   1. Shortness of breath
   2. Dyspnea
   3. Rapid respirations
   4. Cough and congestion
   5. Fever and chills
   6. Decreased ability to perform activities
   7. Extreme fatigue

TUBERCULOSIS

A. **Teach medication regimen and importance of adherence to treatment because resistant disease is more likely in individuals who are noncompliant with therapy** (Whitty & Dombrowski, 2009).
B. **Explain mechanism of transmission for tuberculosis.**

SYSTEMIC LUPUS ERYTHEMATOSUS AND ANTIPHOSPHOLIPID ANTIBODY SYNDROME

INTRODUCTION

A. **Systemic lupus erythematosus (SLE) is a chronic multisystem inflammatory disorder characterized by autoimmune antibody production resulting in inflammation of connective tissue in various organs or systems in the body that primarily affects women of childbearing age** (Molad, 2006). **Development of an antibody to autologous deoxyribonucleic acid (DNA) and other cell components leads to the deposition of antigen-antibody complexes and resultant inflammatory responses in target tissues** (Cunningham et al, 2001; De Swiet, 1999). **Pregnancy outcome for women with SLE is inconsistent and often unpredictable, necessitating careful monitoring** (Williams & Davidson, 2009).

1. Incidence of SLE is approximately 1 per 1000; 90% of cases occur in women during their childbearing years; incidence is higher among U.S. African Americans, Asian Americans, and Native Americans (Cunningham et al, 2001; De Swiet, 1999).
2. SLE is characterized by remissions and exacerbations.
3. Etiology is unknown, but evidence suggests genetic, environmental, hormonal, and immunologic factors (Cunningham et al, 2001; De Swiet, 1999; Wenstrom & Malee, 1999).
4. SLE is considered a syndrome, and diagnosis is usually based on symptoms. The American College of Rheumatology has proposed a list of 11 criteria for diagnosis; 4 or more of these clinical manifestations should be present to confirm the diagnosis of SLE (Cunningham et al, 2001; Ramsey-Goldman, 2001).
   a. Malar rash (butterfly rash)
   b. Discoid rash
   c. Photosensitivity
   d. Oral ulcers (usually painless)
   e. Arthritis (involving two or more peripheral joints)
   f. Serositis (pleuritis or pericarditis)
   g. Renal disorder (persistent proteinuria over 0.5 g or cellular casts)
   h. Neurologic disorder (seizure or psychosis)
   i. Hematologic disorder (hemolytic anemia, leukopenia, lymphopenia, or thrombocytopenia)
   j. Immunologic disorder (positive lupus erythematosus cell preparation, anti-DNA, anti-Sm, or false-positive serologic test result for syphilis)
   k. Antinuclear antibody (ANA)
5. SLE and pregnancy
   a. Lupus can be life-threatening to mother and fetus; the pregnancy outcome is better if (Cunningham et al, 2001; Molad, 2006):
      (1) SLE has been in remission for at least 6 months.
      (2) There is no active renal involvement.
      (3) Superimposed preeclampsia does not develop.
      (4) There is no evidence of antiphospholipid antibody activity.
   b. There is an increased risk of the following adverse outcomes:
      (1) Spontaneous abortion
      (2) Stillbirth
      (3) Preterm labor and potential preterm birth
      (4) Neonatal death
      (5) IUGR (Cunningham et al, 2001; De Swiet, 1999)
   c. SLE disease flare should be actively managed.
6. Neonatal lupus erythematosus (NLE) is a rare and often transient syndrome caused by passage of maternal autoantibodies across the placenta to the fetus and manifested by dermatologic lesions and cardiac abnormalities such as congenital heart block (Cunningham et al, 2001; De Swiet, 1999; Wenstrom & Malee, 1999).

B. **Antiphospholipid syndrome (APS) is an autoimmune disorder characterized by the presence of specific clinical features and specified levels of circulating antiphospholipid antibodies (aPLs); several aPLs have been identified, but the lupus anticoagulant (LA) and anticardiolipin antibody (aCL) are the most widely accepted for clinical use** (Cunningham et al, 2001; Silver & Branch, 1999; Wenstrom & Malee, 1999).
   1. The information on APS is new and evolving and there remains some controversy and uncertainty.
   2. The most frequent medical problems include arterial and venous thrombosis, autoimmune thrombocytopenia, and pregnancy loss (Silver & Branch, 1999; Wenstrom & Malee, 1999).
   3. APS can coexist with other autoimmune conditions, especially SLE; the prevalence of aPLs in patients with SLE is 30% to 40%.
   4. The fetal loss rate in SLE patients with aPLs is 73% compared with 19% in SLE patients without aPLs (Scott & Branch, 1999).
   5. Clinical and laboratory criteria for APS are listed below; one clinical and one laboratory finding are needed for clinical diagnosis (Cunningham et al, 2001; Silver & Branch, 1999; Tincani, Bazzani, Zingarelli, & Lojacono, 2008; Wenstrom & Malee, 1999).
      a. Recurrent early pregnancy loss before the tenth week of pregnancy
      b. Fetal death (second and third trimesters)

      c. Venous thrombosis

      d. Arterial thrombosis including stroke

      e. Autoimmune thrombocytopenia

      f. Autoimmune hemolytic anemia

      g. Livedo reticularis

      h. False-positive serologic test for syphilis

      i. Lupus anticoagulant

      j. Anticardiolipin antibody

  6. Obstetric disorders associated with APS (Tincani et al, 2008)

      a. Preeclampsia especially if early and severe

      b. IUGR

      c. Uteroplacental insufficiency

      d. Preterm delivery

CLINICAL PRACTICE

A. Assessment

  1. History

      a. Duration and presence of signs and symptoms listed by the American College of Rheumatology

      b. Race: higher incidence among African Americans, Asian Americans, and Native Americans

      c. Family history of SLE or other connective tissue disorder

      d. Obstetric history

         (1) Stillbirth

         (2) Miscarriage

         (3) Neonatal death

         (4) IUGR

         (5) Preterm labor and/or preterm birth

      e. Duration of exacerbations and remissions

  2. Physical findings (Cunningham et al, 2001; Ramsey-Goldman, 2001; Silver & Branch, 1999)

      a. Constitutional symptoms

         (1) Fatigue

         (2) Fever

         (3) Weight loss

         (4) Malaise

      b. Musculoskeletal

         (1) Arthralgia

         (2) Polyarthritis

         (3) Myalgia

         (4) Myopathy

      c. Mucocutaneous

         (1) Butterfly rash

         (2) Discoid rash

         (3) Oral and nasal ulcers

         (4) Photosensitivity

      d. Gastrointestinal

         (1) Anorexia

         (2) Nausea/vomiting

         (3) Abdominal pain

         (4) Diarrhea

         (5) Constipation

      e. Liver

         (1) Hepatomegaly

         (2) Enzyme elevation

         (3) Chronic hepatitis

     f. Cardiac disease
       (1) Pericarditis
       (2) Myocarditis
       (3) Endocarditis
       (4) Ischemia
       (5) Hypertension
       (6) Tachycardia
     g. Pulmonary
       (1) Pleuritis
       (2) Pleural effusion
       (3) Pneumonitis
       (4) Dyspnea
     h. Hematologic
       (1) Anemia
       (2) Leukopenia
       (3) Thrombocytopenia
     i. Renal
       (1) Nephritis
       (2) Nephrotic syndrome
       (3) Urinary tract infection
       (4) Glomerular nephritis
     j. Nervous system
       (1) Seizures
       (2) Headaches
       (3) Irritability
       (4) Depression
       (5) Cognitive dysfunction
       (6) Psychosis
  3. Laboratory and diagnostic studies
     a. Laboratory value abnormalities found in patients with SLE
       (1) Anemia
       (2) Leukopenia
       (3) Thrombocytopenia
       (4) Positive direct Coombs' test result
       (5) Positive ANA test result
       (6) Lupus erythematosus cells
       (7) Decreased complement levels
       (8) Increase in gamma globulin
       (9) Positive rheumatoid factor
       (10) False-positive serologic test for syphilis
       (11) Positive lupus anticoagulant
       (12) Prolonged prothrombin and thrombin time
       (13) Positive anticardiolipin antibody
       (14) Anti-DNA and anti-Sm antibodies
     b. Critical laboratory tests to be performed are:
       (1) CBC
       (2) Platelet count
       (3) Electrolytes
       (4) BUN
       (5) 24-hour urine for protein and creatinine clearance
       (6) Urinalysis
       (7) Urine culture
       (8) Serum glutamate pyruvate transaminase (SGPT)
       (9) Serum glutamic-oxalo-acetic transaminase (SGOT)
       (10) Bilirubin
       (11) Erythrocyte sedimentation rate (ESR)
       (12) Total serum complement for C3 and C4
       (13) Fluorescent antinuclear antibodies
       (14) ECG

B. **Interventions**
1. Observe for varied signs and symptoms indicating exacerbation of SLE.
2. Distinguish between the symptoms of SLE and preeclampsia.
    a. Monitor patient closely for preeclampsia; assess blood pressure (BP), edema, proteinuria, deep tendon reflexes, and clonus
3. Protect patient from infection.
    a. Use aseptic technique for all potential sites of infection.
    b. Perform and instruct patient in proper handwashing technique.
4. Maintain patient's hydration with fluids.
5. Observe skin, joints, and extremities for areas of redness and swelling.
6. Encourage patient to maintain caloric and protein intake.
7. Observe type, amount, and odor of discharge or drainage.
8. Assess patient for:
    a. Fundal tenderness
    b. Pain, burning, and frequency of urination
    c. Flank pain
9. Assess for fever and chills.
10. Monitor vital signs, especially temperature, every 4 hours and as needed.
11. Monitor laboratory results, especially white blood cell count.
12. Assess fatigue levels and activity tolerance.
    a. Encourage expression of feelings regarding effects of fatigue on life.
    b. Provide and encourage rest periods and a restful environment.
    c. Assist patient in modifying her schedule and spacing her activities to allow time for more rest.
13. Teach energy conservation techniques.
14. Assist patient with ADLs and ambulation as necessary.
15. Assess pain-precipitating factors, quality, region radiation, severity, duration, and relieving factors; document deviation from baseline.
    a. Have patient evaluate pain intensity on a 1 to 10 scale (10 being most severe).
    b. Observe, report, and record verbal and nonverbal expressions of pain, fear, and anxiety.
    c. Medicate patient with analgesics as ordered.
    d. Assess effectiveness of pain medications.
    e. Teach patient and family about factors that contribute to pain experience.
16. Administer prescribed medications and observe for side effects of:
    a. Corticosteroids
    b. Salicylates
    c. Nonsteroidal antiinflammatory agents
    d. Analgesics
    e. Antipyretics
    f. Immunosuppressants
    g. Antimalarials
    h. Heparin
17. Assist patient in improving her self-esteem.
18. Refer patient to self-help groups and local and national SLE organizations.
19. Assist patient in using alternative coping strategies: relaxation techniques, meditation.
    a. Set short-term coping goals with patient.
20. Monitor the patient for placental competency and fetal well-being.
21. Observe patient for signs and symptoms of glucose intolerance due to steroids.
22. Observe patient for signs and symptoms of deteriorating cardiovascular and renal status.
23. Observe patient for signs and symptoms of thrombosis formation.
24. Observe patient for signs and symptoms of arterial occlusion, including stroke.
25. Observe patient closely for worsening condition in the postpartum period; might need intensive nursing observation for the first 24 to 48 hours after delivery.
26. Observe patient for early signs and symptoms of psychosis.
    a. Restlessness
    b. Distractibility
    c. Emotional sensitivity
    d. Confusion
    e. Vague personality changes
    f. Disorientation

HEALTH EDUCATION

A. **Preconceptual counseling**
   1. Advise patient to postpone conception until at least 1 to 2 years after the diagnosis of SLE, when the disease has been in remission for at least 6 months and doses of corticosteroids are low (Molad, 2006).
   2. Provide reassurance that SLE patients with mild to moderate renal disease who are in remission before conception have a successful live birth rate of 80% to 90%.
B. **Discuss the increased incidence of spontaneous abortions, stillbirths, IUGR, and premature birth.**
C. **Discuss the illness as a pathologic process.**
D. **Discuss the increased incidence of maternal nephritis, placental insufficiency, preeclampsia, and venous and arterial thrombosis.**
E. **Encourage patient to keep appointments with her internist or rheumatologist and her obstetrician or perinatologist.**
F. **Teach patient importance of frequent monitoring of creatinine clearance, proteinuria, and hematologic parameters.**
G. **Teach patient self-monitoring of weight gain, edema, and blood pressure.**
H. **Teach patient about signs and symptoms to report.**
   1. Chest pain
   2. Bleeding
   3. Confusion
   4. Decreased ability to perform activities
   5. Fever
   6. Extreme fatigue
   7. Edema
   8. Anorexia
   9. Vomiting
   10. Abdominal pain
   11. Weight loss
   12. Leg pain, tenderness, color change, or edema
I. **Educate patient about prescribed medications and side effects.**
J. **Inform the patient that corticosteroids, a strong immunosuppressant, can mask the symptoms of infection.**
K. **Teach patient to avoid exposure to infection, including persons with known infectious processes.**
L. **Plan with patient how she can avoid periods of fatigue or stress.**
M. **Teach patient to take 1200 mg of calcium and vitamin D to decrease the risk of osteoporosis if she is receiving corticosteroids or heparin.**
N. **Discuss the importance of early and frequent monitoring of patient's condition during pregnancy and encourage the patient to be in the care of an obstetrician and rheumatologist.**
O. **Discuss the importance of a multidisciplinary team including rheumatology, obstetrics, nursing, dietary, social service, and pediatric/neonatology.**
P. **Discuss the need for frequent and close monitoring of fetal well-being.**

HEMATOLOGIC COMPLICATIONS

INTRODUCTION

A. **Anemias**
   1. Anemia complicates 15% to 60% of all pregnancies (Kilpatrick, 2009; Wenstrom & Malee, 1999).
   2. Pregnancy results in an intravascular volume expansion, with the increase in plasma volume larger than the rise in erythrocyte volume, resulting in hemodilution of pregnancy; the net result is a physiologic drop in the hemoglobin and hematocrit.
   3. According to the Centers for Disease Control and Prevention (CDC, 1998), anemia is present in pregnant women if the hemoglobin concentration drops below 11 g/dL in the first and third trimesters, or lower than 10.5 g/dL in the second trimester.

4. Iron deficiency anemia
   a. Approximately 75% of all anemias in pregnancy result from iron deficiency, related to suboptimal iron content of the average U.S. diet and insufficient iron stores in women of reproductive years (Kilpatrick, 2009; Long, 1995; Wenstrom & Malee, 1999).
   b. Signs and symptoms
      (1) Pallor
      (2) Fatigue
      (3) Reduced exercise tolerance
      (4) Anorexia
      (5) Weakness
      (6) Malaise
      (7) Dyspnea
      (8) Edema
      (9) Pica
   c. Might be prevented by iron supplementation during pregnancy of 60 mg of elemental iron per day, the amount contained in 300 mg of ferrous sulfate (Wenstrom & Malee, 1999)
   d. Is treated by oral administration of ferrous sulfate 325 mg one to three times per day (Kilpatrick, 2009)
   e. Oral iron therapy might be associated with gastrointestinal intolerance, requiring a reduction in dose to a tolerable level.
   f. Constipation can be a side effect of iron therapy.
5. Megaloblastic anemia
   a. Occurs in up to 1% of pregnant women; usually the result of folic acid deficiency and occasionally the result of vitamin B_{12} deficiency
   b. Is often found in combination with iron deficiency
   c. Folic acid deficiency is treated with 1 mg/day of folic acid. Parenteral administration may be required for individuals with malabsorption.
   d. Treatment of B_{12} deficiency is parenteral cyanocobalamin (vitamin B_{12}) (Kilpatrick, 2009; Wenstrom & Malee, 1999).
6. Sickle cell anemia (Cunningham et al, 2001; Wenstrom & Malee, 1999)
   a. Recessive inheritance: Sickle cell trait is the heterozygous form of the condition, whereas sickle cell disease or anemia is the homozygous form of the condition (occurs when the gene for the production of S hemoglobin is inherited from both parents).
   b. When deoxygenated, the sickle cell hemoglobin molecule becomes rigid and dehydrated and assumes an abnormal sickled shape; these sickled erythrocytes are not deformable and cannot squeeze through the microcirculation; obstruction results in local hypoxia causing progressive tissue and organ damage (especially kidneys, lungs, and bone), painful vaso-occlusive crises, and increased susceptibility to infection (Cunningham et al, 2001; Wenstrom & Malee, 1999).
   c. Pregnancy is associated with more severe anemia and more common vaso-occlusive crises, and increased maternal and perinatal morbidity and mortality.
   d. Management during pregnancy includes:
      (1) Frequent prenatal visits
      (2) Careful screening for infections
      (3) Folic acid supplementation
      (4) Hospitalization at the earliest signs of crisis, and treatment with analgesics, oxygen, and hydration
      (5) Intensive fetal surveillance
      (6) Transfusion therapy for severe maternal anemia
7. Thalassemia
   a. This hemoglobinopathy is characterized by a defect in the ability to synthesize alpha or beta-globin chains at a normal rate.
   b. Alpha thalassemia minor is characterized by hypochromic microcytic erythrocytes but little or no anemia; pregnancy usually is uncomplicated; incidence is highest in Southeast Asians.
   c. Beta thalassemia minor is characterized by a mild hypochromic microcytic anemia, with hematocrit between 32% and 35% (Wenstrom & Malee, 1999).

B. Thrombocytopenia
1. Thrombocytopenia can be a consequence of the following:
   a. Inadequate production of platelets
   b. Increased peripheral consumption of platelets
   c. Destruction of platelets
2. The body can develop an antiplatelet antibody that is responsible for destruction of platelets; this immune process is called idiopathic thrombocytopenic purpura (ITP), also known as primary immune or autoimmune thrombocytopenic purpura (Kilpatrick, 2009).
3. The most common causes of thrombocytopenia in pregnancy are ITP, preeclampsia or eclampsia, and SLE.
4. Therapy of choice for pregnant women with ITP is glucocorticoids or IV immunoglobulin (American Society of Hematology ITP Practice Guideline Panel, 1997; Kilpatrick, 2009).
5. The signs and symptoms of thrombocytopenia include the signs and symptoms of bleeding.
   a. Petechiae and ecchymoses
   b. Oozing from IV site or wound
   c. Hematuria
   d. Hematemesis
   e. Hemoptysis
   f. Signs of cerebral hemorrhage

C. Thromboembolic disease
1. During pregnancy there is an increased potential for thromboses resulting from increased levels of coagulation factors and decreased fibrinolysis, venous dilation, and obstruction of the venous system by the gravid uterus.
2. Thromboembolic diseases occurring most frequently during pregnancy include deep vein thrombosis (DVT) of the lower extremities and pulmonary embolism.
3. Thromboembolism is reported to occur during pregnancy at a rate of approximately 0.5 to 3 in 1000; events occur with equal frequency during antepartum and postpartum (Laros, 1999).
4. Patients at high risk for thromboembolic disease during pregnancy include those with the following:
   a. Previous venous thromboembolism
   b. Advanced maternal age
   c. Increased parity
   d. Artificial heart valves
   e. Thrombophilia syndrome
   f. Obesity
   g. Cesarean delivery
   h. Prolonged immobilization or bedrest
   i. Dehydration
5. Anticoagulation therapy with heparin is the mainstay of therapy for DVT, with or without pulmonary embolism (Laros, 1999).

D. Fetal implications
1. Chronic anemia limits the amount of oxygen available for fetal oxygenation and increases the risk for the following:
   a. Spontaneous abortion
   b. Premature birth
   c. Small for gestational age (SGA) neonates
2. With ITP the fetus is at risk for hemorrhage in utero or after birth because the antiplatelet antibodies are actively transported across the placenta, causing thrombocytopenia.

CLINICAL PRACTICE

A. Assessment
1. History
   a. Iron deficiency anemia
      (1) Evidence of decreased dietary iron intake
      (2) Risk factors, such as a history of poor nutritional status, close spacing of pregnancies, multiple gestation, excessive bleeding, adolescence, eating disorders, and personal or family history of anemia

     b. Megaloblastic anemia
       (1) History of bariatric surgery
       (2) Evidence of inadequate dietary folate intake
     c. Sickle cell anemia
       (1) Family history
       (2) African American or Mediterranean ancestry
     d. Thrombocytopenia: family history
     e. Thromboembolic disease
       (1) DVT
       (2) Pulmonary embolus
       (3) Artificial heart valve
       (4) Hypercoagulable disorder
       (5) Prolonged immobilization
       (6) Obesity
2. Physical findings: signs and symptoms specific to the diagnosed hematologic disorder
     a. Iron deficiency anemia
       (1) Pallor
       (2) Fatigue
       (3) Decreased exercise tolerance
       (4) Anorexia
       (5) Weakness
       (6) Malaise
       (7) Dyspnea
       (8) Edema
       (9) Pica
     b. Megaloblastic anemia
       (1) Folate deficiency presents with typical symptoms of anemia plus roughness of skin and glossitis
       (2) Vitamin B_{12} deficiency may present with neurologic deficits (Kilpatrick, 2009).
     c. Sickle cell anemia or sickle cell crisis
       (1) Pain in the abdomen, chest, vertebrae, joints, or extremities
       (2) Sudden anemia
       (3) Marked pallor
       (4) Cardiac failure
     d. Thalassemia: mild persistent anemia with no unusual systemic problems
     e. Thrombocytopenia: signs and symptoms of bleeding
       (1) Petechiae
       (2) Oozing from IV site or wound
       (3) Hematuria
       (4) Hemoptysis
       (5) Signs of cerebral hemorrhage
     f. DVT
       (1) Pain
       (2) Tenderness
       (3) Edema (difference between leg circumference of > 2 cm)
       (4) Change in limb color
       (5) Calf pain with dorsiflexion (Homans' sign)
3. Diagnostic and laboratory studies: evaluate laboratory data for indicators or presence of specific disorder (Table 26-5)
     a. Iron deficiency anemia
       (1) Hemoglobin less than 10 g/dL
       (2) Hematocrit less than 30%
     b. Megaloblastic anemia
       (1) Elevated mean cell volume
       (2) Reduced serum levels of folate or vitamin B_{12}
     c. Sickle cell anemia; hemoglobin electrophoresis
     d. Thalassemia
       (1) Mild persistent anemia

■ TABLE 26-5
■ ■ **Indices of Iron Homeostasis**

	Normal Nonpregnant	Normal Pregnant	Iron Deficiency Anemia in Pregnancy
Hemoglobin (g/dL)	12.5-14	11.5-12.5	<10
Hematocrit (%)	37-45	33-38	<30
Mean corpuscular hemoglobin concentration	32-36	32-36	<30
Mean corpuscular volume (cubic micrometers)	80-100	70-90	
Mean corpuscular hemoglobin (pg/cell)	27-34	23-31	
Serum iron (mcg/dL)	50-110	35-100	<30
Unsaturated iron-binding capacity (mcg/dL)	250-300	280-400	>400
Transferrin saturation (%)	25-35	16-30	<16
Serum ferritin (mcg/L)	75-100	55-70	<10

From Scott, J., DiSaia, P., Hammond, C., & Spellacy, W. (1994). *Danforth's obstetrics and gynecology* (7th ed., p. 384). Philadelphia: Lippincott Williams & Wilkins.

      (2) Hypochromic microcytic RBCs
      (3) Elevated hemoglobin A_2 concentrations with normal serum iron and ferritin levels (Wenstrom & Malee, 1999)
    e. Thrombocytopenia
      (1) Low platelet count (less than $150/mm^3$)
      (2) Prolonged bleeding time
      (3) ITP is diagnosed by presence of antiplatelet antibodies in maternal serum.
    f. DVT
      (1) Doppler ultrasonography
      (2) Impedance plethysmography (IPG)
      (3) Contrast venography
B. Interventions (Carpenito, 1997; Kilpatrick, 2009)
  1. Treat causative or contributing factors (anemia) as ordered.
  2. Refer to dietitian for nutritional counseling.
  3. Assess fatigue levels: onset, precipitating factors, pattern, and whether relieved by rest.
  4. Encourage expression of feelings regarding the effects of fatigue on patient's life.
  5. Assist patient to identify energy patterns and the need to schedule activities.
  6. Assist patient to identify what tasks can be delegated.
  7. Teach energy conservation techniques.
  8. Assist patient with ADLs and ambulation as required.
  9. Assess extremity for adequate tissue perfusion related to DVT or thrombophlebitis for:
    a. Temperature
    b. Color
    c. Pulses
    d. Capillary refill
    e. Swelling sensation
    f. Movement
    g. Strength
 10. Elevate or position leg on pillows or use foot cradle as indicated.
 11. Reduce or remove external compression that impedes flow: pillows, leg crossing, and so on.
 12. Change patient's position every 2 hours while she is on bedrest.
 13. Measure and record calf and thigh circumference.
 14. Assess skin integrity.

15. Assess for complications of DVT (i.e., pulmonary embolism).
    a. Sudden chest pain
    b. Cough
    c. Dyspnea
    d. Change in level of consciousness
16. Administer anticoagulant medications as ordered.
17. Give instructions to patient concerning medications and side effects of bleeding.
18. Assess for signs and symptoms of bleeding if patient is on anticoagulants.
    a. Petechiae
    b. Hematemesis
    c. Hematuria
    d. Epistaxis
    e. Blood in stool
    f. Bleeding from gums
    g. Vaginal bleeding
19. Monitor for signs and symptoms of anemia.
20. Monitor laboratory values, including CBC with reticulocyte count.
21. Monitor for signs and symptoms of infection.
    a. Fever
    b. Pain
    c. Chills
    d. Increased white blood cells (WBCs)
22. Teach patient with sickle cell anemia to avoid factors that can initiate a vaso-occlusive crisis.
    a. Viral and bacterial infections
    b. Fever
    c. Acid-base imbalance
    d. Dehydration
    e. Severe emotional disturbance
    f. Strenuous physical activity
    g. Exposure to cold
    h. Alcohol intoxication
    i. Extreme fatigue
    j. Air travel
    k. Drug overdose
    l. Anesthesia
    m. Trauma or blood loss
23. Instruct patient with sickle cell anemia to report symptoms of vaso-occlusion.
    a. Any acute illness
    b. Severe joint or bone pain
    c. Chest pain
    d. Abdominal pain
    e. Headaches, dizziness
    f. Gastric distress
24. Initiate therapy per physician order (e.g., antisickling agents, analgesics, oxygen, hydration, transfusions, antibiotics).
25. Avoid events that might precipitate a sickle cell crisis during the intrapartum period.
    a. Promote rest and relaxation to reduce oxygen demands extraneous to the labor process.
    b. Provide a calm, quiet atmosphere.
    c. Control environmental temperature to prevent hypothermia.
26. Monitor for hemorrhage related to altered clotting factors secondary to heparin therapy or thrombocytopenia (Carpenito, 1997).
    a. Monitor CBC, coagulation tests, and platelet counts.
27. Assess for signs and symptoms of spontaneous or excessive bleeding.
    a. Petechiae, ecchymoses, hematomas
    b. Bleeding from nose or gums
    c. Prolonged bleeding from venipuncture or IV sites
    d. Hemoptysis
    e. Hematemesis or "coffee grounds" emesis

  f. Hematuria

  g. Vaginal or rectal bleeding

  h. Change in vital signs

 28. Observe color, consistency, and amount of stool and urine.

 29. Administer blood products per physician order following hospital protocol.

HEALTH EDUCATION

A. Preconceptual counseling: inheritance patterns for sickle cell trait/disease; implications for offspring

B. Encourage patient to keep appointments with her internist or hematologist and obstetrician.

C. Teach patient how to prevent conditions that cause sickling and other exacerbations of hematologic disorders.

D. Teach patient to report signs and symptoms of bleeding and report any observed.

E. Ensure adequate nutrition with prescribed diet and iron supplements as appropriate.

F. Teach subcutaneous administration of heparin as required.

GASTROINTESTINAL COMPLICATIONS OF PREGNANCY

INTRODUCTION

A. Hyperemesis gravidarum

 1. Hyperemesis gravidarum occurs in 3.3 to 10 in 1000 pregnancies and is defined as persistent vomiting unresponsive to outpatient treatment and severe enough to cause weight loss and disturbed nutritional status; it is associated with altered electrolyte balance, dehydration, weight loss, acidosis from starvation, alkalosis from loss of hydrochloric acid, ketonuria, and hypokalemia (Cunningham et al, 2001; Heppard & Garite, 2002; Scott, 1999).

 2. The cause of hyperemesis gravidarum remains unclear and is most likely multifactorial; theories include hormonal, endocrine, psychologic, or metabolic (Goodwin, 2008).

 3. Pregnancy outcome in hyperemesis gravidarum depends on the severity and duration of the nutritional deficit; significant weight loss might be associated with intrauterine growth restriction of the fetus, low birthweight, and preterm birth (Goodwin, 2008; Scott, 1999).

 4. Interventions might begin with dietary adjustment and lifestyle alterations, proceed to oral nutritional supplementation or pharmacologic preparations, alternative therapy, and continue on to IV vitamin-mineral therapy and either parenteral or enteral nutrition; supportive psychotherapy might be indicated (Cunningham et al, 2001; Goodwin, 2008; Scott, 1999).

 5. In severe cases, persistent dehydration, acetonuria, and ketosis might occur with potential neurologic, hepatic, and renal damage.

B. Inflammatory bowel disease

 1. Inflammatory bowel disease (IBD) refers to ulcerative colitis and Crohn's disease, which are inflammatory conditions of the luminal gastrointestinal tract (Kelly & Savides, 2009).

 2. The peak incidence of these immunologically mediated disorders is during the woman's reproductive period.

 3. Mothers with IBD have an increased risk of preterm delivery and low-birthweight babies (Habel & Ravindran, 2008).

 4. If IBD is quiescent at the time of conception, the pregnancy outcome is essentially normal; active disease at conception has a worse prognosis (Cunningham et al, 2001; Kelly & Savides, 2009; Wenstrom & Malee, 1999).

 5. Pregnancy does not increase the likelihood of an attack of IBD; if the disease is quiescent in early pregnancy, flares are uncommon, but if they do occur they might be severe (Cunningham et al, 2001).

 6. Active disease poses a greater risk to the fetus than most therapies; therefore, when disease is active, aggressive management is essential (Cappell, 2007; Kelly & Savides, 2009; Wenstrom & Malee, 1999).

7. Diagnostic evaluations, including radiologic studies, should not be postponed if their results are likely to affect management.

8. Many of the usual medications may be continued and pregnant patients with IBD should stay on medications that are maintaining their remission (Kelly & Savides, 2009).

9. If indicated, surgery done for emergencies should be performed (Cunningham et al, 2001; Kelly & Savides, 2009; Wenstrom & Malee, 1999).

CLINICAL PRACTICE

A. **Assessment**
   1. History
      a. Duration and course of IBD or hyperemesis gravidarum
      b. Prescribed medications
      c. Any contributing or precipitating factors
   2. Physical findings
      a. Signs and symptoms of gastrointestinal disturbances
         (1) Anorexia
         (2) Nausea and vomiting
         (3) Indigestion
         (4) Abdominal pain or distention
         (5) Diarrhea
         (6) Weight loss
         (7) Passage of blood or mucus per rectum
      b. Signs and symptoms of fluid and electrolyte imbalance and nutritional deficiencies
         (1) Dry mucous membranes
         (2) Poor skin turgor
         (3) Malaise
         (4) Low blood pressure
      c. Symptoms of severe fluid and electrolyte imbalance and nutritional deficiency
         (1) Weight loss
         (2) Acetonuria
         (3) Ketosis
   3. Laboratory and diagnostic studies
      a. Serum electrolytes
      b. Renal and liver function studies
      c. Acid base and pH
      d. Hemoglobin and hematocrit
      e. Urine dipstick for specific gravity, ketones, and glucose
      f. Serum glucose
      g. Abdominal ultrasonography
      h. Colonoscopy
   4. Nutrition-related factors (Carpenito, 1997)
      a. Prepregnancy weight and height; current weight
      b. Diet recall for 24 hours
      c. Appetite: usual and any changes
      d. Dietary patterns
         (1) Food and fluid likes and dislikes, preferences, food allergies, and taboos
         (2) Religious dietary practices
      e. Activity level
         (1) Occupation
         (2) Exercise: type and frequency
      f. Food procurement and preparation (and by whom)
         (1) Functional ability
         (2) Kitchen facilities
         (3) Income adequate for food needs
      g. Knowledge of nutrition
         (1) Basic four food groups/nutrition pyramid

     h. Nutrition supplements
       (1) Folic acid
       (2) Vitamins
       (3) Iron

B. Interventions

1. Monitor patient's vital signs.
2. Monitor patient's intake and output.
3. Assess patient's skin turgor, color, and temperature.
4. Observe patient's urine for color and amount.
5. Assess amount, color, and consistency of patient's vomitus and stool.
6. Assess patient's oral mucous membranes.
7. Assess level of consciousness.
8. Weigh patient daily, noting loss or gain.
9. Assess patient for edema of the legs, arms, hands, or sacral region.
10. Auscultate patient's lungs every shift and as needed.
11. Observe patient for cough, dyspnea, tachypnea, and sputum.
12. Monitor serum electrolytes, BUN, creatinine, urine osmolality, hematocrit, and hemoglobin.
13. Administer parenteral fluids, electrolytes, antiemetics, and supplements as prescribed and as needed.
14. Administer prednisone and sulfasalazine as ordered for management of IBD.
15. Assess patient's nutritional status by monitoring the following:
    a. Weight
    b. 24-hour diet recall
    c. Calorie counts
    d. Intake and output
    e. Appetite
    f. Nausea and vomiting
    g. Diarrhea
16. Reduce or eliminate factors that contribute to anorexia, nausea, vomiting, and diarrhea.
    a. Maintain an odor-free, well-ventilated room.
17. Consult with nutritionist and dietitian to establish appropriate daily caloric and food-type requirements for the patient.
18. Determine the patient's food preferences and arrange to have these foods provided, as appropriate.
19. Administer progressive diets according to the patient's tolerance.
    a. Provide small, frequent feedings.
    b. Restrict liquids with meals and avoid fluids 1 hour before and after meals.
20. Help patient maintain good oral hygiene before and after ingestion of food.
21. Give patient instructions according to proper diet.
    a. Foods and liquids to avoid
    b. Specific times to eat specific foods
    c. Alternative sources of foods
22. Provide oral nutrient supplementation as ordered.
23. Administer IV vitamin-mineral therapy and enteral tube feedings or parenteral nutrition as required and as prescribed.
24. Assess the patient's affect and response to her family, environment, and pregnancy.
25. Assess pain-precipitating factors, quality, region radiation, severity, duration, and relieving factors; document any deviation from baseline.
    a. Have patient evaluate pain intensity on a 1 to 10 scale (10 being the most severe).
    b. Observe, report, and record verbal and nonverbal expressions of pain, fear, and anxiety.
    c. Medicate patient with analgesics or antiemetics as ordered.
    d. Assess effectiveness of pain medications and antiemetics.
    e. Teach patient and her family about factors that contribute to the pain experience.
26. Assess patient's activity tolerance.
    a. Assist patient in modifying her schedule and spacing her activities to allow for more rest.
    b. Maintain patient's activity level just short of fatigue.
    c. Provide and encourage rest periods and a restful environment.
    d. Provide long periods for sleep at night and frequent rest periods during the day.
    e. Assist patient with ADLs and ambulation as required.
27. Initiate health teaching and referrals as indicated.

HEALTH EDUCATION

A. Pregnancy planning should be discussed prior to conception, and the patient should be advised to avoid pregnancy until the disease (IBD) is quiescent.

B. Discuss the importance of early and frequent monitoring of the patient's condition during pregnancy and encourage the patient to be in the care or an obstetrician and gastroenterologist.

C. Include the woman and her family in care conferences.

D. Give specific diet and nutritional information and directions: amount, type, and time for food and liquid.

E. Explain the physiologic changes and nutritional needs during pregnancy.

F. Discuss signs and symptoms of hypoglycemia.

G. Teach patient signs and symptoms to report.
   1. Anorexia
   2. Nausea
   3. Vomiting
   4. Weight loss
   5. Abdominal pain or distention
   6. Diarrhea or constipation
   7. Decreased ability to perform activities
   8. Extreme fatigue
   9. Decreased urine output
   10. Dry mucous membranes
   11. Poor skin turgor

H. Plan with the patient how she can get adequate sleep and take frequent rests.

I. Teach patient to avoid fatigue or stress.

J. Teach patient medication regimen and importance of adherence to treatment.

HEPATIC COMPLICATIONS—HEPATITIS

INTRODUCTION

A. **Viral hepatitis occurs in at least six distinct forms (A, B, C, D, E, and G)** (Williamson & Mackillop, 2009).
   1. Viral hepatitis is the most common cause of jaundice during pregnancy (Heppard & Garite, 2002; Williamson & Mackillop, 2009).
   2. The incubation periods vary and are followed by anorexia, nausea, and weight loss with variable jaundice and laboratory evidence of hepatocellular dysfunction lasting for weeks or months (Varner, 1994; Williamson & Mackillop, 2009) (Table 26-6).
   3. Diagnosis requires serologic markers for acute and chronic infection.
   4. The clinical course of viral hepatitis is not affected by pregnancy, but clinical implications of each virus and its effect on maternal, fetal, and neonatal outcomes vary.

B. **Hepatitis A**
   1. Accounts for 30% to 35% of cases of acute hepatitis in the United States; course and management are the same as in nongravid patients.
   2. There is no evidence that hepatitis A is teratogenic (Cunningham et al, 2001).
   3. Spread by fecal-oral route; associated with poor hygiene and poor sanitation
   4. Perinatal transmission is rare and occurs when fecal contamination occurs during delivery (Williamson & Mackillop, 2009).
   5. Symptoms are nonspecific and include malaise, headache, fatigue, anorexia, nausea, vomiting, and diarrhea (Williamson & Mackillop, 2009).
   6. Treatment with immune globulin used prophylactically and after exposure appears to be safe during pregnancy (Heppard & Garite, 2002; Williamson & Mackillop, 2009).

C. **Hepatitis B** (Cunningham et al, 2001; Freitag-Koontz, 1996; Heppard & Garite, 2002; Williamson & Mackillop, 2009)
   1. Accounts for 40% to 45% of all cases of hepatitis in the United States; acute hepatitis B occurs in 1 to 2 of 1000 pregnancies, and chronic infection occurs in 5 to 15 of 1000 pregnancies
   2. Approximately 20,000 infants are delivered of hepatitis B surface antigen (HBsAg)–positive women each year in the United States (Williamson & Mackillop, 2009).

▒ TABLE 26-6
▒ ▒ **Forms of Viral Hepatitis**

Characteristics	Hepatitis A	Hepatitis B	Hepatitis C
Older name	Infectious hepatitis	Serum hepatitis	Non-A, Non-B
Virus type	RNA	DNA	RNA
Virus size	27 nm	42 nm	30-60 nm
Incubation period	15-50 days	30-180 days	30-160 days
Transmission	Fecal-oral	Parenteral or body fluids	Parenteral, sporadic
Vertical transmission to fetus	Not observed	Common	Uncommon
Immunologic diagnosis	HA antibody, IgM and IgG types	HBsAg; HBcAb; HbsAb; HBeAg; Ab	HC antibody
Maximum infectivity	Prodrome	Prodrome or HBeAg positive; HbsAg carriers	Probably prodrome and carriers
Carrier state	None	5%-10%	50%
Acute clinical forms	Asymptomatic to fulminant	Asymptomatic to fulminant	Asymptomatic to fulminant; relapsing
Chronic clinical forms	None	Chronic persistent hepatitis; chronic active hepatitis	Chronic persistent hepatitis; chronic active hepatitis

From Burrow, G., & Ferris, T. (1995). *Medical complications during pregnancy* (4th ed., p. 322). Philadelphia: Saunders.

3. Transmitted primarily through direct contact with the blood or sexual fluid of an infected person
4. Hepatitis B virus (HBV) infections are readily transmitted from an infected mother to her infant. Infants infected at birth have a 90% risk of becoming chronically infected with HBV (carrier) and an approximate 25% risk of developing significant liver disease or cancer as an adult. If these infants receive postexposure prophylaxis at birth and complete the series of HBV vaccinations, more than 95% of these HBV infections can be prevented. Key to the prevention of perinatal HBV infection is the screening of all pregnant women, because approximately 50% of the women thus identified do not fall into established high-risk groups (Freitag-Koontz, 1996).
5. Weinbaum, Mast, and Ward of the CDC recommend screening of all pregnant women for HBsAg, immunoprophylaxis of all infants born to women identified as HBsAg-positive with hepatitis B immunoglobulin (HBIG), and routine immunization of all infants against HBV.
6. There is no evidence that breastfeeding increases the risk of HBV transmission in infants, provided they have received HBIG prophylaxis at birth and completed their HBV immunizations on schedule.

D. **Hepatitis C**
1. Accounts for 5% of all cases of hepatitis (Heppard & Garite, 2002); approximately 4 million individuals in the United States are affected (Williamson & Mackillop, 2009), and 40,000 births occur to hepatitis C virus (HCV)–infected women each year (Airoldi & Berghella, 2006)
2. The prevalence of HCV infection in pregnant women is approximately 1% (Airoldi & Berghella, 2006).
3. The greatest risk factor is a history of blood exposure.
4. Perinatal outcome is not adversely affected in HCV-positive women (Cunningham et al, 2001) and pregnancy does not affect the clinical course of hepatitis C (Airoldi & Berghella, 2006).
5. Perinatal transmission of HCV is relatively rare, except in women who are immuno-compromised, such as those coinfected with HIV.

6. There is no recommendation at present to test pregnant women routinely for HCV. However, women with certain risks should be offered anti-HCV testing during pregnancy (Airoldi & Berghella, 2006).
7. Of all acute infection, 50% progress to chronic liver disease (Heppard & Garite, 2002).

CLINICAL PRACTICE

A. **Assessment**
   1. History
      a. Exposure to contaminated food or water
      b. Travel to high-prevalence areas for hepatitis A
      c. Risk factors for HBV infection
         (1) Sexual or household exposure to an HBV-infected person
         (2) Homosexual activity
         (3) Illicit parenteral drug use
         (4) Occupational exposure to blood
         (5) Heterosexual activity with multiple partners
      d. Long-term sequelae of hepatitis: chronic hepatitis, cirrhosis, primary hepatocellular carcinoma
   2. Signs and symptoms of hepatic dysfunction
      a. Jaundice
      b. Anorexia, indigestion, nausea, and vomiting
      c. Petechiae, ecchymoses
      d. Clay-colored stools
      e. Malaise
   3. Diagnostic and laboratory tests
      a. Elevated liver function test results
      b. Prolonged prothrombin time
      c. Hepatitis A: immunoglobulin M (IgM) antibody levels
      d. Hepatitis B (Cunningham et al, 2001)
         (1) HBsAg
         (2) Hepatitis Be antigen (HBeAg)
         (3) Antibody to viral core antigen (anti-HBc)
         (4) Antibody to e antigen (anti-HBe)
         (5) Antibody to HB surface antigen (anti-HBs)
      e. Hepatitis C
         (1) Hepatitis C antibody

B. **Interventions**
   1. Identify susceptible newborns through prenatal screening of mother for HBsAg.
   2. Implement universal precautions for blood and body fluids when caring for mother or newborn.
   3. Bathe newborns of HbsAg-positive mothers as soon as possible after delivery to remove maternal blood and bodily fluids; after bathing, newborns can be managed without special precautions while in the nursery.
   4. Administer HBIG immunoprophylaxis and hepatitis B vaccine to newborn as ordered.
   5. Monitor for any adverse reactions to vaccine and teach parents about potential adverse reactions.
   6. Monitor for signs and symptoms of hepatic dysfunction.
   7. Monitor for hemorrhage.
   8. Teach the patient to report any unusual bleeding.
   9. Monitor for electrolyte and acid-base disturbances.

HEALTH EDUCATION

A. **Discuss the importance of early and frequent monitoring of the patient's condition during pregnancy and encourage the patient to be in the care or an obstetrician and gastroenterologist or hepatologist.**

B. Teach patient and family about risks, pathophysiology, plan of care, and infectivity.
C. Teach patient about immunization schedule for hepatitis vaccines and prophylaxis.
D. Teach patient good personal hygiene:
   1. Handwashing technique
   2. Advise patient not to prepare or serve food to others.
E. Teach patient about transmission precautions until period of infectivity has passed.

CASE STUDIES AND STUDY QUESTIONS

Ms. M., a 30-year-old G3, P2002, woman is admitted to Labor and Delivery for preterm labor at 32 weeks' gestation. Her pregnancy had been normal, with the exception of increasing dyspnea and easy fatigability. Her past medical history includes surgery to repair a ventricular septal defect in infancy. Her vital signs at admission are temperature 37° C (98.6° F), pulse 84, respirations 20, and blood pressure 110/64. Her assessment reveals the following: 1+ + bilateral pedal edema, no proteinuria, and breath sounds clear to auscultation.

1. What would you include in obtaining a history from Ms. M.?
   a. Previous pregnancy history
   b. Course of heart disease
   c. Prescribed medications
   d. Chest pain or syncope with fatigue
   e. All of the above
2. According to the New York Heart Association Functional Classification of Cardiac Disease, she would be categorized as:
   a. Class I
   b. Class II
   c. Class III
   d. Class IV

Ms. S. is a 21-year-old G1, P0 woman at 20 weeks' gestation. She calls your office at 1 PM with complaints of pain on her right side, fever, chills, nausea, and vomiting.

3. Your recommendation to her is:
   a. Drink plenty of fluids and the physician will call at the end of the day.
   b. Have her come to the office as soon as possible.
   c. Make an appointment first thing the next morning.
   d. Go to the nearest emergency room.
4. The most common cause of pyelonephritis is:
   a. *Klebsiella pneumoniae*
   b. *Proteus mirabilis*
   c. *Escherichia coli*
   d. *Staphylococcus saprophyticus*

5. Pyelonephritis might cause further complications, which include all of the following *except:*
   a. Preterm labor
   b. Renal insufficiency
   c. Septicemia
   d. Chorioamnionitis

Ms. B. is a 28-year-old G1, P0 woman at 6 weeks' gestation, based on her last menstrual period. She presents to the clinic today for a new obstetric visit. She has a history of asthma since childhood and is very concerned about the effect this will have on her baby. She has considered stopping her medications. She is currently under good control and has not had an exacerbation in 4 months. Her vital signs are temperature 37° C (98.6° F), pulse 68, respirations 16, and blood pressure 96/68.

6. Education for Ms. B. should include all of the following *except:*
   a. Well-controlled asthma during pregnancy allows women to continue a normal pregnancy.
   b. Pregnancy has variable effects on the course of asthma.
   c. Most of the commonly used asthma medications are considered safe during pregnancy.
   d. Asthma is not treated aggressively in a pregnant woman.
7. Poorly controlled asthma during pregnancy is associated with an increase in all of the following *except:*
   a. Preterm birth
   b. IUGR
   c. Neonatal hypoxia
   d. Postdate pregnancy

Ms. G. is a G4, P0 woman at 28 weeks' gestation. Her pregnancy history includes two first-trimester and one second-trimester pregnancy losses. She has been diagnosed with antiphospholipid antibody syndrome and is receiving subcutaneous heparin. She is admitted to Labor and Delivery for decreased fetal movement.

8. The most frequent medical problem associated with antiphospholipid antibody syndrome is:
    a. Polyarthritis
    b. Photosensitivity
    c. Malar rash
    d. Arterial or venous thrombosis

9. Patient teaching for Ms. G. should include all of the following *except:*
    a. Signs and symptoms to report, including bleeding and leg pain or edema
    b. The need for 1200 mg of calcium and vitamin D
    c. Antiphospholipid antibody syndrome will not affect all of her pregnancies
    d. The importance of continued daily fetal movement counting

Ms. P. is a 17-year-old primigravida at 28 weeks' gestation. She is in obstetrics triage for preterm labor. Her vital signs are temperature 37° C (98.6° F), pulse 88, respirations 16, and blood pressure 100/64. She has a weight gain this pregnancy of 25 pounds and states she is not very hungry. You notice that she frequently chews ice. Her hemoglobin count is 9.6 g/dL.

10. Which objective information in her history is indicative of iron deficiency anemia?
    a. Temperature of 37° C (98.6° F) and her age
    b. Her age and chewing ice
    c. Poor weight gain and elevated blood pressure
    d. Preterm labor and her poor weight gain

11. What is the best indicator of nutritional status?
    a. Current weight
    b. 24-hour diet recall
    c. Good skin turgor
    d. Ability of patient to eat three meals and two snacks

12. All of the following require long-term follow-up due to the high rate of chronic hepatitis *except:*
    a. Hepatitis A
    b. Hepatitis B
    c. Hepatitis C
    d. Hepatitis D

ANSWERS TO STUDY QUESTIONS

1. e	4. c	7. d	10. b
2. a	5. d	8. d	11. b
3. b	6. d	9. c	12. a

REFERENCES

Airoldi, J., & Berghella, V. (2006). Hepatitis C and pregnancy. *Obstetrical and Gynecological Survey, 61*(10), 666–672.

American Society of Hematology ITP Practice Guideline Panel. (1997). Diagnosis and treatment of idiopathic thrombocytopenic purpura: Recommendations of the American Society of Hematology. *Annals of Internal Medicine, 126*(4), 319–326.

American Thoracic Society and the Centers for Disease Control & Prevention. (1994). Treatment of tuberculosis and tuberculosis infection in adults and children. *American Journal of Respiratory and Critical Care Medicine, 149*(5), 1359–1374.

Arafab, J. M., & McMurtry Baird (2006). Cardiac disease in pregnancy. *Critical Care Nursing Quarterly, 29*(1), 32–52.

Arias, F. (1993). *Practical guide to high-risk pregnancy and delivery* (2nd ed.). St. Louis: Mosby.

Blanchard, D. G., & Shabetai, R. (2009). Cardiac diseases. In R. K. Creasy, R. Resnik, J. D. Iams, C. J. Lockwood, & T. R. Moore (Eds.), *Creasy & Resnik's maternal-fetal medicine: Principles and practice* (6th ed., pp. 797–824). Philadelphia: Saunders.

Cappell, M. (2007). Hepatic and gastrointestinal diseases. In S. Gabbe, J. L. Simpson, J. R. Niebyl, H. Galan, L. Goetzel, E. Jauniaux, & M. Landon (Eds.), *Obstetrics: Normal and problem pregnancies* (5th ed., pp. 1105–1117). Philadelphia: Churchill Livingstone.

Carpenito, L. (1997). *Nursing diagnosis: Application to clinical practice* (7th ed.). Philadelphia: Lippincott Williams & Wilkins.

Centers for Disease Control and Prevention (CDC). (1998). PNSS Health Indicators, Maternal Health Indicators, Anemia. www.cdc.gov/PEDNSS/what_is/pnss_healthindicators.htm.

Cruickshank, D. (1994). Cardiovascular, pulmonary, renal, and hematologic diseases in pregnancy. In R. Scott, P. DiSaia, C. Hammond, & W. Spellacy (Eds.), *Danforth's obstetrics and gynecology* (7th ed., pp. 367–392). Philadelphia: Lippincott Williams & Wilkins.

Cunningham, F. G., Gant, N. F., Leveno, K. J., Gilstrap, L. C., III, Hauth, J. C., & Wenstrom, K. D. (2001). *Williams obstetrics* (21st ed.). New York: McGraw-Hill.

De Swiet, M. (1999). Rheumatologic and connective tissue disorders. In R. K. Creasy, & R. Resnik (Eds.), *Maternal-fetal medicine* (4th ed., pp. 1082–1090). Philadelphia: Saunders.

Dobbenga-Rhodes, Y. A., & Privé, A. M. (2006). *Journal of Perinatal & Neonatal Nursing, 20*(4), 295–302.

Dombrowski, M. P., & Schatz, M. (2008). Asthma in pregnancy. ACOG practice bulletin No. 90. American College of Obstetricians and Gynecologists. *Obstetrics & Gynecology, 111*(2), 457–464.

Freitag-Koontz, M. (1996). Prevention of hepatitis B and C transmission during pregnancy and the first year of life. *Journal of Perinatal & Neonatal Nursing, 10*(2), 40–55.

Gei, A., & Hankins, G. (2001). Cardiac disease in pregnancy. *Obstetrics and Gynecology Clinics of North America, 28*(3), 465–512.

Gilbert, E. S. (2007). *Manual of high risk pregnancy & delivery* (4th ed.). St. Louis: Mosby.

Goodwin, T. M. (2008). Hyperemesis gravidarum. *Obstetrics and Gynecology Clinics of North America, 34*(3), 401–417.

Habel, F. M., & Ravindran, N. C. (2008). Management of inflammatory bowel disease in the pregnant patient. *World Journal of Gastroenterology, 14*(9), 1326–1332.

Heppard, M. C., & Garite, T. J. (2002). *Acute obstetrics* (3rd ed.). St. Louis: Mosby.

Kelly, T. F., & Savides, T. J. (2009). Gastrointestinal disease in pregnancy. In R. K. Creasy, R. Resnik, J. D. Iams, C. J. Lockwood, & T. R. Moore (Eds.), *Creasy & Resnik's maternal-fetal medicine: Principles and practice* (6th ed., pp. 869–884). Philadelphia: Saunders.

Kilpatrick, S. J. (2009). Anemia and pregnancy. In R. K. Creasy, R. Resnik, J. D. Iams, C. J. Lockwood, & T. R. Moore (Eds.), *Creasy & Resnik's maternal-fetal medicine: Principles and practice* (6th ed., pp. 869–884). Philadelphia: Saunders.

Lake, M. F. (2001). Tuberculosis in pregnancy. *AWHONN Lifelines, 5*(5), 35–40.

Laros, R. K. (1999). Thromboembolic disease. In R. K. Creasy, & R. Resnik (Eds.), *Maternal-fetal medicine* (4th ed., pp. 821–831). Philadelphia: Saunders.

Long, P. (1995). Rethinking iron supplementation during pregnancy. *Journal of Nurse-Midwifery, 40*(1), 36–40.

Luskin, A. T., & Lipkowitz, M. A. (2000). The diagnosis and management of asthma during pregnancy. *Immunology and Allergy Clinics of North America, 20*(4), 745–761.

Molad, Y. (2006). Systemic lupus erythematosus and pregnancy. *Current Opinions in Obstetrics and Gynecology, 18*(6), 613–617.

Murdock, M. P. (2002). Asthma in pregnancy. *Journal of Perinatal & Neonatal Nursing, 15*(4), 27–36.

National Asthma Education Program. (1993). *Report of the Working Group on Asthma and Pregnancy. Management of asthma during pregnancy (NIH Publication no. 93-3279A)*. Bethesda, MD: National Institutes of Health.

National Asthma Education and Prevention Program (NAEPP). (2007). *Guidelines for the diagnosis and management of asthma* (NIH Publication No. 97-4051). Bethesda, MD: National Institutes of Health.

National Heart, Lung, and Blood Institute, National Asthma Education and Prevention Program. *Working group report on managing asthma during pregnancy, update 2004.* (NIH Publication No. 05-3279). Internet document available at: wwwnhlbi.gov/health/prof/lung/asthma/astpreg.htm. Retrieved February 14, 2009.

Ramin, S. M., Vidaeff, A. C., Yeomans, E. R., & Gilstrap, L. C. (2006). Chronic renal disease in pregnancy. *Obstetrics & Gynecology, 108*(6), 1531–1539.

Ramsey-Goldman, R. (2001). Connective tissue disorders. In L. Robbins, C. Burckhardt, M. Hannan, & R. De Horatius (Eds.), *Clinical care in the rheumatic diseases* (pp. 97–103). Atlanta: Association of Rheumatology Health Professionals.

Rey, E., & Boulet, L. P. (2007). Asthma in pregnancy. *British Journal of Medicine, 334*(7595), 582–585.

Scott, L. (1999). Gastrointestinal disease in pregnancy. In R. K. Creasy, & R. Resnik (Eds.), *Maternal-fetal medicine* (4th ed., pp. 1038–1053). Philadelphia: Saunders.

Scott, J., & Branch, D. (1999). Immunologic disorders in pregnancy. In J. R. Scott, P. J. DiSaia, C. B. Hammond, & W. N. Spellacy (Eds.), *Danforth's obstetrics and gynecology* (8th ed., pp. 363–391). Philadelphia: Lippincott Williams & Wilkins.

Shabetai, R. (1999). Cardiac diseases. In R. K. Creasy, & R. Resnik (Eds.), *Maternal-fetal medicine* (4th ed., pp. 793–819). Philadelphia: Saunders.

Silver, R., & Branch, D. W. (1999). Immunologic disorders. In R. K. Creasy, & R. Resnik (Eds.), *Maternal-fetal medicine* (4th ed., pp. 465–483). Philadelphia: Saunders.

Simpkins, S., Hench, C., & Bhatia, G. (1996). Management of the obstetric patient with tuberculosis. *Journal of Obstetric, Gynecologic and Neonatal Nursing, 25*(4), 305–312.

Sui, S. C., & Coleman, J. M. (2001). Heart disease and pregnancy. *Heart, 85*, 710–715.

Thorsen, M. S. (2002). Renal disease in pregnancy. *Journal of Perinatal & Neonatal Nursing, 15*(4), 13–26.

Tincani, A., Bazzani, C., Zingarelli, S., & Lojacono, A. (2008). Lupus and the antiphospholipid syndrome in pregnancy and obstetrics: Clinical characteristics, diagnosis, pathogenesis, and treatment. *Seminars in Thrombosis and Hemostasis, 34*(3), 267–273.

Varner, M. (1994). General medical and surgical diseases in pregnancy. In J. Scott, P. DiSaia, C. Hammond, & W. Spellacy (Eds.), *Danforth's obstetrics and gynecology* (7th ed., pp. 427–463). Philadelphia: Lippincott Williams & Wilkins.

Vidaeff, A., Yeomans, E., & Ramin, S. (2008). Pregnancy in women with renal disease Part 1. General principles. *American Journal of Perinatology, 25,* 385–397.

Weinbaum, C., Mast, E., & Ward, J. (2009). Recommendations for identification and public health management of persons with chronic hepatitis B virus infection. *Hepatology, 49*(5 Suppl), 535–544.

Wendel, P. (2001). Asthma in pregnancy. *Obstetrics and Gynecology Clinics of North America, 28*(3), 537–551.

Wenstrom, K., & Malee, M. (1999). Medical and surgical complications of pregnancy. In J. R. Scott, P. J. DiSaia, C. B. Hammond, & W. N. Spellacy (Eds.), *Danforth's obstetrics and gynecology* (8th ed., pp. 327–361). Philadelphia: Lippincott Williams & Wilkins.

Whitty, J. E., & Dombrowski, M. P. (2009). Respiratory diseases of pregnancy. In R. K. Creasy, R. Resnik, J. D. Iams, C. J. Lockwood, & T. R. Moore (Eds.), *Creasy & Resnik's maternal-fetal medicine: Principles and practice* (6th ed., pp. 927–952). Philadelphia: Saunders.

Williams, D. J., & Davidson, J. M. (2009). Renal disorders. In R. K. Creasy, R. Resnik, J. D. Iams, C. J. Lockwood, & T. R. Moore (Eds.), *Creasy & Resnik's maternal-fetal medicine: Principles and practice* (6th ed., pp. 905–926). Philadelphia: Saunders.

Williamson, C., & Mackillop, L. (2009). Diseases of the liver, biliary system, and pancreas. In R. K. Creasy, R. Resnik, J. D. Iams, C. J. Lockwood, & T. R. Moore (Eds.), *Creasy & Resnik's maternal-fetal medicine: Principles and practice* (6th ed., pp. 869–884). Philadelphia: Saunders.

27 Labor and Delivery at Risk

Elizabeth Gilbert

OBJECTIVES

1. Identify factors in a patient's prenatal history that put her at risk for preterm labor.
2. Describe important assessment parameters for patients who are at high risk for preterm labor.
3. Summarize treatments for the patient in preterm labor.
4. Discuss side effects of tocolytic therapy.
5. Describe methods commonly used for pregnancy dating.
6. Define postterm pregnancy.
7. Differentiate between a postterm pregnancy and a postmature infant.
8. Identify early signs and symptoms of chorioamnionitis.
9. List potential complications for the patient with premature rupture of membranes (PROM).
10. Identify risk factors associated with multiple gestation.
11. Describe delivery room preparation and added precautions for a multiple birth.
12. Discuss physical findings that lead to a diagnosis of a stillbirth.
13. Describe the stages of grief.
14. Differentiate between perinatal grief and other grieving responses.
15. Describe possible intervention strategies for delivery management.
16. Explain the pathophysiology of anaphylactoid syndrome of pregnancy.
17. Describe the signs and symptoms that lead to a diagnosis of anaphylactoid syndrome of pregnancy.
18. Discuss the mortality and morbidity associated with anaphylactoid syndrome of pregnancy.
19. Identify patients at high risk for uterine rupture.
20. Discuss life-threatening complications that may result from uterine rupture.
21. Classify the types of uterine rupture.
22. Rank emergency actions in order of priority for a patient presenting with traumatic uterine rupture.

PRETERM LABOR

INTRODUCTION

A. Preterm labor is defined as regular uterine contractions and cervical dilation before completion of the 36th week of gestation.
B. Certain factors are associated with a high incidence of preterm labor; recurrent preterm labor is related to a short cervix, bacterial infection, or short interval between pregnancies; bacterial infection accounts for 25% to 40% of all preterm births because endotoxins have a preinflammatory effect and stimulate prostaglandin production. Other factors are stress, uterine anomalies or cervical trauma; uterine stretch caused by multiple gestation or polyhydramnios; smoking, drug, or alcohol use; and maternal age extremes or low socioeconomic and educational status or an uncontrolled medical condition.
C. Preterm labor has increased in the past few years in spite of all the efforts to identify patients at risk and provide patient education. Therefore, the focus is shifting to prophylactic treatment for at risk patients.

CLINICAL PRACTICE

A. Assessment

1. History

   a. Signs and symptoms of uterine contractions, low back pain, menstrual-like cramps, or pelvic pressure

   b. Increased vaginal discharge or bloody show

   c. Presence of risk factors associated with spontaneous preterm labor, accounting for 75% of cases (Ananth & Vintzileos, 2006; Morken, Kallen, & Jacobsson, 2007)

      (1) Prior preterm birth

      (2) Preterm premature rupture of the membranes (PPROM)

      (3) Bacterial infections including mycoplasma of the genital track, pyelonephritis, asymptomatic bacteriuria, and pneumonia (Goldenberg, Culhane, & Johnson, 2005)

      (4) Uterine stretch caused by hydramnios and multiple gestation

      (5) Uterine anomalies (Zlopasa, Skrablin, & Kalafatic, 2007)

      (6) Stress (Dole et al, 2003)

      (7) Drug or alcohol use (Behrman & Stith, 2007)

      (8) Low socioeconomic and educational status (Smith, Draper, Manktelow, Dorling, & Field, 2007; Thompson, Irgens, Rasmussen, & Daltveit, 2006)

      (9) African American (Behrman & Stith, 2007)

      (10) Trauma including domestic violence

      (11) Maternal age extremes (younger than 16 or older than 40 years) (Smith et al, 2007; Thompson et al, 2006)

      (12) Cervical injury from an elective abortion (Virk, Zhang, & Olsen, 2007) or prior cervical surgery (Jakobsson, Gissler, Sainio, Paavonen, & Tapper, 2007; Nohr, Tabor, Frederiksen, & Kjaer, 2007; Sjoborg et al, 2007)

   d. Presence of risk factors associated with indicated preterm labor, accounting for 25% of cases

      (1) Placental hemorrhage

      (2) Hypertensive disorders of pregnancy

      (3) Inadequate control of diabetes

      (4) Poor nutrition as measured by low body mass index (Hendler et al, 2005)

      (5) Smoking (Cnattingius, 2004; Nabet, Lelong, Ancel, Saurel-Cubizolles, & Kaminski, 2007; Tikkanen, Nuutila, Hiilesmaa, Paavonen, & Yikorkala, 2006)

      (6) Fetal anomalies

2. Physical findings

   a. Uterine contractions (painful or painless) palpable or evident on external fetal monitor

   b. Cervical changes: softening, effacement, dilation, or shortening of cervical length

   c. Engagement of fetal presenting part

   d. Fetal heart rate (FHR): tachycardia (may indicate maternal infection)

   e. Elevated temperature or tachycardia (may indicate dehydration or infection)

   f. Costovertebral angle (CVA) tenderness

   g. Evidence of nitrites, leukocytes or white blood cells (WBCs), and/or red blood cells (RBCs) in urine

3. Risk screening for preterm birth

   a. Presence of fetal fibronectin in cervicovaginal secretions; fibronectin is a glycoprotein that adheres the maternal decidua to the fetal membranes; when uterine contractions are stimulated the adherence is disrupted and fetal fibronectin is released indicating a risk of preterm delivery

   b. Cervical length is measured, preferably with transvaginal ultrasound (TVU) (Burwick, Lee, Benedict, Ross, & Kjos, 2009; Matijevic, Grgic, & Vasili, 2006; Owen, 2003; Romero, 2007) or U.S. Food and Drug Administration (FDA)–approved CervilLenz cervical length measuring device (Ross et al, 2007) because the risk of preterm delivery increases as the cervical length in the second trimester declines.

   c. Clinical markers of an inflammatory cascade resulting from an ascending genital tract infection or a systemic infection such as pyelonephritis, asymptomatic bacteriuria, or pneumonia may indicate a risk for preterm labor; bacterial vaginitis is an example of a clinical marker of preterm labor because its presence correlates with an increased risk of preterm birth, but treatment and eradication do not decrease its risk; periodontal disease may be another marker (Klebanoff & Searle, 2006).

    4. Diagnostic procedures of related risk factors

        a. Complete blood count (CBC): elevated WBC count may indicate infection (WBC count is normally elevated in pregnancy and in labor, but a WBC count greater than 18,000 is considered significant for infection)

        b. Urinalysis: Note presence of WBCs, RBCs, bacteria, nitrites, or leukocytes.

        c. Urine culture and sensitivity testing

        d. Amniotic fluid

            (1) Gram stain

            (2) Culture and sensitivity

            (3) Amniotic fluid for lecithin-sphingomyelin (L/S) ratio to assess fetal lung maturity

        e. Cervical cultures

            (1) Group B streptococcus (GBS)

        f. Wet mount; assess for bacterial vaginosis or trichomonas vaginalis

        g. Ultrasound examination to assess:

            (1) Gestational age

            (2) Presenting part

            (3) Cervical length

            (4) Multiple gestation

            (5) Placenta location

            (6) Evidence of fetal or uterine anomalies

            (7) Amniotic fluid volume

B. Interventions to prevent preterm labor

    1. Interventions indicated by research reviews that decrease the risk of preterm labor are:

        a. Smoking cessation program (Lumley, Oliver, Chamberlain, & Oakley, 2004)

        b. Routine screening and treatment for asymptomatic bacteriuria (Smaill & Vasquez, 2007)

        c. Use of a laminaria for women undergoing second-trimester dilation and evacuation (Kalish, Chasen, Rosenzweig, Rashbaum, & Chervenak, 2002)

        d. Preconception medical management of medical conditions such as diabetes, seizures, asthma, or hypertension (Haas et al, 2005)

    2. Interventions once thought to lower the risk of preterm labor but not proven by research

        a. Early access to care (Healy, Fergal, Malone, & Sullivan, 2006)

        b. Nutritional supplements such as protein (Kramer & Kakuma, 2003), calcium (Hofmeyr, Atallah, & Duley, 2006), and vitamins C and E (Rumbold et al, 2006)

        c. Periodontal care (Michalowicz et al, 2006)

        d. Routine screening and treatment of bacterial vaginosis (BV) (Centers for Disease Control and Prevention [CDC], 2006)

C. Intervention for women at risk for preterm labor

    1. Progestational supplementation: Current research indicates that progesterone vaginal gel or cream may be beneficial in reducing preterm labor by 40%, especially in women with a history of preterm birth and a short cervical length verified by vaginal ultrasound (DeFranco et al, 2007; Dodd, Flenady, Cincotta, & Crowther, 2006; Farine et al, 2008; Fonseca, Celik, Parra, Singh, & Nicolaides, 2007; Romero, 2007; Weiner & Buhimschi, 2009).

        a. Physiologic benefits of progesterone (Sfakianaki & Norwitz, 2006)

            (1) Reduces gap junction formation in the uterus

            (2) Antagonizes oxytocin receptors

            (3) Maintains cervical integrity

            (4) Antiinflammatory

        b. Contraindications (Weiner & Buhimschi, 2009)

            (1) Peanut allergy

            (2) Thromboembolism

    2. Screen and treat at risk women for BV

D. Interventions to treat preterm labor

    1. Treat presence of bacterial infections such as pyelonephritis, asymptomatic bacteriuria, and pneumonia.

    2. Hydrate patient with oral (PO) or intravenous (IV) fluids (uterine contractions or irritability may result from dehydration).

    3. Monitor intake and output (I&O); avoid volume overload.

    4. Monitor maternal vital signs.

5. Continuous external fetal monitoring for:
   a. FHR pattern
   b. Frequency, duration, and approximate intensity of uterine contractions
6. Palpate patient's abdomen to assess strength of uterine contractions.
7. Administer tocolytic therapy as ordered to delay delivery long enough to administer therapy.
   a. Corticosteroids to treat fetal lung maturity
   b. Complete maternal transport to a Level III center prior to delivery.
   c. Treat with antibiotics to prevent neonatal GBS infection
8. Type of tocolytic therapy
   a. No medication has been identified to effectively stop preterm labor.
   b. No one drug is approved in the United States or has been proven superior as a tocolytic agent. Medication selection is individualized based on efficacy, risks, and side effects.
   c. The following drugs are used as tocolytics per FDA as "off-label" use.
      (1) Nifedipine: calcium channel blocker that works primarily by blocking the flow of calcium ions through the cell membrane, thereby decreasing the activation of smooth muscle contractile proteins. According to a Cochrane Review (King, Flenady, Papatsonis, Dekker, & Carbonne, 2003) and several meta-analyses (Weiner & Buhimschi, 2009), nifedipine can delay delivery by 2 to 7 days and has a favorable ratio of risk-to-benefit related to decreased adverse side effects. Also, nifedipine is more cost-effective than terbutaline or magnesium sulfate (Weiner & Buhimschi, 2009).
         (a) Dosage and administration
            [i] Initial loading dose: 10 to 40 mg PO, followed by 30 to 60 mg of a long-acting preparation PO every 8 to 12 hours for maximum of 48 hours
         (b) Side effects: usually mild, less common with long-acting preparations
            [i] Insignificant decrease in blood pressure (no change in heart rate)
            [ii] Facial flushing
            [iii] Headache
            [iv] Nausea
            [v] Dizziness
            [vi] Fetal effects: minimal randomized, controlled studies at this time; however, clinical evidence indicates beneficial effects of decreased respiratory distress syndrome (RDS), intracranial bleeding, and neonatal jaundice
         (c) If nifedipine is given with magnesium sulfate or erythromycin, sudden cardiac arrest can occur (Weiner & Buhimschi, 2009).
         (d) Contraindicated in the presence of an intrauterine infection, maternal hypertension, or cardiac disease
      (2) Indomethacin: prostaglandin synthetase inhibitor; a Cochrane Review concludes that indomethacin significantly reduces contractions for 48 to 72 hours but has greater adverse fetal effects following 1 week of use as compared to nifedipine (King, Flenady, Cole, & Thornton, 2005). Both nifedipine and indomethacin are more cost-effective then terbutaline or magnesium sulfate (Weiner & Buhimschi, 2009).
         (a) Dosage and administration
            [i] Initial dose: 50 mg PO; then 25 mg PO every 6 hours for 2 days maximum
         (b) Side effects
            [i] Maternal: increased bleeding time; potential to exacerbate hypertensive disorders
            [ii] Fetal: after 1 week or more exposure, oligohydramnios, premature closure of the ductus arteriosus, increased risk of necrotizing enterocolitis (NEC), increased risk of intraventricular hemorrhage (IVH) and renal dysfunction
         (c) Contraindications (maternal)
            [i] If labor is imminent within 24 hours, the initial 50-mg dose may prolong maternal bleeding time.
            [ii] Poorly controlled maternal hypertension
            [iii] Asthma
            [iv] Renal disease
            [v] Active peptic ulcer disease

        [vi]   Vaginal bleeding
        [vii] Coagulation disorder
        [viii] Liver disease
    (d) Contraindications (fetal)
        [i]   Intrauterine growth restriction (IUGR)
        [ii]   Oligohydramnios
        [iii] Chorioamnionitis
        [iv] Ductal dependent cardiac defect
        [v]   Twin-twin transfusion syndrome

(3) Terbutaline sulfate: beta-adrenergic agonist; a Cochrane Review concludes that beta-mimetic drugs can delay delivery by 48 hours but have greater maternal side effects than other tocolytic agents. Its long-term use is not supported (Anotayanonth, Subhedar, Neilson, & Harigopal, 2004).

    (a) Dosage and administration
        [i]   Subcutaneous (SC) dosage: 0.25 mg times one to arrest contractions to facilitate maternal transport or initiate tocolysis while another agent with a slower onset of action is started.

    (b) Side effects
        [i]   Tachycardia
        [ii]   Nervousness
        [iii] Tremors
        [iv] Nasal congestion
        [v]   Headache
        [vi] Nausea and vomiting
        [vii] Hyperglycemia
        [viii] Decrease in serum potassium level
        [ix] Palpitations
        [x]   Cardiac dysrhythmias
        [xi] Pulmonary edema

    (c) Contraindications
        [i]   Placental abruption
        [ii]   Chorioamnionitis
        [iii] Pre-viable gestation
        [iv] Fetal demise
        [v]   Fetal anomalies incompatible with life

    (d) Relative contraindications
        [i]   Maternal diabetes
        [ii]   Severe preeclampsia
        [iii] IUGR
        [iv] Maternal cardiac disease
        [v]   Hyperthyroidism
        [vi] History of migraine headaches

    (e) Nursing actions
        [i]   Baseline electrocardiogram (ECG) is recommended.
        [ii]   Monitor pulse rate: Hold medication for resting pulse rate greater than 120 beats per minute (bpm).

(4) Magnesium sulfate ($MgSO_4$): relaxes smooth muscle by competing with calcium at the motor end plate (reducing the release of acetylcholine) or at the cell membrane decreasing calcium influx into the cell. A Cochrane Review concludes that magnesium sulfate has limited effect as a tocolytic agent, with severe risk factors such as pulmonary edema and cardiovascular problems (Crowther, Hiller, & Doyle, 2002). However, research indicates that magnesium sulfate may have a neuroprotective benefit, protecting the brain of the very preterm infant by possibly reducing the risk of cerebral palsy (Marret et al, 2007; Rouse et al, 2008).

    (a) Dosage and administration
        [i]   Loading dose: 4 to 6 g/hr IV piggyback (IVPB) over 20 to 30 minutes
        [ii]   Maintenance dose: 1 to 3 g/hr IVPB
        [iii] Medication should be administered by infusion pump.

(b) Side effects
- [i] Sweating
- [ii] Flushing
- [iii] Nausea and vomiting
- [iv] Depressed deep tendon reflexes (DTRs)
- [v] Flaccid paralysis
- [vi] Hypocalcemia
- [vii] Depressed cardiac function
- [viii] Respiratory depression

(c) Nursing actions
- [i] Monitor vital signs.
- [ii] Monitor DTRs (generally graded on a scale of 0 to 4)
  - 4+: very brisk, hyperactive; associated with clonus (clonus is the series of rhythmic contractions or convulsive movements of the ankle when the foot is sharply dorsiflexed; it is measured in beats [e.g., "two beats of clonus"])
  - 3+: brisker than average
  - 2+: average; normal reflex response
  - 1+: diminished
  - 0: absent (Seidel, Ball, Dains, & Benedict, 2006)
  - The patellar tendon is most commonly used to assess reflexes because it is easiest to elicit, but biceps or triceps reflexes may also be used.
- [iii] Monitor serum magnesium levels.
  - Although laboratory values may vary slightly from one institution to another, approximate values are as follows:
    - ○ 4 to 7 mEq/L = therapeutic
    - ○ 10 mEq/L = loss of DTRs
    - ○ 15 mEq/L = respiratory depression
    - ○ 25 mEq/L = cardiac arrest
  - Discontinue magnesium sulfate in the presence of elevated serum levels or of signs and symptoms of central nervous system (CNS) or cardiovascular depression.
  - Be prepared to administer antidote (calcium gluconate) if necessary.

9. Interventions related to unknown pregnancy outcome
   a. Encourage patient to verbalize her feelings and assist her in identifying specific concerns.
   b. Provide realistic information about preterm labor and delivery.
   c. Provide information about premature infants; be as detailed as possible, giving information related to her specific gestational age. (See Chapter 17 for complete discussion.)
   d. Visit neonatal intensive care unit (NICU) with patient to familiarize her with that environment.
   e. Allow patient and family to participate in plan of care whenever possible.

HEALTH EDUCATION

A. **Teach patient to recognize signs and symptoms of preterm labor.**
   1. Uterine contractions, cramping, and low back pain
   2. Feeling of pelvic pressure or fullness
   3. Change in amount or character of vaginal discharge
   4. Bloody show; discharge of mucus plug
   5. GI upset: nausea, vomiting, and diarrhea
   6. General sense of discomfort or unease

B. **Teach patient how to palpate uterine contractions.**
   1. Tell patient to sit up from a reclining position and to palpate her abdomen immediately. (This action will usually induce a uterine contraction.)
   2. Patient may also palpate the sensation of a muscular contraction by placing her hand over her biceps and flexing her arm.

3. Describe contraction intensity; compare the feeling of firmness to the following:
   a. Tip of nose: mild
   b. Tip of chin: moderate
   c. Forehead: strong
4. If any preterm labor symptoms occur, teach patient to:
   a. Empty bladder.
   b. Lie down on side.
   c. Drink two to three glasses of fluid.
   d. Palpate for uterine contractions.
   e. Notify her health care provider if symptoms persist or she experiences four or more contractions in 1 hour.
C. **Review timing of contractions with the patient; time contractions from onset to onset.**
D. **Patient should call health care provider or go to the hospital if contractions are coming regularly.**
E. **Discuss treatment routines with the patient.**
   1. Try bedrest in the lateral position. (Mild uterine activity may subside with increased uterine blood flow.)
   2. Maintain adequate hydration. (Uterine activity or irritability may result from dehydration.)
   3. If uterine activity persists, the patient should call her health care provider or go to the hospital for further evaluation; hospitalization for IV tocolytic therapy may be required.

POSTTERM PREGNANCY

INTRODUCTION

A. **Definitions**
   1. Term pregnancy: 37 to 42 completed weeks from the last menses or 35 to 40 weeks from the time of conception
   2. Posterm pregnancy (prolonged pregnancy): exceeds 42 completed weeks of menstrual age
   3. Postmaturity: a diagnosis that cannot be made in the antepartal period but is made by recognizable clinical findings in the infant that are associated with dysmaturity
B. **Decreased amniotic fluid after 42 weeks' gestation is the most frequently associated factor, reducing the cushioning effect and increasing the risk for umbilical cord compression.**

CLINICAL PRACTICE

A. **Assessment**
   1. History: pregnancy dating
      a. Nägele's rule: Add 7 days to the first day of the last menstrual period (LMP), count back 3 months, and adjust year (assumes regular 28-day menstrual cycle).
      b. Timing of positive pregnancy test result
      c. Timing of quickening
      d. When fetal heart rate can be auscultated
      e. Ultrasound examination provides a more accurate gestational age date; by measuring crown-rump length (CRL), fetal biparietal diameter, femur length, abdominal circumference, or chest circumference; or by using a formula involving the ratio of these values; ultrasound dating is most accurate when done in the first trimester of pregnancy using the CRL (see Chapter 8 for complete discussion of antepartum testing).
   2. Physical findings
      a. Gestational age by ultrasound examination
      b. Fundal height
         (1) Measurement from symphysis pubis to top of fundus correlates approximately with the number of weeks of gestation (e.g., 28 cm indicates approximately 28 weeks' gestation).
         (2) If fetal presenting part is engaged, the fundal height is less accurate.
      c. Decreased amniotic fluid volume (AFV) occurs most commonly and can cause fetal distress related to cord compression.
      d. Macrosomia, another common finding, can lead to shoulder dystocia and birth trauma.

      e. Dysmaturity syndrome in response to uteroplacental insufficiency occurs in only 1% to 2% of the cases and is characterized by (see Chapter 17 for complete discussion):

        (1) Long, lean bodies

        (2) Long fingernails

        (3) Abundant hair growth

        (4) Parchment-like skin (dry, peeling)

      f. Higher incidence of meconium aspiration and asphyxia

    3. Psychosocial findings

      a. Stress factors

        (1) Anxiety

        (2) Fear of unknown: Expectations of delivery by estimated date of confinement (EDC) have not been fulfilled.

      b. Behavioral response: impatience with normal discomforts of pregnancy

    4. Antepartum fetal surveillance testing (see Chapter 8 on antepartum testing)

      a. Biophysical profile (BPP)

      b. Nonstress test (NST)

      c. Amniotic fluid volume or index (AFV or AFI)

      d. Fetal movement counts (FMC)

      e. Contraction stress test (CST) (seldom used today)

B. Interventions: Antepartum

    1. Antepartum intervention is still controversial.

    2. According to the Cochrane Review, there is no conclusive evidence that one protocol affords greater benefit or greater risk to low-risk patients (Gulmezoglu, Crowther, & Middleton, 2006).

    3. According to the Society of Obstetricians and Gynaecologists of Canada (SOGC) clinical practice guideline, women should be offered induction at 41 to 42 weeks' gestation (SOGC, 2008).

    4. If expectant management is chosen by the patient, antepartum fetal surveillance should be used. BPP or a modification of BPP such as NST and AFI is preferred (Resnik & Resnik, 2009; SOGC, 2008).

    5. Fetal membrane sweeping has been shown to reduce the number of pregnancies exceeding 41-plus weeks by increasing production of prostaglandins (Boulvain & Irion, 2004). Risks of the procedure are discomfort at the time of the procedure and bleeding.

    6. Prostaglandin gel may be used for cervical ripening.

      a. Explain methods of induction to patient.

      b. Discuss indications and risks.

      c. Assist with insertion of prostaglandin gel intracervically.

      d. Continuous fetal monitoring should be performed after patient receives prostaglandin gel to observe for uterine contractions and to monitor FHR pattern.

C. Interventions: Intrapartum

    1. Perform continuous fetal monitoring during labor and delivery.

    2. Maintain patient in the lateral position as much as possible to maximize placental blood flow.

    3. Keep patient well hydrated to maximize placental perfusion.

    4. Administer amnioinfusion to relieve repetitive deep variable decelerations secondary to low fluid volume. However, amnioinfusion is not beneficial for the treatment of meconium-staining as was once thought (Fraser et al, 2005).

HEALTH EDUCATION

A. Define terms of normal gestation.

B. Explain function of amniotic fluid.

    1. Delivery of oxygen

    2. Cushioning effect to umbilical cord

    3. Normal levels at term 800 to 1000 mL

    4. Gradual decreasing levels after 40 weeks

C. Explain function of placenta.

    1. Delivery of oxygen and gas exchange

    2. Delivery of nutrients for fetal growth

    3. Efficiency may decrease after 40th week.

D. **Review fetal growth and development.**
  1. Organ development and maturation are complete by the 36th week.
  2. Last 4 weeks of gestation are primarily for weight gain. (See Chapter 17 for a complete discussion of late preterm infant.)
  3. Vernix caseosa, the oily substance that protects the fetal skin in utero, begins to disappear after the 36th week, making the infant's skin appear dry and peeling.
E. **Discuss physiology of labor.**
  1. Precise mechanism for initiation of labor is unknown.
  2. Cervix may require ripening with prostaglandin gel.
    a. Gel is inserted intracervically to induce softening and effacement.
    b. Continuous fetal monitoring is recommended after the insertion of prostaglandin gel because it may induce uterine contractions; assess for uterine activity and FHR patterns.
  3. Induction or augmentation of labor may be necessary and is commonly done with oxytocin (Pitocin); it should not be done without continuous FHR monitoring.
F. **Discuss effect of postterm pregnancy on the fetus.**
  1. Meconium passage into the amniotic fluid occurs with higher frequency in postterm pregnancy.
  2. Meconium aspiration at delivery causes a chemical pneumonitis and alveolar obstruction in newborn lungs.
    a. Infant will be aggressively suctioned at delivery.
    b. Infant will most likely be intubated and suctioned after delivery to make every attempt to avoid aspiration of meconium into lungs.
    c. Oligohydramnios further complicates meconium aspiration related to the consistency of the meconium.

PREMATURE RUPTURE OF MEMBRANES

INTRODUCTION

A. **Premature rupture of membranes (PROM) refers to the spontaneous rupture of the amniotic membrane before the onset of labor; this may occur at or before term.**
B. **Gestational age usually determines the plan and intervention.**
C. **The patient at or near term generally benefits from expedited delivery if fetal pulmonary maturity is documented; patients with PROM remote from term are at much greater risk for increased neonatal morbidity related to gestational age.**
D. **Induction or augmentation of labor may be necessary.**
E. **For the purpose of this section, PROM refers to the rupture of membranes (ROM) before term; often called preterm PROM.**
F. **Strong clinical evidence links PROM to intrauterine infection; clinical trials with antibiotic therapy have demonstrated a delay in the onset of infection, as well as a delay in delivery, decreased postpartum maternal endometritis, and decreased infant morbidity related to sepsis, pneumonia, and RDS.**

CLINICAL PRACTICE

A. **Assessment**
  1. History
    a. Gestational age
      (1) By last normal menstrual period (LNMP)
      (2) By ultrasound dating
    b. Date and time of ROM
    c. Associated labor symptoms, cramping, or feeling of pelvic pressure or back pain
    d. Any event that immediately preceded ROM (e.g., trauma)
    e. History of urinary tract infections (UTIs): signs and symptoms of urinary frequency, urgency, dysuria, or flank pain
    f. History of vaginal or pelvic infection; signs and symptoms of change in vaginal discharge; pelvic pain
    g. Nutritional status

    2. Physical findings
        a. Sterile speculum examination findings
            (1) Evidence of fluid pooling in vaginal vault
            (2) Nitrazine test result positive
            (3) Ferning positive
            (4) Appearance of cervix
            (5) Any discharge
            (6) Inflammation or lesions
            (7) Protrusion of membranes
            (8) Presenting part visible
            (9) Umbilical cord prolapse
        b. Amount, color, and consistency of fluid
            (1) Odor
            (2) Presence of vernix, blood, or meconium in fluid
        c. Vital signs: Elevated temperature or tachycardia may indicate presence of infection.
        d. CBC: Elevated WBC count greater than 18,000 may indicate presence of infection.
        e. External fetal monitoring
            (1) Uterine contractions
            (2) Uterine irritability
            (3) FHR tachycardia: may be an early indication of infection
   3. Psychosocial findings
        a. Stress factors
            (1) Anxiety
            (2) Fear of pregnancy loss
            (3) Feeling unprepared for delivery
            (4) Guilt
        b. Behavioral factors
            (1) Difficulty communicating
            (2) Expression of fears
            (3) Coping mechanisms
   4. Diagnosis confirmed
        a. Sterile speculum vaginal examination to check for evidence of fluid pooling in the posterior fornix
        b. Nitrazine test: paper turns blue in the presence of amniotic fluid (alkaline); however, false-positive results are common in the presence of alkaline antiseptics, bacterial vaginosis, or blood or semen contamination.
        c. Ferning: Amniotic fluid on a slide crystallizes into a characteristic fern pattern as it dries, which can be readily identified under a microscope.
        d. AFV: as measured by ultrasound examination, AFV may help to confirm a questionable diagnosis of ROM (decreased if membranes are ruptured).
   5. Rule out infection
        a. Amniocentesis to obtain amniotic fluid for:
            (1) Gram stain and glucose levels: positive result indicates infection.
            (2) Culture and sensitivity testing to identify specific organisms
        b. WBC count and C-reactive protein
   6. Fetal maturity studies
        a. Collect amniotic fluid from the vaginal pool; if phosphatidylglycerol (PG) is found in the pooled fluid, provides considerable reassurance of fetal pulmonary maturity.
        b. Collect amniotic fluid through amniocentesis; L/S ratio 2:1 or greater indicates fetal pulmonary maturity in a nondiabetic woman.
        c. If tests indicate fetal pulmonary maturity, delivery should be considered.
B. Interventions
   1. Risk for infection related to break in amniotic membrane barrier and proximity to vaginal and enteric flora
        a. Monitor maternal vital signs: elevated temperature or increased pulse rate may indicate infection.
        b. Monitor CBC values: Elevation in WBC count (greater than 18,000) may indicate infection.
        c. Observe amniotic fluid for purulence or odor.

      d. Observe vaginal discharge: purulence or foul odor may indicate infection.

      e. Monitor FHR: Observe for fetal tachycardia, which may develop with maternal infection.

      f. Monitor uterine activity; note contractions or uterine irritability.

      g. Palpate abdomen to assess for uterine tenderness.

      h. Do not perform any vaginal examinations.

      i. Administer antibiotics as ordered.

2. Risk for fetal compromise or neonatal RDS or infection

      a. Initiate bedrest with FHR monitoring.

        (1) Recommend continuous fetal monitoring for the first 48 hours.

        (2) Follow with bedrest with fetal heart check every 4 hours and fetal well-being studies such as NST, AFV, BPP, and ultrasound studies.

      b. Evaluate fetal presenting part by Leopold's maneuvers or ultrasound examination.

        (1) Nonvertex presentations are at higher risk for umbilical cord prolapse.

        (2) Patient with nonvertex presentations may be put in a slight Trendelenburg position to decrease the chance of umbilical cord prolapse.

        (3) Observe for evidence of cord compression: variable decelerations visible on fetal monitor

        (4) If severe variables are observed, amnioinfusion may be ordered according to institutional protocol.

      c. Antenatal corticosteroids for preterm PROM in the absence of intraamniotic infection to decrease neonatal respiratory distress and intraventricular hemorrhage

      d. Intrapartum antibiotic prophylaxis if group B streptococcus (GBS) positive or in the presence of ROM for 18 hours or more, with GBS status unknown

3. Fear of possible preterm delivery

      a. Provide patient with as much information as possible about PROM.

      b. Discuss fetal growth and development, and focus on gestational age of this fetus.

      c. Visit NICU if possible to prepare patient for intensive care environment.

      d. Include patient in plan of care and decision-making whenever possible.

      e. Encourage verbalization of patient's feelings and help her identify specific concerns.

      f. Identify coping mechanisms most helpful during times of stress.

      g. Identify patient's support system.

      h. Contact social service if necessary to assist patient.

4. Effective therapeutic regimen management related to PROM

      a. Review anatomy and physiology with patient; describe fetal membranes.

      b. Discuss potential complications and their treatments.

        (1) Development of infection usually necessitates delivery.

        (2) FHR variable decelerations warrant continuous fetal monitoring, possible amnioinfusion, and possible delivery for fetal distress.

        (3) Prolapse of umbilical cord requires emergency cesarean section.

        (4) Developmental anomalies such as skeletal compression deformities, amniotic band syndrome, and pulmonary hypoplasia can result if PROM occurs before 26 to 28 weeks' gestation.

HEALTH EDUCATION

A. **Review anatomy and physiology of pregnancy.**

  1. Enlarging uterus: appropriate for gestational age

  2. Function of placenta: to provide oxygen and nutrients to the fetus

  3. Umbilical cord: attaches fetal placental unit to mother

  4. Fetal membranes

      a. Provide protective barrier to fetus

      b. Contain amniotic fluid to provide cushioning and flotation for fetus

      c. Eliminate compression of any fetal part, including the umbilical cord

B. **Review fetal growth and development.**

  1. Use growth charts to give patient a realistic idea of fetal size.

  2. Focus on key landmarks of fetal development.

      a. 28 weeks: fetal anatomic development complete; maturity needed

      b. 34 weeks: approaching pulmonary maturity

   3. Discuss care in the NICU.

C. Teach patient signs and symptoms of infection; instruct her to report any of the following symptoms:

   1. Elevated temperature

   2. Foul-smelling amniotic fluid

   3. Significant increase in vaginal discharge

   4. Abdominal pain or tenderness

   5. Onset of uterine contractions

D. Instruct patient to go to the hospital immediately for decreased fetal movement or prolapse of umbilical cord; explain significance of each and the need for emergency cesarean section.

MULTIPLE GESTATION

INTRODUCTION

A. Multiple-gestation pregnancies are more common now because of the increased use of assisted reproductive technology (ART) such as in vitro fertilization (IVF) and embryo transfers, and increasing maternal age.

B. Approximately 3% of all live births in the US are multiples (Martin et al, 2007). **The majority of multiples are twins and approximately one fourth of twins are monozygotic, and two thirds are dizygotic (resulting from the fertilization of two eggs).**

C. Pregnancy risk factors, such as discordant growth and twin-to-twin transfusion syndromes, arise from carrying more than one fetus who share the placenta.

D. The patient with a multiple gestation is also at higher risk for many of the complications of pregnancy such as preterm labor, IUGR, preeclampsia, and antepartum hemorrhage.

E. In the United States, the mean gestational age at delivery is 35 weeks for twin gestations, 32 weeks for triplets, and 29 weeks for quadruplets (Martin et al, 2007).

CLINICAL PRACTICE

A. Assessment

   1. History

      a. Pregnancy dating: Diagnosis is often preceded by the observation that size is greater than dates.

      b. Fertility enhancement: use of ovulation-stimulating drugs or other assisted reproductive technologies

      c. Family history of multiples

   2. Physical findings

      a. Fundal height measurement greater than number of weeks of gestation

      b. Leopold's maneuvers may distinguish more than one fetus.

      c. Auscultation of more than one fetal heartbeat

      d. Ultrasound examination gives evidence of more than one fetus or gestational sac.

      e. Laboratory data

         (1) Beta–human chorionic gonadotropin (hCG) greatly elevated

         (2) Other placental hormones such as progesterone, estradiol, estriol, and human chorionic somatomammotropin (hCS) (formerly human placental lactogen [HPL]) significantly elevated

         (3) Maternal serum alpha-fetoprotein (MSAFP) elevated

      f. Once the diagnosis of multiple gestation is made, the patient should be considered as high risk; assessment for pregnancy complications should include the following:

         (1) Congenital anomalies

         (2) Preterm labor

         (3) Preterm PROM

         (4) IUGR

        (5) Maternal anemia

        (6) Preeclampsia

        (7) Gestational diabetes

        (8) Acute fatty liver disease of pregnancy

        (9) Antepartum hemorrhage, such as abruptio placentae

      (10) Stillbirth

   g. Assessment for complications specific to multiple gestation

        (1) Discordant growth

        (2) Twin-to-twin transfusion syndrome

        (3) Vanishing twin syndrome; the prognosis for the remaining twin is good

  3. Psychosocial responses

   a. Stress factors

        (1) Fear related to high-risk pregnancy

        (2) Fear of pregnancy loss

        (3) Anxiety related to parenting more than one infant

   b. Behavioral factors

        (1) Fear of upcoming events

        (2) Compulsiveness in preparing for children

  4. Diagnostic procedures

   a. Ultrasound examination

        (1) Most reliable test for making diagnosis

        (2) Can identify separate placenta sites, dividing membranes, relationship, and gender

        (3) Assessment of congenital anomalies

        (4) Serial ultrasound scans to follow fetal growth curves

        (5) Used to estimate fetal weight and to diagnose discordance

        (6) Assessment of AFV: hydramnios more common in multiple-gestation pregnancies

   b. Amniocentesis to diagnose chromosomal anomalies

   c. Antepartum surveillance for early detection of risks

        (1) NST and AFI

        (2) CST

        (3) BPP

B. Antepartum interventions

  1. Increase patient's caloric intake, folic acid, iron, calcium, magnesium, and zinc to support growth and development of multiple fetuses.

  2. Provide nutritional consultation to evaluate specific dietary needs and assist patient in planning to meet these needs.

  3. Monitor hemoglobin levels and hematocrit for maternal anemia.

  4. Discuss importance of additional rest; ideally in 1- to 2-hour segments in the morning, afternoon, and evening.

  5. Explain reasons for risk factors to patient.

   a. Increased placental demands for two or more developing fetuses

   b. Overdistention of uterus, which may lead to uterine irritability or premature contractions

  6. List signs and symptoms of which the patient should be aware, and report immediately.

  7. Prepare patient for various fetal assessments.

  8. Visit NICU before births if possible to prepare patient for intensive care environment.

  9. Encourage verbalization and assist patient in identifying specific concerns.

 10. Assist patient in identifying support system and other resources available.

C. Intrapartum interventions

  1. Review delivery room practices and added precautions for multiple infants.

   a. On admission, an IV line is placed for administering fluids and treatment in the event of hemorrhage or the need for emergency delivery and anesthesia.

   b. Continuous or simultaneous FHR monitoring

   c. Ultrasound scan on admission to assess the presentation and estimated fetal weight of each infant

   d. Double set-up: having equipment for cesarean section available and ready in the room at the time of delivery

   e. Extra personnel are likely to be present at delivery to attend to needs of each newborn (especially if preterm).

2. Mode of delivery for twins is usually based on fetal presentation as well as medical indications
   a. For vertex-vertex presentations, vaginal delivery regardless of gestational age is supported by research (Cruikshank, 2007; Hogle, Hutton, McBrien, Barrett, & Hannah, 2003).
   b. For vertex-nonvertex presentations, mode of delivery is based on obstetric experience, size of the second twin, and presence of growth discordance (Malone & D'Alton, 2009).
   c. If first twin is nonvertex, the standard of delivery is by cesarean.
3. Cesarean delivery is standard practice for higher-order multiple gestations.
4. Cesarean delivery may be necessary for the second twin even after successful vaginal delivery of the first.
   a. Ultrasound examination is often performed after the delivery of twin A to reassess position of twin B, as well as to guide external version if needed to facilitate vaginal delivery.
   b. Oxytocin administration may be necessary to augment uterine activity and to enhance descent of the second twin.
   c. Twin B is at considerably higher risk for delivery-related complications such as umbilical cord prolapse, malpresentation, and abruptio placentae; therefore, intensive monitoring must be continued until twin B is delivered.
D. **Postpartum interventions**
1. Provide a list of resources and services available (e.g., Mothers of Twins support group, lactation consultants).
2. Discuss aspects of normal newborn infant care; assess learning needs.
3. Explore patient's specific concerns.

HEALTH EDUCATION

A. **Twins**
1. Monozygotic: identical twins; originate from one zygote that divided around the end of the first week of pregnancy.
   a. Accounts for one third of all twins
   b. Genetically identical; very similar in appearance
2. Dizygotic: fraternal twins; result from the fertilization of two ova
   a. Accounts for two thirds of all twins
   b. Tends to repeat in families
   c. Increased risk with advancing maternal age
   d. May result from induction of ovulation by fertility drugs and procedures
B. **Other multiple births**
1. Triplets occur once in every 6900 pregnancies.
2. Multiple births of more than three babies are rare.
C. **Nutritional requirements**
1. Caloric intake must be greatly increased to support the growth of multiple fetuses (3000 to 40000 kcal/day).
2. Outline a dietary plan for patient.
D. **Inform patient of high-risk status.**
E. **Instruct patient to be aware of any developing symptoms of complications.**
1. Preterm labor
   a. Uterine contractions, cramping, or low back pain
   b. Feeling of pelvic pressure or fullness
   c. Change in amount or character of vaginal discharge
   d. Gastrointestinal (GI) upset: nausea, vomiting, or diarrhea
2. PROM: Report any leaking of fluid.
3. Precautionary measures
   a. Increase patient's rest periods.
   b. Have patient lie in the lateral position to maximize blood flow to the uterus.
   c. Teach patient to palpate uterine contractions (see discussion of health education under Preterm Labor).

STILLBIRTH

INTRODUCTION

A. Perinatal death, whether it occurs before delivery as a stillbirth or after delivery as a neonatal death, presents a unique set of physical and psychosocial problems.
B. The developmental task of attachment and preparing for parenthood is abruptly interrupted; parents are shocked and confused, and they suddenly find themselves faced with issues of grief and mourning.
C. The physical process of labor and delivery, as well as the handling of the infant after delivery, requires extreme sensitivity on the part of the nurse.

CLINICAL PRACTICE

A. Assessment
  1. History
     a. Loss of fetal movement
     b. Diminishing signs of pregnancy
        (1) Maternal weight gain ceases.
        (2) Mother may even lose weight.
        (3) Breast changes begin to reverse.
     c. Associated high-risk factors
        (1) Advanced diabetes in pregnancy
        (2) Hypertensive disorders of pregnancy
        (3) Systemic vascular disease
        (4) Autoimmune disease
        (5) Thrombophilia, inherited or acquired
        (6) Obesity
        (7) Sickle cell disease
        (8) Previous unexplained loss of fetus
  2. Physical findings
     a. Cessation or decrease in uterine growth
     b. Absence of fetal heart tones by auscultation or Doppler
     c. Ultrasound findings
        (1) Lack of cardiac activity
        (2) Spalding's sign: overlapping of the fetal skull bones
     d. Vaginal examination: observe for the following:
        (1) Bleeding
        (2) Umbilical cord prolapse
        (3) ROM: Amniotic fluid often appears cloudy and brownish-red if the fetus has been dead for several days.
        (4) Note any cervical dilation or effacement.
        (5) Note fetal presenting part or presence of any softening or overlapping of skull bones.
  3. Psychosocial findings
     a. Stress factors
        (1) Fear for self
        (2) Anxiety related to labor and delivery process
        (3) Confusion
     b. Behavioral factors
        (1) Difficulty in communicating
        (2) Shock and numbness (first stage of grief)
        (3) Demonstration of some attachment behaviors
        (4) Expression of significance of this pregnancy
        (5) Expression of significance of this loss
        (6) Expression of guilt
  4. Diagnostic procedures
     a. Ultrasound examination: most accurate to identify absence of fetal cardiac activity

      b. Radiologic signs of fetal death

         (1) Significant overlap of skull bones (process takes several days to develop)

         (2) Exaggerated curvature of the fetal spine (depends on the degree of maceration of sacral ligaments)

         (3) Evidence of gas in the fetus (uncommon but reliable sign)

      c. Palpation of collapsed fetal skull through the cervix

B. Interventions

   1. Delivery management

      a. Allow patient choices relating to labor and delivery (e.g., induction of labor immediately after diagnosis is made or waiting until the spontaneous onset of labor; patients often benefit from having a few days to deal with this issue before going through delivery).

      b. Prior to 28 weeks' gestation, choices include:

         (1) Second-trimester dilation and evacuation (American College of Obstetricians and Gynecologists [ACOG], 2009)

         (2) Vaginal misoprostol 200 to 400 mcg vaginally every 4 to 12 hours (Dickinson & Evans, 2005; Tang, Lau, Chan, & Ho, 2004)

         (3) Intravenous high-dose oxytocin infusions (ACOG, 2009)

      c. Induction with oxytocin is most often used for fetuses at 28 weeks' gestation or beyond using normal obstetric protocols.

      d. Analgesia or anesthesia

         (1) More liberal use is possible when the drug effect on the fetus is not considered.

         (2) Avoid oversedation because it may interfere with the grieving process.

   2. Grief support related to stillbirth (preferred term over fetal demise or death)

      a. Encourage patient and her family to verbalize feelings.

      b. Discuss the grieving process with the patient and her family (see Health Education).

      c. Allow patient choices relating to labor and delivery (e.g., induction of labor immediately after diagnosis is made or waiting until the spontaneous onset of labor; patients often benefit from having a few days to deal with this issue before going through delivery).

      d. Offer patient and family the opportunity to see, touch, and hold the infant.

      e. Provide tangible remembrances (e.g., photographs, footprints, infant identification bands, locks of hair).

      f. Offer support from clergy members.

      g. Offer baptism or blessing.

      h. Discuss plans for funeral or memorial services.

      i. Prepare patient and her family for appearance of the infant.

      j. Provide patient and her family with information about support groups.

      k. Provide reading materials to the patient and her family to take home because information may be overwhelming during hospitalization.

      l. Provide materials or references to address specific areas of grieving, such as siblings' responses, grandparents' responses, and so forth.

      m. Follow-up after delivery may be performed by a bereavement counselor, a social worker, or the nurse who cared for the patient; follow-up should assess the progress of the patient and her family in the grieving process after discharge and should continue to provide support.

   3. Identification of cause

      a. Goal: to provide appropriate family counseling to answer why the death occurred, if possible, and provide future family planning

      b. Fetal examination

         (1) Assess fetus for dysmorphic features.

         (2) Obtain measurements such as weight, length, head circumference, and possible foot size (if less than 23 weeks' gestation) to aid in dating (ACOG, 2009).

         (3) Photograph fetus to document abnormalities.

      c. Discuss autopsy with patient and her family; explain its benefits.

      d. Assist with karyotype analysis; most valuable tissue for karyotyping is placenta or segment of umbilical cord close to placenta (ACOG, 2009). If delivery is not imminent, amniocentesis is most effective.

HEALTH EDUCATION

A. **Stages of grief**
1. Shock, numbness, and yearning
2. Searching (includes anger)
3. Disorientation and depression
4. Reorganization

B. **Normal grief responses**
1. Preoccupation with the dead infant
2. Guilt and self-blame
3. Anger and hostility
4. Parents may grieve at a different pace, and therefore may seem not to be available to each other for support.
5. Strange dreams related to the infant
6. Aching arms
7. Hearing an infant cry
8. Still feeling the infant move

C. **Appearance of dead infant**
1. Maceration (peeling) of the skin
2. Discoloration of areas that had pressure on them, which look grossly ecchymotic
3. Areas of swelling and fluid retention
4. Discussion of any specific abnormalities
5. Amniotic fluid often reddish-brown and more viscous than normal
6. Delivery may cause trauma more readily (e.g., skull bones may collapse and cause unusual facial appearance).

ANAPHYLACTOID SYNDROME OF PREGNANCY (FORMERLY KNOWN AS AMNIOTIC FLUID EMBOLISM)

INTRODUCTION

A. **Anaphylactoid syndrome of pregnancy is a rare but extremely dangerous obstetric complication; the exact incidence is unknown; the complication is unpreventable and unpredictable. It is thought that the entry of amniotic fluid and fetal cells into the maternal circulation in certain patients triggers an anaphylactic reaction, causing an acute onset of maternal dyspnea and hypotension, followed quickly by cardiopulmonary collapse; of patients who survive the acute event, 40% develop adult respiratory distress syndrome (ARDS), left-sided heart failure, as well as severe disseminated intravascular coagulation (DIC) and multisystem organ failure.**

B. **The mortality rate for this complication has been reported to be as high as 80%. Of the patients who survive, most (85% to 92%) have permanent neurologic impairment.**

CLINICAL PRACTICE

A. **Assessment**
1. Physical findings
   a. Acute onset of respiratory distress, often during labor, delivery, or within 30 minutes following delivery
      (1) Unexpected, rapid onset dyspnea
      (2) Facial erythema
      (3) Cough
      (4) Cyanosis
      (5) Chest pain
      (6) Seizures
      (7) Restlessness
      (8) Pulmonary edema

      b. Acute onset of circulatory collapse
         (1) Severe hypoxia
         (2) Severe hypotension
         (3) If patient does not die from the initial respiratory insult, she needs to overcome the severe hemorrhage and coagulopathy that follow.
      c. Acute onset of coagulopathy
         (1) Uterine bleeding at delivery is not easily controlled.
         (2) Oozing may begin from puncture sites.
  2. Psychosocial findings
      a. Fear of death
      b. Fear on the part of the family in response to the rapid onset of life-threatening complications
  3. Diagnostic procedures
      a. The diagnosis of anaphylactoid syndrome of pregnancy must be made from the clinical picture.
      b. A definitive diagnosis is made only by ruling out other possible diagnoses such as:
         (1) Septic shock
         (2) Pulmonary embolism
         (3) Eclampsia
         (4) Placental abruption
         (5) Uterine rupture
         (6) Uterine atony
         (7) Myocardial infarction
         (8) Aortic dissection
         (9) Anaphylactic reaction to local anesthetic

B. Interventions
  1. Recognize this life-threatening diagnosis.
  2. Provide supportive therapies of oxygen, maintaining cardiac output and organ perfusion, and correct DIC.
  3. Ensure IV access; if patient does not have an IV line, start one immediately because a delay of even a few minutes may result in circulatory collapse and make IV access more difficult; consider having two IV lines in place.
  4. Initiate cardiopulmonary resuscitation (CPR) if indicated. If fetus is undelivered, be prepared for a perimortem cesarean delivery after 5 minutes of unsuccessful CPR.
  5. Administer oxygen to maintain normal saturation.
  6. Prepare for and assist with intubation and ventilation if patient loses consciousness.
  7. Administer crystalloid IV fluids rapidly if patient is hypotensive; if blood pressure is maintained, do not overload with fluids because it can result in pulmonary edema resulting from developing ARDS.
  8. Monitor vital signs, pulse oximetry, skin color, temperature, and moisture frequently.
  9. Have emergency medications to assist in patient stabilization, according to Moore (2008):
      a. Dopamine (Intropin) to maintain perfusion by increasing myocardial contractility, increase systolic blood pressure, dilate renal vasculature, increase renal blood flow, and increase glomerular filtration rate (GFR).
      b. Digoxin (Lanoxin) to improve myocardial contractility
      c. Hydrocortisone (Hydrocort, Cortef) to treat the immune response
      d. Uterotonics postdelivery to enhance myometrial contractility to decrease uterine atony such as:
         (1) Oxytocin (Pitocin) to enhance myometrial contractions and decrease capillary permeability
         (2) Methylergonovine (Methergine) to promote stronger myometrial contractions by acting directly on the uterine smooth muscle
         (3) Carboprost tromethamine (Hemabate), a prostaglandin that promotes longer lasting myometrial contractions
 10. Chest radiograph and 12-lead ECG can assist in hemodynamic management.
 11. Observe for signs and symptoms of shock.
 12. Observe for signs and symptoms of coagulopathy (inability to control intrapartum or immediate postpartum vaginal bleeding or bleeding from IV site or puncture or trauma sites).

13. Send laboratory work.
    a. Arterial blood gases
    b. CBC
    c. Platelet count
    d. Fibrinogen
    e. Fibrin degradation products
    f. Partial thromboplastin time
    g. Tryptase
14. Prepare for and assist with placement of central line (a pulmonary artery catheter may be useful for further hemodynamic management).
15. Administer blood; blood products such as packed RBCs, platelets, fresh-frozen plasma, and cryoprecipitate; or volume expanders as ordered.
16. Prevent hypothermia by using warmed blankets and intravenous fluids.
17. If fetus is undelivered, continuously monitor fetal heart rate and position mother to prevent vena cava syndrome.
18. Inform and reassure patient and family as much as possible during crisis.

HEALTH EDUCATION

A. Amniotic fluid embolism or anaphylactoid syndrome of pregnancy is so rare an obstetric complication that preparing a patient for its possibility is not needed.
B. After a patient has survived such an incident, the nurse may explain to her and her family what is known about this disorder.

UTERINE RUPTURE

INTRODUCTION

A. Uterine rupture is rare; the incidence ranges from 0.07% to 0.013% (Nahum, 2008) and is considered an obstetric emergency.
B. Clinical conditions associated with uterine rupture are uterine scar, uterine anomalies, uterine trauma, prior invasive molar pregnancy, excessive uterine stimulation during attempted vaginal birth after cesarean (VBAC), history of placenta percreta or increta, obstructed labor, mid- to high-operative vaginal delivery, and malpresentation.
C. Sudden fetal bradycardia or prolonged late or variable decelerations are the most common signs and symptoms even before the onset of abdominal pain or vaginal bleeding.
D. A normal uterus with no prior surgery contracting spontaneously is unlikely to rupture unless significant trauma exists.
E. The most common risk factor of uterine rupture is a trial of labor after cesarean.

CLINICAL PRACTICE

A. Assessment for risk factors. If the patient has a history of any of the following, the risk for uterine rupture increases to 1 in 200 deliveries.
    1. Previous cesarean delivery; more than one, interval less than 2 years, without previous history of vaginal delivery (Hibbard, Ismail, & Wang, 2001)
    2. Uterine incision; classic or low transverse cesarean with a single-layer hysterotomy closure (Blanchette, Blanchette, McCabe, & Vincent, 2001; Ravasia, Wood, & Pollard, 2000)
    3. VBAC needing labor induction with prostaglandins (ACOG, 2004) or labor induction or augmentation with oxytocin greater than 20 mU/min (Cahill et al, 2008).
    4. Estimated fetal weight greater than 4000 g (Elkousy, Sammel, & Stevens, 2003)
    5. Uterine anomalies (Erez et al, 2007; Nahum, 2008)
    6. Abdominal trauma: sharp or blunt
    7. Previous uterine trauma, such as perforation at the time of dilation and curettage (D&C), instrumented abortion, or previous myomectomy (Serrachioli et al, 2006)

B. **Signs of uterine rupture**
   1. Most classic sign is bradycardia or late/variable decelerations at a time in labor when they are usually unlikely to occur (Bujold & Gauthier, 2002).
   2. Decreased baseline uterine pressure or loss of uterine contractility
   3. Abdominal pain
   4. Vaginal bleeding
   5. Signs of shock
C. **Interventions**
   1. Recognize early signs of uterine rupture.
   2. Immediately notify attending physician.
   3. Assist in the stabilization of mother.
   4. Maintain IV access with large bore catheter.
   5. Prepare for emergency cesarean delivery if any evidence of uterine rupture is present; response time is critical to decrease fetal and maternal morbidity; goal is 10 to 37 minutes (Bujold & Gauthier, 2002; Nahum, 2008).
      a. Alert operating room and anesthesia provider.
      b. Alert patient's physician.
      c. Alert neonatal team, pediatrician, or both.
      d. Perform abdominal shave and skin preparation.
      e. Insert Foley catheter.
      f. Have patient sign consent forms.
   6. Maintain continuous FHR monitoring.
   7. Maintain patient on her side to maximize uterine blood flow.
   8. Inform patient that this condition is serious and that hospital staff will be working quickly to ensure her health and that of her infant.
   9. Encourage patient and family to verbalize feelings and to identify specific concerns.
   10. Provide as much information as possible to patient and family.
   11. Reassure patient and family as often as possible during any emergency procedures.

HEALTH EDUCATION

A. **Definitions**
   1. Uterine rupture is classified as complete disruption of all layers of the uterus (endometrium, myometrium, and perimetrium).
   2. Uterine scar dehiscence: previous scar begins to separate; this condition usually happens gradually, and if the fetal membranes are intact, no protrusion of fetal parts into the peritoneal cavity occurs.
B. **Types of scar**
   1. Low transverse
      a. Transverse or horizontal incision into the lower uterine segment
      b. Because of the way the muscle fibers are arranged, low transverse scars are under relatively little tension when the uterus contracts.
   2. Classical incision
      a. Uterine scar vertically placed on the body of the uterus and may extend up as far as the fundus
      b. This area is under a great deal of stress with contractions.
      c. Classical incisions are used if cesarean delivery is indicated before term because the lower uterine segment is not yet well enough developed, but they may also be used for an urgent cesarean delivery; this is why it is important to ask the reason for any previous cesarean delivery.

CASE STUDIES AND STUDY QUESTIONS

Mrs. C. is a 22-year-old gravida 3, para 2 (G3, P2) woman. She delivered her first child spontaneously at 34 weeks' gestation, and the child has subsequently done well. Her second child underwent cesarean delivery at 29 weeks and died 10 days later from complications of prematurity.

Mrs. C. is at 25 weeks' gestation and has been feeling pelvic pressure and a vague sense of cramping since 7 AM. It is now 11 AM, and she has called the labor and delivery unit because of concerns about her cramping.

1. Your best response to her is:
   a. Maintain bedrest in the lateral position and drink plenty of fluids.
   b. Go to the hospital immediately for further evaluation.
   c. Do not be concerned because the cramping is probably Braxton Hicks contractions and is normal at this gestational stage.
2. Mrs. C. is at risk for preterm labor because:
   a. She is a young multipara.
   b. She has previously undergone cesarean delivery.
   c. She has had previous preterm labors and births.
   d. She is not at risk for preterm labor.

Postterm Pregnancy

Ms. H. is a 26-year-old G1, P0 patient. She has had no prenatal care, but her LMP puts her at 42 weeks' gestation. She came into the hospital with possible ROM. She is not sure whether her membranes have ruptured because, although she felt a gush, she saw only a small amount of brownish fluid.

3. The labor and delivery nurse is concerned about Ms. H. because:
   a. She is probably in preterm labor.
   b. Her history indicates the risk for oligohydramnios and the probable presence of meconium.
   c. She is at risk because she is an older primipara.
   d. She is in active labor at this time.

After Ms. H. has been on the external fetal monitor for 40 minutes, the tracing shows minimal FHR variability but no evidence of decelerations. No fetal movement and no spontaneous FHR accelerations are present.

4. Appropriate nursing interventions at this time include:
   a. Preparing her for emergency cesarean delivery
   b. Allowing her to ambulate to stimulate the onset of contractions
   c. Maintaining her on bedrest in lateral position, starting an IV, and continuing the FHR monitoring
   d. Discharging her home to return when contractions are 5 minutes apart

Premature Rupture of Membranes

Mrs. L. is a 30-year-old G3, P2 woman at 31 weeks' gestation. She presents to the labor and delivery suite complaining of leaking fluid for the last couple of hours. Her vital signs are blood pressure 108/60 mm Hg, pulse 70 bpm, respirations 20, and a 36.4° C (97.6° F) temperature. She is monitored for 1 hour, and the FHR tracing is in the range of 130 to 145 bpm, reactive with no decelerations. No uterine contractions are perceived by Mrs. L. or recorded on the monitor.

5. Mrs. L. is a candidate for expectant management because:
   a. She is afebrile and has no other symptoms of infection.
   b. Her fetus is in the vertex position.
   c. A normal amount of amniotic fluid by ultrasound examination is present.
   d. She is not a candidate for expectant management.
6. In your initial assessment of Mrs. L. you note that she is nitrazine-negative but positive for vaginal pooling and ferning. These findings would lead you to believe that she is:
   a. Probably not ruptured because nitrazine is the most accurate test
   b. Most likely ruptured because many factors may interfere with nitrazine testing
   c. Definitely ruptured because ferning is 100% accurate
   d. Most likely infected because that causes a positive fern test result

Multiple Gestation

Mrs. D. is a 30-year-old G1, P0 patient. She has a history of infertility for 4 years and conceived while taking fertility drugs. She is carrying twins at 33 weeks' gestation and presents to the labor and delivery unit with complaints of cramping and a feeling of pelvic pressure. After 30 minutes on the fetal monitor, you note that Mrs. D. has mild uterine contractions every 5 to 6 minutes. Her cervical examination reveals a long, closed posterior cervix.

7. Uterine activity at 33 weeks is particularly significant for Mrs. D. because:
   a. She is at high risk for preterm labor.
   b. She has been contracting and her cervix has not changed.
   c. She is at high risk for chorioamnionitis.
   d. No reason for concern exists; uterine contractions are common at this gestational age.
8. Mrs D. is also at high risk for which other pregnancy complications?
   a. Preeclampsia
   b. Antepartum hemorrhage
   c. Preterm PROM
   d. All of the above

Stillbirth

Ms. T. is a 34-year-old G3, P1 woman with class C diabetes. She had a previous stillborn at 36 weeks' gestation with an undetermined cause of fetal death. She is at 35 weeks' gestation. She has had an uneventful pregnancy so far but now calls the labor and delivery unit because she has not felt the infant move since early this morning. It is now 1 PM.

9. Your best response to Ms. T. is to tell her:
   a. Go to Labor and Delivery as soon as possible for further evaluation.
   b. Wait at least 10 to 12 hours, then call her physician if she still has not felt movement.
   c. Her anxiety is most likely related to her previous loss at this gestation and therefore no need for concern exists.
   d. Maintain bedrest in the left lateral position.
10. When Ms. T. arrives in the labor and delivery unit, you are unable to auscultate a fetal heart rate. You suspect she may have experienced intrauterine fetal death. The most definitive way to confirm this diagnosis is to:
    a. Document the absence of fetal cardiac activity by ultrasonography.
    b. Send her for pelvic radiographs.
    c. Find an elevation in serum fibrinogen.
    d. Obtain an L/S ratio.

Anaphylactoid Syndrome of Pregnancy

Ms. N. is a 25-year-old primigravida at term who arrives in the labor and delivery unit at 2 AM. Her contractions started at midnight, and their frequency and intensity increased so rapidly that she was no longer able to tolerate the pain and came to the hospital. On examination, her cervix is 6 cm dilated and completely effaced. The presenting part is at zero station. She continues in very active labor with uterine contractions every 1 to 2 minutes over the next 30 minutes, at the end of which she is completely dilated and effaced. She pushes for 10 minutes and is prepared for delivery.

11. Immediately after the delivery of the infant, Ms. N. complains of dyspnea and shortness of breath. Within minutes, she becomes cyanotic and lethargic and seems to be losing consciousness. Recognizing this clinical picture as most likely an anaphylactoid syndrome of pregnancy, appropriate nursing actions are to:
    a. Prepare a loading dose of magnesium sulfate for seizure precaution.
    b. Open her IV line and administer oxygen at high concentrations.
    c. Notify the NICU and prepare for possible neonatal transfer because the newborn is at great risk for RDS.
    d. Perform an abdominal shave and skin preparation to get Ms. N. ready for emergency surgery.
12. Ms. N. is intubated and ventilated by the anesthesiologist for 10 minutes. She is fighting the endotracheal tube and breathing on her own. Blood for laboratory work is drawn, and her arterial blood gas values are within normal limits. She is extubated and resumes spontaneous respirations. Her color is good, but nasal oxygen is kept on at 10 L/min. Her oxygen saturation is 96% to 97%. She has survived the initial insult of anaphylactoid syndrome of pregnancy. Ms. N. is still at great risk for which subsequent complications?
    a. Preeclampsia
    b. ARDS
    c. Postpartum endometritis
    d. Deep vein thrombosis

Uterine Rupture

Mrs. P. is a 30-year-old G2, P1 woman with class B diabetes who is at term. She had a previous cesarean delivery at 27 weeks' gestation for an abruptio placentae 6 years earlier.

13. Mrs. P. is not a candidate for trial of labor because:
    a. This infant is likely to be much bigger than her previous one.
    b. She has diabetes and therefore requires another cesarean delivery.
    c. A cesarean delivery at 28 weeks' gestation was likely to have involved a classical incision.
    d. She is a good candidate for trial of labor.

14. If Mrs. P. arrived in the labor and delivery unit and told you she had been having contractions for the last 8 hours, and now the pain "just won't go away," you might consider the possibility of uterine rupture. Other assessment parameters consistent with uterine rupture are:

a. Systolic hypertension
b. Bleeding
c. Fetal bradycardia
d. Excess fetal movement

ANSWERS TO STUDY QUESTIONS

1. b	5. a	9. a	13. c
2. c	6. b	10. a	14. c
3. b	7. a	11. b	
4. c	8. d	12. b	

REFERENCES

Agency for Healthcare Research and Quality (AHRQ). (2002). *Management of prolonged pregnancy, Evidence report/technology assessment, No. 23.* Durham, NC: Duke Evidence-Based Practice Center.

American College of Obstetricians and Gynecologists (ACOG). (2000). *Management of postterm pregnancy.* Practice bulletin, No. 6. Washington, DC: ACOG.

American College of Obstetricians and Gynecologists (ACOG). (2004). *Vaginal birth after previous cesarean delivery.* Practice bulletin, No. 54. Washington, DC: ACOG.

American College of Obstetricians and Gynecologists (ACOG) (2007). *Premature rupture of membranes.* Practice bulletin, No. 80. Washington, DC: ACOG.

American College of Obstetricians and Gynecologists (ACOG). (2009). *Management of stillbirth.* ACOG clinical management guidelines for obstetrician-gynecologists. No. 102. Washington, DC: ACOG.

Ananth, C., & Vintzileos, A. (2006). Epidemiology of preterm birth and its clinical subtypes. *Journal of Maternal Fetal & Neonatal Medicine, 19,* 773–782.

Anotayanonth, S., Subhedar, N. V., Neilson, J. P., & Harigopal, S. (2004). Betamimetics for inhibiting preterm labour. *Cochrane Database of Systematic Reviews,* (4), Art. No.: CD004352.

Behrman, R., & Stith, B. (Eds.), (2007). *Institute of Medicine committee on understanding preterm birth and assuring healthy outcomes, preterm birth: Causes, consequences, and prevention* Washington, DC: National Academies Press.

Blanchette, H., Blanchette, M., McCabe, J., & Vincent, S. (2001). Is vaginal birth after cesarean safe? Experience at a community hospital. *American Journal of Obstetrics & Gynecology, 184*(7), 1478–1484.

Boulvain, M., & Irion, O. (2004). Stripping/sweeping the membranes for inducing or preventing postterm pregnancy. *Cochrane Database Systematic Reviews, Oct 18*(4), CDC001328.

Brown, J. E., & Carlson, M. (2000). Nutrition and multifetal pregnancy. *Journal of the American Dietetic Association, 100*(3), 343–348.

Bujold, E., & Gauthier, R. (2002). Neonatal morbidity associated with uterine rupture: What are the risk factors? *American Journal of Obstetrics & Gynecology, 186*(2), 311–314.

Burwick, R., Lee, G., Benedict, J., Ross, M., & Kjos, S. (2009). Blinded comparison of cervical portio length measurements by digital examination versus CerviLenz. *American Journal of Obstetrics & Gynecology, 200*(5), e37–e39.

Cahill, A., Waterman, D., Stamilio, D., Odibo, A., Allsworth, D., Evanoff, B., & Macones, G. (2008). Higher maximum doses of oxytocin are associated with an unacceptably high risk for uterine rupture in patients attempting vaginal birth after cesarean delivery. *American Journal of Obstetrics & Gynecology, 199*(1), e1–e5.

Centers for Disease Control and Prevention (CDC) (2006). Sexually transmitted diseases treatment guidelines 2006. *MMWR Morbidity & Mortality Weekly Report, 55*(No RR-11), 1–100. Retrieved from http://depts.washington.edu/nnptc/online_training/2006%20STD%20Treatment%20Guidelines.pdf.

Cnattingius, S. (2004). The epidemiology of smoking during pregnancy: Smoking prevalence, maternal characteristics, and pregnancy outcome. *Nicotine & Tobacco Research, 6*(Suppl 2), S125–S140.

Crowther, C. A., Hiller, J. E., & Doyle, L. W. (2002). Magnesium sulphate for preventing preterm birth in threatened preterm labour. *Cochrane Database of Systematic Reviews,* (4), Art. No.: CD001060.

Cruikshank, D. (2007). Intrapartum management of twin gestations. *Obstetrics & Gynecology, 109,* 1167.

Dalziel, R. (2006). Antenatal corticosteroids for accelerating fetal lung maturation for women at risk of preterm birth. *Cochrane Database of Systematic Reviews*(Issue 3).

Dare, M. R., Middleton, P., Crowther, C. A., Flenady, V. J., & Varatharaju, B. (2006). Planned early birth versus expectant management (waiting) for prelabour rupture of membranes at term (37 weeks or more). *Cochrane Database of Systematic Reviews,* (1), Art. No.: CD005302.

DeFranco, E., O'Brien, J., Adair, C., Lewis, D., Hall, D., Fusey, E., et al. (2007). Vaginal progesterone is associated with a decrease in risk for early preterm birth and improved neonatal outcome in women with a short cervix: A secondary analysis from a randomized, double-blind, placebo-controlled trial. *Utrasound in Obstetrics & Gynecology, 30,* 697–705.

DeJong, M., & Fausett, M. (2003). Anaphylactoid syndrome of pregnancy. *Critical Care Nurse, 23,* 42–48.

Dickinson, J., & Evans, S. (2005). The optimization of intravaginal misoprostol dosing schedules in second-trimester pregnancy termination. *American Journal of Obstetrics & Gynecology, 193,* 597.

Dodd, J., Flenady, V., Cincotta, R., & Crowther, C. (2006). Prenatal administration of progesterone for preventing preterm birth. *Cochrane Database of Systematic Reviews,* (1):CD004947.

Dolan, S., Gross, S., Merkatz, I., et al. (2007). The contribution of birth defects to preterm birth and low birth weight. *Obstetrics & Gynecology, 110,* 318–324.

Dole, N., Savitz, D., Hertz-Picciotto, I., Siega-Riz, A., McMahon, M., & Buekens, P. (2003). Maternal stress and preterm birth. *American Journal of Epidemiology, 157,* 14–24.

Elkousy, M., Sammel, M., & Stevens, D. (2003). The effect of birth weight on vaginal birth after cesarean delivery success rates. *American Journal of Obstetrics & Gynecology, 188*(3), 824–830.

Erez, O., Dukler, d, Novack, L., Rozen, A., Zolotnik, L., & Bashiri, A. (2007). Trial of labor and vaginal birth after cesarean section in patients with uterine Mullerian anomalies: A population-based study. *American Journal of Obstetrics & Gynecology, 196*(6), 537. e1-537.e11.

Farine, D., Dodd, J., Basso, M., Delisle, M. F., Farine, D., Grabowska, K., Hudon, L., Menticoglou, S. M., Mundle, W. R., Murphy-Kaulbeck, L. C., Ouellet, A., Pressey, T., & Roggensack, A. Maternal Fetal Medicine Committee, & Society of Obstetricians and Gynaecologists of Canada (SOGC). (2008). The use of progesterone for prevention of preterm birth. *Journal of Obstetrics & Gynaecology Canada, 30*(1), 67–71. Retrieved from www.guideline.gov.

Fonseca, E., Celik, E., Parra, M., Singh, M., Nicolaides, K., for The Fetal Medicine Foundation Second Trimester Screening Group (2007). Progesterone and the risk of preterm birth among women with a short cervix. *New England Journal of Medicine, 357,* 462–469.

Fraser, W., Hofmeyr, J., Lede, R., Garon, G., Alexander, S., Goffinet, F., Ohlasson, A., Goulet, C., Turcot-Lemay, L., Pendiville, W., Marcoux, S., Laperriere, L., Roy, C., Petrou, S., Xu, H., & Wei, B. for the Amnioinfusion Trial Group. (2005). Amnioinfusion for the prevention of the meconium aspiration syndrome. *New England Journal of Medicine, 353,* 909–917.

Gilbert, E. (2011). *Manual of high risk pregnancy & delivery* (5th ed.). St. Louis: Mosby.

Gilmore, D., Wakim, J., Secrest, J., & Rawson, R. (2003). Anaphylactoid syndrome of pregnancy: A review of the literature with latest management and outcome data. *AANA Journal, 71*(2), 120–126.

Goldenberg, R., Culhane, J., & Johnson, D. (2005). Maternal infection and adverse fetal and neonatal outcomes. *Clinics in Perinatology, 32,* 523–559.

Grobman, W., Gilbert, S., Landon, M., Spong, S., Leveno, K., & Rouse, D. (2007). Outcomes of induction of labor after one prior cesarean. *Obstetrics & Gynecology, 109*(2 Pt 1), 262–269.

Gulmezoglu, A., Crowther, C., & Middleton, P. (2006). Induction of labour for improving birth outcomes for women at or beyond term. *Cochrane Database of Systematic Reviews, Oct 18*(4), CDC004945.

Haas, J., Fuentes-Afflick, E., Stewart, A., Jackson, R., Dean, M., Brawarsky, P., & Escobar, G. (2005). Prepregnancy health status and the risk of preterm delivery. *Archives of Pediatric & Adolescent Medicine, 159,* 58–63.

Healy, A., Fergal, D., Malone, F., & Sullivan, L. (2006). Early access to prenatal care: Implications for racial disparity in perinatal mortality. *Obstetrics & Gynecology, 107,* 625–631.

Hendler, I., Goldenberg, R., Mercer, B., Iams, J., Meis, P., Moawad, A., MacPherson, C., Caritis, S., Miodovnik, M., Menard, K., Thurnau, G., & Sorokin, Y. (2005). The preterm prediction study: Association between maternal body mass index (BMI) and spontaneous preterm birth. *American Journal of Obstetrics & Gynecology, 192*(3), 882–886.

Hibbard, J., Ismail, M., & Wang, Y. (2001). Failed vaginal birth after a cesarean section: How risky is it? Maternal morbidity. *American Journal of Obstetrics & Gynecology, 184*(7), 1365–1371.

Hofmeyr, G. J. (1998). Amnioinfusion for potential or suspected umbilical cord compression in labour. *Cochrane Database of Systematic Reviews,* (Issue 1), Art. No.: CD000013.

Hofmeyr, G., Atallah, A., & Duley, L. (2006). Calcium supplementation during pregnancy for preventing hypertensive disorders, and related problems. *Cochrane Database of Systematic Reviews,* (3), CD001059.

Hogle, K., Hutton, E., McBrien, K., Barrett, J., & Hannah, M. (2003). Cesarean delivery for twins: A systematic review and meta-analysis. *American Journal of Obstetrics & Gynecology, 188*, 220.

Jakobsson, M., Gissler, M., Sainio, S., Paavonen, J., & Tapper, A. (2007). Preterm delivery after surgical treatment for cervical intraepithelial neoplasia. *Obstetrics & Gynecology, 109*(2, Part 1), 309–313.

Kalish, R., Chasen, S., Rosenzweig, L., Rashbaum, W., & Chervenak, F. (2002). Impact of midtrimester dilation and evacuation on subsequent pregnancy outcome. *American Journal of Obstetrics & Gynecology, 187*, 882–885.

Kenyon, S., Boulvain, M., & Neilson, J. (2004). Antibiotics for preterm rupture of membranes: A systematic review, *Obstetrics & Gynecology, 104*(5 Pt 1), 1051–1057.

King, J. F., Flenady, V. J., Papatsonis, D. N. M., Dekker, G. A., & Carbonne, B. (2003). Calcium channel blockers for inhibiting preterm labour. *Cochrane Database of Systematic Reviews*, (1), Art. No.: CD002255.

King, J., Flenady, V., Cole, S., & Thornton, S. (2005). Cyclo-oxygenase (COX) inhibitors for treating preterm labour. *Cochrane Database of Systematic Reviews*, (2), Art. No.: CD001992.

Klebanoff, M., & Searle, K. (2006). The role of inflammation in preterm birth: Focus on periodonitis. *BJOG: An International Journal of Obstetrics & Gynaecology, 113*(Suppl. 3), 43–45.

Kramer, M., & Kakuma, R. (2003). Energy and protein intake in pregnancy. *Cochrane Database of Systematic Reviews*, (4), DC000032.

Limbo, R., & Wheeler, S. (1995). *When a baby dies: A handbook for healing and helping*. LaCrosse, WI: Resolve Through Sharing.

Luke, B., & Eberlein, T. (1999). *When you're expecting twins, triplets, and quads*. New York: Harper & Row.

Lumley, J., Oliver, S. S., Chamberlain, C., & Oakley, L. (2004). Interventions for promoting smoking cessation during pregnancy. *Cochrane Database of Systematic Reviews*, (4), Art. No.: CD001055.

Malone, F., & D'Alton, M. (2009). Multiple gestation: Clinical characteristics and management. In R. Creasy, R. Resnik, J. Iams, C. Lockwood, & T. Moore (Eds.), *Creasy & Resnik's maternal-fetal medicine: Principles and practice* (6th ed.). Philadelphia: Saunders.

Marret, S., Marpeau, L., Zupan-Simunek, V., Eurin, D., Leveque, C., Hellot, M., Benichou, J. for the PREMAG Trial Group (2007). Magnesium sulfate given before very-preterm birth to protect the infant brain: The randomised controlled PREMAG trial. *BJOG: An International Journal of Obstetrics & Gynaecology, 114*, 310–318.

Martin, J., Hamilton, B., Sutton, P., Ventura, S., Menacker, F., Kirmeyer, S., & Munson, M. (2007). Births: Final data for 2005. *National Vital Statistics Report, 56*(6), 1–103.

Matijevic, R., Grgic, O., & Vasili, O. (2006). Is sonographic assessment of cervical length better than digital examination in screening for preterm delivery in a low-risk population? *Acta Obstetricia et Gynecologica Scandinavica, 85*, 1342–1347.

Mesiano, S. (2001). Roles of estrogen and progesterone in human parturition. *Frontiers of Hormone Research, 27*, 86–104.

Michalowicz, B., Hodges, J., DiAngelis, A., Lupo, V., Novak, M., Ferguson, J., Buchanan, W., Bofill, J., Papapanou, P., Mitchell, D., Matseoane, S., & Tschida, P. for the OPT Study (2006). Treatment of periodontal disease and the risk of preterm birth. *New England Journal of Medicine, 355*, 1885–1894.

Moore, L. (2008). Amniotic fluid embolism. *eMedicine Obstetrics and Gynecology*, 1–13. Retrieved from: http://emedicine.medscape.com/article/253068-overview.

Morken, N., Kallen, K., & Jacobsson, B. (2007). Outcomes of preterm children according to type of delivery onset: A nationwide population-based study. *Paediatric & Perinatal Epidemiology, 21*, 458–464.

Nabet, C., Lelong, N., Ancel, P., Saurel-Cubizolles, M., & Kaminski, M. (2007). Smoking during pregnancy according to obstetric complications and parity: Results of the EUROPOP study. *European Journal of Epidemiology, 22*, 715–721.

Nahum, G. (2008). Uterine rupture in pregnancy. *eMedicine Obstetrics and Gynecology, 2008*. Retrieved from: http://emedicine.medscape.com/article/275854-overview.

National Colaborating Centre for Women's and Children's Health (2007). *NICE clinical guidelines: Intrapartum care*. London: National Institute for Health and Clinical Excellence. Retrieved from: http://guidance.nice.org.uk/CG55.

Nohr, B., Tabor, A., Frederiksen, K., & Kjaer, S. (2007). Loop electrosurgical excision of the cervix and the subsequent risk of preterm delivery. *Acta Obstetricia Gynecologica Scandinavica, 85*, 596–603.

Owen, J. (2003). Evaluation of the cervix by ultrasound for the prediction of preterm birth. *Clinics in Perinatology, 30*(4), 735–755.

Ravasia, D., Wood, S., & Pollard, J. (2000). Uterine rupture during induced trial of labor among women with previous cesarean delivery. *American Journal of Obstetrics & Gynecology, 183*(5), 1176–1179.

Resnik, J., & Resnik, R. (2009). Post-term pregnancy. In R. Creasy, R. Resnik, J. Iams, C. Lockwood, & T. Moore (Eds.), *Creasy & Resnik's maternal-fetal medicine: Principles and practice* (6th ed.). Philadelphia: Saunders.

Robinson, J., & Abuhamad, A. (2002). Determining chorionicity and amnionicity in multiple pregnancies. *Contemporary OB/GYN, 6*, 94–108.

Romero, R. (2007). Prevention of spontaneous preterm birth: The role of sonographic cervical length in identifying patients who may benefit from progesterone treatment. *Ultrasound in Obstetrics & Gynecology, 30*(5), 675–686.

Ross, M., Cousins, L., Baxter-Jones, R., Bemis-Heys, R., Catanzarite, V., & Dowling, D. (2007). Objective cervical portio length measurements: Consistency and efficacy of screening for a short cervix. *Journal of Reproductive Medicine, 52*(5), 385–389.

Rouse, D., Hirtz, D., Thom, E., Varner, M., Spong, C., Mercer, B., Iams, J., Wapner, R., Sorokin, Y., Alexander, J., Harper, M., Thorp, J., Jr., Ramin, S., Malone, F., Carpenter, M., Miodovnik, M., Moawad, A., O'Sullivan, M., Peaceman, A., Hankins, G., Langer, O., Caritis, S., & Roberts, J. for Eunice Kennedy Shriver NICHD Maternal-Fetal Units Network. (2008). A randomized, controlled trial of magnesium sulfate for the prevention of cerebral palsy. *New England Journal of Medicine, 359*(9), 895–905.

Rumbold, A., Crowther, C., Haslam, R., Dekker, G., & Robinson, J. for the ACTS Study Group (2006). Vitamins C and E and the risks of preeclampsia and perinatal complication. *New England Journal of Medicine, 354*, 1796–1806.

Seidel, H., Ball, J., Dains, J., & Benedict, G. (2006). *Mosby's guide to physical examination.* St. Louis: Mosby.

Serrachioli, R., Manuzzi, L., Vianello, F., Gualerzi, B., Savelli, L., & Paradisi, R. (2006). Obstetric and delivery outcome of pregnancies achieved after laparoscopic myomectomy. *Fertility & Sterility, 86*(1), 159–165.

Sfakianaki, A., & Norwitz, E. (2006). Mechanisms of progesterone action in inhibiting prematurity. *Journal of Maternal Fetal & Neonatal Medicine, 19*, 763–772.

Sjoborg, K., Vistad, I., Myhr, S., Svenningsen, R., Herzog, C., Kloster-Jensen, A., Nygard, G., Hole, S., & Tanbo, T. (2007). Pregnancy outcome after cervical cone excision: A case-control study. *Acta Obstetricia et Gynecologica Scandinavica, 86*, 423–428.

Smaill, F., & Vazquez, J. (2007). Antibiotics for asymptomatic bacteriuria in pregnancy. *Cochrane Database of Systematic Reviews,* (2), CD000490.

Smith, L., Draper, E., Manktelow, B., Dorling, J., & Field, D. (2007). Socioeconomic inequalities in very preterm birth rates. *Archives of Disease in Childhood: Fetal & Neonatal Edition, 92*, F11–F14.

Society of Obstetricians and Gynaecologists of Canada (SCOG) Clinical Practice Obstetrics Committee & Maternal Fetal Medicine Committee. (2008). Guidelines for the management of pregnancy at 41+0 to 42+0 weeks. *Journal of Obstetrics & Gynaecology Canada, Sep 30*(9), 800–810, Retrieved from: www.guideline.gov.

Spong, C. (2007). Amnioinfusion: Indications and controversies. In J. Queenan, C. Spong, & C. Lockwood (Eds.), *Management of high-risk pregnancy: An evidence-based approach* (5th ed.). Oradell, NJ: Wiley-Blackwell Publishing.

Tang, O., Lau, W., Chan, C., & Ho, P. (2004). A prospective randomised comparison of sublingual and vaginal misoprostol in second trimester termination of pregnancy. *BJOG: An International Journal of Obstetrics & Gynaecology, 111*, 1001–1005.

Thompson, J., Irgens, L., Rasmussen, S., & Daltveit, A. (2006). Secular trends in socio-economic status, and the implications for preterm birth. *Paediatric & Perinatal Epidemiology, 20*, 182–187.

Tikkanen, M., Nuutila, M., Hiilesmaa, V., Paavonen, J., & Yikorkala, O. (2006). Clinical presentation and risk factors of placental abruption. *Acta Obstetricia et Gynecologica Scandinavica, 85*, 700–705.

U.S. Department of Health and Human Services (USDHHS). (2000). *Healthy People 2010: Understanding and improving health.* Washington, DC: USDHHS.

Virk, J., Zhang, J., & Olsen, J. (2007). Medical abortion and the risk of subsequent adverse pregnancy outcomes. *New England Journal of Medicine, 357*, 648–658.

Weiner, C., & Buhimschi, C. (2009). *Drugs for pregnant and lactating women* (2nd ed.). Philadelphia: Saunders.

Word, R., Li, X., Hnat, M., & Carrick, K. (2007). Dynamics of cervical remodeling during pregnancy and parturition: Mechanisms and current concepts. *Seminars in Reproductive Medicine, 25*, 69–79.

Zlopasa, G., Skrablin, S., & Kalafatic, D. (2007). Uterine anomalies and pregnancy outcome following resectoscope metroplasty. *International Journal of Gynaecology & Obstetrics, 98*, 129–133.

28 Postpartum Complications

Mary Ann Rhode

OBJECTIVES

1. Recognize the causes of four types of postpartum complications: hemorrhage, infection, venous disorders, and postpartum mood disorders.
2. Assess factors for increased risk for the selected complications.
3. Define specific treatments for selected postpartum complications
4. Analyze assessment data and select appropriate actions to prevent or minimize effects of selected postpartum complications.
5. Design health education strategies to prevent, minimize the effects of and/or enhance recovery from postpartum hemorrhage, infection, venous disorders, and postpartum mood disorders.
6. Select strategies to provide care to the high-risk postpartum woman and her family based on analysis and synthesis of her needs in her particular situation.

POSTPARTUM HEMORRHAGE

INTRODUCTION

A. **Definition: Postpartum hemorrhage has classically been defined in several ways:**
   1. Blood loss greater than 500 mL in the first 24 hours after delivery (greater than 1000 mL blood loss after cesarean delivery)
   2. A change in postpartum hemoglobin concentration
   3. Blood loss requiring transfusion (Smeltzer, Bare, Hinkle, & Cheever, 2008)
   4. Accurate estimates of blood loss are not easily obtained and have made estimates of the incidence of postpartum hemorrhage difficult (Francois & Foley, 2007).
B. **Incidence: The overall incidence of postpartum hemorrhage is 4% to 6% of deliveries** (Francois & Foley, 2007).
C. **Types**
   1. Primary or early postpartum hemorrhage: occurring within the first 24 hours after delivery
   2. Secondary or delayed postpartum hemorrhage: occurring 24 hours to 12 weeks after delivery
      a. More commonly due to placental site subinvolution, infection, and retained placental tissue
      b. May be associated with von Willebrand disease
D. **Causes** (Francois & Foley, 2007; Lowdermilk, 2007)
   1. Uterine atony most common
   2. Lacerations of the upper or lower genitourinary tracts
      a. May result in hematoma formation, which are collections of blood in the pelvic tissue (may involve the vulva, vaginal or retroperitoneal area) resulting from damage to a vessel wall without laceration of the tissue
      b. Episiotomy, instrumental delivery, and primigravidity increase the risk of vaginal hematoma formation (Cunningham et al, 2005).
   3. Retained products of conception
   4. Invasive placental implantation: placenta accreta, placenta increta, placenta percreta
   5. Uterine inversion or rupture
   6. Blood coagulation disorders

      a. Disseminated intravascular coagulation (DIC) can cause or be a result of postpartum hemorrhage.

      b. Abruptio placentae, fetal demise, or amniotic fluid embolism may be the underlying cause of DIC (see Chapter 21 for a complete discussion of hemorrhagic disorders).

  7. Infection

  8. Placental site subinvolution

CLINICAL PRACTICE

A. Assessment

  1. Risk factors: Despite many known risk factors, postpartum hemorrhage is unpredictable and may occur when no risk factors are present (Burtelow et al, 2007; Francois & Foley, 2007). Known risk factors are:

    a. Precipitous or prolonged first or second stage of labor or both

    b. Overstretching of the uterus (large fetus, hydramnios, or multiple gestation)

    c. Drugs (general anesthesia, magnesium sulfate, prolonged use of oxytocin)

    d. Trauma through the use of forceps or other intravaginal manipulations, such as internal podalic version or forceps rotation

    e. Previous postpartum hemorrhage, uterine rupture, or uterine surgery (cesarean section or dilation and curettage)

    f. Past placenta previa; placenta accreta, increta, or percreta. The incidence of placenta accreta may be increasing due to a higher cesarean section rate.

    g. Current diagnosis of placenta previa

    h. Uterine malformation or uterine fibroids

    i. Maternal exhaustion, malnutrition, anemia, or pregnancy-induced hypertension (PIH)

    j. Coagulation disorders, such as idiopathic thrombocytopenia, purpura, or von Willebrand disease

    k. Grand multiparity

    l. Uterine infection

  2. Physical findings (Lowdermilk, 2007)

    a. General symptoms

      (1) Dizziness, fainting, lightheadedness

      (2) Tachycardia, tachypnea, weak pulse, decreasing blood pressure

      (3) Oliguria, profound hypotension, and signs of shock (weak pulse, increased respirations, shallow respirations, and pale, clammy skin) do not appear until hemorrhage is advanced because of increased fluid and blood volume of pregnancy (Lowdermilk, 2007).

      (4) Altered level of consciousness

    b. Uterine atony/retained placental fragments

      (1) Boggy, large uterus

      (2) Expelled clots

      (3) Excessive vaginal bleeding

      (4) Bleeding may be slow and steady or sudden and massive.

    c. Lacerations

      (1) Firm uterus with bright red blood

      (2) Steady stream or trickle of unclotted blood

    d. Hematoma

      (1) Firm uterus with bright red blood

      (2) Extreme perineal or pelvic pain

      (3) Bluish bulging area just under the skin surface

      (4) Difficulty in voiding

      (5) Unexplained tachycardia

      (6) Hypotension

      (7) Anemia

    e. DIC

      (1) Petechiae

      (2) Ecchymosis

      (3) Prolonged bleeding from gums and venipuncture sites

        (4) Uncontrolled bleeding during childbirth
        (5) Tachycardia
        (6) Oliguria
        (7) Signs of acute renal failure
        (8) Convulsions
        (9) Coma
  3. Psychosocial response
    a. Fear
    b. Anxiety and restlessness
    c. Fatigue

INTERVENTIONS

A. Anticipated medical intervention (Francois & Foley, 2007)
  1. Prompt response to request for evaluation of excessive bleeding
  2. Medical orders
    a. Uterotonic agents
    b. Fluid replacement and blood component replacement
    c. Laboratory evaluation
        (1) Complete blood count (CBC)
        (2) Coagulation studies: prothrombin time (PT), partial thromboplastin time (PTT), fibrinogen, D-dimer
  3. Examination for vaginal or cervical lacerations
  4. Removal of retained products of conception
  5. Depending on clinical situation, institution, available personnel and available equipment, other interventions may include:
    a. Uterine tamponade techniques
    b. Arterial embolization
    c. Surgery techniques
        (1) Bleeding site ligation
        (2) Ligation of uterine artery
        (3) Uterine compression sutures
        (4) Hysterectomy
  6. After initial postdelivery assessment
    a. Continue to assess the height and position of the fundus at least each shift.
        (1) If uterus is soft and boggy, perform uterine massage.
        (2) For mild uterine bogginess, in addition to fundal massage, put infant to breast if mother is breastfeeding.
    b. Monitor lochia for color, odor, amount, consistency, or clots. Weigh used pads whenever there is a question of continued heavy bleeding (1 g equals 1 mL).
    c. Monitor and record vital signs.
    d. Guard against inaccurate assessment of postpartal bleeding (due to pooling unnoticed underneath the mother or poor lighting (Pillitteri, 2007).
  7. In the presence of continued or new onset of excessive bleeding:
    a. Continue uterine massage.
    b. Activate postpartum hemorrhage response team, if available within institution (massive transfusion protocols for hemorrhage anticipated to require more than 10 units of packed red blood cells) (Burtelow et al, 2007; Chichester, 2005).
        (1) Quickly assemble a multidisciplinary care team.
        (2) Provide for rapid availability of blood products.
        (3) Optimize outcomes by rapid, early intervention.
    c. Notify care provider.
    d. Ensure intravenous (IV) access for fluid replacement, medications, and blood product replacement.
    e. Administer oxygen.
    f. Continue assessments and interventions previously listed.
    g. Administer uterotonic drugs as ordered (Francois & Foley, 2007).

(1) Oxytocin (Pitocin): 10 to 40 units in 500 to 1000 mL of crystalloid solution, by IV infusion (Ladewig, London, and Davidson, 2010)
  (a) DO NOT give undiluted oxytocin as an IV bolus.
  (b) Doses of oxytocin higher than 20 units will be ordered only for short amounts of time.
(2) Methylergonovine (Methergine): 0.2 mg intramuscularly (IM) every 2 to 4 hours, unless contraindicated by maternal hypertension (Ladewig et al, 2010)
(3) Carboprost tromethamine (Hemabate): 0.25 mg IM every 15 to 90 minutes, 8-dose maximum, contraindicated with active cardiac, pulmonary (asthma), renal, or hepatic disease (Ladewig et al, 2010)
(4) Misoprostol (Cytotec): 800 to 1000 mcg per rectum as a single dose (Ladewig et al, 2010)
  h. Administer blood component products as ordered.
  i. Monitor for signs of transfusion reaction or reaction to oxytocic agents (fever, chills, diarrhea, nausea or vomiting with carboprost tromethamine, and tachycardia or fever with misoprostol.
  j. Keep woman flat to supply blood to heart and brain.
  k. Catheterization of distended bladder if indicated. Indwelling catheter may be ordered to monitor mother's condition.
  l. Keep accurate intake and output (I&O).
  m. Facilitate arrangements for adequate anesthesia, if required.
  n. Assist care provider during examination for lacerations and retained placental fragments if indicated by continued hemorrhage.
  o. Facilitate arrangements for surgical intervention if medical control of hemorrhage is unsuccessful.
  p. Stay with woman and use physical touch if appropriate.
  q. Offer reassurance and support to mother and family.
  r. Give information to woman and her family in clear, brief statements.
8. Following stabilization of the woman after a postpartum hemorrhage:
  a. Coordinate nursing interventions with the mother's schedule to allow for rest periods that are undisturbed.
  b. Assist mother with activities of daily living (ADLs).
  c. Encourage appropriate nutritional intake and increased fluids.
  d. Encourage woman to take vitamins and iron tablets.
  e. Encourage techniques for standing and moving slowly to minimize orthostatic hypotension.
  f. Mobilize support system or resources.
  g. Administer antibiotics as ordered.

HEALTH EDUCATION

A. **Explain normal lochia changes and encourage mother to report any episodes of recurrent excessive bleeding or unusual blood clots, especially after discharge from the hospital.**
B. **Review danger signs and when to call care provider: excessive bleeding, signs of infection.**
C. **Identify self-care measures to facilitate recovery from postpartum hemorrhage: increased rest, ways to minimize orthostatic changes, need for adequate nutrition and fluid intake, and arrangements for help with infant care** (Lowdermilk, 2007).
D. **Educate mother about need for iron supplementation, importance of compliance, duration of treatment, possible side effects, and measures to control side effects.**
E. **Encourage mother to share history of postpartum hemorrhage with future care providers.**

POSTPARTUM INFECTIONS

CLINICAL PRACTICE

Introduction
A. Definition
  1. Postpartum febrile morbidity is defined by the U.S. Joint Commission on Maternal Welfare as an oral temperature of greater than or equal to 38° C (100.4° F) on any two of the first 10 days postpartum or 38.7° C (101.6° F) or higher during the first 24 hours, taken by a standard technique at least four times a day.

2. Short-term temperature elevations not requiring antibiotic therapy are common and may be due to:
   a. Dehydration from fluid loss during labor and delivery
   b. Breast engorgement, if temperature elevation occurs 48 to 72 hours after delivery
   c. Postoperative elevation immediately after a cesarean birth
B. **Types of postpartum infection**
   1. Genitourinary tract
      a. Endometritis
         (1) Usually a mixture of several aerobic and anaerobic organisms from the genital tract
         (2) *Chlamydia trachomatis* infection more common when onset is 2 or more weeks after delivery.
         (3) Incidence (Duff, 2007)
            (a) 1% to 3% after vaginal delivery
            (b) 5% to 15% after elective cesarean section without rupture of membranes
            (c) 15% to 20% after cesarean section following extended labor with rupture of membranes with antibiotic prophylaxis
            (d) 30% to 35% after cesarean section in the same situation without antibiotic prophylaxis
         (4) Use of single-dose perioperative antimicrobial prophylaxis has dramatically reduced the incidence and severity of postcesarean endometritis and wound infection (Cunningham et al, 2005).
      b. Cesarean section wound infection
         (1) Occurs after the third or fourth postoperative day
         (2) Can be masked by early postoperative fever
         (3) Often associated with endometritis
      c. Perineal wound infection: rare progression to necrotizing fasciitis can be life threatening and require aggressive surgical debridement
      d. Urinary tract infection
   2. Breast infection
   3. Other: viral infection, upper respiratory infection, appendicitis, etc.

CLINICAL PRACTICE

A. **Assessment**
   1. Risk factors (Duff, 2007; Lowdermilk, 2007)
      a. Cesarean birth: most important risk factor
      b. Young age
      c. Low socioeconomic status
      d. Prolonged labor
      e. Prolonged rupture of membranes
      f. Multiple vaginal examinations during labor
      g. Severe anemia or diabetes
      h. Traumatic delivery, intrauterine manipulation, manual removal of placenta
      i. Postpartum hemorrhage
      j. Malnutrition, general debilitation
      k. Preexisting infection or colonization of the lower genital tract such as bacterial vaginosis, herpes, etc.
      l. Hematoma
      m. Droplet infection from personnel, breaks in aseptic technique
      n. Foley catheter in place more than 24 hours
      o. Perineal lacerations (third or fourth degree)
      p. Internal monitoring
      q. Meconium-stained amniotic fluid (Tran, Caughey, & Musci, 2003)
   2. Physical findings
      a. Infections of the genital tract: varies by site
         (1) Fever
         (2) Uterine tenderness

        (3) Foul-smelling lochia (amount can be normal, scant, or profuse)

        (4) Edema

        (5) Lower abdominal pain

        (6) Malaise/lethargy

        (7) Anorexia

        (8) Chills

        (9) Headache

       (10) Backache

       (11) Increased pulse rate (100 to 140 beats per minute [bpm])

       (12) Diaphoresis

       (13) Increased pain, redness, drainage, induration, or poorly approximated edges of episiotomy of perineal lacerations

    b. Urinary tract infections (Lowdermilk, 2007)

        (1) Small voiding volume or inability to void

        (2) Pain with urination

        (3) Frequency or urgency

        (4) Fever

        (5) Hematuria

        (6) Overdistended bladder

        (7) Backache

        (8) Restlessness

    c. Infections of the breast/mastitis (Betzold, 2007)

        (1) Temperature elevated up to 40° C (104.1° F)

        (2) Chills

        (3) Malaise, myalgia

        (4) Hard, red, and tender irregular mass in one or both breasts

        (5) Severe to acute pain and tenderness in one or both breasts

        (6) Cracked nipples

        (7) Breast engorgement

    d. Wound infections from cesarean section or dehiscence (Duff, 2007)

        (1) Elevated temperature on third or fourth postpartum day

        (2) Drainage of pus or blood from the wound

        (3) Red and inflamed appearance of repaired edges

        (4) Presence of cellulitis

        (5) Wound opened and abdominal contents exposed to air

  3. Psychosocial findings

    a. Anxiety

    b. Stress

    c. Pain

INTERVENTIONS

A. Intravenous antibiotics

  1. Usually until the mother is improved and afebrile for 24 hours

  2. Continued oral antibiotic therapy after IV antibiotics does not improve outcome and is considered unnecessary (Duff, 2007)

B. Cultures (Cunningham et al, 2005)

  1. Due to difficulty obtaining specimens and the need to treat prior to the availability of results, endometrial cultures are no longer routinely performed.

  2. Blood cultures are usually reserved for when there is a failure to respond to treatment.

C. Prevention of postpartum infection (Lowdermilk, 2007)

  1. Encourage proper handwashing by staff, mother, family, and visitors.

  2. Provide for adequate nutrition, fluids, and rest.

  3. Facilitate complete bladder emptying.

  4. Assess breastfeeding initiation to ensure proper technique and adequate breast emptying and to minimize nipple trauma.

5. Encourage use of brassiere for the non-breastfeeding mother to minimize stimulation of lactation response.
6. Ensure proper breast and perineal hygiene.
D. **Minimizing the effects of infection to enhance recovery**
1. Administer antibiotics as ordered.
   a. Traditional dosing schedules may be changing.
   b. Once daily dosing has been shown to have a similar success rate as more frequent dosing regimens (Livingston et al, 2003).
2. Timely administration of analgesics and antipyretics as needed
3. Alleviate discomforts associated with fever and diaphoresis.
   a. Change gown and bed linen when damp.
   b. Offer bed bath or shower.
   c. Offer back rub or application of cool cloth to forehead.
4. Monitor woman's condition for signs of improvement or decline—assess vital signs, fundus, perineum, and/or abdominal wound and report deviations from expected findings.
5. Encourage adequate oral fluid intake.
6. Monitor and record I&O, if ordered.
7. Assist mother to balance her need for rest with her need to care for her newborn.
   a. Assist woman to place limits on visitors and telephone calls if she does not have sufficient energy.
   b. Assist woman to care for her infant if she has the energy to do so.
   c. Facilitate infant care by other caregivers when the mother is unable to provide the care herself.
8. Allow mother time to discuss feelings and concerns.
9. Help mother focus on normal aspects of her situation

HEALTH EDUCATION

A. **Teach patient about signs of recurrent infection after discharge.**
B. **Emphasize need for increased rest, fluids, and adequate nutrition to continue recovery.**
C. **Teach patient about transmission of infection and ways to prevent complications and further infections.**
D. **Teach signs and symptoms of mastitis to all breastfeeding mothers and encourage mothers to call their care provider immediately if any signs of mastitis appear.**

VENOUS DISORDERS

INTRODUCTION

A. **Definition: A variety of terms are used for venous thromboembolic disorders.**
1. Superficial phlebitis
2. Venous thromboembolism (VTE); acute pulmonary embolus is a form of VTE
3. Deep vein thrombosis (DVT)
4. Phlebothrombosis
5. Thromboembolic disease
6. Thrombophlebitis: an infection of the lining of a vessel in which a clot attaches to the vessel wall, often accompanied by thrombus formation (Smeltzer et al, 2008)
B. **Incidence:**
1. Early ambulation after delivery has decreased the incidence but it still remains the leading cause of maternal mortality in the United States.
2. DVTs are more commonly diagnosed in the antepartum period, whereas pulmonary emboli are more frequently diagnosed in the postpartum period, often with cesarean delivery.
3. Onset is usually between the 10th and 20th postpartum days
C. **Types**
1. Superficial phlebitis, not involving thrombus formation
2. DVT

3. Septic pelvic thrombophlebitis (SVT) (Klima & Snyder, 2008)
   a. Deep pelvic septic thrombophlebitis: onset usually within a few days
   b. Ovarian vein thrombophlebitis: onset usually within 1 week
   c. These two types may be variant of a similar disease process.
D. **Causes: Virchow's triad** (Smeltzer et al, 2008)
   1. Vessel wall damage
   2. Venous stasis
   3. Altered coagulation

CLINICAL PRACTICE

A. **Assessment**
   1. Intrapartum and postpartum risk factors (Smeltzer et al, 2008)
      a. Related to venous wall damage
         (1) Lower extremity trauma
         (2) Operative delivery
         (3) Prolonged labor with potential pelvic vein endothelial damage
      b. Related to venous stasis
         (1) Prolonged hospitalization or bedrest
         (2) Obesity
         (3) Advanced age
         (4) Varicosities
      c. Related to altered coagulation
         (1) Pregnancy and postpartum status
         (2) Prior history or prior family history of venous thromboembolism
         (3) Infection/septicemia
         (4) Inherited or acquired hypercoagulation condition (protein S deficiency, antiphospholipid antibody syndrome, lupus anticoagulant, factor V Leiden defect, etc.)
B. **Physical findings**
   1. Evaluation and diagnosis are complicated by lack of sensitivity and specificity of signs and symptoms (Lowdermilk, 2007; Pettker & Lockwood, 2007; Smeltzer et al, 2008).
      a. Patient reports pain in the leg or groin. NOTE: Homans' sign is no longer considered a reliable or valid sign for assessment (Gupta & Stouffer, 2001).
      b. Nonspecific back pain or right lower quadrant pain
      c. Tenderness with palpation or palpable cordlike segment
      d. Difference in leg circumference bilaterally from thigh to ankle
      e. Increase in surface temperature of leg, especially of the calf or ankle
      f. Coolness of entire extremity associated with edema and pain (symptoms of iliofemoral venous thrombosis)
      g. Edema or ankle engorgement
      h. Erythema or discoloration of extremity
      i. Unexplained fever or fever unresponsive to antibiotics
      j. Signs and symptoms of pulmonary embolus (Urden, Stacy, & Lough, 2006)
         (1) Tachypnea
         (2) Tachycardia
         (3) Chest pain
         (4) Dyspnea
         (5) Hemoptysis
   2. Diagnostic procedures (Pettker & Lockwood, 2007)
      a. First diagnostic step is to assess level of risk for DVT
      b. Testing for D-dimer, a product of the degradation of fibrin by plasmin
      c. Imaging studies appropriate to the suspected type of venous disorder: venous compression ultrasonography, magnetic resonance imaging (MRI), or contrast venography (most invasive)
      d. Complete blood count to evaluate for leukocytosis
      e. Blood cultures possible for persistent fever
      f. Screening for an inherited thrombophilia may be considered in some circumstances

INTERVENTIONS

A. **Superficial phlebitis**
   1. Bedrest
   2. Elevation of extremity
   3. Analgesics and antiinflammatory medication
   4. Compression therapy
B. **DVT—anticoagulants**
C. **Septic pelvic thrombophlebitis**
   1. Antibiotics
   2. Anticoagulants—use of anticoagulants is considered by some to be controversial due to the lack of prospective, randomized treatment trials (Duff, 2007; Pettker & Lockwood, 2007)
D. **Prevention of venous disorders** (Lowdermilk, 2007; Smeltzer et al, 2008; Urden et al, 2006)
   1. Application of graduated elastic compression stockings or pneumatic compression devices, when ordered. Pneumatic compression devices are especially recommended during and after cesarean section.
   2. Encourage adequate hydration.
   3. Positioning to minimize stasis: elevate extremities and discourage prolonged sitting, and/or crossed legs
   4. Encourage early ambulation.
   5. Active and passive leg exercises when ambulation is not possible
E. **Minimizing complications of venous disorders to enhance recovery**
   1. Ensure bedrest as ordered.
   2. Administer anticoagulants (Pettker & Lockwood, 2007; Smeltzer et al, 2008)
      a. Unfractionated heparin, warfarin (Coumadin), and low-molecular-weight heparin (LMWH) such as dalteparin, enoxaparin, and tinzaparin are all considered safe for use during lactation.
      b. Heparin side effects: hemorrhage, osteoporosis (usually reversible), and heparin-induced thrombocytopenia (occurring in 3% of patients)
      c. LMWH anticoagulants have fewer side effects.
   3. Administer oxygen as necessary.
   4. Administer sedatives and pain relief medication, as needed (inflammation and arterial spasm contribute to pain).
   5. Observe for signs and symptoms of pulmonary embolism.
   6. Administer antibiotics that may be ordered if infectious process persists.
   7. Ensure frequent rest periods.
   8. Assess vital signs at each shift.
   9. Apply continuous, moist heat to extremity to relieve pain and promote circulation.
   10. Explain the importance of treatment.
   11. Avoid pillows behind knees or raising the knee gatch of the bed.
   12. Teach relaxation or distraction techniques.
   13. Elevate extremities on pillows for relief of venous aching and to increase venous return.
   14. Use a bed cradle to keep linens and blankets off of extremities.
   15. Provide emotional support as necessary.
       a. Stay with the woman when she is anxious.
       b. Provide occupational therapy or diversion.
       c. Assure mother that infant has appropriate care.
       d. Allow infant's siblings to visit.
       e. Explain thrombophlebitis to the family.
       f. Refer mother to a social worker if necessary.

HEALTH EDUCATION

A. **Instruct patient regarding proper application and use of compression stockings.**
B. **Teach patient passive and active leg exercises; encourage an exercise or daily walking program.**
C. **Explain purpose of anticoagulants, need for strict compliance with dosage ordered and timing of doses, and importance of follow-up blood tests.**

D. Review signs of anticoagulant overdose: faintness, dizziness, severe headaches or abdominal pain, reddish or brownish urine, nosebleeds or bleeding from any part of the body, bruises, or red or black bowel movements. Emphasize need to promptly report any spontaneous bleeding from anywhere in the body.

E. Encourage woman to check with a physician or pharmacist before taking other prescribed or over-the-counter medications that may negatively interact with sodium warfarin (Coumadin), such as those containing acetylsalicylic acid formulations (aspirin-based products).

F. Educate patient about risks of future venous disorder episodes, need to avoid contraceptive methods containing estrogen, and medications that affect the action of anticoagulants.

G. Educate patient about need to minimize venous stasis to prevent further thrombotic episodes.

   1. Avoid dehydration in warm weather.
   2. Wear warm clothes during cold weather to maintain adequate circulation.
   3. Avoid periods of prolonged sitting at work, while traveling, or while watching television; getting up to walk around every 30 to 60 minutes prevents venous pooling in the legs by increasing circulatory return to the heart.
   4. Avoid crossing the legs while seated, which decreases circulation to the legs because of pressure on the popliteal space behind the knee.
   5. Elevate the legs whenever possible when sitting, but avoid pressure under the knees when legs are elevated.
   6. Avoid garters, knee-high stockings, and trauma to legs.

POSTPARTUM MOOD DISORDERS

INTRODUCTION

A. Three types of recognized postpartum mood disorders: postpartum blues, postpartum depression, and postpartum psychosis (Payne, 2007)

B. "Baby blues" or adjusted reaction with depressed mood
   1. Mildest form of postpartum mood disorder
   2. Occurs on the third to eighth postpartum day, usually at home because of early postpartum discharge
   3. Has an incidence of 60% to 80% of all postpartum women (Payne, 2007)
   4. Symptoms disappear spontaneously by the second postpartum week with support and adequate rest. May progress to postpartum depression.

C. Postpartum depression is a major mood disorder, not a separate diagnosis, the onset of which occurs within the first 4 weeks after delivery.
   1. Has an incidence of approximately 10% to 20% of all postpartum women (Payne, 2007)
   2. Greatest risk occurs around fourth postpartum week, but can occur at any time during the first postpartum year (60% to 70% in the first 3 weeks to 3 to 6 months).
   3. Diagnosis is based on presence of five symptoms of major depression recognized in the *Diagnostic and Statistical Manual of Mental Disorders,* one of which must be either depressed mood or decreased interest or pleasure in activities, most of the day nearly every day for 2 weeks or more (Wisner, Parry, & Piontek, 2002).
   4. Effective screening tools to assess for postpartum depression are readily available.
      a. Edinburgh Postnatal Depression Scale (EPDS): most data available (Cox, Holden, & Sagovsky, 1987)
      b. Beck Depression Inventory (Beck, 2002)
      c. Others screening tools such as Zung Depression Scale, Center for Epidemiological Studies Depression Scale
   5. Etiology unknown, but likely to be multifactorial, including psychological, biological, hormonal, and social factors
   6. Negative effects (Payne, 2007; Wisner et al, 2002)
      a. Impaired mother-child relationship
      b. Impaired emotional development, language development, attention and cognitive skills in child
      c. Increased risk of long-term behavioral problems in child
      d. Marital relationship difficulties
      e. Increased risk of further episodes of depression

7. Can be disabling and last for prolonged periods
8. New-onset postpartum depression may represent the first manifestation of previously undiagnosed bipolar disorder.

D. Postpartum psychosis
1. Symptoms include hallucinations, bizarre behavior, delusions, extreme disorganization of thought, and phobias; often a manifestation of bipolar disorder.
2. Has an incidence of 0.1% or 1 per 1000 postpartum women (Payne, 2007)
3. Onset usually occurs within the first 2 weeks after delivery (Wisner et al, 2002).
4. Women with postpartum psychosis should not be left alone with their infants.

CLINICAL PRACTICE

A. Assessment
1. History
   a. Risk factors (Payne, 2007; Wisner et al, 2002)
      (1) History of major depression or postpartum depression
      (2) Depression during pregnancy
      (3) Diagnosis of neurosis or psychosis (schizophrenia, bipolar disorder)
      (4) Family history of depression or other psychiatric disorders
      (5) Premenstrual or oral contraceptive-associated mood changes
      (6) Stressful life events
         (a) Lack of social, emotional, or financial support
         (b) Increased child care responsibilities
         (c) Marital conflict, single, separated, or divorced status
      (7) Substance use or abuse
      (8) Metabolic disorders, especially hypothyroidism or hyperthyroidism, thyroiditis
      (9) Rapid decline in levels in reproductive hormones after delivery may be a contributor in susceptible women; however, this is somewhat controversial (Wisner et al, 2002).
   b. Symptoms associated with postpartum mood disorders, some of which may also be seen in postpartum women not experiencing mood disorders
      (1) Mood swings
      (2) Weepiness, sadness
      (3) Irritability, anxiety, restlessness
      (4) Fatigue, difficulty sleeping, exhaustion
      (5) Feeling of being overwhelmed
      (6) Decreased concentration
      (7) Decreased libido
      (8) Extreme anxiety about infant's feeding, sleeping, or crying
      (9) Inability to complete activities of daily living (ADLs) or care adequately for infant
      (10) Guilt
      (11) Anorexia
      (12) Helplessness, feelings of inadequacy
      (13) Avoidance of family or friends
2. Physical findings
   a. Hyperthyroidism or hypothyroidism
   b. Difficulty in breathing
   c. Heart palpitations
   d. Tremors
3. Psychosocial findings
   a. Poor social support networks
   b. Expression of concern about difficult labor and delivery
   c. Unplanned pregnancy
   d. Unwanted pregnancy
   e. Feelings of being unloved
   f. Poor relationship with mother
   g. Detachment from reality
   h. Disturbances in thinking, feeling, and behavior

        i. Poor interactions with infant, family, and staff

        j. Inability to relax

    4. Diagnostic procedures

        a. Hormonal level determinations, including thyroid testing

        b. Blood tests for drugs and alcohol

        c. Psychological profile/evaluation

INTERVENTIONS

A. Data collection

    1. Observe mother with infant, by herself, and with family and friends.

    2. Discuss mother's plans for her infant and for herself.

    3. Assess sleeping, eating, resting, and coping behaviors.

    4. Assess psychosocial factors, mood, and support systems.

B. Interventions

    1. Request psychiatric evaluation whenever indicated.

        a. Expressed thoughts about suicide or thoughts of harming her infant should always be taken seriously and require urgent referral.

        b. Women with one of the three types of postpartum mood disorders, depending on the specific diagnosis, may require one or more of the following:

            (1) Referral to support groups

            (2) Antidepressants

                (a) Antidepressant treatment may trigger the onset of hypomania or mania (Payne, 2007).

                (b) Antidepressants that are considered safe for use during breastfeeding are available.

        c. Referral for psychotherapy: individual, group, or both

        d. Transfer to psychiatric inpatient service.

    2. Confirm correct use of any antidepressant medication ordered.

    3. Support coping mechanisms.

        a. Allow mother time for herself and encourage her to have time away from infant.

        b. Reinforce mother's self-care activities.

        c. Encourage and allow mother to ventilate her feelings.

        d. Provide reality orientation.

    4. Support and facilitate parent-infant interaction.

        a. Encourage mothering behaviors and assumption of the maternal role.

        b. Assist mother to learn parenting skills.

        c. Praise the woman's positive actions of mothering.

    5. Support efforts of significant other and family to care for mother.

        a. Encourage family support for mother.

        b. Listen to family's concerns and take them very seriously.

        c. Determine when significant others can be present to learn about infant's needs and infant care.

        d. Follow through with resources to help family.

        e. Explain psychologic changes during the postpartum period.

        f. Assist family to identify ways to keep home environment safe.

            (1) Remove potentially harmful objects and weapons.

            (2) Arrange for someone to be at home to help mother.

HEALTH EDUCATION

A. Teach woman and significant others the signs and symptoms of depression and mania (decreased ability to sleep, psychosis, and agitation) and encourage them to call a care provider if symptoms occur, persist, or worsen (Payne, 2007).

B. Assist family to develop plans to provide a safe and secure environment for mother and infant.

C. Discuss benefits of contraception during the period of depression.

D. Instruct woman how to avoid crisis situations and develop coping skills.

E. Instruct woman in stress reduction techniques.
F. Increase family awareness that postpartum depression and psychosis need professional intervention.

CASE STUDIES AND STUDY QUESTIONS

Ms. H. is a 34-year-old woman gravida 5, para 5 (G5, P5) who delivered a healthy boy weighing 4800 g (10 pounds, 9.5 ounces) after 16 hours of labor. Her pregnancy was complicated by chronic hypertension. She is breastfeeding her infant in the recovery room when she is assigned to your care. Her vital signs are stable, although her blood pressure is mildly elevated at 130/90. Her lochia is bright red and heavy, and it has a clot approximately 2 cm (0.79 inch) in diameter.

1. The *most* important assessment that needs to be performed is:
   a. Checking her vital signs every 5 to 15 minutes for the first hour after delivery
   b. Checking location and firmness of the fundus
   c. Charting the amount and saturation of menstrual pads every hour
   d. Continuing to support her breastfeeding efforts
2. Ms. H. is considered to be at high risk for uterine atony because:
   a. She is a grand multipara.
   b. The size of her infant
   c. The length of her labor
   d. All of the above
3. You notice that Ms. H. has saturated four menstrual pads with bright red blood during a 1-hour period. Her vital signs are stable. The most likely cause for her bleeding is:
   a. Subinvolution related to retained placental fragments
   b. Ruptured hematoma
   c. Uterine atony
   d. Lacerated cervix
4. Considering Ms. H.'s history, it would be important to question the physician's order for which medication to control her uterine hemorrhage?
   a. Misoprostol
   b. Oxytocin
   c. Methylergonovine
   d. Carboprost tromethamine
5. Postpartum hemorrhage uncontrolled by uterotonic medication may require all of the following *except:*
   a. Tamponade
   b. D-dimer assays
   c. Selective arterial embolization
   d. Hysterectomy

6. You receive a telephone call from Ms. H. about 2 weeks after delivery, reporting continued small amounts of bleeding since discharge, but the bleeding has suddenly increased. She reports saturating four menstrual pads in the past hour. You recognize she may be having a late postpartum hemorrhage and instruct her to call her care provider immediately for emergency treatment. The cause of her current bleeding is most likely to be:
   a. Uterine atony
   b. DIC
   c. Retained placental fragments
   d. Hematomas and lacerations
7. Vaginal hematomas are associated with all of the following except:
   a. Forceps delivery
   b. Episiotomy
   c. Excessive fundal pressure on the uterus
   d. Nulliparity

Ms. P. is a 24-year-old woman who is G1, P1. She was in labor for 28 hours. A cesarean section was performed because of failure to progress. She delivered a 3629-g (8-pound) boy in good health. After delivery her vital signs were stable, and lochia was slight, red, and contained no clots. A Foley catheter has been inserted to straight drainage. Her dressing is clean and dry. Forty-eight hours after delivery, her temperature is 38° C (100.4° F) and continues to rise.

8. What factors have predisposed her to a postpartum infection?
   a. Age and type of delivery
   b. Length of labor and type of delivery
   c. Parity and type of delivery
   d. Age and number of vaginal exams during labor
9. Which type of puerperal infection does she likely have?
   a. Breast
   b. Bladder
   c. Vaginal
   d. Uterine
10. Which medication regimen would you anticipate being ordered for Ms. P.?
   a. Oral antibiotics if temperature is less than 101° F
   b. IV antibiotics until afebrile for 24 hours

c. IV antibiotics until discharge, then oral antibiotics at home

d. IV antibiotics until afebrile for 24 hours, then oral antibiotics until discharge

11. Daily inspection of the perineum may reveal problems with an episiotomy, such as:
    a. Hematoma
    b. Infection
    c. Edema
    d. All of the above

12. To promote healing of an episiotomy and prevent infection, the nurse should:
    a. Teach the mother perineal care.
    b. Teach the mother about how infections are transmitted.
    c. Teach the mother about the importance of rest, nutrition, and fluid intake.
    d. All of the above are correct.

Ms. G. is a 27-year-old overweight woman who is a G1, P1 who delivered a girl weighing 2800 g (6 lb, 3 oz) by cesarean section. She underwent a prolonged labor of 27 hours.

13. Which factors contribute to the risk of Ms. G. developing septic pelvic thrombophlebitis?
    a. Obesity, type of delivery, pregnancy
    b. Type of delivery, parity, length of labor
    c. Length of labor, obesity, age
    d. Pregnancy, age, length of labor

14. Ms. G. is prescribed warfarin for anticoagulation. You advise her to avoid:
    a. Aspirin
    b. Massage of extremities
    c. Oral contraceptives
    d. All of the above

15. Ms. G. asks if her children may come see her in the hospital. You respond that:
    a. Her condition is very serious and she needs to rest right now.
    b. Only children older than age 14 years can visit the unit.
    c. Her children may visit when she wants.
    d. You will call the social worker and the children will be cared for so she does not have to worry about them.

16. Which symptom is *most* indicative of development of a pulmonary embolism?
    a. Generalized pallor
    b. Dyspnea
    c. Absence of peripheral pulses
    d. Positive Homans' sign

17. What is *not* useful for the prevention of thrombophlebitis?
    a. Compression stockings
    b. Early ambulation
    c. Antiinflammatory medication
    d. Pneumatic compression devices

18. LMWH is preferable to unfractionated heparin because:
    a. Heparin is contraindicated in breastfeeding women.
    b. LMWH has fewer side effects.
    c. Length of treatment is less.
    d. Risk for recurrence is decreased.

Ms. Q. is a 21-year-old woman who is G1, P1. At 39 weeks' gestation, she vaginally delivered an infant girl late last night who is in good health. Ms. Q. was excited about being pregnant and felt well throughout her pregnancy. She is eager to breastfeed but feels anxious about being a new mother. You enter her room and she is crying because her husband cannot come to visit because he must work overtime.

19. Based on her history, what is correct?
    a. She is not exhibiting any specific symptoms of a postpartum mood disorder.
    b. She suffering from mild depression based on her pregnancy course.
    c. She should be evaluated for psychosis because she has phobias.
    d. She is severely depressed based on social and personal history.

20. Puerperal depression:
    a. Usually resolves spontaneously in a short period of time
    b. Rarely recurs after treatment
    c. Is likely to be caused by many factors
    d. Has few long-term effects on the children of the affected mother

21. Use of antidepressants in the postpartum period:
    a. Is contraindicated in breastfeeding mothers
    b. May trigger a manic episode
    c. Is usually not necessary due to postpartum hormone changes
    d. Requires a different dosage until 6 weeks postpartum

22. Treatment for postpartum depression includes:
    a. Active empathic listening
    b. Psychiatric care
    c. Antidepressive agents
    d. All of the above

23. Postpartum psychosis includes which symptom?
    a. Fear
    b. Tearfulness
    c. Delusions
    d. Elation

24. When taking a history for depression, it is important to assess for:
    a. Depressed mood
    b. Decreased interest or pleasure in activities
    c. Duration of symptoms
    d. All of the above

ANSWERS TO STUDY QUESTIONS

1. b	7. c	13. a	19. a
2. d	8. b	14. d	20. c
3. c	9. d	15. c	21. b
4. c	10. b	16. b	22. d
5. b	11. d	17. c	23. c
6. c	12. d	18. b	24. d

REFERENCES

Austin, M. P., & Mitchell, P. B. (1998). Use of psychotropic medications in breast-feeding women: Acute and prophylactic treatment. *Australian-New Zealand Journal of Psychiatry, 32*(6), 778–878.

Beck, C. T. (2002). Revision of the postpartum depression predictors inventory. *Journal of Obstetric, Gynecologic, and Neonatal Nursing, 31*(4), 394–402.

Betzold, C. M. (2007). An update on the recognition and management of lactational breast inflammation (review). *Journal of Midwifery and Women's Health, 52*(6), 595–605.

Burtelow, M., Riley, E., Druzin, M., Fontaine, M., Viele, M., & Goodnough, L. T. (2007). How we treat: Management of life-threatening primary postpartum hemorrhage with a standardized massive transfusion protocol. *Transfusion, 47*, 1564–1572.

Chichester, M. (2005). When your patient is from the obstetric department: Postpartum hemorrhage and massive transfusion. *Journal of Perianesthesia Nursing, 20*, 167–176.

Cox, J. L., Holden, J. M., & Sagovsky, R. (1987). Detection of postnatal depression. Development of the 10-item Edinburgh Postnatal Depression Scale. *British Journal of Psychiatry, 150*, 782–786.

Cunningham, F., Leveno, K., Bloom, S., Hauth, J., Rouse, D, & Spong, C. (Eds.). (2010). Puerperal infection. In *Williams obstetrics* (23rd ed.). New York: McGraw-Hill Medical.

Duff, P. (2007). Maternal and perinatal infection—Bacterial. In S. G. Gabbe, J. L. Simpson, & J. R. Niebyl (Eds.), H. Galan, L. Goetzl, Eric R.M. Jauniaux, M. Landon (associate eds), *Obstetrics: Normal and problem pregnancies* (5th ed., pp. 1233–1248). New York: Churchill Livingstone.

Francois, K. E., & Foley, M. R. (2007). Antepartum and postpartum hemorrhage. In S. G. Gabbe, J. R. Niebyl, & J. L. Simpson (Eds.), *Obstetrics: Normal and problem pregnancies* (5th ed., pp. 456–485). New York: Churchill Livingstone.

Gupta, R., & Stouffer, G. A. (2001). Deep venous thrombosis: A review of the pathophysiology, clinical features, and diagnostic modalities. *American Journal of the Medical Sciences, 322*(6), 358–364.

Klima, D. A., & Snyder, T. E. (2008). Postpartum ovarian vein thrombosis. *Obstetrics & Gynecology, 111*(2 Part 1), 431–435.

Ladewig, P., London, M., & Davidson, M. (2010). *Contemporary maternal-newborn nursing care* (7th ed., p. 888). Upper Saddle River, NJ: Pearson.

Livingston, J. C., Llata, E., Rinehart, E., Leidwanger, C., Mabie, B., Haddad, B., & Sibai, B. (2003). Gentamicin and clindamycin therapy in postpartum endometritis: The efficacy of daily dosing versus dosing every 8 hours. *American Journal of Obstetrics & Gynecology, 188*, 149–152.

Lowdermilk, D. L. (2007). Postpartum complications. In D. L. Lowdermilk, & S. E. Perry (Eds.), *Maternity & women's health care* (9th ed., pp. 975–990). St. Louis: Mosby.

Payne, J. L. (2007). Antidepressant use in the postpartum period: Practical considerations. *American Journal of Psychiatry, 164*(9), 1329–1332.

Pettker, C. M., & Lockwood, C. J. (2007). Thromboembolic disorders. In S. G. Gabbe, J. R. Niebyl, & J. L. Simpson (Eds.), *Obstetrics: Normal and problem pregnancies* (5th ed., pp. 1067–1077). New York: Churchill Livingstone.

Pillitteri, A. (2007). *Maternal & child health nursing care of the childbearing and childrearing family* (5th ed., pp. 654–678). Philadelphia: Lippincott Williams & Wilkins.

Rhode, M. A. (2009). Medication considerations for women during the postpartum period. In M. C. Brucker, & T. L. King (Eds.), *Pharmacology for women's health,* Sudbury, MA: Jones and Bartlett.

Smeltzer S., Bare B., Hinkle J., & Cheever, K. (Eds.), (2008). Assessment and management of patients with vascular disorders and problems of peripheral circulation. In *Brunner & Suddarth's textbook of medical-surgical nursing* (11th ed., pp. 1004–1010). Philadelphia: Lippincott Williams & Wilkins.

Tran, S. H., Caughey, A. B., & Musci, T. J. (2003). Meconium-stained amniotic fluid is associated with puerperal infections. *American Journal of Obstetrics & Gynecology, 189*, 747–750.

Urden, L., Stacy, K., & Lough, M. (2006). Cardiovascular disorders. In *Thelan's critical care nursing: Diagnosis and management* (5th ed., pp. 427–502). St. Louis: Mosby.

Wisner, K. L., Parry, B. L., & Piontek, C. M. (2002). Postpartum depression. *New England Journal of Medicine, 347*(3), 194–199.

Yonkers, K. A. (2009). Management of depressions and psychoses in pregnancy and the puerperium. In R. Creasy, R. Resnik, J. Iams, C. Lockwood, & T. Moore (Eds.), *Creasy & Resnik's maternal-fetal medicine: Principles & practice* (6th ed., pp. 1113–1122). Philadelphia: Saunders.

ETHICS AND ISSUES

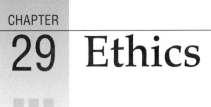

CHAPTER

29 Ethics

Charlotte Stephenson

OBJECTIVES

1. Define common terms used in ethical discussions.
2. Identify three theories or approaches to ethical thinking.
3. Discuss the principle of autonomy and the concept of informed consent.
4. Discuss the principles of beneficence and nonmaleficence and the concept of paternalism.
5. Discuss the principle of justice and the concepts of microallocation and macroallocation.
6. Discuss proxy decision-makers for care of the newborn.
7. Explain the influences of spirituality and culture on ethical decision-making by parents and professionals.
8. Explain the female versus male and nursing versus medical perspectives brought to ethical discussions.
9. Distinguish among autonomy, substituted judgment, and best interests as a basis for ethical decisions.
10. Define the purpose and goals of palliative care and infants for whom this type of care may be chosen by parents.
11. Identify five clinical issues that commonly lead to ethical dilemmas for nurses.
12. Identify two professional issues that commonly lead to ethical dilemmas for nurses.
13. Outline key points of a teaching plan for patients and families regarding ethics and ethical dilemmas.

INTRODUCTION

A. **Terminology**
  1. Morals: from the Latin word *mores*, which means "custom" or "habit"; the moral principles that guide nursing practice are respect, autonomy, beneficence, nonmaleficence, veracity, confidentiality, fidelity, justice, and privacy (American Nurses Association [ANA], 2001)
  2. Morality: one's belief about what is right or the best thing to do; general rules of conduct and standards for evaluating behavior; learned through socialization and association with groups such as family, religious, ethnic groups
  3. Moral agent: one who has the power to act; one who is making a moral decision
  4. Values: standards that are a person's basic beliefs about the self and relationships to others
  5. Value system: a learned, organized set of principles and beliefs concerning conduct and behavior that helps a person choose options, make decisions, and resolve conflicts
  6. Ethics: from the Greek word *ethos*, meaning "custom" or "character"; established by Socrates, the discipline dealing with what is good or bad and with moral duty and obligation
  7. Bioethics: a subdivision of ethics to determine the most morally desirable course of action in health care when there are conflicting values inherent in varying treatment options (American Hospital Association, 1985)
  8. Ethical-moral dilemma: a difficult choice between two alternatives when there is a conflict of values, no clear consensus about what is right and wrong, and all options are morally justifiable and equally defendable
  9. Law: set of rules for social behavior; enforced by the police, courts, and prisons
  10. Quality of life: total well-being, including both physical and psychosocial determinants (Hack, 1999) so that the individual can lead his or her life and function as part of the human family, individually and collectively (Kirschbaum, 1996; Swaney, English, & Carter, 2006); to ensure that quality of life decisions not be reduced to arbitrary judgments based on personal preference or the perceived social worth of the patient, justified criteria of benefits and burdens must be considered (Beauchamp & Childress, 2008)

B. **Ethical approaches and theories**
1. Non-normative ethics: an approach to ethics that denies that universal principles exist to guide behavior
   a. Descriptive ethics: represents the work of sociologists, anthropologists, psychologists, historians, and others who describe or attempt to explain moral behaviors (Beauchamp & Childress, 2008)
   b. Metaethics: from the Greek word *meta*, meaning "behind, beyond, higher"; the division of ethics wherein professional ethicists or philosophers attempt to analyze reasons behind the principles
2. Principle-based ethics: an approach to ethics that identifies and defines fundamental principles to guide behavior and decision-making
   a. Duty and obligation–based approach: deontology
      (1) From Greek word *deonteis*, meaning "duty"
      (2) Devises norms or rules from duties human beings owe one another because of commitments made
      (3) Duty to follow universally accepted rules of what is right and wrong
      (4) Looks at motives behind an action.
      (5) Related principles (and the moral principles guiding nursing practice) (ANA, 2001)
         (a) Autonomy
            [i] From Greek words *auto*, meaning "self," and *nomos*, meaning "law"
            [ii] Respect for the unconditional worth of people; for their thoughts and actions; and for their free choice and personal decisions (Joffe, Manocchia, Weeks, & Cleary, 2003)
            [iii] The right of people to be left alone and to define their own destiny without interference; self-determination
            [iv] In health care, based on the doctrine of informed consent, making deliberate choices about an option (Beauchamp & Childress, 2008)
         (b) Beneficence
            [i] From the Hippocratic oath; a duty to help others; to balance good and harm; to prevent harm, to remove harm, and to not inflict harm
            [ii] An obligation to accomplish good in service to others through acts such as mercy, kindness, and generosity
            [iii] In health care, providing information on the benefits as well as risks of an intervention (Beauchamp & Childress, 2008)
         (c) Nonmaleficence
            [i] From the Hippocratic oath; an obligation to "first, do no harm" to others; the duty to avoid intending, causing, permitting, or imposing harm or the risk of harm to another person
            [ii] Harm must be ultimately justified to achieve some greater good or to prevent a greater harm
         (d) Justice
            [i] Rule derived from Aristotle; the obligation to treat individuals equally or comparably; to distribute benefits and burdens equally throughout society
            [ii] Must guard against arbitrary, inconsistent decision-making
            [iii] Macroallocation: distribution at a societal level; example: which program is funded?
            [iv] Microallocation: distribution at a personal level; example: who receives the transplant?
         (e) Veracity: obligation to tell the truth and to give full, complete, and truthful information to patient and parents for decision-making
         (f) Fidelity: obligation to keep promises or commitments; to remain loyal
         (g) Privacy: right of an individual or group to decide when and to what extent information about themselves can be revealed to others; freedom from intrusion
         (h) Confidentiality: an extension of privacy; right to limit the access of others to private information revealed by a patient to his or her provider
         (i) Respect: reverence for persons and for human dignity
   b. Goal outcome consequences–based approach: teleology, utilitarianism, or consequentialism
      (1) The rightness or wrongness of an act depends on its utility or usefulness.
      (2) Rights consist of actions that have good consequences, and wrong consists of actions that have bad consequences; acts are judged according to their value.

(3) Achieving the greatest good or happiness for the greatest number of people by balancing the good that is possible with the harm that might result from performing or not performing an action; the end justifies the means.

(4) Related principles (Lagana & Duderstadt, 1995)

(a) Allocation of resources versus cost-effectiveness; relates to the distribution of scarce resources

(b) Quality of life versus sanctity of life; addresses the question of a good life compared with life at all costs.

(c) Paternalism versus autonomy; addresses the question of who knows best and who should make the decision for an individual.

(d) Withholding of care versus starting care; relates to the delivery of care to individuals and society; questions when care should be initiated, withheld, or withdrawn.

c. Virtue character–based approach

(1) Traced to Aristotle; decisions about actions are based on what a virtuous person would do

(2) Ethics is not about following rules, but about character and virtues (e.g., respect, fidelity, honesty, benevolence); rules and principles come later.

d. Case-based approach (casuistry)

(1) The claims or grounds of a particular case are compared with similar cases.

(2) Casuistry is about how a general moral principle should be understood in a similar set of circumstances.

e. Story-based approach (narrative)

(1) The narrative story is a method of ethical reasoning.

(2) Specific narratives for each case, such as the person or people involved, the subjective experience, the illness and caring, are the focus of consideration.

f. Care-based approach (feminist)

(1) Related to virtue theory; not based on fixed rules, principles, or theories, but on regard for the person; in health care is relationship-based and stresses the context of a situation: a person has a life before and after the illness, and caregivers should ensure continuity and connectedness to that life

(2) Nurses have looked at this model carefully as a basis for their practice because it stresses holism, connectedness, hearing the patient's story, and the ethics of care (Anderson, 2007).

g. Social ethics (Swaney et al, 2006)

(1) Concern for the individual and for the common good of all; moral judgments affect the larger social community of which the individual and institutions are a part; example: society may bear the financial, physical, educational, and social costs of severely disabled infants.

(2) How individual moral behavior and the range of moral responsibility and accountability are influenced by social context, social structures, and public policy issues

h. Protection of human subjects in research (Swaney et al, 2006)

(1) Introduction of interventions or treatments without appropriate research into safety, efficacy, and long-term outcomes

(2) Professional responsibility to evaluate the quality of evidence regarding the use and benefit of both traditional and newer clinical practices; evidence-based practice (Orleans, Tappero, Glicken, & Merenstein, 2002)

(3) Importance of empirical studies to contribute to the ethical aspects of clinical practice and the effect of ethical decision-making (McHaffie, Laing, Parker, & McMillan, 2001)

C. **Related principles and concepts**

1. Informed consent: based on principle of autonomy or the right to make decisions without coercion (Joffe et al, 2003)

a. The fundamental right of a person to determine what happens to his or her own body; to decide what is harmful or beneficial in treatment and care; should be interfered with only to prevent harm to others

b. Supported by considerable court decisions in the United States; stresses patient rights; to accomplish informed consent, the reasonable person standard may be applied: "What would the reasonable person want in this circumstance?"

    c. Requires that professionals have a positive attitude about autonomy

    d. Rests on an assumption of competence and capacity

      (1) Competence

        (a) A legal status; decided by the courts, usually based on age of majority; definition of adult

        (b) All adults are competent unless a court decides otherwise.

      (2) Capacity

        (a) A clinical judgment; decided by caregivers based on patient's ability to understand alternatives and consequences of treatment and no treatment, to weigh options, to think about life goals and values, to choose the best option for self, and to communicate the decision

        (b) Levels of capacity

          [i] Decisional capacity: ability to make decisions

          [ii] Executional capacity: ability to carry out decisions

        (c) Nuances to capacity

          [i] Capacity may come and go, depending on such factors as time of day, effects of medication and anesthesia, environment, stress, and pain.

          [ii] Must use caution when determining capacity; should not manipulate or control patient's capacity; should not judge quickly; should not assume anyone who disagrees does not have capacity; be careful about words used, time of day, condition of patient

          [iii] Consider ways to restore capacity so patient can make own decision (e.g., hold medications temporarily to restore capacity).

          [iv] Determine whether the decision can be delayed while patient regains capacity.

    e. The process of informed consent

      (1) Process is important; paper is often used as evidence that process occurred

      (2) The right to consent also includes the right to refuse.

      (3) Components of informed consent are defined by each state, but usually include:

        (a) A health care professional's recommendation for treatment

        (b) Determination of competence and capacity

        (c) Truthful and honest disclosure of information such as medical condition, nature and purpose of procedure, consequences, risks, alternatives, and name and qualifications of person performing treatment

        (d) Patient understanding of information

        (e) Voluntary consent or refusal, with a lack of coercion

        (f) Documentation of process

      (4) Responsibility for obtaining consent remains with the person performing procedure or care.

      (5) Types of consent

        (a) Blanket consent: signed on admission to a hospital

        (b) Battery consent: signed for a procedure such as surgery

        (c) Detailed consent: signed for such things as a research drug or treatment

      (6) Who gives consent

        (a) Competent adult: age of majority; determined by state law

        (b) Incompetent adult: court-appointed guardian; person close to adult who knows wishes if no court-appointed guardian is available

        (c) Minors: parent or guardian

        (d) Emancipated minor: when no longer subject to parental control (e.g., after marriage)

        (e) Mature minor: age limits and scope determined by state law; usually applies to consent for situations such as pregnancy care, sexually transmitted disease care, and substance abuse treatment

      (7) Research consent requires detailed information and a lengthy, special process

2. Concept of paternalism-maternalism-parentalism

    a. A competent, capable adult being treated as if he or she were a child by a person or people acting as if they had the authority and concern of a parent (Cahill, 2001)

      (1) Paternalism or patriarchal health care system: fathering behaviors (Woodward, 1998)

      (2) Maternalism: mothering behaviors

      (3) Parentalism: nonsexist term; parenting behaviors

    b. Person or people claim they are acting on behalf of the patient; they know what is best and good for the patient (Cahill, 2001).

    c. Is based on the assumption that a patient's lack of technical or medical expertise justifies the provider in making the decision for the patient (Cahill, 2001)

    d. A way to induce, coerce, or direct others to do what one wants them to do (Cahill, 2001)

    e. May include a variety of behaviors such as nonverbal pretenses, withholding of relevant information, lying, and coercion, with the goal being that the patient complies with what the provider wants to do.

    f. Anyone can be parental: spouse, family, friends, clergy, provider, or administrator.

3. Proxy decision-makers

    a. Newborns are incompetent and unable to make their own decisions.

    b. Parents have primary authority (parental autonomy) to act as proxy or surrogate decision-makers for their infants.

    c. Legally, through court rulings, society has designated parents as primary decision-makers because they love the infant and are concerned for the infant's well-being; they have the best interests of their infant in mind; they know the values of the family culture and environment in which the infant will be raised; and generally are interested in the welfare of their children. As a general matter of law, except in cases of abuse and neglect, courts have ruled that parents have the right to make medical decisions about their children (Annas, 1994; Purdy & Wadhwani, 2006; Rushton & Hogue, 1993).

    d. Some professional guidelines state that parental autonomy should not be absolute and that the decisions made by parents of premature infants should not be considered absolute (American Academy of Pediatrics [AAP], and American College of Obstetricians and Gynecologists [ACOG], 1995; ACOG, 1989) and that "physicians should not be forced to undertreat or overtreat an infant if, in their best medical knowledge, the treatment is not in compliance with the standard of care for that infant" (AAP, 1995); in protecting the rights of nonautonomous patients, guidelines to facilitate decision-making, establish a standard of care and support health care professionals in making the decision to remove life-sustaining support have been published (AAP, Committee on Bioethics, 1994).

    e. Double effect: principle that asserts that an action is considered good if the intent has positive value, even if secondary effects of the action might be considered harmful if undertaken as a primary goal (e.g., using narcotics for a dying newborn [the positive goal is relief of suffering, even at the expense of shortening life]) (Swaney et al, 2006).

    f. Problem of uncertainty (Swaney et al, 2006)

        (1) Medical uncertainty about the long-term prognosis or quality of life of a newborn infant complicates decision-making about what is in the best interests of the child and family (Stutts & Schloemann, 2002a; Zeigler, 2003)

        (2) Parental question: "Will my infant be OK when he [she] grows up?" Professional responses: A statistical approach gives probabilities about similar babies, but not about the parent's individual infant; "I don't know" response about their individual infant's outcome may be the most honest answer.

        (3) How prognostic uncertainty is (or is not) communicated to parents before delivery will influence decision-making when the prognosis or quality of life becomes more certain over time.

    g. Treatment versus nontreatment

        (1) Treatment goals should be established by parents (parental autonomy) with input or participation from health care professionals so that both are working toward the same goals (Culver et al, 2000; Glassford, 2003; Harrison, 1993; McHaffie et al, 2001; Swaney et al, 2006).

        (2) For parents to be decision-makers, they must be fully informed to consent to or refuse treatment for their newborn infant or infants (Culver et al, 2000; Purdy & Wadhwani, 2006; Zeigler, 2003).

            (a) Professionals have an ethical and legal obligation (AAP, 1995; Clark, 1996; Doroshow et al, 2000; Tyson, 1995) to inform parents with facts about the neonate's condition, illnesses, outcomes, risks, and benefits of various interventions or noninterventions so they are able to give informed consent or refusal (Culver et al, 2000; Siegel, Gardner, & Merenstein, 2002).

(b) Professional attitudes or intuition that interfere with open, honest communication of information to parents include (Harrison, 1993; McHaffie et al, 2001):

[i] Assuming that parents are too emotional to assimilate information or make a rational decision

[ii] Assuming that information about poor outcomes or complications may disrupt parental attachment to the infant

[iii] Assuming that parental guilt or psychological harm will result from decision-making and that the final decision is too much for the parents to bear

[iv] Health care providers' efforts to persuade parents: a difficult question between a respect for parental autonomy or an attempt to overcome it; professionals must be careful not to usurp parental authority

(c) Use of an evidence-based table of the likely outcomes (e.g., mortality, ventilator or oxygen use, brain scan results, long-term neurodevelopmental outcomes) may be useful for parental decision-making (Koh, Casey, & Harrison, 2000; Koh, Harrison, & Morley, 1999).

(d) In several studies, prenatal consultation with a neonatologist for the woman has been found to be useful (Neufeld, Woodrum, & Tarczy-Hornoch, 2000; Paul et al, 1999).

(e) Research (McHaffie et al, 2001) has indicated that parents believe:

[i] They can or should accept responsibility for making difficult decisions; the majority state that the ultimate decision should be theirs.

[ii] They are able to understand medical issues or information and to assess consequences for their own child.

[iii] They can make a decision and do so without guilt, doubt, or adverse consequences and believe that the right decision was made.

(f) Decisions are often based on the infant's medical condition and less by the parent's wishes (Brinchmann, Forde, & Nortwedt, 2002; Partridge, Freeman, Weiss, & Martinez, 2001); parental choices can be limited by:

[i] A lack of information on options for limited resuscitation

[ii] Differing resuscitation thresholds and an unwillingness by physicians to accept parental requests not to resuscitate above these thresholds

[iii] Parental indecision, uncertainty, and guilt for making a wrong choice

(3) In addition to what kind of treatment is in the best interests of the infant, the appropriateness of any treatment must be considered.

(a) A nontreatment decision is withholding or withdrawing of treatment.

(b) A nontreatment decision should not be referred to as withholding or a withdrawing care.

(c) Care, whether curative (with treatment) or palliative (with comfort care), is always provided.

(d) Nonbeneficial: treatment considered not to benefit the patient may be withheld or withdrawn.

[i] No ethical obligation exists to provide nonbeneficial treatment, but a standard definition of nonbeneficial is lacking.

[ii] A medical effect may be obtained without a medical benefit as determined by family goals for the newborn or child; may include physiologic, psychologic, social, and religious reasons (Lantos et al, 1989).

4. Creating an ethical environment: one that promotes ethical practice and preserves integrity (Rushton & Scanlon, 1995)

a. When faced with a moral or ethical dilemma, there are four elements necessary to ensure an integrity-preserving compromise (Winslow & Winslow, 1991):

(1) Sharing a common moral language

(2) Developing a mutual respect

(3) Understanding and acknowledging moral complexity

(4) Defining the compromise's limits

b. Legal versus ethical perspective

(1) Legal means something fulfills the terms of the law.

(a) Types of laws:

[i] Constitutional law: source of the law is the federal or state constitution; it guarantees individuals certain rights or freedom (e.g., right to free speech).

            [ii] Statutory law: source of the law is the federal or state legislature; law is made by men and women in legislature (e.g., a living will, Health Insurance Portability and Accountability Act [HIPAA] regulations) (Chesney, 2001; Gotlieb, 2002; Welch, 2001).

            [iii] Common law, judicial law, decisional law, and case law: source is the decision handed down by courts on a particular case and the opinion that is written to accompany the decision; helps shape conduct in future cases of same type; for example, the Cruzan decision: surrogate decision-makers' expression of an incompetent patient's wishes should be respected

            [iv] Administrative law (agency rules and regulations): source is the federal or state legislature; rules and regulations are made by men and women in legislature (e.g., board of nursing rules and regulations)

        (b) Case law's importance to ethics: increasing recognition in court decisions of importance of individual autonomy with regard to treatment decisions, even if treatments are lifesaving and the patient is not suffering from a terminal illness (Nelson, 1989)

    (2) Ethical means something fulfills the terms of ethics and is higher than the law.

        (a) Actions are in one of four categories:

            [i] Ethical and legal

            [ii] Ethical and illegal

            [iii] Legal and unethical

            [iv] Illegal and unethical

        (b) In ethical discussions, the individual focuses on what is ethical, not on what is legal.

        (c) If an individual chooses an option that is ethical and illegal, he or she must be aware of the effect and have a plan to deal with it.

        (d) Courts do not decide questions of ethics, courts decide questions of law.

        (e) Attempts should be made to keep ethical dilemmas out of the courts.

        (f) Ethical codes

            [i] Religious codes

            [ii] Professional codes developed by professional organizations:

                • The International Council of Nurses Code for Nurses (2006)

                • American Nurses Association Code for Nurses (2001)

            [iii] Medical codes

c. Cultural and spiritual influences

    (1) Culture: beliefs and values that impart a sense of identity, security, and belonging; a guide for emotional expression, behavior, and experiencing of life events (Kagawa-Singer, 1998; Stutts & Schloemann, 2002a)

    (2) Spirituality: the dynamic, interpretive relationship between oneself and a higher power that is an integral part of human life (De Marco, 2000); also defined as a belief system that transmits meaning to life's events by focusing on intangible elements expressed through religious or ritual practices and inner piety (Daaleman & VandeCreek, 2000; Maugans, 1996; Stutts & Schloemann, 2002a)

    (3) Every culture and religious tradition has its own ways of defining, celebrating, ritualizing, and acknowledging:

        (a) The two major life passages of birth and death

        (b) The meaning of health, illness, and disability (Dyer, 2005; National Perinatal Association, 2001; Ott, Al-Khadhuri, & Al-Junaibi, 2003; Stutts & Schloemann, 2002a, 2002b)

    (4) The belief systems of all participants in decision-making and providing care for a patient should be considered.

        (a) Pastoral care services may be needed by both parents and the health care team (Milstein & Raingruber, 2007).

        (b) Spiritual distress can be a commonly unrecognized consequence for professionals (Catlin et al, 2001).

    (5) Parental cultural differences can influence their:

        (a) Emotional response to and perceptions of illness, disability, and death

        (b) Use of community and professional services

    (c) Interactions with health care providers (Dyer, 2005; National Perinatal Association, 2001; Ott et al, 2003; Stutts & Schloemann, 2002b)

  (6) Innovative strategies to offer culturally or spiritually sensitive care include (Catlin & Carter, 2002; Dyer, 2005; Stutts & Schloemann, 2002b):

    (a) Assess the needs of parents and health care professionals.

    (b) Educate professionals about their own culture and the culture of others.

    (c) Provide translation services for verbal encounters and written culturally sensitive materials in primary language.

    (d) Encourage parent-to-parent support from parents of familiar religious, cultural, language, and customs backgrounds.

    (e) Identify and link the family with community services (e.g., outpatient health care provider who speaks family's own language).

    (f) Using culturally sensitive practices to facilitate grief and loss: viewing or touching dead body as desired, appropriate use of eye contact and touch, autopsy, grief counseling, establishing trust among different cultures

d. Female versus male perspective; according to Gilligan's (1982) viewpoint:

  (1) Men and women have different approaches to ethical questions, so there is a need to appreciate and understand both perspectives.

  (2) Men tend to focus on the concept of justice and:

    (a) See the world as separate individuals in competition for everything

    (b) Believe the goal is to equalize the playing field and give everyone an equal opportunity.

    (c) Emphasize the application of universal rules to ensure fairness and justice.

  (3) Women, in general, tend to focus on relationships and

    (a) See relationships as more desirable than competition

    (b) Strive to establish and preserve relationships

    (c) Allow individuals to be different

    (d) Bend the rules and try to find a way to accommodate differences among people

    (e) Focus on feelings and interactions of the people involved

    (f) Look for resolution in the details of the problem

  (4) Female physicians, according to Gilligan (1982), tend to be:

    (a) Guided by their feelings of responsibility and concern for others

    (b) Less paternalistic and somewhat less directive than male physicians (Gilligan, 1982)

  (5) A research study on parental decision-making in clinical genetics supports Gilligan's viewpoint (Anderson, 2007). Men used analytical and rational thinking and ethical certainty when making decisions. Women engaged in ethical, moral, and practical thinking while experiencing private emotional struggles and uncertainty.

e. Nursing versus medical perspective

  (1) The foundation of medical practice is curing; medical intervention treats disease in a patient.

  (2) The foundation of nursing practice is caring; nursing interventions protect and restore health and prevent disease in a patient.

f. Standard of best interest

  (1) Best interest standard, advocated by the President's Commission (1983) and others (Weil, 1984; Weir, 1984), obliges decision-makers for newborns "to try to evaluate benefits and burdens from the infant's own perspective" (President's Commission, 1983).

  (2) Preservation of life without the benefit of the human capabilities to think, be self-aware, and relate to others is controversial and challenged in quality-of-life decisions (Arras, 1984; Kuhse & Singer, 1985; Weir, 1984).

  (3) Two models of determining best interest have been proposed (Leuthner, 2001).

    (a) Expertise model: The best outcome data are presented to the parents and used in a directive counseling approach based on the best medical judgment; limited moral weight is given to the views of the parents when they are the opposite of the views of the responsible physician.

    (b) Negotiated model: maximizes parental input, recognizes physicians as moral agents, and incorporates the moral values of both the parents and the physician into the decision.

g. Ethics and infant bioethics committees (AAP, 2001a; Stutts & Schloemann, 2002b; Swaney et al, 2006)

  (1) Promotes quality decisions regarding difficult ethical issues by being a resource for consultation and advice; may or may not be a decision-making committee

  (2) Confirms the plan of care when the parents and professionals agree

  (3) Clarifies ethical principles, values, and various treatment options that are consistent with ethical and legal standards

  (4) Educates families and professionals; provides a venue for expressing views and feelings; may be a mediator or liaison between the health care providers and the family

  (5) Develops policy statements for the institution

  (6) Retrospectively reviews case management

  (7) Has a multidisciplinary membership (nurses, physicians, administrators, lawyers, parents and families, clergy, ethicists, consumer or community representatives); any interested party, including parents or families, may request a consultation from the committee

5. Ethical decision-making

  a. The decision-makers need to be determined and need to comprehend (Swaney et al, 2006; Thompson & Thompson, 1990):

    (1) Their philosophy of relationship to the patient and to each other

    (2) Their interpretation of ethical principles and values

    (3) The theoretical basis of ethics (utilitarian, feminist, deontologic, and so forth) used in the decision-making process

    (4) The source from which morality is derived

  b. Steps in ethical decision-making (Swaney et al, 2006)

    (1) Consider all people who are involved in making and implementing the decision.

    (2) Decide who makes the final decision and whether a referral to an ethics committee is indicated.

    (3) Consider and clarify all medical facts in the case: all indications, alternatives, and consequences of every action and inaction.

    (4) Understand significant human factors and values for all participants in the process, as well as the patient.

    (5) Identify the moral or ethical conflict or dilemma.

    (6) Decide: List options as problem solutions; weigh and prioritize values and then make a decision.

    (7) Reevaluate for moral and rational defensibility.

CLINICAL PRACTICE

Nurses are closer to patients and families than any other health provider. Nurses spend more time with the patient and family, and they are usually the first to identify an ethical dilemma. Once a dilemma is identified, assessment begins.

A. Assessment

1. Assess the situation for time constraints.

  a. Is an immediate decision needed?

  b. How much time is available for discussion?

2. Assess the possible treatment options.

  a. Do everything.

  b. Do some thing or things selectively.

  c. Do nothing but comfort.

  d. Withdraw and comfort.

3. Assess the basis for decision-making and who will be the decision-maker.

  a. Autonomy (based on competence and capacity)

    (1) The competent, capable person makes the decision about his or her own care, including refusing or discontinuing treatment; permission is needed to treat; verbal refusal can occur at any time for any aspect of care.

    (2) The person continues to exercise autonomy even after capacity is lost through the written document called a living will.

        (a) Legal document

        (b) Providers are obligated to follow it.

        (c) Goes into effect only after the patient is no longer competent, capable, or both.

    (3) Parental autonomy in decision-making for the newborn

  b. Substituted judgment (based on former competence and capacity)

    (1) A surrogate stands in the place of the patient and states what the patient would want to say if the patient had capacity.

    (2) The durable power of attorney for health care decisions allows patients to name a surrogate to make decisions for them after they lose capacity.

    (3) If a surrogate has not been established, search for someone who had discussion with the patient, knows the values, lifestyle, and choices of the patient, and can likely speak for patient.

    (4) Parents are the proxy decision-makers for their newborns or infants.

  c. Best interests (based on no competence, no capacity, or no surrogate available)

    (1) Decision is made in the context of what is best for the patient in current circumstances through an analysis of benefits and burdens

    (2) Question: What would a reasonable person in these circumstances do?

    (3) Examples of situations

        (a) Patient is never able to communicate preferences (e.g., a retarded adult).

        (b) Patient has not yet developed a value system or ability to communicate (e.g., a newborn).

        (c) Patient was competent and capable but is no longer, and no one is available who knows the patient or can speak for the patient (e.g., a homeless person who is now in a vegetative state).

4. Assess patient and family's ethnic, cultural, and spiritual background, and understand how these influence communication and collaboration, decision-making, and ethical dilemmas (Leininger, 1997, 2001; National Perinatal Association, 2001; Ott et al, 2003).

B. Interventions/Outcomes

  1. Ethical decision-making process:

    a. Select and follow a recognized process.

    b. Focus the discussion with participants according to the selected process.

    c. Do a complete data collection according to selected process.

    d. Maintain objectivity and depersonalize issues according to selected process.

  2. Use an ethics committee as an available resource to assist in providing interventions for patients, families, and providers.

    a. Determine whether an ethics committee exists in the agency or institution.

    b. Determine how to access the ethics committee.

  3. Provide culturally sensitive patient and family support during the decision-making and while the plan is being implemented.

  4. Perform the roles of advocate, communicator, facilitator, coordinator, and planner (Monterosso et al, 2005).

    a. Prepare the family for what will happen and how it will appear.

    b. Work with key players, other professionals, and family to develop a plan for implementing the decision—what, when, how, by whom, and so forth—in a culturally sensitive manner.

    c. Encourage all participants to follow the plan.

    d. Assist the patient and family to identify and cope with "unfinished business."

    e. Assess coping abilities, and make referrals as needed.

    f. Identify a primary contact person who will communicate and coordinate the decision-making.

  5. Provide palliative or comfort care as needed.

    a. A family-centered, interdisciplinary, holistic, comprehensive approach to the care of patients with life-threatening or life-limiting conditions and their families is best (Purdy & Wadhwani, 2006; Romesberg, 2007; Swaney et al, 2006; Toce et al, 2007).

    b. A shift from rescue or cure mode to comfort care should occur at the earliest recognition of life-threatening or life-limiting conditions—futile technologic support is withheld or withdrawn (Catlin & Carter, 2002; Glicken & Merenstein, 2002); may be combined with efforts to prolong life (Levetown, 2001; Swaney et al, 2006).

    c. Newborn infants with the following conditions may be candidates (Catlin & Carter, 2002; Glassford, 2003; Glicken & Merenstein, 2002):

        (1) Those at the threshold of viability (very low birthweight; less than 500 g and less than 24 weeks' gestation; less than 750 g and less than 27 weeks' gestation may initially do well but may develop life-limiting complications)

        (2) Those with complex or multiple congenital anomalies that are incompatible with any substantial length of life (e.g., trisomy 13, 15, 18; thanatophoric dwarfism; anencephaly, encephalocele; hypoplastic left heart syndrome) (Zeigler, 2003)

    d. Palliative care may be provided in the community hospital, in a community hospice, at home, or in the neonatal intensive care unit (NICU) where the family has social, familial, and spiritual support (Catlin & Carter, 2001, 2002; Glassford, 2003; Glicken & Merenstein, 2002).

E. Outcomes: The patient, family, or significant others will:

    1. Identify and discuss their beliefs or values that affect decision-making.

    2. Verbalize knowledge of the situation and what is causing the dilemma.

    3. Express feelings and emotions appropriately and freely.

    4. Participate or collaborate in decision-making and problem-solving.

    5. Visit regularly and participate in care.

    6. Demonstrate ability to relate to one another and support one another in coping.

    7. Express some sense of control over the outcome.

    8. Adjust lifestyle by initiating changes that help them deal with the crisis.

    9. Identify their needs; identify support systems available; use outside resources as needed.

    10. Acknowledge that the infant's life is limited and provide for a pain-free dignified death (Glicken & Merenstein, 2002).

    11. Integrate psychologic, spiritual, cultural, and physiologic aspects of care into their decision-making (Catlin & Carter, 2001, 2002; Glicken & Merenstein, 2002; Swaney et al, 2006).

    12. If needed, receive aggressive management of pain, discomfort, and any other distressing symptoms (Catlin & Carter, 2001, 2002; Glicken & Merenstein, 2002; Swaney et al, 2006).

    13. Seek and receive social, emotional, physical, spiritual, and cultural support during illness or in the event of death (Catlin & Carter, 2001, 2002; Glicken & Merenstein, 2002; Swaney et al, 2006).

HEALTH EDUCATION

A. Inform patients and families about the Patient Self-Determination Act and the need to prepare for important decisions before a crisis occurs.

    1. Explain the purpose of written documents, what is included, and how to complete them (e.g., living will or durable power of attorney for health decisions).

    2. Encourage patients and families to discuss their wishes and decisions with family members and to give copies of written documents to appropriate persons.

B. Discuss the importance of being involved in decision-making regarding their health care: how to be involved, what questions to ask, and how to ask them.

C. Explain other important patient rights.

    1. The right to change providers to find one who will honor their values, beliefs, or decisions

    2. The right to information about their diagnosis, treatment, other options, and anticipated outcomes

    3. The right to say no to anything or anyone at any time

D. If an ethics committee exists, explain the purpose and how to access it, if needed.

DILEMMAS COMMON IN MATERNAL-NEWBORN NURSING PRACTICE

CLINICAL ISSUES

A. Reproductive choice or freedom

    1. Contraception or sterilization: voluntary or involuntary

    2. Abortion: first trimester or second trimester (Garel, Gosme-Seguret, Kaminiski, & Cuttini, 2002)

    3. Lesbian motherhood (Chan, Fox, McCormick, & Murphy, 1993)

   B. Assisted reproductive technology
     1. Artificial insemination
     2. Surrogate motherhood
     3. Cytoplasmic transfer
     4. In vitro fertilization
       a. Frozen embryos
       b. Orphaned embryos
     5. Gamete intrafallopian transfer
     6. "Made-to-order babies": preimplantation genetic diagnosis
     7. Cloning
   C. Prenatal screening, testing, and diagnosis: the option to consent or decline (AAP, 2001b; Anderson, 2007; Fioravanti, 2002; Zechmeister, 2001)
     1. Maternal serum alpha-fetoprotein
     2. Amniocentesis
     3. Chorionic villus sampling
     4. Ultrasound
     5. Genetic counseling, testing, and therapy
     6. Drug screening
     7. Human immunodeficiency virus (HIV) screening
   D. Human fetal tissue research or transplant donation
   E. Healthy pregnancy
     1. Elective induction and active medical management
     2. Elective cesarean: issue of autonomy in birthing decision, maternal mortality/morbidity, risk for premature birth, neonatal complications, issues of justice in use of resources (ACOG, 2003; McFarlin, 2004)
     3. High cesarean birth rate: consumer demand, litigation, medical convenience, medicalization of birth (Lee & Kirkman, 2008)
   F. High-risk pregnancy
     1. Intrauterine fetal treatment or surgery
     2. Substance abuse
     3. Treatments for preterm labor
     4. Pregnancy (selective) reduction
   G. Court-ordered obstetric treatment: cesarean section and other therapies (Cahill, 1999)
   H. Neonatal intensive care issues (Hurst, 2005; Swaney et al, 2006)
     1. Resuscitation of infants at the threshold of viability (low birthweight, very low birthweight)
     2. Rights of infants as individuals
     3. Parents as decision-makers; parental autonomy; proxy decision-makers
     4. Application of experimental or invasive technologies (Zeigler, 2003)
     5. Neonates as research subjects
     6. Pain management in neonates
     7. Palliative or comfort care (Kain, 2006)
       a. Withholding or withdrawing of resuscitation or life support
       b. Nutrition, hydration, and pain relief
       c. Supportive care
       d. Futility
     8. Organ transplant and donating organs

GENERAL PROFESSIONAL NURSING ISSUES

A. A majority of surveyed nurses confront ethical issues daily or weekly, yet they reported that they did not receive sufficient ethics content in their education (Scanlon, 1994a).

B. Resources for nurses with ethical problems were identified as literature or journals (44%), ethics committees (42%), and continuing education (39%); 11% were unable to identify any available resources (Scanlon, 1994a).

C. The most frequently occurring (more than 50%) ethics and human rights issues were cost containment, end-of-life decisions, and confidentiality (Scanlon, 1994b); other important issues were pain management, use of advance directives, informed consent, access to health care, care of patients with HIV or acquired immunodeficiency syndrome (AIDS), and futile care (Scanlon, 1994b).

D. Barriers in providing palliative care in the NICU including: sense of failure with an infant's death; difficulty to change from curative to palliative care; communication with parents; frequent stress associated with neonatal death; conflicting decision-making; physical environment of NICU; lack of support and formal training in palliative care (Kain, 2006).

E. Moral distress from situational binds in which the nurse's core beliefs are in conflict with providing care

1. Distress comes from the philosophic and theoretical differences between nursing and medical professions, how end-of life care is delivered, and feelings that care is causing suffering and "torture" to the infant (Catlin et al, 2008).

2. Moral distress contributes to potential loss of nurses' integrity and diminished work satisfaction as well as affecting nursing care provided (Nathaniel, 2006).

F. Code of Ethics (ANA, 2001) should provide the basis for care.

1. Practices with compassion and respect for the dignity, worth, and uniqueness of every individual

2. Has a primary commitment or responsibility to patient: an individual, family, group, or community

3. Promotes, advocates, and protects the health, safety, and rights of the patient

4. Is responsible and accountable for individual nursing practice and delegation of tasks to others

5. Owes same duties to self as to others: responsibility to preserve integrity, provide safety, maintain competence, and to grow personally and professionally

6. Through individual and collective action, nurses establish, maintain, and improve health care environments and conditions of employment necessary to provide quality care and that are consistent with the values of the profession

7. Participates in the advancement of the profession by contributions to practice, knowledge development, education, and administration, in accord with national practice standards and guidelines

8. Collaborates with other health professionals and members of the community to promote local, national, and international health efforts

9. Profession, through associations and members, is responsible for articulating nursing values, maintaining professional and practice integrity, and shaping social policy

---

CASE STUDY AND STUDY QUESTIONS

After 4 years of infertility treatments, Mr. and Mrs. S. had their first child. Within hours of the infant's birth, complications developed. Over several days, the following diagnosis was made: multiple congenital anomalies involving the cardiac, neurologic, and renal systems. Baby S. is in the NICU under the care of a neonatologist. She is on a ventilator with high pressures, has a central line, and is on multiple intravenous medications to maintain the function of her kidneys and heart and to prevent seizures. Decisions about dialysis will need to be made in the next 24 hours. The oximeter reads in the low 70s. She has frequent seizure activity in spite of the medications. She is unresponsive except to painful stimuli. The infant will not live much longer, and no therapy is available to resolve the multiple problems. The physician has been talking with the parents constantly to prepare them for the inevitable and to provide information they will need to make the tough decisions. Until now, the parents have refused to acknowledge the infant's condition and are convinced that a cure must be available. Both parents are educated

professionals, they are financially stable, and they are committed to having a family. Grandparents on both sides are supportive and involved. The family has no specific church affiliation.

One of the NICU residents told the parents about an article he read that discussed experimental surgical procedures on babies such as Baby S. The article said only one infant had survived the procedures. An hour ago, Mr. and Mrs. S. angrily confronted the neonatologist and demanded that their infant be sent for the experimental surgery immediately.

1. In this situation, the patient:
   a. Has competence and capacity
   b. Has competence but no capacity
   c. Has capacity but no competence
   d. Has neither capacity nor competence

2. In this dilemma, the conflicting principles are:
   a. Justice and fidelity
   b. Beneficence and nonmaleficence
   c. Veracity and confidentiality
   d. Beneficence and privacy

3. The decision is being made from the perspective of:
   a. Autonomy
   b. Substituted judgment
   c. Best interests
4. The physician has an obligation and duty to:
   a. Do everything the parents demand.
   b. Offer all experimental procedures available.
   c. Do good for the infant.
   d. Follow the legal advice of the hospital attorney.
5. The *best* way to handle this conflict between physician and parents is to:
   a. Let the court decide.
   b. Petition the court to appoint a guardian.
   c. Ask for an ethics committee consultation.
   d. Not allow the residents to talk with families.
6. The nurse can assist and support the family by:
   a. Testifying at the court hearing
   b. Encouraging them to get another physician
   c. Giving them time with the infant and making sure they understand the issues and information
   d. Restricting visiting hours

7. The family acknowledges the terminal condition of the infant, and a decision is made not to pursue experimental surgery. What is the immediate next step?
   a. Develop a plan of what will happen, when it will happen, how it will happen, and who will be involved.
   b. Tell the NICU residents to stop talking with the families about experimental procedures.
   c. Discontinue the ventilator and all intravenous medications.
   d. Move the infant to an isolation room to discontinue care.
8. The decision not to offer experimental surgery is:
   a. Illegal and unethical
   b. Legal and unethical
   c. Ethical and illegal
   d. Ethical and legal
9. Which type of law would offer the *most* support for this decision?
   a. Administrative rules and regulations
   b. Case law
   c. Statutory law
   d. Constitutional law

ANSWERS TO STUDY QUESTIONS

1. d	6. c
2. b	7. a
3. c	8. d
4. c	9. b
5. c	

REFERENCES

American Academy of Pediatrics (AAP). (1995). The initiation or withdrawal of treatment for high-risk newborns. *Pediatrics, 96*(2 Pt 1), 362–363.

American Academy of Pediatrics, Committee on Bioethics. (1994). Guidelines on forgoing life-sustaining medical treatment. *Pediatrics, 93*(3), 532–536.

American Academy of Pediatrics, Committee on Bioethics. (2001a). Institutional ethics committees. *Pediatrics, 107*(1), 205–209.

American Academy of Pediatrics, Committee on Bioethics. (2001b). Ethical issues with genetic testing in pediatrics. *Pediatrics, 107*(6), 1451–1455.

American Academy of Pediatrics (AAP) and American College of Obstetricians and Gynecologists (ACOG). (1995). Perinatal care at the threshold of viability. *Pediatrics, 96*(5), 974–976.

American Academy of Pediatrics (AAP) and American College of Obstetricians and Gynecologists (ACOG). (2002). *Guidelines for perinatal care* (5th ed.). Washington, DC: AAP and ACOG.

American College of Obstetricians and Gynecologists (ACOG). (1989). *Ethical decision-making in obstetrics and gynecology.* ACOG Technical Bulletin, *136*, 1–7.

American College of Obstetricians and Gynecologists Committee Opinion. (2003). Surgery and patient choice: The ethics of decision making. *Obstetrics and Gynecology, 102*, 1101–1106.

American Hospital Association (AHA). (1985). *Report of the Special Committee on Biomedical Ethics: Values in conflict: Resolving ethical issues in hospital care.* Chicago: American Hospital Publishing.

American Nurses Association (ANA). (2001). *Code for nurses with interpretative statements (brochure)*. Washington, DC: ANA.

Anderson, G. (2007). Patient decision-making for clinical genetics. *Nursing Inquiry, 14*(1), 13–22.

Annas, G. (1994). Asking the courts to set the standard of emergency care. *New England Journal of Medicine, 330*(21), 1542–1545.

Arras, J. (1984). Toward an ethic of ambiguity. *Hastings Center Report, 14*(2), 25–33.

Beauchamp, T., & Childress, J. (2008). *Principles of biomedical ethics* (6th ed.). New York: Oxford University Press.

Brinchmann, B. S., Forde, R., & Nortwedt, P. (2002). What matters to the parents? A qualitative study of parents' experiences with life-and-death decisions concerning their premature infants. *Nursing Ethics, 9*(4), 388–404.

Cahill, H. (1999). An Orwellian scenario: Court-ordered caesarean section and women's autonomy. *Nursing Ethics, 6*(6), 494–505.

Cahill, H. (2001). Male appropriation and medicalization of childbirth: An historical analysis. *Journal of Advanced Nursing, 33*(3), 334–342.

Catlin, A., & Carter, B. (2001). Creation of a neonatal end of life protocol. *Journal of Clinical Ethics, 12*(3), 316–318.

Catlin, A., & Carter, B. (2002). Creation of a neonatal end of life protocol. *Journal of Perinatology, 22*(3), 184–195; reprinted in *Neonatal Network, 21*(4), 37–49.

Catlin, A., Armigo, C., Volat, D., Valle, E., Hadley, M. A., Gong, W., Bassir, R., & Anderson, K. (2008). Conscientious objection: A potential neonatal nursing response to care orders that caused suffering at the end of life. Study of a concept. *Neonatal Network, 27*(2), 101–108.

Catlin, E. A., Guillemin, J. H., Thiel, M. M., Hammond, S., Wang, M. L., & O'Donnell, J. (2001). Spiritual and religious components of patient care in the neonatal intensive care unit: Sacred themes in a secular setting. *Journal of Perinatology, 21*(7), 426–430.

Chan, C., Fox, J., McCormick, R., & Murphy, T. (1993). Lesbian motherhood and genetic choices. *Ethics Behavior, 3*(2), 211–222.

Chesney, R. (2001). Privacy and its regulation: Too much too soon, or too little too late? *Pediatrics, 107*(6), 1423–1424.

Clark, F. (1996). Making sense of *State v Messenger*. *Pediatrics, 97*(4), 579–583.

Culver, G., Fallon, K., Londner, R. B., Montalvo, N., Vila, B., Ramsey, B. J., Ramsey, C. S., Trebaol, G., Houle, L., Williams, A., Williams, H., & Wolding, T. (2000). Informed decisions for extremely low birth weight infants. *Journal of the American Medical Association, 283*(24), 3201–3202.

Daaleman, T., & VandeCreek, L. (2000). Placing religion and spirituality in end-of-life care. *Journal of the American Medical Association, 284*(19), 2514–2517.

De Marco, D. G. (2000). Medicine and spirituality. *Annals of Internal Medicine, 133*(11), 920–921.

Doroshow, R. W., Hodgman, J. E., Pomerance, J. J., Ross, J. W., Michel, V. J., Luckett, P. M., & Shaw, A. (2000). Treatment decisions for newborns at the threshold of viability: An ethical dilemma. *Journal of Perinatology, 20*(6), 379–383.

Dyer, K. A. (2005). Identify, understanding, and working with grieving parents in the NICU, Part II: Strategies. *Neonatal Network, 24*(4), 27–40.

Fioravanti, J. (2002). Issues related to prenatal diagnosis of congestive heart disease. *Neonatal Network, 21*(6), 23–29.

Garel, M., Gosme-Seguret, S., Kaminiski, M., & Cuttini, M. (2002). Ethical decision-making in prenatal diagnosis and termination of pregnancy: Qualitative survey among physicians and midwives. *Prenatal Diagnosis, 22*(9), 811–817.

Gilligan, C. (1982). *In a different voice: Psychological theory and women's development*. Cambridge, MA: Harvard University Press.

Glassford, B. (2003). A case study in caring: Trisomy 18 syndrome. *American Journal of Nursing, 103*(7), 81–83.

Glicken, A., & Merenstein, G. (2002). A neonatal end-of-life protocol—An evolving new standard of care? *Neonatal Network, 21*(4), 35–36.

Gotlieb, E. (2002). Privacy rights, HIPAA, and the AAP: About right, about time. *Pediatrics, 109*(1), 146–149.

Hack, M. (1999). Consideration of the use of health status, functional outcome, and quality-of-life to monitor neonatal intensive care practice. *Pediatrics, 103*(1 Suppl E), 319–323.

Harrison, H. (1993). The principles of family-centered neonatal care. *Pediatrics, 92*(5), 643–650.

Holmes, H., & Prudy, L. (Eds.). (1992). *Feminist perspectives in medical ethics*. Indianapolis: Indiana University Press.

Hurst, I. (2005). The legal landscape at the threshold for viability for extremely premature infant: A nursing perspective, part II. *Journal of Perinatal & Neonatal Nursing, 29*, 253–264.

International Council of Nurses (ICN). (2006). *ICN code for nurses—Ethical concepts applied to nursing (brochure)*. Geneva: International Council of Nurses.

Joffe, S., Manocchia, M., Weeks, J., & Cleary, P. (2003). What do patients value in their hospital care? An empirical perspective on autonomy centered bioethics. *Journal of Medical Ethics, 29*(2), 103–108.

Kagawa-Singer, M. (1998). The cultural context of death rituals and mourning practices. *Oncology Nursing Forum, 25*(10), 1752–1756.

Kain, V. J. (2006). Palliative care delivery in the NICU: What barriers do neonatal nurses face? *Neonatal Network, 25*(6), 387–392.

Kirschbaum, M. (1996). Life support decisions for children: What do parents value? *Advances in Nursing Science, 19*(1), 51–71.

Koh, T. H., Casey, A., & Harrison, H. (2000). Use of an outcome by gestation table for extremely premature babies: A cross-sectional survey of the views of parents, neonatal nurses and perinatologists. *Journal of Perinatology, 20*(8 Pt 1), 504–508.

Koh, T. H., Harrison, H., & Morley, C. (1999). Gestation versus outcome table for parents of extremely premature infants. *Journal of Perinatology, 19*(6 Pt 1), 452–453.

Kuhse, H., & Singer, P. (1985). *Should the baby live?* New York: Oxford University Press.

Lagana, K., & Duderstadt, K. (1995). *Ethical decision making for perinatal nurses.* White Plains, NY: March of Dimes Birth Defects Foundation.

Lantos, J. D., Singer, P. A., Walker, R. M., Gramelspacher, G. P., Shapiro, G. R., Sanchez-Gonzalez, M. A., Stocking, C. B., Miles, S. H., & Siegler, M. (1989). The illusion of futility in clinical practice. *American Journal of Medicine, 87*(1), 81–84.

Lee, A., & Kirkman, M. (2008). Disciplinary discourse: Rates of cesarean section explained by medicine, midwifery and feminism. *Health Care for Women International, 2*(5), 448–467.

Leininger, M. (1997). Future directions in transcultural nursing in the 21st century. *International Nursing Review, 44*(1), 19–23.

Leininger, M. (2001). *Culture care diversity and universality: A theory of nursing.* New York: National League for Nursing Press.

Leuthner, S. R. (2001). Decisions regarding resuscitation of the extremely premature infant and models of best interest. *Journal of Perinatology, 21*(3), 193–198.

Levetown, M. (2001). Pediatric care: The inpatient/ICU perspective. In G. Ferrell, & N. Coyle (Eds.), *Textbook of palliative nursing.* New York: Oxford University Press.

Maugans, T. (1996). The spiritual history. *Archives in Family Medicine, 5*(1), 11–16.

McFarlin, B. L. (2004). Elective cesarean birth: Issues and ethics of an informed decision. *Journal of Midwifery and Women's Health, 49*(5), 421–429.

McHaffie, H. E., Laing, I. A., Parker, M., & McMillan, J. (2001). Deciding for imperiled newborns: Medical authority or parental autonomy? *Journal of Medical Ethics, 27*(2), 104–109.

Milstein, J. M., & Raingruber, B. (2007). Choreographing the end of life in a neonate. *American Journal of Hospice and Palliative Medicine, 24*(5), 343–349.

Monterosso, L., Kristianson, L., Sly, P. D., Mulcahy, M., Holland, B. G., Grimwood, S., & White, K. (2005). The role of the neonatal intensive care nurse in decision-making: Advocacy, involvement in ethical decisions and communication. *International Journal of Nursing Practice, 11*(3), 108–117.

Nathaniel, A. K. (2006). Moral reckoning in nursing. *Western Journal of Nursing Research, 28*(4), 419–438.

National Perinatal Association. (2001). *Transcultural aspects of perinatal care: A resource manual: Part I.* Tampa, FL: National Perinatal Association.

Nelson, L. J. (1989). Bioethics in the courts: Summaries of selected judicial decisions. *Clinical Ethics Report, 3*, 1–16.

Neufeld, M., Woodrum, D., & Tarczy-Hornoch, P. (2000). Prenatal and postnatal counseling for parents of infants at the limits of viability. *Pediatric Research, 47*, 420A.

Omnibus Reconciliation Act of 1990, Sections 4206 and 4751. (The Patient Self-Determination Act, 1990).

Orleans, M., Tappero, E., Glicken, A., & Merenstein, G. (2002). Evidence-based clinical practice decisions. In G. B. Merenstein, & S. L. Gardner (Eds.), *Handbook of neonatal intensive care* (5th ed., pp. 1–8). St. Louis: Mosby.

Ott, B., Al-Khadhuri, J., & Al-Junaibi, S. (2003). Preventing ethical dilemmas: Understanding Islamic health care practices. *Pediatric Nursing, 29*(3), 227–230.

Partridge, J. C., Freeman, H., Weiss, E., & Martinez, A. M. (2001). Delivery room resuscitation decisions for extremely low birth weight infants in California. *Journal of Perinatology, 21*(1), 27–33.

Paul, D. A., Leef, K. H., Epps, S., & Stefano, J. L. (1999). Usefulness of the prenatal consult: Mothers' response. *Pediatric Research, 45*(4), 218A.

President's Commission for the Study of Ethical Problems in Medicine and Biomedical and Behavioral Research (1983). *Deciding to forego life-sustaining treatment.* Washington, DC: Public Health Service, U.S. Department of Health and Human Services.

Purdy, I., & Wadhwani, R. (2006). Embracing bioethics in neonatal intensive care, Part II: Case histories in neonatal ethics. *Neonatal Network, 25*(1), 43–53.

Raeside, L. (1997). Ethical decision-making in neonatal intensive care. *Professional Nurse, 13*(3), 157–159.

Romesberg, T. L. (2007). Building a case for neonatal palliative care. *Neonatal Network, 26*(2), 111–115.

Rushton, C., & Hogue, E. (1993). When parents demand everything. *Pediatric Nursing, 19*(2), 180–183.

Rushton, C., & Scanlon, C. (1995). When values conflict with obligations: Safeguards for nurses. *Pediatric Nursing, 21*(3), 260–261, 268.

Scanlon, C. (1994a). Survey yields significant results. *American Nurses Association Center for Ethics and Human Rights Communique, 3*(3), 1–3.

Scanlon, C. (1994b). Ethics survey looks at nurses' experiences. *American Nurse, 26*(10), 22.

Siegel, R., Gardner, S., & Merenstein, G. (2002). Families in crisis: Theoretic and practical considerations. In G. B. Merenstein, & S. L. Gardner (Eds.), *Handbook of neonatal intensive care* (5th ed., pp. 725–753). St. Louis: Mosby.

Stutts, A., & Schloemann, J. (2002a). Life-sustaining support: Ethical, cultural, and spiritual conflicts. Part I: Family support—a neonatal case study. *Neonatal Network, 21*(3), 23–29.

Stutts, A., & Schloemann, J. (2002b). Life-sustaining support: Ethical, cultural, and spiritual conflicts. Part II: Staff support—A neonatal case study. *Neonatal Network*, *21*(4), 27–34.

Swaney, J., English, N., & Carter, B. (2006). Ethics in neonatal intensive care. In G. B. Merenstein, & S. L. Gardner (Eds.), *Handbook of neonatal intensive care* (6th ed., pp. 801–821). St. Louis: Mosby.

Thompson, J., & Thompson, H. (1990). *Professional ethics in nursing*. Malabar, FL: Robert Krieger.

Toce, S., Leuthner, S. R., Dokken, D., Carter, B. S., & Catlin, A. (2004). The high risk newborn. In B. S. Carter, & M. Levetown (Eds.), *Palliative care for infants, children and adolescents* (pp. 247–272). Baltimore: Johns Hopkins University Press.

Tyson, J. (1995). Evidence-based ethics and the care of premature infants. *Future of Children*, *5*(1), 197–213.

U.S. Department of Health and Human Services (USDHHS). (1991). *Federal policy for the protection of human subjects: Notice and rules* (45 C.F.R. 11 [a]). Washington, DC: USDHHS.

Weil, W. B. (1984). Issues associated with treatment and non-treatment decisions: Special reference to newborns with handicaps. *American Journal of Diseases of Children*, *138*(6), 519–522.

Weir, R. (1984). *Selective nontreatment of handicapped newborns*. New York: Oxford University Press.

Welch, C. A. (2001). Sacred secrets: The privacy of medical records. *New England Journal of Medicine*, *345*(5), 371–372.

Winslow, B., & Winslow, G. (1991). Integrity and compromise in nursing ethics. *Journal of Medicine and Philosophy*, *16*(3), 307–323.

Woodward, V. (1998). Caring, patient autonomy and the stigma of paternalism. *Journal of Advanced Nursing*, *28*(5), 1046–1052.

Zechmeister, I. (2001). Fetal images: The power of visual technology in antenatal care and the implications for women's reproductive freedom. *Health Care Analysis*, *9*(4), 387–400.

Zeigler, V. (2003). Ethical principles and parental choice: Treatment options for neonates with hypoplastic left heart syndrome. *Pediatric Nursing*, *29*(1), 65–69.

Index

A

Abbreviations
for charting electronic fetal
monitoring, 264b
ABCs (Airway, Breathing,
Circulation), 536, 541, 541f
Abdomen
extension and stretch marks, 83
fetal development of,
pain
and placenta previa, 480
and uterine rupture, 642
physical examination of
newborn's, 350
postpartum muscle changes, 304
trauma to, 537f–538f, 538
Abdominal wall defects
description and risks in
newborns, 401–402
Abortion, 679; *See also* spontaneous
abortion
Abruptio placentae, 485–489
assessment of, 485–489
complications, 487
definition of, 485
diagnostic procedures, 487
health education, 489
interventions and outcomes, 488
and maternal drug/ alcohol
abuse, 573, 578b
risk factors, 485
and small for gestational age
(SGA) newborns, 363
transfer disorder, 45
Abstinence
as method of contraception,
337t–339t
Abuse; *See also* alcohol and drug
abuse; intimate partner
violence (IPV)
assessment screens, 425
cycle of violence, 418, 418f
intimate partner violence (IPV),
417
substance, 573
Abused women
characteristics of, 422f, 423–424
during pregnancy, 423
Abusers
characteristics of, 421, 422f
power and control wheel, 422, 422f
Accelerations
pattern of fetal heart rate (FHR),
261–262, 261f, 267–268, 268f

Acceptance
of child, 103
of one's own body image, 119
Acid-base balance
changes during pregnancy, 82
normal values, 285t
postpartum changes in, 304
Acidosis
and persistent pulmonary
hypertension of newborn
(PPHN), 389–391
causing respiratory distress in
newborns, 380–381
Acquired cardiac disease
during pregnancy, 589
Acquired immunodeficiency
syndrome (AIDS), 454–461,
455t–458t, 461f
assessment of, 462
causes and transmission of,
454–459, 455t–458t
characteristics of, 455t–458t
counseling and early diagnosis
of, 460
ethical issues regarding care, 680
ethnic, race and age statistics, 461f
human immunodeficiency virus
(HIV), 459
statistics, 454–460, 459f–461f
Acrocyanosis, 349
Acrosomal reactions, 35
Active transport
in placental transfer, 44, 45t
Acyanotic defects, 403–404
Addison's disease, 527
Administrative law, 674
Adnexa, 14
Adolescents
pregnancy, 117–121
clinical assessment procedures,
117
health education, 124
interventions/outcomes, 120
maternal mortality risks, 117
nutrition risks and education
in, 86, 117–121
prenatal care education,
117–121
and preterm labor, 624–629
risk-taking and sexual behaviors
of, 118–119
and small for gestational age
(SGA) newborns, 363
statistics, 117

Adoption grief, 107, 111
Adrenal gland
changes during pregnancy, 84
disorders, 523–525
adrenal hyperfunction, 523
adrenal insufficiency, 525–526
assessment of, 524
Cushing's syndrome, 523–525
effects on pregnancy, 523
fetal/neonatal effects, 524
health education, 525
hyperadrenocorticism, 523–525
interventions and outcomes,
524
Adrenal hyperfunction, 523
Adrenal insufficiency, 525–526
assessment of, 526
definition and classification of,
525
effects on fetus/ neonates, 526
effects on pregnancy, 525
interventions and outcomes, 526
and steroid replacement therapy,
527
Adrenocorticotropic hormone
(ACTH), 523–524
Adrenogenital syndrome, 524
Advanced maternal age
assessment of, 121
assisted reproductive technology
(ART), 121
fertility rates, 121–122
health education, 125
interventions and outcomes, 123
risks of, 117, 121–124
and small for gestational age
(SGA) newborns, 363
statistics, 121
African Americans
childbearing cultural
considerations, 64
ethnocultural "Quick Reference
Guide," 75t–79t
HIV/AIDS statistics among, 461,
461f
intimate partner violence among,
420
maternal mortality rates in, 478
preterm infant risks among, 372
sickle cell trait in, 79t
Age
adolescent pregnancies, 117–121
clinical assessment procedures,
117

Age (*Continued*)
  health education, 124
  interventions/outcomes, 120
  maternal mortality risks, 117
  nutrition education, 117–121
  prenatal care education, 117–121
  risk-taking and sexual
      behaviors of, 118–119
  statistics, 117
  advanced maternal age
    assessment of, 121
    assisted reproductive
        technology (ART), 121
    fertility rates, 121–122
    health education, 125
    interventions and outcomes, 123
    risks of, 117, 121–124
    statistics, 121
  childbearing cultural
      considerations, 64
  and preterm labor, 624–629
Aggression
  in children witnessing domestic
      violence, 421
Alba stage, 302
Albumin
  affected by preeclampsia and
      HELLP, 439t
Alcohol abuse
  by abused women, 420, 424
  assessing maternal, 55, 581–582
  during breastfeeding, 330
  complications due to, 578b
  and cycle of domestic violence,
      418, 418f, 576
  during fetal development
      process, 57
  fetal risk factors, 548
  fetus/newborn disorders
      associated with, 580
  health education regarding fetal
      health and, 57
  and intimate partner violence
      (IPV), 576
  issues and variables associated
      with, 583–584
  maternal risk factors, 548
  obstetric complications of, 573
  patient education, 582–583
  physical signs of, 580–581
  postpartum, 660
  pregnancy nutritional deficiency
      risks of, 86
  causing preterm infants, 372, 374,
      624–629
  resources, 583b
  and small for gestational age
      (SGA) newborns, 363–366
  statistics regarding, 580–583
  and trauma, 536
Alcoholism; *See* alcohol abuse
Alcohol-related birth defects,
    580–581
Alcohol-related neurodevelopment
    disorder (ARND), 580–583
Alkaline phosphatase
  affected by preeclampsia and
      HELLP, 439t
Allele
  definition of, 20

Alpha-fetoprotein, 129
Altered secondary sex ratio
  and toxin exposure, 166–177
Amenorrhea
  description of, 10
American Academy of Pediatrics
    (AAP)
  on high-risk pregnancy
      conditions, 129
American College of Obstetricians
    and Gynecologists (ACOG)
  on high-risk pregnancy
      conditions, 129
Amish
  childbearing cultural
      considerations, 64
Amniocentesis
  to determine fetal lung maturity,
      139
  diagram illustrating, 133f
  to evaluate fetal status with
      diabetes, 504
  in fetal/placental assessment, 55
Amnioinfusion, 263
Amnion, 53
  development of, 36, 36f–37f
Amniotic bands, 50, 52t
Amniotic fluid
  abnormalities, 54
  altered, 56
  anaphylactoid syndrome, 640
  circulation illustration, 53f
  composition of, 54
  description of, 53
  evaluation
    during antepartum fetal
        assessment, 138, 146
    in fetal development process,
        53, 53f
  function of, 630–632
Amniotic fluid embolism, 640
Amniotic fluid index (AFI), 138
Amniotic membrane
  premature rupture of membranes
      (PROM), 632–635, 637
  premonitory signs preceding
      birth, 226
Ampulla
  fertilization in, 35, 36f
  part of fallopian tubes, 5f, 7
Anaphylactoid syndrome, 640
  description and high mortality
      rates with, 640
  interventions, 641
  signs of, 640
Ancillary tools
  for intrapartum fetal assessment,
      283–288
    fetal pulse oximetry, 284
    fetal scalp sampling, 283
    fetal scalp stimulation, 284
    umbilical cord blood
        sampling, 284–286, 285t
    vibroacoustic, 284
Android pelvis, 196f, 197
Anemia
  iron deficiency, 609–614
  iron homeostasis indices, 612t
  megaloblastic, 609–614
  prevalence of, 608

Anemia (*Continued*)
  causing respiratory distress in
      newborns, 380–381
  sickle cell, 609–614
  and small for gestational age
      (SGA) newborns, 363
  tests, 14
  thalassemia, 609–614
  types of, 608
Anencephaly
  development during embryonic
      stage, 40, 40f
Anesthesia
  cardiovascular changes, 557
  changes in maternal physiology,
      557
  fetal risks, 557–558
  gastrointestinal system changes,
      558
  hematologic system changes, 558
  maternal morbidity risks, 557
  respiratory changes, 558
Aneuploidies, 35
Aneuploidy/polyploidy
  and toxin exposure, 166–177
Anger
  in children witnessing domestic
      violence, 421
  in substance abusers, 576
Ankle dorsiflexion
  in newborn neurological
      assessment, 354b
Announcement phase
  expectant father's, 104
Anorexia nervosa, 106, 111, 660
Anovulatory cycles, 11
Antepartum fetal assessment
  ancillary antenatal tests, 141–155
    biophysical profile (BPP),
        145–148, 148t
    contraction stress test (CST), 153
    Doppler ultrasound blood
        flow assessment, 149–151,
        150f
    Doppler velocimetry, 149–151,
        150f
    fetal movement counting
        (FMC), 141–142
    modified biophysical profile,
        148–149
    nonstress test (NST), 142–144
    oxytocin administration,
        154–155
    three-dimensional (3D) view,
        planes or 4D, 151–153
    vibroacoustic stimulation
        (VST), 144–145
  biochemical assessments
    amniotic fluid evaluation, 138
    anomalies, 139
    bleeding, 138
    ectopic pregnancies, 135
    fetal maturity scoring, 135t
    fetal viability, 138
    multiple gestation, 136
    placental grading level, 135, 136f
    placental positions, 136
    presentation/positioning, 137
    ultrasonography, 134, 135t,
        136f–137f

Antepartum fetal assessment
    (*Continued*)
    clinical practice procedures,
        132–155
        alpha-fetoprotein, 129
        biochemical assessments,
            132–133
        delta OD 450, 133, 133f
        triple and quad screening, 132
    fetal behavioral states, 128–130,
        137f
    fetal growth and development,
        130–131, 130b, 137f
    fetal response to hypoxemia,
        131–132
    goals of, 129
    health education regarding, 155
    high-risk conditions, 129
    importance of, 128–132
Antepartum period; *See also*
    antepartum fetal assessment
    ethnocultural considerations
        during, 64, 75t
    interventions with multiple
        gestation, 636
Anthropoid pelvis, 196f, 197
Antiarrhythmic agents
    use and adverse effects during
        pregnancy, 593t
Antibiotics, 655–656
Antibody screens
    during pregnancy assessment, 94
Anticoagulant therapy, 592
Anticoagulants
    strict dosage compliance,
        658–659
    use and adverse effects during
        pregnancy, 593t
Antineoplastic drugs
    as occupational environmental
        hazard, 167
Antiphospholipid antibody
    syndrome, 129, 604–605
Antithyroid drugs
    for hyperthyroidism, 519
Antituberculosis drugs
    and toxicity, 602t
Anxiety
    with abruptio placentae, 487–488
    in abused women, 420, 424–425
    due to diabetes, 508
    ethnocultural considerations
        regarding, 65
    and heart disease, 592
    regarding HIV and AIDS, 462
    interventions for different
        cultures, 69
    during labor, 214, 217
    and latching-on problems, 324,
        326
    monitoring during surgery, 557,
        559, 562
    in older pregnant women, 123
    in placenta previa cases, 481
    postpartum, 660
    regarding preexisting conditions,
        587
    in substance abusers, 576
    regarding surgery, 562
    with thyroid disorders, 518, 521

Aorta
    coarctation of, 405
Apgar scores
    components of, 348t
    improvements in SGA newborns,
        366
    of newborns, 146, 348, 348t
Appearance
    indicating alcohol abuse in
        mothers, 581–582
    indicating mother's nutritional
        status, 92, 93t
Appendectomy, 564–566, 565f
Appropriate for gestational age
    (AGA), 351
Arabic heritage
    ethnocultural "Quick Reference
        Guide," 75t–79t
Areola
    anatomical illustration of, 316f
    changes in during pregnancy, 84
    characteristics of preterm infant,
        374
Arm recoil
    in newborn neurological
        assessment, 354b
Arnold-Chiari syndrome, 400
Arrhythmias
    causes and patterns, 273
    definition and characteristics of
        fetal, 273
    interventions, 282
    as preexisting maternal
        condition, 588–594
Arsenic, 171
Arterial blood gases
    and asthma, 599
    metabolic acidemia ranges, 285,
        285t
Artificial insemination, 680
Asherman syndrome, 12
Asians
    childbearing cultural
        considerations, 64
    ethnocultural "Quick Reference
        Guide," 75t–79t
    higher rate of hyperbilirubinemia
        in, 394–397
    HIV/AIDS statistics among, 461,
        461f
Aspartate aminotransferase (AST)
    affected by preeclampsia and
        HELLP, 439t
Asphyxia
    amniotic fluid volume and BPP
        assessing, 146–147
    fetal
        dangers in surgery, 556, 558, 570
        related to maternal diabetes,
            505
        intrauterine risk during surgery,
            558
    perinatal, 370
    causing respiratory distress in
        newborns, 380–381
Aspiration syndromes
    meconium aspiration syndrome,
        387–389
    causing respiratory distress in
        newborns, 380–381

Assaults, 535, 539
Assisted hatching, 122
Assisted reproductive technology
    (ART)
    ethical dilemma for nurses, 679
    and multiple gestation, 635
    trends and types of, 121, 635–637
Asthma
    preexisting maternal, 599,
        602–603, 603b
    and small for gestational age
        (SGA) newborns, 363
Asymptomatic bacteriuria,
    465–467
Atrial fibrillation, 278, 283
Atrial flutter, 277, 278f, 283
Atrial septal defects (ASDs)
    description and risks in
        newborns, 404
Atrioventricular (AV) block,
    279–280, 281f, 283
Attachment
    definition of, 305
    malattachment behaviors, 310
    paternal, 309
    during postpartum period, 305,
        309–310
Attention-deficit hyperactive
    disorder
    in children witnessing domestic
        violence, 421
Auscultation
    for fetal heart rate assessment,
        249
Autoimmune diseases
    antiphospholipid antibody
        syndrome (APS), 604
    systemic lupus erythematosus
        (SLE), 603–605
Autonomy
    defining in ethics, 670, 677–679
Autosomal dominant inheritance,
    24, 24f
Autosomal recessive inheritance,
    25, 25f
Awake states
    examining in newborns, 351

B

Babinski reflex
    examining in newborns, 350, 350t
Baby blues, 305, 308, 659–662
Back
    physical examination of
        newborn's, 350
Bacterial infections; *See also*
    infections
    and preterm labor, 624–629
Bacterial vaginosis, 455t–458t, 464
Baroreceptors
    influencing fetal heart rate
        (FHR), 253
Bartholin's glands, 4, 4f
Basal metabolic rate
    changes during pregnancy, 82
    postpartum changes in, 304
Baseline FHR
    bradycardia, 256, 256f
    characteristics of, 253–260, 254f
    tachycardia, 254, 254f

Baseline monitoring
electronic fetal monitoring
(EFM), 253–260
Bathing
ethnocultural considerations
regarding, 62
Battering; See intimate partner
violence (IPV)
Battledore, 53
Behavioral disorders
in small for gestational age
(SGA), 365
and toxin exposure, 166–177
Behavioral state system
of newborns, 350
Belief systems
of different cultures, 61
and ethics, 669
Beneficence
defining in ethics, 670, 677–679
Benign ovarian tumors, 564
Best interest standards, 676, 678
Beta-blocking agents
use and adverse effects during
pregnancy, 593t
Bicornuate uterus
affecting labor passage, 195
Bilateral tubal ligation
as method of contraception,
337t–339t
Bilirubin
affected by preeclampsia and
HELLP, 439t
production and conjugation, 391
rate of increase, 392
"Binding-in," 103–104
Biochemical disorders
assessing antepartum fetal,
132–133
risk factors, 29
Bioethics, 669, 677
Biophysical profile (BPP)
during antepartum fetal
assessment, 145–148, 148t
to evaluate fetal status with
diabetes, 504
modified, 148–149
and placenta previa, 483
Birth; See childbirth; labor and
delivery
Birth defects
complications due to alcohol
abuse, 580
genetic screening procedures,
28–29
intrauterine fetal surgery,
568–569
and toxin exposure, 165–166
Birth positions
ethnocultural "Quick Reference
Guide," 76t
Birth trauma
related to maternal diabetes, 505
Birthweight
classifying newborn's, 351
and gestational age
large for gestational age
(LGA), 367, 367–370
late preterm infants, 379–380
postterm infants, 370–372

Birthweight (Continued)
preterm infants, 372–380
small for gestational age
(SGA), 363–367
low
and maternal asthma, 599
in preterm infants, 373
and toxin exposure, 166–177
of newborns
large for gestational age (LGA),
367–370
of SGA versus IUGR, 363
Bishop scores, 238, 239t
Bladder
assessing postpartum, 306
extravasation during embryonic
stage, 41
fetal development of, 43, 46–49, 51f
Blastocyst
development of, 36, 36f–37f
in placenta development process,
37
Blastogenic period, 36, 36f–37f
Bleeding
assessing placental, 138
with disseminated intravascular
coagulation (DIC), 489–492
duration of menstrual, 12
hemorrhagic disorders, 478
postpartum hemorrhages,
650–651
causes of, 650
classification of, 650
health education, 653
interventions, 652–653
risk factors, 651
signs and symptoms of, 651
reporting of unusual, 653
tests during antepartum fetal
assessment, 138
Bleeding time tests
to test for hypertensive
disorders, 438, 439t
Blood; See also hemorrhagic
disorders
changes during pregnancy
clotting factor, 82
red blood cells, 82
white blood cells, 82
characteristics in preterm infants,
376
disorders
causing respiratory distress in
newborns, 380–381
maternal flow to fetus, 44, 44f
postpartum hemorrhages,
650–651
causes of, 650
classification of, 650
health education, 653
interventions, 652–653
risk factors, 651
signs and symptoms of, 651
Blood cells
development of primitive, 39,
40f
primitive development during
embryonic stage, 39, 40f, 44f
Blood chemistry
testing, 14

Blood clots
reporting of unusual, 653
Blood glucose
control and monitoring, 503
values, 501t
Blood group
incompatibility, 304
Blood loss
hemorrhagic disorders, 478
with trauma, 548
Blood pressure
assessing postpartum, 305
changes during pregnancy, 82
examining for hypertension,
436
monitoring during surgery, 557,
559
postpartum changes in, 303
Blood tests; See also complete blood
count (CBC) tests
during pregnancy assessment,
94
Blood transfusions
intrauterine, 259
Blood vessels
changes in during pregnancy, 84
Blood volume
changes during postpartum
period, 303
changes during pregnancy, 82
Blunt trauma, 535
Body image, 108, 119
Body mass index (BMI), 85
Body temperature
instability in postterm infants,
371
instability in preterm infants,
373–374
measures to regulate in preterm
infants, 376
postpartum changes in, 303
regulation of newborn in
delivery room, 352
thermoregulation during fetus/
neonate transition, 346
Bony diseases
affecting labor passage, 196
Bony pelvis, 8, 8f
parts of
coccyx, 8f, 9
ilium, 8, 8f
ischium, 8f, 9
pubic bone, 8f, 9
sacrum, 8f, 9
true versus false pelvis, 9, 9f
physical examination of, 14
supporting female reproductive
organs, 8, 8f
Bottle-feeding, 347
Bowels
assessing postpartum, 306
complications during
postpartum period, 304, 307
Brachycephalism
development during embryonic
stage, 43
Bradley method, 108
Bradycardia
cause of fetal, 256, 256f
sinus, 256f, 274, 283

Brain
   fetal development, 43, 46–49, 51f
Braxton Hicks contractions, 80,
   85, 225
Brazelton Neonatal Assessment
   Scale (BNAS), 350
Breast size
   scoring newborn's, 353t
Breastfeeding
   adequate milk supply, 329
   assessing maternal, 317
   and contraception, 336
   by drug abusers, 577
   ethnocultural "Quick Reference
      Guide," 78t
   with gestational diabetes, 514
   health education, 331–332
   inspecting nipples and breasts,
      318
   latching-on problems
      anxiety, 324, 326
      engorgement pain, 325
      mastitis, 326
      multiple births, 328
      nipple confusion, 323
      nipple pain, 324
      physiologic jaundice, 327
      plugged ducts, 326
      preterm or hospitalized infant,
         328
      sleepy or reluctant infant, 327
   maternal/infant positions,
      318–319
      cradle-hold position, 318–319,
         319f–320f
      cross-cradle position, 318, 320,
         320f–321f
      football-hold position, 318,
         321, 322f
      side-lying position, 318, 321,
         322f
   nutritional recommendations,
      330
   physiology of, 315, 316f
      hormonal influences, 315, 316f
      human milk stages, 317
      milk production, 315, 316f
Breasts
   anatomical illustration of, 316f
   assessing postpartum, 305
   changes during postpartum
      period, 302
   changes during pregnancy, 81
   characteristics of preterm infant,
      374
   inspecting nipples and, 318
   mastitis infections, 655
   postpartum infections, 654–655
Breathing
   ABCs (Airway, Breathing,
      Circulation), 536, 541, 541f
   education for childbirth, 108
   following trauma, 536, 547–548
Breech presentation, 137, 204f
   Elkins procedure, 203
   increased fetal morbidity and
      mortality, 203
Bulimia nervosa, 106, 111
Bulk flow
   in placental transfer, 44, 45t

Burns
   fetal/maternal trauma caused
      by, 539

C

Caffeine
   during breastfeeding, 330
Calcium
   function and needs for pregnant
      women, 86–87
Calcium channel blockers
   use and adverse effects during
      pregnancy, 593t
Caldeyro-Barcia, 195
Calm stage
   in cycle of violence, 418f, 419
Calorie needs
   during lactation, 330
   during pregnancy, 85–86
   of twins, 637
Capacitation, 35
Capacity
   and competence, 672, 677–679
Capillary hemangiomas, 349
Caput succedaneum, 208, 349
Carbohydrate metabolism
   interventions and outcomes, 507
   maternal changes with
      pregnancy, 501, 512
Carbon dioxide
   changes during pregnancy, 82
Carbon monoxide poisoning, 539
Carcinogens
   definition of, 164
Cardiac diseases
   classification, 590t
   versus normal pregnancy
      changes, 591t
   preexisting and maternal
      mortality, 588–594
   causing respiratory distress in
      newborns, 380–381
Cardiac output
   changes during pregnancy, 81
   following trauma, 548
   monitoring during surgery, 557
Cardiac system
   physical examination of
      newborn's, 349
Cardinal movements, 208
Cardiopulmonary compromise
   in newborn in delivery room,
      352
Cardiorespiratory disease
   and small for gestational age
      (SGA) newborns, 363
Cardiovascular drugs
   recommendations during
      pregnancy, 593t
Cardiovascular system
   adaptation of fetus to neonate,
      346
   changes during anesthesia, 557
   changes during postpartum
      period, 303
      blood volume, 303
      heart, 303
   changes during pregnancy
      arterial blood pressure, 82
      blood volume, 82

Cardiovascular system (Continued)
      cardiac output, 81
      heart, 81
      heart rate, 81
      in hemodynamic system, 81
      stroke volume, 82
      vasodilation, 82
      venous pressure, 82
   changes with preeclampsia, 434,
      435f
   congenital disorders/defects
      acyanotic defects, 403–404
      atrial septal defects, 404
      coarctation of the aorta, 405
      congenital cardiac lesions, 403
      cyanotic defects, 405–406
      hypoplastic left heart
         syndrome, 406–407
      patent ductus arteriosus,
         403–404
      tetralogy of Fallot, 405–406
      transposition of great arteries,
         406
      ventricular septal defects,
         404–405
   considerations with trauma, 536
   development of primitive, 39,
      40f
   developmental problems
      in preterm infants, 372, 375
   drug group recommendations
      during pregnancy, 593t
   heart disease classification, 590t
   indicating mother's nutritional
      status, 92, 93t
   normal adaptations to
      pregnancy, 433
   preexisting maternal disorders
      classification of, 590t
      complications with, 588–594
      drugs used during pregnancy,
         593t
      interventions, 591
      mortality risks, 589b
      patient education, 594
      signs and symptoms common
         to, 590, 591t
   status and hypertension, 437
Care-based ethical approach, 671
Carpal ablation
   development during embryonic
      stage, 41
Case law, 674
Case-based ethical approach, 671
Cells
   division of, 20
   mitosis and meiosis, 20
   zygotes, 20
Central nervous system (CNS)
   changes with preeclampsia, 434,
      435f
   damage in children witnessing
      domestic violence, 421
   influencing fetal heart rate
      (FHR), 253
   and respiratory distress in
      newborns, 380–381
Cephalhematoma, 349
Cephalic presentation, 202, 203f
Cervical cerclage, 566–567

Cervical dilation
  and preterm labor, 624–630
Cervical smears
  during initial pregnancy
    assessment, 95
Cervical spine
  stabilization following trauma,
    547f
Cervical trauma
  affecting labor passage, 196
Cervix
  anatomical description and
    illustration of, 5, 5f
  changes during labor, 201
  changes during postpartum
    period, 302
  changes during pregnancy, 81
  changes with fetal head
    progression, 210f
  dilation of, 201, 201f
  incompetent, 12
  during menstrual cycle, 10
  physical examination of, 14
  short and preterm labor, 624–629
  trauma affecting labor passage,
    196
Cesarean section
  assessing incision site, 306
  for multiple gestations, 637
  and uterine rupture, 642–644
  wound infection, 654–655
Chemical abuse
  assessing maternal, 55
  and fetal development process,
    57
Chemical agents
  as occupational environmental
    hazard, 167
  antineoplastic drugs, 167
  colorants, 168
  ethylene oxide, 168
  nanoparticles, 169
  organic solvents, 169
  pesticides, 170
  phthalates, 171
  polychlorinated biphenyls
    (PCBs), 171
  toxic (heavy) metals, 171
  waste anesthetic gases, 173
Chemical stimuli
  during fetus/ neonate transition,
    345
Chemicals
  health education regarding fetal
    health and, 57
Chemistry panels
  to test for hypertensive
    disorders, 438, 439t
  to test for placenta previa, 482,
    487, 490
Chemoreceptors
  influencing fetal heart rate
    (FHR), 253
Chest
  injuries, 544, 547, 547f
  physical examination of
    newborn's, 349
Chickenpox, 468t–471t
Child abuse
  characteristics of abusers, 421, 422f

Childbearing
  ethnocultural considerations
    in, 61
  maternal age-related concerns,
    117
  possible complications with
    hemorrhagic disorders, 478
    hypertensive disorders, 432
    intimate partner violence, 417
    maternal infections, 449
Childbirth
  Bradley, 108
  dysfunctional labor, 241–243
    abnormal Friedman curve,
      241, 241f
    assessing, 241
    Cesarean birth, 243–244
    interventions, 242
  ethnocultural definitions of, 62,
    63f
  Lamaze, 108
  pain management during, 230
  positions in ethnocultural
    "Quick Reference Guide,"
    76t
  premonitory signs preceding,
    225–227
    amniotic sac rupture, 226
    Bishop scores, 238, 239t
    Braxton Hicks contractions,
      225
    energy burst, 226
    gastrointestinal symptoms, 226
    intervention procedures, 226
    lightening, 225
    vaginal discharge/ show,
      225–226
  preparation education, 107, 244
  psychological preparation, 107,
    111
  stages of
    dilation stage of labor, 227–232
    immediate postpartum period,
      237–238
    infant expulsion, 232–235
    placental expulsion, 235–237,
      236f
  trauma related to maternal
    diabetes, 505
  variables influencing labor and
    delivery, 238–241
    dysfunctional labor, 241–243,
      241f
    induction augmentation,
      238–241, 239t
Children
  witnessing intimate partner
    violence (IPV), 421, 422f
Chlamydia, 95, 455t–458t, 464
Chloasma, 84
Cholecystectomy, 562–564
Chorioamnionitis, 363, 472–473
Choriocarcinoma, 493
Chorionic cavity
  illustration of, 37f
Chorionic villi
  development of, 38, 38f
Chorionic villus sampling (CVS)
  description of, 137
  in fetal/ placental assessment, 55

Chromosomal aberration
  pregnancy risk factors, 29
  and toxin exposure, 166–177
Chromosomal abnormalities
  and small for gestational age
    (SGA) newborns, 363
Chromosomes
  abnormalities, 23
  diploid number (46), 35, 36f
  genetic blueprints, 22–23
  parent cell, 20, 21f
Chronic hypertension
  and pregnancy, 433, 444
Chronic maternal conditions; See
  preexisting conditions
Chronic renal disease
  as high-risk pregnancy/ fetal
    condition, 129
Circulation
  supporting female reproductive
    organs, 7
Circumcision
  ethnocultural considerations
    regarding, 62
Cirrhosis, 548
Cleft lip, 41, 400
Cleft palate, 43
Clitoris, 3, 4f
Clotting factors
  changes during pregnancy, 82
  with disseminated intravascular
    coagulation (DIC), 489–492
  in trauma cases, 545
Clotting studies
  to diagnose placenta previa, 482,
    487, 490
  to test for hypertensive
    disorders, 438, 439t
Coagulation disorders
  causing postpartum
    hemorrhages, 650
Coarctation of the aorta
  description and risks in
    newborns, 405
Coccygeal muscles, 8f
Coccyx, 8f, 9
Codes of ethics, 681
Cold and hot beliefs, 66, 68, 77t
Colic, 331
Colorants
  as occupational environmental
    hazard, 168
Common law, 674
Communication
  SBAR technique, 287
Competence
  and capacity, 672, 677–679
Complete blood count (CBC) tests
  to diagnose placenta previa, 482,
    487, 490
  for hypertensive disorders, 438,
    439t
  during pregnancy assessment,
    94
  for TORCH diseases, 454
  in trauma cases, 545
Compound presentation, 204
Compression stockings, 658–659
Computed tomography
  for trauma cases, 546

Concentration gradients
  in placental transfer, 45, 45t
Conception
  and menstrual cycle, 10
  problems with older maternal
    age, 121–124
  stage in fetal development
    process, 35, 36f
Condoms, 337t–339t
Cone biopsies
  to cervix, 12
Confidentiality
  defining in ethics, 670, 677–680
Congenital anomalies
  and breech presentation, 203
  formation during embryonic
    stage, 50
  interventions and outcomes, 55
  and intrauterine fetal surgery,
    568–569
  in newborns
    abdominal wall defects, 401–402
    acyanotic defects, 403–404
    atrial septal defects (ASDs), 404
    cleft lip/ palate, 400
    coarctation of the aorta, 405
    congenital cardiac lesions, 403
    congenital diaphragmatic
      hernia (CDH), 402–403
    cyanotic defects, 405–407
    gastrointestinal system,
      400–401
    hydrocephalus, 399
    hypoplastic left heart
      syndrome, 406–408
    neural tube defects, 399–400
    patent ductus arteriosus,
      403–404
    small for gestational age
      (SGA), 364
    spina bifida, 399
    tetralogy of Fallot (TOF),
      405–406
    transposition of the great
      arteries (TGA), 406
    ventricular septal defects
      (VSDs), 404–405
  related to maternal diabetes, 505
  and toxin exposure, 166–177
Congenital cardiac disease
  during pregnancy, 589
Congenital cardiac lesions
  description and risks in
    newborns, 403
Congenital diaphragmatic hernia
  (CDH), 402–403
Congenital heart disease (CHD)
  during pregnancy, 589
  causing respiratory distress in
    newborns, 380–381
Congenital hyperthyroidism,
  380–381
Congestive heart failure (CHF)
  as preexisting maternal
    condition, 588–594
  causing respiratory distress in
    newborns, 380–381
  signs and symptoms of, 591
Constipation, 307
Constitutional law, 674

Contraception, 118
  and breastfeeding, 336
  emergency, 337t–339t
  and ethics, 679
  health conditions that affect, 335
  interventions and outcomes, 336,
    337t–339t
  methods and choices of, 336,
    337t–339t
  postpartum, 335
  psychosocial issues, 336
  risks/disadvantages/benefits of,
    337t–339t
Contracted pelvis
  affecting labor passage, 195
Contraction stress test (CST)
  during antepartum fetal
    assessment, 153
Contractions
  with coupling, 271f
  description and illustration of,
    192, 193f
  diagnostic evaluation of, 195
  duration of, 195
  examining and monitoring, 194
  false labor, 194
  fetal factor theories, 192
  frequency of, 195
  maternal factor theories, 192
  onset of, 192
  physiology of, 192
    intensity, 193
    myometrium, 192
    pacemakers, 193
    retractions, 192
    shortening contractions, 192
    tonus, 193
  power of, 192
  strength of, 194
    expulsive activity, 194
    myometrial activity, 194
  therapeutic and diagnostic
    interventions, 216
  true labor, 194
Convulsions
  eclampsia, 443
Coping abilities
  of abused women, 423
  with hypertensive disorders, 446
  during labor, 215, 218
  with postpartum mood
    disorders, 661–662
  for pregnancy, 108, 110–111
Copper intrauterine device (IUD),
  337t–339t
Cordocentesis, 259
Corpus (body)
  of uterus, 5, 5f
Corpus luteum cysts, 564
Costs
  versus ethics, 674, 680
Couvelaire uterus, 487
Cradle-hold position, 318–319,
  319f–320f
Cramps; *See* menstrual cramps
Cranial bones
  of fetal skull, 207
Creatinine
  affected by preeclampsia and
    HELLP, 439t

Cross-cradle position, 318, 320,
  320f–321f
Crown-rump length, 130b
Cryosurgery, 12
Cultural assessment
  in antepartum period, 64
  defining and steps, 64
  during history-taking, 13
  in intrapartum period, 65
  postpartum period, 66
Cultural competence
  balancing, 62
  defining in transcultural nursing,
    62
Cultures
  biological variations, 68, 79t
  and childbearing, 61
  ethnocultural "Quick Reference
    Guide," 75t–79t
  and spiritual influences on
    ethics, 675
Culture-specific, 61
Culture-universal, 61
Cushing's syndrome, 523–525
Cutis marmorata, 349
Cyanosis
  as preexisting maternal
    condition, 588–594
Cyanotic defects
  description and risks in
    newborns, 405–406
Cyanotic heart disease
  as high-risk pregnancy/ fetal
    condition, 129
Cycle of violence
  in intimate partner violence
    (IPV), 418, 418f, 422f
Cyclopia, 40, 40f
Cystitis, 465–467
Cystocele, 13
Cytomegalovirus (CMV), 449–454,
  450t–453t
Cytoplasmic transfer, 680
Cytotrophoblast, 37–38, 38f

D

Danger assessment questionnaire
  for intimate partner violence
    (IPV), 425–426, 426f
Decelerations
  forces, 535
  prolonged or variable, 642
Decidua
  description and illustration of,
    37, 37f
  maternal changes during
    pregnancy, 80
  three layers of, 37f, 38
Decidua basalis, 37f, 38
Decidua capsularis, 37f, 38
Decidua parietalis, 37f, 38
Decision-making process
  in ethics, 677–679
  patient's right to be involved in,
    679
  proxy decision-makers, 673,
    677–679
Deep tendon reflexes
  examining for hypertension, 436
Deep vein thrombosis, 656–658

Dehydration
    regulating in preterm infants, 378
Dehydroepiandrosterone sulfate
    (DHEAS), 15
Delayed growth and development
    due to maternal nutrition, 56
Delivery; *See* labor and delivery
    ethnocultural considerations
        regarding, 62
    expectant father's role in, 104
    expected delivery date (EDD)
        calculation, 92
Delivery room
    assessment of newborns, 352
    care of neonates, 357
Delta OD 450
    testing during antepartum fetal
        assessment, 133, 133f
Deontology, 670, 677–679
Deoxyribonucleic acid (DNA)
    chromosome composition and, 22
    definition and components of, 22
    and genetic blueprints, 23
    National Human Genome
        Project, 20
    sequences of, 20
    testing on fetus, 29
Depression
    in children witnessing domestic
        violence, 421
    postpartum, 659–662
    in substance abusers, 576
Developmental defects
    due to genetic disorders, 56
    and toxin exposure, 166–177
Developmental (maturational)
    crisis, 102
Developmental tasks
    fetal embodiment and
        distinction, 103
    pregnancy validation, 102
    role transition, 103
Developmental toxicity
    definition of, 164
Diabetes ketoacidosis (DKA), 503
Diabetes mellitus, 500–502
    assessment of, 502
    blood glucose values, 501t
    classifications of, 500, 503, 503t,
        514t
    definition of, 500, 502–509
    diagnostic procedures, 506
    fetal complications associated
        with, 505
    gestational diabetes mellitus
        (GDM), 501, 510–515
    health education, 509–510
    as high-risk pregnancy/ fetal
        condition, 129
    impaired fasting glucose (IFG),
        501, 501t, 503t
    impaired glucose tolerance
        (IGT), 501, 501t, 503t
    interventions and outcomes, 507
    nutritional deficiency risks of, 86
    pathophysiology with
        pregnancy, 501
    pregestational, 502–509
    and small for gestational age
        (SGA) newborns, 363

Diabetes mellitus *(Continued)*
    symptoms of, 500
    type 1, 500, 502–509
    type 2, 501–509
    White's classification of, 503t
Diagnostic peritoneal lavage
    (DPL), 547
Diagnostic tests
    for female reproductive health, 14
    for genetic disorder screening,
        28–29
Diaphoresis, 304
Diaphragm
    contraceptive device with
        spermicide, 337t–339t
    fetal development of, 43, 46–49,
        51
Diaphragmatic hernia
    development during embryonic
        stage, 42
Diet; *See* nutrition
Diffusion
    in placental transfer, 45, 45t
Digital stunting, 43
Dilation stage of labor, 227–232
Diploid number (46)
    of chromosomes, 35, 36f
Disseminated intravascular
    coagulation (DIC), 489–492
    definition of, 489
    health education, 491
    interventions and outcomes, 491
    signs indicating, 490, 651
Diuretics
    use and adverse effects during
        pregnancy, 593t
Dizygotic twins, 637
Doctors
    ethnocultural considerations
        regarding, 62
Documentation
    examples of EFM, 287b
    intimate partner violence (IPV),
        417, 427
    during intrapartum fetal
        assessment, 286–287,
        286b–287b
Domestic violence; *See* intimate
    partner violence (IPV)
Donor oocytes, 122
Dopamine
    for neonatal resuscitation, 356t
Doppler ultrasound
    blood flow assessment
        during antepartum period,
            149–151, 150f
    electronic fetal monitoring (EFM)
        during intrapartum period, 250
    to evaluate fetal status with
        diabetes, 504
Doppler velocimetry
    during antepartum fetal
        assessment, 149–151, 150f
Doptone
    to assess fetal heart rate (FHR),
        249
Down syndrome
    maternal serum alpha-
        fetoprotein (MS-AFP)
        testing for, 55

Down syndrome *(Continued)*
    nuchal translucency screening, 29
    screening with maternal serum
        alpha-fetoprotein (AFP), 28
Drug abuse
    by abused women, 420, 424
    assessing maternal, 55, 575–579,
        581
    during breastfeeding, 330
    drugs
        cocaine, 574
        heroin, 574
        marijuana, 575
        methadone hydrochloride, 575
    and fetal development process, 57
    health education regarding fetal
        health and, 57
    and HIV/AIDS, 460–462, 461f
    physical signs of, 576, 579, 581
    pregnancy nutritional deficiency
        risks of, 86
    and preterm labor, 372, 374,
        624–629
    psychosocial signs of, 576, 579, 582
    causing respiratory distress in
        newborns, 380–381
    and risks during surgery, 558
    and small for gestational age
        (SGA) newborns, 363–366
    statistics concerning, 573
Drugs
    abuse of (*See* drug abuse)
    as environmental hazard,
        177–178
        FDA pregnancy risk
            categories, 177
        fetal pharmacology drugs, 178
        iPledge risk management, 178
        prescriptions, 178
    used to treat hypertensive
        disorders, 441t–442t, 443
Ductal sprouting, 315, 316f
Duodenal atresia, 43
Duty and obligation-based ethics,
    670, 677–679
Duvall's stages, 102
Dysfunctional grieving, 111
Dysfunctional labor, 241–243
    abnormal Friedman curve, 241,
        241f
    assessing, 241
    Cesarean birth, 243–244
    interventions, 242
Dysrhythmias
    causes and patterns, 273
    definition and characteristics of
        fetal, 273
    interventions, 282

E
Ears
    fetal development of, 43, 46–49,
        51
    physical examination of
        newborn's, 349
    scoring newborn's, 353t
Eating disorders
    in abused women, 420, 424
    adolescent, 118
    postpartum, 660

Eclampsia
  seizure activity with, 433, 443
  and small for gestational age
      (SGA) newborns, 363
Economic abuse
  and intimate partner violence
      (IPV), 420–421, 422f
Ectoderm
  development of, 37
Ectopia, 40, 40f
Ectopic pregnancies, 135
Ectromelia
  development during embryonic
      stage, 40, 40f
Edema
  examining for hypertension, 437
  postpartum changes in, 304
  scoring newborn's external signs
      for, 353t
Egg
  donors, 117
  during menstrual cycle, 10
Electronic fetal monitoring (EFM),
      248–249, 264b
  abbreviations for charting, 264b
  baseline monitoring, 253–260
  Doppler ultrasound, 250
  fetal spiral electrode (FSE), 251
  importance in intrapartum fetal
      assessment, 248–249
  intrauterine pressure catheter
      (IUPC), 251
  tocodynamometer, 251
  in trauma cases, 546
Elimination, 304, 307
Elkins procedure
  for breech presentation, 203
Embryo
  development stages, 39, 40f–42f,
      57
  early development of, 36, 36f–37f
  illustration of, 37f
Embryo cryopreservation, 122
Embryo donation, 122
Embryo transfers
  ethical dilemma concerning, 680
  and multiple gestation, 635–637
Embryolethality
  definition of, 164
Embryonic stage
  in fetal development process, 39,
      40f–42f
  toxin exposure during, 165
Embryotoxicity
  definition of, 164
Emergency contraception, 337t–339t
Emotional abuse; See intimate
      partner violence (IPV)
Emotions
  ethnocultural "Quick Reference
      Guide," 75t
  expression in different cultures, 66
Endocrine disorders
  Addison's disease, 527
  adrenal disorders, 523–525
    adrenal hyperfunction, 523
    assessment of, 524
    Cushing's syndrome, 523–525
    effects on pregnancy, 523
    fetal/neonatal effects, 524

Endocrine disorders (*Continued*)
    health education, 525
    hyperadrenocorticism, 523–525
    interventions and outcomes,
        524
  adrenal insufficiency, 525–526
    assessment of, 526
    definition and classification
        of, 525
    effects on fetus/neonates, 526
    effects on pregnancy, 525
    interventions and outcomes,
        526
    and steroid replacement
        therapy, 527
  diabetes mellitus, 500–502
    assessment of, 502
    blood glucose values, 501t
    classifications of, 500, 503,
        503t, 514t
    definition of, 500, 502–509
    diagnostic procedures, 506
    fetal complications associated
        with, 505
    gestational diabetes mellitus
        (GDM), 501, 510–515
    health education, 509–510
    impaired fasting glucose (IFG),
        501, 501t, 503t
    impaired glucose tolerance
        (IGT), 501, 501t, 503t
    interventions and outcomes,
        507
    pathophysiology with
        pregnancy, 501
    pregestational, 502–509
    symptoms of, 500
    type 1, 500, 502–509
    type 2, 501–509
    White's classification of, 503t
  gestational diabetes mellitus
      (GDM), 510
    definition and incidence of, 510
    diagnostic testing, 511, 514t
    fetal and neonatal effects, 510
    glucose screening, 511
    health education, 514–515, 514t
    macrosomia, 513
    maternal effects, 510
    nutritional planning, 513
    OGTT, 511, 511t, 515
    risk factors, 510
    self-care planning, 513
  Graves' disease, 515–516
  hyperthyroidism, 515–516
    antithyroid drugs, 519
    assessment of, 517–520
    health education, 520
    thioamides, 516
    thyroid function test changes,
        516t
    thyroid storm, 516
    treatment of, 518
  hypoadrenocorticism (Addison's
      disease), 527
  hypothyroidism
    assessment of, 521–522
    definition of, 520
    etiology of, 520
    Hashimoto's thyroiditis, 520

Endocrine disorders (*Continued*)
    health education, 522–523
    prognosis for mother/fetus, 520
    thyroid function tests, 516t
    treatment of, 521
  maternal phenylketonuria,
      528–529
    assessment of, 529
    definition and incidence of,
        528
    effects on pregnancy and fetus,
        529
    health education, 531
    interventions and outcomes,
        530
    management of, 528
    nutritional planning, 530
  types to identify in health
      histories, 12
Endocrine disrupters
  definition of, 164
Endocrine system; *See also*
      endocrine disorders
  changes during postpartum
      period, 303
    pituitary hormones, 303
    placental hormones, 303
  changes during pregnancy
    in ovaries and hormones, 84
    in pancreas, 84
    in pituitary gland, 84
    in thyroid gland, 84
  fetal development of, 43, 46–49
  normal adaptations to
      pregnancy, 433
  pituitary hormones
    changes during postpartum
        period, 303
    follicle-stimulating hormone
        (FSH), 303
    luteinizing hormone (LH), 303
    serum prolactin, 303
  placental hormones
    changes during postpartum
        period, 303
    human chorionic
        gonadotropin (HCG), 303
    human chorionic
        somatomammotropin
        (HCS), 303
    plasma estrogen, 303
    plasma progesterone, 303
Endoderm
  development of, 37
End-of-life decisions, 680
Endometrial biopsy, 15
Endometriosis
  fertility problems due to, 122
  identifying in health histories, 12
Endometritis, 654
Endometrium, 10, 81
Endoscopic gastrointestinal
      procedures, 567–568
Engorgement pain
  and latching-on problems, 325
Environmental hazards, 163
  assessment procedures, 179–180
  definition of terms, 163
  interventions and outcomes,
      180–184

Environmental hazards *(Continued)*
occupational risks, 167–177;
See also (occupational
environmental hazards)
patient education, 180, 181b
pharmaceuticals, 177–178
FDA pregnancy risk
categories, 177
fetal pharmacology drugs, 178
iPledge risk management, 178
prescriptions, 178
referrals, 183
reproductive risks and outcomes,
166–167
resources, 181b
scope of, 163
teratology principles, 165–184
embryonic stage, 165
fetal stage, 166
pre-embryonic stage, 165
timing, 165
toxicology principles, 164–165
air pollution, 164
definition of, 164
dermal and direct contact, 164
dose toxicity variables, 164
dose-response relationship, 165
exposure duration, 164
ingestion, 164
inhalation, 164
routes of exposure, 164
target organs, 165
Enzyme-linked immunosorbent
assay (ELISA), 94, 454, 463
Epinephrine
for neonatal resuscitation, 356t
Episiotomy
healing of, 302
postpartum assessment and care
of, 306
Episodic patterns
pattern of fetal heart rate (FHR),
267, 269f
Ergonomic hazards, 174
ionizing radiation, 174
noise, 175
physical tasks, 174
second hand smoke, 176
temperature extremes, 176
Erythema toxicum, 349
Esophageal atresia, 41
Estimated date of confinement
(EDC), 130–131
Estimation of gestational age
(EGA)
normal length of, 130–131
Estrogen
changes during pregnancy, 84
and ductal sprouting, 315, 316f
levels during ovulation, 35
during menstrual cycle, 10
within ovarian feedback loop, 11
Ethical
definition of, 675
Ethical decision-making
process, 677–679
proxy decision-makers, 673,
677–679
Ethical-moral dilemmas
definition of, 669

Ethics
approaches and theories
care-based approach, 671
case-based approach, 671
goal outcome consequences-
based, 670
non-normative, 670
principle-based, 670
research and human subject
protection, 671
social ethics, 671
story -based approach, 671
virtue character-based
approach, 671
best interest standards, 676, 678
codes of ethics, 681
competence and capacity, 672,
677–679
creating ethical environment, 674
cultural and spiritual influences,
675
definition of, 669
ethical decision-making process,
677–679
ethical dilemmas in nursing
assisted reproductive
technology (ART), 679
intensive care issues, 679
reproductive choices/
freedom, 679
informed consent, 671–672,
677–679
interventions and outcomes, 678
versus law, 674
patient education and rights, 679
terminology, 669
treatment *versus* nontreatment
issues, 673, 677–679
Ethnic groups, 63, 68, 79t
Ethnocultural considerations
biological variations, 68, 79t
regarding breastfeeding, 78t
and care of newborns, 67, 78t
childbearing customs and beliefs,
62
clinical practice applications,
64–68
components of, 63f
cultural assessment
in antepartum period, 64
defining and steps, 64
in intrapartum period, 65
postpartum period, 66
cultural/linguistic competence, 62
data collection, 61
and ethics, 675
health education regarding,
69–70
HIV/AIDS statistics, 461, 461f
interventions and outcomes,
68–69
regarding labor process, 62
during postpartum period, 62,
66, 77t
and preterm infants, 372
psychological aspects of, 105
"Quick Reference Guide," 75,
75t–78t
transcultural nursing, 61
and violence against women, 420

Ethylene oxide
as occupational environmental
hazard, 168
Eunice Kennedy Shriver National
Institute of Child Health
and Development (NICHD),
248–249
Excretion
during placental transfer, 46
Expectant fathers
phases of tasks, 104
psychological issues with, 104
Expectant grandparents, 105
Expectant siblings
psychological issues with, 105
Expected confinement date (ECD),
92
Expected date of birth (EDB)
calculation of, 92
Expected delivery date (EDD)
calculation of, 92
External cephalic version (ECV),
137–138
External female genitalia, 3, 4f
characteristics of preterm infant,
374
clitoris, 3, 4f
fetal development of, 43, 46–49
fourchette, 4, 4f
labia majora, 3, 4f
labia minora, 3, 4f
mons pubis, 3, 4f
perineum, 4, 4f
physical examination of, 13
prepuce of clitoris, 3, 4f
vestibule, 4, 4f
External genitals
physical examination of
newborn's, 350
External physical characteristics
scoring system of newborn's,
353t
Extrachorial placentas, 50
Extravasation of bladder, 41
Extremities
assessing maternal trauma to, 544
indicating mother's nutritional
status, 92, 93t
physical examination of
newborn's, 350
Eyes
assessing maternal trauma to, 543
changes with preeclampsia, 434,
435f
indicating mother's nutritional
status, 92, 93t
physical examination of
newborn's, 349

F

Facial clefts, 41
Facial dysmorphia
with alcohol abuse, 548, 580
Facilitated diffusion
in placental transfer, 45, 45t
Fallopian tubes, 5f, 7
anatomical description and
illustration of, 5f, 7
changes during pregnancy, 81
fertilization in, 35, 36f

Fallopian tubes *(Continued)*
  parts of
    ampulla, 5f, 7
    infundibulum, 5f, 7
    interstitial, 5f, 7
    isthmus, 5f, 7
Falls, 535, 539
Families
  structure and violence, 421, 422f
  taking health histories of, 90
Fathers
  attachment factors, 309
  phases of tasks for expectant, 104
  psychological issues with, 104
  taking health histories of, 90
Fatigue
  with anemia, 609–614
  of labor, 215
Fear
  with abruptio placentae, 487–488
  in abused women, 420, 424–425
  ethnocultural considerations
      regarding, 65
  regarding HIV and AIDS, 462
  during labor, 214, 217
  in placenta previa cases, 481
  regarding preexisting conditions,
      587
  psychological issues with
      pregnancy, 102, 110
Feeding
  adaptation of fetus to neonate, 346
  ethnocultural considerations
      regarding, 62
Feet
  fetal development of, 43, 46–49
Female attendants
  preference in ethnocultural
      "Quick Reference Guide,"
      75t–76t
Female condoms, 337t–339t
Female genitalia; *See* external and
      internal female genitalia
Female gonads; *See* ovaries
Female reproductive system
  anatomy of, 3–11, 4f–6f, 8f–9f
  changes during postpartum
      period, 301
    assessment of, 305
    breasts, 302
    cervix, 302
    menstrual cycle return, 302
    perineum, 302
    uterus, 301
    vagina, 302
  changes during pregnancy
    breasts, 81
    cervix, 81
    fallopian tubes, 81
    ovaries, 81
    uterus, 80
    vagina, 81
    vulva, 81
  clinical assessment procedures,
      12–16
  diagnostic procedures, 14
  external genitalia, 3, 4f
    clitoris, 3, 4f
    fourchette, 4, 4f
    labia majora, 3, 4f

Female reproductive system
      (Continued)
    labia minora, 3, 4f
    mons pubis, 3, 4f
    perineum, 4, 4f
    prepuce of clitoris, 3, 4f
    vestibule, 4, 4f
  health education, 16
  history-taking regarding, 12
  hormones, 11
  hypothalamic-pituitary-ovarian
      axis, 11
  internal organs, 4, 5f
    fallopian tubes, 5f, 7
    ovaries (female gonads), 5f, 7
    oviducts, 5f, 7
    uterus, 5, 5f
    vagina, 4, 5f
  interventions/outcomes, 15
  menstruation, 9
    anatomy and physiology of, 9
    menarche, 9
    menstrual cycles, 9
  physical examinations, 13, 14f
  support for organs in, 7
    bony pelvis, 8, 8f
    circulation, 7
    motor and sensory nerves, 9
    pelvic floor and perineum, 7, 8f
Female sterilization
  as method of contraception,
      337t–339t
Fertility
  awareness and periodic
      abstinence, 337t–339t
  conditions affecting, 122
  and toxin exposure, 166–177
Fertility rates
  with advanced maternal age,
      121–122
Fertilization process
  in fetal development process,
      35, 36f
Fetal alcohol syndrome (FAS),
      580–581
Fetal asphyxia
  dangers in surgery, 556, 558, 570
  related to maternal diabetes, 505
Fetal attitude
  during labor, 202
Fetal bradycardia, 642
Fetal death
  and maternal morbidity
      trauma leading to, 535–540
Fetal development, 35
  amniotic fluid, 53, 53f
  antepartum assessment of,
      130–131, 130b, 137f
  chemical and substance abuse
      issues, 57
  clinical practice associated with,
      54–56
  conception, 35, 36f
  fertilization process, 35, 36f
  health education regarding, 57
  implantation process, 36, 36f
  nutritional needs for adequate, 57
  overall stages of
    embryonic stage, 39, 40f–42f
    fetal stage, 43, 44f, 45t, 43

Fetal development *(Continued)*
    pre-embryonic stage, 36, 36f
    placental abnormalities, 50, 52t
    pregenesis, 35
    umbilical cord, 50
    weekly stages
      week 1, 36–37
      week 2, 37–38, 37f, 41f
      week 3, 39, 40f
      week 4, 40, 41f–42f
      week 5, 41, 42f
      week 6, 41, 42f
      week 7, 41, 42f
      week 8, 42f, 43
      week 9 to 12, 46
      week 13 to 16, 47
      week 17 to 20, 47
      week 21 to 24, 48
      week 25 to 29, 48
      week 30 to 34, 49
      week 35 to 38, 49
      week 39 to 40, 49
      postterm, 49
Fetal gas exchange, 56
Fetal heart rate (FHR)
  arrhythmias and dysrhythmias,
      249, 273, 275f–276f
  assessment methods, 249–252
    electronic methods, 250
    nonelectronic methods, 249
  factors that influence
    baroreceptors, 253
    central nervous system (CNS),
        253
    chemoreceptors, 253
    hormones, 253
    parasympathetic nervous
        system, 252
    sympathetic nervous system,
        252
  interpreting patterns, 272–283
    fetal arrhythmias and
        dysrhythmias, 249, 273,
        275f–276f
    three-tier categorization
        system, 272
  monitoring during surgery, 557,
      559, 561
  patterns
    accelerations, 261–262, 261f,
        267–268, 268f
    early accelerations, 267, 267f
    episodic patterns, 267, 269f
    late accelerations, 264–267,
        265f–266f
    periodic patterns, 260–283
    prolonged decelerations,
        268–269, 270f
    uterine activity, 269–272, 271f
    variable accelerations, 262–264,
        262f–263f, 268, 269f
  with placenta previa, 480–481,
      483
Fetal hyperinsulinemia
  related to maternal diabetes,
      505
Fetal lie
  during labor, 202
Fetal lung maturity
  amniocentesis to determine, 139

Fetal maturity scoring
   during antepartum fetal
      assessment, 135t
Fetal movement counting (FMC)
   during antepartum fetal
      assessment, 141–142
   and breathing characteristics, 146
   and high-risk pregnancy/ fetal
      conditions, 129
Fetal oxygenation
   and FHR with placenta previa,
      480–481, 483
Fetal pulse oximetry, 284
Fetal scalp sampling, 283
Fetal skull, 207
Fetal spiral electrode (FSE)
   electronic fetal monitoring
      (EFM), 251
Fetal station
   asynclitism, 206f, 207
   designations, 205
   engagement, 205
   floating, 206
   synclitism, 206, 206f
Fetal tissue perfusion, 550
Fetal viability
   confirming, 138
   definition of, 131
   testing during antepartum fetal
      assessment, 138
Fetoscope
   to assess fetal heart rate (FHR),
      249
Fetoscopic laser ablation, 569
Fetotoxins
   definition of, 163
Fetus
   abruptio placentae, 485–489
   actual or potential loss with
      trauma, 550
   anemia influences on, 610
   anesthesia risks to, 557
   antepartum fetal assessment
      ancillary antenatal tests,
         141–155
      biophysical profile (BPP),
         145–148, 148t
      contraction stress test (CST),
         153
      Doppler ultrasound blood
         flow assessment,
         149–151, 150f
      Doppler velocimetry,
         149–151, 150f
      fetal movement counting
         (FMC), 141–142
      modified biophysical profile
         (BPP), 148–149
      nonstress test (NST), 142–144
      oxytocin administration,
         154–155
      three-dimensional view,
         planes or 4D, 151–153
      vibroacoustic stimulation
         (VST), 144–145
   biochemical assessments
      amniotic fluid evaluation,
         138
      anomalies, 139
      bleeding, 138

Fetus (Continued)
   ectopic pregnancies, 135
   fetal maturity scoring, 135t
   fetal viability, 138
   multiple gestation, 136
   placental grading level, 135,
      136f
   placental positions, 136
   presentation/ positioning,
      137
   ultrasonography, 134, 135t,
      136f–137f
   clinical practice procedures,
      132–155
      alpha-fetoprotein, 129
      biochemical assessments,
         132–133
      delta OD 450, 133, 133f
      triple and quad screening,
         132
   fetal behavioral states,
      128–130, 137f
   fetal growth and development,
      130–131, 130b, 137f
   fetal response to hypoxemia,
      131–132
   health education regarding, 156
   high-risk conditions, 129
   importance of, 128–132, 248
   assessing following trauma, 544
   complications with renal disease,
      594–596
   determining size of during labor,
      207
   development of (See fetal
      development)
   diagnostic tests
      for genetic disorder screening,
         28
   effects of endocrine and
      metabolic disorders on, 500
   effects of maternal diabetes on,
      505
   effects of substance abuse on, 574
   embryo development stage, 39,
      40f–42f
   environmental hazards, 163
   fetal alcohol syndrome (FAS),
      580–581
   fetal embodiment and
      distinction, 103
   fetal heart rate (FHR)
      assessment methods, 249–252
      baseline FHR, 253–260, 254f,
         256f
      documentation, 286–287,
         286b–287b
      electronic fetal monitoring,
         248–249
      factors that influence, 252–253
      patterns, 260–283, 261f–263f,
         265f–271f
   fetal pulse oximetry, 284
   fetal scalp sampling, 283
   fetal scalp stimulation, 284
   full term timing, 49
   health education, 288
   hypertensive disorders, 438
   illustration of development
      stages, 51

Fetus (Continued)
   infections, 129
   intrapartum fetal assessment
      abbreviations, 264b
   intrauterine fetal surgery,
      568–569
   and maternal morbidity due to
      trauma, 535–540
   maternal nutritional needs for
      healthy, 88
   mortality associated with breech
      presentation, 203
   percutaneous umbilical blood
      sampling (PUBS), 140, 140f
   and placenta previa, 478–485
   position during labor, 205, 205f
   potential loss with trauma, 550
   presentation and position, 137
   at risk with maternal cardiac
      disease, 589b, 590
   safety concerns
      with intimate partner violence
         (IPV), 423, 425
   stillbirths, 638–640
      delivery management, 639
      description of, 638
      grief support, 639–640
      interventions, 639
      possible causes of, 639
      signs indicating, 638
   TORCH diseases affecting, 449,
      450t–453t
   toxin exposure, 166
   transition to neonate, 345, 352
      cardiovascular system
         adaptation, 346
      feeding, 346
      gastrointestinal system
         adaptation, 346
      respiratory system adaptation,
         345
      thermoregulation, 346
   umbilical cord blood sampling,
      284–286, 285t
   variability, 254f, 257–258,
      258f–260f
   vibroacoustic, 284
Fibrinogen
   affected by preeclampsia and
      HELLP, 439t
   and placenta previa tests, 482,
      487, 490
   in trauma cases, 545
Fibroid tumors
   fertility problems due to, 122
   identifying in health histories, 12
Fidelity
   defining in ethics, 670, 677–679
Fingers
   fetal development of,
First trimester
   health education regarding, 96
   psychological changes during,
      103, 112
Focusing phase, 104
Folic acid
   deficiency causing neural tube
      defects, 88
   function and needs for pregnant
      women, 87

Follicles, 10
Follicle-stimulating hormone
    (FSH), 303
    diagnostic tests, 15
    within ovarian feedback loop, 11
Follicular phase
    of menstrual cycles, 10
Fontanelles
    of fetal skull, 208
Food; *See also* nutrition
    childbearing cultural
        considerations, 64
    cravings, 102
    ethnocultural "Quick Reference
        Guide," 76t
Football-hold position, 318, 321, 322f
Foremilk, 317
Four P's
    of alcohol-use assessment, 581
Fourchette
    anatomical description and
        illustration of, 4, 4f
Fraternal twins, 637
Fruits and vegetables
    needs for pregnant mothers, 87
Fundal height
    evaluation of, 95, 95f
    postpartum, 301
Fundus
    anatomical description and
        illustration of, 5, 5f

G

Gallbladder
    changes during pregnancy, 83
Gamete intrafallopian transfer
    (GIFT), 122, 680
Gametes
    formation of, 35
Gametogenesis, 21, 22f
Gastrointestinal system
    adaptation of fetus to neonate, 346
    changes during postpartum
        period, 304
        assessment of, 306
        bowels/ elimination
            complications, 304, 307
        weight loss, 304
    changes during pregnancy
        in gallbladder, 83
        in gastrointestinal tract, 83
        mouth, saliva and gums, 83
    changes with anesthesia, 558
    cleft lip/ palate risks for
        newborns, 400–401
    considerations with trauma, 537
    fetal development of, 43, 46–49
    of fetus
        affected by maternal substance
            abuse, 574
        indicating mother's nutritional
            status, 92, 93t
    preexisting maternal disorders
        assessment of, 615
        complications with, 614–616
        hyperemesis gravidarum, 614
        inflammatory bowel disease, 614
        interventions and outcomes,
            616
    symptoms preceding birth, 226

Gastrointestinal tract
    changes during pregnancy, 83
Gastrulation, 39
Gender
    ethical approaches according
        to, 676
    roles and intimate partner
        violence, 421, 422f
Genes
    composition of, 22
    definition of, 20
    modes of inheritance
        autosomal dominant
            inheritance, 24, 24f
        autosomal recessive
            inheritance, 25, 25f
        complex disorders, 27
        polygenic or multifactorial
            disorders, 27
        sex-linked dominant
            inheritance, 26
        sex-linked recessive
            inheritance, 26, 26f
    mutation
        and toxin exposure, 166–177
Genetic blueprints, 23
Genetic diseases
    blood tests, 95
    developmental defects due to, 56
Genetics
    clinical practice guidelines,
        27–31, 28f
    complex disorder causes, 27
    definitions of key terms, 20
    ethical issues with, 680
    genogram symbols, 27, 28f
    health education regarding, 31
    inheritance
        foundations of, 20, 21f, 23f–24f
        modes of, 24, 24f–26f
    Internet genetic reference sites,
        30t
    The National Human Genome
        Project, 20
    polygenic or multifactorial
        disorders, 27
    useful Internet reference sites
        regarding, 30t
Genital tract infections
    postpartum, 654
Genitalia; *See* external female
    genitalia; internal female
    genitalia
Genitourinary system
    considerations with trauma, 538
    fetal development of, 43, 46–49
Genograms
    elements of, 27
    symbols, 28f
Genome
    definition of, 20
    The National Human Genome
        Project, 20
Genotypes
    definition of, 20
Gestation period
    defining, 630
    normal length of, 130–131
Gestational age
    classifications of newborns, 351

Gestational age *(Continued)*
    conditions related to
        large for gestational age
            (LGA), 83, 367–370
        late preterm infants, 379–380
        postterm infants, 370–372
        preterm infants, 372–380
        small for gestational age
            (SGA), 363–367
Gestational carriers, 122
Gestational diabetes mellitus
    (GDM), 501, 510–515
    definition and incidence of, 510
    diagnostic testing, 511, 514t
    fetal and neonatal effects, 510
    glucose screening, 511
    health education, 514–515, 514t
    macrosomia, 513
    maternal effects, 510
    nutritional planning, 513
    OGTT, 511, 511t, 515
    risk factors, 510
    self-care planning, 513
Gestational hypertension, 432
Gestational lengths
    and toxin exposure, 166–177
Gestational trophoblastic disease
    (GTD), 492–494
    definition of, 492
    hydatidiform mole, 492–494
Gestational trophoblastic neoplasia
    (GTN), 492–495
Glasgow coma scale, 545, 545t
Glucose levels
    criteria for diagnosis, 514t
    in fetus related to maternal
        diabetes, 505
    instability in postterm infants, 371
    screening
        for gestational diabetes
            mellitus (GDM), 511
        of newborns, 357
Glucose-6 phosphate
    dehydrogenase deficiency
    (G6PD)
    in different ethnic groups, 79t
Glucosuria, 83
Goal outcome consequences-based
    ethics, 670
Gonorrhea, 95, 455t–458t, 464
Goodell's sign, 81, 85
Graafian follicles, 10–11
Graves' disease, 515–516
Great vessel transposition
    development during embryonic
        stage, 41
Grief
    and loss issues, 107, 111
    maternal with preterm infants,
        107, 111
    over spontaneous abortion, 107,
        111
    over stillbirths, 639–640
Group B streptococcus, 468t–471t
Growth disturbances
    related to maternal diabetes, 505
Growth parameters
    of newborns, 348
Gums
    changes during pregnancy, 83

Gunshot wounds, 535, 540
Gynecoid pelvis, 196f, 197

H

Hair
    changes in during pregnancy, 84
    fetal development of, 43, 46–49
    indicating mother's nutritional
        status, 92, 93t
Hands
    fetal development of, 43, 46–49,
        51f
Hashimoto's thyroiditis, 520
Head
    assessing maternal trauma to, 543
    characteristics of preterm infant,
        374
    development of primitive, 39,
        40f
    physical examination of
        newborn's, 349
Head circumference
    of SGA *versus* IUGR, 363
Head lag
    in newborn neurological
        assessment, 354b
Head to tail regions
    development of, 41f
Hearing
    evaluating newborn's, 351
Heart
    changes during postpartum
        period, 303
    changes during pregnancy, 81
    fetal development of, 43, 46–49
Heart disease
    classification, 590t
    as preexisting maternal
        condition, 588–594
Heart rate
    changes during pregnancy, 81
Heel-to-ear maneuver
    in newborn neurological
        assessment, 354b
Hegar's sign, 85
HELLP syndrome, 434, 435f, 439t
Helplessness
    felt by abused women, 420,
        424–425
    in placenta previa cases, 481
Hematocrit
    affected by preeclampsia and
        HELLP, 439t
    changes during postpartum
        period, 303
    decreases with obstetric
        hemorrhages, 478
    normal *versus* pregnancy ranges
        of, 612t
    testing, 14, 94
Hematologic system
    changes during postpartum
        period, 303
        hematocrit and hemoglobin,
            303
        white blood cell count, 303
    changes during pregnancy
        clotting factor, 82
        red blood cells, 82
        white blood cells, 82

Hematologic system *(Continued)*
    changes with anesthesia, 558
    considerations with trauma,
        538
    disorders causing respiratory
        distress in newborns,
        380–381
    preexisting maternal disorders,
        608–610
        anemia, 608
        assessment of, 610
        fetal implications, 610
        interventions and outcomes,
            612
        patient education, 614
Hematoma, 651
Hemodynamic system
    changes during pregnancy, 81
    changes with placenta previa,
        480
    changes with preeclampsia, 434,
        435f, 440
    normal adaptations to
        pregnancy, 433
Hemoglobin
    abnormal in different ethnic
        groups, 79t
    changes during postpartum
        period, 303
    normal *versus* pregnancy ranges
        of, 612t
    tests, 14
        affected by preeclampsia and
            HELLP, 439t
        during pregnancy assessment,
            94
Hemoglobin electrophoresis, 482
Hemoglobinopathy
    as high-risk pregnancy/fetal
        condition, 129
Hemolysis
    affected by preeclampsia and
        HELLP, 439t
Hemorrhages
    postpartum, 650–651
        causes of, 650
        classification of, 650
        health education, 653
        interventions, 652–653
        risk factors, 651
        signs and symptoms of, 651
    causing respiratory distress in
        newborns, 380–381
Hemorrhagic disorders
    abruptio placentae, 485–489
        assessment of, 485–489
        complications, 487
        definition of, 485
        diagnostic procedures, 487
        health education, 489
        interventions and outcomes,
            488
        risk factors, 485
    disseminated intravascular
        coagulation (DIC), 489–492
        definition of, 489
        health education, 491
        interventions and outcomes,
            491
        signs indicating, 490

Hemorrhagic disorders *(Continued)*
    gestational trophoblastic disease
        (GTD), 492–494
        definition of, 492
        gestational trophoblastic
            neoplasia (GTN), 492–494
        hydatidiform mole, 492–494
    maternal morbidity and
        mortality rates, 478
    obstetric hemorrhages, 478
    placenta previa, 478–479
        assessment of, 479–485
        classifications of, 479
        complications associated with,
            480–481
        definition of, 478
        fetal oxygenation and FHR,
            480–481, 483
        health education, 484
        interventions and outcomes,
            482
        risk factors, 479
        signs indicating, 479–485
Hemorrhoids, 306–307
Hepatic system
    changes with preeclampsia, 434,
        435f
    preexisting maternal disorders
        complications with, 617–619,
            618t
        hepatitis A, B, and C, 617–619,
            618t
        patient education, 619–620
        signs and symptoms of, 619
        treatment of, 619
        viral hepatitis, 617–619
Hepatitis
    blood tests, 95
    characteristics of, 618t
    as preexisting maternal
        disorders, 617–619, 618t
    in TORCH maternal infections,
        449–454, 450t–453t
Heredity; *See also* genetics
    genes as smallest unit of, 22
Herpes simplex virus (HSV), 95,
    449–454, 450t–453t
Hindmilk, 317
Hispanics
    childbearing cultural
        considerations, 64
    ethnocultural "Quick Reference
        Guide," 75t–79t
    HIV/AIDS statistics among, 461,
        461f
    intimate partner violence among,
        420
Homan's sign, 306
Homelessness
    in substance abusers, 576
Honeymoon stage
    in cycle of violence, 418f, 419
Hormones
    affecting thyroid gland,
        515–516
    changes during pregnancy, 84
    and hypothalamic-pituitary-
        ovarian axis, 11
    influence on milk production,
        315, 316f, 317

Hormones *(Continued)*
  influencing fetal heart rate
    (FHR), 253
  during menstrual cycle, 10
  within ovarian feedback loop, 11
  during placental transfer, 46
Hot and cold
  ethnocultural beliefs concerning,
    66, 68, 77t
  regulating in preterm infants,
    375–376
Human chorionic gonadotropin
  (HCG), 28, 303
Human chorionic
  somatomammotropin (HCS),
  303
Human immunodeficiency virus
  (HIV); *See also* acquired
  immunodeficiency virus
  (AIDS)
  in pregnancy, 459
Human milk
  adequate supply for
    breastfeeding, 329
  production of, 315, 316f
  stages of, 317
Human papilloma virus (HPV),
  455t–458t
Hyaline membrane disease, 374
Hyaluronidase, 35
Hydatidiform mole, 492–494
Hydralazine hydrochloride,
  441t–442t
Hydramnios, 54
  as high-risk pregnancy/fetal
    condition, 129
  and preterm labor, 625
Hydrocephalus
  description and risks in
    newborns, 399
  surgery, 557
Hymen, 4, 4f, 13
Hyperadrenocorticism, 523–525
Hyperbilirubinemia
  assessing and treating, 394–397
  description and risks in
    newborns, 391–399, 394f
  in fetus related to maternal
    diabetes, 505
  health education and discharge
    planning, 397–399
  phototherapy for, 393
  and physiologic jaundice, 393
Hyperglycemia
  maternal, 501
  causing respiratory distress in
    newborns, 380–381
Hypermagnesemia, 380–381
Hyperpigmentation, 84, 304
Hyperplasia
  and maternal nutrition habits,
    88
Hypertension
  as high-risk pregnancy/fetal
    condition, 129
  as preexisting maternal
    condition, 588–594
  with renal disease, 595
  and small for gestational age
    (SGA) newborns, 363

Hypertensive disorders
  chronic hypertension, 433, 444
  classification of, 432
  eclampsia, 433, 443
  gestational hypertension, 432
  as most common pregnancy
    complication, 432–434
  normal physiologic adaptations
    to, 433
  postpartum, 444
  preeclampsia, 432–433
    assessment of, 436, 439t
    etiology of, 433
    HELLP syndrome, 434, 435f,
      439t
    lab tests, 438, 439t
    mild, 438, 445
    pathophysiology stages, 433,
      435f
    pharmacology therapy, 440,
      441t–442t
    physiologic alterations with,
      434
    predicting and preventing, 436
    risk factors, 433
    severe, 440
    treatment of, 438–445,
      441t–442t
  self-care education, 438, 445–446
Hyperthermia
  as occupational hazard, 176
  causing respiratory distress in
    newborns, 380–381
Hyperthyroidism, 515–516
  antithyroid drugs, 519
  assessment of, 517–520
  health education, 520
  as high-risk pregnancy/fetal
    condition, 129
  thioamides, 516
  thyroid function test changes,
    516t
  thyroid storm, 516
  treatment of, 518
Hypoadrenocorticism (Addison's
  disease), 527
Hypocalcemia
  in fetus related to maternal
    diabetes, 505
  in preterm infants, 374
  causing respiratory distress in
    newborns, 380–381
Hypoglycemia
  in fetus related to maternal
    diabetes, 505
  in preterm infants, 374–376
  causing respiratory distress in
    newborns, 380–381
Hypoplastic left heart syndrome,
  406–408
Hypothalamic-pituitary-ovarian
  axis, 11
Hypothermia
  as occupational hazard, 176
  causing respiratory distress in
    newborns, 380–381
Hypothyroidism
  assessment of, 521–522
  definition of, 520
  etiology of, 520

Hypothyroidism *(Continued)*
  Hashimoto's thyroiditis, 520
  health education, 522–523
  prognosis for mother/fetus,
    520
  thyroid function tests, 516t
  treatment of, 521
Hypoxemia
  antepartum fetal assessment of,
    131–132
  and persistent pulmonary
    hypertension of newborn
    (PPHN), 389–391

I

Identical twins, 637
Ilium
  description and illustration in
    bony pelvis, 8, 8f
Immune system
  changes during postpartum
    period, 304
  changes during pregnancy, 84
  developmental problems in
    preterm infants, 373
  maternal transfer to infant, 46
  in preterm infants, 373
  in small for gestational age
    (SGA) newborns, 364
Immunoglobulin G (IgG)
  to test for TORCH diseases, 454
Impaired fasting glucose (IFG), 501,
  501t, 503t
Impaired glucose tolerance (IGT),
  501, 501t, 503t
Implantation process
  in fetal development process,
    36, 36f
In vitro fertilization (IVF), 122
  ethical dilemma concerning, 680
  and multiple gestation, 635–637
Incompetent cervix, 12
Indomethacin, 627
Infant expulsion
  stage of childbirth, 232–235
Infants; *See* newborns
Infections
  acquired immunodeficiency
    syndrome (AIDS), 454–461,
    455t–458t, 461f
  causes and transmission of,
    454–459, 455t–458t
  characteristics of, 455t–458t
  counseling and early diagnosis
    of, 460
  statistics, 454–460, 459f–461f
  chorioamnionitis, 472–473
  group B streptococcus, 468t–471t
  health education regarding, 454,
    459–460, 463, 465, 472–473
  influenza, 468t–471t
  listeriosis, 468t–471t
  Lyme disease, 468t–471t
  measles, 468t–471t
  mumps, 468t–471t
  parvovirus B19, 468t–471t
  postpartum, 653–654
    breast/mastitis infections, 655
    cesarean section infections, 655
    definition of, 653

Infections *(Continued)*
   genital tract infections, 654
   risk factors, 654
   treatment of, 655–656
   types of, 654
   urinary tract infections, 655
  and preterm labor, 624–629
  prevention of newborn, 357
  causing respiratory distress in
    newborns, 380–381
  sexually transmitted diseases
    (STDs), 455t–458t, 464–465
  and small for gestational age
    (SGA) newborns, 363
  TORCH, 449–454, 450t–453t
  tuberculosis, 468t–471t
  urinary tract and pyelonephritis,
    465–467
  varicella zoster, 468t–471t
Infertility
  conditions predisposing, 122
  in older women, 117
Influenza, 468t–471t
Informed consent, 671–672,
  677–679
Infundibulum, 5f, 7
Inhalation, 539
Inheritance
  modes of
    autosomal dominant
      inheritance, 24, 24f
    autosomal recessive
      inheritance, 25, 25f
    complex disorders, 27
    polygenic or multifactorial
      disorders, 27
    sex-linked dominant
      inheritance, 26
    sex-linked recessive
      inheritance, 26, 26f
    single/ paired genes, 24
Injuries; *See* trauma
Inotropic agents
  use and adverse effects during
    pregnancy, 593t
Insensible water losses (IWLs), 377
Insulin
  control and monitoring, 503
Integumentary system
  changes during postpartum
    period, 304
    diaphoresis, 304
    hyperpigmentation
      disappears, 304
  changes during pregnancy, 84
  physical exam of newborn's, 349
  problems in postterm infants,
    370
Intensive care
  ethical dilemmas, 679
Intercourse
  contraindications with
    pregnancy, 109
Intergenerational cycle of violence,
  421
Internal cervical os, 478–479
Internal female genitalia; *See also*
  external female genitalia
  characteristics of preterm infant,
    374

Internal female genitalia *(Continued)*
  fetal development of, 43, 46–49,
    51f
  physical examination of
    newborn's, 350
  scoring newborn's, 353t
Internal organs
  of female reproductive system,
    4, 5f
    fallopian tubes, 5f, 7
    ovaries (female gonads), 5f, 7
    oviducts, 5f, 7
    uterus, 5, 5f
    vagina, 4, 5f
Interstitial
  part of fallopian tubes, 5f, 7
Intestines
  fetal development of, 43, 46–49, 51f
Intimate partner violence (IPV)
  abused women characteristics,
    422f, 423–424
  abuser characteristics, 421
  assaults, 535, 539
  assessment of, 423, 425
  children witnessing, 421, 422f
  common injuries associated
    with, 419
  cultural influences on awareness
    of, 420
  cycle of abuse, 418, 418f, 422f
  danger assessment
    questionnaire, 425–426,
    426f
  emotional abuse, 422, 422f
  intergenerational cycle of
    violence, 421
  interventions and prevention, 425
  mandatory reporting and
    documentation of, 417, 427
  possible causes of verbal and
    physical, 422, 422f
  power and control wheel, 422f
  during pregnancy, 423
  and preterm labor, 624–629
  prevalence of, 417
  resources and abuse education,
    427–429
  safety plans, 426–427, 426f
  signs and indicators of, 422f,
    423–424
  socioeconomic and ethnic issues,
    420
  and substance abuse, 576
  types of, 417–418, 422, 422f
Intracytoplasmic sperm injection
  (ICSI), 122
Intraembryonic coelom, 39
Intrapartum fetal assessment
  abbreviations
    for charting electronic fetal
      monitoring, 264b
  ancillary tools, 283–288
    fetal pulse oximetry, 284
    fetal scalp sampling, 283
    fetal scalp stimulation, 284
    umbilical cord blood
      sampling, 284–286, 285t
    vibroacoustic, 284
  baseline FHR
    bradycardia, 256, 256f

Intrapartum fetal assessment
  (Continued)
    characteristics of, 253–260, 254f
    tachycardia, 254, 254f
  documentation, 286–287,
    286b–287b
  electronic fetal monitoring,
    248–249
  factors that influence FHR
    baroreceptors, 253
    central nervous system (CNS),
      253
    chemoreceptors, 253
    hormones, 253
    parasympathetic nervous
      system, 252
    sympathetic nervous system,
      252
  fetal heart rate (FHR) assessment
    methods, 249–252
    electronic methods, 250
    nonelectronic methods, 249
  fetal heart rate (FHR) patterns
    accelerations, 261–262, 261f,
      267–268, 268f
    early accelerations, 267, 267f
    episodic patterns, 267, 269f
    late accelerations, 264–267,
      265f–266f
    periodic patterns, 260–283
    prolonged decelerations,
      268–269, 270f
    uterine activity, 269–272, 271f
    variable accelerations, 262–264,
      262f–263f, 268, 269f
  health education, 288
  importance of, 248
  interpreting FHR patterns,
    272–283
    fetal arrhythmias and
      dysrhythmias, 249, 273,
      275f–276f
    three-tier categorization
      system, 272
  variability
    categories, 254f, 258, 258f–259f
    definition of, 257
    sinusoidal patterns, 258, 260f
Intrapartum period; *See also*
  intrapartum fetal assessment
  ethnocultural considerations
    during, 65, 76t
  interventions with multiple
    gestation, 636
Intrauterine asphyxia
  risk during surgery, 558
Intrauterine blood transfusions, 259
Intrauterine environment
  contributing to small for
    gestational age (SGA)
    newborns, 363
Intrauterine fetal surgery, 568–569
Intrauterine growth restriction
  (IUGR)
  characteristics of, 363
  as high-risk pregnancy/ fetal
    condition, 129
  and maternal asthma, 599
  and maternal drug/alcohol
    abuse, 573

Intrauterine growth restriction *(Continued)*
in multiple gestation cases, 635–637
and nutrition, 88
related to adrenal disorders, 524
related to maternal diabetes, 505
with renal disease, 595
Intrauterine pressure catheter (IUPC), 216
electronic fetal monitoring (EFM), 251
Ionizing radiation, 174
IPledge program, 178
Iron
needs for pregnant women, 86–87
Iron deficiency anemia, 609–614
Iron homeostasis
indices of, 612t
Ischemic cardiac disease
during pregnancy, 589
Ischium
description and illustration in bony pelvis, 8f, 9
Isthmus
of fallopian tubes, 5f, 7
of uterus, 5, 5f

J

Jaundice
breastfeeding, 391, 395
and hyperbilirubinemia, 391–399
Joints
changes during postpartum period, 304
changes during pregnancy, 83
Justice
defining in ethics, 670, 677–679

K

Kaposi's sarcoma, 462
Karyogamy, 35
Kernicterus, 392
Kidneys
acute nephrolithiasis, 595
acute pyelonephritis, 595
acute renal failure, 595
changes during pregnancy, 83, 594
nephrotic syndrome, 595
postpartum changes in, 304
renal stones, 595
Kleihauer-Betke test, 259
to diagnose placenta previa, 482
in fetal/placental assessment, 55
Kyphoscoliosis
affecting labor passage, 196

L

Labetalol hydrochloride, 441t–442t
Labia majora
anatomical description and illustration of, 3, 4f
scoring newborn's, 353t
Labia minora
anatomical description and illustration of, 3, 4f
scoring newborn's, 353t

Labor; *See also* labor and delivery
cervical changes during, 201
contraction power, 192
examining and monitoring, 194
false labor, 194
fetal factor theories, 192
maternal factor theories, 192
physiology of, 192
therapeutic and diagnostic interventions, 216
true labor, 194
diagnostic studies, 201
pelvic capacity exam, 201
vaginal exam, 201
dilation stage of, 227–232
dysfunctional; *See* (dysfunctional labor)
ethnocultural considerations regarding, 62
expectant father's role in, 104
forces affecting, 191
four P's of, 191
health education regarding, 219–220
maternal postures and positions, 199
passage, 195
history-taking, 195
physical examination, 196
passenger (infant)
breech presentation, 202, 204f
cardinal movements, 208
cephalic presentation, 202, 203f
compound presentation, 204
diagnostic studies of, 209, 209f, 217
fetal attitude, 202
fetal lie, 202
fetal position, 205, 205f
fetal size, 207
fetal skull, 207
fetal station, 205, 205f; (*See also* fetal station)
Leopold's maneuver, 209, 209f, 217
transverse presentation, 204, 205f
ultrasonography, 210
vaginal examination, 210, 210f
pelvic shapes, 196, 196f
android pelvis, 196f, 197
anthropoid pelvis, 196f, 197
and dimensions, 197, 197f–198f
gynecoid pelvis, 196f, 197
platypelloid pelvis, 196f, 197
pelvic tilt, 219, 219f
power of contractions, 192
preterm labor, 624–630
psyche stage
anxiety, 214, 217
coping abilities, 215, 218
cultural considerations, 211
expectations and preparations, 211–212
fatigue and weariness, 215
fear, 214, 217
interventions, 217
maternal history and experience, 211
personality styles, 215

Labor *(Continued)*
psychological reactions to, 214, 217
psychosocial responses, 213
support system, 212
therapeutic and diagnostic procedures, 216
variables influencing, 238–241
dysfunctional labor, 241–243, 241f
induction augmentation, 238–241, 239t
Labor and delivery; *See also* labor
amniotic fluid embolism, 640
anaphylactoid syndrome, 640
description and high mortality rates with, 640
interventions, 641
signs of, 640
ethnocultural considerations regarding, 63f, 65
maternal positions, 199
sitting, 200
squatting, 199
standing, 200
multiple gestation, 635–637
antepartum interventions, 636
and assisted reproductive technology (ART), 635
health education regarding, 637
indications of, 635–637
intrapartum interventions, 636
postpartum interventions, 637
statistics and increases in, 635
postterm pregnancy, 630–632
premature rupture of membranes (PROM), 632–635, 637
preterm labor, 624–630
definition of, 624
factors associated with, 624–625
health education, 629–630
indications of, 625
interventions, 626
risk factors for, 625
tocolytic drug therapy, 627
at risk, 624
stillbirths, 638–640
delivery management, 639
description of, 638
grief support, 639–640
interventions, 639
possible causes of, 639
signs indicating, 638
uterine rupture, 642–643
Laboratory tests
to test for hypertensive disorders, 438, 439t
in trauma cases, 545
Lactate dehydrogenase (LDH)
affected by preeclampsia and HELLP, 439t
Lactation; *See* breastfeeding
Lactogenesis stages, 317
Lactose intolerance, 94
Lamaze method, 108
Lamellar body count (LBC), 139
Languages
barriers and interpreters, 68
and cultural competence, 62

Lanugo
scoring newborn's external signs for, 353t
Large for gestational age (LGA), 351, 363, 367–370
Laser surgery
to cervix, 12
Last menstrual period (LMP)
normal length of, 130–131
Latching-on problems
anxiety, 324, 326
engorgement pain, 325
mastitis, 326
multiple births, 328
nipple confusion, 323
nipple pain, 324
physiologic jaundice, 327
plugged ducts, 326
in preterm infants, 328
preterm or hospitalized infant, 328
sleepy or reluctant infant, 327
Late accelerations
pattern of fetal heart rate (FHR), 264–266, 265f–266f
Late preterm infants
description and risks in newborns, 379–380
discharge criteria, 379
Latinos
childbearing cultural considerations, 64
Law
versus ethics, 674
ethics definition of, 669
Lead
exposure to, 172
Leg recoil
in newborn neurological assessment, 354b
Length
of SGA *versus* IUGR, 363–364
Leopold's maneuver, 209, 209f, 217, 635
Levator ani muscles, 8f
Levonorgestrel intrauterine system (LNG-IUS), 337t–339t
Libido
changes during pregnancy, 108
Lightening, 225
Limb defects
and toxin exposure, 165–166
Linea alba, 84
Linguistic competence
and cultural competence, 62
Lipid levels, 14
Listeriosis, 468t–471t
Liver
fetal development of, 43, 46–49
hyperbilirubinemia, 391–399, 394f
immaturity in preterm infants, 373
Liver enzyme tests
to test for hypertensive disorders, 438, 439t
to test for TORCH diseases, 454
Local anesthetics, 560
Lochia
assessing postpartum, 306
explaining normal, 653
stages of, 302

Loop electrosurgical excision procedure (LEEP)
to cervix, 12
Low prepregnancy weight
nutritional deficiency risks of, 86
Low-Phe diet, 530
Lungs
fetal development of,
physical examination of newborn's, 349
transient tachypnea of the newborn (TTN), 385–387
Lupus; *See* systemic lupus erythematosus (SLE)
Luteal phase
of menstrual cycles, 10
Luteinizing hormone (LH), 303
diagnostic tests, 15
within ovarian feedback loop, 11
Lyme disease, 468t–471t

M

Macrosomia, 513
Magnesium sulfate
for seizure prophylaxis, 441t–442t, 443
for tocolytic therapy, 441t–442t, 443
Magnetic resonance imaging
for trauma cases, 546
Malattachment behaviors, 310
Male/ female relationships
and intimate partner violence (IPV), 417
Male genitalia
characteristics of preterm infant, 374
physical exam/ scoring of newborn's, 350, 353t
Male sterilization, 337t–339t
Malignant ovarian tumors, 564
Malnutrition
as risk factor for preterm infants, 372
Mania, 659–662
March of Dimes
abuse danger assessment tool, 426, 426f
on preventing violence during pregnancy, 418f
Marginal insertion, 53
Marked sinus arrhythmias, 274, 275f
Marriage
childbearing cultural considerations, 64
Mastitis
infections, 655
and latching-on problems, 326
Maternal age
adolescent pregnancies, 117–121
clinical assessment procedures, 117
health education, 124
interventions/outcomes, 120
maternal mortality risks, 117
nutrition education, 117–121
prenatal care education, 117–121

Maternal age (Continued)
risk-taking and sexual behaviors of, 118–119
statistics, 117
advanced
assessment of, 121
assisted reproductive technology (ART), 121
fertility rates, 121–122
health education, 125
interventions and outcomes, 123
and multiple gestation, 635–637
and preterm labor, 624–629
risks of, 117, 121–124
statistics, 121
Maternal conditions; *See* preexisting conditions
Maternal dwarfism
affecting labor passage, 195
Maternal/ infant breastfeeding positions, 318–319
cradle-hold position, 318–319, 319f–320f
cross-cradle position, 318, 320, 320f–321f
ethnocultural "Quick Reference Guide," 76t
football-hold position, 318, 321, 322f
side-lying position, 318, 321, 322f
Maternal infections
acquired immunodeficiency syndrome (AIDS), 454–464, 455t–458t, 461f
assessment of, 462
causes and transmission of, 454–459, 455t–458t
characteristics of, 455t–458t
counseling and early diagnosis of, 460
ethnic, race and age statistics, 461f
human immunodeficiency virus (HIV), 459
statistics, 454–460, 459f–461f
chorioamnionitis, 472–473
group B streptococcus, 468t–471t
health education regarding, 454, 459–460, 463, 465, 472–473
influenza, 468t–471t
listeriosis, 468t–471t
Lyme disease, 468t–471t
measles, 468t–471t
mumps, 468t–471t
parvovirus B19, 468t–471t
sexually transmitted diseases (STDs), 455t–458t, 464–465
TORCH
cytomegalovirus (CMV), 449–454, 450t–453t
hepatitis B, 449–454, 450t–453t
herpes simplex virus (HSV), 449–454, 450t–453t
rubella, 449–454, 450t–453t
toxoplasmosis, 449–454, 450t–453t

Maternal infections *(Continued)*
  tuberculosis, 468t–471t
  urinary tract and pyelonephritis, 465–467
  varicella zoster, 468t–471t
Maternal morbidity
  and mortality rates for hemorrhagic disorders, 478
  risks with anesthesia, 557
  trauma leading to, 535–540
Maternal phenylketonuria, 528–529
  assessment of, 529
  definition and incidence of, 528
  effects on pregnancy and fetus, 529
  health education, 531
  interventions and outcomes, 530
  management of, 528
  nutritional planning, 530
Maternal serum alpha-fetoprotein (AFP)
  for Down syndrome screening, 28
Maternal serum alpha-fetoprotein (MS-AFP), 55
  to evaluate fetal status with diabetes, 504
Maternal trauma algorithm, 541f
Mature milk, 317
Measles, 468t–471t
Meconium aspiration syndrome
  description and risks in newborns, 387–389
Meconium passage, 370
Medications
  during breastfeeding, 330
  as environmental hazard, 177–178
    FDA pregnancy risk categories, 177
    fetal pharmacology drugs, 178
    iPledge risk management, 178
    prescriptions, 178
Megaloblastic anemia, 609–614
Meiosis
  process of, 21, 22f
Melasma, 84
Menarche
  minimum height and weight issues, 9
Mendelian inheritance, 24, 30t
Meningocele
  with spina bifida, 399
Menopause
  average age of, 10
  and toxin exposure, 166–177
Menses
  cessation of, 10
  during menstrual cycle, 10
Menstrual ages
  per crown-rump length, 130b
Menstrual cramps
  taking histories regarding, 12
Menstrual cycle
  amenorrhea, 10
  anovulatory cycles, 11
  description of, 9
  phases of
    follicular phase, 10
    luteal phase, 10
  return during postpartum period, 302
  taking histories regarding, 12

Menstruation, 12
Mental retardation
  due to substance abuse, 580
Mercury
  exposure to, 172
Mesenchyme, 39, 40f
Metabolic acidemia ranges, 285, 285t
Metabolic acidosis
  monitoring with renal conditions, 597
  and persistent pulmonary hypertension of newborn (PPHN), 389–390
Metabolic disorders
  causing respiratory distress in newborns, 380–390
Metabolism
  affecting thyroid gland, 515–516
  maternal changes with pregnancy, 501
Microphthalmia
  development during embryonic stage, 41
Microsurgical epididymal sperm aspiration (MESA), 122
Milk; *See also* human milk
  needs for pregnant mothers, 86
Milk duct
  anatomical illustration of, 316f
Mitosis
  process of, 20, 21f
Modes of inheritance
  autosomal dominant inheritance, 24, 24f
  autosomal recessive inheritance, 25, 25f
  complex disorders, 27
  polygenic or multifactorial disorders, 27
  sex-linked dominant inheritance, 26
  sex-linked recessive inheritance, 26, 26f
  single/ paired genes, 24
Modified biophysical profile, 148–149
Molimina, 13
Mongolian spots, 349
Monosomy, 23
Monozygotic twins, 136, 637
Mons pubis
  anatomical description and illustration of, 3, 4f
Montevideo units, 195, 271
Mood disorders
  in abused women, 420, 424–425
  in children witnessing domestic violence, 421
  interventions, 310
  postpartum, 106, 308, 310, 659–662
    baby blues, 659–662
    depression, 659–662
    health education, 661–662
    psychosis, 659–662
    treatment of, 661
  in substance abusers, 576
Mood swings
  in abused women, 420, 424

Mood swings *(Continued)*
  postpartum, 660
  during pregnancy, 102
Moral agents
  ethics definition of, 669
Morality
  ethics definition of, 669
Morals
  ethics definition of, 669
Moratorium phase, 104
Moro (startle) reflex
  examining in newborns, 350, 350t
Mortality rates
  with preexisting cardiac disease, 588–594
  risks associated with pregnancy, 589b
  risks in pregnant adolescents, 117
Morula, 36, 36f–37f
Motor nerves
  supporting female reproductive organs, 9
Motor vehicle collisions, 535, 539
Mouth
  changes during pregnancy, 83
  fetal development of, 43, 46–49
  physical examination of newborn's, 349
Multifactorial disorders, 27, 29
Multiparity
  associated with breech presentation, 203
Multiple gestations, 635–637; *See also* twins
  antepartum interventions, 636
  and assisted reproductive technology (ART), 635
  health education regarding, 637
  as high-risk pregnancy/ fetal condition, 129
  indications of, 635–637
  intrapartum interventions, 636
  and latching-on problems, 328
  nutritional deficiency risks of, 86
  postpartum interventions, 637
  and preterm labor, 624–629
  and small for gestational age (SGA) newborns, 363–364
  statistics and increases in, 635
  testing during antepartum fetal assessment, 136
  twin-twin transfusion syndrome, 569
Mumps, 468t–471t
Muscles
  changes during pregnancy, 83
  indicating mother's nutritional status, 92, 93t
Musculoskeletal system
  changes during postpartum period, 304
    abdominal muscles, 304
    joints, 304
  changes during pregnancy, 83
  deformities
    affecting labor passage, 195
  fetal development of, 43, 46–49
Mutagens, 163

Mutation
    definition of, 20
Myelomeningocele
    development during embryonic
        stage, 41
    intrauterine fetal surgery, 569
    with spina bifida, 399
Myeloschisis, 400
Myometrium
    physiology of during
        contractions, 192, 193f

N

Nagele's rule, 92
Nails
    formation of, 47–48, 50
Naloxone hydrochloride
    for neonatal resuscitation, 356t
Nanoparticles
    as occupational environmental
        hazard, 169
National Domestic Violence Hot
    Line, 427
Native Americans
    childbearing cultural
        considerations, 65
    ethnocultural "Quick Reference
        Guide," 75t–79t
    higher rate of hyperbilirubinemia
        in, 394
    HIV/AIDS statistics among, 461,
        461f
    intimate partner violence among,
        421
Natural family planning, 337t–339t
Neck
    assessing maternal trauma to,
        544
    physical examination of
        newborn's, 349
Necrotizing enterocolitis (NEC),
    373
Neonatal deaths
    and toxin exposure, 166–177
Neonatal hypoxia
    and maternal asthma, 599
Neonatal lupus erythematosus
    (NLE), 604
Neonatal substance-withdrawal
    syndrome, 380–390
Neonates; See newborns
Nervous system
    fetal development of,
Neural crest, 39
Neural thermal environment
    (NTE), 346
Neural tube
    development process, 39–40, 41f
Neural tube defects
    description and risks in
        newborns, 399–400
    in fetus
        and Downs syndrome, 28
        risk factors, 29
    intrauterine fetal surgery, 569
    and nutrition, 88
Neurological system
    fetal development of, 43, 46–49
    physical examination of
        newborn's, 350

Neurological system (Continued)
    techniques to assess newborn's,
        354b
Neurulation, 39
Newborns
    breastfeeding of (See
        breastfeeding)
    complete assessment of
        Apgar scores, 348, 348t
        behavioral state system, 350
        in delivery room, 352
        gestational age classifications,
            351
        glucose screening, 357
        growth parameters, 348
        infection prevention, 357
        neurological system
            techniques, 354b
        physical exam, 348–349
        resuscitation steps and
            summary, 355f
        scoring system of external
            physical characteristics,
            353t
        sensory capabilities, 351
        vital signs, 348
    complications due to substance
        abuse, 577, 578b, 580
    diseases/congenital anomalies
        abdominal wall defects,
            401–402
        acyanotic defects, 403–407
        atrial septal defects (ASDs),
            404
        cleft lip/palate, 400
        coarctation of the aorta, 405
        congenital cardiac lesions,
            403–408
        congenital diaphragmatic
            hernia (CDH), 402–403
        cyanotic defects, 405–407
        gastrointestinal system,
            400–403
        hydrocephalus, 399
        hyperbilirubinemia, 391–399,
            394f
        hypoplastic left heart
            syndrome, 406–408
        large for gestational age (LGA),
            363, 367–370
        late preterm infants, 379–380
        meconium aspiration
            syndrome, 387–389
        neural tube defects, 399–400
        patent ductus arteriosus,
            403–404
        persistent pulmonary
            hypertension of newborn
            (PPHN), 389–390
        postterm infants, 370–372
        preterm infants, 372–380
        respiratory distress, 380–390
        respiratory distress syndrome,
            380–390
        small for gestational age
            (SGA), 363–366
        spina bifida, 399
        tetralogy of Fallot (TOF),
            405–406
        transient tachypnea, 385–387

Newborns (Continued)
    transposition of the great
        arteries (TGA), 406
    ventricular septal defects
        (VSDs), 404–405
    ethnocultural considerations for
        care of, 62, 67, 78t
    infants at risk, 362
    latching-on problems (See
        latching-on problems)
    as passengers (See passenger
        [infant])
    physical signs of maternal
        alcohol abuse, 580–581
    positioning for breastfeeding
        cradle-hold position, 318–319,
            319f–320f
        cross-cradle position, 318, 320,
            320f–321f
        football-hold position, 318,
            321, 322f
        side-lying position, 318, 321, 322f
    presentations
        breech presentation, 202, 204f
        cardinal movements, 208
        cephalic presentation, 202, 203f
        compound presentation, 204
        diagnostic studies of, 209, 209f,
            217
        fetal attitude, 202
        fetal lie, 202
        fetal position, 205, 205f
        fetal size, 207
        fetal skull, 207
        fetal station, 205, 205f (See also
            fetal station)
        Leopold's maneuver, 209, 209f,
            217
        transverse presentation, 204,
            205f
        ultrasonography, 210
        vaginal examination, 210, 210f
    sleepy or reluctant
        and latching-on problems, 327
    transition from fetus to, 345, 352,
        362
        cardiovascular system
            adaptation, 346
        feeding, 346
        gastrointestinal system
            adaptation, 346
        respiratory system adaptation,
            345
        thermoregulation, 346
    transitional care of, 345
Nicotine, 55, 86
Nifedipine, 441t–442t, 627
Night terrors
    in abused women, 420, 424
Nipple confusion
    and latching-on problems, 323
Nipple formation
    scoring newborn's, 353t
Nipple pain
    and latching-on problems, 324
Nipple Stimulation (NST) test, 129
Nipples
    anatomical illustration of, 316f
    assessing postpartum, 305
    changes in during pregnancy, 84

Nipples *(Continued)*
  changes in postpartum period, 302
  characteristics of preterm infant, 374
  inspecting breasts and, 318
  latching-on problems, 323
Noise, 175
Nonelectronic FHR assessment, 249
Nonmaleficence
  defining in ethics, 670, 677–679
Non-normative ethics, 670
Nonobstetric surgery, 556–557
Nonstress tests (NST)
  during antepartum fetal assessment, 142–144
  to evaluate fetal status with diabetes, 504
  and placenta previa, 483
Normal childbirth; *See* childbirth
Normal gestation
  defining, 630
Nose
  physical examination of newborn's, 349
Notochordal process, 39
Nuchal translucency, 29
Nuclear cataracts
  development during embryonic stage, 41
Nursing
  and ethics, 669
Nutrition
  adolescent, 118
  during breastfeeding, 330
  education for pregnant adolescents, 117–121
  ethnocultural considerations regarding, 62, 64
  ethnocultural "Quick Reference Guide," 75t, 77t
  during fetal development process, 57
  health education regarding fetal health and, 57
  and hypertensive disorders, 446
  interventions in preterm infants, 376
  low-Phe diet, 530
  newborn, 358
  physical assessment of mother's status, 92, 93t
  during placental transfer, 46
  during pregnancy, 85–86
  and preterm labor, 624–629
  problems in postterm infants, 371
  in substance abusers, 576
  taking maternal histories concerning, 89
  and twins, 637

O

Obesity
  adolescent, 118
  as preeclampsia risk, 433
  pregnancy recommendations for maternal, 86
Obstetric capacity
  of pelvis, 197
Obstetric conjugate, 197, 197f
Obstetric hemorrhages, 478

Obstructive uropathy, 569
Occupational environmental hazards
  chemical agents, 167
    antineoplastic drugs, 167
    colorants, 168
    ethylene oxide, 168
    nanoparticles, 169
    organic solvents, 169
    pesticides, 170
    phthalates, 171
    polychlorinated biphenyls (PCBs), 171
    toxic (heavy) metals, 171
    waste anesthetic gases, 173
  ergonomic hazards, 174
    ionizing radiation, 174
    noise, 175
    physical tasks, 174
    second hand smoke, 176
    temperature extremes, 176
  statistics, 167
Ogita, 482
Older mothers; *See* advanced maternal age
Oligohydramnios, 54, 146
Oocyte, 35, 36f
  donor, 122
  in vitro fertilization (IVF), 122
Oogenesis, 22
Oophorectomy, 564
Open laparotomy
  versus laparoscopic, 560
Opthalmic system
  changes with preeclampsia, 434, 435f
Optic nerves
  fetal development of, 43, 46–49
Oral cavity
  indicating mother's nutritional status, 92, 93t
Oral contraceptives
  types of, 337t–339t
Oral glucose tolerance test (OGTT)
  gestational diabetes mellitus (GDM), 511, 511t, 515
Organ system
  developmental problems, 372
  fetal development of, 43, 46–49
Organic solvents
  as occupational environmental hazard, 169
Organized newborns, 351
Ova
  fertility span, 35
  and meiosis, 21, 22f
  during menstrual cycle, 10
  and twins, 637
Ovarian cystectomy, 564
Ovarian tumors, 564
Ovaries
  anatomical description and illustration of, 5f, 7
  changes during pregnancy, 90
  and hormone changes during pregnancy, 84
Overweight women
  pregnancy recommendations for, 86

Oviducts; *See* fallopian tubes
Ovulation
  estrogen levels during, 35
  during menstrual cycle, 10
Ovum membrane, 35
Oxytocin
  during antepartum fetal assessment, 154–155
  and oxytocin-induced tachysystole, 288
  role in milk production, 316, 316f

P

Pacifiers, 347
Pain
  from episiotomy, hemorrhoids or cesarean section, 307
  ethnocultural considerations regarding, 62, 63f, 65
  ethnocultural "Quick Reference Guide," 76t
  and latching-on problems, 324
  management
    during normal childbirth, 230
  nipple and breast, 317
Palliative care
  ethical issues with, 678, 680
Palmar grasps
  examining newborn, 350, 350t
Pancreas
  changes during pregnancy, 84
Papanicolaou tests, 95
Parasympathetic nervous system
  influencing fetal heart rate (FHR), 252
Parathyroid gland
  changes during pregnancy, 84
Parenting
  attachment factors and behaviors, 309–310
  education, 111
Partial thromboplastin time (PTT)
  to test for hypertensive disorders, 438, 439t
  in trauma cases, 545
Parvovirus B19, 468t–471t
Passage
  defining in labor 4 P's, 191
Passenger
  defining in labor 4 P's, 191
Passenger (infant)
  during labor
    breech presentation, 202, 204f
    cardinal movements, 208
    cephalic presentation, 202, 203f
    compound presentation, 204
    diagnostic studies of, 209, 209f, 217
    fetal attitude, 202
    fetal lie, 202
    fetal position, 205, 205f
    fetal size, 207
    fetal skull, 207
    fetal station, 205, 205f (*See also* fetal station)
    Leopold's maneuver, 209, 209f, 217
    transverse presentation, 204, 205f
    ultrasonography, 210
    vaginal examination, 210, 210f

Patent ductus arteriosus (PDA)
    description and risks in
        newborns, 403–404
    indications in preterm infants,
        375
    causing respiratory distress in
        newborns, 380–381
Paternalism-maternalism-
    parentalism ethical concept,
    672
Patient education
    concerning infants at risk,
        407–408
    on newborn care, 357–358
Patient Self-Determination Act, 679
Patient's rights, 679
Pedal ablation, 41
Pelvic abnormality
    associated with breech
        presentation, 203
Pelvic capacity
    manual determination of, 201
Pelvic cavity planes, 198, 198f
Pelvic diaphragm, 8f
Pelvic floor
    muscles of, 7, 8f
    supporting female reproductive
        organs, 7, 8f
Pelvic inflammatory disease (PID)
    fertility problems due to, 122
Pelvic shapes, 196, 196f
    android pelvis, 196f, 197
    anthropoid pelvis, 196f, 197
    and dimensions, 197, 197f–198f
    gynecoid pelvis, 196f, 197
    platypelloid pelvis, 196f, 197
Pelvic tilt
    during labor, 219, 219f
Pelvis
    dimensions, 197, 197f–198f
    infections, 12
    trauma
        affecting labor passage, 196
        maternal, 536, 538f, 544
Penetrating trauma, 535
Percutaneous umbilical blood
    sampling (PUBS)
    description and illustration of,
        140, 140f
Perimenopause, 10
Perinatal asphyxia
    in postterm infants, 370
Perinatal mortality
    and maternal asthma, 599
    stillbirth, 638–640
Perineum
    anatomical description and
        illustration of, 4, 4f
    assessing postpartum, 306
    changes during postpartum
        period, 302
    muscles of, 7, 8f
    supporting female reproductive
        organs, 7, 8f
Peripheral smear
    affected by preeclampsia and
        HELLP, 439t
Peritonitis, 565
Periventricular intraventricular
    hemorrhage (PIVH), 373

Persistent pulmonary hypertension
    of newborn (PPHN), 389–391
Personality styles
    and labor, 215
Pesticides
    as occupational environmental
        hazard, 170
Pet abuse, 422f, 424
PH balance
    changes during pregnancy, 82
    metabolic acidemia ranges, 285,
        285t
    normal values, 285t
    postpartum changes in, 304
Pharmaceuticals
    defining, 177
    as environmental hazard,
        177–178
        FDA pregnancy risk
            categories, 177
        fetal pharmacology drugs, 178
        iPledge risk management, 178
        prescriptions, 178
Phenotypes
    definition of, 20
Phosphatidylglycerol (PG), 139
Phthalates
    as occupational environmental
        hazard, 171
Physical abuse
    behaviors common in, 418f, 419
    injuries commonly seen with,
        419–420
    possible causes of, 422, 422f
Physical activity
    ethnocultural considerations
        regarding, 62, 64
    ethnocultural "Quick Reference
        Guide," 75t, 77t–78t
Physical examinations
    of female reproductive system,
        13
    of newborns, 348–349
    during pregnancy, 92
Physical tasks
    as ergonomic hazard, 174
Physical violence; See intimate
    partner violence (IPV)
Physiologic jaundice
    and hyperbilirubinemia, 391–399
    and latching-on problems, 327
Pica, 65, 87, 94
Pinocytosis
    in placental transfer, 45, 45t
Pituitary gland
    changes during pregnancy, 84
Pituitary hormones
    changes during postpartum
        period, 303
    follicle-stimulating hormone
        (FSH), 303
    luteinizing hormone (LH), 303
    serum prolactin, 303
Placenta; See also abruptio
    placentae; placenta previa
    abnormalities in fetal
        development process, 50, 52t
    description of, 37
    development process, 38
        abnormalities, 50

Placenta (Continued)
    growth periods, 43, 44f
        placenta circulation, 44, 44f
    evaluating for abnormalities, 138
    functions, 45, 630–632
        excretion, 46
        hormonal production, 46
        nutrition, 46
        protection, 46
        respiration, 45
        storage, 46
    grading with ultrasonography,
        135
    and maternal blood flow, 44, 44f
    placental transfer, 44, 45t
    during pre-embryonic stage,
        36, 36f
    process of, 36f, 37–38
Placenta previa, 45, 478–479
    assessment of, 479–485
    associated with breech
        presentation, 203
    classifications of, 479
    complications associated with,
        480–481
    definition of, 478
    fetal oxygenation and FHR,
        480–481, 483
    health education, 484
    interventions and outcomes, 482
    and maternal drug/ alchohol
        abuse, 573
    risk factors, 479
    signs indicating, 479–485
    and small for gestational age
        (SGA) newborns, 363
Placental degeneration
    in postterm infants, 370
Placental expulsion
    stage of childbirth, 235–237, 236f
Placental grading level
    testing during antepartum fetal
        assessment, 135, 136f
Placental hormones
    changes during postpartum
        period, 303
    human chorionic gonadotropin
        (HCG), 303
    human chorionic
        somatomammotropin
        (HCS), 303
    plasma estrogen, 303
    plasma progesterone, 303
Placental infarcts, 45
Placental insufficiency
    and intrauterine growth
        restriction (IUGR), 363
    in postterm infants, 370
Placental membrane
    defects in, 44, 45t
Placental migration, 136
Placental perfusion
    with preeclampsia, 433, 435f
Placental positions
    testing during antepartum fetal
        assessment, 136
Placental transfer
    description of, 44
    disorders, 45
    functions of, 45, 45t

Placental transfer (*Continued*)
 and maternal blood flow, 44, 44f
 problems associated with impaired, 55
 products transferred, 44, 45t
Plantar creases
 scoring newborn's, 353t
Plantar grasps
 examining newborn, 350, 350t
Plasma estrogen, 303
Plasma progesterone, 303
Platypelloid pelvis, 196f, 197
Plugged ducts
 and latching-on problems, 326
Pneumatic antishock garments, 549, 549f
Pneumonia
 with meconium aspiration syndrome, 387–389
 causing respiratory distress in newborns, 380–381
Pneumonitis, 387–389
Poisoning, 539
Polychlorinated biphenyls (PCBs), 171
Polycythemia
 in fetus related to maternal diabetes, 505
 causing respiratory distress in newborns, 380–381
Polydrug use, 573
Polyhydramnios
 and maternal drug/alchohol abuse, 573
Polymorphism
 definition of, 20
Popliteal angle
 in newborn neurological assessment, 354b
Positions; *See also* presentations
 maternal during labor passage, 199
  sitting, 200
  squatting, 199
  standing, 200
 maternal/infant breastfeeding, 318–319
  cradle-hold position, 318–319, 319f–320f
  cross-cradle position, 318, 320, 320f–321f
  football-hold position, 318, 321, 322f
Posterior sagittal diameters, 198, 198f
Postmaturity
 defining, 630
Postpartum depression (PPD), 64, 308, 659–662
Postpartum febrile morbidity
 definition of, 653–654
Postpartum mood disorders, 106, 111, 659–662
 baby blues, 659–662
 depression, 659–662
 health education, 661–662
 psychosis, 659–662
 treatment of, 661

Postpartum period
 cardiovascular system changes, 303
  blood volume, 303
  heart, 303
 complications, 650
  infections, 653–656
  mood disorders, 659–662
  postpartum hemorrhages, 650–653
  venous disorders, 656–659
 endocrine system changes, 303
  pituitary hormones, 303
  placental hormones, 303
 ethnocultural considerations during, 62, 66, 77t
 gastrointestinal system changes, 304
  assessment of, 306
  bowels/ elimination complications, 304, 307
  weight loss, 304
 health education, 307–311
 hematologic system changes, 303
  hematocrit and hemoglobin, 303
  white blood cell count, 303
 hemorrhages, 650–651
  causes of, 650
  classification of, 650
  health education, 653
  interventions, 652–653
  risk factors, 651
  signs and symptoms of, 651
 hypertensive disorders in, 444
 immune system changes, 304
 infections, 653–654
  breast/ mastitis infections, 655
  cesarean section infections, 655
  definition of, 653
  genital tract infections, 654
  risk factors, 654
  treatment of, 655–656
  types of, 654
  urinary tract infections, 655
 integumentary system changes, 304
  diaphoresis, 304
  hyperpigmentation disappears, 304
 interventions with multiple gestation, 637
 musculoskeletal system changes, 304
  abdominal muscles, 304
  joints, 304
 psychological changes, 304, 308–311; (*See also* postpartum mood disorders)
  attachement, 305, 309–310
  baby blues, 305, 308
  developmental stages, 305
  mood changes, 106, 310, 659–660
  role changes, 304
 reproductive system physical changes, 301
  assessment of, 305
  breasts, 302
  cervix, 302

Postpartum period (*Continued*)
  menstrual cycle return, 302
  perineum, 302
  uterus, 301
  vagina, 302
 respiratory system changes, 304
  acid-base balance, 304
  basal metabolic rate, 304
  pulmonary function, 304
 urinary system changes
  edema, 304
  kidney function, 304
  urinary retention, 306
 venous thromboembolic disorders, 656–659
  description and types of, 656–659
  prevention of, 658
  risk factors, 657
  signs of, 657
  treatment of, 658
 vital signs, 303
  blood pressure, 303
  pulse rate, 304
  temperature, 303
Postterm infants
 description and risks in newborns, 370–372
 problems associated with, 370–371
Postterm pregnancy, 630–632
 defining, 630
Posttraumatic stress disorders
 in children witnessing domestic violence, 421
Postures
 during labor passage, 199
 maternal during labor passage
  horizontal, 199
  kneeling, 200
  upright, 199
  walking and changing positions, 199
 newborn
  neurological assessment of, 354b
  physical examination of, 350
Poverty
 and domestic violence, 420
 pregnancy nutritional deficiency risks of, 86
 as risk factor for preterm infants, 372
Power
 defining in labor 4 P's, 191
Power and control wheel
 and intimate partner violence (IPV), 422f
Preeclampsia, 432–433
 assessment of, 436, 439t
 etiology of, 433
 HELLP syndrome, 434, 435f, 439t
 as high-risk pregnancy/ fetal condition, 129
 lab tests, 438, 439t
 mild, 438, 445
 monitoring with renal conditions, 597
 pathophysiology stages, 433, 435f

Preeclampsia (Continued)
pharmacology therapy, 440,
441t–442t
physiologic alterations with, 434
predicting and preventing, 436
risk factors, 433
severe, 440
and small for gestational age
(SGA) newborns, 363
treatment of, 438–445, 441t–442t
Pre-embryonic stage
in fetal development process,
36, 36f
toxin exposure during, 165
Preexisting conditions
antiphospholipid antibody
syndrome (APS), 604
assessment of, 605
cardiovascular system diseases
classification of, 590t
complications with, 588–594
drugs used during pregnancy,
593t
interventions, 591
mortality risks, 589b
patient education, 594
signs and symptoms common
to, 590, 591t
gastrointestinal system disorders
assessment of, 615
complications with, 614–616
hyperemesis gravidarum,
614
inflammatory bowel disease,
614
interventions and outcomes,
616
hematolic disorders, 608–610
anemias, 608
assessment of, 610
fetal implications, 610
interventions and outcomes,
612
patient education, 614
hepatic system disorders
complications with, 617–619,
618t
hepatitis A, B, and C, 617–619,
618t
patient education, 619–620
signs and symptoms of, 619
treatment of, 619
viral hepatitis, 617–619
renal system diseases
adverse consequences, 595
assessment of, 596
chronic renal disease, 595
complications with, 594–596
interventions, 597
kidney changes during
pregnancy, 594
new onset of, 595
preconceptual counseling and
education, 598
respiratory system diseases
assessment of, 600
asthma, 599, 602–603, 603b
complications with, 598–600
interventions and outcomes,
601

Preexisting conditions (Continued)
patient education, 602–603
tuberculosis, 599, 602t, 603
systemic lupus erythematosus
(SLE)
assessment of, 605
description of, 603–605
symptoms of, 605
Pregenesis, 35
Pregestational diabetes mellitus,
502–509
Pregnancy
changes in maternal physiology
during, 80–88
clinical practice guidelines, 88–96
maternal history-taking, 88
physical examination, 92
prenatal health assessment, 88
complications
due to substance abuse, 577,
578b
diagnostic procedures, 94
blood tests, 94
cervical smears, 95
fundal height, 95f
laboratory tests, 96
pregnancy tests, 94
urinalysis tests, 95
endocrine and metabolic
disorders in, 500
environmental hazards, 163
ethnocultural considerations
in, 61
expected confinement date
(ECD) calculation, 92
expected date of birth (EDB)
calculation, 92
expected delivery date (EDD)
calculation, 92
fetal development weekly stages
week 1, 36–37
week 2, 37–38, 37f, 41f
week 3, 39, 40f
week 4, 40, 41f–42f
week 5, 41, 42f
week 6, 41, 42f
week 7, 41, 42f
week 8, 42f, 43
week 9 to 12, 46
week 13 to 16, 47
week 17 to 20, 47
week 21 to 24, 48
week 25 to 29, 48
week 30 to 34, 49
week 35 to 38, 49
week 39 to 40, 49
postterm, 49
health education, 96–98
health education regarding,
96–98
and intimate partner violence
(IPV), 417
maternal cardiovascular system
changes during
arterial blood pressure, 82
blood volume, 82
cardiac output, 82
heart, 81
heart rate, 81
in hemodynamic system, 81

Pregnancy (Continued)
stroke volume, 82
vasodilation, 82
venous pressure, 82
maternal endocrine system
changes during
in ovaries and hormones,
84
in pancreas, 84
in pituitary gland, 84
in thyroid gland, 84
maternal gastrointestinal system
changes during
in gallbladder, 83
in gastrointestinal tract, 83
mouth, saliva and gums,
83
maternal hematologic system
changes during
clotting factor, 82
red blood cells, 82
white blood cells, 82
maternal immune system
changes during
in ovaries and hormones, 84
maternal infections during
acquired immunodeficiency
syndrome (AIDS),
454–461, 455t–458t, 461f
chorioamnionitis, 472–473
cytomegalovirus (CMV),
449–454, 450t–453t
group B streptococcus,
468t–471t
health education regarding,
454, 459–460, 463, 465,
472–473
hepatitis B, 449–454,
450t–453t
herpes simplex virus (HSV),
449–454, 450t–453t
influenza, 468t–471t
listeriosis, 468t–471t
Lyme disease, 468t–471t
measles, 468t–471t
mumps, 468t–471t
parvovirus B19, 468t–471t
rubella, 449–454, 450t–453t
sexually transmitted diseases
(STDs), 455t–458t,
464–465
toxoplasmosis, 449–454,
450t–453t
tuberculosis, 468t–471t
urinary tract and
pyelonephritis, 465–467
varicella zoster, 468t–471t
maternal integumentary system
changes during, 84
maternal musculoskeletal system
changes during, 83
maternal reproductive system
changes during
breasts, 81
cervix, 81
fallopian tubes, 81
ovaries, 81
uterus, 80
vagina, 81
vulva, 81

Pregnancy *(Continued)*
  maternal respiratory system
    changes during
    carbon dioxide, 82
    tidal volume, 82
  maternal urinary system changes
    during
    renal and kidney function, 83
  maternal-fetal well-being
    age-related concerns, 117
    antepartum fetal assessment,
      128
  normal cardiac changes *versus*
    cardiac disease, 591t
  nutritional considerations, 85, 91f
    body mass index, 85
    for fetal health, 88
    MyPyramid nutritional chart,
      91f
    special needs during, 86
    weight gain, 85
  physical examinations, 92
  physiology of, 80
  psychology of, 101
    adoption grief, 107, 111
    anorexia nervosa, 106, 111
    assessment of, 101
    bulimia nervosa, 106, 111
    childbirth preparation classes,
      107, 111
    coping strategies, 108, 110–111
    as developmental
      (maturational) crisis, 102
    developmental tasks, 102
    Duvall's stages, 102
    ethnocultural considerations,
      105
    expectant father's issues, 104
    expectant siblings and
      grandparents, 105
    fears, 102, 110
    grief and loss issues, 107, 111
    importance of health
      education, 112
    intercourse contraindications,
      109
    interventions and outcomes,
      108
    libido changes, 108
    mood swings, 102
    overview of, 101
    postpartum mood disorders,
      101, 106, 111
    preterm or ill child grief, 107,
      111
    psychosocial findings, 102
    reactions to news of, 102
    Rubin's tasks, 103
    self-esteem, 108
    single expectant mothers, 105
    spontaneous abortion, 107, 111
    stress, 109
    thoughts and desires, 102
  signs and symptoms indicating,
    85
Pregnancy tests, 94
Preimplantation loss
  and toxin exposure, 166–177
Premature atrial contractions
  (PACs), 274, 275f–277f

Premature labor and delivery
  and maternal drug/ alchohol
    abuse, 573
Premature rupture of membranes
  (PROM)
  description and possible causes
    of, 632–635, 637
  and maternal drug/ alchohol
    abuse, 573
  and preterm labor, 624–629
Premature ventricular contractions
  (PVCs), 278, 279f–281f
Prematurity; *See also* preterm
  infants
  associated with breech
    presentation, 203
  integumentary system skin
    problems, 374, 377
  organ immaturity, 372
  related to adrenal disorders, 524
  related to maternal diabetes,
    505
Prenatal care education
  for pregnant adolescents,
    117–121
Prepuce of clitoris, 3, 4f
Prescriptions
  assessing maternal, 55
Presentations
  breech presentation, 202, 204f
  cephalic presentation, 202, 203f
  compound presentation, 204
  fetal, 137
  fetal attitude, 202
  fetal lie, 202
  of multiple gestations, 637
  testing during antepartum fetal
    assessment, 137
  transverse presentation, 204,
    205f
Preterm infants
  body temperature issues with,
    373
  description and risks for, 372–380
  developmental problems
    cardiovascular system, 372,
      375–376
    immune system, 373, 376
    organ system, 372, 376
    renal system, 373, 376–378
    respiratory system, 372,
      375–376
  health education, 379–380
  hypocalcemia in, 374
  hypoglycemia in, 374, 376
  interventions and outcomes,
    376, 378
  latching-on problems, 328
  and maternal asthma, 599
  maternal grief concerning, 107,
    111
  necrotizing enterocolitis (NEC),
    373, 376
  periventricular intraventricular
    hemorrhage (PIVH) in, 373
  physical characteristics of, 374
  with renal disease, 595
  risk screening for, 625
  and toxin exposure, 166–177
  weight issues with, 373, 376

Preterm labor, 624–630
  definition of, 624
  factors associated with, 624–625
  health education, 629–630
  indications of, 625
  interventions, 626
  risk factors for, 625
  tocolytic drug therapy, 627
Principle-based ethics, 670, 677–679
Privacy
  defining in ethics, 670, 677–679
Progesterone
  changes during pregnancy, 84
  and lobular formation, 315, 316f
  within ovarian feedback loop, 11
  testing levels of, 15
Progesterone implants, 337t–339t
Prolactin, 15, 315, 316f
Prolonged decelerations
  pattern of fetal heart rate (FHR),
    268–269, 270f
Protein metabolism
  interventions and outcomes, 507
  maternal changes with
    pregnancy, 501
Proteinuria, 83, 595
Prothrombin time (PT)
  to diagnose placenta previa, 482,
    487, 490
  to test for hypertensive
    disorders, 438, 439t
  in trauma cases, 545
Proxy decision-makers, 673
Psyche stage
  defining in labor 4 P's, 191
  of labor
    anxiety, 214, 217
    coping abilities, 215, 218
    cultural considerations, 211
    expectations and preparations,
      211–212
    fatigue and weariness, 215
    fear, 214, 217
    interventions, 217
    maternal history and
      experience, 211
    personality styles, 215
    psychological reactions to,
      214, 217
    psychosocial responses, 213
    support system, 212
Psychological abuse; *See* intimate
  partner violence (IPV)
  behaviors constituting, 418f, 419
  injuries commonly seen with,
    420
  possible causes of, 422, 422f
Psychological disorders
  postpartum, 659–662
    baby blues, 659–662
    depression, 659–662
    health education, 661–662
    psychosis, 659–662
    treatment of, 661
Psychology
  issues during postpartum
    period, 304, 308–311
    attachment, 305, 309–310
    baby blues, 305, 308
    developmental stages, 305

Psychology (Continued)
  mood changes, 106, 310
  role changes, 304
  issues with pregnancy, 101
    adoption grief, 107, 111
    anorexia nervosa, 106, 111
    assessment of, 101
    bulimia nervosa, 106, 111
    childbirth preparation classes,
      107, 111
    coping strategies, 108, 110–111
    as developmental
      (maturational) crisis, 102
    developmental tasks, 102
    Duvall's stages, 102
    ethnocultural considerations,
      105
    expectant father's issues, 104
    expectant siblings and
      grandparents, 105
    fears, 102, 110
    grief and loss issues, 107, 111
    importance of health
      education, 112
    intercourse contraindications,
      109
    interventions and outcomes,
      108
    libido changes, 108
    mood swings, 102
    overview of, 101
    preterm or ill child grief, 107,
      111
    psychosocial findings, 102
    Rubin's tasks, 103
    self-esteem, 108
    single expectant mothers, 105
    spontaneous abortion, 107,
      111
    stress, 109
    thoughts and desires, 102
Psychosis
  postpartum, 659–662
Psychosocial responses
  regarding labor, 213
Puberty
  characteristics associated with,
    12
Pubic bone
  description and illustration in
    bony pelvis, 8f, 9
Pulmonary diseases
  complications with pregnancy,
    598–600
  as high-risk pregnancy/ fetal
    condition, 129
Pulmonary edema
  as preexisting maternal
    condition, 588–594
Pulmonary hypertension,
  588–594
Pulmonary stenosis
  development during embryonic
    stage, 43
Pulmonary system
  status and hypertension, 436
Pulse rate
  following trauma, 548
  monitoring during surgery, 557
  postpartum changes in, 304

Purification rituals
  ethnocultural "Quick Reference
    Guide," 77t
Pyelonephritis, 465–467

Q

Quality of life
  ethics definition of, 669
  versus sanctity of life, 670

R

Radiation
  exposure to, 174
Radioactive iodine, 515–516, 521
Radioimmunoassay (RIA), 94
Radiology
  for trauma cases, 546
Rapid compression forces, 535
Rectal atresia
  development during embryonic
    stage, 42
Rectocele, 13
Rectum
  fetal development of, 43, 46–49,
    51f
Red blood cells (RBCs)
  changes during pregnancy, 82
  testing placenta previa, 482, 487,
    490
Reflex late deceleration, 265
Reflexes
  physical examination of
    newborn's, 350, 350t
Regional anesthesia, 560
Relaxin, 84
Religion
  ethnocultural considerations
    regarding, 63
Renal insufficiency, 597
Renal system
  changes during pregnancy, 83
  changes with preeclampsia, 434,
    435f
  developmental problems
    in preterm infants, 373,
      377–378
  infections during pregnancy,
    465–467
  normal adaptations to
    pregnancy, 433
  preexisting maternal disorders
    adverse consequences, 595
    assessment of, 596
    chronic renal disease, 595
    complications with, 594–596
    interventions, 597
    kidney changes during
      pregnancy, 594
    new onset of, 595
    preconceptual counseling and
      education, 598
    status and hypertension, 436
Reproductive choices/ freedom, 679
Reproductive risks
  definition of environmental
    hazard, 181
Reproductive system; See female
  reproductive system
Reproductive toxins
  definition of, 163

Research
  and human subject protection, 671
Respect
  defining in ethics, 670, 677–679
Respiratory distress
  description and causes in
    newborns, 380–381
  in newborn in delivery room, 352
  in postterm infants, 371
Respiratory distress syndrome
  assessment of, 382
  description and risks in
    newborns, 380–385
  interventions and outcomes, 383
  and maternal diabetes, 505
  surfactant deficiency, 381
  type II, 385–387
Respiratory system
  adaptation of fetus to neonate,
    345
  changes during postpartum
    period, 304
    acid-base balance, 304
    basal metabolic rate, 304
    pulmonary function, 304
  changes during pregnancy
    carbon dioxide, 82
    tidal volume, 82
  changes with anesthesia, 558
  conditions posing risks to
    newborns
    meconium aspiration
      syndrome, 387–389
    persistent pulmonary
      hypertension of newborn
      (PPHN), 389–391
    respiratory distress, 380–381
    respiratory distress syndrome,
      380–385
    transient tachypnea, 385–387
  considerations with trauma, 536
  developmental problems
    in preterm infants, 372, 375
  fetal development of, 43, 46–49
  of fetus
    affected by maternal substance
      abuse, 574
  during placental transfer, 45
  preexisting maternal disorders
    assessment of, 600
    asthma, 599, 602–603, 603b
    complications with, 598–600
    interventions and outcomes,
      601
    patient education, 602–603
    tuberculosis, 599, 602t, 603
Resuscitation
  ABCs (Airway, Breathing,
    Circulation), 536, 541, 541f
  following trauma, 536
  medications for neonate, 356t
  steps for newborns, 352, 355f
Retained lung fluid (RLF), 385–387
Retractions, 192, 193f
RH factor tests, 94
Rh isoimmunization, 129
Rh sensitization, 44, 45t, 304
Risk-taking
  and sexual behaviors of
    adolescents, 118–119

Ritual beautification, 67
Rooting reflex, 350, 350t
Rubella, 449–454, 450t–453t
Rubella titer, 95, 304
Rubin's tasks, 103
Rubra stage, 302

S
Sacrum
    description and illustration in
        bony pelvis, 8f, 9
Safe passage, 103
Safety
    newborn, 358
Safety plans
    and intimate partner violence
        (IPV), 426–427, 426f
Saliva
    changes during pregnancy, 83
SBAR technique, 287
Scarf sign
    in newborn neurological
        assessment, 354b
Scoring system of external physical
        characteristics
    of newborns, 353t
Seat belts
    proper use during pregnancy,
        535, 551f
Second hand smoke, 176
Second trimester
    physiological changes during
        health education regarding, 97
    psychological changes during,
        103, 112
Seizures
    eclampsia, 443
    in fetus
        and maternal substance abuse,
            574
Self-blood glucose monitoring
        (SBGM), 503
Self-esteem
    issues in abused women,
        420, 424
    low in substance abusers, 576
    and pregnancy, 108
Sensory capabilities
    of newborns, 351
Sensory nerves
    supporting female reproductive
        organs, 9
Sensory stimuli
    during fetus/neonate transition,
        345
Septic pelvic thrombophlebitis, 658
Serosa stage, 302
Serum ferritin
    normal *versus* pregnancy ranges
        of, 612t
Serum iron
    normal *versus* pregnancy ranges
        of, 612t
Serum prolactin, 303
Sex glands
    fetal development of, 43, 46–49
Sex-linked dominant inheritance,
        26
Sex-linked recessive inheritance,
        26, 26f

Sexual abuse
    characteristics of abusers, 421,
        422f
Sexual behaviors
    after childbirth, 331
    and risk-taking of adolescents,
        118–119
Sexual violence; *See* intimate
        partner violence (IPV)
Sexually transmitted diseases
        (STDs), 119, 455t–458t,
        464–465
Shearing forces, 535
Shingles, 468t–471t
Shock
    with placenta previa, 480
    pneumatic antishock garments,
        549, 549f
Sickle cell anemia, 609–614
Sickle cell trait
    in native Americans and African
        Americans, 79t
Side-lying position, 318, 321, 322f
Single expectant mothers
    psychological issues with, 105
Sinus bradycardia, 256f, 274, 283
Sinus tachycardia, 255f, 274
Sirenomelia, 52
Skene's glands, 4, 4f
Skin
    changes during pregnancy, 84
    characteristics of preterm infant,
        374
    indicating mother's nutritional
        status, 92, 93t
    interventions in preterm infants,
        376
    physical exam of newborn's, 349
    problems in postterm infants,
        370–371
    scoring newborn's, 353t
    toxins absorbed through, 164
Skin color
    scoring newborn's external signs
        for, 353t
Skin opacity
    scoring newborn's external signs
        for, 353t
Sleep states
    examining in newborns, 351
Small for gestational age (SGA),
        351
    description and risks in
        newborns, 363–367
    health education, 366–367
    immediate post-birth problems
        with, 364
    physical indications of, 365
Smegma, 3
Smell
    evaluating newborn's sense of,
        351
Smoking
    and abruptio placentae, 485
    during breastfeeding, 330
    health education regarding fetal
        health and, 57
    and placenta previa, 484
    pregnancy nutritional deficiency
        risks with, 86

Smoking *(Continued)*
    and preterm infants, 372, 374
    as risk factor for preterm infants,
        372
    second-hand smoke, 176
    and small for gestational age
        (SGA) newborns, 363
Social ethics, 671
Sociocultural system
    chart illustrating, 63f
    taking histories regarding, 13
Socioeconomic factors
    associated with small for
        gestational age (SGA)
        newborns, 364
    and intimate partner violence
        (IPV), 420
    as risk factor for preterm infants,
        372, 624–629
Sodium
    function and needs for pregnant
        women, 88
Sodium bicarbonate
    for neonatal resuscitation, 356t
Somites, 39
Spermatogenesis, 22
Spermatozoa
    count and toxin exposure,
        166–177
    in fertilization and conception
        process, 35, 36f
    and meiosis, 21, 22f
Spermicide
    with condom or alone, 337t–339t
Spina bifida
    description and risks in
        newborns, 399
    surgery, 557
Spinal anesthesia, 560
Spine
    physical examination of
        newborn's, 350
    stabilization following trauma,
        547f
Spinnbarkeit, 10
Spontaneous abortions
    with drug/ alcohol abuse, 548, 573
    psychological issues with, 107, 111
    related to adrenal disorders, 524
    with renal disease, 595
    and toxin exposure, 166–177
Square window
    in newborn neurological
        assessment, 354b
Stab wounds, 535, 540
Statutory law, 674
Steroid replacement therapy
    and adrenal insufficiency, 527
Stillbirths, 638–640
    with alcohol/ drug abuse, 548
    delivery management, 639
    description of, 638
    grief support, 639–640
    interventions, 639
    possible causes of, 639
    psychological issues with, 111
    related to adrenal disorders, 524
    related to maternal diabetes, 505
    with renal disease, 595
    signs indicating, 638

Stomach
  fetal development of, 43, 46–49
Story-based ethical approach, 671
Stress
  and heart disease, 592
  psychological issues with
    pregnancy, 109
Stretch marks, 84
Stroke volume
  changes during pregnancy, 82
  monitoring during surgery, 557
Substance abuse
  alcohol abuse
    assessing in mothers, 581–582
    fetus/newborn disorders
      associated with, 580–583
    patient education, 582–583
    physical signs of, 581
    resources, 583b
    statistics regarding, 580–583
  assessing maternal, 55, 575–579,
    581
  complications due to, 578b
  diagnostic studies, 577, 579, 582
  drugs
    cocaine, 574
    heroin, 574
    marijuana, 575
    methadone hydrochloride,
      575
  effects on fetus, 57, 574
  interventions, 577, 579, 582
  and intimate partner violence
    (IPV), 576
  issues and variables associated
    with, 583–584
  obstetric complications of, 573
  physical signs of, 576, 579, 581
  polydrug use, 573
  postpartum, 660
  causing preterm infants, 372, 374
  psychosocial signs of, 576, 579,
    582
  causing respiratory distress in
    newborns, 380–381
  and small for gestational age
    (SGA) newborns, 363–366
  statistics concerning, 573
  tobacco
    adverse effects of, 578–580
    patient education, 579–580
Succenturiate placenta, 481
Sucking reflex, 350, 350t
Suckling, 315
Sudden fetal bradycardia, 642
Sudden infant death syndrome
  (SIDS), 574
Superficial phlebitis, 656
Supplemental nursing systems,
  328, 329f
Supraventricular tachycardia
  (SVT), 276, 277f, 282
Surgery
  in pregnancy
    anesthesia considerations,
      557–562
    anxiety, 562
    appendectomy, 564–566, 565f
    cervical cerclage, 566–567
    cholecystectomy, 562–564

Surgery (Continued)
    endoscopic gastrointestinal
      procedures, 567–568
    fetal heart rate monitoring, 561
    fetal risk, 557–558
    interventions and outcomes,
      561
    intrauterine fetal surgery,
      568–569
    maternal morbidity risk, 557
    nonobstetric, 556–557
    obstructive uropathy, 569
    oophorectomy, 564
    open laparotomy versus
      laparoscopic, 560
    ovarian cystectomy, 564
    ovarian tumors, 564
    patient education and prep,
      569–570
    preoperative maternal
      assessment, 559
    for spina bifida/
      hydrocephalus, 557
    twin-twin transfusion
      syndrome, 569
    types of procedures, 557
Surrogacy, 117, 680
Sutures
  of fetal skull, 207
Swaddling
  ethnocultural considerations
    regarding, 62
Swallowing reflex, 350, 350t
Sympathetic nervous system
  influencing fetal heart rate
    (FHR), 252
Syncytiotrophoblast, 37–38, 38f
Syphilis, 95, 455t–458t, 464
Systemic lupus erythematosus (SLE)
  assessment of, 605
  description of, 603–605
  as high-risk pregnancy/fetal
    condition, 129
  symptoms of, 605

T

T-ACE questions, 581
Tachycardia
  cause of fetal, 254, 254f
  sinus, 255f, 274
Tachysystole, 272, 288
Tanner stages, 12–13, 14f
Taste
  evaluating newborn's sense of,
    351
Teen pregnancy; See adolescents
Temperature
  extremes as ergonomic hazard,
    176
  hot and cold beliefs, 66, 68, 77t
  instability in postterm infants, 371
  instability in preterm infants, 374
  postpartum changes in, 303
  regulation in delivery room, 352
  thermoregulation during fetus/
    neonate transition, 346
Tentative pregnancy, 105
Teratogenicity
  of alcohol, 581
  risks during surgery, 558

Teratogens
  congenital malformations due
    to, 55
  definition of, 163
  TORCH, 449, 450t–453t
Teratology
  principles of, 165–184
    embryonic stage, 165
    fetal stage, 166
    pre-embryonic stage, 165
    timing, 165
Terbutaline sulfate, 628
Term pregnancy
  defining, 630
Testicular sperm extraction (TESE),
  122
Testosterone
  testing levels of, 15
Tetralogy of Fallot (TOF),
  405–406
The National Human Genome
  Project, 20, 30t
Thermoregulation
  during fetus/neonate transition,
    345–346
  in preterm infants, 374
Thioamides
  for hyperthyroidism, 516
Third trimester
  bleeding
    as high-risk pregnancy/fetal
      condition, 129
  physiological maternal changes
    during
    health education regarding,
      98
  psychological changes during,
    103, 112
Thoracic circumference
  changes during pregnancy, 82
Thrombocytopenia, 610–614
Thromboembolic disease, 610–614,
  656–659
Thrombophlebitis, 306, 656–659
Thyroid function tests, 15, 516t
  for hyperthyroidism, 516t
  for hypothyroidism, 516t
Thyroid gland
  changes during pregnancy, 84
  Graves' disease, 515–516
  hyperthyroidism, 515–516
    antithyroid drugs, 519
    assessment of, 517–520
    health education, 520
    thioamides, 516
    thyroid function test changes,
      516t
    thyroid storm, 516
    treatment of, 518
  hypothyroidism
    assessment of, 521–522
    definition of, 520
    etiology of, 520
    Hashimoto's thyroiditis,
      520
    health education, 522–523
    prognosis for mother/fetus,
      520
    thyroid function tests, 516t
    treatment of, 521

Thyroid storm, 516
Thyroidectomy, 521
Thyroid-stimulating hormone (TSH), 515–516
Tidal volume, 82
Tobacco
  adverse effects of, 578–580
  during breastfeeding, 330
  patient education, 579–580
Tocodynamometer
  electronic fetal monitoring (EFM), 251
Tocolytic drug therapy
  for preterm labor, 627
Toes
  fetal development of, 43, 46–49
TORCH
  cytomegalovirus (CMV), 449–454, 450t–453t
  hepatitis B, 449–454, 450t–453t
  herpes simplex virus (HSV), 449–454, 450t–453t
  rubella, 449–454, 450t–453t
  toxoplasmosis, 449–454, 450t–453t
Touch
  evaluating newborn's sense of, 351
Toxic (heavy) metals
  as occupational environmental hazard, 171
Toxicology
  definition of, 164
  principles of, 164–165
    air pollution, 164
    definition of, 164
    dermal and direct contact, 164
    dose toxicity variables, 164
    dose-response relationship, 165
    exposure duration, 164
    ingestion, 164
    inhalation, 164
    routes of exposure, 164
    target organs, 165
Toxins
  definition of, 163
  and preterm infants, 166–177, 624–629
Toxoplasmosis, 449–454, 450t–453t
Tracheoesophageal fistulas, 41
Transcultural nursing; See also ethnocultural considerations
  goals of, 61
Transdermal contraceptive skin patches, 337t–339t
Transient tachypnea of the newborn (TTN)
  description of, 385–387
  causing respiratory distress in newborns, 380–381
  risk factors, 386
  treatment of, 386
Transitional milk, 317
Translocation process, 23, 23f
Transposition of the great arteries (TGA), 406
Transverse fetal presentation, 138, 204, 205f

Trauma
  assessing seriousness of, 540, 541f, 545t
  causes of, 539
  domestic violence
    common physical injuries, 419–420
    common psychological injuries, 420
  health education regarding, 551–552
  interventions and outcomes, 547
    blood loss, 548
    breathing difficulties, 547–548
    chest injuries, 547, 547f
    fetal tissue perfusion, 550
    fetus potential loss, 550
  maternal algorithm, 541f
  and postpartum hemorrhages, 651
  in pregnancy
    cardiovascular system considerations, 536
    dangers to pelvis, 538
    emergency treatment goals for maternal/fetal, 536
    fetal death risk factors, 536
    gastrointestinal system considerations, 537
    genitourinary system considerations, 538
    hematologic system considerations, 538
    incidence and epidemiology of, 535
    PaO₂ system considerations, 537
    respiratory system considerations, 536
    types of forces, 535
    uterus size and location, 538, 538f
  and preterm labor, 624–629
  preventing, 551–552
  types of fetal and maternal injuries, 539
Treatment
  versus nontreatment issues, 673, 677–679
Trichomonas, 455t–458t, 464
Triple and quad screening, 132
Triplets, 637
Trisomy, 23
Trophoblast, 36, 36f–37f
True pelvis
  versus false pelvis, 9, 9f
Tubal embryo transfer (TET), 122
Tuberculosis
  antituberculosis drugs and toxicity, 602t
  characteristics of, 468t–471t
  preexisting maternal, 599, 602t, 603
Twins; See also multiple gestation
  assessment of fetal health of, 136
  Doppler ultrasound comparison of, 150f
  labor and delivery risks with, 635–637
  monozygotic versus dizygotic, 637
  and small for gestational age (SGA) newborns, 363

Twin-twin transfusion syndrome, 569, 635

U

Ultrasonography
  during antepartum fetal assessment, 134, 135t, 136f–137f
  to calculate expected date of birth, 92
  to diagnose placenta previa, 482
  equipment and safety, 134
  to evaluate fetal status with diabetes, 504
  fetal genetic screening with, 29
  during labor process, 210
  of ovarian tumors, 564
  for trauma cases, 546
  used in fetal/placental assessment, 55
  uses as assessment and diagnostic tool, 134
Umbilical cord
  ethnocultural considerations regarding, 62
  in fetal development process, 50
  metabolic acidemia ranges, 285, 285t
Umbilical cord blood sampling, 284–286, 285t
Urethral meatus, 4, 4f
Uric acid
  clearance affected by preeclampsia and HELLP, 439t
  increased levels during pregnancy, 594
Urinary output
  assessing postpartum, 306
Urinary retention
  interventions and outcomes, 306
  postpartum changes in, 306
Urinary system
  changes during postpartum period
    edema, 304
    kidney function, 304
    urinary retention, 306
  changes during pregnancy
    renal and kidney function, 83
Urinary tract infections (UTIs)
  postpartum, 654
  and pyelonephritis, 465–467
  and renal disease, 596
Urogenital diaphragm, 8f
U.S. Food and Drug Administration (FDA)
  on pregnancy risk categories, 177
Uterine activity (UA)
  definition of, 269–272
  importance of monitoring, 248–249
  pattern of fetal heart rate (FHR), 269–272, 271f
  tracings illustrating, 271f
Uterine atony
  causing postpartum hemorrhages, 650
  signs of, 651

Uterine contractility
    changes during pregnancy, 80
Uterine contractions; *See*
    contractions
Uterine fibroids
    fertility problems due to, 122
    identifying in health histories, 12
Uterine irritability, 271f
Uterine monitoring
    in trauma cases, 546
Uterine neoplasms
    affecting labor passage, 195
Uterine prolapse, 13
Uterine resting tone, 251, 272
Uterine rupture, 642–644
Uterine stretch, 625
Uterine wall
    anatomical description of, 6
    layers of
        endometrium, 6
        myometrium, 6
        parietal peritoneum, 7
    placenta previa, 478–485
Uteroplacental insufficiency, 264
Uteroplacental perfusion
    changes with preeclampsia, 434,
        435f
    with hypertensive disorders, 438
Uterus
    and abruptio placentae, 478
    anatomy of
        cervix, 5, 5f
        corpus (body), 5, 5f
        fundus, 5, 5f
        isthmus, 5, 5f
        positions, 6, 6f
        support, 5f, 6
        uterine wall, 6
    assessing postpartum, 305
    changes during postpartum
        period, 301
    changes during pregnancy, 80
    description and illustration of,
        5, 5f
    physical examination of, 14
    size and location and trauma,
        537f–538f, 538
    uterine rupture, 642–644

V

Vagina
    anatomical description and
        illustration of, 4, 5f
    changes during postpartum
        period, 302
    changes during pregnancy, 81
    examination during labor
        process, 201
    physical examination of, 13
Vaginal birth after cesarean
    (VBAC), 642
Vaginal bleeding
    with abruptio placentae, 478,
        485–489
    with placenta previa, 479–485
Vaginal discharge/show
    preceding birth, 225–226
Vaginal rings, 337t–339t
Value systems
    ethics definition of, 669

Values, 669
Variability
    categories, 254f, 258, 258f–259f
        absent, 258, 258f
        marked, 258, 259f
        minimal, 258, 259f
        moderate, 254f, 258
    definition of, 257
    sinusoidal patterns, 258, 260f
Variable accelerations
    pattern of fetal heart rate (FHR),
        262–264, 262f–263f, 268, 269f
Varicella zoster, 468t–471t
Vasa previa, 52, 481
Vasectomy, 337t–339t
Vasodilation
    changes during pregnancy, 82
Vasodilators
    use and adverse effects during
        pregnancy, 593t
VATERS syndrome, 52
Vegetarian diets, 86
Velamentous cord insertion, 52, 481
Venous pressure
    changes during pregnancy, 82
Venous thromboembolic disorders
    postpartum, 656–659
        description and types of,
            656–657
        prevention of, 658
        risk factors, 657
        signs of, 657
        treatment of, 658
Venous thromboembolism (VTE), 656
Ventral suspension
    in newborn neurological
        assessment, 354b
Ventricular septal defects (VSDs)
    description and risks in
        newborns, 404–405
    development during embryonic
        stage, 42
Ventricular tachycardia, 279, 283
Veracity
    defining in ethics, 670, 677–679
Verbal abuse, 422, 422f
Vernix caseosa, 37, 48–49
Vertex presentation, 137
Vestibule
    anatomical description and
        illustration of, 4, 4f
    Bartholin's glands, 4, 4f
    hymen, 4, 4f
    Skene's glands, 4, 4f
    urethral meatus, 4, 4f
Viability
    definition of, 131
Vibroacoustic stimulation (VST)
    during antepartum fetal
        assessment, 144–145
    for intrapartum fetal assessment,
        284
Violence; *See* intimate partner
    violence (IPV)
Viral hepatitis
    characteristics of, 618t
Virtue character-based ethical
    approach, 671
Vision
    evaluating newborn's, 351

Vital signs
    changes during postpartum
        period, 303
        blood pressure, 303
        pulse rate, 304
        temperature, 303
    following trauma, 536, 543, 548
    monitoring during surgery, 557,
        559, 561
    of newborns, 305, 348
Vitamins
    and fetal health, 88
    function and needs for pregnant
        women, 87
Volume expanders
    for neonatal resuscitation, 356t
Vulva
    changes during pregnancy, 81

W

Waddle gait, 83
Waste anesthetic gases
    as occupational environmental
        hazard, 173
Weight; *See also* birthweight
    maternal, 55, 85
    of newborns
        classification of, 351
        issues in preterm infants,
            372–380
        large for gestational age
            (LGA), 367–370
        late preterm infants, 379–380
        postterm infants, 370–372
        small for gestational age
            (SGA), 363–367
Weight loss
    during postpartum period, 304
Weight management
    and diabetes, 503, 507, 513, 515
    and heart disease, 592
    and hypertension, 436
Wet lung syndrome, 385–387
Wharton jelly, 52
White blood cells
    changes during postpartum
        period, 303
    changes during pregnancy, 82
White's classification, 503t
Withdrawal
    of fetus from alcohol and drugs,
        574
    of mothers from alcohol and
        drugs, 582
Withdrawal contraception,
    337t–339t
Women
    abused (*See* intimate partner
        violence [IPV])

X

Xenobiotics
    definition of, 164
X-linked inherited disorders, 29

Y

Yolk sac
    development of, 36, 36f–37f
    illustration of, 37f

Z

Zidovudine (ZDV), 463
Zona pellucida, 35, 36f
Zygote intrafallopian transfer
    (ZIFT), 122

Zygotes
    development of, 35, 36f
    division of, 36, 36f–37f
    mitosis and meiosis, 20
    and twins, 637